THE
ILLUSTRATED
FAMILY DOCTOR

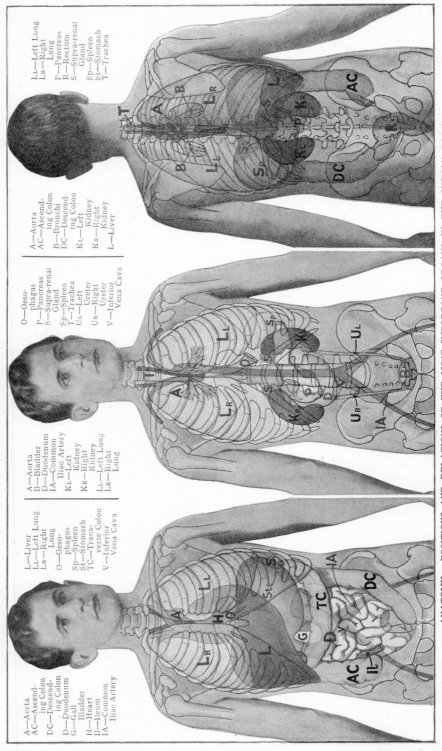

ANATOMY: POSITIONS AND RELATIONS OF THE MOST IMPORTANT ORGANS IN THE HUMAN BODY

On left the internal organs are shown much as they might be revealed by removal of the covering integuments. In central figure the intestines are removed with the exception of the duodenum, in the loop of which the head of the pancreas is now seen lying. From behind (right) the kidneys, spleen and liver are seen in their positions nearer the dorsal surface, while the much greater mass of the lungs towards the back, as compared with the front, of the chest will also be noted.

Frontispiece

THE ILLUSTRATED FAMILY DOCTOR

A Handy and Authoritative Guide
to Essential Medical Knowledge and
the Maintenance of Good Health

By
A GENERAL PRACTITIONER
Medical Editor of The Home Doctor
and The Household Encyclopedia

LONDON :: MCMXXXIV

Printed in Great Britain by Waterlow & Sons Limited, London and Dunstable.

INTRODUCTION

THE purpose of this book is to provide the lay reader with a simple and concise account of the present position of medical science. Technical terms have been avoided as far as possible in the description of diseases and methods of treatment, but at the same time an explanation has been given of current names and expressions as these crop up in discussions of medical topics. The alphabetical arrangement of subjects, supplemented by cross-references, should make it possible to find any desired information easily and quickly.

There would appear to be a growing interest among people generally in the problems of health, and it is desirable that this interest should be extended and deepened, as there is no subject about which the public could more profitably be informed. In the preparation of this book practical needs have been consistently kept in view, and no more than necessary has been said about medical theories, however fascinating many of these may be.

A FACT upon which it is constantly necessary to insist is that a very large amount of the disease that afflicts us is by no means inevitable and could be prevented by the utilisation of medical knowledge. Doubtless considerable responsibility for taking measures designed to promote health is assumed by the various public health authorities, but it is well recognized that satisfactory progress in this direction requires the intelligent co-operation of the individual citizen. It cannot be said that up to the present there has been any conspicuous help from people generally, beyond that exacted by the law, and the majority have still to learn how to keep healthy, even when they have made up their minds to take pains about it.

Fresh information relevant to the prevention and cure of disease has been accumulating rapidly, for example, on the rôle of vitamins in food, the effects of the ultra-violet rays in light, the part played by local irritation of one kind and another in the causation of cancer, and the extent to which infection may be prevented by the use of vaccines. A great deal is therefore said in these pages about the causes of disease and the means of avoiding them. The treatment of the various diseases and injuries is also discussed.

IT cannot be pretended that the perusal of this or any book will fit a layman for being his own doctor. The manifestations of disease are frequently elusive and puzzling, and a correct interpretation of them can only be made by one whose business it is to deal with sickness and who has therefore the necessary experience. Training and experience are also needed for the proper treatment of sickness.

Nevertheless it must be recognized that emergencies often arise and have to be dealt with, at any rate in the first instance, by persons who have had no professional training. It may be taken for granted that, when someone is injured or suddenly becomes ill, those about him will wish to do something for his relief. In such circumstances the treatment has often been quite wrong, the condition of the patient has been aggravated and not infrequently his life has been jeopardised. Similar untoward results have happened when the by-standers have been ignorant about what to do and have done nothing. Many lives have been lost through ignorance of the proper way to arrest bleeding, to restore a suffocated person, and so on.

THEREFORE it is not only the interest but the duty of everyone to acquire some knowledge of the characteristics and correct first-aid treatment of accidents of this kind. The scope of the information given in this book goes, however, beyond what would be sufficient for a first-aid manual, as it is considered that a description of the treatment usually adopted for the various complaints may be useful to the layman in several ways. It is desired, for example, to help those whose lot is cast in out-of-the-way parts of the world, missionaries, traders and others, who are unable to obtain the services of a doctor, or only do so after considerable delay. Such will be able to avail themselves of the instructions given in this book according to the experience thay may have had. Moreover, information about the course of diseases and their treatment may be useful to those who can readily procure medical advice, as it should enable them to co-operate more intelligently in the care of the patient, more particularly as descriptions are given of the many duties which must be undertaken by those who are nursing the sick.

THE attention of the reader is drawn to the accounts given in these pages of the early symptoms of grave diseases that often come on insidiously, for example, those of consumption or cancer. Many valuable lives are lost through persons suffering from such complaints failing to consult a doctor until successful treatment is hopeless. It is sometimes alleged that the perusal of medical literature by a layman may do harm by making him unduly fidgety about his health. Yet the nett result would be pure gain if the perusal of a book of this kind induced uneasy people to consult a doctor, and symptoms apparently trivial, but actually the early manifestations of serious diseases, received skilled attention.

In the treatment of minor maladies it is desirable that reliance, when possible, should be placed on a correction of habits as regards diet, exercise, rest and so on, rather than on drugs. The fact remains, however, that very many people habitually dose themselves with one nostrum or another. It is hoped that such persons will be shown how to dispense with drugs or, at any rate, be enabled by an intelligent appreciation of the accounts given here regarding the actions and doses of drugs, to employ only such as are safe, with advantage at once to health and pocket.

LIST OF PLATES

List of Plates *(continued)*

SPECIAL COLOUR FRONTISPIECE

Three Views Showing Position of Organs in the Human Body

The Illustrated
FAMILY DOCTOR

A. **B.C. LINIMENT.** Compound liniment of aconite, consisting of equal parts of the liniments of aconite, belladonna, and chloroform, is known by this name. It is used for relieving lumbago, sciatica, neuralgia, etc., and may be rubbed over the part or applied on lint covered with oiled silk. The bottle should be shaken well and the liniment used with caution to begin with, as it may irritate the skin in some people.

See Aconite ; Liniment.

ABDOMEN. Abdomen is the technical name for the belly. It is often popularly referred to as the stomach, and we say that a man has been hit in the stomach when we should say abdomen. The stomach is merely one of the most important organs inside the abdomen.

The abdomen is separated from the chest, which lies above it, by a great muscle called the diaphragm, or midriff. This is the second most important muscle in the body, the heart being, of course, the most important. The diaphragm is a flat, thin dome of muscle and membrane which stretches right across the middle of the body. It is arched upwards, towards the chest. It is attached all round to the ribs and the spinal column, and when it contracts it flattens itself so that the contents of the abdomen are compressed and the size of the chest is increased by what amounts to a temporary sinking of its floor. This contraction of the diaphragm is an essential part of the act of breathing, and occurs constantly night and day, without our being aware of it, from the moment of birth until that of death.

When it contracts it compresses the organs that lie beneath it, and thus assists in maintaining their activity. This is one of the reasons why breathing exercises are so valuable. It is, further, a reason why what is called the diaphragmatic method of breathing should be practised by everyone. All children breathe in this fashion, and so do all men to a large extent. Formerly most women breathed by the upper part of the chest mainly, and this was considered to be a natural characteristic of the sex, but it became apparent, when women discarded tight corsets, that they had not used the diaphragm more in breathing simply because they were prevented from doing so by the constriction of the corset. This change to rational clothing has improved the health of women enormously.

The abdomen is bounded in front by a thick wall of flat muscles which normally keep up a gentle pressure on the contents. These are attached above to the lower ribs, behind to the spinal column, and below to the hip bones or pelvis. The cavity of the abdomen is continuous below with that of the pelvis, the bony basin forming the lowest part of the trunk.

The abdominal contents must now be considered. (These are well shown in the frontispiece.) The cavity in which they are contained is lined by a smooth membrane, which is also spread out upon the surface of all the organs, so that there is no friction and they can move freely against one another. This important and complicated membrane is called the peritoneum.

Amongst other important structures inside the abdomen is the alimentary canal, including the stomach and the bowels. In the diaphragm there is a large opening through which the gullet passes into the stomach. The stomach lies immediately under the diaphragm on the left side and leads into the first portion of bowel, which is called the small intestine, or small gut. This, after a coiled-up and complicated course of 20 to 25 feet, passes into the large intestine, or large gut. The large gut, about 4½ feet long, starts in the

1

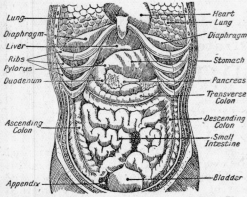

Abdominal organs shown diagrammatically. The pancreas is actually situated more behind the stomach and the transverse colon higher

In considering the remaining organs of the abdomen, it will be found convenient to divide it up into nine areas, three rows of three. The middle area of the top row corresponds very exactly to what is known as the pit of the stomach. It is called the epigastrium, and the sense of "sinking" which is often felt there is thus known to the doctor as "epigastric sinking." The areas on either side of this are called the right and left hypochondrium, a word which simply means that they lie under the cartilaginous or gristly parts of the ribs. The greater part of these three regions is occupied by the liver and the stomach, but in the left hypochondrium there is also another organ called the spleen. This lies very far behind, under cover of the back parts of the lower ribs

right-hand lower corner of the abdomen and passes up the right side, then across to the left and down the left side, ending in a straight part called the rectum. Close to the junction of the large and small intestines is the appendix.

The liver, which is the largest gland in the body is situated immediately under the diaphragm, most of its bulk lying to the right. Underneath the liver is a small bag called the gall bladder, which acts as a reservoir for part of the bile secreted by the liver. The bile coming from the liver or gall bladder passes through a small tube which opens into the small intestine some four or five inches from its beginning. If the ribs are counted on the right side until the ninth is reached, and a finger is put on the inner end of that rib (the end nearest the front), the position of the gall bladder is indicated.

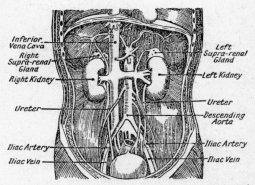

By removing the liver, the kidneys and supra-renal glands come completely into view. The left kidney is situated slightly higher than the right

on the left side. Right across this region of the abdomen also there lies a long, narrow organ called the pancreas. This produces a secretion which passes through a narrow tube or duct into the small intestine, making use of the same opening as that which serves for the entry of the bile.

Behind the stomach also there is a large collection of nervous tissue called the solar plexus. A blow from a fist or a football on the pit of the stomach seriously affects the solar plexus and gives rise to the sensations known as being "winded."

In the middle zone of the abdomen the most important organs besides the bowels, which are found in all the areas of the abdomen, are the two kidneys, which lie one on each side against the back wall

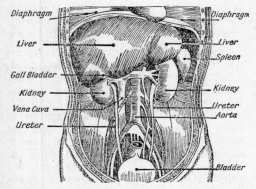

The stomach and bowel have here been removed, revealing the liver, spleen and kidneys, and the large blood vessels, the aorta and the vena cava

of the abdomen, rather close to the middle line. At the top end of each kidney is a much smaller gland which is nevertheless exceedingly important, and is known as the supra-renal or adrenal gland These

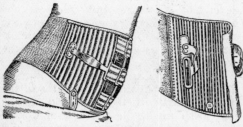

Abdominal Belt for supporting a displaced kidney; right, showing inflatable inner pad

adrenal glands, like some others in the body, are peculiar in that they have no duct or tube leading any secretion from them, but they form a secretion which is most important in keeping up the blood pressure, and this is taken up by the veins leaving them. The secretion of each kidney passes downwards from it through a long and narrow tube called the ureter. The two ureters open into the lower part of the urinary bladder.

Leaving now the abdominal cavity, the important contents of which are described each in its own place, special attention must be paid to the abdominal wall. This mainly consists of a number of flat muscles. Every muscle has the property of elasticity, and the elasticity of the abdominal wall is a most important factor in the health of the body. It permits the contents of the abdomen to vary in amount without inconvenience; and it constantly exercises a gentle pressure on all the abdominal contents. In rational systems of physical exercise the muscles of the abdominal wall are recognized to be as important as the muscles of the calf or arm.

At various points in the abdominal wall there are partial gaps or openings. It is obvious that the existence of any such gap offers an opportunity for the escape or partial escape of one or other of the organs which lie inside, under

very considerable pressure. Thus when the pressure is very suddenly increased, as it sometimes is during violent physical exertion, a portion of the abdominal contents may make its way through one of these weaker places. This is called a hernia, or rupture. Many ruptures are due to a weakness or defect in the abdominal wall which is present at birth, but many are not. One of the useful results of keeping in good condition is that the abdominal wall remains firm and elastic, and far less likely to permit of a rupture than the flabby and inelastic abdominal walls of people who lead sedentary or self-indulgent lives. Increased pressure in the abdomen, due to the accumulation of fat and sagging of the abdominal contents, may also lead to rupture.

Another important peculiarity of the abdominal wall is the tendency for fat to accumulate there, even in persons who have no particular tendency to accumulate it anywhere else.

See Abdominal Exercises; Appendicitis; Breathing Exercises; Hernia; Indigestion; Intestine; Respiration; Tympanites; Visceroptosis; and under the headings of the various organs mentioned.

ABDOMINAL BELT. It is sometimes desirable to give support to the abdominal wall by wearing a belt; for example, during pregnancy or after labour, after abdominal operations, in abdominal hernia, and in visceroptosis or sagging of

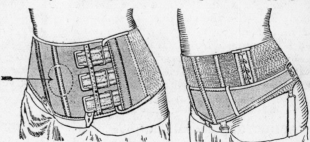

Left, belt for umbilical hernia, with position of inner pad indicated by arrow. Right, maternity belt with side lacings
Courtesy of Salt & Son, Ltd.

the abdominal contents. A steady pressure is obtained by including in the belt a woven elastic fabric, and this may be reinforced by straps or lacing. Where pressure is required, more particularly on certain parts of the abdominal wall, for example, to keep up a kidney which tends to drop, or to retain a hernia, a pad of an appropriate size and shape is fixed to the inside of the belt. This may be solid, or an air-filled bag, and the pressure it exerts may be increased by incorporating a spring arrangement of some kind. It is important that a belt be properly fitted, otherwise it may be not only uncomfortable but ineffective.

See Truss.

ABDOMINAL EXERCISES. The functional activity of the abdominal organs is promoted by deep breathing, and breathing exercises are therefore also abdominal exercises. Vigour in the muscles which form the anterior abdominal wall is required for correct breathing and also for giving support to the abdominal contents, and the regular performance of certain simple exercises will increase this vigour. The easiest exercise of this type consists, when lying on the back, in pressing the flat of the hands against the abdominal wall and then raising the hands by causing the muscles of the wall to contract. By varying the pressure of the hands the effort required from the muscles can be graduated.

A more strenuous type of exercise is, when lying on the back, to rise into the sitting posture without any help from the arms ; or the legs may be raised into a vertical position. Each of these movements should be done slowly, and for a beginning it would suffice to raise first the body and then the legs five times, adding a movement each day until twenty of each is being performed. If these exercises cause any pain in the groins it will be safer to content oneself with the easy exercise first mentioned. Both are illustrated in Plate I, 1 and 2.

See Breathing Exercises ; Exercise.

ABDUCTOR. Literally meaning drawing away, abductor is the name applied to muscles which move the structures to which they are attached away from the middle line of the body or of a limb. For instance, there are abductor muscles which tend to separate the fingers and toes, abductor muscles which move the eyeballs outwards, and others which move the limbs outwards.

See Adductor.

ABORTION. The expulsion of the product of conception or immature child from the womb before the end of the twenty-seventh week constitutes abortion. This period roughly marks the point when the child becomes capable of independent existence, but survival has followed birth earlier than this, and by the aid of an incubator and gavage, or forcible feeding, even as early as the end of the sixth month.

It would appear that abortion is more likely to occur in the later months of the period stated with the first child, and in the earlier months in the case of women who have already been pregnant, and this latter fact would be explained by the existence of uterine disease, dating in all probability from a prior abortion or confinement. The greater the mother's age the more likely abortion is to occur.

There is a large number of possible causes. It may follow any violent shock or emotion, or excessive physical exertion, as in lifting weights, walking too far or too fast, dancing and so on, or may be caused by a fall. Illnesses, as, for example, infectious fevers, are dangerous in this respect, and kidney diseases are particularly so. It is not safe for pregnant women to suffer from severe or prolonged diarrhoea, and strong purgatives should never be used. Displacements of the womb and other diseases of the genital organs are responsible in some cases.

It may happen that when grave danger threatens the life of the mother a doctor may consider it necessary to terminate pregnancy, but the induction of abortion apart from such circumstances is, of course, criminal, and the drugs and manipulations used for this purpose are likely to make the mother very ill and often cause her death.

Abortion occurring early in pregnancy may be mistaken for a menstrual discharge, and women who may be pregnant and have a period when they lose more blood than usual would often save themselves much subsequent trouble by resting and taking care, or even consulting their doctor at such a time. When abortion is threatening, the patient may feel weary and depressed, and have a weight in the lower part of the abdomen ; the hands and feet may be cold. Then bleeding occurs, and may be accompanied by pain in the back, loins and hips. The pains may be severe, resembling labour pains, especially when abortion occurs well on in pregnancy.

On the first hint of abortion the patient should be put to bed and the doctor summoned. Strict rest will be necessary, and if the signs are definite it is better to use a bed pan and retain the recumbent position when the bladder or bowels are being relieved. Food should be light, and nothing should be taken hot. The bowels should be kept regular with small doses of castor oil, one or two teaspoonsful, and repeated if necessary. Should clots come away they should be kept for inspection by the doctor.

The abortion may be incomplete—that is, portions of placenta or membranes may be left in the womb. These may come away without interference, but, on the other hand, the doctor may have to remove them. If left, they may give rise to severe bleeding, or may putrefy and cause blood poisoning ; and this risk of retained materials makes it desirable to have medical assistance in cases of abortion. The patient should keep her bed for at least a week afterwards, and the external parts should be washed with antiseptic lotions, and the same careful attention paid to her as after an ordinary confinement. If she becomes pregnant again, she should keep in close touch with her doctor for observation of the urine and guidance regarding the régime she must follow.

See Childbirth ; Ectopic Gestation ; Embryo ; Pregnancy.

ABRASION. This name is applied to a superficial injury of the skin or the membrane lining the mouth, nose, etc. Abrasions usually bleed only slightly. They should be kept clean, and an abrasion of the skin may be painted over with flexible collodion or new skin, or dabbed with iodine and, if the occupation is a dirty one, covered with a dressing. Exceptional care should be taken in the case of elderly and debilitated people in whom the circulation is poor, especially in the fingers and toes. Abrasions of the toes, for instance, in old people may lead to the attack of germs on tissues which are imperfectly supplied with blood, and thus there ensues what is called mortification or gangrene. Many an abrasion of the toe in very old people has led to the loss of limb or life.

See Antiseptic ; Collodion ; Gangrene ; Wound.

ABSCESS. An abscess is a localised collection of pus or matter separated from the healthy tissues by a more or less definite layer of altered tissues known as the abscess wall. It is due to the invasion of the tissues by microbes, which may be introduced through a wound of some sort, or may reach the tissues from within, as when microbes are brought to a particular spot by the blood.

An abscess may be acute or chronic. In a very few instances a chronic abscess differs from an acute one only in being less intense and of longer duration, but much more usually it differs from the other in character, cause and course. An acute abscess, which is due to one of the pus-forming microbes, may be an exceedingly disagreeable and painful affair, and if it occurs in internal organs—for example, the appendix, brain, etc.—its significance may be very serious indeed.

The signs of an acute abscess are at first those of inflammation, and when one forms where it can be observed, say, on a limb, it is seen that the part becomes reddened, it feels hard and hot, and the patient complains of pain. These are the signs of inflammation, and they may disappear and the part regain its normal condition, or they may increase in intensity, and about the centre of the hard area an elasticity develops which points to the presence of fluid. Moreover, it may be noticed that where the skin has been pressed little depressions have been left which take some time to fill up again. This is known as pitting, and is due to the skin over the abscess becoming dropsical.

At the beginning, if the inflamed area is of any size, the patient merely feels feverish and out of sorts, but if pus forms the temperature shoots up, and he may suffer from what is known as a rigor. Although the thermometer shows that the temperature is raised, perhaps to 103°F. or more, the patient feels cold and shivery and his teeth may actually chatter ; then, after a time, he feels a hot glow come over him, which lasts till he sweats profusely, when his temperature will have fallen to a varying extent.

The pus in the abscess may spread in different directions, but it usually works its way to the surface, and one spot will probably be found where the redness has become darker and where the pain is greater. The abscess is said to point at this spot, and sooner or later the skin gives way and the pus gushes out. This is a thick, creamy fluid, generally of a yellow colour and without smell. With the discharge the pain is relieved, and the patient's general state is usually much improved. The discharge goes on for some days, gradually diminishing till it ceases ; the signs of inflammation disappear, and the parts regain their normal appearance. While the pus is forming, the part should be put at rest, and, in the case of a limb, elevated on a pillow or sling. Hot fomentations or poultices may be put on to hasten the process.

But when the pus has formed it should be let out by the doctor as soon as possible instead of waiting for the abscess to burst. There is not only much unnecessary suffering involved in the delay, but some danger of blood poisoning.

Besides, the opening made by the doctor will give free vent to the pus and diminish the danger of the opening closing up unduly before the abscess is cleaned out. Poultices should not be applied after the abscess has been opened.

Origin of a Cold Abscess

A chronic abscess in the great majority of cases is due to the tubercle bacillus, the microbe of tuberculosis. From the fact that it forms without the usual signs of inflammation being present, it is also known as a " cold " abscess. There may be little or no general disturbance and no pain, though pain may be caused at times by pressure on nerves, and when the pus is just beneath the skin the latter may be reddened. When tubercle bacilli invade the tissues new cells form round them for the purpose of walling them off, but, owing to the poisonous effects of the microbes, these cells undergo fatty degeneration and die, so that a cheesy mass develops.

In the course of the fight between the tissues and the microbes this mass becomes bigger, though sometimes the tissues prevail, and there results a scar simply or a hard nodule owing to lime being deposited in the mass. If the bacilli prevail, however, the mass is liquefied, resulting in a " cold " abscess. This forms commonly in connexion with bones, joints or glands.

Extension Determined by Gravity

The fluid is surrounded by a wall of granulation tissue or proud flesh, and as the contents of the cavity increase the fluid extends from its first site along the lines of least resistance. This is sometimes determined by gravity, and an abscess which begins in front of the spine, somewhere about the middle of the body, while it may come to the surface just above the small of the back, may, instead, travel downwards inside the sheath of the psoas muscle, which lies by the side of the spine on each side. This is called a psoas abscess, and it may open at the lower part of the abdominal wall or in the thigh ; it has even been known to point at the ankle.

The treatment of such an abscess is the treatment of tuberculosis, namely rest, fresh air, sunlight, an abundant nutritious diet and cod-liver oil, combined with such surgical interference as may be necessary. Such an abscess should not be allowed to burst of itself, as when it is open there is a great risk of the cavity becoming infected with the ordinary pus-forming microbes, with a resulting chronic discharge. This will produce some degree of fever and prove a serious drain on the patient's strength. It not infrequently leads to amyloid or lardaceous disease affecting the liver, spleen, bowel, etc.

When an abscess of any kind continues to discharge along a narrow track the latter is known as a sinus, and where an abscess has formed between two hollow organs and has left a communicating passage between them it constitutes a fistula. This may occur, for example, between the lower bowel and the bladder, and a fistula may also form between a hollow organ and the surface of the skin. *See* Degeneration ; Dressing ; Fistula ; Inflammation ; Sinus ; Tuberculosis.

ABSINTHE. The liqueur known as absinthe is obtained from the artemisia or wormwood plant and from several other species. It contains a large proportion of alcohol, about 60 per cent, and in addition to the volatile oil of absinthium, to which some of its effects are due, it contains oil of anise and other aromatic oils.

Poisoning by Absinthe. Chronic poisoning by absinthe is known as absinthism, and is more serious even than that produced by excessive drinking of whisky or other spirits. The physical powers are sapped, moral force declines rapidly, and the deleterious effect on the intellect is more rapid than is the case with the ordinary spirit drinker. Convulsions like those of epilepsy are a characteristic feature. Hallucinations may be present, and the person may become violently delirious.

The treatment must be on the lines followed in cases of chronic alcoholism. Absinthe and other forms of alcohol must be withheld. Plenty of good, easily digested food must be taken, and as much easy open-air exercise as possible.
See Alcohol.

ABSORBENT. Substances which, like a sponge, easily take up liquid are known as absorbents. The most important absorbent substance used in medicine is cotton wool. Wood charcoal absorbs gases, and it may be given inwardly for flatulence in dyspepsia and other diseases. It may also be sprinkled on foul sores or applied as a poultice.
See Charcoal ; Cotton Wool ; Dressing ; Gamgee Tissue ; Sphagnum.

ACARUS. This is the technical name for the kind of parasite or mite which causes the troublesome skin disease known as the itch or scabies (*q.v.*).

ACCIDENT. *See* Antidote ; Asphyxia ; Bleeding ; Fainting ; First Aid ; Fit ; Fracture ; Poisoning ; Transport of the Sick and Wounded.

ACCIDENTAL HAEMORRHAGE. The accoucheur applies this term to bleeding which occurs, during pregnancy, from a partial separation of the placenta or afterbirth from the upper part of the wall of the womb, on which it is normally placed. When the placenta is situated in the lower part of the womb, in the condition known as placenta praevia, the bleeding which occurs is known as unavoidable haemorrhage.

Accidental haemorrhage may be due to a strain, to falls or other injuries, and to other causes. Blood may flow from the patient in larger or smaller amounts, but sometimes the blood does not leave the cavity of the womb, when the bleeding is said to be concealed. Its occurrence may, however, be indicated by the patient becoming very pale and collapsed. Frequently also there is very severe pain of a tearing or bearing-down character. The doctor should be sent for at once, and meanwhile the patient must be kept as quiet and still as possible. She should be kept warm, but alcoholic stimulants should not be given.
See Placenta Praevia ; Pregnancy.

ACCLIMATISATION. Human beings, when removed from the environment in which they and their ancestors have been born and brought up, to one which has widely different climatic conditions of temperature, moisture, etc., and new diseases, require to be acclimatised if they are to survive and multiply. This means a readjustment of their physiological processes to meet the new circumstances.

Suitability for a particular climate is largely a matter of heredity. The white man is healthier in temperate climates, the negro in Africa. When the negro is transported to England he runs a very considerable risk of contracting tuberculosis, whilst the white man suffers far more seriously from malaria than does the native of malarious regions. Nevertheless, men have the power, in common with all living organisms, of adapting themselves, at any rate in some measure, to new conditions, and the process of acclimatisation is just one aspect of this power of adaptation to the environment.

True acclimatisation is an exceedingly gradual process and a costly one, since many individuals die by the way. In general it may be said that only the healthy should emigrate to climates very different from those in which they were born.

As Virchow pointed out, acclimatisation has two aspects, individual and racial, and of these the latter is by far the more important. Probably the most remarkable instances of acclimatisation are furnished by the Jews, but in their case, as in every case of racial acclimatisation, the process has been very slow, and doubtless natural selection has weeded out the many unable to survive in the new environment.

ACCOMMODATION. The process by which the focussing apparatus of the eye is modified in order to produce on the retina a distinct image of objects at varying distances is known as accommodation. For clear vision of objects at $16\frac{1}{2}$ feet or beyond, no change in the eyes is necessary, but for nearer objects the lens must become more convex. How this is accomplished will be understood by a reference to the illustration.

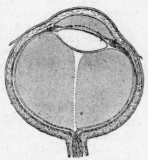

Horizontal section of eye, dotted line showing convexity of lens obtained by accommodation

The lens is within a capsule which is supported all round its circumference by a suspensory ligament, seen here in section. The ligament is tense and drags on the capsule so that the anterior surface of the lens is more or less flattened. The ciliary muscle is attached to the front of the suspensory ligament all round, and when its fibres contract it draws the ligament forwards, thus easing the tension, and the anterior surface of the lens bulges forward. The greater the bulge the more powerfully must the muscle be contracting. When the muscle relaxes, the elasticity of the suspensory ligament restores this to its original position and the lens resumes its first shape.

It follows, then, that in doing near work —for example, reading—one is undergoing muscular exertion, and if too much near work is done, or if the general health is below par, the eyes may be easily tired. The power of accommodation diminishes as one gets on in life, generally after the age of 40, through hardening of the lens,

and this is why glasses become necessary for near work.

Accommodation may be lost from paralysis of the ciliary muscle, a not infrequent occurrence in diphtheria, and inability to read print in people who have suffered from slight sore throats should always raise suspicion of this disease. Belladonna and similar drugs paralyse the ciliary muscle and accommodation is lost. The effort to read small print is very tiring to young children, and before the age of eight it should be avoided, as also similar occupations like threading needles and fine sewing. Headache is not infrequently due to strain of this kind.

See Asthenopia ; Eye ; Spectacles.

ACCOUCHEMENT. This is a French word meaning a confinement. A male doctor who attends a confinement is referred to as an accoucheur.

See Childbirth.

A.C.E. MIXTURE. A mixture of alcohol, chloroform and ether, which is often used to produce unconsciousness for surgical operations, is known by this term. It is taken easily by children.

See Anaesthetic.

ACETABULUM. The rounded, cupshaped cavity on each side of the pelvis, into which the head of the thigh bone fits, is called the acetabulum.

See Hip ; Pelvis.

ACETANILIDE. Also known as antifebrin, acetanilide is a crystalline substance which was one of the first powerful drugs introduced to lower the temperature in fever. It is now recognized, however, that active measures to lower the tempera-

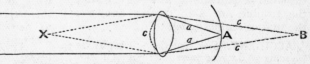

Accommodation. Rays from near object (X) are, through accommodation (c), focussed (a, a) on retina (A) instead of behind (B)

ture are not desirable unless it is dangerously high, and that then the best remedy is the application of cold water by sponging baths or packs. Acetanilide, moreover, is dangerous when used for this, or, indeed, for any other purpose. It has been used for headache and neuralgia, and is contained in some proprietary headache cures. It is not safe, therefore, to indulge in such preparations without knowing what is in them.

Acetanilide may produce serious collapse and difficulty of breathing, even when given in moderate doses. The patient should lie down, and vomiting may be induced by a tablespoonful of mustard in half a glass of water. Hot drinks should then be given and the patient kept warm with hot-water bottles. The doctor should be sent for at once.

See Antipyretic ; Fever.

ACETIC ACID. The essential constituent of vinegar is simply a dilute and somewhat impure solution of acetic acid in water. The acid is formed from alcohol by the action of certain bacteria, the process being known as acetic fermentation. Glacial acetic acid acts as a caustic and may be employed for the removal of warts. It should be applied by a glass rod or on a small brush, or by rolling a little piece of cotton wool on the end of a match. Care must be taken that the acid does not trickle over the surrounding skin, or it will cause irritation and pain. As a precaution against this the skin round the wart may be smeared with vaseline. The application is made each day ; if redness and pain occur it should be discontinued till signs of irritation disappear, and then resumed.

If glacial acetic acid is drunk accidentally it will cause a burning pain in the mouth, throat and stomach. An antidote such as chalk or whiting mixed in water should be given at once, and later white of egg, olive oil or other demulcents. Acetic acid or vinegar is sometimes taken by young women with the object of reducing stoutness. It may do so sometimes, but it is at the expense of the digestion and of good health, so that the practice is entirely wrong.

Toilet vinegars consist of pure acetic acid combined with perfumes. One or two teaspoonsful are added to the water when washing, and this produces an astringent effect on the skin. Dilute acetic acid is a five per cent. solution of the strong acid. It makes a good antidote for poisoning by strong alkalies, such as caustic potash or soda, washing soda or strong ammonia. Two or three table-spoonsful should be given in a little water. If it is added to cold or tepid water in sponging a patient it contributes greatly to his refreshment, and relieves heat and itching. For this purpose add two table-spoonsful to a pint of water. Vinegar can be substituted for dilute acetic acid for any of these purposes.

Acetic acid is used as a solvent for drugs to form the aceta or vinegars—for example, vinegar of squills and of cantharides.

ACHE. Ache is the term particularly applied to a kind of pain—an " aching pain." It denotes a continuous, dull and sometimes throbbing pain. It occurs in a variety of conditions. Thus there is usually a general aching of all the muscles after hard exercise when one is out of training, and pain of the same sort is common in muscular rheumatism. In both cases massage is very effective in restoring comfort. Stomach-ache is a term which is rather loosely applied. Aching in the pit of the stomach is common in indigestion, but the term is sometimes used to describe colicky pains anywhere in the belly.

See Backache ; Headache ; Pain ; Toothache.

ACHILLES TENDON. This is the name given to the tendon or sinew at the back of the ankle, by which the muscles of the calf are attached to the heel bone. It is the strongest tendon in the body. It occasionally snaps, as in the case of an elderly gentleman dancing. In such a case the patient usually thinks that someone has kicked him. It easily heals with rest. Short of snapping the tendon, an undue strain may give rise to inflammatory conditions about its attachment to the bone and cause a painful heel. Here also rest, and the use of a boot with a raised heel when the patient begins to get about, is usually sufficient.

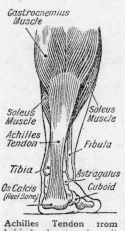

Achilles Tendon from behind, showing how it connects the heel and calf

See Foot ; Leg.

ACID. Most of the substances described as acids are sour ; they turn blue litmus red, form salts with alkalies and have other chemical properties in common. Two classes may be distinguished : (1) inorganic or mineral acids, such as sulphuric, nitric and hydrochloric acids ; and (2) organic acids, of which examples are lactic, citric and uric acids. Both classes of acids are formed within the human body.

Strong mineral acids act as corrosive poisons—that is to say, they destroy living tissues with which they come into contact. Signs of their having been taken will be apparent on the lips and within the mouth. They produce a burning sensation within the mouth, throat, and stomach when swallowed, and this is followed by great pain in the abdomen, by vomiting and perhaps purging. There may also be difficulty in breathing from irritation of the larynx. The patient is more or less collapsed. The doctor should be summoned at once. In the meantime, no attempt should be made to cause vomiting by the use of an emetic or otherwise.

Water may be given to dilute the poison, and then some alkaline substance, baking soda, soap, whiting, chalk or magnesia in water. Thereafter demulcents such as white of egg, arrowroot, salad oil, etc., will be useful. Hot fomentations or poultices will help to relieve the pain, and sponges or cloths wrung out of hot water and applied to the throat may make the breathing easier.

See Antidote ; Poisoning ; the various acids.

ACIDITY. An acid or burning taste or sensation at the back of the throat and tongue is termed acidity, or more popularly heartburn. The term acidity is also used for acid dyspepsia, where there is undue or improper formation of acid in the stomach. Of this there are two distinct kinds which must be carefully distinguished. The first consists in the excessive secretion of gastric juice, including the normal acid of the stomach —hydrochloric acid—and is known as hyperacidity (*q.v.*).

The other form of acidity is due to the opposite cause. Here the stomach is incapable of producing the right amount of hydrochloric acid. This normal acid of the gastric juice is a powerful antiseptic, habitually destroying innumerable bacteria which are constantly taken in with the food. When, therefore, owing to causes which are discussed in the article on digestion, the secretion of hydrochloric acid is diminished or absent, these germs may flourish in the stomach.

The characteristic symptoms of fermentative acid dyspepsia are easy to recognize. They have the special features due to the fact that the fermentation takes some time to occur. About half an hour after a meal these acids may begin to be formed ; together with them there is produced a large amount of gas which tends to distend the stomach and increase the discomfort of the patient. In addition there is the frequent bringing up into the back of the throat of an acid, acrid, burning fluid. This symptom is given the technical name of pyrosis, from the Greek word for fire, and was first used to describe the burning sensation in the pit of the stomach and behind the breast bone known as heartburn. When the fluid has very much less taste the symptom is popularly known as water-brash.

Acidity due to fermentation may be relieved in various ways, though they can never replace the treatment of the original cause of the condition. The most common way is to give something which neutralises the acids which are formed. This is usually baking soda—that is, bicarbonate of soda—or magnesia, or some other alkali. The following is a useful combination of alkalies with bismuth which acts as a sedative :

Bismuth carbonate ..	..	5 grains
Bicarbonate of soda	..	10 ,,
Light magnesium carbonate	10	,,

To be taken stirred up in a little milk or water when necessary.

The B.P. compound lozenges of bismuth provide another good remedy, and can be carried about and used at any time.

A more desirable method of treating fermentative acidity is to give the stomach something which enables it to kill the germs which produce the acids. For this purpose hydrochloric acid itself is often given and is very useful. But the best treatment is that which restores the health of the stomach

See Digestion ; Hyperacidity ; Indigestion.

ACIDOSIS. In the late stages of diabetes, in starvation, in the severest form of vomiting in pregnancy, and in the form of chloroform poisoning which does not come on for a considerable number of hours after the administration of the anaesthetic, and in other conditions, the blood is found to contain certain acids, among them diacetic acid and acetone. This condition is referred to as acidosis. The acids are derived from the fats of the body breaking down in an unusual way, and they do so because the tissues are not being supplied with a sufficiency of glucose.

The presence of these acids in the blood produces several symptoms, two of the most striking being the drowsiness, perhaps leading on to coma, observed in diabetes, and a form of dyspepsia or difficulty in breathing in which the patient appears to suffer from " air-hunger." If carbohydrate food, starch and sugar, and fat are withheld from a person, acidosis is likely to result from the breaking down of the person's own fat, but it is much more likely to be pronounced and dangerous if, while carbohydrate is withheld, the person goes on taking fat.

Herein lies the danger of treating diabetes by rapidly or completely cutting carbohydrates out of the diet while the patient is allowed fat. At the same time the carbohydrates must be sufficiently reduced if the disease is to be held in check. The " fasting " treatment was introduced to meet this dilemma. The patient is at first put on what is virtually a starvation diet, but more food is added by degrees and, if the urine is free from sugar after about twelve days, carbohydrate (bread) is added and increased to about the full amount which can be taken without sugar appearing in the urine.

Acidosis in diabetics is treated by insulin, glucose and, sometimes, bicarbonate of soda. Insulin has also been used when the disorder had a different origin. *See* Diabetes.

ACNE or ACNE VULGARIS. This is the technical name for the very common ailment of the skin which is sometimes referred to as pimples and sometimes as blackheads. The special feature of the disease is the development of little painful pimples which become filled with matter and burst, leaving more or less scarring. It is commonly seen on the face, but may also be found on the chest, the back or elsewhere. It usually occurs somewhere between the ages of fifteen and twenty-five, and is very apt to annoy boys when they start to shave.

Its association with the period of puberty, the stage when the adult phase of life is beginning, is due to the fact that at this time there is an increase in the development and activity of all glands. The oil glands of the skin share in this, and, as a result, the skin may become greasy and of a sallow tint. Later on firm plugs form in the orifices of these glands and develop blackheads. Then inflammation takes place round the plugs and papules or pimples appear.

The disease is due to the invasion of the glands by a microbe, but there are certain conditions which seem to predispose, notably anaemia, constipation, dyspepsia, and genital disorders in women.

People with dark, greasy skins should be very thorough in their ablutions. Night and morning the face should be washed with very hot water and a superfatted soap. Plenty of lather should be produced and rubbed vigorously into the skin all over. An ether soap might then be used if there is any difficulty in getting rid of the grease on the skin. In drying the skin should be rubbed very briskly with the towel. If blackheads are present, the face after washing should be covered for a few minutes with a towel wrung out of water as hot as can be borne, and an attempt should then be made to squeeze out as many of the blackheads as possible. For this purpose a comedo extractor (obtainable from a chemist) may be used, or the finger-nails protected by a thin silk handkerchief. The removal of blackheads is illustrated in Plate I, 3-6.

When papules are present, in addition to the foregoing, treatment should include the application of sulphur. At bedtime the following lotion should be applied and allowed to dry and remain on :

Precipitated sulphur	..	1	drachm
Rose water ..	.. ..	3	ounces
Lime water ..	.. ..	3	"

Sop on with a little cotton wool.

A good method is to use a lotion by day and an ointment by night. The following ointment might be employed :

Precipitated sulphur	..	1 drachm
Starch powder	.. ..	2 drachms
Powdered zinc oxide	..	2 ,,
Vaseline or soft paraffin	..	4 ,,

Where acne occurs on the back, if, as usually happens, the patient also suffers from dandruff of the scalp, this must be cleaned off if progress is to be made. It is also necessary to deal with any of the predisposing conditions mentioned above, anaemia, etc. The bowels should be kept regular, if necessary by the use of an aperient or saline. Sugar and starchy foods should be taken very moderately, and such things as pastry, pickles, greasy food or baked meats, beer and other malt liquors and sweet wines, should not be taken at all. When the patient suffers from flatulent indigestion, the following mixture should be taken three times a day about an hour after meals :

Bismuth carbonate	.. ..	2 drachms
Sodium bicarbonate	..	2 ,,
Mucilage of tragacanth	..	1 ounce
Peppermint water	.. to	6 ounces

General fitness should be aimed at by a sufficiency of sleep and of open-air exercise. The treatment takes a long time, and it may be necessary to try other drugs and applications which the doctor will prescribe. If little abscesses form on the face it is better that the matter should be let out, as pain and subsequent scarring will be lessened. X-rays have done good in some cases, and in others vaccines, and where the acne proves obstinate it may be an advantage to resort to such treatment. *See* Dandruff ; Indigestion ; Skin.

ACNE ROSACEA. The skin complaint known as acne rosacea owes its name to the fact that it begins with flushing, usually of the face, and that later on papules or pimples, resembling those of acne vulgaris, may appear on the affected skin. Unlike the latter disease, which begins in early life, acne rosacea is a disease of middle age, and more often affects women. Disorders of the stomach and of the genital organs in women are prominent amongst its causes. It may occur in those who have always abstained from alcohol, but alcohol and also tea and coffee have much to do with it in other cases. Exposure of the face to heat or to cold winds are amongst the possible causes.

The flushing, which is at first transitory, becomes more lasting and its colour becomes darker. Later dilated blood vessels are always present. Papules or pimples may appear and very commonly suppurate. In some cases the nose may become greatly enlarged and deformed, a condition known as rhinophyma.

Treatment should be directed to the cause, but in all cases alcohol, coffee and probably tea must be avoided. The bowels should be regulated, cascara being a suitable drug for the purpose. The diet should be plain and moderate in quantity, and if dyspepsia is present the following might be taken thrice daily before, or if there is much acidity after, food :

Bismuth carbonate	.. ..	2 drachms
Sodium bicarbonate	..	4 ,,
Heavy magnesium carbonate	6	,,

A small teaspoonful in a little milk.

The affected skin may be painted twice daily with the following lotion :

Strong solution of lead subacetate	4 drachms
Liquor carbonis detergens	.. 4 ,,
Rectified spirits of wine	.. 4 ,,

Or the following paste may be applied :

Resorcin	.. .. ..	15 grains
Zinc oxide powder	.. ..	2 drachms
Powdered talc	.. ..	2 ,,
Vaseline	.. .. to	1 ounce

When, however, the disease is of long standing and the skin is thickened, it is necessary to resort to treatment by light or X-rays, or to surgical measures.

ACONITE. This powerful drug is obtained from the root of the aconite plant (aconitum napellus) or monkshood. The active principle of the drug is the alkaloid aconitine, a most dangerous poison. Aconite slows the action of the heart, reduces the temperature and increases perspiration. It was formerly much used with the idea of cutting short inflammatory disorders, such as tonsillitis and pleurisy. It paralyses nerve-endings, and is used to relieve pain, in neuralgia, etc., occasionally in the form of aconitine ointment, but much more frequently as the liniment. The latter is one of the constituents of A.B.C. liniment (*q.v.*).

The root has been eaten in mistake for horseradish with fatal consequences. The two can be readily distinguished, however, if attention is given to the matter. The root of horseradish is cylindrical, that of aconite conical. Horseradish root is of a yellow or light buff colour on the outside, while that of aconite is dark brown. When chewed, aconite root causes a numbness and tingling of the mouth, while horseradish has a sweetish, pungent taste.

Poisoning by Aconite. The symptoms of poisoning include tingling in the mouth, pain in the pit of the stomach and severe vomiting, an icy wet skin, prostration and a feeble, irregular pulse. The doctor should be sent for at once, and meanwhile an emetic, consisting of a tablespoonful of mustard in a glass of water, should be given. The patient should be kept lying down in bed, and warmth promoted by hot-water bottles and chafing of limbs. Hot, strong tea or coffee should be given freely, and if there is difficulty in swallowing they should be given as an enema.

See Antidote ; Poisoning.

ACRIFLAVINE. Some of the aniline dyes, and among them acriflavine, which is a reddish brown powder, are used as antiseptics. It is generally accepted as being useful, in proper dilution, for wounds and for such infections as gonorrhoea. It was formerly known as flavine.

See Antiseptic.

ACROMEGALY. In this rare disease, as the derivation of the name implies, the extremities of the body become enlarged. The feet and hands and head, and notably the bone of the lower jaw, become overgrown. It is due to the alterations in nutrition caused by disease of a small gland inside the head which is known as the pituitary body (*q.v.*). Besides the bony changes, headache and other symptoms may be troublesome. Sometimes, in consequence of the pressure of the pituitary growth on the optic nerve, there is a serious loss of vision. Thyroid extract benefits some cases, whilst in others removal of a portion of the growth by surgical operation has proved of value. Treatment only affects the symptoms, however, and not the bone changes.

ACROMION. The acromion is practically the summit of the shoulder and is a bony projection from the shoulder blade or scapula. It is sometimes injured by a fall on the point of the shoulder, but more often the force is transmitted through it to the collar bone or clavicle, which is attached to it, and which is thus very frequently broken.

See Collar Bone ; Shoulder.

ACTINOMYCOSIS. This disease sometimes occurs in man and not infrequently in some of the lower animals. It is due to the growth in various parts of the body of a fungus called the actinomyces or ray fungus. It may be acquired by chewing raw grain or by inhaling the dust when this is being ground. It commonly attacks the jaw, but it may also affect the tongue, the lungs (inducing symptoms like those of consumption), the intestines, the skin, and other parts. It gives rise to chronic inflammatory swellings which may break down into pus. This is discharged and the parasite may be found in it along with little yellow gritty masses which are characteristic of the disease. When important organs are affected the outlook is generally bad.

People who handle raw grain should avoid putting it into their mouths and should wash their hands before taking food. If they are exposed to dust in grinding, winnowing, etc., respirators should be worn, a desirable precaution in any case as dust irritates the lungs. The disease is treated by giving large doses of potassium iodide, though surgical measures may also be necessary.

ACTUAL CAUTERY. This term is used for the white-hot iron used for producing blisters, stopping bleeding from a vessel, and for other purposes. Generally the metal is only heated to a dull red glow.

See Cautery.

ACUTE. Those illnesses which have a rapid onset and which run a short course with marked symptoms are termed acute. They are nearly all due to microbes. The other terms which are usually contrasted with acute are subacute and chronic. Rheumatism may be acute, as in rheumatic fever ; when the fever and other symptoms are less pronounced and more prolonged it is said to be subacute ; and in the chronic form pain and stiffness may affect joints for months or years.

ADAM'S APPLE. The projection in the front of the throat of the larynx or voice box is popularly known as the Adam's apple. The larynx is much larger in men than in women, apparently accounting for the lower pitch of their voices and also for the fact that in them the projection is usually much more prominent.

See Larynx.

ADDER BITE. The bite of the variety of adder or viper found in Great Britain is rarely fatal, except in children and weakly persons. Symptoms and treatment are discussed under the heading Bite.

ADDISON'S DISEASE. The chief symptoms of this disorder are bronzing of the skin, profound muscular weakness and vomiting. They result from the lack of the internal secretions of the supra-renal capsules, two glands which are perched on the upper ends of the kidneys, and notably of adrenalin. The failure of the secretions follows degeneration of the capsules, which is nearly always due to tuberculosis, and the subjects of Addison's disease often develop general tuberculosis. The treatment is not at all satisfactory, and the most that can be done is to ensure warmth and rest, with a light, easily digested diet including plenty of milk. Sunshine and fresh air are also important. In advanced cases rest in bed is necessary as there is a constant danger of heart failure.

See Adrenal.

ADDUCTOR. Muscles which move the structures to which they are attached towards the middle line of the body or of a limb are called adductors. For instance, there are adductor muscles which move the eyeball inwards, and very powerful adductor muscles which move the legs together, and are much used in riding.

See Abductor.

ADENITIS. This word denotes inflammation of a gland. A common form of adenitis is inflammation of the lymph glands of the neck due to their invasion by the tubercle bacillus, and commonly known as " glands in the neck."

See Lymphatic System.

ADENOIDS. The lining membrane of that part of the pharynx which lies behind the nose is studded with a considerable amount of lymphoid tissue the same as that which composes the tonsils. It is an overgrowth of this tissue which constitutes adenoids. These exist as finger-like processes or bosses on the walls of

the naso-pharynx and are usually associated with enlarged tonsils. The processes, especially if of recent formation, may be soft and easily torn, but they may be tough and firmly attached. On account of their position they readily obstruct the passage of air from the nose into the throat and sometimes they encroach on the openings of the Eustachian tubes and prevent the passage of air through these tubes into the ears, causing deafness and perhaps earache. This happens more readily because adenoids act as a constant source of irritation and set up catarrh which extends into the nose and may also pass into the ears.

Although they are most commonly noticed between the ages of three and ten, they may occur shortly after birth, and by interfering with easy breathing through the nose may impede suckling and seriously affect an infant's nutrition. At a later age, say between three and four, adenoids will be found to produce a constant " wet nose," the discharge perhaps containing matter and on occasion being blood-stained. The mouth always seems to be open, and the child is a " mouth breather." This has grave drawbacks in that the air which is taken in through the nose is warmed and to a large extent filtered before it passes into the lower air passages, while that which passes through the mouth, in addition to the dust and other impurities which it contains, is liable to pick up infective material from the mouth, particularly if this contains decayed teeth or is otherwise septic.

It is not surprising then that children with adenoids frequently suffer from catarrh of the throat and air tubes. For this reason, and through the irritation caused by the adenoids, an irritating hacking cough is common. The voice may become thick and of a nasal quality, and it is usual to find snoring at night. If this condition is allowed to persist a characteristic change takes place in the face, the nose is compressed, and the upper teeth become prominent like those of a rabbit.

The difficulty of filling the lungs with air produces changes in the shape of the chest. This may take the form of pigeon breast, in which the chest is flattened from side to side and the breast bone is prominent, or it may be flattened from front to back. The chest becomes fixed in this position, with the result that the patient is always a shallow breather and is prone to chest complaints, including consumption. In quite a considerable number of cases it is found that tonsils and adenoids are infected with tuberculosis, which they pass on to the glands of the neck or to other glands or organs.

The sleep of a child with adenoids is apt to be disturbed and bed-wetting is common. Such a child is also apt to be peevish and irritable when awake. The expression is often dull and stupid and the child may be inattentive at school, sometimes no doubt because of deafness, and this interferes with mental development. The wonderful effects of treatment on the mental and bodily health of such a child are illustrated in Plate II, 1.

As regards the form which treatment should take, it may be said that if the adenoids are small and recent it is possible that correct habits of breathing, the maintenance of a clean nose, and tonic treatment, including plenty of fresh air, may bring about their disappearance; but if the adenoids are firm and tough nothing short of an operation will be of the slightest use in bringing about a proper cure, nor should the other method be tried too long in the absence of signs of improvement. The operation is usually simple, and generally it is advisable to remove enlarged tonsils at the same time.

After the operation the child should be put to bed and kept there for two or three days, and it should be kept indoors for an equal time. For the pain which follows the operation ice may be given to suck and this will also help to restrict bleeding. If there is much bleeding at any time the doctor should be sent for. The diet for the first few days will be liquid or semi-liquid and bland, and a return to solid food will depend on the comfort in swallowing and the appetite. No hot food should be given to begin with.

A simple mouth wash is useful and may consist of a weak solution of permanganate of potash, or a mixture of equal parts of borax, common salt, bicarbonate of soda and white sugar, a teaspoonful of which is to be dissolved in a glass of tepid water. If there is a nasty discharge from the nose these lotions may be used for gently syringing it out.

Even after the operation there is still something to be done, and failure to carry out this after-treatment is nearly always the cause of incompleteness in the cure.

This after-care consists in supervising the child each day in keeping the nose clean and in practising nose breathing. A beginning should be made in a week to ten days after the operation. For clearing the nose the following drill has been suggested. The child should stand erect and grasp the bridge of the nose, not the compressible part, with the finger and thumb of the right hand. It then takes a long breath through the nose and then blows down forcibly through the nose on to a piece of soft paper held in the left hand. This is repeated several times.

It may be pointed out here that few people blow the nose correctly. Their habit is to compress the nostrils and only let go when the pressure within the nose is high enough to bulge out the drums of the ears. If there is any infectious material in the nose it may easily be carried up into the ears; the proper way is to compress one nostril at a time.

Breathing exercises should be done in the open air if possible. A simple one is to make the child stand erect with his

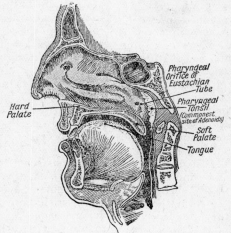

Hard Palate — Pharyngeal Orifice of Eustachian Tube — Pharyngeal Tonsil (Commonest site of Adenoids) — Soft Palate — Tongue

Adenoids : their most usual site

mouth closed. He should then stoop forward about ten or twelve times a minute, breathing out as he descends and in as he raises himself. The exercise should last from five to ten minutes, with rests if necessary, and may be done several times a day. Breathing exercises should be kept up for at least four or five months. If the tendency to sleep with the mouth open persists, it will be necessary to bandage up the lower jaw to prevent it.

To increase the general vigour a tonic may be taken for three or four weeks. The following is a good one :

Iron and ammonium citrate   1 drachm
Cod-liver oil emulsion, B.P.C.   8 ounces

Dissolve the iron in sufficient water and mix. Dose : one-half to one tablespoonful three times a day, after meals.

Instead of this, or alternately with it, one might give syrup of the iodide of iron, in doses of 10 to 20 minims, in water. The food should be plain and nourishing. The child should be as much in the open air as possible, taking such exercise as it is capable of without fatigue. It may be necessary to take it away from school, and if convalescence is slow the feasibility of a month at the seaside or in the country should be considered.

See Breathing Exercises; Deafness; Tonsil, etc.

ADENOMA. A tumour composed of tissue resembling that of the secreting gland in which it occurs, *e.g.* the breast, the thyroid, etc., is called an adenoma. Such tumours usually grow slowly and if completely removed do not recur.

ADHESIONS. The undesirable attachments that occur in the course of recovery from any injury or inflammation are called adhesions. The commonest are those that follow upon a sprain. Their result is that the joint becomes stiff and its range of movement limited. When such adhesions are allowed to form they are very persistent, and if they are allowed to continue for a long period it is often necessary to give the patient an anaesthetic and forcibly break them down. Sometimes they even require to be cut by the knife.

Adhesions may follow inflammation of the smooth membranes which cover the heart, the lungs, and the abdominal viscera and line the cavities in which they are respectively contained. Adhesions in the abdomen may cause obstruction of the bowels, and those in the neighbourhood of the heart may greatly hamper its movements.

See Appendicitis ; Inflammation ; Sprain ; Visceroptosis.

ADHESIVE PLASTER. The older form of adhesive plaster consists of resin, lead plaster and hard soap, melted together and spread on strips of linen. Mead's plaster, which can be obtained in various widths, has a rubber basis, and does not require warming before application, as the other does. These plasters are useful, for example, in bringing the edges of a wound together, strapping on dressings (*see* Plate II, 2), putting limbs up in extension, covering boils, etc. In using adhesive plaster for the last purpose, a circular opening is made, through which the point of the boil projects and the discharge comes away freely. The plaster hastens the resolution of the boil and helps to prevent extension of the infection to sound skin. In strapping wounds several narrow strips are better than one broad one, so that if there is any discharge it has free exit.

See Plaster.

ADIPOSE TISSUE. *See* Fat.

ADOLESCENCE. The period between the time at which a boy or girl begins to undergo the subtle changes of puberty and the time at which full-grown manhood or womanhood is reached is termed adolescence. A boy or girl from about the age of thirteen until a year or two over twenty is an adolescent. It is a period characterised by an outburst of activity of all the glands of the body. A girl's shape begins to assume womanly lines and a boy's voice " breaks " and his beard and moustache begin to sprout. The physical changes have their mental counterpart. Several diseases are prone to make their appearance at this stage, among them being acne, chlorosis, dementia praecox, epilepsy, hysteria, and acute rheumatism. Chlorosis, it may be noted, however, is a relatively rare disease nowadays.

ADRENAL. The supra-renal capsules or adrenals are two small bodies placed on the upper poles of the kidneys. They are of immense importance to health in virtue of their secretions, which are taken up by the blood as it passes through them. Each adrenal consists of two parts, one enclosing the other. The inner is known as the medulla, and the outer is the cortex, and each has its peculiar function. The secretion of the medulla, or adrenalin, has marked influence in maintaining muscular tone, and the lack of adrenalin owing to disease of the gland accounts for the profound muscular weakness in Addison's disease (*q.v.*).

A secretion of the cortex appears to affect the development of sexual characteristics. Tumours of this part have resulted in a woman losing female attributes and developing those of the male.

See Endocrine ; Kidney.

ADULTERATION. The addition of any substance to an article of food may constitute a fraud on our pockets without causing us other injury, but in many cases adulteration of food and drugs is hurtful to the health. Milk, for example, may be the sole food of infants or invalids and these will run the risk of malnutrition if, as is sometimes done, some of the cream is removed and water added to bring down the specific gravity of the milk to that of milk which retains the whole cream. Milk containing preservatives may not be sold.

Preservatives are frequently added to other forms of food, meat, fruit pulp, etc., which is too stale to be wholesome. The usual adulteration of beer is to dilute with water and add salt or a mixture of salt and alum to bring up its density. Beer which has been treated in this way readily becomes sour and heady. Cheap wines are frequently concoctions of potato spirit with chemical or other flavouring and colouring ingredients. Whenever a purchaser has reason to suspect that he has been supplied with adulterated food or drugs, he should bring the circumstance to the notice of the medical officer of health.

See Food.

AEROBIC. Microbes or bacteria which can live only in the presence of air are called aerobic. Pasteur showed that other microbes cannot live in the presence of air, but get their oxygen by the decomposition of compounds in which it occurs. These, in order to distinguish them, are called anaerobic ; the germ of tetanus, the drum-stick bacillus, is an anaerobe.

See Bacteria.

AFFERENT. This term is applied to structures in the body that carry something towards a centre, for example, an artery conveying blood to the tissues, a nerve carrying an impulse to the brain.

See Efferent.

AFFUSION. Pouring water on the whole body or a part of it in the treatment of disease is known as an affusion. The cold affusion may be used in fevers to reduce the temperature. The patient lies in a bath and cold water is poured on him. It is easier to sponge the patient with cold or tepid water and this is usually effective ; or, if necessary, a cold pack or bath is employed. In cases of sun or heat stroke a cold affusion is a rapid and useful remedy.

See Baths ; Cold Pack ; Fever.

AFRICAN LETHARGY. In certain parts of Africa there is an endemic disease in which the patient progressively becomes lazier and drowsier, and which has therefore been called African Lethargy or Sleeping Sickness (*q.v.*).

AFTER-BIRTH. This is the popular name for the placenta, the spongy mass by which the unborn child is attached to the inner surface of the womb, and through which the circulation of blood in the child is carried on. The name has its origin in the fact that the placenta comes away some time after the birth of the child. It is of great importance that the whole placenta should be expelled, as if a portion is left behind either after birth at term or a miscarriage, it is likely to decompose and give rise to blood poisoning.

See Accidental Haemorrhage ; Childbirth ; Placenta Praevia ; Sapraemia.

AFTER-PAINS. During two or three days after childbirth women are liable to suffer pains which resemble, though they are not so severe as, those of labour. They are generally due to the presence in the womb of retained portions of placenta or membrane or of blood clot. The attention of the doctor should be called to their existence. The dose of castor oil which is commonly given on the third day may lead to their disappearance, but if severe, relief may be obtained by the application of hot turpentine stupes to the abdomen, or by the use of an antiseptic douche.

AGE CHANGES. There are certain changes in the tissues of the body which are associated with advancing years and which appear progressively when middle life has been passed, though individuals, families and even races show wide differences in the date of the appearance and the rapidity of the evolution of such traits.

Life is maintained by a struggle against forces of various kinds, bacterial, chemical and physical, and notably in the case of the heart, which has to go on pumping blood night and day for year after year against the resistance of the blood vessels and of gravity. While the blood vessels maintain their elasticity this is accomplished without much difficulty, but when through wear and tear and the influence of noxious substances circulating in the blood the vessels become harder, the effect appears in degenerative changes in the heart and in a poorer blood supply and consequent retrogressive changes in the tissues and organs of the body. The body loses bulk, though in some cases it is rather corpulence which develops, the bones become hard and brittle, the hair becomes grey and falls out, the capacity for muscular and mental effort diminishes, and disease changes may become manifest in the kidneys, the lungs and other organs.

Sour Milk as an Antiseptic

Metchnikoff attached a paramount importance in the production of these changes in the blood vessels to poisonous substances formed in the intestinal tract by certain bacteria which are always found there except in very young infants, and his object in advocating the consumption of milk soured by the Bulgarian bacillus was that the latter might multiply in the bowel and reduce the numbers of other bacteria and therefore the amount of poisonous material produced by them. In that way he argued the incidence of senile changes would be postponed.

Other organs which are subjected to severe mechanical strain are the teeth and jaws, and old age brings a change in the shape of the latter and almost always the loss of the former. The loss of teeth may be compensated by the use of artificial dentures, but it is wise to remember that the digestive powers also wane, and as age advances the diet should become more simple and easily digested, while a smaller amount of food is necessary ; much less protein food is taken up for tissue repair, though a sufficiency of heat-giving food is

called for. Alcohol, unless taken in strict moderation, has a marked effect in producing arterial disease.

The joints are other points on which stress falls, and this, in combination with a poorer blood supply, is largely responsible for the diseased and stiffened joints to which old people are prone. Other things being equal, the man lives longest who maintains a vital interest in life, and it is a common story that when a man's business is his life, his life is curtailed when he passes into retirement.

To return to the subject of blood supply, this depends certainly on the heart and blood vessels, but it depends also on the claims made by the tissues, and if the latter are exercised they are likely to be better nourished than when the body and mind are largely put out of commission and laid up in dock. But the exercise should be proportioned to the capacity to stand strain, and too vigorous exertion may overstrain the heart, or by an apoplectic seizure cut short the activities, and too often life itself. No more is an old brain capable of withstanding the assaults of rush and worry.

In conclusion, while the inimical factors above mentioned are of the greatest importance in unrolling the picture of old age, they do not furnish a full explanation. The various glands of the body which provide the internal secretions upon which the health of so many functions depends become less active, and even when all these things have been taken into account as causative agents, there would appear to be limits set for the existence of every living thing, to which the living tissues of the body can form no exception.

See Blood Pressure ; Diet ; Exercise ; Food ; Rejuvenation.

AGGLUTINATION. The clumping together of blood corpuscles or bacteria is called agglutination. When blood is shed, the red blood corpuscles tend to run together and adhere to one another, as if their body wall had acquired a certain stickiness, and the same phenomenon may be seen to occur with bacteria in certain circumstances. It accompanies dissolution of the bacteria and is brought about by substances known as agglutinins which are produced by the cells of the body in the scheme of resistance to microbic invasion. This forms the basis of what is known as the Widal test for enteric and allied fevers. A little blood is taken from a suspected case and a small quantity of the serum is added to a culture of the microbe of the disease in question. If clumping takes place the test is said to be positive, and the existence of that disease is accepted

See Blood ; Enteric Fever ; Serum.

AGORAPHOBIA. A morbid fear of open places is termed agoraphobia. It literally means " fear of the market place." The opposite condition is claustrophobia, or a morbid fear of a closed space, for example, being alone in a room. These symptoms are common in psychoneuroses.

See Hysteria ; Neurasthenia ; Neurosis.

AGRAPHIA. In learning to write, memories of the movements necessary to form the letters are stored in the brain. In some brain diseases, for example, a haemorrhage damaging the left side of that organ, the ability to reproduce such memories is lost and the patient cannot write spontaneously or from dictation, though sometimes he can copy. Along with this there may be a want of understanding of the significance of written or printed words, while the sound of the words may be understood and expressed.

See Aphasia.

AGUE. This is a popular name for malaria (*q.v.*).

AGUE CAKE. In malarial countries the spleen is often chronically enlarged, and may extend far down in the abdominal cavity. Ague cake is a popular name for this condition, which is common, among other places, in China. In that country its presence is said to be taken advantage of sometimes by men who are fighting, as by striking smartly over the ague cake with the edge of the hand a man may rupture the spleen and inflict what is probably a fatal injury on his opponent.

See Malaria ; Spleen.

AIR. Air is a mixture of gases : 78 per cent. of nitrogen, 1 per cent. of argon, 20·96 per cent. of oxygen, and about 0·04 per cent of carbonic acid gas. Minute quantities of rarer gases may also be present. It contains a varying amount of water vapour. It is quite pure far out at sea and high in the mountains, but elsewhere it holds in suspension organic and mineral impurities, vegetable fibre, dust, pollen, carbon, as well as a variety of microbes. The amount of such substances is high in towns, especially manufacturing centres, in mines, unless means are taken to prevent it, in quarries and in workshops of various kinds.

When polluted air is constantly breathed the carbon and other mineral dust is deposited in the lungs and imparts a grey colour to them, while an excess of dust is likely to result in chronic inflammatory disease, and may predispose to consumption. In a badly ventilated room air becomes impoverished in oxygen, the carbonic acid gas and water vapour are increased and it becomes loaded with particles of animal matter from the air passages of the occupants. Professor Leonard Hill has, however, demonstrated that the bad effects formerly attributed to vitiated air are really due to insufficient circulation of air about the bodies of the occupants, whereby perspiration from the body is diminished and the stimulating effect of air currents on the skin is lost.

See Climate ; Damp ; Fog ; Humidity ; Ventilation.

ALBINISM. Especially amongst the coloured races, children are sometimes born in whom there is a failure of development of pigment in the situations in which it naturally occurs in the body. In some cases parents or other ancestors have shown a similar defect. The condition, which is known as albinism, persists throughout life and cannot be benefited by any treatment. The skin is light in colour, the hair quite white, the iris of the eye pink and the pupil red. Through the absence of pigment in the texture of the eye the retina is unduly sensitive to light. Most albinos are mentally defective and are physically weak, showing a tendency to develop tuberculosis.

See Skin.

ALBUMEN WATER. *See* Beverages.

ALBUMIN. Albumins are substances of complex character which form a class of proteins. They contain carbon, hydrogen, nitrogen, oxygen and sulphur. They are soluble in water and are coagulated by heat. Albumin enters very largely into the composition of protoplasm which forms living cells and has been defined as the physical basis of life. Egg albumen consists almost entirely of albumin, which is also found dissolved in the blood fluid as serum albumin.

See Protein.

ALBUMINURIA. In certain circumstances albumin appears in the urine and the patient is said to exhibit albuminuria. Its discovery always gives rise to misgiving, owing to the possibility of its being due to inflammation of the kidneys or Bright's disease, which is the most common cause. But it is also found in other kidney disorders, such as amyloid disease, congestion in cases of heart disease, irritation from drugs, as well as in anaemia, and temporarily in febrile conditions. In the more definite forms of kidney disease, along with albumin in the urine one usually finds casts of the kidney tubules. Inflammation of the urinary tract, for example, the bladder or urethra, also gives rise to albumin in the urine.

A constant albuminuria will usually be found a bar to acceptance for life assurance.

The occurrence of albuminuria in pregnant women should always be looked upon as a danger signal pointing to the possibility of eclampsia, and it is a wise precaution for expectant mothers to have the urine examined periodically by the doctor.

In young people, and especially boys, albumin is sometimes found in the urine, apart from the presence of kidney disease ; it is found at some time in the day—for example, the evening—while it is absent at others, and may occur only after a cold bath or a meal, much standing or severe exercise. It is only, however, after repeated tests throughout a long period that one can establish the harmlessness of the albuminuria in such cases.

A simple test for albuminuria is to boil a little urine in a spoon or a test tube. The urine may become cloudy, but as this may be due to phosphates a few drops of vinegar or acetic acid should be added. The acid will cause turbidity from phosphates to disappear, but will not affect that due to albumin. In the latter event no time should be lost in consulting a doctor.

See Bright's Disease.

ALCOHOL. By alcohol is generally meant ethyl alcohol, a liquid obtained from the distillation of sugary solutions, either natural sugar derived from malted grain, sugar cane or beet root, or artificial, formed by the action of dilute mineral acids on starch obtained from the potato or other sources. Absolute alcohol may contain a small amount of water, but not more than 1 per cent. by weight ; rectified spirit contains 10 per cent. of water by volume, and proof spirit 43 per cent. by volume. Spirits are " overproof " when they contain less water, and " underproof " when they contain more water, than this.

The percentage of alcohol by volume in the various spirituous liquors is as follows : Brandy, 40–50 per cent. (in good Cognac it may be 60 per cent. and in liqueur brandy as high as 70 per cent.) ; whisky and rum, 40–50 per cent. ; gin, 25–50 per cent. ; beer, light 2–5 per cent., heavy 6–9 per cent. ; claret, hock, burgundy, 8–16 per cent. or a little more ; sherry or port, 15–20 per cent., or more ; liqueurs, about 40–50 per cent. ; champagne, 9–14 per cent. ; stout, 2–5 per cent. ; cider, less than 4 per cent.

About $1\frac{1}{2}$ ounces of pure alcohol can be burnt up in the body, and therefore act as a food, in the course of 24 hours. What this represents in the case of the various alcoholic beverages can easily be calculated by reference to the foregoing list. It is said that when doing active open-air exercise, and in fevers, the amount so consumed is increased.

Alcohol increases the flow of the salivary and gastric juices, and in small quantities may stimulate the appetite and digestion ; but in large quantities it irritates the stomach, and more than a small quantity taken for any length of time tends to cause chronic gastritis, and may result in degenerative changes in the liver and kidneys (cirrhosis), as well as in the heart, blood vessels, brain and other tissues.

The first effect of a dose of alcohol on the brain and circulation is stimulation, but that effect quickly wears off and later becomes narcotic. When used as an emergency stimulant, as in accidents, only small doses should be given, and hot tea or coffee and sal volatile can do as much good without the risk of untoward after-effects.

However much it may appear to increase vigour, it has been found that its use does not increase the amount of work done, while it diminishes the accuracy of the finer movements and impairs the judgement. Its power in warming the body is equally fallacious. The surface capillaries of the body are dilated and a pleasant warm glow is felt, but if rigours of weather have to be faced immediately afterwards this means that the blood in the body is readily cooled. It is for this reason that alcohol is avoided by workers in very cold climates where an excess might easily lead to a fatal result. On account of its dilating the arteries, however, its use in small quantities may add to the comfort of some old people.

A serious drawback to the use of alcohol is the risk of a craving being formed, when it is easy for the bounds of moderation to be overpassed.

Poisoning by Alcohol. The effects of an excess of alcohol constitute alcoholism, which may be acute or chronic. The symptoms of the former are more or less known to everyone : the loss of emotional control resulting in pugnacity or a maudlin sentimentality, the impairment of memory and judgement, the submergence of the higher, and the liberation of the animal, instincts, impairment of muscular co-ordination resulting in a reeling gait, thick and slurring speech, awkward movements of the upper limbs and perhaps double vision, nausea and sickness, and then drowsiness which may deepen into coma.

Some of the results of chronic excess have already been mentioned ; amongst others are obesity, sterility, multiple neuritis causing paralysis of the limbs, a tendency to apoplexy and insanity. Chronic alcoholics also are always liable to develop delirium tremens. The children of drunkards may inherit an unstable nervous system.

In the treatment of acute alcoholism the first thing to be done is to empty the stomach. An emetic of a tablespoonful of mustard in a glass of water may accomplish this, or the doctor may use a stomach pump or siphon tube. Then hot coffee should be given freely. Aromatic spirit of ammonia, a drachm in a wineglass of water, and 30 grains of ammonium chloride dissolved in water, are other remedies. The patient should be kept warm, and if he is comatose he should be watched, as when he begins to come round he may be sick and some of the vomited matter may get into the air passages.

The treatment of chronic alcoholism is very difficult, and will fail unless the victim can be induced to give up alcohol altogether. It will assist his weakened will-power if he consents to begin his cure in an institution, or to live in a part of the country where liquor is not easily obtainable.

See Delirium Tremens ; Dipsomania.

ALIMENTARY CANAL. The digestive tube extending from the mouth to the anus is known as the alimentary canal or tract. These names also connote the glands which pour their juices into the canal, namely, the salivary glands, the pancreas and the liver.

See Digestion ; Intestine ; Stomach, etc.

ALKALI. This name, derived from the Arabic, is applied to certain chemical substances, of which bicarbonate of soda, or baking soda, and carbonate of soda, or washing soda, are perhaps the most familiar examples. These and other alkalies are often used in medicine, most frequently in cases of acidity ; for when an alkali encounters an acid the two unite and form a new substance known in chemistry as a salt, which has the characteristic properties of neither ; in other words, they neutralise each other.

Poisoning by Alkalies. The strong alkalies, caustic soda, caustic potash, strong ammonia, and the corresponding carbonates, act as corrosive poisons, destroying the tissues with which they come into contact. Emetics should not therefore be given, but while awaiting the doctor give an antidote in the form of weak acids, vinegar, lemon, or lime juice, in about half a pint of water. Follow this up with bland liquids, such as milk, the white of an egg beaten up in water, barley water, thin arrowroot, gruel, or olive or linseed oil. A fomentation or poultice may be placed over the abdomen for the relief of pain, and, if there is difficulty in breathing, sponges or cloths wrung out in hot water should be applied to the throat. The patient should be kept warm, and hot-water bottles put to the feet. *See* Antidote ; Poisoning.

ALKALOID. A large number of important substances are called alkaloids because chemically they resemble ammonia in acting as bases and forming salts with acids. Some alkaloids, ptomaines, are found in decomposing animal tissues, and poisonous symptoms occurring after the consumption of bad meat or fish have been attributed to ptomaines, though, as a matter of fact, these are rarely, if ever, the actual cause of food poisoning.

The most important alkaloids are obtained from plants, many of which are invaluable. The active principles of nearly all the important drugs derived from the vegetable world are alkaloids. Tea and coffee owe their virtues to the presence of an alkaloid, theine or caffeine ; opium or laudanum contains, amongst other alkaloids, morphia or morphine ; nux vomica contains strychnine ; belladonna, atropine ; and cinchona bark, quinine. Nearly all alkaloids are highly poisonous except when taken in minute doses. Warm, strong tea is a handy antidote in poisoning by alkaloids, the tannic acid which it contains forming insoluble tannates with these substances. *See* Poisoning.

ALMOND. The sweet almond is very nutritious, and is often used as a food in diabetes, for it contains no starch, and can be made into a sort of flour which produces palatable biscuits and bread. The bitter almond contains a special kind of oil called the essential oil of bitter almonds, which is formed when the substance of the almond is mixed with water. This is quite distinct from the ordinary oil obtained from both the sweet and the bitter almond, which is known as almond oil, and is a bland, harmless, pleasant substance often used in ointments. The oil of bitter almonds is not in itself poisonous. It has a very delicate flavour, and is often used to flavour sweets. It must, however, be very carefully purified before being used in confectionery, for during the course of its production there is also produced the deadly poison, prussic acid, and this is why death has so often followed the eating of bitter almonds.

Poisoning by Bitter Almonds. In a case of poisoning the doctor should be summoned and cold water dashed on the patient's face and chest. As soon as he is roused he should be given a tablespoonful of mustard in half a glass of water. While the emetic is being prepared vomiting may be induced by tickling the back of the throat with a feather or with a paper spill. The patient is then undressed, dried, and put to bed, being kept warm by hot-water bottles or by chafing the limbs. Ammonia or smelling-salts should be held below the nose, and a teaspoonful of whisky or brandy given every ten minutes for a few doses. If breathing has stopped, artificial respiration should be started and kept up till the doctor arrives. *See* Hydrocyanic Acid.

ALOES. Among purgative medicines few have been so widely used as aloes, for in addition to pharmacopoeial preparations it is very largely used in patent medicines of this nature. It consists of the dried-up juice which has flowed out from the cut leaves of the aloe plant that grows in the West Indies and in Africa, and the drug is known as Barbadoes aloes or Socotrine aloes, according to its source. The active principle of this juice is called aloin, and is often used by itself in medicine.

The chief use of aloes and aloin is in constipation. When the drug enters the intestine it stimulates the movements of the muscular tissue that is included in the walls of the intestine, its principal effect being on the large bowel ; and it also increases the flow of the intestinal juices. As the use of aloes by itself usually causes griping, it is generally given in combination with some other substance which prevents this, for example, hyoscyamus, belladonna, or a carminative. In addition to moving the bowels, aloes has a tonic effect on the digestion.

It produces its purgative effect in about twelve hours, so that if it is desired that the bowels should move about 8 o'clock in the morning the dose should be taken about 7 o'clock the previous evening. The movement may be expedited by taking a saline just after getting up, for example, a heaped teaspoonful of Rochelle salts in half a glass of warm water. The drug may be taken as the pill of aloes in a dose of 5 grains.

Aloes is a good remedy for chronic constipation, as it can be used in diminishing doses ; thus it has been recommended that a pill containing 1 grain of the extract of aloes and 2 grains of iron sulphate be taken thrice daily for a week, twice during the next fortnight, and thereafter once daily. Aloes, or its active principle aloin, is found in most " dinner " pills. The following is an example :

Aloin	..	..	..	..	12 grains
Extract of nux vomica			..	6	,,
Extract of belladonna			..	6	,,

Make into 24 pills. Take one in the evening when necessary.

Besides the pill of aloes, there are the pill of aloes and asafoetida, pill of aloes and myrrh, and pill of aloes and iron, the dose of each being 4 to 8 grains. Aloes is also found in the colocynth pills and in the compound rhubarb pill.

See Cathartic ; Constipation.

ALOPECIA. *See* Baldness.

ALSTONIA BARK. The bark of Alstonia constricta is used in Australia as a remedy for fevers, and that of Alstonia scholaris, or Dita bark, which is obtained from India and the Philippines, as a bitter tonic and anthelmintic mainly, though it also has been used for recurring fevers. Tinctures of these barks are official in the British Pharmacopoeia and are given in doses of about 10 minims.

ALTERATIVE. Drugs which improve the nutrition of the tissues and act as general tonics to the body, though we cannot say how they do it, are known as alteratives. They include arsenic, sulphur, phosphorus, the iodides, some preparations of mercury, sarsaparilla (possibly), guaiacum and colchicum, etc.

ALUM. Alum is a crystalline substance which is often valuable in medicine. It is an astringent, and is useful as a gargle in cases of sore throat. The strength in which it should be used is about as much as will lie on a sixpence to two tablespoonful of warm water. Glycerin of alum may be painted on enlarged tonsils or over the back of the throat, but the mouth should be rinsed quickly, as alum may injure the teeth. Powdered alum will often arrest bleeding, such as occurs from piles, from cuts inflicted during shaving, or from the gums or the nose. Alum very rapidly and certainly causes vomiting when given in large doses, say a teaspoonful of the powder in water or syrup every quarter of an hour. It is one of the few drugs which cause vomiting without causing depression, and hence it is of value in the treatment of children. For this reason, and also because it is so often found ready to hand, alum may be of signal use if freely administered in urgent cases of poisoning. A lotion consisting of a teaspoonful of alum dissolved in a pint of warm water may be injected in leucorrhoea or " whites."

See Antidote ; Poisoning.

ALVEOLUS. The socket in which a tooth is fixed is known as an alveolus ; hence an abscess occurring in one of these sockets is called an alveolar abscess, or, more commonly, a gumboil. It should be opened as soon as possible, or an ugly scar may be left on the surface of the cheek or neck by the pus or matter burrowing through. While the abscess is discharging, the mouth should be kept clean by the frequent use of a mouth wash, for instance, compound solution of thymol B.P.C., or hydrogen peroxide solution, a dessertspoonful of either in two tablespoonsful of warm water. After a gumboil a dentist should attend to the offending tooth or teeth.

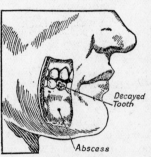

Alveolar abscess or gumboil

See Gum.

AMAUROSIS. Now rarely used, this word means blindness.

AMBLYOPIA. This term is used to indicate in general all forms of defective or weak vision that are not due to errors of refraction or to gross changes in the structure of the eye. The kind of weakness that consists in inability to use the eyes for long is called asthenopia (*q.v.*).

AMBRINE. A waxy preparation, known as ambrine, is used in the treatment of burns, frostbite, chilblains, ulcers or whenever it is desirable to cover a surface with a protective layer. It is painless in its application, and as, unlike collodion, it does not adhere closely to a broken skin surface, it is easy to remove when the parts are again dressed, and discharges from the wound are able to make their way out at the margin of the dressing.

For use it should be melted in a water bath, that is to say, the wax, cut into small pieces, is put into a tin or enamel cup which is then placed in a stew pan or similar vessel containing a little water. The water must be kept at the boil for ten minutes, and during this time care must be taken to prevent the water from spurting into the wax, as although ambrine can be applied without discomfort at a temperature of 140°-150° F. there will be burning if water is allowed to mix with it. The ambrine should be allowed to cool a little before applying.

It is dabbed on with a camel's hair brush which has been soaked in some antiseptic solution and thoroughly dried with a clean cloth. A thin layer of absorbent cotton wool is applied as soon as the ambrine is on, and should overlap the edge of the latter all round. Over this is placed a layer or two of gauze. The dressing should not be left on for longer than 24 hours in the first few days, but it may be left for 48 hours when the discharge becomes less.

The makers of ambrine supply a water bath for convenience in melting it, and they also supply candles of the material for use when the surface to be covered is small.

See Bandage ; Burn ; Chilblain ; Dressing ; Ulcer, etc.

AMENORRHOEA. The absence of the normal menstrual or monthly flow in women is called amenorrhoea. Physiological amenorrhoea occurs before puberty, after the change of life, and during pregnancy and lactation or nursing. Morbid amenorrhoea occurs in many diseases. When the flow fails to appear at the age when one would expect it to do so, there may be some congenital defect or malformation of the internal genital organs. The discharge may in some cases be actually produced but be prevented from leaving the body by a membrane closing the passage. In such event a small operation will be effective.

The flow may fail to appear from chill through getting the feet wet and cold a day or two before the expected period. Mental shock may cause it, and sometimes even a change of residence, as from town to country or vice versa. It occurs in serious diseases and is common in consumption and in anaemia. In such cases the condition is obviously desirable, since it economises the patient's strength by averting the periodical loss of blood. The treatment will vary with the causes, so medical advice should be obtained.

See Anaemia ; Menstruation.

AMMONIA. Really a gas, ammonia is generally used in medicine dissolved in water, so that for practical purposes it is a colourless liquid. The gas is obtained by thoroughly mixing quicklime and sal-ammoniac and heating. It is employed in the preparation of a great many drugs both for external and for internal use.

It makes one of the best applications to insect bites or stings. When applied to the skin, ammonia is an irritant and is very often used in liniments. It is contained in the old-fashioned liniment, oil of hartshorn, and in the liniment of camphor and ammonia, either of which may be used after sprains or in chest complaints. When taken internally or inhaled in gaseous form, ammonia is an exceedingly powerful and rapid stimulant. Hence it is extremely useful in the form of smelling salts in cases of fainting or sudden collapse from any cause.

Ammonium carbonate, dose 3 to 10 grains, is a valuable stimulant and is contained in sal volatile. It is often included in mixtures for chronic bronchitis. In doses of 8 to 10 grains it may act as an emetic and is to be preferred, as a rule, when it is desired to induce vomiting in elderly or debilitated persons. Ammonium chloride, dose 5 to 20 grains, also relieves cough when taken in a mixture, a lozenge, or as a vapour formed by mixing the vapours of ammonia and hydrochloric acid in a special inhaler.

Ammonium bromide, dose 5 to 30 grains, may often be used with advantage

PLATE I

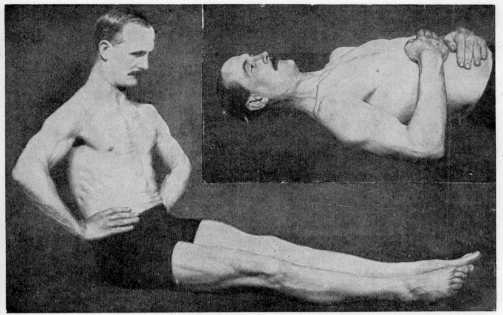

1 and 2. Abdominal exercises. Rising from supine to sitting posture; inset, contraction against pressure

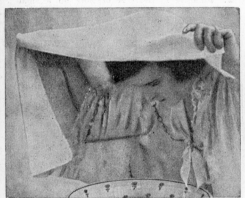

Acne. 3. Treatment begins by steaming the face

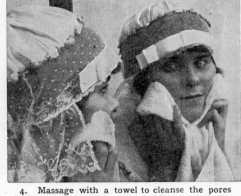

4. Massage with a towel to cleanse the pores

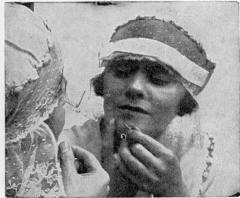

5. Sterilised needle used to pierce the skin

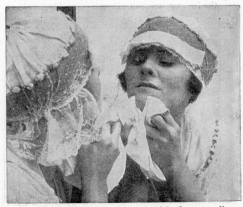

6. Blackheads squeezed out with finger nails

PLATE 11

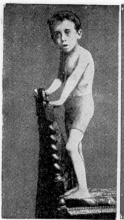
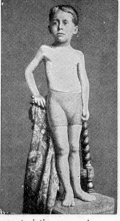

1. Adenoids. Left, characteristic expression, attitude and chest constriction Right, same boy seven months after removal of adenoids

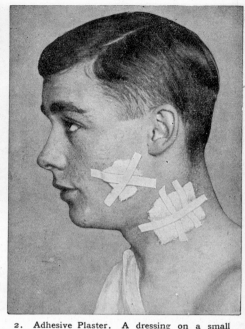

2. Adhesive Plaster. A dressing on a small wound can be kept in place by strips of adhesive plaster arranged crosswise over it

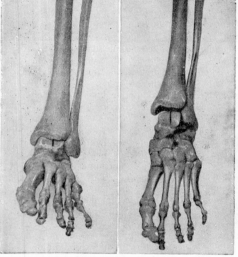

3. Ankle. In low (left) and high heeled shoes, the latter causing displacement of the joint

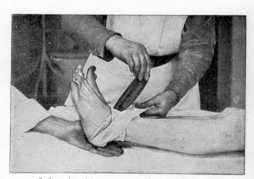

4. Injured ankle strapped with adhesive plaster, the strips being applied to overlap each other

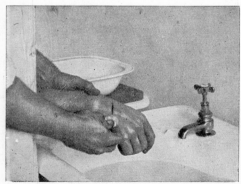

5. Antiseptic. Cleansing wound and surrounding surface with a swab dipped in lysol solution

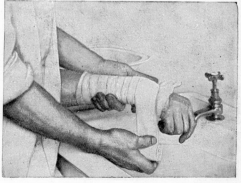

6. After careful drying the wound is covered with a layer of lint held in place by a bandage

instead of potassium bromide, as it is less depressing. Ammonium benzoate, dose 5 to 15 grains, is frequently used as an antiseptic in chronic inflammation of the bladder; it also increases the flow of urine. Liquor ammonii acetatis, or solution of Mindererus, dose 2 to 6 drachms, is a simple and safe diaphoretic, and is much used for a common cold and other feverish affections. A wineglassful may have a sobering effect in drunkenness. Liquor ammonii citratis has the same actions and is given in the same doses.

Strong ammonia is a corrosive poison, and the treatment is to give vinegar or lemon juice in water.

AMNESIA. This is the technical name for loss of memory.

AMNION. The amnion is a bag-like structure, which is of great importance in the early stages of human development before birth. It produces a fluid in which the unborn child floats. The amniotic fluid constitutes the "waters" which escape at an early stage in childbirth (q.v.).

AMOEBA. In the lowest division of the animal kingdom there are minute one-celled organisms, specks of protoplasm or living matter, which in an active state are constantly changing their form and so have been called amoebae, from a Greek word meaning "changing." They are found both in the sea and in fresh water, and have an importance in medicine because species of the organism may be found in the body. In decayed teeth one may find the amoeba buccalis. The entamoeba coli may be present in the bowel and appear in the stools, but it gives rise to no trouble. Its chief importance is that it has to be distinguished from the entamoeba histolytica, which is the cause of amoebic dysentery and of an amoebic liver abscess.
See Dysentery.

AMPUTATION. The removal of a limb or part of a limb is known as amputation, though the term is sometimes also used for removal of the breast and other parts. When a limb is taken off through a joint the operation is often called disarticulation. Amputation may be necessary in the case of severe injuries or of certain diseased conditions of the limb, for example, gangrene, malignant tumours,

incurable ulcers, spreading infections, etc. The operation may produce severe shock in the case of disarticulation at the hip or where it has to be performed on old or weak people. Septic poisoning and haemorrhage, owing to modern methods, are not anything like so frequent as they once were.

The surgeon aims at securing as large a pad of soft tissues for the end of the stump as possible. A conical stump, which is one in which the end of the bone is not well covered, may result from growth in length of the bone in young people, or from sloughing or death of part of the amputation flaps of skin and muscle, and the bone may actually project through the end of the stump. This necessitates re-amputation. The operation has to be planned also so that the pressure of an artificial limb will not fall on a scar. Pain in the stump may be due to septic inflammation of the bone or of the nerves, or to a nerve ending being caught in the scar, and a further operation may be necessary.

A kineplastic stump is one in which the surgeon has manipulated the bones and soft parts, by making artificial joints and loops in the skin and muscles, so that the patient is able to produce more or less movement in his artificial limb.
See Artificial Limb; Operation.

AMYL ALCOHOL. This form of alcohol, also known as fusel oil or potato spirit, has been used to adulterate whisky and to fabricate wines. It is extremely unwholesome.

AMYL NITRITE. A drug of very considerable importance, amyl nitrite is a fluid with the flavour of pear drops and a very penetrating and not unpleasant odour. It is very effective in treating the severest form of pain of the heart, angina pectoris (q.v.), and is also sometimes used in asthma, in haemoptysis, in epilepsy and for other purposes. It lowers the blood pressure by dilating the small arteries, and its use is followed by flushing of the face and body generally. Amyl nitrite is usually supplied in small glass capsules, which are crushed in a handkerchief, and when the handkerchief is held to the nose the drug is inhaled.
See Ethyl Nitrite; Nitrite; Nitroglycerin.

AMYLOID DISEASE. In cases of long-standing suppuration, in advanced cases of tuberculosis and syphilis, and in rare instances of other diseases, a peculiar degeneration is found in some of the tissues of the body, notably the liver, spleen, kidneys, bowels and blood vessels. Other names are lardaceous disease and waxy disease, based on the fact that the material formed is translucent, like wax. See Blood Vessel ; Degeneration ; Intestine ; Kidney ; Liver, etc.

ANAEMIA. The popular description of the conditions included under this heading, namely, bloodlessness, is a literal translation of the word anaemia ; but, as a matter of fact, except for a short time after a considerable bleeding, anaemia does not mean a diminution in the quantity of blood in the body, but a deficiency of some of its important constituents. After a loss of blood fluid pours into the blood vessels from the tissues, so that the bulk of circulating blood is soon made up, though it will be thinner in quality for some time.

Some degree of anaemia is found in debilitating diseases ; for example, in consumption and other forms of tuberculosis, after fevers, in advanced kidney disease, cancer, malaria, syphilis, etc. It may be marked in cases of hookworm disease, in which much blood is lost, and for the same reason in gastric or duodenal ulcer, from bleeding piles or excessive menstruation. It results also from faulty hygienic conditions of life and work, too little exercise in the open air, badly ventilated homes and workshops, under-feeding, as in a diet consisting mostly of bread and tea, septic mouths and so on.

The subjects of the disease become pale, and in particular there is blanching of the mucous membranes, observable easily in the gums and in the lining of the lower eyelids. The bodily and mental vigour become impaired, work and exercise are felt to overtax the strength, and exertion, as in climbing hills or going upstairs, easily produces breathlessness and perhaps palpitation. The poor blood supplied to the digestive organs soon leads to dyspepsia, which increases the drowsiness and irritability already resulting from the insufficiently nourished nervous system.

When the cause of anaemia has been obscure, it has been customary to call it primary anaemia. The two principal forms of this type are chlorosis and pernicious or Addisonian anaemia.

Chlorosis is generally found in girls, usually first between the ages of fifteen and twenty, though it may sometimes appear later. The name is derived from a Greek word meaning green, and in Great Britain the disease used to be called green sickness. These names have their origin in the fact that in typical cases of the disease the face has a greenish-yellow tinge. The face is usually fairly plump and the skin clear. Sometimes the patient may have pink cheeks, due to flushing, and this is sometimes apt to conceal the fact of her bloodlessness. She is apt to have headache, easily to become giddy and to faint, but her first and most characteristic complaint is breathlessness on exertion. The monthly periods may become scanty and irregular, or may cease altogether.

Principal Symptoms of Chlorosis

Generally the appetite is poor, though some of these girls eat well and are apt to become stout. The patient may, however, develop a fondness for highly spiced foods, such as pickles for the sake of the vinegar, and perhaps for unusual things like raw oatmeal or dried tea leaves. The tongue is usually large, pale and flabby, and often shows the marks of the teeth along its edges. Constipation is the general rule. Vomiting of blood is not uncommon, and in some cases may be due to ulceration of the stomach. When chlorosis is marked there may be a little swelling of the ankles.

If an examination of the blood be made it will be found that the red blood cells are fewer than they should be, but the characteristic feature of the blood in this disease is that the red blood cells show a marked deficiency in their content of red colouring matter or haemoglobin, an organic compound of iron. It is in virtue of their containing this substance that the red blood cells can take up oxygen in the lungs for the use of the body.

As to its causes, it is significant that chlorosis has become a relatively uncommon disease in recent years, and that this remarkable diminution has coincided with an increase of open-air exercise amongst girls and the consequent adoption of a more natural type of clothing, in particular, the disuse of tight corsets.

There is scarcely any disease more satisfactory to treat than this. If proper care is taken every case without exception should be easily and completely cured, though it is often apt to recur. All cases should be treated by as much sunlight and fresh air as can be obtained. It is also very important that the girl should get rest, and when the circulation is weak and the ankles are swollen she should be sent to bed for a week or two. She should be well fed, though the diet at first may have to be light, but plenty of milk should be given and she should take meat.

No form of alcohol should be given. The notion that claret and other red wines make blood is quite incorrect.

The bowels must be carefully attended to. Constipation is often relieved when the patient is taking enough iron, but laxatives may be necessary and aloes or cascara sagrada will be found very suitable.

The essential part of the treatment is to give iron in some form and in sufficient quantity. Blaud's pills or tablets, or capsules corresponding to these, provide a convenient preparation. It is usual to begin with one three times a day and gradually increase by one a day until four are being taken thrice daily. The doses are taken after the three main meals. There will be a quick response, and if this is not so when pills are used, it may be that they are not fresh and are passing through the bowel unchanged. This can easily be verified by an examination of the stools. Iron may also be given in liquid form, as in the following prescription :

Sulphate of iron .. .. 16 grains
Magnesium sulphate .. 1 ounce
Dilute sulphuric acid .. 1 drachm
Peppermint water .. to make 8 ounces
Dose : a tablespoonful in a glass of water three times a day after meals.

When using liquid preparations of iron it is desirable for the sake of the teeth to rinse the mouth out immediately after taking the dose, or the medicine may be sucked through a glass tube. The organic preparations of iron which are recommended as being more easily absorbed and less likely to upset digestion, do not appear to possess any real advantage over the others.

In whatever form iron is taken it should be continued for at least two months before a cure can be certain, and in spite of the fact that the patient has now a sense of well-being.

Although she feels well her blood has not regained its normal state, and there will be a relapse if the treatment is too soon interrupted. If symptoms of indigestion appear when taking a preparation of iron, another may be tried, for example, a liquid form instead of the pills, or the iron may be stopped for a few days, and one or two tablets of bismuth and soda taken thrice daily, after which iron will be resumed, at first in half doses.

Pernicious anaemia, as contrasted with chlorosis, is more frequent in men, and usually after the age of 40, though it may occur in women. In this disease, which is very deadly, there is an active degeneration of the red blood cells themselves. Its predisposing cause would appear to be absorption of poison from a septic mouth or from the stomach and bowels, but it is considered that in addition to this there must be the liberation of another poison of obscure origin, which breaks down the blood cells. Examination of the blood shows that these cells are greatly reduced in number, perhaps 40 to 70 per cent. below normal, while the colouring matter, instead of being decreased as in chlorosis, may be relatively increased. Many deformed red cells are seen and unusual cells are also present.

Subjects of the disease suffer from progressive weakness and increasing pallor of the mucous membranes and skin, the latter commonly assuming a lemon yellow tint. Sickness, vomiting and diarrhoea occur sooner or later, and some degree of fever, chiefly in the evening. Dropsy appears in the legs and elsewhere, and sometimes there is pain in the bones of the legs and other long bones.

The treatment must be supervised by a doctor, who should be called in without delay. Rest in bed on a light and easily digestible diet, attention to the bowels, thorough cleansing of the mouth by the use of antiseptic washes and the extraction of foul stumps, and the administration of bone marrow and arsenic, are the usual lines of treatment. Large doses of hydrochloric acid have also been given because it is found that the victims of pernicious anaemia lack this acid in the gastric juice. Complete recovery has been rare, though numbers of cures have been reported. Treatment by feeding with about half a pound of liver, raw and cooked, each day, has now come into vogue, and the results much surpass anything that has hitherto obtained. The raw liver is given in sandwiches as a rule, or a reliable extract may be chosen.

Anaemia due to debilitating disease and faulty hygiene presents a similarity to chlorosis in that the haemoglobin is deficient, but at the same time the number of blood cells is greatly reduced, and some cases resemble the pernicious type.

Anaemia is a much more common complaint in children than most mothers realise, and may result from the child being cooped up and deprived of sufficient fresh air, sunshine and exercise. The diet is often at fault, consisting mainly of starchy food and tea, or it may be that the child has a foul mouth or septic tonsils. All such possibilities should be considered in treatment. The diet should be plain and include meat, oatmeal, milk, vegetables, fresh fruit and fresh butter. The bowels should be kept regular. Iron may be given in the form of chemical food (compound syrup of iron phosphate B.P.C.), a fourth to one teaspoonful thrice daily. Plenty of exercise in the open air and a sufficiency of sleep are all-important.

See Blood ; Diet ; Iron ; Leukaemia.

ANAESTHESIA. Strictly speaking, anaesthesia means a loss of sensibility for touch, but it is used frequently when other forms of sensation are lost or impaired, for example, pain (analgesia) and heat or cold (temperature sense). It occurs in various diseases of the nervous system, for example, following apoplexy, locomotor ataxia, neuritis and functional conditions like hysteria. It is produced by the use of anaesthetics either general, when consciousness is also lost, or local, when a limited area of the body is affected.

See Sensation.

ANAESTHETIC. Any drug used to produce insensibility to pain is an anaesthetic. General anaesthetics act on the brain and spinal cord, producing unconsciousness, insensibility to pain and other sensations and relaxation of muscles. In sufficient doses they also prevent and may diminish shock. They are used to prevent the pain of operations or in conditions like gallstone or renal colic, and to relieve local or general spasm, for example, convulsions. Volatile substances are generally used by inhalation, and the principal examples are chloroform, ether, ethyl chloride and nitrous oxide or laughing gas.

Local anaesthetics act on the nerve endings. Cocaine, eucaine and stovaine are examples ; these are injected into or under the skin or mucous membrane. Another method is to chill the skin with an ethyl chloride spray. Local anaesthetics are also injected into the spinal canal and produce anaesthesia of large portions of the body so that abdominal operations, amputations, etc., can be satisfactorily performed while the patient remains conscious.

See Inhalation.

ANALGESIA. Insensibility to pain is known as analgesia. Drugs which relieve pain by numbing the brain centres and sensory nerves are called analgesics, for example, opium, chloroform, antipyrine, phenacetin, belladonna, etc.

See Anaesthesia.

ANAPHRODISIAC. This is the name applied to drugs which diminish the desires of sex. Of these by far the most useful is bromide of potassium, which may be taken in doses of ten grains, dissolved in water, three or four times a day.

ANAPHYLAXIS. The injection into the body of foreign protein substances, for example, the blood serum of a horse into a human being, produces an antibody to the foreign protein, which is gradually formed and reaches its height apparently within about a fortnight, the period for horse serum in human beings being about eight days. If a second injection of the same protein is made after this time certain phenomena may occur which have been called anaphylaxis. A rash may come out rapidly over the body, with high fever, difficulty of breathing, blueness of the face and hands, shivering or convulsions, and the patient may collapse, and may die.

The sensitiveness produced by injection may last for many months and confers a certain danger on the use of antitoxin. For example, a person who at one time receives diphtheria antitoxin and after the lapse of eight days up to an unknown number of months or even years again receives diphtheria antitoxin, or say, tetanus antitoxin, may possibly develop anaphylaxis. Therefore, in such cases and also in asthmatics it is necessary to give antitoxins very carefully. Serum sickness is regarded as being of the nature of anaphylaxis, as are asthma, hay fever, nettle-rash and other conditions.

See Antibody; Antidiphtheritic Serum; Antitoxin; Serum Therapy.

ANASARCA. This name is applied to dropsy, or the accumulation of water in the body, when this accumulation occurs just under the skin and is thus easily visible. Its presence can be established by pressing firmly on the skin, preferably over a bone, when a depression will be felt which will take some time to fill up.

See Ascites; Bright's Disease; Dropsy, etc.

ANASTOMOSIS. Intercommunication through transfer of two blood vessels is called anastomosis, a word derived from the Greek stoma and meaning literally that they are applied mouth to mouth. A number of operations also go by this name, such as making one part of the bowel open into another, when there is some permanent obstruction to the natural course of the bowel.

ANEURYSM. An aneurysm is the swelling of an artery due to the stretching of its walls. In some cases the inner coat is broken through. It may be due to injury or weakening of the arterial walls by degenerative changes in chronic alcoholism, Bright's disease, syphilis and other

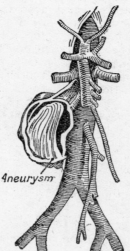

Aneurysm situated in the abdominal aorta. It contains several successive layers of blood clot

diseases. Its most common site is the aorta, the great artery that runs immediately from the heart.

The symptoms depend on the position of the aneurysm and its size, many of them being caused by the pressure of the swelling on nerves and other structures. If in a leg or arm or anywhere near the surface, a rounded swelling may be felt which expands with each beat of the heart; there may be little or no pain. When it occurs in the chest, the patient may complain of shortness of breath, of pain, which may be continuous and severe, of huskiness of the voice, or of a hard metallic cough. Apart from injury, aneurysm occurs most often in men of middle age who have lived strenuously.

In some aneurysms a spontaneous cure results from the laying down of clot along the walls of the dilatation, but unless treated, and often in spite of this, the swelling usually increases in size until it bursts. This ending may be precipitated by blows or by sudden physical or emotional strain, and the subjects of the disease must be careful to avoid anything of the kind.

Any treatment must be supervised by a doctor. When the aneurysm is accessible—for example, in a limb—a speedy cure may be wrought by ligaturing the vessel, and electrolysis and other surgical methods may be adopted for aneurysms in which ligaturing is out of the question. General treatment consists of rest in bed and limitation of the diet in quality and quantity, so as to encourage the formation of clot. Alcohol, strong tea and coffee must be given up. People who are willing to regulate their lives carefully in all such matters may do much to prolong them. Among drugs, iodide of potassium has proved most useful.

See Artery; Thrombosis; Tuffnell's Diet.

ANGINA. Derived from a Latin word meaning to strangle, the term angina is applied to certain disorders attended by a sensation of choking or suffocation.

Ludwig's angina is an inflammation of the loose cellular tissue of the neck which occurs from infection arising in the mouth, frequently during the course of disorders such as scarlet fever. There is considerable swelling and the formation of pus, or matter. Early operation is necessary.

Vincent's angina is a disorder in which ulcers, covered with dirty grey membrane, form on the tonsils. A bacteriological examination must be made to exclude the presence of diphtheria. The patches are cleansed with solutions of potassium chlorate, but swabbing with tincture of iodine or another antiseptic, or even the use of a cautery, may be required. Inhalation of steam impregnated with Friar's balsam or eucalyptus oil helps to relieve the feeling of choking.

See Larynx ; Mouth ; Tonsil.

ANGINA PECTORIS. Breast pang, or angina pectoris, consists in the sudden occurrence of severe pain under the breast bone, which may pass into the arms and elsewhere. The patient feels as if the chest were being powerfully compressed. He suffers from great anxiety and feels that he is about to die. A first attack may be fatal, but more often it passes off after a short time, though it tends to recur and the attacks increase in severity, while the intervals between them shorten. The disease is more common in men than in women, and occurs usually after middle life.

Different opinions are held regarding the cause of the pain, but the general view is that it depends on morbid changes of the heart muscle, at any rate in the cases of greatest severity. The most useful remedy is amyl nitrite, and no one who has suffered from an attack of angina pectoris should be without a supply of the small glass capsules containing the drug, which may be obtained from any chemist. A capsule is broken in a handkerchief, and the contents are inhaled. The doctor should be summoned at once, and meanwhile the patient is placed in the position which is easiest for him ; a hot-water bag may be placed over the heart and he may be given sips of brandy and hot water.

After an attack the greatest care must be taken to avoid physical strain. The patient must not climb hills, rush to catch a train, try to walk against a strong wind, or do anything similar. He must also avoid mental and emotional strain. A fit of anger may prove fatal to him. His diet should be plain, with a great reduction in starchy foods, and the meals should be moderate in amount. If alcohol and tobacco are taken at all it should be very moderately, and so also with tea and coffee. The bowels should be well regulated.

False Angina Pectoris. Not every pain in the region of the heart develops into the disease first described ; in fact, in the great majority of cases it does not, and to cases which have a superficial resemblance to it, the name false and pseudo angina pectoris is given. These roughly comprise two main groups : first, those resulting from neurasthenia, hysteria, or other nervous conditions, and second, those due to the excessive use of tobacco, tea, coffee, and other drugs.

While the pain, as in the other condition, comes on suddenly and the patient is pale and possibly covered with a clammy sweat, the stillness which characterises the sufferer from angina pectoris is replaced by great restlessness. The patient throws himself about or may even move about. He pants for air and may wish to get to an open window. The diagnosis must be made by the doctor, however, and he should be sent for without loss of time.

For immediate treatment a teaspoonful of sal volatile in a wineglass of water, or sips of very hot water, should be given. A hot-water bag may be applied over the heart, and sometimes a large mustard plaster is very efficacious. Other sufferers get relief from the application of an ice-bag. The underlying cause will demand investigation and neurasthenia or hysteria will be dealt with appropriately. Where tea, coffee, or tobacco are suspected as being responsible, they must, of course, be given up.

See Amyl Nitrite ; Heart ; Hysteria ; Neurasthenia.

ANGIOMA. This is the technical name for a tumour or swelling which consists of a mass of any kind of blood-vessel. Perhaps the commonest kind of angioma is that usually called a birthmark (*q.v.*).

ANILINE. Aniline, also known as aniline oil, which is a colourless fluid with a faint aromatic odour, can be prepared from coal-tar, from benzene, and from indigo. From it are derived the aniline dyes and other important substances, among them being acetanilide and exalgin, remedies which lower the temperature in fevers, and which relieve pain. Acriflavine, methylene blue, malachite green, brilliant green and others of the dyes are used as antiseptics.

Poisoning by Aniline. Aniline oil has been swallowed, and has caused death. In cases of poisoning the doctor should be sent for, and an emetic of a tablespoonful of mustard in half a glass of water should be given at once. The patient should be kept warm, by using hot-water bottles, and one of these, or a mustard plaster, should be placed over the heart. If breathing stops, artificial respiration (*q.v.*) should be at once begun.

ANIMAL HEAT. The heat of the body, or the animal heat, is produced entirely by the burning or combustion of the food. When we speak of warm clothing we really mean clothing that keeps the heat of the body in. No clothes add warmth to the body : they merely retain it. The temperature of the body has to be kept at one level in all warm-blooded animals, and so the heat of the body is constantly being disposed of, at various rates, mainly by the skin. The rate at which the heat leaves the surface depends on the amount of blood that circulates through the skin, where it is rapidly cooled. The heat radiates from the skin, and warms air, clothing, etc., in contact with it. Heat is also lost by perspiration, the secretion of which is constantly taking place. The nervous system controls the amount of blood that circulates through the skin and the activity of the sweat glands. It is the circulation of the warm blood that constantly equalises the temperature of different parts of the body.

See Circulation of the Blood ; Clothing ; Fever ; Food ; Temperature.

ANISE. The preparations of anise are derived from the dried fruits of anise plants, and owe their properties to the volatile oil of anise, the dose of which is $\frac{1}{2}$ to 3 minims. Other preparations are the water of anise, $\frac{1}{2}$ to 1 ounce (a teaspoonful for a child of one year) and the spirit, 5 to 20 minims. Anise may be used for flatulence and colic, the water being a convenient remedy for children. The drug is included in many cough preparations, as it helps in the expulsion of sputum from the bronchial tubes. It is included in the following cough balsam :

Liquorice juice	..	..	1 ounce
Ipecacuanha wine	..	..	$\frac{1}{2}$,,
Oxymel of squills	..	..	4 ounces
Oil of anise	..	..	20 drops
Treacle	..	..	1 pound
Gum arabic	..	..	1 ounce

First boil the liquorice juice and gum arabic (both broken up into small pieces) in half a pint of water, then add the treacle. Allow it to cool, and add the other ingredients, adding sufficient water to make two pints. The dose is one to two teaspoonful three or four times a day.

See Carminative.

ANKLE. The ankle joint is of the hinge variety, normally permitting of two movements only, namely, elevation of the fore part of the foot (dorsiflexion) and its depression (plantarflexion). The main ligaments attaching the foot to the lower ends of the leg bones are the internal and external lateral ligaments. It should be possible to dorsiflex the foot so that the angle it makes with the leg is less than a right angle. Walking is more or less impeded, when, as the result of injury, the ankle joint is ankylosed, or fixed with the foot at a greater than a right angle, and also in cases of foot drop.

The ankle joint is constantly subjected to considerable, or sudden, strain, and it is frequently sprained. This is caused by a twisting movement of the foot, which tears the ligaments, and is sometimes due to the wearing of high heels and the consequently abnormal position of the bones (*See* plate II, 3). Bleeding results, and is responsible for the discoloration which ensues, while the ankle swells up and becomes hot and painful. Movement at the joint is fairly full, but causes much pain. When greater force has been applied to the parts, the tips of the lower ends of the tibia and fibula to which the ligaments are attached may be torn. Considerable force may cause displacement of the foot. When, as is most frequently the case, the foot is displaced outwards, it usually results in a Pott's fracture, that is to say, fracture of the fibula about three inches above the tip at the lower end of the external prominence of the ankle. Other fractures and dislocations may also occur in this region.

A sprain is treated by placing the limb at rest, the foot being elevated on a pillow. Cloths wrung out of cold water are applied to the ankle in the first instance, in order to limit bleeding and afford ease. Bleeding may be limited by maintaining pressure on the ankle, and if possible the boot should be kept on and may be supplemented by a bandage applied over it, or a flannel bandage may be applied firmly and evenly to the naked foot (*see* Plate II, 4). Later on, hot fomentations or bran poultices may be used if they are found to be more comfortable.

For fracture or dislocation, if the patient has to be removed before being seen by a doctor, the foot is placed as far as possible in its correct position by gently pulling on it, and well padded splints are then applied to the outer and inner sides of the leg in order to fix the ankle. The legs are then tied together and placed on a pillow or cushion. A bed cradle, or similar contrivance, should be used to keep the weight of the bedclothes off the toes. The reduction of a dislocation or the setting of a fracture should be left to the doctor, as unskilled handling may do much harm. A radiogram of a dislocated ankle is shown in Plate XIV, 6.

When the sprain is slight the patient may be able to get about after two days, nd in all cases, after the acute symptoms have lessened, perhaps in three or four days, the part should be massaged, and as the swelling subsides gentle movements should be performed. These, to begin with, are passive, that is, they are

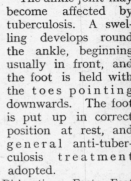

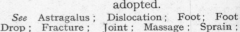
Bones of the right ankle from the left side

done by the nurse, and then the patient is encouraged to do them for himself. Such after-treatment is very necessary for the avoidance of subsequent stiffness in the joint.

The ankle joint may become affected by tuberculosis. A swelling develops round the ankle, beginning usually in front, and the foot is held with the toes pointing downwards. The foot is put up in correct position at rest, and general anti-tuberculosis treatment adopted.

See Astragalus; Dislocation; Foot; Foot Drop; Fracture; Joint; Massage; Sprain; Tuberculosis.

ANKYLOSIS. This name is applied to stiffness of the joints, and may result from inflammation in or about the joints and from other causes. If the bones forming the joint have united we get bony ankylosis, permitting of no movement, but if the stiffness is due to the soft parts, the formation of fibrous bands or contraction of ligaments, etc., it is fibrous ankylosis, and a certain amount of movement may be present.

When it is evident that ankylosis is going to occur in a joint, an attempt is made to secure this in the very best position for function. These positions are described under the heading Joint (*q.v.*).

ANKYLOSTOMIASIS. This disease is due to a species of small worm called the ankylostoma, or hook-worm. It is not uncommonly found in miners; hence its synonym, miner's anaemia. It is also called brickmaker's disease and tunnel disease. The eggs are discharged in the stools of an infected person, and the larvae, when hatched out, get into water. Infection generally takes place through the skin, the point of entrance of the parasite being marked by itching and subsequently the appearance of a blister containing matter. The parasites make their way into the veins and are carried to the lungs, where they escape into the bronchial tubes and thence into the gullet and stomach. At other times the parasites may be taken into the body in drinking-water. The mature forms of the worm have hooked teeth by which they attach themselves to the walls of the duodenum and jejunum, the upper parts of the small gut, and from which they suck blood. This leads to anaemia, which may be very severe. Where the disease exists, drinking-water should be filtered. Treatment consists in giving drugs to kill the worms, a favourite being carbon tetrachloride, perhaps with oil of chenopodium. This must only be taken under medical observation, however.

ANODYNE. This name is applied to any drug or treatment that relieves pain. *See* Analgesia.

ANOPHELES. Some of the mosquitoes or gnats are known to be carriers of certain diseases, and the anopheles is the genus which carries malaria. Like other mosquitoes, it breeds principally in marshy districts, but may do so on stagnant water anywhere, so that pools of water or fire buckets or other vessels containing water in the neighbourhood of dwellings are always dangerous in malarious districts. The adult of the species which is the common malaria carrier, has three or four black marks along or near the front borders of the wings, but another distinction is that when resting the insect cocks the hind part of its body high in the air. On the other hand, the culex mosquito, which is very common, remains with its body parallel to the surface on which it rests, or it may be somewhat depressed.

The female insect lays 40 to 400 eggs on the surface of the water These may be single, but more commonly they adhere together as boat-shaped rafts. The larvae of the anopheles have to be parallel to the surface of the water, but those of the culex hang head downwards. Adults and larvae are shown in Plate XXVI, 1-3. Mosquitoes seldom fly further than a quarter of a mile from their breeding places, but they may fly or be blown by the wind over a much wider range.

When an anopheles sucks the blood of a person infected with malaria, the parasite of the disease undergoes development in the body of its host and finally reaches the salivary glands of the insect. If then the mosquito bites another person the malaria parasite is inoculated with the saliva, but, as development within the mosquito takes ten or twelve days for its completion, the insect may have fed off various people two or three times in the interval without doing them any harm.

The measures to be taken against mosquitoes are detailed under that heading. *See* Bite; Malaria; Mosquito; Tropical Hygiene.

ANT BITE. The pain of an ant bite is due to formic acid which the creature injects when biting. Treatment is discussed under the heading Bite.

ANTERIOR. This term is used to describe any structure or part of the body that is in front of any other part when a man is standing upright. Its opposite is posterior. Thus we speak of the anterior and posterior aspects of the chest, and so forth.

ANTHELMINTIC. Any drug that kills intestinal worms is called by this name. Examples are oil of male fern, santonin, thymol and turpentine. *See* Worms.

ANTHRAX. A very important disease which often occurs amongst the lower animals, anthrax is sometimes communicated to man by contact with the hides or skins of infected animals. Hence it is popularly known as woolsorters' disease. It is due to a special germ or microbe called the anthrax bacillus. This bacillus is of interest as having been the very first that was demonstrated by Pasteur to be the actual cause of a disease. If the bacillus gains entry to the skin it is apt to cause a very severe and dangerous swelling which is usually called malignant pustule, and requires the most energetic and early surgical treatment. On the other hand, if a workman, whilst engaged in handling hides that are infected with the anthrax

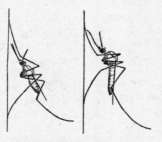
Anopheles (left) and culex in resting position

bacillus, inhales some of the bacilli, he develops a still more serious kind of anthrax which almost invariably proves fatal. The microbes invade the blood (anthracaemia) and the blood poisoning is accompanied by a form of pneumonia.

Once the cause of this disease is absolutely known, there is no excuse whatever for neglecting to take the obvious precautions to prevent its communication to a human being, for this bacillus, like all others can be killed by processes of disinfection. Anthrax has been contracted from shaving brushes imported from abroad.

ANTI-ACID or ANTACID. This name is given to drugs which relieve acidity, for example, sodium bicarbonate, or liquorice.

ANTIBODY. The entrance of microbes into the body provokes the living tissues to produce protective substances which are collectively known as antibodies. They are of various kinds and their functions differ, but all are directed to destroying the invaders and neutralising the poisons produced. The substances responsible for dealing with the poisons are known as antitoxins; the other antibodies produce clumping of the microbes, or render the latter an easier prey for the cells (phagocytes) which eat up microbes, or break down the protoplasmic substance of which bacteria are composed.

When a person or animal is immune to an infectious disease it means that the blood contains the antibodies which deal with the microbe causing the disease. In treatment by antitoxins and vaccines we seek to imitate the natural defensive mechanism. The injection of a foreign protein into an animal, including man, leads to the formation of an antibody known as a precipitin. Thus, if white of egg be injected into a human being, his blood after a certain period will be found to precipitate white of egg. It is then said to be sensitised to white of egg.

See Anaphylaxis; Immunity.

ANTIDIPHTHERITIC SERUM. This contains diphtheria antitoxin and is prepared from the blood of horses which have been rendered immune against diphtheria. Since its introduction into medical practice in 1891 it has enormously diminished the death rate from diphtheria, but its efficacy depends largely on whether or not it is given early in the disease, and on the dose given. This is calculated in units, and for a mild case, seen on the first day of the disease, 6000 units are considered to be sufficient, but in severer cases larger doses are given, and the dose has to be progressively increased for each day which has elapsed since the first, so that 20,000 units may be required. Smaller doses are used as a preventive measure when children have been exposed to infection, more especially when the application of Schick's test has shown them to be susceptible to the disease. The serum is usually injected into the muscle on the outer side of the thigh, though it may be injected under the skin of the abdomen or between the shoulders.

In certain circumstances the injection may be followed by what are known as anaphylactic phenomena, which may appear at once or in a day or two, or after the lapse of about eight days as serum sickness, marked by the appearance of a rash like nettle-rash, by pain in the joints and by a rise of temperature. The former condition requires energetic treatment, but serum sickness usually disappears in a few days.

See Anaphylaxis; Diphtheria; Immunity; Serum Therapy.

ANTIDOTE. A substance which may be used to neutralise a poison or counteract its effects is known as an antidote. It may act by converting the poison into a harmless substance, as when chalk, given as an antidote for oil of vitriol, forms with the latter the insoluble sulphate of lime. The tannic acid in strong tea has the same effect on morphine and other alkaloids, forming with them insoluble tannates. Coffee acts as an antidote in opium poisoning by combating the narcotic action of the latter. The main poisons and their appropriate antidotes are given in the table in the opposite page.

See Poisoning.

ANTIFEBRIN. *See* Acetanilide.

ANTIMONY. Antimony, which was formerly much used, chiefly as antimonial wine or as tartar emetic, in bronchial and other affections, but had fallen more or less into disuse, has again assumed importance in the treatment of certain parasitic diseases, namely, leishmaniasis

COMMON POISONS GROUPED ACCORDING TO THEIR ANTIDOTES

POISON	ANTIDOTE
Sulphuric acid (oil of vitriol) .. .. Hydrochloric acid (spirit of salt) .. Nitric acid (aqua fortis) .. .. Oxalic acid (salt of sorrel or lemon) ..	Alkalies : magnesia ; chalk ; whitening ; plaster from the wall or ceiling, one or two tablespoonsful ground and mixed with water. For all except oxalic acid, bicarbonate of soda, or weak washing soda solution, or weak ammonia.
Washing soda .. .. Caustic soda .. .. Caustic potash (pearl ash) .. .. Ammonia (spirits of hartshorn) ..	Acids : two or three tablespoonsful of vinegar, lemon or lime juice in water.
Carbolic acid .. .. Creosote	Epsom salts.
Corrosive sublimate (perchloride of mercury)	White of egg.
Phosphorus (match heads, rat poison)	Oil of turpentine ; copper sulphate ; these should be given by the doctor.
Iodine	Weak solution of washing soda : starch.
Arsenic (rat poison, weed killer, Fowler's solution)	Dialysed iron, two tablespoonsful in half a glass of water, or calcined magnesia freely mixed with water.
Antimony (tartar emetic, antimonial wine)	Strong warm tea.
Sugar of lead	Epsom salts.
Copper (bluestone, verdigris)	White of egg.
Poisonous fungi	Atropine given by the doctor.
Hydrocyanic or prussic acid, cherry laurel water, oil of bitter almonds, cyanide of potassium	If unconscious, inhalation of ammonia ; otherwise spirits of sal volatile freely.
Opium (laudanum, morphia, paregoric, chlorodyne, Dover's powder, soothing syrups)	A small pinch of permanganate of potash crystals thoroughly dissolved in half a tumbler of warm water. Strong coffee by the mouth, or half a pint given as an enema. Strong warm tea.
Deadly nightshade, belladonna (atropine, liniment of belladonna) .. .. Hyoscyamus (henbane) .. .. .. Black nightshade .. .. Woody nightshade (bittersweet) ..	Strong warm tea.
Alcohol	Hot strong coffee ; sal volatile.
Cocaine .. .. Ether .. .. Chloroform .. .. Chloral .. .. Nitrobenzene (spirit of mirbane) .. Phenacetin, antipyrine, exalgen, antifebrin, headache powders	Stimulants : whisky or brandy ; hot strong coffee ; sal volatile.
Strychnine (nux vomica, Easton's syrup)	Strong warm tea.
Digitalis (foxglove) .. .. .. Aconite (monkshood, wolfsbane) .. Tobacco	Sal volatile ; strong warm tea.

or infection by some species of Leishman–Donovan body, as in Baghdad or oriental sore ; infection by trypanosomes, as in African sleeping sickness ; bilharzia disease, and others.

Poisoning by Antimony. Preparations of antimony in large doses act as irritant poisons, causing violent vomiting and diarrhoea and great depression of the heart. In cases of poisoning, if vomiting has not set in it should be induced by an emetic of a tablespoonful of mustard in half a glass of water. Strong warm tea should then be given freely, and later white of egg and milk. The patient should be kept lying down, with hot-water bottles at his feet and by his side.

ANTIPARASITIC or PARASITICIDE. This is a drug that kills parasites, and the term is usually applied to those which kill parasites in the skin. Sulphur preparations are used to kill the itch insect, kerosene, stavesacre and other substances to kill lice, iodine to kill the fungus of ringworm, and so on. All antiseptics (*q.v.*) are more or less useful for this purpose.

ANTIPYRETIC. Any drug or method of treatment which lowers the temperature is an antipyretic, a word derived from the Greek pur, fire. Quinine, salicin, and the coal-tar derivatives, phenacetin, antipyrine, acetanilide, and other drugs have this effect, but there is much less tendency now to use them for this purpose, and especially the coal-tar products, on account of the depression produced. Moreover, it is recognized that fever is but a symptom of disease which, unless it is somewhere in the neighbourhood of 103°F, or associated with sleeplessness or delirium, need not be interfered with, unless, as in using quinine in malaria, the cause of the disease is actually being combated.

Fever of moderate degree can be controlled by keeping the skin active, by giving liquids freely and perhaps remedies like sweet spirits of nitre and spirit of Mindererus, and by tepid or cold sponging. Should the temperature be dangerously high, about 106°F or over, cold baths or iced packs will become necessary. In some circumstances one may have to fall back on antipyretic drugs.

See Fever.

ANTIPYRINE or PHENAZONE. Antipyrine is one of the coal-tar antiseptic remedies, though it is little used now for this purpose, as it depresses the heart. A dose of 5 grains may be taken by an adult for pain like that of neuralgia, and depression may be counteracted by lying down for half an hour after the dose or by taking a teaspoonful of sal volatile in a wineglass of water. In cases of overdose the doctor should be sent for and the patient kept warm and lying down. He should also be given stimulants.

ANTISCORBUTIC. Scurvy or scorbutus is due to an absence from the food or a deficiency of a vitamin or accessory food factor known as " water soluble C." Substances which contain this vitamin, and thus may be given to prevent or cure scurvy, are known as antiscorbutics. Of these orange and lemon juice are perhaps the best. The juice of swede turnips can be used and fresh green vegetables. The vitamin may also be contained in potatoes rapidly boiled in their skins. It is present in fresh milk, but is destroyed by sterilising. Bottled lime juice is not now believed to have an antiscorbutic effect.

See Scurvy.

ANTISEPTIC. Any substance which hinders the growth and activities of the microbes which produce putrefaction is an antiseptic. It is a matter of practical importance to distinguish between an agent which acts as an antiseptic and one which is a disinfectant or deodorant. A disinfectant kills the microbes which produce communicable diseases, for example, scarlet fever, and a deodorant destroys or covers disagreeable smells. Carbolic acid, if used in sufficient strength and for a sufficient length of time, will disinfect, but when used as an antiseptic it must be in greater dilution, or it will injure or destroy the body tissues. Eau de Cologne and the fumes of tobacco or of brown paper are sometimes used as deodorants, but of course they exert neither a destructive nor a restraining effect on microbes. Chloride of lime and similar preparations can be used for all three purposes.

The introduction of antiseptics by Lord Lister has revolutionised surgical practices, and in saving life and preventing suffering the importance of the discovery is only approached by that of anaesthetics. It made possible the performance of a large number of operations, for example, abdominal operations, which previously, owing to the risk of infection, were considered indefensible. A further advance has been taken in what is known as aseptic surgery. Recognizing the injurious effects of antiseptic solutions on the delicate tissues of the body, an attempt, and usually a successful one, is made to prevent the access of germs to any wound which the surgeon may make. To this end, dressings, instruments, operating gloves, and everything which can come near the wound are thoroughly disinfected.

In rendering first aid in the case of accidental wounds, however, and in dealing with suppurating or dirty wounds, antiseptics are necessary (*see* Plate II, 5-6). Much is accomplished if the person who handles the wound cleanses his hands thoroughly with soap and water, washes the wound with clean water which has been boiled, and covers it up with a clean bit of linen, but the use of an antiseptic is desirable, and some such should be available in houses and workshops. Some of the commonest antiseptics are :

PERCHLORIDE OF MERCURY (corrosive sublimate) and BINIODIDE OF MERCURY. Solutions in water in a strength of 1 in 2,000 for wounds to 1 in 10,000 for an eye lotion. These preparations are extremely poisonous, and if obtained from the chemist as a lotion are coloured in order to prevent their being mistaken for and drunk as water. They may be obtained in coloured tablets, and this is very convenient, as it is easy from the directions accompanying the tablet to make solutions of the required strength. Corrosive sublimate should not be brought into contact with metal instruments, as it destroys them.

CARBOLIC ACID. In water, 1 part in 20, 40 or 60. In mixing, the water should be hot. If a wound is to be covered by gutta-percha tissue or oiled silk, the weaker solutions only should be used to moisten the dressing.

TINCTURE OF IODINE. This can be painted on, the sharp smarting produced when applied to broken skin quickly

passing off ; or it may be used as a lotion, a teaspoonful to a pint of water. This makes a useful vaginal douche.

POTASSIUM PERMANGANATE. Dissolve sufficient crystals in the water to produce a light port wine tint, or obtain from the chemist solution of potassium permanganate B.P. and use a tablespoonful to a pint of water. When wounds or ulcers are foul-smelling this is very effective. Weak solutions (pink) are used as injections and lotions in gonorrhoeal affections.

HYDROGEN PEROXIDE SOLUTION. Diluted with five parts of water, this makes a good mouth wash, and is used in pyorrhoea. The compound solution of thymol B.P.C. also makes a good mouth wash or gargle, and can be used for a nasal douche. It is diluted with 3 or 4 parts of water.

BORACIC ACID. A saturated solution is used, which is obtained by dissolving in hot water as much of the powder as can be taken up and pouring off the clear liquid after cooling. This will serve as a lotion, gargle or mouth wash. For an eye wash dilute the above with 5 parts of warm water. Boracic acid powder may also be dusted over wounds.

IODOFORM. A yellow powder with a somewhat disagreeable smell. It is chiefly used for tubercular affections or venereal sores. As a dusting powder for sores it may be mixed with 4 parts of boracic acid powder.

CRESOL SOAP SOLUTION OR LYSOL. A teaspoonful in a pint of warm water.

EUSOL AND DAKIN'S SOLUTIONS. These are hypochlorite solutions, and are good also as deodorants. The latter rarely irritate, if at all.

There are also many reliable proprietary antiseptics.

Antiseptics are of value internally in gastric fermentation, diarrhoea, enteric fever, dysentery, and other affections, but should only be used under the supervision of a doctor.

See Acriflavine ; Benzoic Acid ; Chloride of Lime ; Corrosive Sublimate ; Creosote ; Cresol ; Disinfectant ; Dressing ; Formalin ; Iodine ; Iodoform ; Manganese ; Mercury ; Sterilisation ; Wound.

ANTISPASMODIC. As the name suggests, antispasmodics are drugs which relieve spasm or a sudden contraction of muscle fibres, whether of skeletal muscles or of those lining arteries, the gut, or the bronchial or other tubes. They include aromatic spirit of ammonia, or sal volatile, and other carminatives, amyl nitrite, belladonna, bromides, chloroform, hyoscyamus, opium, valerian, etc. The application of warmth has often the same effect, as when a hot-water bag or a fomentation is applied to the abdomen to relieve colic. In spasm of the arteries, as in angina pectoris, the inhalation of amyl nitrite may relieve the spasm very greatly; stramonium and belladonna are useful in asthma, the bromides in preventing epileptic fits, and valerian in hysteria.

ANTITOXIN. Among the defensive measures undertaken by the living tissues of the body against microbic invasion is the formation of an antitoxin, that is, a substance which neutralises the toxin or poison produced by the microbe. This action resembles the neutralisation of an acid by an alkali, but differs in this respect, that whereas any alkali will neutralise any acid, the antitoxin for any disease only neutralises the toxin of that disease; the antitoxin of diphtheria is thus useless against the toxin of tetanus, and vice versa. Antitoxins may be used either in cure or prevention.

See Anaphylaxis; Antidiphtheritic Serum; Diphtheria; Immunity; Tetanus.

ANTRUM. The literal meaning of the word antrum is a cavern or cavity, and thus it is used to describe a large cavity in the upper jaw bone on either side, known as the antrum of Highmore, and a cavity in the mastoid process, the mastoid antrum. The former communicates

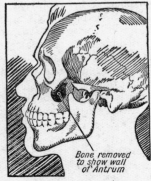

Antrum in upper jaw

Bone removed to show wall of Antrum

with the cavity of the nose through a narrow opening, and when the antrum becomes infected from the nose, or perhaps more frequently from certain diseased upper teeth, pus has difficulty in draining away. The surgeon must then provide for drainage by drilling through the socket of a tooth or by making an opening beneath the cheek. Suppuration, or, as it is often called, empyema of the antrum, may cause pain in the jaw and swelling of the cheek. The condition is to be suspected if a discharge of offensive pus takes place into the nose when a person lies on one side of his head. The mastoid antrum communicates with the middle ear, from which it may become infected.

See Ear.

ANUS. The external opening of the rectum, or lowest part of the large bowel, is called the anus. When, in consequence of obstruction of the lower bowel by a cancerous growth or otherwise, a surgeon has to establish an exit through an opening in the lower part of the belly or the back, the opening is called an artificial anus. The diseases most commonly found in this region include piles, abscess, fistula, fissure, pruritus, and prolapse and stricture, which are discussed under these headings.

ANXIETY. It is common knowledge that worry may depress the bodily functions and seriously affect health. Few people are fortunate enough to escape a personal experience of its truth. Indigestion is a common result, and instances have occurred where jaundice appeared, seemingly entirely due to worry. Individuals differ in the extent to which the unpleasant or difficult incidents of life affect them; but in abnormal conditions, like hysteria and neurasthenia, there may be evidence of worry out of all proportion to any apparent reason for it. Such people may be tremulous, restless and apprehensive and unduly preoccupied about their health or their circumstances.

In neurasthenia, overstrain is generally responsible, and rest is imperative whatever other treatment is adopted. In the condition called anxiety hysteria, the anxiety is assumed to be evidence of a mental conflict between repressed organic cravings or fears and the conventions which the individual feels constrained to obey. The remedy is pyscho-therapy.

See Hysteria; Neurasthenia; Pyscho-therapy.

APERIENT. The milder purgatives are known as aperients or laxatives. Their effect is to produce one or two soft motions. The doses of those most commonly used are as follows :

Dry extract of cascara sagrada..2 to 8 grains
in pills or tablets
Liquid extract of cascara sagrada .. ½ to 1
drachm
Aromatic syrup of cascara .. ½ to 2 drachms
This affords an agreeable way of taking cascara which will appeal to children ; about a half-teaspoonful for a child of eight
Castor oil .. .. 1 to 2 teaspoonsful
This is the best aperient during pregnancy in teaspoonful doses, repeated if necessary. The taste may be concealed by an equal quantity of glycerin and some lemon juice.
Castor oil mixture ..2 to 4 tablepoonsful
Flowers of sulphur .. 20 to 60 grains in
molasses
Confection of sulphur .. 1 to 2 teaspoonsful
Milk of sulphur .. 20 to 60 grains in
molasses
Sulphur lozenges .. 1 or 2 at bedtime
Compound liquorice powder .. 1 to 2
teaspoonsful
Syrup of figs .. 1 teaspoonful for children
Liquid paraffin .. 1 teaspoonful to 1
tablespoonful
Powder of magnesia or magnesia carbonate
5 to 30 grains, repeated doses ; 30 to 60 grains as a single dose
May be mixed in milk, plain water or soda-water.
Solution of magnesium citrate .. 5 to 10
ounces
Olive oil .. 1 to 2 tablespoonsful
Tamar indien lozenges .. 1, less or more
Useful for old people

The more active purgatives, such as senna, rhubarb and aloes, act as aperients when given in sufficiently small doses.

See Cathartic ; Constipation ; Diarrhoea.

APEX. As applied to the lung, the apex means the upper extremity which reaches to a point about 1½ inches above the first rib in front. The apex beat of the heart is normally felt in adults in the space between the fifth and sixth ribs inside the nipple line, which is one drawn downwards from the nipple or, more accurately, the middle of the collar bone. The apex beat alters its situation in enlargement of the heart and other conditions.

See Heart ; Lung.

APHASIA. The communication of our ideas to others implies, first, mental processes in which thoughts are shaped, things and qualities being correctly named and associated in the form of propositions ; and, secondly, mechanisms to reproduce these propositions whether by speech, writing or gesture. After an apoplectic seizure and in other brain diseases certain disorders of speech may be found,

in which, although the mechanisms for reproduction are in order, they cannot be utilised properly or at all, because of some impairment of the intellectual processes. Aphasia is the name under which such disorders are grouped.

People who become aphasic are not always affected in the same way, and Sir Henry Head recognizes at least four varieties of the disease, which are discriminated by their response to a series of tests. To put the matter briefly, sufferers from the first understand what is said to them, but in speaking and writing they have difficulty in expressing themselves, the pronunciation is defective and their vocabulary appears to be small ; the second variety pronounce words properly, but appear to have lost their knowledge of what written and spoken words stand for ; the third talk jargon, having a poor sense of the grammar and rhythm of sentences and of balance in the enunciation of words ; and the fourth, while they can read and write, tend to become confused, and if told to do something, do not appear to understand clearly what the ultimate aim of the action is.

Dr. Hughlings Jackson pointed out that the words which pass out of currency for the aphasiac are those used in intellectual operations rather than those evoked by emotional states, and in human development it would be the latter, cf course, which would be possessed first.

APHONIA. Loss of voice is termed aphonia. It is usually due to inflammation of the vocal chords, but sometimes it is due to hysteria.

See Speech.

APOMORPHINE. This drug is derived from opium. It causes vomiting more quickly and certainly than any other known drug, and may thus, if at hand, be very useful in cases of poisoning. It is injected under the skin in doses of $\frac{1}{20}$ to $\frac{1}{10}$ of a grain, though it may also be given by the mouth.

APONEUROSIS. This is the name of a flat sheet of fibrous tissue by means of which many muscles, especially of the trunk, are attached to the bones which it is their duty to move, or which covers or encloses muscles.

APOPLEXY. When a person becomes suddenly unconscious from bleeding caused by rupture of an artery in the brain or from the blocking of such an artery, he is said to suffer from apoplexy. Cerebral haemorrhage is not common before middle life, when the effects of age are apparent in the arteries ; and, as strain is an important cause of these arterial changes, it occurs most often in men. The arteries tend to become more brittle with advancing years, but more so and more quickly in people who over-eat or who constantly take more alcohol than is good for them. Kidney disease, syphilis and lead poisoning cause thickening and degeneration of arteries and may precipitate a cerebral haemorrhage at an unusually early age.

Blocking of an artery, or embolism, is brought about by a clot or other foreign body which is carried to the brain by the blood stream. Any person with a diseased heart is liable to the accident, which may therefore occur in quite young persons. In old people with degenerate arteries the blood may clot in the arteries and apoplexy may result, but more usually the development of symptoms is gradual. An attack of apoplexy may follow physical or mental strain, from an increase in the blood pressure, but it may occur without apparent provocation, and may happen during sleep. It may prove fatal, either immediately or after the lapse of some hours or days, but this is not usual in first attacks, and the patient gradually becomes conscious, though paralysis of muscles on one side of the body and perhaps mental impairment or disturbances of speech will remain for some time and in some degree may persist indefinitely.

The word apoplexy is derived from a Greek one meaning to strike down or to stop, and describes exactly what takes place in the seizure. The patient suddenly loses consciousness and becomes completely helpless. His face may be pale, but more commonly is flushed, and the head and eyes may be turned to one side, generally that on which the brain has been damaged. The breathing is laboured and sterterous, the lips are blown out, and the cheeks flap with each expiration. The eyeballs are insensitive to touch and the pupils are contracted, one being bigger than the other. The bladder may be emptied and the bowels may move.

Those who witness such a seizure should have little difficulty in recognizing its nature, but, when, as sometimes happens, the victim of an attack is not seen until some time later, it may be necessary to distinguish the condition from some others. The pupils may be very small as in opium poisoning, and the flushed face and noisy breathing may suggest acute alcoholism. The latter impression may be heightened by the fact that the patient smells of alcohol.

An important sign of apoplexy, if it can be elicited, is paralysis of one side of the body.

If the arms of the patient are lifted up one after the other and allowed to fall, it will be found that on one side the arm drops just like a dead thing, and the muscles of this limb will feel looser and more flaccid than those of the other. The doctor will have to make the diagnosis, of course, but it is necessary to emphasise the distinction between alcoholism and apoplexy, because it has sometimes been too readily assumed that a man was drunk when actually he was suffering from apoplexy, and he has been left to die in a police cell. Whenever there is the slightest doubt about it, the case should be treated as if it were apoplexy.

Unconsciousness usually passes off in three or four hours, but in cases of haemorrhage there is likely to be some mental confusion and perhaps a complaint of headache. In cases of embolism, consciousness is usually recovered earlier and more completely. If unconsciousness lasts longer than twelve hours the outlook is grave. The paralysis of the face and limbs usually improves, and also the speech if this has been impaired, but some time must elapse before one can form an opinion as to how complete the recovery will be. One attack is liable to be followed by others ; as a physician said in his own case, " the archer has other arrows in his quiver."

The treatment of an attack consists in laying the patient on his back or, if his breathing is especially difficult in this position, turned a little to one side. His head should be a little raised, and clothing about the neck and chest should be loosened.

The greatest gentleness must be exercised in handling the patient, and no one should be allowed to do more than this till a doctor comes. Lives have been lost through over-zealous helpers lifting up such cases, carrying them upstairs to bed and undressing them.

Any but the slightest movements may further increase the escape of blood from the ruptured vessel. Hot-water bottles may be placed at the patient's feet and between his thighs, and if an ice-bag is available it may be placed on his head. While the patient is lying helpless in bed it will be necessary to prevent his bladder from going too long unemptied, and enemata may be required to clear the bowel. Should unconsciousness be prolonged, it may be necessary to feed the patient with nutrient enemata. While limbs remain paralysed their position should be changed frequently, to avoid their becoming flexed and stiff at the joint. Care must be taken to avoid the formation of bedsores (*q.v.*).

When the patient begins to take nourishment this should be restricted at first to small quantities of milk and beaten-up eggs, and the advice of the doctor should be followed with regard to any increase in the diet. At no time should alcohol be given unless prescribed by the doctor. During convalescence the doctor may order massage or electrical treatment for the paralysed limbs. When the patient is up and about he must lead a quiet, retired life, free from worry and excitement. He should take gentle exercise daily. The diet should be plain and easily digested. Alcohol should be avoided, and if tobacco is used at all it must be in strict moderation. The skin should be kept active by warm baths followed by a rub down, and regularity of the bowels must be maintained.

See Artery; Embolism; Paralysis; Thrombosis.

APOTHECARIES' WEIGHTS AND MEASURES. In prescribing solid drugs doctors may order so many grains, or they may use the apothecaries' scale and symbols for quantities up to a drachm;

in the case of larger quantities, 1 ounce and 1 pound, the avoirdupois scale is used. There is a material difference in the two scales for these quantities. In the Apothecaries' scale a pound consists of 12 ounces of 480 grains each, or in all 5,760 grains, while a pound avoirdupois consists of 16 ounces of 437·5 grains each, or in all 7000 grains. In describing liquids the apothecaries' measures are used for quantities up to an ounce and beyond this the imperial measures. The composite scales would therefore appear as follows:

APOTHECARIES'		
DRY		WET
20 grains (gr.)	=1 scruple (℈)	
3 scruples	=1 drachm or dram (ℨ)	60 minims (♏) =1 fluid drachm or dram (ℨ) 8 fluid drachms= 1 fluid ounce (℥)

IMPERIAL		
437·5 grains	=1 ounce (oz.)	
16 ounces	=1 pound (lb.)	20 fluid ounces = 1 pint 8 pints = 1 gallon

It is to be noted that a drop varies in size and does not correspond to a minim. The doses of drugs are given in the British Pharmacopoeia also according to the metric system, and there are very good reasons for the universal adoption of the latter.

See Domestic Measures; Dose; Drug; Medicines; Prescription.

APPENDICITIS. Inflammation of the vermiform appendix is known as appendicitis. The vermiform appendix is a narrow tube which emerges from the wall of the caecum, or first part of the large intestine, near the point where the latter is joined by the small intestine. In an adult its average length is about 4 inches, and it is not very thick; hence its description as vermiform, which means worm-like. Appendicitis may occur at any age, but is commoner in young people, and especially in males.

The appendix communicates with the bowel, but is closed at the other end. Its lumen is narrow, and if there is a slight swelling of the lining at the entrance, or if the appendix is kinked, secretions may be imprisoned and decompose. The walls contain a large amount of lymphoid tissue similar to that of which the tonsils are composed, and this is readily liable to inflammatory swelling. Foreign bodies, such as grape seeds and fruit pips, are not found in the appendix so frequently as was at one time supposed, but what is found quite frequently is a little piece of hardened faeces, probably resulting from chronic constipation, and this may irritate the appendix lining or ulcerate into or even through the wall of the organ. Besides irritation produced by bodies of this kind, the tissues of the organ may be infected in such diseases as rheumatism or tuberculosis, and, of course, the appendix may share in catarrhal conditions affecting the adjoining bowel.

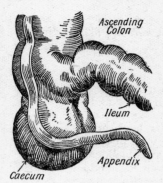

Appendix. How it is attached and opens into the caecum

Whatever may be the cause of the inflammation, the lining or the whole organ swells and becomes painful. It is evident that the walls of the little tube are very vulnerable and allow microbes and their products a fairly ready access to the peritoneum, which covers the organ like the finger of a glove and is continuous with that lining the interior of the abdomen and covering the bowels and other organs. When infection reaches this membrane through the appendix it becomes inflamed, and lymph, a soft substance like colourless blood clot, forms on its surface. By means of this the appendix becomes glued to adjoining structures ; it may even be entirely surrounded by a mass of matted tissue and thereby cut off from the general cavity of the abdomen.

This device of Nature may succeed in forthwith bringing the disease to an end by allowing the curative forces to operate in a delimited area, or the infection may be sufficient to produce an abscess within the matted tissues. In other cases the inflamed appendix may become gangrenous, that is to say, its tissues die, and if it could be seen it would appear as a dull dark red or green mass. Even then Nature does not relinquish her efforts to wall in the disease, but, unfortunately, very often the infection is able to reach the general cavity, where it produces general peritonitis. This may occur with a very virulent infection, with rapid perforation of the appendix or with the bursting of an abscess.

The symptoms of the disease in the first instance are nausea, sickness, a sense of pain around the navel, a rise of temperature, perhaps to 101° or 102°F, a quickened pulse and constipation. After some hours there is tenderness at a point to the right of and below the navel, and the muscles of the abdominal wall become rigid and resist any attempt to press in with the fingers. To ease the pain the patient often lies with the right leg bent up. These symptoms may indicate the earlier degrees of inflammation, but one cannot be sure of this, and the surgeon is not infrequently surprised to find the appendix gangrenous when the general condition of the patient has not appeared particularly serious. In general peritonitis the whole belly becomes swollen, hard and painful, and the general condition of the patient is much aggravated.

With regard to treatment, uncertainty as to the real state of affairs within the belly makes it imperative that the patient be placed in the care of the surgeon at the earliest possible moment.

Many cases have got better without operation, but a deplorable number of people lose their lives because operation has been delayed until too late.

For relief of pain till the doctor comes a hot-water bottle may be laid by the side of the patient, or an ice-bag may be applied to the part, and, as this should not press on the belly, it is suspended from a bed cradle (*q.v.*) placed under the bedclothes, so that the bag merely touches the patient (Plate IX, 1).

Dating from an attack of appendicitis perhaps so slight as to be overlooked, there may be a recurrence of attacks, and these also may be slight in character. When an attack has subsided, the exudate which has been mentioned above as forming on the peritoneal covering of the organ becomes converted into tough strings or bands, called adhesions, tethering the appendix to the body wall or to other organs. The result may be interference with the movements of the bowel and constipation or actual obstruction of the gut. Another result may be the production of dyspeptic symptoms which are not relieved till the general condition is dealt with, and in duodenal ulcer there is generally also associated appendix trouble.

In these cases the absence of signs in the neighbourhood of the appendix is far from negativing the reality of disease of this organ as a factor in producing the gastric symptoms; in fact, it is probably found oftener without signs than with them. Some people have symptoms which suggest appendicitis and cause them a lot of worry, but which have nothing to do with the appendix. For example, the accumulation of gas or faeces in the caecum may cause considerable pain in the right lower abdomen, but this will be relieved by the passing of flatus or a motion. If, however, such a condition tends to persist, a doctor should certainly be consulted.

See Adhesion; Constipation; Peritonitis.

APPETITE. When the body requires nourishment there arises automatically the natural craving for food which we call appetite. It is this and the sight, taste and smell of food which start the flow of the gastric juices. The appetite may be affected psychically, and an ill-cooked and badly served meal may do much to reduce it, as may any depressing emotion.

To a certain extent appetite is a measure of the quantity, and a guide to the nature, of the food one should take; what we fancy is likely to be good for us. But there are exceptions to this, as a poor appetite may not represent the needs of the body, but only be due to faulty hygiene, such as sedentary habits, too little exercise, or the abuse of tobacco, tea, alcohol or other drugs. On the other hand, a good appetite may be misleading, as in the case of a convalescent from enteric fever, when the satisfaction of his desire for particular articles of food is likely to produce haemorrhage or perforation of the bowel. Also, it is not uncommon to have an unusually good appetite as an early symptom of gastric catarrh, and its satisfaction will precipitate the symptoms of this disorder.

In cases of duodenal ulcer the pain is usually worst when the patient is beginning to feel hungry; this is sometimes called " hunger pain," and at first it is relieved by the taking of food. In acute fevers the appetite disappears, and in this instance it is desirable that it should, as the patient is not able to digest much, especially solid food. A poor appetite is also found in debilitating diseases such as anaemia or tuberculosis, and it may be an indication of cancer of the stomach. Where it is a symptom of such a disease its treatment is included in that of the particular disease.

In cases where personal habits are at fault the obvious thing to do is to correct the habit. However, something may be done to improve the appetite by the use of " bitters " or " aromatic bitters " such as calumba, gentian, quassia, cascarilla, or bitter orange peel. The preparations employed are the infusions of these drugs in doses of $\frac{1}{2}$ to 1 ounce, and the tinctures in doses of $\frac{1}{2}$ to 1 drachm. The following is an example of an appetiser:

Compound tincture of carda-moms	$1\frac{1}{2}$ drachms
Concentrated compound solution of sarsaparilla ..	1 drachm
Spirit of chloroform.. ..	$1\frac{1}{2}$ drachms
Tincture of calumba ..	4 ,,
Water	to make 6 ounces

Take a small wineglassful ten minutes before dinner.

Increased appetite is found in diabetes, some cases of chronic gastritis, gastric ulcers and other maladies. In some conditions there is a depraved appetite for injurious or unusual things, such as indigestible apples or ashes; for example, in pregnancy, chlorosis, and hysteria.

See Bitters; Diet; Digestion; Eating; Invalid Cookery.

APPLE. Many people pin their faith to apples as a means to keeping fit, and probably there is something in the theory, as raw apples provide fresh fruit juice and keep the teeth clean, and in any form they help to keep the bowels regular. But a raw apple must be ripe and sound, otherwise it may produce indigestion.

ARACHNOID MEMBRANE. So named in allusion to a spider's web, the arachnoid is one of the three membranes which cover the central part of the nervous system, that is, the brain and spinal cord.

ARCUS SENILIS. The white rim that appears at the edge of the iris or coloured part of the eye, usually in elderly people, is called the arcus senilis. Its appearance in younger people is usually a sign of premature old age or senility.

ARECA NUT. The seeds of the catechu palm, an Eastern tree, are known as areca, or betel, nuts. The powder made by grinding them is used as an anthelmintic, and is also put into tooth powders. Mixed with a little quicklime and rolled in a leaf of the piper betel, it is often chewed by Orientals, but this is a dangerous practice, as it may cause cancer in the mouth.

AREOLAR TISSUE. This is the technical name for the loose tissue that lies beneath the skin and mucous membranes, between the muscles, and in general fills up all the odd corners of the body.

ARGYROL. One of the organic silver compounds is known as argyrol. It is used as an antiseptic in eye affections and in gonorrhoea. A few drops of a 5 to 10 per cent. solution dropped into the eyes of a newly-born child prevents the development of ophthalmia neonatorum.

ARM. The upper limb of the body between the shoulder and the wrist is known as the arm, and consists of the upper arm (sometimes referred to simply as the arm) above the elbow and the forearm below it. The former has one bone, the humerus, and the latter two, the radius on the outer or thumb side and the ulna on the inner. The upper arm is jointed on to the scapula or shoulder blade, and is moved by muscles coming from this bone, from the collar bone and from the trunk.

The main artery of the limb, the brachial, runs on the inner side of the humerus in its upper half but comes in front of the bone below this. In compressing the artery to stop bleeding it is necessary therefore to compress above the middle of the bone, and from within outwards. The inner seam of the coat roughly indicates the position ; the limb is grasped from behind and pressure applied by the four fingers (Plate VI, 8). Three main nerves pass down the arm, the median, the ulnar, and the musculo-spiral. The latter winds round the back of the humerus, and is liable to be compressed when the back of the upper arm is pressed on a hard edge, for example, of the bed when one is asleep. This may result in wrist drop. An injured arm should be rested in a greater arm sling, except in fractures of the humerus when the lesser sling is used.

See Artificial Limb ; Elbow ; Humerus ; Median Nerve ; Radius ; Shoulder ; Ulna ; Wrist.

ARMPIT. The axilla or armpit contains the large blood vessels and nerves supplying the arm, and is therefore a dangerous situation for a wound. Care has to be taken in the use of crutches and in applying splints that undue pressure is not made on the armpit, lest crutch palsy be the result. It also contains a number of lymphatic glands, which may become enlarged and inflamed from poisoned wounds on the arm, the hand or the breast. In addition to treatment of the wound, the arm should be rested in a sling. The glands also enlarge in chronic inflammation and in cancer of the breast, and must be removed with the latter for the extirpation of cancer.

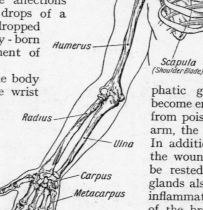

Bones of the arm and forearm

Excessive sweating of the armpits is often met with in forms of debility. The copious sweating in large droplets, which sometimes occurs in the armpits when a person strips, has usually no special significance, however, being merely due to chilling of the skin. Excessive sweating may prove annoying from its amount and the smell caused by its decomposition. The armpits should be washed daily with soap and water, and after drying may be dusted with a powder consisting of equal parts of boracic acid

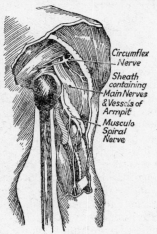

Armpit. Crutch paralysis induced by pressure on nerves

and starch or with this more elegant preparation:

Oil of rose geranium	..	6 minims
Salicylic acid powder	..	1 drachm
Zinc oleate powder ..	..	3 ounces
Starch powder	..	3 ,,

If necessary the hairs should be removed by shaving or by a depilatory. Eczema of the armpit responds well to an ointment consisting of equal parts of diachylon plaster and soft paraffin.

See Lymphatic System ; Shoulder.

ARNICA. This plant yields tincture of arnica, very popular as an external remedy for bruises and sprains. The remedy, however, probably owes all its virtues to the alcohol it contains. It may produce disagreeable rashes, and should never be used when the skin is broken. Other effective remedies are easily available which have none of its risks.

See Bruise ; Sprain ; Tincture.

AROMATIC. This name is applied to substances which have a particular kind of pleasant odour. Many aromatics are used to flavour prescriptions, but in addition to this they act as carminatives, relieving flatulence and aiding digestion. They are also nearly all powerful antiseptics. They include anise, camphor, cardamom, cinnamon, dill, ginger, peppermint, thymol, etc.

See Carminative.

ARROWROOT. Cooked arrowroot makes a bland food for invalids. As it consists almost of pure starch, it must be supplemented by milk, eggs and other foods. To prepare it, mix a dessertspoonful of the powder with two tablespoonsful of milk or water and pour over it a half-pint of boiling milk or water. Stir briskly, then add a teaspoonful of sugar. If ordered, a teaspoonful of brandy or cream may also be added.

See Invalid Cookery.

ARSENIC. The metal arsenic, which has important industrial uses, is often a valuable medicine in some of its various preparations. As it is highly poisonous, it should not be taken except under medical supervision. It is contained in some preparations sold as rat poisons or weed-killers, in fly-papers and some anti-fly mixtures, and in arsenical sprays for trees and plants. It may also be sold as white arsenic (arsenious acid) tinted with soap or indigo, or another compound, for the home preparation of any of these. There is always, therefore, a danger of poisoning from such preparations, and care must be exercised as to their disposal.

Fowler's solution, or liquor arsenicalis, is a favourite method of exhibiting the drug in medicine. Arsenic acts as an alterative (*q.v.*) and as a blood tonic. It is usefully employed in some forms of anaemia, either alone or in combination with iron, and is largely used in the anaemia and debility accompanying malaria. Chronic skin affections may be greatly benefited by its use, and it is added to bromide mixtures when there is a tendency to the development of a bromide acne. It finds another useful sphere in the treatment of some chronic nervous complaints, for example, disseminated sclerosis. Arsenic is a powerful remedy in destroying blood parasites, and one or other of its organic preparations is usually employed for the purpose ; thus galyl has been largely given in malaria and trypanosomiasis, and salvarsan or some of its modifications in syphilis.

Poisoning by Arsenic. Should redness and smarting of the eyes, sneezing and running of the nose develop when arsenic is being taken, the medicine should not be continued without reference to the doctor. Acute poisoning by arsenic results in vomiting, severe diarrhoea, abdominal pain and great weakness. The stomach should be emptied by an emetic of a tablespoonful of mustard in a half-glass of water. Then an antidote should be given, dialysed iron if possible, in two-tablespoonful doses ; or, if this is not available, large quantities of magnesia in milk or water. The white of two eggs beaten up in milk will follow. The patient should be kept warm in bed with hot-water bottles at his feet and by his side. Hot fomentations or a poultice on the abdomen will relieve pain and diarrhoea.

Chronic poisoning may occur in workers whose occupation involves the use of arsenic, for example, in the manufacture of aniline dyes. Formerly it was not infrequent from arsenical pigments used to colour wallpaper, artificial flowers or fabrics. The outbreak of chronic poisoning among beer drinkers which occurred in England in 1900 was shown to be due to the presence of arsenic in the glucose and sugar used in making the beer. The earliest symptoms are those of irritation of the eyes and nose, with which there may be loss of appetite, nausea, vomiting and diarrhoea. Inflammation of the nerves, or neuritis, may lead to increased sensitiveness of the skin, weakness, and foot and wrist drop. The skin may become thickened and deeply pigmented.

The occurrence of such symptoms should of course lead to an instant and thorough investigation into the source of the poisoning, so that the patient and others may be protected from further doses. Potassium iodide will probably be prescribed by the doctor to aid in the elimination of the poison from the system. The diet will have to be light, and tonics may be necessary. The time taken in recovery, and its completeness, will depend on the amount of arsenic which has been absorbed and on the extent and nature of the tissue changes which have resulted.

See Anaemia ; Poisoning ; Salvarsan.

ARTERIO - SCLEROSIS. The literal meaning of arterio-sclerosis is hardening of the arteries, and this is what happens in the disease. Degenerative changes occur in the walls of the vessels which impair their elasticity, and a deposit occurs in the inner coat which narrows the lumen of the vessel. The vessels are weaker also and tend to rupture when exposed to strain, thus giving rise to aneurysm or haemorrhage. A change of this kind is apt to appear in the arteries after middle life, and in old age they may be more or less rigid tubes. In some people, as a part of their physical inheritance, the arteries may harden at an unusually early age. Increase in the blood pressure is an important cause, and, unfortunately, the blood pressure may be abnormally high for a long time without giving any marked hint of its presence. Strenuous muscular toil is another cause, and a large number of cases are due to immoderation in eating and drinking, particularly in those who take insufficient outdoor exercise. Lead poisoning, syphilis and kidney disease are amongst other causes which should be mentioned. Arterio-sclerosis may also give rise to kidney disease, and it may result in enlargement of the heart.

It gives rise to a large variety of symptoms, depending to some extent on the site of the vessels affected. Some of these are : giddiness, especially on altering one's position ; headache ; impairment of the power of attention ; weakness or paralysis of muscles ; coldness of the hands and feet ; insomnia ; noises in the head ; shortness of breath and pain over the heart. The possibility of its occurrence should be borne in mind by those who have passed middle life and especially by those who live freely.

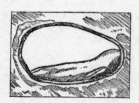

Arterio - sclerosis. Lime deposit in artery

Whether the disease is to be cured or only moderated, if even that, depends upon the stage at which it is discovered and treated. Treatment involves a tranquil life, strict moderation in eating and drinking and in the use of tobacco, and attention to the bowels and to the activity of the skin. It is necessary for such people to keep in touch with their doctor.

See Aneurysm · Angina Pectoris ; Apoplexy ; Artery ; Endarteritis ; Gangrene.

ARTERY. The blood vessels that carry blood from the heart are termed arteries. The name literally means " air bearer," because when arteries are opened after death they are all found to be empty. But the great physician Galen, who practised under Marcus Aurelius, opened an artery in a living animal and found it to contain blood. The blood in the pulmonary artery which is being pumped by the heart into the lungs is dark or impure blood, but with this exception the blood in an artery is always bright red from the presence of oxygen.

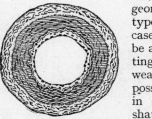

Artery. Cross section showing the three coats

An artery has three coats: an inner smooth, elastic coat; a middle muscular; and an outer supporting coat, composed of connective tissue. The muscular coat is relatively thicker in the smaller arteries, and when it contracts and narrows the lumen of these vessels the resistance to the blood flow is, of course, increased and the blood pressure is raised. The contraction of this coat serves in arresting bleeding from a divided artery, the curling inwards of the elastic inner coat likewise contributing to this effect.

See Aneurysm; Arterio-sclerosis; Circulation of the Blood; Embolism; Endarteritis; Infarction; Pulse; Thrombosis.

ARTHRITIS. When all the tissues of a joint are involved in inflammation, the term arthritis is used to describe the condition. Inflammation of the synovial membrane is known as synovitis. Arthritis may be due to gout, to rheumatism, to tuberculosis, to injury and to many other causes.

See Joint; Osteo-arthritis; Rheumatism; Rheumatoid Arthritis.

ARTICULATION. In ordinary speech articulation means the process of speaking distinctly. It is also the technical name for a joint.

ARTIFICIAL LIMB. Strength, lightness and comfortable adaptation to the stump of the amputated limb are qualities not one of which can be dispensed with in an artificial limb. The mechanical construction should also be sound; the part nearer the body should be the heavier, in order to secure better balance; joints and locking parts should be secure, yet work smoothly, and braces and straps

should be fitted so as not to compress the chest and interfere with breathing.

Artificial limbs are to be had in great variety, some being illustrated in Plate III, and the advice of a surgeon should be taken as to the type suitable in a particular case, while a good maker should be asked to attend to the fitting. It is desirable to begin wearing a limb as soon as possible after the amputation in order to hasten a proper shaping of the stump and the restoration of bulk and tone to the muscles which move it. As a rule it will be only a temporary limb which will be suitable for the purpose.

When first worn, an artificial limb may prove irksome and tiring, but ease in wearing will increase with use. Persevering practice with movable fingers and tools may in time make an artificial arm a fair compensation for the lost one, although the initial awkwardness may appear to be an insuperable difficulty.

For heavy work a hook is the most suitable attachment for an arm, and should be fixed as near the end of the stump as possible; many ingenious tools and appliances are provided for taking food, writing and doing various kinds of light work; these, and hooks also, should be fitted to the limb by a spring attachment rather than by screwing.

A peg leg is more suitable than a full artificial limb for one who has to do much tramping over moist earth, as damp very quickly destroys the various types of artificial foot. In amputations below the knee it may be difficult to prevent the end of the stump from rubbing on the limb casing, or socket, and becoming chafed. A satisfactory method of doing this is to use what is called a slip-socket. This is applied over the end of the stump and firmly attached by strapping; any friction then taking place will only affect the slip-socket. Increased lightness in limbs is secured by the use of composition materials.

Care should be taken to keep joints oiled with a light machine oil, and to keep other parts of the limb as clean as possible. The inside of a bucket, the part which takes the stump, should be washed periodically with warm water to which lysol or sanitas has been added, and dried quickly and thoroughly with a soft rag, and the outer surfaces of leather or metal fittings should be rubbed over with an appropriate polishing material.

See Amputation.

ARTIFICIAL RESPIRATION. In cases of gas poisoning, apparent drowning, etc., when breathing has stopped, it is often possible to resuscitate the· patient by performing movements which alternately expand and contract the chest, so that air is drawn into and expelled from the lungs. This imitation of natural breathing is known as artificial respiration, and may be done in several ways ; Professor Schäfer's is the method now usually adopted and this is illustrated in Plate IV. Before commencing this or any other method, a rapid examination should be made to ensure that the chest and neck are in no way constricted, and that the mouth and throat are clear.

The patient, in Professor Schäfer's method, is then placed face downward on the ground, his head being turned to one side to free his mouth and nose, and his arms stretched out in front. The operator kneels astride him, facing forward, his knees being about the level of the patient's hips. He places his hands over the lower ribs on either side, the thumbs being parallel and nearly touching and the fingers spread out. A common mistake of the inexperienced is to place the hands too low ; they should be on the ribs, not on the loins. Keeping his arms straight, the operator now leans forward, and his weight presses the ribs forwards and inwards. The result is that air is expelled from the lungs and perhaps water, if any has been swallowed. Still keeping his hands on the chest, the operator then springs back, releasing the pressure on the chest, and this is accompanied by an inrush of air to the lungs.

The first movement should occupy the time necessary to count slowly one, two, three, and the second to count one, two. The combined movements take about five seconds to accomplish, and should be continued rhythmically until there are signs of recovery. This will be marked by gasping inspirations taking place at short intervals, followed by a resumption of breathing.

In any event efforts should be persisted with till a doctor arrives, and for at least an hour. Resuscitation has been successful when artificial respiration had to go on for considerably longer than this.

Once breathing has started, an energetic attempt is to be made to help the circulation. The patient should be covered with coats and warmth fostered by rubbing or chafing the limbs, the movements being made towards the heart. As soon as possible wet clothes must be removed and the patient covered with a sufficiency of warm blankets, properly protected hot-water bottles being placed at his feet and by his sides. When he can swallow he should be given sips of hot water, hot tea or coffee, or a teaspoonful of spirits of sal volatile in a small wineglassful of water. He should be closely observed for some time as he may again cease breathing, when artificial respiration must be at once resumed.

Making a New-born Baby Breathe

When childbirth occurs in the absence of a doctor it may be necessary for some one present to carry out artificial respiration should the child show no signs of beginning to breathe. Usually breathing begins after a few gasps, and oftener than not the baby announces its arrival by yelling lustily. Should it be quite still, the nurse must put her finger into its mouth as far as the back of the throat and hook forward so as to bring away any mucus that may be there. She should then slap the child smartly two or three times on the back with the flat of the hand, or sprinkle some cold water on the chest. This usually suffices, but if not the child may be dipped several times alternately into basins of cold and hot water. Care should be taken that the latter is not made over-hot.

Should this also fail, the lungs may be inflated by blowing into its mouth through a thin handkerchief, as in exhaling cigarette smoke, and the air is then expelled by compressing the chest, these manoeuvres being repeated in about the same times as recommended in Schäfer's method, or rather faster, and continued for a few minutes. Another method is to grasp the tip of the baby's tongue with the fingers and thumb through a handkerchief and pull the tongue forward. Still holding on, allow it to slip back, and again draw forward, repeating this about fifteen times a minute. This is known as Laborde's method.

See Asphyxia.

ARYTENOID. This is the name of two very small pieces of cartilage or gristle which are found at the back of the voice box or larynx, and to which the vocal cords are attached.

See Larynx.

ASAFOETIDA. The gum resin known as asafoetida owes its name to its intensely disagreeable odour. It is sometimes of use in hysteria and is a remedy for flatulence, especially for flatulent colic. For the latter purpose it may be given in an enema, one or two teaspoonsful of tincture of asafoetida in about a teacupful of soapy water. It is contained in the pill of aloes and asafoetida, of which a 5-grain pill may be taken in the evening. Another preparation is the spiritus ammoniae foetidus, of which the dose is 60 to 90 minims, or, if several doses are to be given, 20 to 40 minims.

ASCARIS. A worm which very often takes up its abode in the alimentary canal, of children chiefly, is known as the ascaris lumbricoides or the roundworm.

See Worms.

ASCITES. The accumulation of dropsical fluid in the abdomen is known as ascites. This may occur in common with dropsy in other parts of the body, but the most marked cases of ascites are a consequence of cirrhosis of the liver, generally the result of chronic alcoholic excess. Treatment is directed to the cause, and diuretics (q.v.) are given to drain off the fluid by the kidneys. Frequently tapping is required.

See Aspiration ; Dropsy.

ASPHYXIA. The literal meaning of asphyxia is absence of the pulse, but the term is usually applied to the effects produced on the body by interference with the aeration of the blood in the lungs. The blood becomes charged with carbonic acid gas, evidenced by the lips and face becoming livid ; the person breathes hurriedly and forcibly and then becomes convulsed. Finally the breathing centre in the brain is paralysed and breathing movements stop, though the heart beats on for a few seconds longer.

Asphyxia may be brought about by disease, for example, by broncho-pneumonia, through diminution of the lung tissue available for the necessary interchange of gases, or by diphtheria, through closure of the air passages by the diphtheritic membrane ; but it may also be brought about accidentally. Thus it occurs (1) in drowning, when water or some other fluid takes the place of air in the lungs ; (2) from closure of the air passages by closing the mouth and nose, strangling, hanging, or choking ; (3) from compression of the chest, as when a person is buried in a fall of earth or is jammed tightly in a crowd ; (4) from inhalation of coal gas, chlorine, sulphurous acid and other poisonous gases ; and (5) from the action of poisons, for example, strychnine or curare.

What to do to a Choking Person

Choking may be due to a piece of meat or some other mass becoming fixed in the air passages, or to compression of the latter by a mass which has stuck in the gullet. It may be due also to swelling of the back of the throat or of the lining of the larynx, produced by stings or by swallowing boiling water or corrosive poisons. Treatment must first be directed to the cause, which should be dealt with as follows :

Strangling : loosen, or if necessary cut, whatever is constricting the neck ; hanging : cut down ; choking : prise open the jaws, if necessary, with the handle of a spoon, which is then thrust between the back teeth and used as a gag ; pass a finger to the back of the throat and try to hook forward the obstruction ; or, especially in children, hang the person head downward and slap the back ; compression of the chest : uncover properly if buried with earth, or, in pressure from a crowd, try to secure space by letting the person down ; poisonous gases : get the person into the open air ; if a gas mask is not available, the rescuer should cover his mouth and nose with a damp cloth. In the case of a gas-filled room it may make the removal of the patient easier if the gas is turned off and the window thrown open or a pane knocked out.

When the cause has been dealt with, if the mouth and throat have not been examined, this should always be done to ensure that they are clear ; tight clothing should be loosened ; and, if breathing has stopped, artificial respiration should be started at once. In cases of choking from stings, boiling water or corrosive poisons, some relief may be given by putting hot cloths to the throat and saturating the air with steam from a bronchitis kettle (q.v.).

When a child suffering from broncho-pneumonia becomes suddenly blue and breathless, it may help, while awaiting the doctor, to put the child in a warm bath and douche the chest with cold water so as to produce long breaths. If choking appears to be threatening in diphtheria or croup, relief may be got if the child can be induced to vomit. For this purpose a teaspoonful of ipecacuanha wine may be given. Also, the air about the child should be saturated with steam.

See Artificial Respiration ; Carbon Monoxide.

ASPIRATION. This is the name of a simple surgical operation which consists in removing fluid from the chest, the abdomen or elsewhere by suction. An aspirator is a large bottle from which the air can be pumped out and from which there passes a tube ending in a hollow needle. This can be plunged, say, between the ribs, and when the stop-cock is turned the fluid in the chest, due perhaps to pleurisy, rushes into the bottle, and the breathing of the patient is relieved.

ASPIRIN. Acetyl-salicylic acid is known more commonly as aspirin. It is a useful remedy in rheumatism and relieves pain in many other conditions. In feverish colds and at the onset of influenza a good combination is a 5-grain tablet each of aspirin and quinine sulphate. This should be taken at bedtime ; if taken at any other time, exposure must be guarded against, as perspiration may be free. Aspirin may also be used to initiate the treatment in malaria, though quinine must always be given at the same time. It often quickly relieves headache. After-effects are not common, but some people find that it upsets the digestion, more particularly if it is taken

regularly for some time. The dose is 5 to 15 grains. As a powder it is best taken in water, and the taste is not unpleasant.
See Salicylic Acid.

ASSES' MILK. This is not infrequently employed as a substitute for human milk. It more closely resembles human milk than does the milk of the cow, and has proved very successful in rearing premature and feeble infants. But it is deficient in fat, and this should be supplemented by adding a teaspoonful of cream to each feeding bottle. It is, however, almost always possible to modify cow's milk to suit the requirements of any infant.

ASTHENOPIA. Asthenopia is the technical name for the particular weakness of vision in which the patient is not able to sustain the act of vision. It is thus quite different from defective vision, or amblyopia. This is a very important condition, and may be due to several different causes. It almost invariably applies only to vision of near objects, but in modern life it is, of course, the vision of near objects that is important as a means of livelihood. Very soon after the patient attempts to read or write or sew, there is an intolerable feeling of tiredness or actual pain in the eyes, or headache, or sometimes an appearance as if everything was turning black, or as if the letters that are being read were running into one another.

Asthenopia is most commonly due to the effort involved in accommodating the eye for near vision, when the shape of the eye is not well adapted for this purpose. Hence it is an almost constant symptom of long-sightedness. In association with this, or independently, there may be weakness in certain of the muscles which move the eyeball. In these cases it may be immediately relieved by the use of proper spectacles. Anaemia may cause it, more particularly in combination with the defects first mentioned, and the administration of iron will prove very beneficial.

A great many cases of asthenopia are less easily curable. They are due to more general and constitutional conditions of the body. They are nervous in their origin and are really a form of neurasthenia (q.v.) or nerve weakness. This kind of asthenopia often occurs in convalescence after a serious illness, and also in hysteria.

The treatment of asthenopia is the treatment of the underlying cause to which it is due ; but at the same time the eyes should be examined by a doctor to determine whether glasses are likely to afford relief.

See Accommodation : Eye ; Vision.

ASTHMA. Sudden attacks of shortness of breath occur from a variety of causes, and to many of these the name asthma, literally panting, is applied. Thus, there are cardiac asthma from heart disease, renal asthma from kidney disease, and so on. When, however, one uses the name asthma without qualification, what is meant is bronchial asthma, in which the difficulty in breathing is due to a spasm of the muscle fibres in the walls of the smaller bronchial tubes.

The disease occurs most frequently in males and not uncommonly begins in childhood. Children of parents who have suffered from asthma are apt to inherit a susceptibility to it. In very many cases there is evidence of what is known as protein sensitisation, and the symptoms of asthma represent a reaction to foreign proteins which have entered the body. This may occur by the inhalation of pollens, of horse dandruff, or of emanations from the fur of cats or dogs, or by the ingestion of white of egg or some other food. In other cases infection by pus-producing microbes appears to be responsible. Irritation by disease within the nose is capable of precipitating attacks in some people.

A neurotic disposition is a factor which has to be taken into account in many cases, and is seen clearly in people in whom the mere suggestion that they are exposed to their provocative cause, for example, the presence of an imaginary cat or dog in a room, is sufficient to bring on an attack. Also, cures of the disease by hypnotism are reported in people in whom it had existed long enough to produce physical changes in the lungs.

An attack may come on during the day, though it is much more frequent at night and after a few hours' sleep. It may do so without warning, or the patient may have been led to expect it from previous depression, indigestion, wheeziness, or some other indication. He wakes up with some difficulty in breathing which increases so that he has to sit up, and throughout his attack he is very anxiously preoccupied with the effort to breathe. To help himself he grasps or rests his hands on the bed, a chair or any other fixed support, and keeps his arms rigid, while his head is thrown back. His inspirations are short and seem hardly to expand the chest, while the expirations are prolonged and wheezing. The face is covered with sweat, and may be pale, flushed or livid. This may go on for a few hours, and then the breathing becomes easier and the patient begins to cough, bringing up first little pellets like sago grains, and later a thin frothy expectoration.

The attack may clear up completely, or some wheeziness may persist for a few days. As time goes on and attacks follow one another frequently, emphysema of the lungs appears, and tends to produce a barrel chest, that is, one in which the ribs are always more or less raised up as they are in normal inspiration. With this there is chronic bronchitis, and in later years the symptoms partake more of the latter complaint and less of the typical asthmatic seizures.

How to Treat the Attack

The treatment during an attack is to provide the patient with as much fresh air as possible and to let him choose the position in which he feels easiest. If the attack follows a heavy meal his sufferings may be shortened if vomiting can be induced by an emetic composed of a tablespoonful of mustard in half a glass of water. A cup of strong coffee is often found beneficial during attacks ; or a capsule of amyl nitrite may be broken and inhaled. The inhalation of the fumes of burning nitre or drugs like stramonium are usually resorted to sooner or later by asthmatics, sometimes as a burning powder, at other times as cigarettes. Nitre paper can be easily made by soaking pieces of thick blotting-paper in a strong solution of nitre and drying. For burning they are folded into a cone and placed on a saucer. Windows should be closed during inhalation of the fumes.

Of powders for fumigation there exist a large number, the ingredients of which, however, are selected from a few drugs, and an asthmatic pins his faith to one or the other. It may be useful to mention a few of them here:

Lobelia, powdered .. .. 1 ounce
Black tea, powdered .. 1 ,,
Stramonium leaves, powdered 1 ,,
   Make two ounces of a saturated solution of potassium nitrate, pour on the powders, mix thoroughly and dry.

Stramonium leaves, coarsely
   powdered .. .. .. 2 ounces
Anise fruit, powdered .. 1 ounce
Nitre, powdered .. .. 1 ,,
   Mix thoroughly.

Lobelia, powdered .. .. 1 ounce
Potassium chlorate, powdered 2 drachms
Potassium nitrate, powdered 3 ,,
White sugar, powdered .. 3 ,,
Stramonium leaves, powdered 1 ounce
   Mix thoroughly.

Black tobacco, dried and
   powdered .. .. .. 1 drachm
Stramonium leaves, powdered 2½ ounces
Potassium nitrate, powdered 10 drachms
Anise fruit, powdered .. 10 ,,
   Dissolve the potassium nitrate in a little water, pour on the powders, mix thoroughly and dry.

These powders are used by putting a little on a plate, pinching it up into a cone and igniting; the patient holds his head over the fumes and inhales deeply. Sprays are sometimes used in preference to fumigations, some of them relatively harmless, but others containing drugs which may induce drug habits. Injections of adrenalin, and of preparations containing this drug, are often very useful in relieving and warding off attacks.

While a resort to fumigations or sprays may appear to be necessary, it will be unfortunate if asthmatics rest content with the relief which they derive from them and make no effort to discover and remedy the underlying cause of their miseries.

By carefully observing and making notes of the circumstances which precede the attacks, for example, the nature of the food eaten, the animals, plants, clothing or furniture of animal origin with which he has been in contact, the patient may be able to throw light on the probable cause of his disorder. His doctor may be able to give him further help by means of experimental inoculations with a variety of protein substances. If he is found to react to any substance he will at least know what to avoid, or it may be possible to increase

his resistance to the substance in question. In some cases good results follow the administration of vaccines. Sometimes a change of residence will be helpful, for example, from the town to the country, or *vice versa*.

The drugs which stand out as remedies for the conditions underlying asthmatic attacks are iodides and arsenic. Five to ten grains of potassium iodide dissolved in a third of a glass of water may be taken thrice daily after meals. The patient should order his life carefully, taking sufficient exercise, being much in the open air, and sleeping in a well aired bedroom. His meals, of moderate size, should include only good plain food, and the evening meal should be small. Strict attention should be given to maintaining regularity of the bowels. He should seek to harden himself by baths as cold as he can bear them, followed by a good rub down, or at least he should douche his neck and shoulders with cold water in the mornings.

To sum up, he must leave no stone unturned in searching out and correcting the cause of his trouble, and he must keep himself as fit as he can. If he does these things early in the disease there is hope for him, but there is little if he accepts a destiny of invalidism in the drug-impregnated atmosphere of a room.

Asthma in Children. The disease is not uncommon in children, and at the outset the real nature of the complaint is not always suspected. A child suffering apparently from a cold in the chest is suddenly seized with breathlessness, and may now be considered to have developed broncho-pneumonia. After a variable time the distressed breathing clears up, and simple bronchitis may persist for a week or two. Such attacks may be repeated, and it has been pointed out that a history of several attacks of pneumonia in childhood should make us think of the possibility of asthma. On the other hand, asthmatic attacks in children may resemble what has been described as occurring in older people. These may cease as the child grows older, but more frequently they persist into adult life.

The treatment is on the lines already described. In looking for a cause the possibility of rickets or adenoids should not be overlooked. During an attack the sudden plunging of the child into a warm bath may do much to relieve the breathlessness. It may help if the stomach is emptied by giving a teaspoonful of ipecacuanha wine, or the bowels cleared by a dose of castor oil. The doctor should be consulted at every turn, and medicinal treatment should be under his supervision. A resort to the use of fumigating powders should be postponed as long as possible.

Asthma is one of those diseases in which the effect of habit is important ; one attack makes the patient more liable to another, so every effort should be made to prevent future attacks or at least to keep them off as long as one can. The child should live a free, active life and be much in the open air, care being taken, however, that his physical and mental capacities are not overtaxed.

See Anaphylaxis ; Bronchitis ; Emphysema ; Hay Fever ; Pneumonia.

ASTIGMATISM. A particular defect of the eye, resulting in defective sight, is known as astigmatism. Small degrees of astigmatism are extremely common, and probably few people are entirely free from it. The front part of the ball of the eye, immediately in front of the pupil, is curved forwards. For perfect vision its curvature should be the same in all directions, that is to say, the same from above downwards as from side to side ; but very frequently the curvature is not the same in all directions. It is bulged forwards, so to speak, more markedly when looked at from side to side than when looked at downwards. The necessary consequence of this will be that external objects cannot be clearly defined on the retina or " photographic plate " at the back of the eye. For instance, if a patient looks at a cross printed on a wall, one limb of the cross will be in focus and the other out of it, so everything is distorted.

Astigmatism may often give rise to what is called eye-strain and cause frequent and severe headaches. Quite small degrees of astigmatism may cause trouble. Glasses are required for its correction.

See Eye ; Vision.

ASTRAGALUS. The large and important bone in the ankle which transfers the weight of the body from the shin bone to the heel bone is called the astragalus. It enters into the formation of the ankle joint, whilst its front surface is jointed to the front part of the foot. This front surface is rounded and ball-shaped, and is called the head of the astragalus ; it forms the keystone of the antero-posterior arch of the foot. The astragalus is easily displaced by wearing high-heeled shoes, as shown in Plate II, 3.

See Ankle.

ASTRINGENT. Drugs that draw the tissues together are called astringents. They act in two ways ; either they actually reduce the size of the blood vessels to which they are applied, and so diminish the swelling by reducing the amount of blood which goes to the part, or else they act by solidifying some of the fluids in the part to which they are applied.

The number of astringent substances is large. Perhaps amongst the most familiar are dilute mineral acids, vinegar or acetic acid, alum, tannic acid, nitrate of silver, sulphate of zinc, copper sulphate, perchloride of iron, acetate of lead, and adrenalin. When an astringent substance is swallowed and exercises its action upon the wall of the stomach it hinders digestion, and if it passes on into the bowel and interferes with its movements and secretions, it causes constipation. The astringent substance most constantly abused in this respect is strong tea, which contains tannic acid.

On the other hand, astringent substances are often of great use in medicine. For instance, they relieve congestion, which means that a part of the body is unduly engorged with blood. Thus alum, tannic acid, or perchloride of iron will relieve congestion or inflammation of the throat ; strong cold tea is a useful eye wash, relieving congestion of the lining membrane of the eye ; and many other astringent substances, most of them containing tannic acid or some modifications of it, such as catechu (*q.v.*) or kino, are very useful in relieving congestion of the bowel and that over-secretion by the wall of the bowel which results in diarrhoea.

See Krameria ; Tannic Acid.

ATAVISM. This is the technical term for a particular kind of heredity in which the child " throws back," as the saying goes, to a distant ancestor, thus resembling not his immediate parents but a grandparent or an ancestor still more remote. The inherited resemblance may take the form of a disease, for example, haemophilia or gout.

ATAXIA or ATAXY. The nervous defect which results in an inability to control accurately the movements of the body is known as ataxia. Thus the inability to thread a needle or to stand upright with the eyes closed, or to walk without swaying or staggering, are examples of ataxia, and are dependent upon the ability of the nervous system to co-ordinate the action of the various muscles. It is quite different from paralysis. Each separate muscle may be quite efficient, but the patient has lost the power of controlling a number of muscles simultaneously so as to produce the action that he wants.

The most familiar tests for ataxia consist in asking the patient to walk along a straight line, heel and toe ; to turn round suddenly and retrace his steps ; to stand with the feet close together and the eyes closed ; to stand with the eyes closed and arms outstretched and then to touch the tip of his nose with the point of a finger. All these feats, of course, can be easily performed in health. In the last mentioned, the patient may have difficulty not because of ataxia but because of tremor, which makes the movement unsteady, but he reaches his goal and the ataxic does not.

The ataxic gait is very characteristic. The patient does not exactly sway ; his gait is quite different from that of a drunken man. But he walks with the legs rather wide apart and throws the feet out rather aimlessly, as if he was not sure where they were going to land. When the patient comes to a standstill he takes care to use a broad base, so as to make the act of balancing easier, and he often remarks that a firm, hard floor feels like thick carpet or velvet to his feet.

Ataxia is a common symptom of many nervous diseases. It may be quite temporary and unimportant, as in hysteria and in various kinds of poisoning, but on the other hand, it may be permanent. It is, perhaps, the most characteristic symptom, especially in relation to the lower limbs, of tabes dorsalis or locomotor ataxia. Just as a baby must learn to co-ordinate its own movements, and also anyone who is mastering a game of skill, so a great deal can be done for the relief of ataxic patients by systematic training.
See Equilibrium ; Friedreich's Ataxia ; Locomotor Ataxia.

ATHEROMA. After middle life, and earlier in those suffering from syphilis, blood poisoning and other diseases, degenerative thickening takes place in the walls of the arteries so that these become narrowed, rigid and at the same time more easily ruptured. This is atheroma, which, when generalised, is known as arterio-sclerosis (*q.v.*).

ATHLETICS. *See* Exercise.

ATOMISER. An atomiser is a spray apparatus which projects liquids in a fine spray or cloud. It is usually worked by a rubber bulb, but may be obtained with a small metal pump. It should be used for liquids only. The instrument, as usually supplied, has two nozzles, one for the nose and another for the throat. By taking deep inspirations and compressing the bulb to time with these, the fluid may reach the back of the nose and the larynx. When the nose or throat are dry and irritated much relief may be got from spraying simply with liquid paraffin, or one may use liquid paraffin with menthol, 10 grains to the ounce. Another formula is :

Menthol	..	..	.. 6 grains
Camphor	..	..	.. 8 ,,
Thymol	..	..	.. ½ grain
Eucalyptol	..	..	.. ½ drachm
Liquid paraffin B.P.		to make 1 ounce

This will be found useful in sore throat and at the beginning of a cold in the head.
See Eucalyptus ; Inhalation ; Spray.

ATROPHY. When the tissues of the body waste or diminish in bulk either from age, disease, injury, lack of nutrition or disuse, they are said to undergo atrophy. In old age all the tissues of the body show this change ; for instance, the skin becomes thin and semi-transparent, and baldness results from atrophy of the hair bulbs. Atrophy may affect muscles in consequence of nerve disease or injury, and is accounted for partly by disuse and partly by the loss of nutritional stimulus. The wasting may be lessened in some cases by moving the patient's muscles for him, when he cannot do this for himself, by stimulating them by electricity, with which is combined massage. At other times muscular atrophy seems to depend on degenerative changes in the muscles themselves, the reasons being obscure.

General wasting in infants and young children may be due to starvation, from insufficient but more often from improper food. In what is known as infantile atrophy no cause may be obvious to account for the wasting, and it may be extremely difficult to improve nutrition. Rickets, congenital syphilis and tuberculosis may give rise to serious wasting in young children, as, indeed, may any serious illness. The opposite condition to atrophy is hypertrophy (*q.v.*).

See Age Changes; Emaciation; Muscle; Myopathy; Progressive Muscular Atrophy.

ATROPINE. The active principle of the plant atropa belladonna, the deadly nightshade, is the important alkaloid called atropine. The virtues of belladonna, so familiar as tinctures and liniment, are due to the atropine which it contains. The chief actions of atropine are upon the skin, the heart and the eye. It arrests perspiration, and, indeed, practically all the secretions of the body; thus it makes the mouth and throat very dry. It may bring out a profuse red rash over the body. The characteristic action of atropine upon the heart is greatly to increase the rapidity of its beating. It also widens all the blood vessels of the body. It has a very striking action upon the eye, causing marked dilatation of the pupils. This action may be obtained by swallowing the atropine, by injecting it, or by placing a few drops of a very weak solution in the eye.

When applied to the skin, atropine and belladonna tend to relieve pain, if it is superficial. The drug has a large number of other actions upon the body, which are of great importance, and it may be noted that in general children are particularly free from dangerous effects of atropine and are particularly likely to benefit by its medicinal use. The doses in which atropine is usually administered vary from $\frac{1}{100}$ to $\frac{1}{200}$ of a grain; it is usually used as atropine sulphate, which has the same dose. The dose usually applied to the eye is $\frac{1}{200}$ grain or less, and it may be prescribed in drops, in an ointment, or in tiny disks.

The oculist frequently uses atropine in order to dilate the pupil so that he may examine the interior of the eye. It is also very valuable in certain inflammatory conditions of the interior of the eye, for example, iritis, in order to break down adhesions or to prevent their formation. There is one not uncommon condition of the interior of the eye, however, in which if atropine is employed the results are disastrous. This is the disease called glaucoma. In this and in all other cases where the pressure inside the eye is increased, giving rise to undue hardness of the eyeball on pressure and to great pain, atropine must never be employed, since one of its characteristic actions is to raise the pressure inside the eye.

Atropine may be administered at night in order to check the excessive perspiration which often occurs in consumption and other diseases. It relieves muscular spasm and thus is useful in asthma, and in renal and biliary colic. It is recommended that when the heart stops during the administration of chloroform, atropine should be injected straight into the heart muscle. Up to a certain point atropine is an invaluable antidote for poisoning by opium or morphia, by supposed mushrooms, by aconite, and by prussic acid.

Poisoning by atropine most commonly occurs as the result of swallowing the leaves of the deadly nightshade. Symptoms and treatment are identical with those of belladonna poisoning (*q.v.*).

AUDITORY. This adjective is applied to the sense of hearing, to the nerve of hearing and to the centre in the brain which is connected with the function of hearing. The eighth pair of nerves that emerge from the brain itself, that is to say, the eighth cranial nerves, are the auditory nerves. Each of these nerves consists of two distinct parts, one of which is connected with the organ and the sense of hearing, and the other with the sense of equilibrium, which enables us to balance our bodies.

See Ear ; Equilibrium ; Hearing.

AURA. Literally meaning a breath, this word is used to describe the slight warning symptoms that often precede attacks of epilepsy or other diseases, though the word is hardly ever used apart from epilepsy. The symptoms are of many different kinds : sometimes the patient is warned by an itching about the chin or some other part of the skin, sometimes by spots before the eyes, by a peculiar taste in the mouth or by similar disturbances of the sense of smell. Such an aura may be of real use in enabling the patient to take measures to stave off the attack. The electric aura is another name for the electric breeze.

See Epilepsy.

AURICLE. The term auricle means literally a little ear and is the name applied to two exceedingly important parts of the heart which from the outside look rather like the ears of some animals. It is also another name for the pinna or expanded portion of the outer ear.

See Ear ; Heart.

AURIST. This name is applied to specialists who deal particularly with the ear. As a rule an aurist is a surgeon, and the disorders of the nose and throat are included in the scope of his work. The adjective aural is applied to anything connected with the ear.

AUSCULTATION. The art of listening to various sounds produced by the healthy or the diseased body is known as auscultation. There are two organs the auscultation of which is very important, namely, the heart and the lungs. Formerly, auscultation used to be practised by the direct application of the ear to the patient's chest. This is known as immediate auscultation and is still often used in the case of children. The stethoscope furnishes the medium of the newer kind of auscultation, which is distinguished from the older by being called mediate.

The advantages of the stethoscope are, first of all, the obvious convenience to the doctor and the patient, and, secondly, the fact that it enables one to study the sounds proceeding from very small areas, instead of the confused combination of sounds that are heard when the ear is directly applied to the chest. In listening to the heart the doctor hears two sounds which indicate the closing of certain of the valves in the heart. He studies the character of these sounds, which are known as the first and second. In addition to them, or replacing them, he often hears other sounds which, in order to distinguish them, are called murmurs, or by the French name bruits.

It used formerly to be thought that whenever one heard a cardiac murmur there was proof of heart disease, but this has been found to be wrong.

The murmur most often heard is due either to the state of the blood or to some temporary disorder in the working of the heart, which can no more be described as disease than one could describe the feeling of limpness as a disease of the muscles.

In listening to the lungs the doctor hears two gentle sounds, one of which accompanies the act of inspiration and the other the act of expiration. The character of these sounds differs over different parts of the chest, and it is quite different in children from that heard in adults. When by long practice the doctor's ear has become accustomed to normal sounds, he is able to distinguish certain accompaniments of them or changes in their character which may indicate disease.

See Heart ; Murmur.

AUTO-INTOXICATION. The effects on the body of toxins or poisons formed within the body itself, and due to faulty metabolism, constitute auto-intoxication. The tissue changes and symptoms produced by constipation provide a good example. These are extraordinarily varied and may be of great consequence. They include headache, giddiness, dyspepsia, anaemia, physical and mental debility, muscular pain, nervousness and mental depression. The toxins proceeding from faulty intestinal digestion may contribute largely to the age changes in arteries known as arterio-sclerosis.

See Constipation ; Diet ; Pyorrhoea.

AUTOMATISM. This is the name applied to that state in which the patient goes through various actions without the

PLATE III

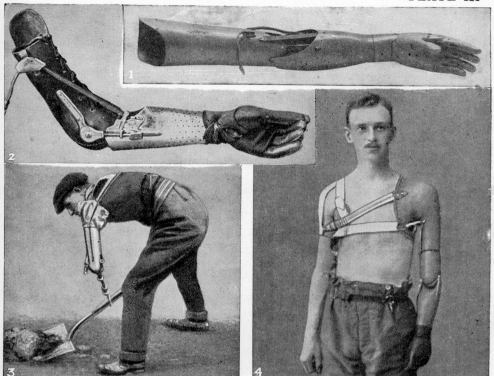

Artificial Arm. 1. For amputation above elbow. 2. For amputation through elbow ; detachable hand in rubber or wood. 3. Hook appliance. 4. Harness and limb for amputation through shoulder

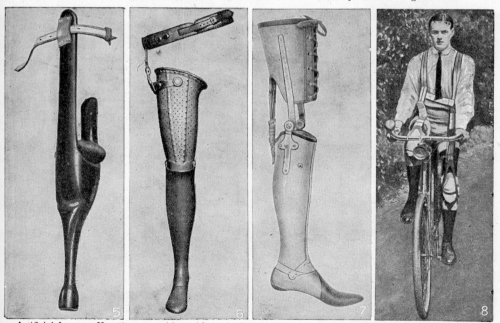

Artificial Leg. 5. Kneeling peg with cushion. 6. Outer casing of metal to match living limb and inner metal socket for shrunken stump. 7. For amputation below knee. 8. Elastic extension to raise limb

Courtesy of Carnes Artificial Limb Co., McKay Artificial Limb Co., Ltd., Blatchford & Sons, Ltd., Horace V. Duncan and J. F. Rowley, Ltd.

PLATE IV

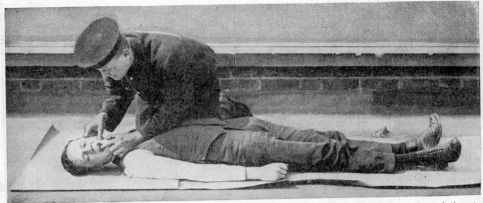

Artificial Respiration: Schäfer's Method. 1. Before starting the manipulations the mouth and throat are examined to ensure that they are clear. This and other preparations must be performed very swiftly

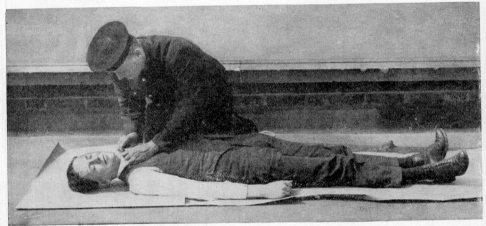

2. Clothing about the neck and chest is loosened and the patient then placed in a prone position, arms extended and face turned sideways. The operator kneels to one side or astride the patient

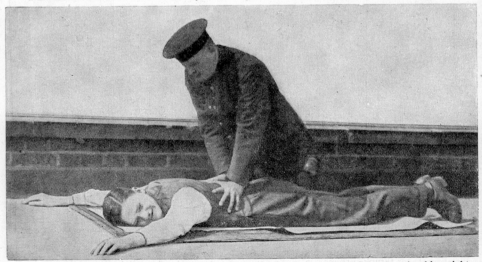

3. Placing his hands on the lower part of the patient's chest, he compresses it by throwing his weight forward. He then springs back, arms still rigid, releasing pressure and so letting the chest expand

aid of the will. Automatic actions occur sometimes in hysteria, in epilepsy, and in some forms of mental disease. Sleep walking might be regarded as a form of automatism.

AUTOPSY. *See* Post-mortem.

AUTO-SUGGESTION. Every one of us is influenced at some time or another by ideas which obtain a firm hold upon us but for which we see no logical basis. Ideas of this kind may be proposed to us by others or may arise from other external circumstances ; for example, if some food substance disagrees with us once, we may conceive that it always will. This may usually happen and seem to justify the notion ; but there may be exceptional occasions when the same food with immaterial differences may be taken with no untoward effect. We may become aware of this, but even then our fixed notion may be proof against a logical demonstration of its baselessness. This is an instance of auto-suggestion, a process which is utilised in treatment.

The method used by the Nancy school, and associated in the minds of most people with M. Coué, is for the patient to take stock of his infirmities and to repeat some such words as " In every respect, and every day, I grow better and better," about twenty times. Later, consideration of the details of the malady becomes unnecessary and it suffices to repeat the formula. The advocates of auto-suggestion lay stress upon the wording used. They say that only the positive formula should be used, never the negative.

The exercise is much more effectual if it is performed just before going to sleep. There should be no effort to convince oneself of the truth of the proposition. It is not a case of forcing betterment by a sheer effort of will. Such hinders rather than helps. It is rather that the ideas enunciated sink into and become part of our sub-conscious mentality, through which they influence our bodily processes and our consciousness. Auto-suggestions, in fact, may originate in these sub-conscious processes from repressed fears and cravings.

See Hypnotism ; Mind ; Pyscho-therapy.

AXILLA. This is the technical name for the armpit (*q.v.*).

BABY. At birth a baby is about 20 inches long, and weighs about 7 lbs., girls being as a rule smaller than boys. The skin is pink in colour, and the head and body may be covered with a greasy material known as the vernix caseosa. This may be somewhat difficult to remove when the baby is having its first bath, and if ordinary soaping does not appear to be successful, olive oil or butter may be rubbed on and washed off with soap. The head may be covered with thick, dark hair, but this comes away sooner or later. The eyes are expressionless and of a dark blue colour, but as time goes on they assume another tint— brown, blue, or grey, as the case may be. The nose is very little developed.

The cranium or brain pan is large as compared with the face, the proportions being 8 to 1 in the infant, as compared with 2 to 1 in the adult. The circumference of the head is about 13 inches ; at six months it is 16 inches, and at one year

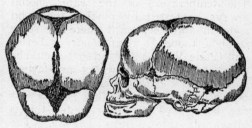

Baby's skull : the fontanelles or soft spaces

18 inches. At two places on the top of the head the skull is open or unprotected by bone. These are known as the anterior fontanelle in front, and the posterior fontanelle behind. The latter closes in about two months, but the former not till about the eighteenth month. During this time it will be seen to pulsate with the heart beats and to become full and tense when the child cries.

At birth a baby should be able to grasp firmly with the hand. Hearing is developed early, but objects are not usually recognized much before six or eight weeks. Babies may contort their mouths in their first weeks of life and mothers may interpret some of their expressions as a smile, but a real smile is not common before the fifth or sixth week. Tears do not appear in the eye till about the third or fourth month, and the fact that an infant's weeping before this time is dry-eyed must not be allowed to throw doubt on the genuineness of the distress.

The motions of the bowels for the first few days are dark green in colour, consisting of a substance known as meconium ; later they become light brown, though this may change to light green, owing to the exposure of the motion to the air. A light green stool may thus be quite normal, but this should not be confused with a stool where the colour is a mixture of yellow, light and dark green ; this should always be regarded as unhealthy. The umbilical cord shrivels up after birth and drops off from the sixth to the eighth day.

How to Bath a Baby

A baby's bath should be of a temperature of 90° to 95° F., though the first bath should be somewhat warmer, 95° to 100°. In its preparation, the cold water should be put in first, and boiling water added to produce the correct temperature. The temperature of the water should always be tested by putting the hand right in and keeping it there for some seconds, though a thermometer is better still (Plate V, 1). A bland soap should be used such as that known as superfatted.

At the first bath the child's eyes must be washed before any other part, a soft rag being used (*see* Plate V, 2) ; this is afterwards thrown into the fire. The object of washing the eyes first is to prevent possible infection from the head or other parts of the child reaching them and giving rise to the serious eye disease known as ophthalmia neonatorum. This is a fruitful source of permanent blindness. As an additional precaution the doctor may put some antiseptic drops into the eyes. After this the head is washed and dried, then the body and limbs are soaped while the baby is on the nurse's knee and the soap is rinsed off by putting the baby into the bath (*see* Plate V, 3,)

Before being put into the bath and afterwards during drying, the body should be covered with a towel. Unnecessary exposure is undoubtedly responsible for some of the indigestion and colic from which babies suffer.

When the baby has been thoroughly but gently dried with a soft towel, the cord is dressed. The old-fashioned dressing was a piece of scorched linen, the scorching being for the purpose of destroying germs ; but a better method is to dust the cord and surrounding skin with powdered boracic acid and wrap up the cord with soft boracic lint or absorbent cotton wool. A square of either of these materials, of suitable size, is cut, a hole is made in the centre through which the cord is passed, and the fabric is then folded over. Fuller's earth should not be used as a dusting powder. The nurse should be careful that her hands are thoroughly clean before she dresses the cord, and should the skin round the cord become inflamed the attention of the doctor should be directed to it at once.

The baby should have a bath in the morning and a sponging in the evening. The clothing should be warm, with high neck and long sleeves. The binders should be soft flannel, four inches wide and long enough to go round the body and overlap about a third. They should be fastened by sewing or with tapes, not with pins. Stiff binders may press unduly on the body and may chafe the armpits and thighs. Knitted woollen socks reaching about as high as the knee should be worn, care being taken to keep the feet warm, as cold feet are a frequent cause of colic.

Time-Table for Infant Feeding

The baby should be put to the breast some hours after its birth, and when the mother is sufficiently rested. For about the first three days the flow from the breast is somewhat scanty, and does not consist of proper milk but of a secretion known as the colostrum. Suckling encourages the formation of milk, and the colostrum appears to assist in clearing the infant's bowels. Until the milk is flowing the baby should therefore be put to the breast at intervals of 6 hours ; if it is not content with this it may be pacified by giving it teaspoonsful of water sweetened with white or with milk sugar. Thereafter between 6 a.m. and 10 p.m. it should be fed at 4-hour intervals, receiving, that is to say, five feeds in the 24 hours, though some babies may require to be fed at 3-hourly intervals, at any rate for a time. In the latter event the first feed might be given at 4 a.m. The feed should last as long as the baby is

AVERAGE HEIGHT & WEIGHT

At Birth	3 Months	6 Months	9 Months	1 Year
21 Inches	22 Inches	24 Inches	27 Inches	30 Inches
7 lbs.	12 lbs.	14 lbs.	17 lbs.	21 lbs.

Baby. Table of growth in height and weight

actually taking milk but no longer; this will be about twenty minutes as a rule. Whichever time-table is adopted, it should be punctually adhered to. On no account should the baby be put to the breast merely to pacify it, but there is no harm in giving it a little plain warm water in a teaspoon. While feeding, and at all other times, the head of a young baby must be well supported (Plate V, 4-5).

It may be assumed that a baby is being properly nourished if it sleeps well and shows a progressive gain in weight. It should be weighed once or twice a week, and the gain each week should be 5 ounces or more. The baby should double its initial weight at five months and treble it at twelve to fifteen months. If it appears that the supply of milk is inadequate, the mother should supplement her diet by extra milk, eggs or meat.

The practice of giving stout or other malt liquors for this purpose is not a sound one ; milk is very much better.

If the breast milk still appears to be insufficient the baby should get a bottle-feed of milk and water proportioned to its age alternately with, and in place of, a breast-feed. Artificial feeding may become necessary, though it has drawbacks. It may be difficult to get an artificial food which the baby can digest easily, as it does its mother's milk, and there is a great risk of dangerous microbes getting into the food. Only the most urgent reasons can, therefore, suffice for taking an infant off the breast. It may have to be done if the mother suffers from tuberculosis or another infectious disease, or from cancer, or if she is very debilitated, for example, from anaemia. Other reasons are abscess of the breast, insufficient development of the nipple, harelip in the child, and the fact that the child is not thriving in spite of everything having been done to improve the mother's milk.

The food which should now be tried, and which is usually quite successful, is cow's milk, though this must be diluted to make it more like human milk and so within the compass of the baby's digestion. It may be diluted with ordinary water, with barley water, or with water and a tablespoonful of lime water. The mixture is sweetened with white sugar or with milk sugar, and a half to one teaspoonful of cream is added to each bottle. The total amounts of the feed for various ages are shown in the following table :—

First week..	..	.. 1 ounce
Second week	..	.. 1–2 ounces
One month	..	.. 2–3 ,,
Two months	..	.. 3–4 ,,
Three months	..	.. 4 ,,
Four months	..	.. 4½–5 ,,
Five months	..	.. 5 ,,
Six months	..	.. 6 ,,
Seven months	..	.. 7 ,,
Eight months	..	.. 8 ,,
Nine months	..	.. 8–9 ,,

For the first week or two the proportions should be one part of milk to two of the diluent, but thereafter, till six months, half and half. Barley water should be strained hot through a thin white cloth which has been boiled. Children vary, of course, in their capacities, and the above figures must be modified accordingly.

During the first six months six feeds are given in the 24 hours, beginning at 6 a.m. and finishing at 9 p.m., and, during the next three months, five feeds. The proportion of cow's milk is increased gradually after six months, and from this time onwards rusks may be allowed.

The cow's milk, which should be received in sealed bottles, is pasteurised for the baby's use. Forms of apparatus are sold for this purpose, consisting of the requisite number of bottles with rubber stoppers, and a tin receptacle in which the bottles, filled with the appropriate milk mixture, are boiled. But the process may be simply done by pouring the milk into a clean jug and placing this in a saucepan of water. In either case the water is brought to the boil and kept thus for twenty minutes. The milk is then put away in the cleanest and coolest place available. In hot weather the bottle should stand in cold water or on ice.

When the feed is not sterilised in the bottles, a boat-shaped bottle with a large teat and a rubber valve stopper should be used, and the most scrupulous cleanliness must be observed in making up the mixture. The opening of the teat should be neither too small nor too large, though the mother or nurse should not test this by putting the teat in her own mouth ; this information can be obtained by observing how the baby gets on with it. Provided the teat is satisfactory the baby should take as long as he wishes.

Meticulous Cleansing of the Bottle

Immediately he has finished the feed, the bottle should be thoroughly washed out with clean water, and the teat and stopper should be cleaned. Preferably two such bottles should be used, so that each may have a thorough soaking in clean water before being again used ; a teaspoonful of baking soda may be added to the water with advantage. Once or oftener during the day the bottles should be scalded after they have been thoroughly washed with cold water.

Artificial foods, such as Allenbury's and Mellin's, can be used advantageously for the night feed and perhaps during the day in place of a milk feed. When on artificial feeding, babies should get a teaspoonful of orange or grape juice once or twice a day between feeds, in order to ensure the requisite vitamin supply.

When the baby is nine months old it should be gradually weaned, though this should be delayed if the weather is hot or if the baby is indisposed from teething or otherwise. To begin with, he gets a meal of arrowroot, ground rice or barley jelly with milk ; then oat-flour rusks, breadcrumb and gravy, bread and milk, veal, chicken or mutton broth from which the fat has been strained, egg custard ; and later he may be given eggs lightly cooked, pounded chicken, mutton or white fish, a mealy potato, cauliflower, milk puddings and bread and butter.

A baby generally cuts its first tooth at six months, though this may be considerably delayed without there being anything wrong. The first teeth to appear are the lower central incisors, then from the eighth to the tenth month the four upper incisors appear, and from the twelfth to the fourteenth month the lower lateral incisors and all the front molars.

The practice of giving a baby a dummy teat or comforter in an attempt to mitigate its teething troubles is very unwise. The teat affords an easy means of conveying dirt and infection to the child, and its use may lead to deformity of the jaws.

A baby should always have its own bed—a crib and not a cradle—as this makes for better rest for both mother and infant and avoids the risk of over-lying. The mattress of the cot should be protected by a waterproof sheet, which should be washed regularly. The baby should be taken out as much as the weather permits, and when indoors should be in a light and well-ventilated room. It should be warmly clothed, care being taken to keep the feet warm, but the opposite error of swathing it in too many clothes must also be avoided.

See Benger's Food ; Birth Paralysis ; Breast Feeding ; Child ; Childbirth ; Condensed Milk ; Fire-guard ; Growth ; Milk ; Teeth ; Vaccination.

BACILLURIA. The presence of any kind of bacillus, the rod-shaped type of microbe, in the freshly voided urine may be described as bacilluria ; the tubercle bacillus, for example, in tuberculosis of the kidney or bladder, or the bacillus of Eberth, during or following an attack of enteric fever. More frequent than any others, however, is an organism which normally inhabits the bowel, the bacillus coli communis. This makes its way to the kidneys, oftener to the right one apparently, and multiplies freely, enormous numbers being passed with the urine. Although their presence may impart a sheen to the urine or even make it turbid, often enough it is quite clear and its appearance suggests nothing abnormal.

Also, while there may be pain, often severe, in the loins, over the bladder or in the urethra, with frequent and painful micturition, in other cases there may be no more than a slight increase in the frequency of passing water or, perhaps in a child, bed-wetting, the true significance of which may be overlooked unless a bacteriological examination of the urine is made. The same difference is noted regarding general symptoms, which may range from high fever, with shivering or perhaps, in a child, convulsions, to merely vague sensations of indisposition and occasional slight rises of temperature.

Children, especially girls, and pregnant women, are the most frequent subjects of bacilluria.

The disorder requires careful medical supervision. The patient is put to bed on a simple light diet, and the bowels are kept freely open. The urine, which is always acid in bacilluria, must be rendered alkaline, and to this end potassium citrate and sodium bicarbonate may be given in liberal doses every two hours. A child might receive 20 grains of the former and 15 grains of the latter, but it may be necessary to increase these doses largely. This treatment is kept up for several days, when it may be possible to reduce the doses. Benefit sometimes accrues from the use of a vaccine prepared from the organisms actually present in the patient's urine.

See Bladder ; Hexamine ; Urine.

BACILLUS. Certain kinds of germs or microbes which are shaped like little rods are known as bacilli (singular bacillus ; Italian, a little rod). They include nearly all the important microbes. The diseases which are known to be due to bacilli include tuberculosis, anthrax, diphtheria, typhoid fever, many kinds of diarrhoea, leprosy, glanders, plague, lockjaw (or tetanus), and very many more. Bacilli, also, are responsible for acid fermentation or acidity (*q.v.*), and for a great many important processes in the making of wines. They are also largely responsible for the putrefaction of dead organic matter everywhere.

See Bacteria.

BACK. The supporting structure of the back is the spinal column or backbone, to which also the back owes its curves. In the dorsal or chest region the curve is backwards and the body wall is supported by the ribs, but the curve is forward in the lumbar region or loins, and the place

of the ribs is taken by sheets of muscle and of strong fibrous tissue or fascia. Fibrositis is common in this part of the back, where it is known as lumbago. The kidneys lie in the back and are partly covered by the lower ribs, but they are not so frequently a direct cause of back-ache as is popularly supposed.

It is important to remember that in protecting the chest from exposure to draughts and cold winds it is very necessary also to safeguard the back, as the bulk of the lung tissue is towards the back. This fact is overlooked in the forms of chest protector ordinarily provided. Sometimes as a result of insufficient or improper food, a lack of open-air exercise or some other debilitating factor, the muscles and ligaments of the back become relaxed. The gait may assume a stooping posture, or the spine may develop lateral curves. In these circumstances a person, usually it is a girl, is said to have a " weak back." When a patient is confined to bed careful watch must be kept on the lowest part of the back, as bed sores are prone to form there

See Backbone ; Fibrositis ; Lumbar Region ; Spinal Curvature.

BACK-ACHE. The back is often the seat of an aching pain which may be very disabling. This may occur to some extent in any febrile disease, but is more marked in influenza and smallpox than in most. A pain between the shoulders is not uncommon in stomach disorders, and in gallstones the pain often strikes up to the back of the right shoulder ; in piles there may be a dull pain at the bottom of the spine. Pain in the back may be due to spinal disease, a fact which should always be borne in mind. A dragging pain often occurs in women from disorders of the womb. Anaemia, hysteria and neurasthenia are amongst numerous conditions in which back-ache may be a feature.

The treatment of back-ache must be directed to the cause, though the application of heat usually produces some benefit, at any rate of a temporary nature. In lumbago the pain is frequently severe, particularly when the patient attempts to move. Rest in bed with a hot-water bottle to the back, and one or two 10-grain doses of aspirin may afford relief.

The following method of dealing with lumbago has been recommended and has proved very effective in many cases. The patient should sit astride a form or a chair and the painful part of his back should be kneaded with the thumbs. This must be done thoroughly, but at the same time the pressure should not be sufficient to cause pain. The two thumbs are then placed on either side of the spine below the painful spot, and the patient is directed to bend forwards and backwards and to turn his body round, first to one side and then the other, these movements being repeated several times. A surprising amount of ease and liberty of movement will often be secured in this way.

See Fibrositis ; Rheumatism.

BACKBONE. The spine, or spinal column, popularly known as the backbone, really consists of a great number of small bones called vertebrae. These are named according to their position : thus the seven vertebrae in the neck are called cervical ; the twelve vertebrae from which the ribs arise are called dorsal : below them are five much larger ones which carry no ribs and are known as the lumbar vertebrae. The next vertebrae have already fused, even in the new-born child, into a single bone called the sacrum, since it was at one time considered to be the seat of the soul. In the lower animals the backbone is continued onwards from this point as the tail, which consists of a number of vertebrae more ; but in man, that is to say, in man after an early stage of development before birth, the tail is

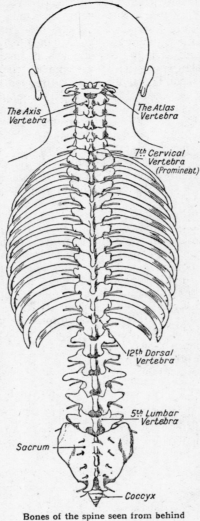

Bones of the spine seen from behind

Labels on figure:
The Axis Vertebra
The Atlas Vertebra
7th Cervical Vertebra (Prominent)
12th Dorsal Vertebra
5th Lumbar Vertebra
Sacrum
Coccyx

represented only by four small, useless and degenerate vertebrae which have fused together into a single bone called the coccyx. This bone is attached to the lower end of the sacrum.

The backbone is, in the first place, the foundation of the skeleton of the body. It supports the head ; it gives rise to the ribs, upon which the arms are attached ; and through the sacrum it is attached to the pelvis or hip bone and thus transmits the weight of the body to the legs. The vertebrae are united to one another by very powerful attachments ; and the backbone is covered behind with a very large and complicated series of powerful muscles which are grouped together under the name erector spinae. Inside the abdomen, also, there are muscles attached to the front of the spine, which bend the body forwards, or if necessary bend the thighs upon the body.

But in addition to all this the backbone has a function which exactly corresponds to the function of the skull ; for whilst the skull contains the brain, the backbone contains that continuation of the brain which is called the spinal cord. So powerful is the backbone, so thick are its bones, and so thickly are they covered by muscular tissue, that the spinal cord is far more completely protected from external injury than is the brain.

The individual vertebrae are separated from each other by elastic disks, so that the spine is not only strong, but is pliable to a considerable degree. Hence, the accidents affecting the backbone are comparatively uncommon. Accidental dislocation is very rare; fracture occurs only as the result of the most violent injuries, such as being run over by a train or crushed in a coal mine. Fractures of the spine,

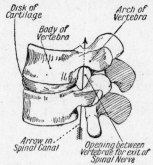

Disk of Cartilage   *Arch of Vertebra*

Body of Vertebra

Arrow in Spinal Canal   *Opening between Vertebrae for exit of Spinal Nerve*

Backbone. Parts of a vertebra

however, are often complicated by dislocation. The injuries to the bone are dangerous because of the liability of the spinal cord to be compressed or injured, leading to paralysis, possibly to death, if the upper part of the spine should be implicated.

The backbone is not uncommonly affected with tuberculosis and other diseases, one effect of which is to produce some alteration in or addition to its natural curves, and this may also happen from muscular weakness and faulty postures, especially in young people.

At birth the spine viewed from the side has only two curves, a long backward curve of the whole spine down to the sacrum and the backward curve of the sacrum itself. Thereafter, from the assumption of the erect posture, two other curves develop, a forward curve of the cervical vertebrae and a forward curve in the lumbar or loin region. If a baby is allowed to sit up too early these curves may not develop properly, and the back will be round.

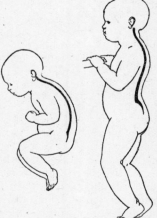

Left, backbone at birth; right, development of normal curves

An increase of the backward curvature of the spine is known as kyphosis. It may arise from a faulty posture, as in stooping over one's work. Tailors are subject to it, and it is common in school children who work at desks which are not sufficiently high. Those who suffer from myopia or short-sightedness are especially prone to it.

When portions of the vertebrae are destroyed, as in tuberculosis, a sharp backward projection occurs at some part of the spine, and is known as an angular curvature. An increase of the forward curve in the loins constitutes lordosis. In addition to the exaggerations of the normal curves, the spine is frequently found to curve to one or other side. This is known as lateral curvature.

See Child; Dislocation; Fracture; Jacket; Pott's Disease; Spinal Cord; Spinal Curvature.

BACTERIA. When Pasteur discovered the existence of numerous minute, living plants which caused disease, he called them microbes, from the Greek words for little and life. The terms microbe and microorganism, which later came into use, are now understood to include not only vegetable parasites but minute animal forms, for example, the malaria parasite. The name applied by botanists to the former is bacteria, a single one being called a bacterium, again from a Greek word meaning a little stick. In botany bacteria are placed in a group by themselves, though formerly they were considered to be forms of fungus; hence the name schizomycetes, or fissionfungi. They exist practically everywhere in Nature, and we could hardly live without them. They are the world's scavengers, destroying dead animal and vegetable matter.

Of the innumerable species of bacteria there is a small number which are able to live within the living body of man. Some of these do him no harm. They live on the skin, but cause no injury there. They live and multiply enormously in the bowel, and ordinarily do no harm; indeed, they actually take part in the process of digestion. Other bacteria are pathogenic, that is to say, they can produce disease in the body.

Bacteria are very minute, from $\frac{1}{5000}$ to $\frac{1}{10000}$ of an inch in length, and various forms are recognized: a rounded form (coccus or micrococcus), such as the germs of suppuration, of pneumonia and gonorrhoea ; a rod-shaped form (bacillus), for example, the germs of tuberculosis, of typhoid fever, and of anthrax ; and a wavy thread-like form (spirillum or spirochaeta), of which the germs of relapsing fever and of syphilis are examples. Such germs are caught by the porcelain candles of a Pasteur-Chamberland filter, but there are very minute forms which pass through, and these are known as filterable viruses. Smallpox and rabies are amongst the diseases which may be caused by such an organism.

Life Cycle of Bacteria

It is also thought likely that bacteria may pass through cycles, in which they assume other forms than those in which they are best known—a bacillus, for instance, may have a coccus and a filterable virus stage—and that a different disease may be produced by the organism according to the stage in which it exists in the body. Bacteria multiply by fission, that is to say, one individual splits up to form two new individuals, and, as this process may take place at short intervals, many millions of descendants may arise from a common ancestor in the course of 24 hours. Some bacilli can also multiply by giving rise to spores or seeds, for example, anthrax and tetanus, and these spores are much more resistant to destructive influences, such as heat and drying, than are the adult forms.

The spirilla and many bacilli, such as that of enteric fever, are capable of moving about in liquids. A sufficiency of moisture is necessary for the activity of all bacteria ; consequently it is desirable, when possible, that the dressings on a wound should be kept dry. Warmth favours their activity ; they may survive freezing, and diseases such as enteric fever and cholera have been carried by ices. They are killed by a sufficient degree of heat, especially moist heat, so surgical instruments, etc., are boiled for at least 15 or 20 minutes before an operation, while dressings are disinfected by steam under pressure. Sunlight inhibits bacterial growth, and in the case of the typhoid bacillus, quickly kills it. Some bacteria require air or oxygen, or are aerobic, while others, the anaerobes, like the bacillus of tetanus, can only flourish in the absence of air.

Bacteria which live on dead organic matter are called saprophytes, but some of those which normally exist in living tissues are capable of maintaining their existence as saprophytes. It is important to keep wounds clear of much blood clot and of dead tissue, as these provide nutriment for the putrefactive bacteria. Like the higher plants, bacteria manufacture a large variety of substances. Thus they may produce acids, as in the souring of milk ; alkalies, as in decomposing urine ; gases, as in gas gangrene ; colouring matter, as in green pus ; phosphorescence and, amongst other things, toxins or poisons. Saprophytes may produce poisons known as ptomaines from food stuffs, or from dead tissues, but poisonous symptoms arising in consequence of the activities of such bacteria are rarely, if at all, due to ptomaines, but to other substances.

The pathogenic bacteria are able to invade and multiply in the living tissues of the body. They do harm by producing poisonous substances, or toxins, which are of two kinds : the first, known as exotoxins, are liberated by the living bacteria, while the second, or endotoxins, are contained in the bacteria themselves, and are not liberated till the bacteria are dissolved or broken up.

Successive Stages of an Infection

The effects of bacterial invasion are well illustrated in the case of the specific fevers. After the actual entry into the body nothing takes place for a certain time, varying in different diseases. This is known as the period of incubation, when the bacteria are multiplying and establishing themselves. This is succeeded by a period of great activity when the bacterial poisons cause constitutional symptoms, such as fever, and local symptoms depending upon the tissue which bears the brunt of the disease, for example, the nervous system in cerebrospinal fever and the bowel in enteric fever.

The patient may succumb, or his tissues may produce protective substances in sufficient amount to repel the attack.

These substances are of different kinds : one counteracts the exotoxin much as an antidote does a poison, another renders the bacteria an easier prey for the phagocytes or white cells, and a third leads to the breaking down or solution of the bacteria.

See Antibody ; Antiseptic ; Antitoxin ; Immunity ; Virus.

BAEL FRUIT. In India the fresh pulp of the bael fruit is used in the treatment of diarrhoea, dysentery, and sprue. It has a pleasant, astringent taste. The dried fruit, which is imported into Europe, and of which a liquid extract is official in the British Pharmacopoeia, does not, however, have the virtues attributed to the fresh fruit.

BAKERS' ITCH. Acute dermatitis of the hands and arms is not uncommon amongst bakers, and is due to the irritation by flour, yeast or sugar, the latter also being responsible for a similar condition amongst grocers. Areas of skin are inflamed, and on these are set numbers of little papules or pimples which may itch intolerably. The tops of the papules break and exude a sticky, clear discharge. There may be some feverishness associated with the local disorder. Strict cleanliness must be observed to prevent the malady in those who are disposed to it. The treatment is that of eczema (*q.v.*).

BALANITIS. An inflammation of the glans penis constitutes balanitis. The usual cause is lack of cleanliness, and this is most likely to occur when the foreskin is long. The foreskin should be retracted and the parts washed regularly, care in this respect being often neglected in little boys. If there is any difficulty about this, circumcision should be performed.

See Circumcision ; Genital System ; Phimosis.

BALDNESS. The loss of the hair of the head may be due to many different causes. The true senile baldness, or the baldness of old age, is doubtless due to a simple atrophy (*q.v.*) or wasting of the hair bulbs, in common with the wasting of many other parts of the body as age advances. It is doubtful whether much can be done by way of arresting this kind of baldness, but anything that increases the flow of blood through the scalp helps the nutrition of the hair. Thus vigorous

brushing, massage of the scalp, perhaps with some mild irritant, such as lotions containing ammonia or alcohol and cantharidin, may be of some use.

Premature baldness in some instances resembles senile baldness, but is usually totally different in causation. It occurs in young people quite often at the age of twenty, and may have given rise to very great loss of hair by the age of thirty. Premature baldness is far more common in men than women. The commonest manner in which premature baldness begins is by thinning of the hair on the crown of the head and also by a thinning on each side of the scalp in front. This spreads backwards, and very often a patch of hair is left running down the middle of the top of the head. Often the hair at the side and top remains quite thick.

As a rule the cause of this premature baldness is bacterial disease of the hair roots, which is known as seborrhoea or scurf, and which may make its appearance at fourteen or fifteen years of age. Sometimes, however, there is no diseased condition of the hair to be detected, but it simply disappears. In such cases it will be found that the disease is hereditary.

Temporary loss of hair is, of course, exceedingly common. The hair of many people falls out excessively during the summer, but soon returns. The hair constantly falls out as a result of various acute diseases, such as typhoid fever or erysipelas, and it tends to become thin in consumption and in other forms of wasting disease. In practically all these cases the hair returns to its former abundance when the hair bulbs have recovered from the weakening influence of the disease. Occasionally the hair may fall out for a time owing to the influence of anxiety or shock upon the nervous system. Many skin diseases cause baldness, such as eczema, and parasitic diseases such as favus and ringworm. It is very frequent in the secondary stage of syphilis.

There is one exceedingly common form of patchy baldness which very much resembles ringworm, and is often confused with it, but is in reality quite distinct. Its technical name is alopecia areata. The patches may be even an inch or more across. Occasionally they occur on the beard. The course of this disease varies in different cases. It is said that if the baldness lasts for over two years the hair is very unlikely to return. Sometimes it may only last for a few weeks. When the hair is about to return it makes the first attempt in the shape of a fine downy growth, such as occurs on the cheek of a girl. This is usually shed and another may appear, but after several attempts the strong hairs appear. The disease may affect several members of a family, and this suggests a parasitic origin, but in many cases it would appear to be due to malnutrition of the skin of nervous origin. Another suggestion is that it is due to the infection of the mouth, tonsils, nose or throat with a streptococcus.

Whenever baldness is due to dandruff (*q.v.*) the essential part of the treatment is to attack and cure that condition.

To encourage the growth of the hair when the scalp has been cleaned in alopecia areata and in baldness due to acute diseases and other debilitating causes, a stimulating lotion will be useful. The following may be used :

Strong solution of ammonia	½ ounce
Chloroform	½ ,,
Oil of sesame	½ ,,
Oil of lemon	½ ,,
Spirit of rosemary ..	2 ounces

The lotion should be rubbed into the roots of the hair night and morning. It should not be forgotten that the massaging of the scalp which accompanies the application of the lotion is an important part of the cure. Stimulating the scalp by the use of electricity is also beneficial. It will often be found that an iron tonic is very helpful in promoting growth of the hair, such as two Blaud's pills thrice daily or a liquid preparation of iron.

As regards alopecia areata, in view of the possibility of its being due to infection in the mouth, nose or throat, it is necessary to search for a focus of infection in these parts and clear it up. Vaccines prepared from swabbings of the nose and throat of patients suffering from this form of baldness have been successfully used. Applications of ultra-violet rays have proved to have a potent influence in promoting hair growth in alopecia areata.

See Anaemia ; Croton Oil ; Dandruff ; Hair ; Jaborandi ; Light ; Seborrhoea.

BALNEOLOGY. Derived from the Latin *balneum*, a bath, balneology is the technical name for the study of baths of all kinds, their effects upon the body under different conditions and their uses in health and disease.

See Baths.

BALSAM. Balm or balsam is the name applied to oily, pleasant-smelling substances which flow out from certain plants, sometimes spontaneously, sometimes after cuts have been made in the stem or leaves. They are mixtures of oil, resin and, as a rule, benzoic acid (*q.v.*).

The most familiar kind of balsam, invented by the friars many centuries ago and popularly known as Friar's Balsam, is powerfully antiseptic in virtue of the benzoic acid which it contains. For this reason it is used as an ingredient in court sticking plaster. When applied to wounds, besides acting as an antiseptic, it aids in the arrest of bleeding. The technical name of Friar's Balsam is compound tincture of benzoin. It is sometimes given by the mouth in doses of about a teaspoonful, but more frequently by inhalation. One or two teaspoonsful may be added to a pint of hot water and the steam inhaled either through an inhaler or from a jug, in cases of sore throat, bronchitis and similar conditions. The fragrant part of the vapour is soothing and so also are the warmth and the water vapour, while the benzoic acid is powerfully antiseptic.

The other balsams used in medicine are copaiba, balsam of Peru, balsam of tolu, and storax or styrax, and all are of value in chronic bronchitis. The chief use of copaiba, however, is in gonorrhoea. Syrup of tolu is often included in cough mixtures for children, the dose for a child of six being 10 to 20 minims. Storax and Peruvian balsam are sometimes used in parasitic skin affections.

See Anise ; Benzoic Acid ; Peruvian Balsam ; Storax ; Tolu.

BANDAGE. There are many different kinds of bandages, most of which can be successfully applied after a short training by any intelligent person. It may be said that the uses of bandages are threefold. In the first place, they may be employed to keep surgical dressings or splints in place. Secondly, they may be used for the sake of their direct pressure upon the part to which they are applied, as in the case of sprain or when they are used to arrest bleeding. Their third use is to give support to the circulation in cases of varicose veins, or to injured parts, as, for example, a broken lower jaw or broken ribs, when the bandages also restrain movements. For varicose veins various other devices are used, such as the elastic stocking, but no elastic stocking is nearly so efficient or so comfortable as a properly applied bandage made of the proper material.

Reef Knot

Granny Knot

Bandages are made of many different shapes. Of these the simplest and the oldest is the triangular bandage, sometimes called the first aid bandage. It is of value in emergencies, but, as a rule, not so efficient as the other kind of bandage usually called the roller bandage.

Triangular Bandage. The triangular bandage is made by taking a piece of fabric, usually calico, 38 inches square and dividing it diagonally, though for some purposes a folded handkerchief will serve. In order to follow a description of the modes of application of this bandage it is necessary to know the names which are given to its various parts. The largest side of the triangle is known as the base or lower border, the other two sides being the side borders. The angle opposite the base is the point and the others form the ends. Reference to the diagram will make these terms clear.

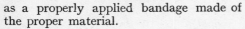

The bandage may be used as the whole cloth, that is, without folding it ; or it may be used as the broad or the narrow fold. The former is made by bringing the point down to the base and folding again ; if folded once more we get the narrow fold. In tying this or any bandage a reef knot must be made, as a granny

knot is liable to slip. The methods of tying these knots will be best understood by reference to the accompanying diagram, but it may be said that when a reef knot is tied the ends lie parallel with the direction of the bandage, whereas in the granny they lie across it. When the knot has been tied the ends should be neatly tucked away under the bandage.

The methods of applying the bandage for various purposes are as follows :

GREATER ARM SLING. This supports the whole forearm, from the elbow to the wrist. Take the whole cloth and place one end over the sound shoulder, with the point towards the injured limb. Carry the forearm across the cloth and bring up the other end over it and over the shoulder on the injured side. Knot off behind the neck. Then take the point, carry it forward in front of the elbow and fasten with a safety pin. The greater arm sling is illustrated in the next page.

LESSER ARM SLING. This supports the forearm at the wrist only. Use a broad or a narrow fold. Place one end over the sound shoulder, bring the other over the wrist, which has been carried across the body at the desired level, over the sound shoulder, and knot off behind the neck. Should the patient complain of the pressure of the knot when using either sling, the position of the knot may be changed and a pad of cotton-wool may be placed beneath it.

The whole cloth is also used in applying to the following parts :

HEAD. For a scalp wound, fold the lower border so as to make a hem an inch wide, and place the centre of the border on the forehead above the root of the nose, the point being thrown backwards over the head. Carry the ends round and cross below the occipital protuberance, the prominence at the back of the head, fixing down the point in doing so. Bring the ends forward and knot over the forehead. Draw down the point so that the bandage is smoothly applied over the head, carry it forward and fix with a safety pin.

SHOULDER. Apply the centre of the lower border to the outside of the upper arm about the middle, the point lying upon the neck. Carry the ends round, cross on the inside, bring out and tie off. Put on a lesser arm sling for the injured limb. Pull the point up beneath this so that the bandage covers the shoulder smoothly. Bring the point down over the sling and pin off.

HAND. Apply the middle of the lower border to the front of the wrist, the fingers being towards the point. Carry the latter back over the fingers to the wrist. Carry the ends to the back of wrist and cross, thus fixing the point. Then cross in front, fixing the lower border. Tie off on the back of the wrist, and pull the point up so as to make the bandage taut. Take the point down over the knot and pin off.

HIP. This is bandaged like the shoulder, except that the point is fixed by a narrow-fold bandage carried round the body and tied off on the opposite side.

FOOT. Place the sole on the bandage, the toes towards the point, and proceed as for the hand.

CHEST. This is for a wound. Place the cloth over the dressing, with the point over the shoulder on the injured side. Carry the ends round the body and tie off so as to leave one end long, this being then brought up and knotted with the point.

PERINEUM OR FORK. Carry the ends round the waist and knot off in front, leaving one end long. Bring the point forward between the thighs and knot off with the end. In some cases the bandage will be applied in front and knotted behind.

For the following parts either the broad or narrow fold is used :

EYE. Place the centre of a narrow fold bandage over the eye. Carry one end obliquely across the brow and another over the ear. Cross below the prominence at the back of the head, bring forward and tie over the dressing.

NECK, ARM AND FOREARM. Place the centre of a narrow fold over the dressing, carry the ends round, cross, bring back and tie over the dressing.

THIGH AND LEG. Proceed as above, using a broad fold.

ELBOW. This is done with the forearm bent up to a right angle. Place the centre of a broad fold over the point of the elbow. Cross in front and carry back round the forearm, overlapping the lower edge of the bandage already applied. Cross again in front, carry back round the arm, overlapping the upper edge, and knot above the elbow.

KNEE. Proceed as above, except that the ends are first carried round the thigh so that the knot is made below the kneecap.

CHEST. Bandage for a broken rib. Place the centre of a broad fold over the fracture, that is, the point where the pain is felt in breathing ; carry the ends round the body and tie. Apply a second broad fold

Greater arm sling completed

Triangular bandage. Left, first stage of greater arm sling ; right, bandage for shoulder combined with lesser arm sling

bandage so as to overlap the first, above or below, according as the fractured rib is a lower or an upper one. The bandages should be just sufficiently tight to restrain the breathing movements somewhat. If the pressure appears to cause pain the bandage should be taken off.

ABDOMEN. Apply the centre of a broad fold bandage over the dressing ; carry the ends round the body and knot off.

Roller Bandage. The roller bandage may be from one to twelve yards long and from one to six inches wide. It is generally made of cotton, bleached or unbleached, but may be of muslin, linen, flannel, crepe, pure rubber, woven elastic, or other material. In preparing most bandages the requisite widths are torn from the piece of material. To roll up, fold up one end two or three times so as to form a tight core or " head," on which the " body " is rolled. The free end of the roll is known as the " tail."

In bandaging a limb always begin on the inside, applying the outer surface of the tail and rolling outwards across the limb. No more than three or four inches should be uncovered at a time. To fix the bandage, a few turns are taken round the limb, then succeeding turns pass obliquely upwards, each turn covering about two-thirds of the preceding one. It will be found that after a few turns, owing to the limb being more or less conical, the bandage will not lie smoothly unless what is known as a reverse is made. The thumb of the free hand is placed in front of the turn which is unrolling, the body of the bandage is twisted round towards the operator, and the turn is completed with the reverse side of the bandage in contact with the skin. Another reverse is made, parallel to the first, when the bandage again comes to the front, and this is continued till the bandage lies evenly without reversing.

The methods just described are the simple spiral and the reversed spiral. Another method is adopted in bandaging

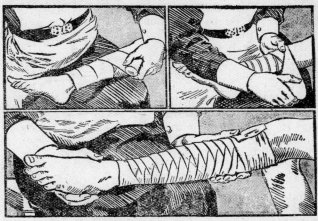

Roller bandage. Three stages in spiral application to leg; top right, a reverse is being made

a joint. A turn is taken round the middle of the joint ; the next turn overlaps the first below, and the next overlaps it above. This is continued till the joint is covered in by alternate loops above and below. This is known as a modified figure of eight.

A simple figure of eight may be used at certain joints ; for example, in bandaging the leg, in order to fix the bandage below, a few turns are taken round the foot. The bandage is then carried up round the ankle and again taken round the foot. After a few turns the bandage is continued up the leg as a reversed or simple spiral. The method is also useful when bandaging the forearm, the first few turns being taken round the wrist.

A variety of figure of eight bandage, known as a spica, is used for bandaging the shoulder, groin, thumb and great toe. As will be seen, it consists of alternate large and small loops.

GROIN. In bandaging the groin, the tail of the bandage is laid along the groin, pointing inwards and downwards. The roll is then carried round the loins just below the edge of the hip bones, brought across the front of the body and thigh and round the latter, as completing the first figure of eight. The others are formed in the same manner, each layer overlapping two-thirds of the preceding one. To bandage both groins, begin as above, and for clearness let it be assumed that the tail of the bandage is laid along the right groin. After taking the roll round the loins, instead of carrying it round the right thigh it is carried back between the thighs and round the left one. It is then carried round across the front of the body and round the loins, but this time it is taken round the right thigh, and so on alternately round each thigh, when the bandage is brought forward from the loins. This is the double spica.

THUMB AND GREAT TOE. In bandaging the thumb a few turns are first made round the wrist, the back of the hand being upwards, and then a turn round the thumb near its tip and back to the wrist. These alternate loops are made till the whole thumb is covered in. The great toe is bandaged similarly.

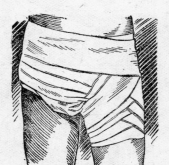

Roller bandage for the groin

FINGER. In bandaging a finger, a few turns are made round the wrist, the hand being held with the back upwards. A few inches of the tail of the bandage are left loose for the purpose of tying off. The bandage is then carried down to near the tip of the finger and continued up the finger by a series of spiral loops till the root of the finger is reached, when the bandage is again carried up to and round the wrist and tied off. If there are more fingers than one to be bandaged, instead of tying, the bandage is taken to the tip of the next finger in order and so on.

BREAST. In applying a supporting bandage to the breast, the left one being taken as an example, the operator stands in front of the patient and, after taking one or two turns from left to right round the body just below the breasts, he raises the breast with one hand and brings the bandage below it from behind forward, continuing over the opposite shoulder to the left armpit and round the waist. A second turn below the breast is then made, and these alternate loops are made until the breast is covered almost to the nipple. In bandaging both breasts the process is begun as above, but instead of making the second turn below the left

breast the bandage is continued on round the waist and then across the back to the left shoulder. It is now carried downwards in front beneath the right breast and round the waist, again lifting the left breast as it comes forward, and so on.

NECK. To bandage the neck the operator stands in front of the patient and lays the tail of the bandage on the front of the shoulder on the injured side, pointing upwards and inwards across the shoulder. While the tail is fixed by one hand, the roll is carried under the armpit and up behind to the root of the neck, in front of which it then passes. It is carried round the neck and again under the armpit. When a sufficient number of turns have been made to fix the bandage, it is carried by spirals up the neck. If necessary, when the neck has been covered, a turn or two may be taken round the head, running up above the ear on the sound side, across the forehead and down over the other ear, round the neck and again round the head.

HEAD. To cover in the scalp the double roller capeline bandage is used. This is simply a long roller bandage, the two ends of which have been rolled in opposite directions till they meet. If the rolls are of the same size, one should be unrolled for a couple of feet, the slack being taken up by the other. The operator stands behind the patient. Taking the larger roll in his left hand and the other in his right, he applies the bandage to the centre of the forehead just above the nose.

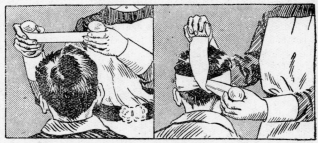

Use of a double roller bandage for a head injury; one roll is brought round the head and the other across the top

The two rolls are then brought round above the ears till they meet below the prominence at the back of the head. The left-hand roll is now taken with the right hand and carried above the right roll, this being carried forward across the middle of the head to the lower part of the brow and fixed there by the original left roll, which is carried round across the forehead for this purpose. The original right roll is then brought to the back of the head to one or other side of the central piece of bandage, but overlapping it. At the back of the head it is again caught by the bandage encircling the head, and then carried across the head on the other side of the central bandage, to be fixed again in front and brought back on the other side. It is thus alternately applied to one side and the other till the scalp is covered in, when both rolls are curved round the head and tied off above the nose.

In applying the capeline, it is necessary to be careful that the bandage is kept low on the forehead and well below the prominence at the back of the head, otherwise it is apt to slip off.

The widths of bandage most suitable for various parts in an adult are as follows : head and neck, 2 to 3 inches ; arm and shoulder, 3 inches ; forearm and hand, 2 inches ; fingers, 1 inch ; chest and abdomen, 4 to 6 inches ; groin, 4 inches ; thigh, 3 to 4 inches ; leg, 3 inches.

In the use of roller bandages certain rules must be carefully observed in addition to those already mentioned. Do not apply a damp bandage, as it will shrink on drying and may constrict the part. Apply the turns with uniform pressure and parallel with each other. Do not reverse over a sharp, bony edge. When bandaging the limbs, the points of the fingers or toes should be left free to make it possible to ascertain that the circulation in the limb is not being impeded. This is done by pressing the nail so as to blanch its bed, and noting whether the blood returns at once, as it should do, when the pressure is removed. In taking off a bandage do not attempt to roll it up in the process, but gather the slack into a bundle, which is carried round and round the limb in unrolling. No attempt should be made to reapply a bandage without removing it completely and again making a firm roll of it. Machines are made for rolling bandages, and are a great convenience when a considerable number of bandages are in use.

T-bandage. A T-bandage is used for supporting a dressing on the perineum. The horizontal portion goes round the pelvis just below the upper rim of the hip bones. A sufficient length of 3 to 4-inch roller is cut off, and to the middle of this the vertical portion is attached. It is better if the latter be slit down as far as the perineum, where its two portions are tied in a half-knot to prevent the slit going further. Each portion is then brought forward and attached to the girdle part at the groin on each side.

Four-tailed Bandage. A four-tailed bandage is used for keeping dressings on the chin. It is made by taking about $1\frac{1}{4}$ yards of a 3-inch roller. A longitudinal slit about

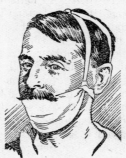

Four-tailed bandage over a chin dressing

3 inches long, is made in the centre, and the bandage is then slit down on either side to about 6 inches from its centre. The central slit is applied over the dressing on the skin. The lower two tails are then taken and knotted in front of the vertex or uppermost part of the head. The other two are taken round, tied over the nape of the neck and the long ends are each tied to the corresponding long end of the upper tails.

Many-tailed Bandage. It is sometimes a convenience to cover in dressings by means of a many-tailed bandage. This is made by taking a piece of 3-inch bandage, sufficiently long for the purpose required, for the leg, for example, from the heel to the back of the knee ; or, for the abdomen, from the bottom of the spine to the top of the small of the back. Along this piece of bandage are attached, by stitching, a succession of cross-pieces, which should be long enough to go round the part and overlap, allowance being made for any dressings which may be necessary. When applying the bandage the central length is placed down the middle of the back of the part, and the lowest two ends are brought forward and crossed, and so on in succession with the other cross-pieces, the ends of the last two being fixed with a safety pin.

Immovable Bandages. Bandages are sometimes impregnated with plaster of Paris, starch and other substances, and applied wet, so that a firm casing for a part of the body is formed when the material hardens. The plaster of Paris bandage is of coarse muslin, the meshes of which are filled with the plaster. It is used on a limb when it is desired to keep a joint at rest or maintain a fracture in position. It is also used to form a jacket to give support to the spine in cases of Pott's curvature.

The part is washed and dried and dusted with boracic acid powder. A flannel bandage is then applied. The plaster of Paris bandage is thoroughly soaked in warm water and laid over the flannel. It should be applied as obliquely as possible, and the more figures of eight there are the better. Three or four layers should be put on, and over all some of the plaster from the vessel in which the bandage has been soaked. The bandage is then allowed to set, the limb or other part meanwhile being kept in the correct position.

See Elastic Bandage; Esmarch's Bandage; First Aid; Fracture; Splint; Tourniquet.

BANTING. A method of treatment of obesity is known as Banting's System. It was popularised by an extremely fat man, so fat as to have to go downstairs backward, named William Banting, who addressed a letter to the public on the subject. Everything else having failed, Banting was advised by a Dr. Harvey to cut out from his diet bread, milk, butter, potatoes and sugar, upon which he had hitherto principally lived. In their place he was recommended to take lean meat and fish, any vegetable but potatoes, plain tea (that is, without milk or sugar), a little fruit and a little wine. The characters of this diet from a physiological point of view will be readily understood when the reader has considered the article on food.

Meanwhile, it may be said that the system was very successful in Banting's case, as he lost over forty pounds of weight in a few months and there was a marked improvement in his general health. In some other reported cases it has proved very satisfactory, but not in all, as while it has reduced the weight the patient has suffered in general health. Some have suffered from indigestion and others from nervous symptoms of one kind and another. The system has been criticised on the ground that the large amount of protein throws an undue strain on the kidneys, and that in the gouty, who are often fat, it is likely to be harmful. Below is given in detail the diet recommended to Banting and regarded as the typical diet of this method.

Breakfast : 4 ounces of beef, mutton, kidneys, broiled fish, or any cold meat except pork ; a large cup of plain tea, and a little biscuit or one ounce of toast. Dinner : 5 to 6 ounces of any lean meat, fish, poultry or game, any vegetable except potatoes ; 1 ounce of dry toast, some fruit out of a pudding, and two glasses of claret, sherry or madeira. Tea : 2 to 3 ounces of fruit, a rusk or two and a cup of plain tea. Supper : 3 to 4 ounces of meat or fish, as at dinner, and a glass or two of claret.

Probably the only improvement that can be suggested on this diet to-day is the substitution of some other drink for the wine, and also the suppression of the tumbler of " grog " which Banting took as a nightcap ; but the cure should only be tried under medical observation, as, like all systems, it cannot satisfy the needs and circumstances of every kind of constitution.

See Diet; Food; Gout; Obesity; Salisbury Treatment.

BARBER'S ITCH. The popular name barber's itch is applied to one variety of " foul shave " contracted by infection in barbers' shops. Its technical name is tinea sycosis or sometimes tinea barbae. The disease is accompanied by a great deal of inflammation, beginning at the roots of the hairs, exceptional rapidity of development and boggy swellings of the skin. A good deal of matter usually forms. This disease is really a severe form of ringworm of the beard. It is well worth noting that the disease is not communicated by the razor but by the brush. This is in general true of all diseases contracted in barbers' shops.

The essential precautions against conveying infection consist in the absolute sterilisation of the implements used in shaving and haircutting, and in the cleanliness of the hands of the operator.

The shaving-brush should be invariably sterilised after each occasion of use, and, as certain other methods of disinfection are apt to make the hairs of the brush fall out, it is usually necessary to employ a powerful disinfecting solution. When the brush has been thoroughly soaked in this for some time, it may be washed in ordinary tap water, and then can be safely employed.

Whether it is necessary for the skin to be actually cut before any risk of infection is incurred we do not very definitely know, but in general it is well to treat all cuts incurred at the barber's by thorough washing and the use of some mild antiseptic. The disease calls for vigorous treatment under medical supervision. Benzoic acid, salicylic acid, mercurial preparations, iodine, and other antiparasitics are used ; and applications of X-rays may be of value.

See Antiseptic ; Ringworm ; Sycosis.

BARIUM. The medical uses of barium, a metal in the same group with calcium and magnesium, are practically restricted to two compounds, namely, barium sulphide, which is occasionally used to remove superfluous hairs, and barium sulphate, which is often used as an opaque substance when making X-ray examinations, for example, of the alimentary tract. The sulphate is a white powder which passes through the tract without being dissolved. Soluble salts of barium are very poisonous.

See Depilatory ; Test Meal.

BARKING COUGH. A loud form of cough is often described as a barking cough on account of its resemblance to the barking of a dog. It is frequently met with in boys of rather nervous temperament about the age of fourteen or fifteen, and is still more frequently heard as a symptom of hysteria. In this last-named disease the patient may cough so loudly and so persistently as to cause real anxiety as to the state of her lungs. A barking cough is a not uncommon event at puberty. In all cases an expert examination should be made of the nose and throat, as a cause for the cough may be found there. The treatment for loud and sensational coughing of this kind, in the absence of a local cause, consists in dealing with the nervous state that underlies it, whether by drugs, discipline, or otherwise.

See Cough ; Hysteria.

BARLEY WATER. This beverage is very frequently used in the sick-room. It has practically no food value at all, but is useful for diluting other foods, such as milk, for it has soothing, demulcent qualities, and interferes with the density of the clot in the stomach when milk is swallowed. Barley water may be made clear or thick. For the clear variety, put two tablespoonsful of pearl barley and sufficient cold water in a saucepan, bring to the boil, and strain. The blanched barley is then returned to the saucepan with 2 pints of cold water. This is brought to the boil, allowed to simmer for half an hour, and strained.

Thick barley water is made in the same way, but after bringing to the boil it is boiled gently till the quantity is reduced to two-thirds or a half. In both cases it is sweetened with sugar if desired, and then allowed to cool. The rind of half a lemon thinly peeled may be boiled with the barley, and after straining the juice is added. When prepared in this way it is not, of course, mixed with milk. Barley water only keeps for a few hours and should not again be brought to the boil.

See Beverages : Invalid Cookery.

BARLOW'S DISEASE. This is the name sometimes given to a disease of infants first described by Sir Thomas Barlow. It is most conveniently considered as a particular form of scurvy (*q.v.*). Alternative names for it are infantile scurvy and scurvy rickets.

BARRENNESS. *See* Sterility.

BASEDOW'S DISEASE. *See* Exophthalmic Goitre.

BASILICON OINTMENT. An ointment composed of 8 parts each of resin, yellow beeswax and olive oil, and 6 parts of lard, is known as basilicon, or resin ointment. It is a slightly antiseptic stimulant, and forms a good application for sluggish ulcers. The addition of 20 grains of salicylic acid to the ounce makes it an effective remedy in many cases of pruritus ani, or itching round the lower end of the bowel.

BATHING. The value of sea bathing lies pre-eminently in its stimulating effect on the nervous system, this being brought about by the sense of adventure, the novelty, the contact of the air, the water with its salt, the breaking of the waves, the sunshine and, where possible, the company. A sea-water bath falls short of open-air sea bathing in some of these respects, and a bag of sea salt in a bath at home, though not to be despised, falls very far short.

There is a general tendency to prolong a sea bath unduly. The length of a bathe must be determined in the first place by the temperature of the water. When it is cold the bather should not stay in more than two or three minutes, whereas in happier climes he may stay all day. Other things being equal, the swimmer may always stay in the water much longer than the non-swimmer, and this for the simple reason that in the act of swimming he is producing a very large amount of heat, which compensates more or less completely for the loss of heat upon the surface of his body.

Important questions arise as to the advisability of sea bathing in various states of disease and under various exceptional conditions. In general it is safer for pregnant women not to indulge in sea baths. On the other hand, it is now known that patients suffering from the early stages of consumption may greatly benefit by sea bathing, though due precautions must be observed. The patient must be absolutely free from fever, and he must not be exhausted by his bathe.

Other conditions in which sea bathing is very beneficial are general lack of tone, nervous indigestion, bloodlessness, asthma, rickets in children, and all forms of tuberculosis. In general, sea baths are very useful in accustoming the skin to changes of temperature and damp. Thus, people who are accustomed to sea bathing will not catch cold or suffer from local rheumatism when subjected to conditions which certainly produce these troubles in other people.

The water should not be entered when the skin is very hot and perspiring, nor when one is very hungry, nor immediately after a meal. An hour or two after a meal is the best time for bathing.

The ideal bathe is when every part of the body is alternately subjected to a sun bath and to a sea-water bath.

In introducing children to sea bathing, care must be taken to respect the natural fear of a child. Nothing annoys the physician more than to see the stupid and cruel performances constantly to be witnessed at the seaside in summer time.

If a child is frightened, not only does he gain no benefit from his bathe, but his nervous system, instead of being stimulated, is made the victim of shock.

This may lead to all sorts of disorders, besides perhaps making him dislike sea bathing for the rest of his life through the effects of early association.

Most fatalities in bathing are probably due to fainting, induced by a state of health which unfits for bathing, to excessive chill or fatigue, or to some other circumstance. Cramp may occur, and when it does the swimmer ought to turn quietly on his back and float. Care must be taken to protect the ears by cotton-wool plugs or otherwise in diving from any height, and the same precaution should be taken by those suffering from chronic discharges from the ears, if, indeed, they bathe at all.

See Exercise; First Aid.

BATHS. Nowadays we hear of sun baths, electric light baths, air baths, sand baths, and so forth, but first place in this article shall be given to the simplest and oldest and most important kind of bath. It consists of water.

A cold bath (32°–70° F.) has very simple properties. It mainly abstracts heat from the surface. This process can only be continued for a very brief time without danger, and in general the law may be laid down that the value of a cold bath is in inverse proportion to its length, that is, the shorter the bath the more useful it is. It stimulates the skin, through the skin the whole nervous system, and through the nervous system the whole body. The effects of this stimulation are familiar to everybody and are often summed up in the single word a " glow." Anyone who takes a cold bath and does not experience this reaction or glow has not benefited by it, but, on the contrary, has been weakened. Each person should be able to decide by this simple and sufficient test whether he ought to take cold baths at all, or at what times of the year he ought to take them, and how often and for how long.

Cold baths are not for the feeble, nor, generally speaking, for elderly people. The bather should not spend longer than two minutes in his cold bath. So long as the water is sufficiently below blood heat, say 40° F. at most, the bath will be stimulating, and the use of unwarmed tap water in freezing wintry weather may be very unwise. For choice, he should employ cold water only as a shower at the end of a warm bath, and then he should dry himself quickly and thoroughly with a very rough towel, so as to assist the coming of the " glow " or reaction. If the hands and feet are blue and cold after the bath, cold sponging while standing in warm water may be tried, but it may be necessary to restrict oneself to cold sponging of the neck and shoulders.

Uses and Dangers of Hot Baths

Water of a warmer temperature is, of course, necessary for cleansing purposes, and it should be combined with a free use of soap and friction. Very hot water, as hot as the skin will permit, has a stimulating effect, if used only for a short time. It soon becomes debilitating, as does a hot bath (about 106° F.) or a warm bath (98°–100° F.). A hot bath should not be continued for longer than ten minutes. Hot baths promote the flow of the sweat, but this is more safely attained by other means, such as the hot-air bath. But a hot bath by the bedside may be used in the treatment of acute Bright's disease, especially when uraemia threatens. The perspiration induced helps to get rid of some of the poison accumulating in the blood owing to the kidneys being more or less out of action. Such treatment should only be given, however, under medical direction.

An important use of a very hot bath is to stimulate the breathing of apparently stillborn babies, who are often made to start breathing for themselves by being dipped alternately in very hot and cold water.

Cold Baths for Treating Fevers

Baths have other important medical uses. Cold water is very frequently and widely used as a means of reducing the temperature in fever. When the temperature shows a tendency to rise above 103° F. the patient may be sponged with cold or tepid water, sponging a part of the body at a time and avoiding unnecessary exposure. In the condition of hyperpyrexia, 105·8° F. or over, when life is endangered, apart from anything else, by the height of the temperature, cold baths are necessary and the water may have to be chilled by the addition of ice. When a patient is in a bath of this kind a close watch must be kept on the temperature and when this has sunk to within two or three degrees of normal, he must be taken from the bath. The temperature continues to sink after removal from the bath, and if he is left too long there is a risk of collapse.

Tepid baths (80° F.) or warm baths are exceedingly valuable in the treatment of the convulsions (q.v.) of children, usually called fits. A warm bath, about 100° F., is an important adjunct in the treatment of severe burns. It helps to mitigate the shock which is frequent in these cases, especially when the burn involves the trunk; and it is a great help in removing clothing. Children should be put into such a bath at once pending the arrival of a doctor. The same applies to the collapse which may occur in infantile cholera and severe diarrhoea.

Very hot baths may be occasionally used for a very short period of time in cases of muscular feebleness, and are sometimes useful in the form of local baths, applied merely to one part of the body, such as a painful joint. Various kinds of douche baths are of real value. They may be employed at various temperatures or with rapidly varying temperatures, as in what is called the Scottish Douche. Many conditions of the joints are often relieved by local douches, as are also various conditions of the lower part of the bowel, such as piles.

The Turkish bath is really a general hot-air bath, and in contrast with it there is the local hot-air bath, which is perhaps more effectual than any other means in relieving the pains of chronic joint disease. The details of the Turkish bath need not be described. The point to remember is that the air of the bath is dry, so that the perspiration can freely escape from the skin. This is the difference between the Turkish bath and the vapour bath. The latter cannot be endured at a temperature higher than about 120° F., whereas the Turkish bath can be endured at a hundred degrees higher than this. In the case of local hot-air baths the temperature may even be raised to 300° F.

Value of a Turkish Bath

Turkish baths are of value for two reasons. First, no other bath is so cleansing. Secondly, a Turkish bath is very valuable as a stimulant to the circulation, especially the circulation through the skin and through the extremities of the body. In a great many diseased conditions, such as gout and Bright's disease (q.v.), in which the body contains poisons which need to be got rid of, Turkish baths are very valuable in enabling the skin to come to the aid of the other organs concerned with the process of expelling the poison. After a Turkish bath the greatest care must be taken against exposure.

A similar bath may be taken at home by using one of the portable baths on the market ; and in the case of people who are bedridden, when it is necessary to induce very free sweating, a cage or bed-cradle (q.v.) is sometimes used. This should be large enough to reach from the neck to the feet, or almost so, and sufficiently wide and high to be quite clear of the body. The patient lies on a waterproof sheet covered by a blanket and the cradle is covered with one or more blankets. The hot air is furnished by a lamp provided with a long tube which passes into the tent, care being taken that the tube is protected where it touches the blanket,

and that the hot air does not blow directly on the patient. Such a bath may last for twenty minutes, but not longer. If during the bath the patient feels faint, the lamp should be removed and he should be dried and placed comfortably in bed. If the faintness persists he should be given a little stimulant, some sal volatile or weak spirits.

Baths of water containing carbonic acid or other gases, represented by those of Nauheim in Germany, appear to have a specially beneficial action upon the heart. Artificial Nauheim baths can be quite easily and cheaply prepared by the addition of certain salts to the ordinary bath. Sulphur baths are made by adding two to six ounces of potassa sulphurata to thirty gallons of water. The sulphur is dissolved in boiling water and then added. Such baths are used in skin diseases and for rheumatism.

Alkaline baths, made by adding six ounces of washing soda to thirty gallons of warm water, may be useful in relieving general pruritis or itching of the skin. They are also used in rheumatism, though it need hardly be said that one cannot introduce drugs into the body by a medicated bath of water.

The addition of mustard to a warm bath adds to its effectiveness in many conditions, for example, in baths for children suffering from convulsions and other complaints. The mustard should be first made into a paste with cold water and then put into the bath, a half to one ounce to the gallon. The addition of a tablespoonful to a footbath is a useful treatment for an oncoming cold, and the same amount added to a hip bath may be of value in some cases of dysmenorrhoea.

Prevention of Rickets by Sun Baths

In many sanatoria for tuberculosis and other diseases, sun baths, or the exposure of the body to sunlight, have been found very valuable in restoring the health of the patient, improving the quality of his sleep, his appetite and his digestion. It has been demonstrated that sunlight can prevent the development of rickets, even when the diet is such as will lead to the disease. The value of sunlight in cases of tuberculosis is enhanced by sea bathing.

The use of baths in many complaints is much more beneficial when combined with massage, the application of electricity in various forms, and a regulated régime of diet, exercise and rest. The advantage of spas is that all these things are provided for and readily available ; and there is also the important factor of a change from the surroundings and responsibilities of everyday life and work. Their only drawback is on the score of expense. There is, of course, no question that a great many people, after a visit to some Continental spa, are found to have lost superfluous fat, to have got rid of twinges of gout or rheumatism, to have recovered their nervous tone, and so forth. Their visit has done them good undoubtedly, but the expense of it could be saved if many of these people would adopt a more healthy mode of life at home. This they will not do, however, and they leave their doctor no alternative to sending them somewhere for the cure.

See Douche ; Electricity in Medicine ; Health Resort ; Light ; Massage ; Mud Bath ; Radiant Heat.

BAY RUM. In cases of greasy scalp and other conditions, bay rum is a useful application. It owes its scent to the leaves of the bay or laurel from which it is prepared, and its cleansing properties to the large quantity of alcohol it contains.

BEARD. Common diseases which affect the beard and whisker area are dealt with under the headings Acne, Barber's Itch and Sycosis.

BED BUG. These insects are of a brownish colour, very flat and from a twelfth to a fifth of an inch long. The female lays her eggs in the beginning of the summer, and these are glutinous at first, so that they readily adhere to whatever they are deposited on. The body of the insect emits an offensive odour when touched. Some people are not affected by the bites, but others suffer from irritation, itching and wheals. It is now known that the bug might be instrumental in conveying relapsing fever, the germs of which, being taken up when biting an infected person, are introduced into others whom it may bite.

Infested premises must have the flooring and skirting-boards sufficiently re- moved to permit of the breeding places and surrounding woodwork being treated with crude creosote or tar. Wood bed- steads and other furniture should be washed thoroughly with soft soap, after which turpentine is applied to the crevices and joints. A thorough sulphur fumigation will dispose of bugs in a room. Clothing may be soaked in disinfecting solutions such as lysol. Kerosene provides another useful means of dealing with bugs. For the irritation of the bites diluted toilet vinegar, ammonia, or a saturated solution of bicarbonate of soda may be used.

See Bite ; Disinfection.

BED CRADLE. In certain cases it is necessary to make use of a cage, known as a bed cradle, to take the weight of the bedclothes off a patient, for instance, in fractures of the lower limbs, in painful abdominal conditions and so on. This consists of three metal or wooden struts to which are attached three or more metal hoops. The cradle can be utilised in giving a hot-air bath to a part, and an ice bag can be suspended from it in appendicitis and other abdominal conditions when any pressure on the part causes pain (Plate IX, 1). In an emergency, stools or some- thing of the kind will serve the purpose.

BED PAN. When patients, either from weakness or other causes, are unable to get up, a bed pan must be employed. There is no doubt that the bed pan is not used frequently enough in cases of heart disease, of extreme weakness due to many causes, and even in certain cases of varicose veins which have become com- plicated by the clotting of the blood in the veins. In such conditions serious harm may be done by the assumption of the erect attitude in getting out of bed, even if it be only for a few seconds. Before use the pan should be warmed and the margin covered with flannel. After use it should be emptied and cleansed as soon as possible, and in many cases it is desirable to use a disinfecting solution for the purpose.

BED REST. It is often necessary to have an appliance to prop up an invalid in bed, for example, in heart disease. This can be improvised in an emergency by putting a chair upside down into the bed and placing cushions or pillows along its

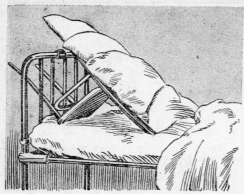
Bed rest improvised from a turned-up chair

back. For a longer use it is more satisfactory to purchase a properly made apparatus (*see* Plate XXVIII, 1).

BED SORE. A bed sore may seem to be a very unimportant and trivial malady, but the beginning of a bed sore very frequently marks the last stage in a chronic illness, its appearance turning the scale against the patient. It is infinitely easier to prevent a bed sore than to cure one ; and there are certain conditions in which it may be said that a bed sore once started is practically incurable. If this be so, it will certainly hasten the fatal termination of the patient's illness.

It may be taken as a good working rule that inefficient nursing is more or less responsible for the occurrence of every bed sore except in the case of patients who are either completely paralysed or who suffer from certain kinds of insanity in which the nutrition of the skin is so lowered that bed sores inevitably form in the later stages of the illness. A bed sore is a state of local inflammation of the skin, the immediate cause of which in every case is pressure.

Attention must be directed to the word immediate, as it is the state of nutrition of the skin that determines whether a given amount of pressure will or will not produce a bed sore.

The patients in whom the occurrence of bed sores is to be guarded against are those in whom the skin is weakened, owing either to general or to local causes. Amongst these are old age, various kinds of fever, especially typhoid, Bright's disease, heart disease and diabetes. In most of the cases named the state of nutrition of the skin has been weakened by the weakness of the circulation through it.

But, on the other hand, there are a large number of cases where the skin has been weakened, not so much by any defect in the circulation as by some defect in the nervous apparatus by which the health of the skin is maintained. Hence it is that in many cases of nervous disease, paralysis and insanity, bed sores are so exceedingly liable to form. The danger is increased by the occurrence of incontinence of urine in paralytic cases, so that the skin and bed tend to be constantly wet with an irritating fluid ; the same condition may occur in some diseases of the bladder. Given these conditions, it only requires pressure continued sometimes for a very short period in order to produce a bed sore.

The most important and perhaps the most frequent site of bed sores is in the skin immediately over the sacrum or termination of the backbone. When a patient is lying in bed on his back, if his skin has been weakened by any of the causes we have named, and if his illness has removed the buffer fat that should lie between his skin and his skeleton, a bed sore is only too likely to form on the site named. The other sites most frequently chosen are in general just those places where the skin lies immediately over a bony point that is subjected to constant or frequent pressure. The tips of the heels, the shoulder blades and the elbows, are frequent sites of bed sores, but the most important bed sore is that which occurs over the sacrum.

Properly speaking, there are two kinds of bed sores, namely, the acute and the chronic. The acute bed sore is far less frequent, and only occurs as a result of grave disease, such as the late stages of general paralysis, apoplexy, etc. It is with the chronic bed sore that we are concerned.

Everyone who has any responsibility in connexion with the nursing of the sick or the care of the aged, should be able to detect the earliest signs of an approaching bed sore, and should be fully aware of the grave responsibility that attaches to their neglect at this early and apparently insignificant stage.

The beginning of a bed sore is simply a local darkening of the skin due to the arrest of the circulation through it. This is scarcely the same as a darkening due to a bruise. It fades away more gradually at its edges, and has a dusky, sullen, purple-red colour which gradually darkens. The skin surrounding the darkened area is boggy and pits on pressure, that is to say, the mark of the pressure of the finger leaves a little pit which takes some time to disappear.

If the condition is not arrested, the injured area of skin will die, and will thereafter be separated, leaving a raw area of very weak vitality, which discharges a little thin matter. There may be little or no pain at this stage. Obviously one great danger of bed sores is that the skin may become infected by microbes, and thus give rise to a blood poisoning which is quite sufficient to carry off a patient already weakened by chronic disease.

Another grave result that frequently follows from the occurrence of a bed sore over the sacrum, or lower part of the backbone, is that the process of local death extends to the backbone itself, and from it also to the spinal cord which it encloses. When this stage is reached, the patient is certain to succumb to a rapidly fatal inflammation of the spinal cord and its coverings.

The prevention of bed sores is to be achieved first of all by the recognition of their liability to occur in certain classes of patient, by the recognition of the causes which produce them, and by the responsible appreciation of their possible consequences.

Whatever the disease or cause for which a patient remains in bed, it is the duty of those who are tending him to see that his position is sufficiently varied.

This is a good general rule to be applied to all cases save those few in which it has been specially ordered that the patient is not to be moved. There is no need to make violent changes of position. A great deal can be done by judicious play with a little cushion, placed now in the small of the back, now under the shoulders, now elsewhere ; even the bending of the knees or the straightening of them may make all the difference ; and of course the patient should be rolled about from side to side at reasonable intervals and in reasonable degree. In the worst cases a water bed may be required. Other local means may be adopted to take pressure off the part. Little rings of cotton-wool, for instance, may be placed upon the bone of the ankle, or water cushions or air cushions may be employed.

At least once a day the parts most liable to suffer must be carefully and gently washed, thoroughly dried and then rubbed—it is assumed, of course, that there is no sign of a bed sore at this stage —with methylated spirits or some other strong preparation of alcohol which is allowed to dry. It must further be remembered that, however dry the skin be kept after washing, it is always perspiring and therefore wetting itself. Perspiration not only softens and weakens the skin, but is apt to constitute an

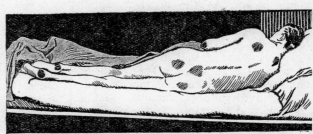

Bed Sores. The sites at which they are most likely to occur

excellent nutrient juice in which microbes may develop. The skin should be kept dusted with some antiseptic dusting powder such as boracic acid. This not only absorbs the moisture which is secreted by the skin, but also interferes with the growth of microbes. Finally should be noted the importance of keeping the sheets dry and free from wrinkles, crumbs and the like.

The treatment of bed sores is a matter for the surgeon, but it may be said that when a bed sore is actually threatening the treatment often is to paint the surface with flexible collodion and to move the patient so as to take pressure off the part. If the skin dies, boracic acid fomentations covered with oiled silk are used frequently to encourage the dead part to separate off. When this has happened the sore may be dressed with Friar's balsam, or with some such ointment as the following : resin ointment and balsam of Peru, one ounce of each ; or ten grains of camphor in one ounce of zinc ointment.

See Nursing.

BED-WETTING. A habit of wetting the bed during sleep, after the age when one expects sufficient control of the bladder to prevent it, say, from three years onwards, calls for the remedying of various causes of possible irritation. Fluids should be restricted or abstained from altogether, in most cases of the complaint, for a few hours before bedtime. Condiments, mustard, pepper and sauces, should be avoided. A tight foreskin or adenoids should be dealt with surgically. Constipation must be corrected, and threadworms cleared out if present.

The child should be made to empty the bladder before going to bed and should be waked to do so again after about an hour's sleep. As the accident usually happens when the child lies on the back, an old-fashioned preventive is to fasten a reel on the small of the back with a tape round the waist, so that the child wakes if it turns on its back. The medicinal remedies for the complaint include belladonna, hyoscyamus, hexamine, alkalies and thyroid extract. In some cases hypnotism effects a cure.

Punishing a child, in the great majority of cases, is about the worst thing to do.

It should be remembered that the habit may be due to such serious disorders as stone in the bladder, tuberculosis of the bladder, kidney disease, diabetes and epilepsy.

See Belladonna.

BEEF EXTRACT. An extract made from lean meat is now amongst the most widely used additions to the diet of convalescents or invalids. It contains a negligible amount of food matter, mainly consisting of what are called extractives, that is, substances of a special chemical class derived from muscular tissue by heating it under pressure with a little water. By exciting the secretion of the digestive juices of the stomach, extract of beef not only aids digestion very markedly, but also stimulates the appetite. Beef extracts are useful flavouring agents in general cookery, and, when giving white of egg to an invalid, the addition of a little meat extract confers palatability on it. They should be avoided by the gouty and those with kidney disease or thickened arteries.

BEEF JUICE. There is a wide difference between a beef extract and a beef juice. The former, while it has an important use as a digestive stimulant, has no food value, but beef juice really consists of the juice of the meat from which it is made, that is to say, consists of the fluid part of the muscular fibres. Beef juice may be prepared by a manufacturer on a large scale, or at home, and constitutes a food which may be of very great value to infants and invalids.

There are several ways of obtaining raw beef juice. The best is to chop up the meat, place it in cold water and leave it to stand in some cool place. The water gradually enters the beef and causes it to swell, and when the pulpy beef is taken and squeezed in muslin the juice is readily obtained. It is, of course, somewhat diluted with water, but there is no loss, and the juice is more completely extracted by this method than by any other that can conveniently be employed at home.

The composition of meat juices varies within somewhat wide limits, according to a great many circumstances. Raw meat juice made at home may contain from 3 to 7 per cent. of valuable food material. The beef juices made by manufacturers—such as Brand's, Valentine's, Armour's, that made by the Bovril Company, Wyeth's and others—may contain very much higher proportions of valuable protein matter or albumin varying between 7 and 30 per cent. or more.

Beef juice is exceedingly expensive, and it is probable that white of egg, at a fraction of the cost, is at least of equal value as a food ; but it is a welcome luxury to many patients, and its use is justified both on the grounds that it is a true food and also because of its stimulant action upon the digestion. A little raw beef juice also may be given—say, a teaspoonful once a week—to babies who are being fed upon sterilised or artificially prepared milk.

See Diet ; Invalid Cookery.

BEEF TEA. There are a number of methods of preparing beef tea, and the character of the beverage varies according to which of these is selected. The worst method is to boil it very quickly, for by this process the albumins, which are the really valuable constituents of the beef, are coagulated or solidified, and are thus prevented from entering the infusion. The best method will be given in detail, following closely the description given by a leading authority, Dr. Robert Hutchison.

The beef must be lean and completely free from gristle and fat. It must be scraped with the back of the knife so as to reduce it to shreds. The object of this is to separate the muscular fibres which contain the nourishment from the nonnutritious connective tissues which hold them together. The shreds are to be placed in a jar and mixed thoroughly with water. The proportions usually suggested are one pint of water to one pound of beef, but this is largely a matter of taste. If this mixture is left alone, there will soon be produced a very dilute beef juice. The jar should now be tightly covered and gradually heated, for at least an hour, in a saucepan of water reaching about three-quarters up the jar. The temperature must be kept below the point at which the valuable constituents of the fibre are apt to solidify, namely, about 167° F.

The tea is now made, but it is not cooked ; it still has the raw red colour and taste, and it must therefore be rapidly boiled and then removed from the fire. The tea must be poured off without straining, and the lumps of beef squeezed in a strainer and the product added to the tea. It is important to note that the tea must not be strained, for the most valuable part of the preparation consists of a number of tiny light particles which settle in a layer as the beef tea cools and which would all have been kept back had the tea been strained.

Beef tea constitutes a change where a patient is confined to a fluid diet, but its percentage of albumin or protein or true food matter is exceedingly small. However carefully the beef tea be made it can never contain even 2 per cent of protein. This fact is one which those in charge of the sick seem to have extreme difficulty in appreciating.

Of somewhat greater food value is what has been called whole beef tea, to which the finely powdered fibres of the meat have been added and in which they are held suspended. Furthermore, actual beef powders may be added to beef tea, and so may various other foods, such as baked flour. In such a case the beef tea is useful in persuading the patient to take more food and also in promoting its digestion.

See Invalid Cookery.

BEER. Many beers are of real food value, quite apart from the alcohol they contain. It has been estimated that a pint of ale contains about as much carbohydrate food as an ounce of bread, but this must not be taken to mean that the food value of the two is equal, as bread also contains a considerable proportion of protein or tissue-forming food in the shape of gluten. Beer is taken usually to help the appetite and to quench thirst. It may serve the former purpose usefully in convalescence from acute diseases, but only the lighter forms should be used. At all times it should be used moderately.

On the Continent there is an affection known as the " beer heart," which is an overstrained condition of the organ produced by the excessive amount of liquid which has to be sent through the circulation of those who drink beer copiously. Chronic gastritis is another and more frequent consequence of an intemperate use of the beverage. It is worth noting that the use of beer and malt liquors in general is highly undesirable in all cases where there is a tendency to obesity, for this tendency is liable to be increased, first of all by the action of the alcohol, and also by the fact that the nutritive part of these liquors is especially suitable for fat formation.

Beer is made by producing fermentation in infusions of sugary subtances, and adding bitters. Stout is beer which has been coloured with burnt malt, or in these days it may be with molasses, caramel or liquorice.

It is a mistake to give stout or other malt liquor to nursing mothers for the purpose of increasing the supply of breast milk. Milk and other wholesome food will accomplish this much better, and if alcoholic liquors are taken the infant's digestion may be upset.

Care must be exercised by beer-drinkers to restrict themselves to a sound brew. A good beer should be clear, transparent and reddish brown in tint, and should not be soured.

See Alcohol.

BEE STING. There is no distinction between the stings of bees and wasps, and what follows should be understood as applying to both. The reason why the sting is painful is that the insect injects into the skin a small quantity of formic acid. It may be noted, in passing, that these insects sting from fear or in order to avenge themselves, a different thing from the bite of insects like the mosquito and the flea, which seek to extract blood for their nourishment.

There are quite a number of cases where bee or wasp stings have caused death, often in under half an hour. The reason for this is by no means clearly understood. It is believed, however, that the cases of serious stinging are due to the production of a special poison by the particular wasp or bee in question, a poison which possibly depends upon a diseased state of the insect. Severe cases of such an accident must be treated according to the symptoms, by the free administration of alcohol and other stimulants, and so forth.

In mild cases the first thing to do is to get rid of the sting, if possible by such delicate manipulation as will not squeeze the poison bag and so introduce more of the poison into the patient's body, and thereafter one should apply any alkaline substance, such as a weak solution of ammonia or soda, in order to neutralise the acid in the poison injected by the insect. When the sting is near the eye, or in a cavity such as the mouth or the ear passage, ammonia would not, of course, be used. Afterwards some antiseptic lotion, containing carbolic acid or any other convenient antiseptic, should be applied, or the part may be painted with tincture of iodine. This last precaution is taken to minimise the risk of infection of the wound by microbes, such as very frequently does occur as a secondary consequence of being stung by a wasp or bee. For the same reason, bleeding should rather be encouraged than the reverse, as poison may be got rid of in this way.

Swelling of the throat from stings in the mouth should be treated by applying hot fomentations to the neck and giving ice to suck, but medical assistance should be sought if relief is not quickly obtained. It is worth noting that bee farmers, especially the elderly ones, suffer on the average far less than other people from the stings of bees. This would appear to be an instance of drug tolerance from repeated doses.

Deliberate stinging with bees is a form of treatment which appears to have been successful in cases of chronic rheumatism.

See Bite; Formic Acid.

BEESWAX. Cera flava, the yellow wax of the honeycomb, and cera alba, or white wax, which is prepared from the yellow by bleaching, are both used in medicine for making ointments. They are bland emollient substances and soothe irritated surfaces of the body. Yellow wax is usually chosen, but the white occurs in two official ointments, that of rose water, commonly known as cold cream, and that of cetaceum or spermaceti.

Preparations, described as cerates, are made by mixing wax with oils, fatty substances or resins, and are used either as emollients or vehicles for applying drugs to body surfaces; they are softer than plasters but stiffer than ointments, so that when spread on linen or muslin, as is usual, they do not melt and disappear so quickly as do the latter.

BELLADONNA. The belladonna plant or deadly nightshade is of much value in medicine, chiefly in virtue of the atropine which it contains. Whilst atropine, however, is very frequently used now by itself, there are still a large number of cases in which preparations made directly from the belladonna leaf or root may be mployed. Of these preparations three nay be noticed. Two of these, the plaster nd the liniment of belladonna, are for xternal application, and are amongst the nost useful of their class. Both relieve pain; often they relieve itching; and very often they relieve local perspiration, such as the tiresome sweating of the feet which bothers many people. In this last case, of course, the liniment would be employed.

The kind of pain which is relieved by the external use of belladonna is that which has its seat very near the surface; the more superficial a pain, the more likely it is to be relieved by belladonna. This definition includes the greater number of cases of neuralgia. In general the liniment is more useful than the plaster, but the latter is very often used for application to the breasts when it is desired to arrest the secretion of milk. Liniment of belladonna is combined with that of aconite and with chloroform in A.B.C. liniment, which is much used as an anodyne. The tincture of belladonna, dose 5 to 10 minims, has many uses; its chief value is in the relief of pain.

Difficult Breathing Relieved by Belladonna

There are several maladies of the breathing organs in the treatment of which belladonna is very valuable. To relieve the spasms of whooping-cough and in the more severe and urgent spasms of asthma, belladonna is frequently employed, and in those cases of chronic bronchitis which tend to assume the asthmatic type much benefit may be derived from it. In whooping-cough, belladonna does not actually shorten the course of the disease, but merely makes it more tolerable. In cases of chronic bronchitis, when there is too much fluid secreted inside the lungs, belladonna tends to dry up the tubes. In oedema of the lungs, which may occur, for instance, in Bright's disease, in which the patient coughs up large quantities of frothy, watery sputum, belladonna is again useful, though the drug is usually given as a hypodermic injection of atropine.

Belladonna has another very important use, namely, in the treatment of bed-wetting in children. Other uses are for the pain of renal colic and gall-stone colic, and in epilepsy.

Poisoning by Belladonna. Belladonna poisoning follows a common type, whether it be due to eating some part of the deadly nightshade, to accidents in the use of belladonna, or even to excessive absorption of atropine from the belladonna plaster or liniment. In general two main facts may be noted. The first is that children are remarkably tolerant of the drug and can take relatively large doses. The second is that there is a wide gap between the dose of belladonna that will cause poisonous symptoms and the dose that will cause death.

The noteworthy symptoms of an over-dose of belladonna are as follows: The throat and mouth are very dry, and hence there is some difficulty in swallowing; the pupils of the eyes are widely dilated, but the sight is blurred, especially the sight of near objects, as in reading or writing; the skin is also very dry. In a short time, if the dose is a very large one, the symptoms are still more marked: the skin becomes flushed and may even display a uniform red rash which has often been mistaken for that of scarlet fever. As in scarlet fever, also, the pulse is very rapid. In such cases the patient's nervous system is often upset: he may become delirious and suffer from hallucinations and illusions.

If the poison has been swallowed, the stomach must be emptied by means of mustard and water or some other emetic. Thereafter strong tea may be given freely, the tannic acid in the infusion acting as an antidote. Alcohol should not be given, but coffee is an excellent stimulant.

See Atropine; Poisoning.

BELL'S PALSY. Facial paralysis is sometimes called Bell's Palsy, after Sir Charles Bell, who described the condition. *See* Facial Nerve.

BELT. *See* Abdominal Belt.

BENGER'S FOOD. As it contains a very small quantity of fat, Benger's Food is made up with milk to make good the deficiency. It is a mixture of wheat-flour and an extract containing the digestive ferments of the pancreatic juice. When a mixture of the food with milk is kept at blood-heat, these juices partly digest the proteins of the milk and the food, and convert the starch in the food into sugar.

This action may be allowed to go on for five to forty-five minutes, and in the end there may be very little starch remaining unconverted. This makes it a very suitable food for babies and invalids. According to the time allowed for preparation, the milk mixture may be graded to the capacity of a child. As the baby grows, and its own pancreatic juice comes into operation, less time will be required.

See Baby; Digestion; Food.

BENIGN. Tumours which only injure neighbouring tissues by pressing upon them and which do not tend to become disseminated throughout the body, *e.g.* a fatty or a fibrous tumour, are said to be benign, as distinguished from the malignant tumours, carcinoma and sarcoma. The milder forms of malaria fever are called benign.

See Malignant.

BENZOIC ACID. Occurring in gum benzoin, which is obtained from an Eastern tree, and in coal tar, benzoic acid and its salts are drugs of great value. It is a valuable antiseptic. When administered internally, either in the form of the acid itself or as ammonium benzoate or sodium benzoate, the drug seems to be rapidly removed from the body by two definite channels, the lungs and the kidneys. In each case it acts as an antiseptic, and also as a stimulant to all the passages with which it comes in contact. Hence it is very largely used in a number of diseased conditions of the lungs and the urinary system. The best form in which to administer the drug is usually considered to be the benzoate of ammonium, dose 5 to 15 grains, which is a salt readily soluble in water and not very disagreeable to take.

See Balsam.

BENZOIN. The balsamic resin, benzoin, is obtained from an Eastern tree. It contains and has the same properties as benzoic acid (*q.v.*).

BENZOL. Also known as benzene, benzol is a colourless liquid obtained from coal tar. It must be distinguished from petroleum benzine or benzoline. Benzol has been used internally in whooping-cough, leukaemia and other disorders. Applied externally it will destroy lice, one application sufficing as a rule. It is

highly inflammable and should not be use near a naked light. In poisoning by benzo give an emetic and stimulants, douch alternately with hot and cold wate and, if breathing fails, employ artificia respiration.

See Poisoning.

BERI-BERI. In tropical countries disease known as beri-beri, and by othe names, occurs in epidemics; its appea ance in temperate climates is limited t isolated cases. It is characterised by multiple neuritis, or inflammation many nerves throughout the body, th result being, in mild cases, muscula weakness or wasting, loss of sensation i various parts, shortness of breath, drops on the front of the legs, and other symp toms. In this form the disease may persis for some weeks.

In other cases it may assume more ser ous proportions, in either of two forms. I may be of the dropsical or wet type, i which there is marked dropsy over th whole body, including its cavities. Palp tation and dyspnoea are troublesome, an dropsy of the lungs and heart weaknes may supervene suddenly, causing intens breathlessness and probably death. In th other or dry type, the muscles waste an lose power progressively, and are ver sensitive to handling. This may drag o for months or years, and death by sudde heart failure or syncope is not infrequent

Amongst various causes for the diseas bacterial infection has been urged. Th disease was observed, however, to have connexion with a diet in which polishe rice bulked largely. This led to the di covery that in polishing the rice a vitami was removed in the husk. This vitami is also contained in whole-grain bread, milk, eggs, yeast extract and other food Beri-beri, it would seem, is prevented o cured by the diet being rearranged in suc a way as to include foods containing thi vitamin.

The administration of such foods i therefore, the first thing in treatment, bu recovery is assisted by removing th patient to roomy, well-ventilated quarter Diuretics (*q.v.*) in dropsical cases, an massage in paralytic cases, are amongs other remedial measures.

See Dropsy; Neuritis; Paralysis; Vitamin

BEVERAGES. In nursing the sick the utmost difficulty is often experienced in persuading the patient to take a sufficiency of nutritious liquids and in satisfactorily quenching his thirst. Variety in food and drink means much to the healthy, but it may be of the greatest importance to the sick. This should be secured by making a judicious selection from the beverages mentioned below. Some of these are nutritive, and when a patient is on a liquid diet an attempt must be made to get him to take a sufficient proportion of his supply of liquid in a form which will also include an adequate amount of food ; some beverages are stimulants mainly or entirely ; some simply relieve thirst ; and imperial drink, a recipe for which is given, not only relieves thirst but has a helpful stimulant action on the kidneys and bowels.

Nutritive Beverages. Of these the most important is milk, and it may be taken undiluted, and either hot or cold. When taken hot it may for some of the feeds be flavoured with a little nutmeg or cinnamon. In fever it is usually desirable to give it diluted, and this may be done by adding hot water, soda water, or such waters as Vichy and Apollinaris. In some circumstances the milk will be peptonised. Fermented milk, Koumiss and Kephir, are sometimes used, and there are times when butter-milk or milk artificially soured by the Bulgarian bacillus prove most grateful to a patient. Butter-milk and ordinary milk in equal quantities is a good combination. Milk may also be given in the form of one of the recipes which follow :

RICE MILK. Cook 2 tablespoonsful of rice in 1 pint of milk very slowly for 1 hour. Pass through a coarse sieve, flavour as desired, add either sugar or a pinch of salt, and serve either hot or cold.

MILK TEA. Into a small, heated teapot put 1 teaspoonful of China tea and over it pour 1 breakfastcupful of boiling milk. Place it by the side of the fire for 20 minutes, care being taken not to let it boil. Pour gently into a heated cup, so as not to disturb the leaves and sediment, and sweeten if liked.

GUM ARABIC MILK. Soak 1 ounce of gum arabic in a teacupful of cold water overnight, then heat slowly till thoroughly dissolved. Add to it a breakfastcupful of boiling milk, add sugar and flavouring, and serve hot.

WHEY. Boil 1 breakfastcupful of milk and add the same quantity of cold milk. Stir into it 1 teaspoonful of rennet and set aside for half an hour. Break up the curd with a fork and strain the whey through a fine muslin. Sometimes a little lemon juice and sugar are added, or two tablespoonsful of cream, sugar, and a few drops of vanilla.

WINE WHEY. Boil 1 teacupful of milk and add to it half a teacupful of sherry and a teaspoonful of sugar. Let it stand for a minute till the curd forms, then strain through muslin into a glass and serve hot.

The following two recipes are most useful for people whose strength is much reduced ; they are highly nutritive and also stimulant.

EGG DRINK. Beat up an egg with a teaspoonful of sugar and a tablespoonful of sherry or a dessertspoonful of brandy. Pour over it a cupful of boiling milk and serve hot.

EGG FLIP. Beat the yolk of an egg with a teaspoonful of sugar and a dessertspoonful of brandy. Pour over it a teacupful of boiling milk, stir briskly, and lastly add the white of egg beaten to a stiff froth. The brandy can be omitted and a few drops of flavouring substituted.

ALBUMEN OR EGG WATER. Mix the white of an egg with a teacupful of cold water, add a pinch of salt and strain through muslin into a glass. Albumen water may be given alternately with milk, but it proves most useful when for some reason milk must be withheld, for example in some forms of infantile diarrhoea

Stimulant Beverages. These include tea, coffee, beef tea, and alcoholic drinks of all kinds. For further particulars see under the respective headings.

Beverages for Relieving Thirst. The most important of this class is, of course, pure water. In some places the water supplied may contain too large a content of mineral matter to suit certain patients. London water, for example, may not agree in some cases of acute eczema. In this case a water may be substituted which has been deprived of these constituents by distillation, such, for example, as the Salutaris waters ; or, instead of plain water, soda or potash or one of the natural table waters may be used.

BARLEY WATER. Apart from water, perhaps the most generally useful beverage in the sick-room is barley water, recipes for which are given under its own heading. Nearly all invalids like barley water, either thick or clear. It is more interesting than plain water and more soothing, for the barley yields a demulcent substance which makes the beverage " smooth." Barley water is largely used to dilute milk. This it does efficiently, and it also has the virtue of making the milk solidify in the stomach in a more readily digestible form than it would otherwise take, though this may be done better by lime water, or by using sodium citrate.

TOAST WATER. Another beverage of the same type is toast water, which is made by breaking in pieces a well-toasted crust of bread into some fresh cold water. After a time the water is strained and is found to have a pleasant flavour and to be of a pale yellow colour.

RICE WATER. To make rice water, put 2 tablespoonsful of rice into a saucepan with 1 pint of cold water. Bring to the boil and simmer slowly for an hour. A piece of cinnamon stick or dry ginger, or a few pieces of lemon rind, can be boiled with it as flavouring, and sugar can be added, if allowed. Strain, and serve either hot or cold.

FRUIT DRINKS. Among fruit drinks, lemonade is the most used. One or two kinds may be noted. The bought lemonades, whether solid or liquid, are inferior to that made from a fresh lemon, and should not be employed for invalids if the latter is available. An ordinary lemonade may be made thus : Use 4 lemons, $\frac{1}{4}$ lb. of loaf sugar and 3 pints of boiling water ; mix the sugar with the juice of the lemons, add the boiling water, and cover until cold. The flavour of the mixture may be much improved by adding to it a number of very thin slices of the surface of the lemon rind, or by first of all rubbing some of the sugar on the rind until it takes up the yellow flavouring matter. It is not generally

known how acceptable this beverage may be when taken hot. It is then an excellent drink for consumptives at bedtime in winter ; the heat gives it some value in inducing sleep and helps to bring out the flavour.

Another form of lemonade may be made by adding lemon juice to water in which sugar has previously been dissolved, beating up the white of an egg and adding this to the mixture. The proportions are 1 lemon to 1 pint of water and 1 ounce of sugar. A tumblerful of such lemonade containing $\frac{1}{2}$ ounce of sugar and half the white of an egg, is of very considerable food value.

For a change apple water may be given. Put into a jug 2 large juicy apples cut into slices, the rind and juice of half a lemon, 3 teaspoonsful of sugar and a pint of boiling water. Let it stand till cold, strain and serve.

IMPERIAL DRINK. This may be made by simply adding cream of tartar to home-made lemonade in the proportion of a teaspoonful to the pint ; or it may consist of $\frac{1}{2}$ ounce of cream of tartar, the rind of a lemon, a heaped teaspoonful of sugar and 3 pints of boiling water. If it is desired to leave out the sugar the drink may be sweetened by the addition of 1 grain of saccharine for each pint. Feverish patients may take imperial drink ad lib.

Beverages that Act as Demulcents. The following beverages are valuable in soothing the throat and the digestive tract.

BLACK CURRANT DRINK. Put into a saucepan 1 tablespoonful of black currant jam, or 1 dessertspoonful of black currant jelly, the juice of half a lemon, 1 tablespoonful of sugar and 1 breakfastcupful of water. Bring to the boil, simmer for 10 minutes, strain and serve hot. This serves as a simple remedy for sore throat and cough proceeding from irritation.

LINSEED TEA. Into a jug put a tablespoonful of whole linseed, a tablespoonful of sugar, the juice of half a lemon and little grated lemon rind. Over it pour pint of boiling water. Cover, and set aside till quite cold. Strain into a glass jug and it is ready for use.

GUM ARABIC WATER. Put into a jar 1 ounce of gum arabic, 1 pint of water, 2 ounces of sugar candy and the juice of alf a lemon. Place in a saucepan of boiling water and stir occasionally till dissolved. Serve very hot.

IRISH OR CARAGEEN MOSS DRINK. This " moss " is in reality a seaweed, found in the northern shores of Ireland. It contains mucilage, and a small proportion of iodine and sulphur. It is procured from chemists in packets in a dry state. Take an ounce of the moss and soak it overnight in 2 quarts of cold water. Bring to the boil, then simmer gently for several hours and the liquid is reduced to about a quart. Strain and sweeten to taste, adding lemon juice or any other suitable flavouring. Carageen moss is commonly supposed to have some nutritious value, but as a fact this is very small.
See Barley Water ; Citric Acid ; Effervescence ; Invalid Cookery ; Lemon.

BICEPS. The name biceps, which literally means two-headed, is applied to the two muscles in the human body which have two distinct origins or upper attachments. One is the large muscle on the front of the upper arm. It has a long head and a short head, attached to the shoulder blade or scapula at two different points. These two heads unite, and as it passes downwards the muscle swells out into the large mass of flesh (technically known as the belly of the muscle) which is so familiar on the arms of muscular people.

From the belly of the muscle there issues a tendon or sinew which is attached to the radius, the outer bone of the forearm. When the muscle contracts it therefore bends the forearm upon the upper arm. It is thus the typical weight-lifting muscle and a notably important one in rowing. It is much less important in swimming, but is, of course, largely used in all gymnastic exercises of the arms. It also supinates the forearm, or, in other words, rotates it so that the palm of the hand comes uppermost. Its antagonist is a large muscle lying on the back of the upper arm, which arises by three heads and is called the triceps. It

is worth noting that when the elbow is slowly bent the movement is not due to the action of the biceps alone, but to the action of the biceps modified and controlled by the balancing action of the triceps.

The other biceps muscle is at the back of the thigh.
See Arm ; Leg ; Muscle.

BIER'S METHOD. Inflammation is a device of Nature to combat bacterial invasion and to promote healing ; these things are accomplished by flooding the diseased or injured tissue with blood, thereby adding to the nutriment available for repair and increasing the number of white blood cells and antibodies which deal with bacteria.

Bier's method of treating various affections is an attempt to imitate the natural mechanism by producing passive congestion. It has been utilised for un-united fractures, chronic joint diseases of all sorts, including tuberculosis, boils, and so on. The method of treating a joint, for example, is as follows :

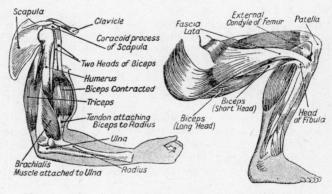

Biceps muscles of arm and thigh that serve to bend the limbs

A bandage must be applied to the limb below the joint, otherwise it will swell unduly ; above the joint there is applied an elastic webbing or a pure rubber bandage outside a layer of lint, and this must be applied tightly enough to produce a bluish tinge of the skin and firmly to press all the superficial veins. Only three turns of the bandage, at most, are necessary. It should be worn for, say, sixteen hours a day, and in the interval the skin and the compressed muscles may be massaged and otherwise attended to.

whilst a light bandage applied directly over the joint is of value in removing the unnecessary superficial swelling occasioned by the treatment.

Glass vessels, known as Bier's cups, are used for creating hyperaemia in smaller parts, such as boils or whitlows, by a process of suction.

See Elastic Bandage ; Hyperaemia ; Inflammation.

BILE. Bile is a secretion produced by the largest gland in the body, namely, the liver. It is a viscid fluid with a very bitter taste, containing mucin, cholesterol, certain salts, and two pigments, bilirubin, which is reddish, and biliverdin, which is green. The colour of bile varies according as one or other of these predominates, but is generally greenish yellow. Cholesterol forms the most important ingredient of gall-stones (*q.v.*). The pigments are derived from effete red blood corpuscles which it is one of the functions of the liver to break down and get rid of. Bile thus is partly an excretion, and it is so also in respect of certain poisonous substances which it extracts from the blood. Sometimes when the bile flows sluggishly these are reabsorbed into the blood, and give rise to depression and the other symptoms connoted by the term biliousness.

The liver produces from 17 ounces to more than twice this amount of bile every day. The bile flows more or less constantly down the common bile duct into the duodenum, or first portion of the bowel ; the pancreatic juice also enters the bowel through the common bile duct, and when it is flowing after a meal the two juices reach the food together, the bile being largely increased in amount a short time after taking food. Part of the bile secreted by the liver enters the gall bladder, its accumulation here permitting of a steady flow into the bowel when necessary.

Bile is of value in digestion in that it aids the pancreatic juice to emulsify and saponify the fats—in other words, to reduce fats into small particles and convert them into drops, a necessary preliminary to their absorption from the bowel. It also stimulates the muscle fibres in the intestinal walls and so assists in moving the contents along. In a slight degree it is antiseptic.

It has been pointed out that biliousness results from a sluggish flow of bile and the reabsorption of some of its poisonous contents. This may be remedied in various ways. Active bodily exercise, for instance, makes the flow more active, and abstinence from rich food diminishes its content of deleterious substances. Alkalies in large doses, for example, bicarbonate of soda, make it more liquid, so that it flows more readily.

Some substances directly stimulate the liver cells to form bile. Amongst them are sodium salicylate and aloes. Others, again, act indirectly by sweeping the bile away from the duodenum, carrying it swiftly through the bowel and preventing reabsorption. These include calomel and podophyllin. Olive oil in large doses appears sometimes to promote the expulsion of gall-stones from the gall bladder.

See Biliousness ; Gall Bladder ; Liver.

BILE DUCT. The channels through which the bile flows from the liver to the bowel are known as bile ducts. The minute channels that pass through the whole substance of the liver join with one another and become larger until finally they emerge from the substance of the liver as two tubes, which are called the right and left hepatic ducts. These join one another, and after joining are themselves joined by another duct which has come from the gall bladder or bile reservoir. The large duct which has been formed by the union of all these is known as the common bile duct, and it terminates by entry into the duodenum or first part of the small bowel about four inches below the lower opening of the stomach. Just before it enters it is joined by the pancreatic duct.

The bile ducts are subject to several important diseases. One is a simple inflammation which naturally interferes with the flow of the bile through them ; this is in any case a matter of some difficulty, since the bile is secreted at very low pressure. This inflammation, or, as it is usually called, catarrh of the bile ducts, is exceedingly common and is usually due to the upward spread of inflammation from the bowel. It results in a varying degree of jaundice. A second disease is blocking by a stone or gall-stone, and a third, very much less common than the

PLATE V

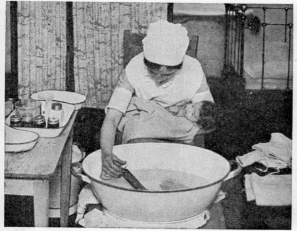

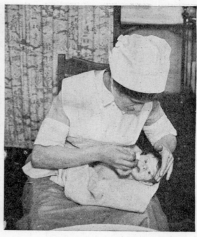

Baby. **1.** The temperature of the bath water (95° F. for a baby six months old) must be tested with a thermometer

2. The baby's eyes, nose and mouth are washed with cold boiled water

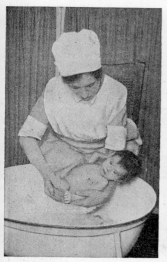

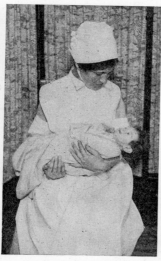

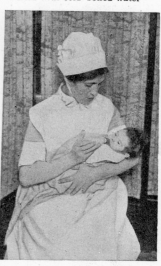

3. How to put the baby into the bath. Very little soap is used

4. A baby should never be held with head and neck unsupported

5. Correct method of holding a baby, the head well supported

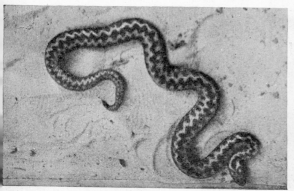

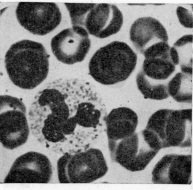

6. Bite. Adder, the only British venomous snake. Note characteristic zig-zag line from head to tail

7. Blood. Microphotograph of red blood cells surrounding a white cell or leucocyte

PLATE VI

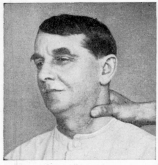
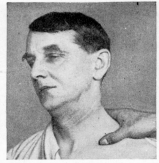
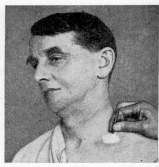

Bleeding. 1. Place for compressing the common carotid artery. 2. Pressure to arrest bleeding from the subclavian artery. 3. Pressure may be applied to the subclavian artery by means of a key handle

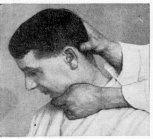
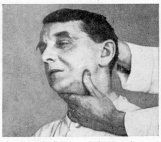
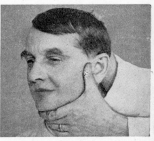

4. When compressing the occipital artery behind the ear the head must be steadied. 5. The facial artery is pressed against the lower border of the jaw. 6. Pressure applied to the superficial temporal artery

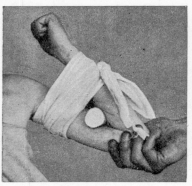
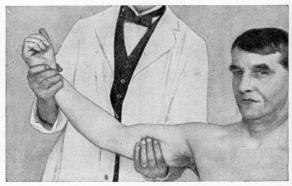

7. Arrest of bleeding from the arm by forced flexion of the elbow joint. 8. Pressure on the brachial artery

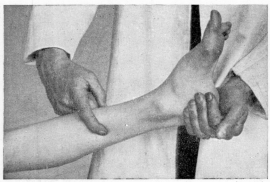
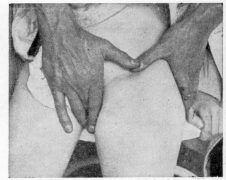

9. Pressure on the posterior tibial artery may arrest bleeding from the sole. 10. Compressing the femoral artery

others, is cancer. It is probable that in very many cases there is a relation between these three diseases ; it is the inflammation of the bile ducts that gives rise to the change in the bile which results in the formation of gall-stones, and it is the chronic irritation set up by the gall-stones that very often seems to be the predisposing cause of the cancer.

BILHARZIASIS. In Africa, especially in Egypt, in Japan and elsewhere, human beings may become infested with small fluke-worms which produce characteristic symptoms. The disease gets the general name of bilharziasis as it results from the presence of bilharzia haematobia, or other varieties of the bilharzia worm. Cases are seen in Great Britain amongst people coming from abroad.

The most usual symptoms are some irritability of the bladder, causing frequency of micturition and the presence of blood and a little pus in the urine. If the urine is examined microscopically the eggs of the worm are seen, each with a sharp spine at one end. In other cases there is irritation in the bowel, occasional diarrhoea with blood and mucus in the stools, and possibly eggs with a lateral spine. When these eggs are shed from the body and reach fresh water the embryos are liberated. They enter the bodies of certain snails, where they undergo development. When again set free from the snail, they swim actively in the water till they reach a human or other host, whose skin they pierce. They then make their way into the portal vein and its tributaries, where they develop into the adult worms. These produce eggs which accumulate in the lining of the bladder and bowel, whence they are discharged.

The invasion with the parasite may be marked by feverishness, abdominal pains, nettle-rash and other symptoms, but the local bladder and bowel symptoms may not occur for many months afterwards. The disease is treated by injection of tartar emetic or of emetine into the veins or muscles. This kills the adult parasites, thereby preventing egg-laying.

BILIARY COLIC. The pain occasioned by the spasmodic contractions of the bile ducts in their attempts to rid themselves of gall-stones is called biliary colic. *See* Gall-stone.

BILIOUSNESS. According to popular usage, the term biliousness is applied to a condition characterised by nausea and possibly sickness, a furred tongue, headache, a dull, heavy feeling in the pit of the stomach, and constipation. The headache is often referred to as bilious headache, and if bouts of this kind occur, accompanied by vomiting, they are called attacks of bile. These conditions have very little to do with the amount of bile produced. It is sometimes thought when bile appears amongst vomited matter that this is because an excess of bile exists. As a matter of fact, however, when vomiting, from whatever cause, has gone on for a short time, bile tends to be drawn into the stomach, so that its presence in the vomit means nothing.

The liver may be implicated in biliousness to this extent, however, that it is not adequately performing its function of clearing the blood of deleterious products of digestion. It will be remembered that all the blood from the stomach and bowels must pass through the liver before it again flows in the general circulation. The default of the liver may be because an overwhelming amount of such substances are being produced owing to a disordered digestion ; or to constipation or a sluggish flow of bile allowing such substances to be reabsorbed into the blood.

Vomiting from a variety of causes is sometimes called a bilious attack. Among possible causes are acute gastritis, following too much or too rich food ; migraine or sick headache ; headache due to eye-strain, either as part of a migrainous attack or separately ; acute glaucoma, due to increase of tension in the eye ; tumours of the brain, etc. It is obvious that a number of possibilities must be excluded before any vomiting attack is accepted and treated simply as a bilious attack. An overhaul is necessary also when attacks of sickness tend to recur. In children the cause of an attack may be acute indigestion, but recurring bouts have in some cases been traced to appendicitis, and in other cases appear to be instances of what is known as cyclical vomiting, which depends mostly on excessive fatigue, excitement or cold. These children appear to suffer from acidosis.

D

The treatment of all these conditions will depend on the cause, but when the digestion has clearly been upset by too much or a wrong kind of food an emetic may do much good, and vomiting should be encouraged by giving long draughts of tepid water, to which may be added a pinch of baking soda. This will wash away the unwholesome stomach contents, but it is desirable also to clear the bowel, which may be done by giving a dose of castor oil or 2 or 3 grains of calomel at bedtime, followed first thing in the morning by 2 drachms of Epsom salts in a half-glass of water or by an ounce of black draught. The diet should be very light for a few days afterwards. When vomiting is persistent and distressing, a mustard plaster may be placed over the patient's stomach, and he may be given chips of ice to suck, though in some cases sips of very hot water are more successful.

A tendency to chronic dyspepsia or chronic gastritis, either of which conditions may be referred to as biliousness, may be counteracted by active bodily exercise, strict moderation in diet, which should be of a plain description, no alcohol, and regularity of the bowels. For the latter purpose cascara may be taken regularly, but it is generally a good thing to take calomel, as suggested above, followed by salts, from time to time, especially if there is a constant feeling of weight about the pit of the stomach and the tongue is always furred. Nausea in these cases may be relieved by doses of bismuth and soda, or of bismuth salicylate, 10 grains, thrice daily, about twenty minutes before food.

See Acidosis ; Gastritis ; Indigestion ; Liver ; Vomiting.

BINOCULAR. The possession of two eyes enables us to judge of the distance of objects and of their form. It makes things appear solid, after the manner of a stereoscopic camera. If we shut one eye, things still appear to have a solid form, but that is because a pure act of visual sensation is not possible after earliest infancy, for in every sensation the mind itself contributes an element derived from its experience and memory of all its past sensations. But one eye may very readily be deceived ; for instance, at breakfast your neighbour hands you a cup of tea for another lump of sugar. If you close one eye, you will as often as not misjudge the distance of the cup and put the lump in the saucer.

Each eye has its own image, which differs in some degree from the image received from the other eye. In the nature of the case it is impossible that the two eyes can see any object at exactly the same angle. Indeed, the distance between the two eyes may count for something in the effectiveness of vision. When they are too near together their possessor does not get the full advantage of having two eyes instead of one, whereas when they are too far apart there is some difficulty in using them in unison.

See Double Vision ; Eye ; Field of Vision ; Squint ; Vision.

BIRTH. Normally a child is born about the end of the 9th calendar or the 10th lunar month. If born after the 27th week but before the 38th, the birth is said to be premature, but the baby can survive. Birth earlier than this but after the 12th week constitutes a miscarriage, and before and including the 12th week an abortion. A still birth is one where the child is born dead. The birth of a child after the 36th week must be notified to the medical officer of health within 36 hours. This includes a still birth, and is in addition to registration. Concealment of birth is a criminal offence.

See Abortion ; Childbirth ; Notification ; Pregnancy.

BIRTH MARK. Certain appearances in the skin, which are more or less visible at birth and popularly known as birth marks, are grouped under the term naevus. This means congenital, and so would include pigmented moles which are present at birth, but in using the term what is almost always in mind is the vascular naevus. This essentially consists of blood vessels of some kind ; veins, as a rule, or dilated blood spaces—the cavernous naevus. A naevus which mainly consists of capillaries is invariably congenital ; even though there is no visible sign of it at birth, it is almost certain to be visible within a fortnight.

A birth mark grows most rapidly when it is young ; after the first few months it usually grows only at the same rate as the child. In the latter case it is very apt to grow smaller as the child grows bigger, and a very large number of birth marks, indeed, undergo a natural cure. The most superficial kind of birth mark, however, often called the port wine stain, is less likely than the others to undergo spontaneous cure. It almost invariably persists throughout life.

The object of treatment, when it is undertaken, is either simply to remove a disfigurement, or to eradicate a birth mark which is being irritated by clothing, etc. Methods include complete removal of the birth mark by the surgeon, or treatment by electrolysis, by liquid air or carbonic acid snow, by radium or by X-rays. Self-treatment of birth marks, including moles, by caustics is a dangerous proceeding.
See Carbonic Acid ; Electrolysis ; Mole.

BIRTH PARALYSIS. Sometimes babies are born with paralysis of one or more limbs, the cause of which, in the majority of cases, is some injury sustained in birth. Paralysis sometimes follows a precipitate birth, but much more usually one that is attended with difficulty and is delayed. Paralysis of an arm may be due to injury to some of the nerve roots forming the brachial plexus ; but, on the other hand, the brain may be injured at birth, generally by a haemorrhage occurring within the skull, and this may be followed by paralysis of both legs, or one side of the body or of both sides of the body.

The paralysis may be present at birth or appear after a few days. The affected muscles are not only weak but they are affected by a spasticity or stiffness, which, when the child begins to walk, causes what is known as " cross-legged progression." Besides this there may be tremor, speech difficulty, epilepsy and mental impairment. Often the mentality is normal, though development may be slow, and this applies also to the learning of movements of affected limbs. This condition has also been called Little's disease. In other cases the paralysis is not accompanied by any rigidity, and in still others the symptoms resemble those of ataxia (*q.v.*).

Surgical measures are required early where there has been damage to nerves, and even in the brain cases operation has done good when performed early. Apart from this the child requires great care and abundance of patience during its training.
See Childbirth ; Paralysis.

BIRTH RATE. In technical language the birth rate is the number of births per thousand per annum. In order, however, to compare properly the birth rates of two communities it is necessary to calculate the birth rate, not per thousand inhabitants, but per thousand women between the ages of fifteen and forty-five, or for certain purposes, per thousand married women of those ages. The outstanding fact about the birth rate is that during many years it has exhibited a steady decline in most civilised countries which collect statistics on the subject. The mean birth rate in England and Wales from 1840 to 1890 was 33·8 per thousand of the total population, while in 1922 it was 20·6, and in 1927, 16·7.

The main reason for this decline, where it occurs, is birth control, the deliberate avoidance, or limitation, of a family. Motives of prudence can be alleged to justify much of this. It is better to have few children if there is going to be any difficulty about rearing them properly. In many cases, however, the duty is in the other direction, as the effects on the nation are sure to be serious sooner or later.
See Death Rate.

BISMUTH. In the form of a large number of salts and other preparations, the heavy metal, bismuth, has many uses in medicine. It acts as an antiseptic, an astringent and a sedative ; and to produce these effects it may be employed either internally or externally. In catarrh or ulceration of the lining membrane of the alimentary tract one of the following preparations may be used : bismuth subnitrate, bismuth carbonate or bismuth salicylate, the dose of each being 5 to 20 grains every 3 or 4 hours ; the solution of bismuth and ammonia citrate, $\frac{1}{2}$ to 1 drachm, which is not so good as the solid preparations ; or the compound bismuth lozenges. The last have the advantage of being easily carried about for use at odd times.

By means of one of the foregoing preparations nausea, gastric pain, vomiting or diarrhœa may often be relieved. If there is much acidity, bismuth carbonate should be used, or, if the stools are offensive, bismuth salicylate. For dyspepsia a good combination is:

Bismuth carbonate	..	10 grains
Sodium bicarbonate	..	20 ,,
Magnesium carbonate	..	10 ,

This is taken in a little milk about 20 minutes before meals, though it will relieve gastric discomfort whenever this occurs.

Any of these salts in fine powder may be used as a snuff for the relief of nasal catarrh. For the sore nipples of nursing mothers a paste consisting of equal parts of bismuth carbonate and castor oil is safe and effective. One drachm of bismuth carbonate, salicylate or oxide, with one ounce of starch powder, is often used for dusting burns or other inflamed skin surfaces; or instead of the starch the bismuth may be made up with an ounce of vaseline. Bismuth, iodoform and paraffin paste, commonly known as B.I.P.P., is largely used in the treatment of wounds and especially those in which bone has been damaged. Bismuth carbonate or oxychloride may be used for a bismuth meal to produce opaque photographs in X-ray investigations of the oesophagus, stomach and bowel. Injections of bismuth are used fairly extensively in the treatment of syphilis. Colloidal bismuth is employed under such names as bismon, collosol bismuth, etc.

Symptoms of poisoning have followed the use of bismuth, but have usually been due to arsenical or other impurities. Chemically pure bismuth will not produce poisoning when given internally, though there would appear to be some danger of poisoning if large quantities are spread on raw surfaces of the body and absorbed into the blood, as, for example, in packing fistulous openings or treating large burns. Poisoning is shown by inflammation of the mouth, a black line along the gums at the roots of the teeth, and patches of white membrane on the gums. The bismuth dressing should be cleaned off the wound, and demulcent mouth washes and drinks used.

Owing to certain chemical changes which take place in the bowel, salts of bismuth almost invariably undergo a change into the sulphide of bismuth, which is black. This naturally imparts its colour to the motions and may lead to great alarm if the patient does not understand the reason.

BITE. A wound made by the teeth of an animal may be infected from the start, or this may happen subsequently. Care should be taken, therefore, to clean the wound and to protect it from contamination by a dressing. Small wounds may be dabbed with tincture of iodine, but a larger one should simply be covered with an antiseptic, or at any rate a thoroughly clean dressing, till it can be attended to by a doctor.

Bites, by a dog particularly, may cause much concern lest the animal should be rabid and the bite possibly result in hydrophobia (*q.v.*). But this is a very rare occurrence.

When a dog, suspected of being rabid, has bitten someone it should on no account be destroyed if it can be safely secured.

If the animal is infected, unmistakable signs of rabies will develop within a few days; if they do not, there need be no further anxiety on the score of hydrophobia.

If the dog has to be killed at once, its spinal cord, packed in glycerin, should accompany the patient to a Pasteur institute, the address of which in Great Britain can be obtained from any police station.

In Great Britain the only dangerous snake bite is that of the viper or adder (*see* Plate V, 6). This may produce at once a burning pain in the part bitten, but sometimes the first warning is the onset of symptoms due to the general action of the venom—faintness, nausea, sickness, diarrhoea perhaps, and a cold, clammy sweat over the body. The patient may actually become unconscious, but death is not likely to occur except, perhaps, in the case of a very young or an old or debilitated person.

In the case of a bite by a possibly rabid animal or a viper, if the bite is on a limb a ligature or tourniquet should be applied above the bite. This is made by folding a handkerchief as a narrow bandage, tying this loosely round the limb, inserting a stick through the loop, and twisting till the bandage is quite tight. The stick may be fixed by tying another handkerchief round the limb, binding down one end of the stick.

When the ligature is applied, or immediately in the case of bites elsewhere than on a limb, the wound should be sucked. There is no danger in doing this if the lips and mouth are free from cracks or abrasions. Afterwards the mouth should be washed out with water or, preferably, a little spirits. The wound is then covered up till a doctor can attend to it. The ligature should be taken off when the wound has been thoroughly cleansed, and in any case should not be left on for longer than half an hour.

The patient should lie down and should be kept as warm as possible ; if out in the open, by overcoats and by chafing the limbs. A little spirits may be given to combat faintness, and he should be reassured as to the consequences of the bite. This last is very important. If the patient is indoors antiseptic lotions, such as a saturated solution of boracic acid, carbolic acid lotion, permanganate of potash solution, etc., should be used to wash the wound, and the general condition may be improved by blankets, hot-water bottles, and by stimulants, such as weak spirits, sal volatile, tea or coffee.

Bites and stings of insects may produce itching, pain and swelling, and there is always the further danger of septic poisoning or of infection by many serious diseases, though the latter is more particularly to be feared in the tropics or during epidemics of typhus, relapsing or some other fevers. The best treatment for the bites is the application of ammonia, or, failing this, of solutions of permanganate of potash, bicarbonate of soda or common salt. Pain may be relieved by rubbing with a menthol cone or by an evaporating lotion.

Insect bites may be prevented by smearing the skin with ointments or lotions containing carbolic acid, kerosene, cinnamon oil, clove oil, etc., or with a bitter infusion, such as infusion of quassia.

See Antiseptic: Bee Sting ; Flies ; Formic Acid ; Hydrophobia ; Mosquito ; Tourniquet, etc.

BITTER ALMOND POISONING. *See* Almond.

BITTERS. The word bitters in popular language indicates alcoholic beverages which contain bitter or aromatic substances added in order to stimulate the appetite and the digestion. In medicine, bitters means the group of drugs of vegetable origin which contain bitter-tasting substances having a characteristic action upon the stomach. Of these there is a large number, including quassia, gentian, cascarilla, calumba, dandelion, orange-peel and chiretta. These all act very similarly and are distinguished from one another by no important differences, save that quassia, chiretta and calumba contain no tannin or tannic acid and can therefore be prescribed together with iron. The objection to the tannin contained in the others is that when it comes into contact with iron it forms a black, inky product, tannate of iron, which is the chief constituent of ink and is unpleasant to look at and to taste. Otherwise there are no objections to it.

Calumba and quassia are examples of pure bitters ; other bitters, like cascarilla and orange-peel, contain also a volatile oil and are known as aromatic bitters. Strychnine and quinine, which are not usually classed with the drugs mentioned, possess the bitter taste and exercise all the actions which these bitters possess, whilst in addition they have distinctive properties of their own. The ordinary bitters have no remote action on the nervous system, for instance, but this is possessed by both strychnine and quinine.

Bitters stimulate the nerves of taste and, by doing so, the appetite. This stimulation increases the amount of the secretion of the salivary glands and also markedly increases, through a reflex nervous action, the amount of digestive juice that is secreted by the wall of the stomach. When the bitter substance reaches the stomach itself a similar action occurs ; not only is the sense of hunger increased and the flow of the digestive juices made more rapid, but the movements of the stomach are also hastened. This stimulation of the muscular wall of the stomach also extends to the muscular wall of the bowel. This greatly aids the digestion of the food, and also tends to relieve pain of a colicky nature that is due to the irregular action of the muscular wall of the bowel, but it must be noticed that strychnine is more effective than any of the ordinary vegetable bitters in stimulating the muscular movements of the alimentary canal.

Generally speaking, the proper time to take a bitter is just before food. The following is an example :

Dilute hydrochloric acid ..	1½ drachms
Tincture of orange	.. 3 ,,
Syrup of lemon ..	.. 4 ,,
Infusion of calumba	to 6 ounces

The dose is a tablespoonful in a wineglass of water.

The desirable action of bitters, however, may very readily be exaggerated into an undesirable irritation ; and this will happen either if the dose is excessively large, or if the doses are repeated for too long a period. A mild chronic inflammation of the stomach is set up.

Bitters must never be employed in cases of ulceration of the stomach or any form of acute inflammation. The cases of dyspepsia in which bitters are of use are those due rather to general bodily weakness than any local malady of the stomach, and thus bitters are typically useful drugs in convalescence and in the general weakness which is associated with the various forms of tuberculosis. They are frequently of value also in treating cases of anaemia.

Bitters such as quassia have the power of killing certain forms of intestinal worm and may be injected into the bowel for this purpose. The usual amount employed in such cases is about half a pint of the infusion ; this is of value not for the roundworm or the tapeworm, but only for the threadworm, which usually inhabits the lower part of the bowel.

See Appetite ; Digestion.

BLACK DRAUGHT. The compound mixture of senna is popularly known as black draught. It is used as a purgative, and owes its effects chiefly to its content of magnesium sulphate and senna. It is taken in a dose of 1 or 2 ounces the first thing in the morning, and is usually preceded by 4 grains of blue pill or 2 or 3 grains of calomel at bedtime.

BLACK EYE. *See* Bruise.

BLACKHEAD. The dark plugs in the sebaceous glands of the skin are popularly known as blackheads. Their presence is often associated with acne vulgaris (*q.v.*).

BLACK MOTIONS. *See* Faeces.

BLACK WASH. The black lotion of mercury is popularly known as black wash. Its composition is as follows :

Calomel	..	..	..	30 grains
Glycerin	..	..	..	4 drachms
Mucilage of tragacanth	..	10	,,
Lime water, enough to make	10 ounces

It is used as a wash for syphilitic sores.

BLACKWATER FEVER. The disease commonly known as blackwater fever is also called bilious remittent fever, haemoglobinuria, and by other names. It occurs in tropical and subtropical countries, and is not seen in England except perhaps as a relapse in people who have been invalided for a recent attack. The common name for the disease is derived from the fact that the red blood cells are destroyed and that their colouring matter, much darkened and changed, passes through the kidneys and gives the urine a characteristic colour.

The disease is now almost generally regarded as a complication of malaria, and it would appear that it may be precipitated by quinine in some cases of neglected malaria, or when the malaria has been inefficiently treated.

Blackwater fever begins with a rigor, the temperature rises rapidly, the urine becomes red or black, and probably the patient is sick. Very soon he is seen to be jaundiced. The urine remains discoloured for a variable time, perhaps twenty hours or for several days, and then clears up ; or the patient may become comatose or convulsed and die. Sometimes death is due to a stoppage of the urine.

Till the patient can be seen by a doctor quinine should be stopped. It is not resumed till the urine is clear, and only then if the patient has malarial parasites in his blood ; it is given in small doses at first, say, three grains. If the temperature is above 103° F., the patient should be sponged regularly with tepid water. A mustard plaster over the stomach may relieve the sickness. The diet should consist of milk diluted with water, and to this a half-teaspoonful of bicarbonate of soda may be added every three hours. Injections into the bowel of warm saline, that is, water containing one teaspoonful of common salt to the pint, will do good, and should be repeated every three or four hours if the urine becomes scanty or the patient becomes unconscious.

See Malaria.

BLADDER. The term bladder is applied to two important organs of the body, the gall bladder (*q.v.*) and the urinary bladder, but it is the latter that is usually meant when the word is used without an adjective.

The secretion of the kidneys reaches the urinary bladder by passing through two long tubes called the ureters, and it leaves the organ through another tube called the urethra. Like nearly all the hollow organs of the body, it consists of four coats : a lining of mucous membrane, a loose fibrous submucous layer, a middle coat of muscular tissue, and a smoother, outer peritoneal coat which enables it to move without friction against the organs which surround it. Urine is expelled by the contraction of the muscular coat. The reader is referred to the illustrations under the headings Abdomen and Kidney.

Diseases of the Bladder. Atony of the bladder, or a loss of power in the muscular coat, may be due to overstretching of the bladder, to inflammatory changes, to old age, or to debilitating diseases. Overstretching is a not uncommon result from failure to obey the call to empty the bladder, or it may result from some obstruction to the flow of urine.

Obstruction, apart from overstretching, may cause retention of urine. It may be due to an enlarged prostate, an impacted stone, inflammatory or spasmodic closure of the urethra, displacements of the womb, and other causes. Retention of urine is not uncommon after childbirth or operations for piles or other disorders about the perineum. It may also occur in nervous and other diseases. The treatment consists in drawing off the urine with a catheter. While awaiting the doctor the condition may sometimes be relieved by putting hot fomentations over the bladder. Inability to hold the water may be due to nervous, inflammatory or other diseases. In some cases there is simply an overflow from the overfilled bladder.

Inflammation of the bladder is called cystitis and may be acute or chronic. It is due to germ infection. Acute cystitis may follow a chill or may develop during influenza, typhoid or other fever ; in other cases it is due to infection introduced on a catheter or some other instrument, and it may result from extension of gonorrhoeal infection of the urethra. Sometimes infection comes downwards from the kidney, or it may come from the bowel or other organ in the neighbourhood of the bladder. There is a frequent and pressing need to pass water, which is thick and turbid and may come away in small quantities. There will be a certain amount of fever, pain over the bladder and possibly in the loins.

Treatment consists in confinement to bed with hot-water bottles at the feet. Hot fomentations may be applied over the bladder, or the patient may be given a hot hip bath once or oftener each day, great care being exercised to avoid exposure and chill. He should be given liquids freely, such as plain water, milk, barley water, gruel, etc. Alcoholic drinks of all kinds must be barred, also spiced foods and condiments till the doctor allows them. Medicinal remedies include bicarbonate of soda or of potash, hyoscyamus, belladonna, morphia or other sedatives, and hexamine or some antiseptic. The bowels should be moved once a day.

Chronic cystitis may follow an acute attack, but it may also result from the presence of a stone or of a tumour in the bladder or from some other cause. In elderly men it is not uncommonly caused by the decomposition of urine which is retained in the bladder in consequence of an enlarged prostate. The symptoms are somewhat similar to what has been described, but the pain is generally less severe than in the acute form. The general health is likely to be seriously depressed by absorption of poisonous materials from the bladder. The urine when passed may be stinking and ammoniacal. Treatment consists in cleaning of the bladder by giving antiseptics by the mouth and by washing out the organ with antiseptic lotions. An enlarged prostate, or other causes, must then be dealt with so far as is practicable.

Tuberculosis usually reaches the bladder from a kidney, though it may originate in the bladder. Besides giving urinary antiseptics and employing every means to build up the general health, tuberculin injections should be tried. When it is certain that the infection is coming from one kidney, while the other is healthy, the diseased kidney should be removed, as the bladder is then likely to clear up.

The bladder may be ruptured by violence, such as a kick or crushing of the pelvis, but this may also result from too long delay in passing water. An immediate operation is necessary. A vesicular calculus or stone in the bladder may be quite minute or as large as a duck's egg; when small, a very large number may be present. Stones usually consist of uric acid, of phosphates or of oxalate of lime. The symptoms resemble those of chronic cystitis. Bed-wetting in children may be due to stone. Surgical treatment is necessary, either crushing the stone and washing it out of the bladder or removal by a cutting operation, though in women it may be possible to effect removal by dilating the urethra.

Of tumours occurring in the bladder the commonest innocent form is a papilloma or villous tumour. Workers in aniline factories seem to be particularly liable to this affection. It causes the occasional presence of blood in the urine and should be removed by operation. Chronic cystitis may also be set up from an innocent tumour. There may be great pain, especially late in the disease. Treatment consists in cleaning up the cystitis, removing the tumour if practicable; otherwise the use of radium is advocated.

See Bacilluria; Bed-wetting; Bilharziasis; Catheter; Kidney; Micturition; Prostate; Strangury; Urine.

BLANCMANGE. When properly made, blancmange is a useful food for invalids and the convalescent. Peptonised milk may be used instead of ordinary milk when the digestive powers are low. Blancmange made with cornflour, one of the numerous invalid foods and milk is even more digestible and more nutritious than ordinary blancmange. The necessary

constituents are ½ pint of prepared food, 3 teaspoonsful of cornflour, 2 teaspoonsful of sugar, 2 tablespoonsful of cream and some flavouring material. The cornflour and sugar should be mixed and the invalid food gradually added, the mixing being vigorously continued. The whole should be poured into a saucepan and stirred over the fire, and allowed to boil for five minutes; the cream and the flavouring are to be added, the whole poured into a wetted mould and allowed to set in a cool place.

See Invalid Cookery.

BLAUD'S PILL. *See* Iron.

BLEACHING POWDER. *See* Chloride of Lime.

BLEB. *See* Blister.

BLEEDER. A person who suffers from a very peculiar and remarkable disease technically known as haemophilia is commonly referred to as a bleeder. The bleeder, who is almost invariably male, inherits his disease, and the symptoms of it may appear in the very earliest moments of life. He is apt to bleed in various parts of his body without any apparent cause, and causes which will produce very slight bleeding in most people, such as a trivial pinprick or the extraction of a tooth, produce the most severe bleeding in such a patient. He is also very apt to undergo large haemorrhages or bleedings into his joints.

The inheritance of this disease is very remarkable: whilst females hardly ever suffer, they constantly transmit the disease from their fathers to their sons, whilst their daughters escape, but may in their turn transmit the disease to their sons. The blood is peculiarly constituted, so that the ordinary clotting which usually arrests bleeding is delayed owing to the slowness with which fibrin ferment is produced. The boy suffers from various bleedings, either apparently spontaneous or in consequence of the slightest accidents; the commonest of these, perhaps, is bleeding from the nose, which is often exceedingly difficult to arrest. Anyone with this tendency should always disclose the fact before he undergoes tooth extraction or any other operation.

When the actual bleeding occurs it must, of course, be treated on the ordinary lines, that is, pressure, very hot or very cold water, the application of perchloride of iron, alum or another styptic (*q.v.*). Transfusion of blood may be called for in desperate cases.

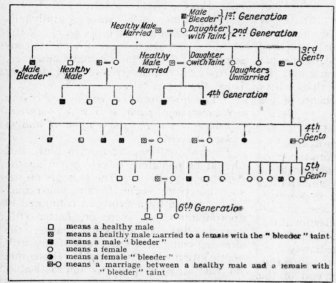

Bleeder. Genealogical tree showing how the taint may be transmitted

A grave question arises as to public duty in cases of haemophilia. It must surely be maintained that in cases of a disease so definite and unmistakable, and one that interferes so seriously with happiness and efficiency, the question arises whether the bleeder or the daughter of a bleeder is justified in having children.

See Blood ; Coagulation ; Transfusion.

BLEEDING. Whenever a blood vessel is injured so that an actual opening is made in its wall there must be a certain amount of bleeding, or, as it is technically described, haemorrhage. The bleeding may be external, that is to say, the blood appears on the surface of the body ; or it may be internal, when the patient may die without any blood being visible, unless it is overflowing into some organ whence it may be ejected by vomiting, coughing or otherwise. There are general signs, however, from which internal bleeding may be suspected, and these will be mentioned later.

In general three kinds of bleeding are distinguished, varying in character according to the kind of blood vessel injured.

Bleeding from an artery—which is more likely to be fatal than any other kind of bleeding—is distinguished in that it comes in jets which correspond to the pulse felt at the wrist, and by the fact that the blood has the character of arterial blood, that is, it is brighter and redder than the blood found in capillaries or veins. Bleeding from a vein is distinguished by the dark colour of the blood as compared with arterial blood, and also by the fact that it flows continuously, since there is no pulsation in the veins. Bleeding from capillaries is easily distinguished, assuming that the site of the bleeding can be seen, by the fact that it is a general ooze from the surface, and not the distinct issue of blood from a single point. When this occurs from the skin it is of small importance, but from mucous membranes. such as the lining of the throat and nose, it may be more difficult to control.

The loss of blood, from whatever source, results in certain symptoms, the severity of which depends, of course, upon the amount of blood lost. Typically, the patient displays a cold, moist skin which, like the lips and finger nails, is abnormally pale ; the pulse, when felt at the wrist, is found to be rapid and small, and when the bleeding has been excessive it is often impossible to feel any pulsation at the wrist at all. The patient breathes more rapidly and often complains of shortness of breath. A very marked and characteristic symptom is extreme restlessness. When the bleeding has reached a certain point the patient becomes unconscious and may ultimately die. There is, however, at this point a certain compensatory action which often saves his life : the immediate cause of the bleeding is the pressure of the blood in the blood vessels, and this may be so reduced by the diminution of the bulk of the blood, and the feebleness of the heart consequent upon this, that bleeding may cease.

Various patients suffer in very varying degree as a result of loss of blood. In general, it may be stated that a woman may lose during childbirth an amount of blood which would entail her death at all other times, but from which she recovers in a few days. Children usually recover very quickly from loss of blood, old people very slowly, but both the young and the old in general are more likely than others to die as an immediate consequence of loss of blood.

Natural Arrest of Bleeding

In the great majority of cases bleeding is arrested by nature long before the compensatory action above mentioned is necessary. In the first place, an artery is an elastic structure ; in fact, it possesses one special coat which is constructed practically of nothing but elastic fibres. Hence, when an artery is completely divided, the opening is immediately contracted, and also, owing to the direction of the elastic fibres, the cut end of the artery tends to turn inwards and so still further to reduce the size of the opening. In the case of very small arteries, which contain a higher proportion of elastic structure, this may suffice to arrest the bleeding. But the most important factor in the natural arrest of bleeding is the coagulation of the blood, which plugs the openings in the injured blood vessels.

The diminished vigour of the heart, by lowering the blood pressure, permits of the arrest of the bleeding by weaker means than would otherwise be necessary. After some hours, when the heart has become stronger, it not infrequently happens that the clots, which were previously sufficient to prevent any bleeding, are forced out, and bleeding begins again. This is known as reactionary haemorrhage, and occurs, as a rule, within 24 hours after the original injury to the blood vessel. It does not occur at a later period, since the clots soon become firmly united with the walls of the blood vessel by permanent union of tissue.

Further bleeding of the blood vessel is impossible unless microbes are present which cause the destruction of the clot. Haemorrhage due to this last cause is known as secondary haemorrhage, and is most likely to occur from the sixth day after the injury or operation until the expiry of a fortnight. In these days of antiseptic surgery, secondary haemorrhage is an extremely rare occurrence.

The treatment of bleeding naturally falls under two heads : attempts to check the bleeding, and attempts to obviate its consequences. Using the ordinary language, we may say that the treatment of bleeding is local and general.

The first thing to do in the case of any haemorrhage from a visible point is firmly to put the finger upon it and to keep it there.

In cases of bleeding from a limb, this should be elevated, thereby securing the assistance of gravity. The pressure on the bleeding point begun by the finger may be continued by a firm pad composed of thoroughly clean linen, or, better still, boracic lint or antiseptic gauze, the dressing being first wrung out of any antiseptic lotion which is available. If pressure on the bleeding point is impracticable, for example, in the case of a large wound, it will be necessary to apply it to the main artery supplying the part, and in order to maintain this pressure an apparatus will have to be used to relieve the fingers. The means for applying this pressure is a tourniquet, which is described under its own heading.

Medical and Surgical Measures

Very cold water, or water as hot as can be borne, arrests haemorrhage, and vinegar, alum, tannic acid, spirits and other substances are helpful ; but these measures are chiefly valuable for capillary bleeding, being useless in bleeding from a large artery. Of the various methods employed by the surgeon for the arrest of bleeding, the most important is the ligature, a thread made of silk or catgut which is firmly tied round the cut blood vessel.

General treatment of haemorrhage may be scarcely less important than local treatment. The patient's head must be kept very low, whilst the arms and legs must be raised in order that the heart, lungs and brain may secure as much blood as possible. This may be further secured by firmly bandaging all four limbs, beginning at the hands and feet and working upwards. The patient must be kept warm and at absolute rest ; and the room in which he is placed must be freely ventilated. If it is absolutely certain that the bleeding has been securely stopped, stimulants may be given, such as spirits well diluted, sal volatile, tea or coffee.

But it has been shown that there is a more important measure than almost any of these. Death from haemorrhage occurs because there is an insufficient amount of fluid in the blood vessels—of fluid, not necessarily of blood—for when the amount of fluid falls below a certain point the heart ceases to contract. Fluid should therefore be freely supplied.

The patient may be urged to drink large quantities of warm fluid, and a pint and a half, or even more, of warm water may be slowly injected into the bowel in the hope, usually justified, that it will be retained. The best fluid to employ is what is called normal saline solution, the composition of which closely corresponds in the percentage of salt (0·9) it contains, to the normal fluids of the body. The desired proportion can easily be remembered, since it closely corresponds to a teaspoonful of salt to a pint of water.

The fluid may also be injected under the skin, in which case it must, of course,

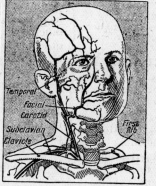

be sterilised. The water must be boiled and then allowed to cool down to a temperature slightly above that of the blood, that is, to about 105° F. It may be injected under the skin into some place where the underlying tissues are loose and can conveniently accommodate a quantity of fluid. In the case of a female patient a very suitable site is furnished by the skin under the breast. In urgent cases the fluid is injected straight into a vein. Sometimes the transfusion of blood has to be undertaken.

It will be useful now to consider in summary form where pressure should be made on main arteries of supply, when bleeding cannot be controlled otherwise. The reader is referred to Plate VI.

FRONT OF SCALP. Press on the superficial temporal artery where it crosses the arch of the zygoma, a finger-breadth in front of the ear-hole. The arch is the rounded bony ridge felt when rubbing the skin up and down in this region.

BACK OF SCALP. Press on the occipital artery at a point two finger-breadths behind, and a little below, the centre of the posterior margin of the ear.

FACE. Press on the facial artery where it crosses the margin of the lower jaw an inch in front of the angle of the jaw.

MOUTH OR SIDE OF HEAD. When bleeding is not controlled by any of the aforementioned procedures, press on the common carotid artery a little below and outside the Adam's apple. The pressure should be exerted backwards and rather inwards.

ARMPIT OR UPPER ARM. Press the subclavian artery down on the first rib in the hollow above and about the middle of the collar-bone. A thumb must be used and its pressure reinforced by the other thumb, or the padded handle of a key may be used.

LOWER PART OF ARM OR HAND. Press the brachial artery out against the humerus in the upper half of the bone. The guide to the direction of the artery is the inner seam of the coat, and the pressure is best applied by gripping the arm from behind, the fingers being inside and exerting the pressure.

THIGH. Press the femoral artery as it passes over the pelvic bone at a point midway between the front end of the upper ridge of the haunch bone and the mid point of the pubis (the bony arch lying in front of the bladder). The pressure must be made with one thumb superimposed on the other. The tendency in this instance is to press too low down ; bone must be felt beneath the thumb, and the pulsation of the artery.

SOLE OF THE FOOT. Press on the posterior tibial artery in the hollow behind the inner prominence of the ankle, the pressure being made forwards and outwards against the foot.

Main arteries of neck and face in relation to the bones

NOSE. In bleeding from the nose, or epistaxis, the patient should half recline and keep still, clothing about his neck being loosened, while cold cloths are applied over the forehead. If bleeding continues, the nostril from which it comes may be stuffed with a fine handkerchief or a long, narrow strip of lint or gauze.

Bleeding from the lungs, or haemoptysis, is recognized by the blood being coughed up. The blood has a bright colour, and is mixed with air. In bleeding from the stomach, haematemesis, the blood is vomited, is generally darker in colour than when from the lungs, and may be mixed with food. In either case the patient must be kept lying down and very quiet. Treatment by the doctor often includes a hypodermic injection of morphia. It is presumed, of course, that when bleeding of any consequence takes place a doctor will be summoned without delay.

See Artery ; Blood ; Calcium ; Coagulation ; Hydrastis ; Ligature ; Styptic ; Tourniquet ; Transfusion.

BLEEDING or BLOOD-LETTING. The term bleeding has a different meaning, in indicating the operation of deliberately removing a certain amount of blood from the patient. This operation may also be called blood-letting or venesection, that is, the cutting of a vein. Bleeding as a remedy has fallen into disrepute, but in certain diseased conditions it is a very valuable means of treatment. One is where, owing to some defect in the action of the heart, there is more fluid in the blood vessels than can conveniently be circulated. As a rule, in cases of heart disease, it is possible to remove the excess of fluid by means of the bowels and kidneys by using purgatives and diuretic remedies, and such means are used in preference to bleeding, unless the need for the withdrawal is urgent, or when the other methods have failed. Another indication for bleeding is the presence in the blood of some noxious substance which is poisoning the patient, and the amount of which must be urgently lessened.

Another method of withdrawing blood from the body, but one which has almost fallen into disuse, was in the employment of leeches.

See Congestion ; Cupping ; Leech.

BLENORRHOEA. Derived from Greek words meaning mucus and to run, blenorrhoea is the technical name for an excessive discharge of mucus or phlegm from any mucous membrane.

BLEPHARITIS. Inflammation or, as it really is, eczema of the margins of the eyelids is known as blepharitis. It may exist as pustules, that is, blisters containing matter, at the roots of the eyelashes ; and sometimes a pustule will involve several eyelashes, which are thus matted together. When the pustules burst or the crusts which they form fall off, ulceration is left at their sites. Many of the eyelashes drop out. As the ulcers heal and form scars they may change the direction of the lashes, which perhaps project inward and rub on the eyeball ; this is known as trichiasis. The whole eyelid margin may be dragged outwards (ectropion) or inwards (entropion), with much resulting disfigurement amongst other troubles. In more chronic forms of the malady the eyelid margins are red, thickened and covered with scales.

The disease is contagious, but tends to occur chiefly in children, naturally weak, or whose health has been lowered by measles or a similar complaint. This is particularly the case if there is some error of refraction present, which, sometimes blamed for causing the disorder, can at least keep it going.

As regards treatment, the eyes should be examined for refractive errors and suitable glasses provided if necessary. The general health should be improved by plenty of open-air exercise and a sufficiency of nourishing food, including cod-liver oil. An iron tonic such as Parrish's syrup may be given three times a day with advantage. If the scalp is scurfy it should be cleaned up with sulphur ointment.

The treatment of the eyelids depends upon the precise condition present, but in all cases great cleanliness is necessary. The eyelids should be washed frequently with a lotion of boracic acid, 10 grains to the ounce of water, and, for the removal of crusts or scales, solutions of sodium bicarbonate as often as may be necessary. Loose eyelashes should be pulled out. The pustular stage may be treated with a mixture of equal parts of yellow oxide of mercury ointment and vaseline, and it is usually necessary to apply nitrate of silver in some form to the ulcers. This, however, should only be done by a doctor's directions. For the scaly stage the above ointment or boracic acid ointment may be used.

The ointments are best applied on a glass rod or with a camel-hair brush, both of which must be kept clean. Much patience and perseverance are often needed to effect a cure. Bearing in mind the contagiousness of the disorder, no other child should sleep with the patient, and no one should use his sponge or towel.
 See Eye; Stye.

BLINDNESS. The education of blind children cannot begin too soon; they must not be kept in bed, nor too sedugously protected from injury. Well-meaning parents must remember that all the other senses of blind children must be given a chance to develop and that they can only do so by experience. In the case of older people, who occasionally suffer from progressive disease which will probably end in blindness, it is a great advantage to begin education for the coming deprivation as soon as possible, since by this means much of the shock entailed by the final loss of sight may be averted.
 See Cataract; Conjunctivitis; Cyclitis; Eye; Glaucoma; Nyctalopia; Optic Nerve.

BLINDNESS, COLOUR. *See* Colour Blindness.

BLISTER. A variety of causes, some acting from within and some from without, may produce blisters, also known as blebs or vesicles, but in every case the blister is due to irritation of the deeper layer of the skin, which is stimulated to pour out a certain quantity of fluid; this fluid accumulates underneath the surface layer of skin and thus a blister is produced. In course of time the surface layer of skin becomes thin and bursts.

Blisters form in certain skin and general diseases, for example, eczema, herpes, pemphigus, impetigo, scabies, vaccinia, chicken-pox, etc., the size of the blister varying in different diseases. The contents may be clear and watery or turbid, but when a blister becomes filled with pus or matter it is called a pustule.

Blisters resulting from external irritants are exemplified in those resulting from burns or scalds, from pressure, or from the action of mustard, Spanish fly, or similar substances.

Blisters on the feet which result from much continuous walking may often be prevented if the boots chosen for the excursion are well-fitting. They should be roomy enough not to pinch the feet but not too big or the movement of the foot inside the boot may cause blistering. Care should be taken that the socks are not creased, and it will be an advantage if the insides of these are dry-rubbed with soap or dusted with boracic acid or some other smooth powder. The skin may be hardened by bathing the feet with weak solution of permanganate of potash or formaldehyde, a solution of alum or some methylated spirit. The boots should always be taken off at the end of the day's excursion, the feet bathed and put into easy slippers.

When blisters of any size form either from pressure or burns, the contents should be let out, and the best way to do this is to thread

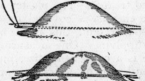

Above, blister with needle run through; below, thread left in

a long needle with white thread and boil it for ten minutes. The needle is then passed through the top layers of the skin a short distance from the blister and carried on through this, a short length of thread being left at either side. This will enable the blister to drain, and will not leave the raw surface which results if the blister bursts. A needle can be sterilised for pricking a small blister by passing it two or three times through a spirit-lamp flame.

Some people are troubled with blisters on the face and neck after exposure to strong sunlight. These may be prevented by using a veil or parasol of a red or orange colour, and powdering may be of use. When blisters form, the skin should be bathed with weak lead lotion and boracic acid ointment applied.

Cheiropompholyx is a skin disorder in which groups of blisters form on the hands and feet. It occurs usually in the spring and autumn and affects women mainly. It gives rise to much itching, which is increased by taking tea, coffee or alcohol. These should therefore be avoided. The health is usually poor and rest and tonics are required. Half a teaspoonful of Easton's syrup, or two teaspoonsful of the simple syrup of hypophosphites, may be taken thrice daily in a little water, after food. The affected parts should be bathed in a warm solution of boracic acid several times daily, and in the intervals be kept covered with long strips of surgeon's lint or linen smeared with zinc ointment or cold cream.

Blistering is often done deliberately with the object of relieving deep-seated congestion or irritation by producing what is known as counter-irritation near the surface of the body; blood is thus drawn away from the deeper parts. This may be accomplished with a hot iron, but is most usually done by applying a blister or blistering fluid, the active constituent of which is Spanish fly or cantharides. Lumbago, sciatica, pleurisy, pericarditis and synovitis are examples of ailments which may be so treated. The plaster as supplied by the chemist is covered by a layer of tissue-paper, and this must be removed before applying. One measuring 3 inches square is a convenient size, but frequently several 1-inch square blisters are put round the area, one after the other, in succession as the vesicles form. Sometimes the blister is left sufficiently long to produce redness only, and then it is known as a flying blister. Ordinarily a blister is left on for eight to ten hours, or where the skin is thick, as on the scalp, it may be left for two hours longer.

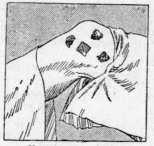

Use of a flying blister

When the vesicle has formed it is pricked with a clean instrument, such as the sharp point of a pair of scissors which have been boiled for twenty minutes, and then the loose skin is snipped off all round, the resulting raw surface being dressed with boracic ointment. Care should be taken that the fluid does not run over adjoining skin, and particularly into the eyes or mouth, etc. To prevent this, and also when painting on a blistering fluid, the area may be ringed with vaseline.

See Burn ; Cantharides ; Counter-irritation.

BLOOD. In the body the blood is contained within a completely closed network of tubes called the blood vessels : arteries, veins and capillaries. From these it never escapes, save by accident ; that is to say, it never escapes in mass, but, on the other hand, various constituents of the blood are incessantly passing through the walls of the blood vessels to every organ and tissue of the body, and other substances pass through the walls of the blood vessels in the opposite direction.

The blood is in the first place a food, or vehicle for food, for every part of the body. The substances required by the various tissues for their health are very numerous, and each of them must be represented in the blood. Furthermore. from the blood are produced all the special fluids which the body forms by means of various organs. Some of these are excretions, getting rid of waste matter, for example, the urine and sweat ; the others are secretions formed to fulfil a specific function, such as the digestive juices, milk, thyroid extract, suprarenal extract, etc. In the case of the two last mentioned and others, not only are they produced from materials brought by the blood, but they are poured by the glands producing them into the blood, in which they circulate.

The blood also carries oxygen from the lungs to the tissues, the oxygen being taken up by the haemoglobin or red colouring matter. Another function of the blood is to distribute heat. This is formed by a process of oxidation, principally in the muscles and in the larger glands, and the blood flowing through these structures is warmed.

Blood also removes the waste or even poisonous substances which have been formed by the process of living. Every living thing, be it animal or vegetable, and every part of every living thing, produces in the course of its life waste substances of which it must get rid if it is to continue to live. The blood is therefore a drainage arrangement as well as a food supply. Carbonic acid gas, formed by combustion going on in the tissues, is carried from the tissues to the lungs, where it is liberated. In the blood the carbonic acid is chiefly carried as bicarbonate of soda and of potash, but part is attached to the red blood corpuscles. Amongst other waste substances is urea which is excreted by the kidneys.

The total amount of blood in the body is about one-twelfth of its weight. The amount is exceedingly constant; thus if there be an excess of water the kidneys will rapidly remove it, and if there be a deficiency of fluid this is made up from that bathing the tissues. Of this total quantity of blood about fourteen per cent. consists of solid elements. The fluid part of the blood is called the blood plasma. It can easily be examined by itself when the solid elements have been removed from a specimen of blood. It is an almost colourless fluid; its most important constituents are a protein substance or albumin which has a very close resemblance to white of egg, a kind of sugar, a certain amount of fat, and another protein substance called fibrinogen which is of great importance in the arrest of bleeding.

Vital Salts in the Blood

In addition, the fluid part of the blood contains the internal secretions already mentioned and at least a dozen poisonous substances which it is carrying to the organs concerned with their removal. The most important of the many salts of the blood (there are at least nine) are common salt, or chloride of sodium, and the phosphate of sodium, each of which is essential to life. Another important salt is phosphate of lime.

The solid constituents of the blood are minute cells, of which there are two kinds, the white and the red. The white blood cells or blood corpuscles are technically known as leucocytes (*q.v.*), literally meaning white cells. Several kinds can easily be distinguished, and most have the character of changing their shape

and of being able to crawl slowly about along the walls of blood vessels, and through the walls into the tissues outside. They play an important part in the clotting of blood; they also attack microbes that enter the blood, and those resulting from disease or injury to various parts of the body which the white cells can reach by emigration through the walls of the blood vessels. The average number of white cells in one cubic millimetre of blood—roughly corresponding to two pinheads—is 10,000.

The average number of red cells in the same space is about 5,000,000; thus the normal proportion, sometimes very much disturbed, of white cells to red cells is about 1 to 500.

Structure of the Red Cells

The red blood cells, the amazing abundance of which has already been stated, are in some ways much simpler to study than are the white cells. In health there is only one kind of red cell to be found in the blood, though in certain kinds of disease there occur many other kinds. The healthy red cell is a circular, flat object rather more than one four-thousandth of an inch across (*see* Plate V, 7). It has a simple network structure and is filled with a yellowish red material which gives its colour to the blood and is known as haemoglobin. The blood in the arteries is bright red because the haemoglobin is combined freely with oxygen; when this oxygen has been lost, as in venous blood, the colour is purple or black.

These cells are incapable of any independent movement except when they are very young; they have but a short life, probably only two or three weeks, and are mainly broken down in the liver. From them is derived the colouring matter of the bile. They are constantly being produced by the red marrow of the bones; few people realise that one of the most important constituents of the blood is manufactured inside their ribs and shin bones.

Unlike the white blood cells, the red cells appear to have only one function, the performance of which depends entirely upon their possession of haemoglobin. As stated above, this has the power of forming a very loose union with oxygen, and as the red blood cells pass through the lungs they take up from the air a quantity of oxygen, which is carried to the tissues and given up to them as they require it, while the carbonic acid is partly conveyed from the tissues by these corpuscles.

In addition to the blood corpuscles, minute bodies called blood platelets are found floating in the plasma. These would appear to have some action furthering the clotting of blood as they are absent in purpura and in some of the specific fevers when bleeding takes place into the skin and from mucous membranes.

See Anaemia ; Circulation of the Blood ; Coagulation ; Cyanosis ; Leucocyte ; Leukaemia ; Plethora ; Secretion ; Transfusion.

BLOOD HEAT. The normal temperature of the blood is about 100° F. When the temperature of the body is ascertained by the means of a thermometer, however, it is not possible to bathe the instrument in the warm blood, and so the normal temperature for practical purposes is about 98·4° F. It is the circulation of the blood that keeps the various parts of the body at the same temperature (*q.v.*).

BLOOD POISONING. When, as a result of a dirty wound or other infection, bacteria or their products, or both, are circulating in the blood and giving rise to fever and other symptoms, the condition is popularly called blood poisoning.

See Pyaemia ; Sapraemia ; Septicaemia.

BLOOD PRESSURE. In order to maintain the circulation of blood through all parts of the body it is necessary that the pressure in the arteries should be kept at a sufficient level. The amount of blood in the vessels affects the pressure, but the main factors in producing it are the action of the heart and the resistance interposed by the smaller arteries ; these contract or dilate according as the pressure requires to be raised or lowered. After large haemorrhages even the veins may contract in order to maintain the flow of the lessened quantity of blood. The blood pressure rises as people grow older. If it is too high giddiness and other symptoms arise, and there is a danger of apoplexy.

See Arterio-sclerosis ; Circulation of the Blood ; Hyperpiesis.

BLOOD VESSEL. The blood vessels are divided into those which carry blood from the heart, the arteries ; those which carry blood to the heart, the veins ; and those which connect the arteries and the veins, the capillaries. The blood vessels are naturally subject to the influence of any poisons that may be present in the blood, and these cause the most common disease of blood vessels, an irregular thickening of their walls, together with a loss of elasticity which renders them liable to break. The technical name for this condition is arterio-sclerosis (*q.v.*).

See Artery ; Blood ; Circulation of the Blood ; Vein.

BLOTCH. Marks on the skin described as blotches may consist of discoloured areas, pimples or groups of pustules. They may be due to various causes, but a common one is constipation. This should be treated by regular doses of cascara or sulphur at night or by salts in the morning. A useful ointment is the following :

Zinc oxide powder	..	1 drachm
Camphor powder ..	..	10 grains
Precipitated sulphur	..	10 ,,
Salicylic acid powder	..	10 ,,
Lanolin ..	..	to 1 ounce

See Acne ; Constipation ; Dyspepsia.

BLUE DISEASE. Congenital cyanosis or lividity of the skin and mucous membranes is sometimes called blue disease.

See Cyanosis ; Heart.

BLUE OINTMENT. Mercury ointment, also called, on account of its colour, blue ointment or blue butter, has been largely used for introducing mercury into the system in the treatment of syphilis. It is also sometimes used for destroying lice on the pubis.

BLUE PILL. The pill of mercury, or blue pill, is an old-fashioned remedy for clearing away bile. It is taken in a dose of 4 to 8 grains, in the evening, followed next morning by a dose of black draught (*q.v.*) or of salts.

BLUE STONE. A sulphate of copper crystal, popularly called blue stone, is often used to reduce exuberant granulations, which are better known as proud flesh, and to stimulate the healing of sluggish ulcers. The part is washed free from discharge, touched lightly with the blue stone, dried and covered with a dressing.

See Caustic ; Copper.

BLUSHING. A blush is due to a widening of the blood vessels of the skin induced by the nervous system in certain mental states. Blushing and flushing of the face are most common and troublesome at the period of puberty and also at the change of life in women. The victim of the habit may be painfully aware of its occurrence. Young people who are shy and self-conscious may diminish this tendency by cultivating a sympathetic interest in the doings of their fellows and by joining heartily in their games whether in or out of doors.

See Adolescence ; Change of Life.

BODY. The science of the structure of the body is Anatomy, and that of its functions Physiology. From the point of view of anatomy, the foundation of the body is the skeleton, which is clothed with the muscles, whilst certain parts, namely, the skull and spinal column, contain the nervous system. The trunk of the body, having its walls formed by bony and muscular tissue, consists of two large cavities, the abdomen and the chest. Lastly, to the trunk of the body are attached two pairs of limbs, as in all animals that possess a backbone ; these are sometimes called the appendages.

See Bone ; Muscle ; Nervous System.

BOIL. A boil is a local inflammation of the skin due to attacks by certain microbes. In general microbes will not cause a boil, unless the power of resistance of the skin has been weakened. The causes of such weakening may be general ; thus boils frequently occur in the course of chronic disease, for example, diabetes and Bright's disease and during convalescence from various fevers. The cause may also be local, the resistance of the skin being weakened by continued irritation or by friction. The commonest site of boils in healthy people is the nape of the neck, which, as a rule, has been irritated by a rough collar.

The smaller boils are usually allowed to follow their own course, though boils about the nose or in the ear should be at once shown to a doctor. Large boils anywhere may be exceedingly painful and require surgical treatment, but in every case it is very desirable to apply some antiseptic ointment— one, for instance, containing 60 grains of boracic acid in one ounce of vaseline—to the skin around the boil, otherwise this is almost certain to become infected, and so one crop of boils will succeed another. Another method is to apply a piece of adhesive plaster with a circular opening over the point of the boil.

The occurrence of boils all over the body demands tonic treatment and change of air, and must not be regarded as merely a disease of the skin. The technical name for this condition is furunculosis. Children may be benefited by chemical food.

See Carbuncle.

BONE. Bones owe their hardness to mineral salts, chiefly phosphate and carbonate of lime, and their elasticity to the fibrous tissue which they contain. In the early stages of their development they consist of cartilage or gristle or of membrane in which mineral matter is gradually laid down, a process known as ossification (*q.v.*). In the bones of a young child there is twice as much animal as mineral matter, so that they do not usually break completely but partly break and partly bend, as with a green twig. As age advances the bones progressively increase their content of mineral

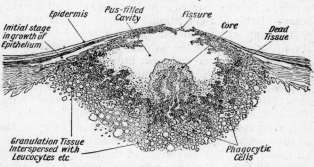

Boil. Sectional diagram of the core surrounded by pus and dead tissue

matter, which becomes so high proportionately in old people that a very slight jar may suffice to break a bone.

In individual bones part of the structure will be found to consist of dense ivory-like bone while the remainder is spongy or cancellous, the spaces being filled with red marrow. Thus a long bone, such as the humerus, consists of a shaft or tube of dense bone containing yellow marrow, while the expanded ends are formed of spongy bone with a thin covering of dense bone. Illustrations of types of bones and bone structure are given in Plate VII.

Every bone has a covering of membrane, known as the periosteum, which takes an important share in nourishing it. When

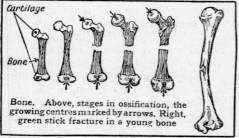

Bone. Above, stages in ossification, the growing centres marked by arrows. Right, green stick fracture in a young bone

bones move on one another the opposing surfaces are covered with cartilage. Bone is tunnelled by an immense number of minute channels (the Haversian canals) along which run its blood vessels (*see* Plate VII, 7). When inflammation occurs in bones it may affect the periosteum (periostitis), the bone (osteitis), the bone marrow (osteomyelitis), or all three. It may be due to injury, for example, a kick on the shin, or microbes may enter through an open wound or be brought by the blood, more particularly after an injury. Acute osteomyelitis is an instance of this last condition.

A young child suffering from a sore throat or having some other source of infection may receive a slight injury to a bone, for instance, the femur, in consequence of which a violent inflammation is set up in the bone and bone marrow. The child may die of blood poisoning, but if it recovers a large portion of the shaft of the bone dies. Death of bone like this, en masse, is called necrosis, and the dead piece of bone is a sequestrum. Death of minute portions, comparable with ulcers of soft tissues, is known as caries.

The bones become softened in rickets (*q.v.*) and osteomalacia (*q.v.*). In consequence they are frequently deformed, as may happen also in osteitis deformans and other diseases. In connexion with bone a variety of tumours may form. These may be of the simple variety, bony, cartilaginous, etc., or they may be malignant and more especially types of sarcoma (*q.v.*). Beginning in a bone a malignant growth may become disseminated throughout the body. One result of such a tumour is that a bone may break without obvious provocation, an event known as spontaneous fracture.

See Caries ; Cartilage ; Epiphysis ; Fracture Joint ; Myeloma ; Necrosis ; Osteitis ; Osteoarthritis ; Osteomalacia ; Osteomyelitis ; Periosteum ; Skeleton ; Tumour.

BORACIC ACID. Boracic, also known as boric powder, has feeble but useful antiseptic properties. The drug is of value because it is so safe, but when a powerful antiseptic action is required it must not be relied upon. It may be used as a lotion, a dusting powder, or an ointment. A saturated solution, made by dissolving in hot water as much of the acid as will dissolve, and allowing to cool, may be used to wash sores ; as an eye lotion, the saturated solution should be mixed with an equal part or more of hot water. The powder may be dusted on sores, or used in eczema and other conditions in the following prescription :

Boracic acid	..	..	1 drachm
Zinc oxide ..	..	..	1 ,,
Starch powder	..	..	1 ounce

To be dusted on.

An ointment may consist of 1 drachm of boracic acid with vaseline to make an ounce. The glycerin of boracic acid may be dropped into the ears to lessen discharge, or it may be diluted with water and used like the acid. The acid is sometimes used as a urinary antiseptic in doses of 10 grains thrice daily.

BORAX. Biborate of soda, commonly called borax, is the usual remedy for destroying the fungus of thrush. The powder may be rubbed on the affected surface, but for infants glycerin of borax should be used. This is better than honey of borax. It is applied to the mouth with a brush or the nurse's finger, and is equally useful in other forms of sore mouth. As a lotion for the eyes, 10 grains are dissolved in an ounce of water, and an ounce in a pint of water may be used as a gargle or as an injection for leucorrhoea or whites. This lotion will often relieve itching of the skin. The glycerin of borax is a good application for sore nipples. The addition of borax softens water and makes it more wholesome for delicate skins ; a strong solution lathers on the scalp and is helpful in getting rid of dandruff. The internal administration of borax, along with bromides, has given good results in epilepsy.

BOTULISM. Cases of poisoning occurring from eating food which has been canned or bottled, usually when this has been done at home, have been traced to the presence of the bacillus botulinus in the food. The ill effects are due to substances manufactured by this microbe. The symptoms include vomiting and purging, abdominal pain, cramp in the limbs, paralysis or weakness of the legs, and perhaps difficulty in speaking. The attacks are often fatal ; in some outbreaks all those affected have died. The danger is avoided by thoroughly cooking the food before use ; it is not enough merely to warm it.
See Food.

BOUGIE. This general name is applied to a rod-like surgical instrument used for the purpose of opening or stretching one or other of the many tubes in the body. It is applied also to thin suppositories used in the treatment of gonorrhoea.

BOWEL. *See* Intestine.

BOW LEG. The usual form of bow leg is more accurately bow knee ; on the other hand, the thigh may be normal in alinement, and the curve occur entirely in the shin. In practically every case bow legs are due to deformity of the bones of the leg caused by former rickets. It is, so to speak, a mere accident whether bow legs or knock knees result in cases where the bones of the leg have been softened by rickets. Not infrequently one leg may be bow, whilst the other exhibits knock knee, and so the curve of one leg fits in with the curve of the other. The condition is due to the weight of the body pressing on the softened bones. When the tendency appears in a young child it may be countered by keeping him in bed and binding the legs to a well-padded splint placed between them. It is essential, at the same time, that attention should be paid to the general health. Children who are allowed to walk about should wear metal splints or braces on the insides of the legs. Bow leg is less disabling than knock knee, but, if the patient desires, the twisted bones may be broken and the legs straightened.
See Rickets.

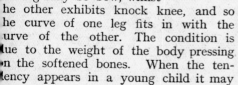
Bow leg compared with normal leg

B.P. The initials B.P. appended to the name of a preparation signify that it is mentioned in the compilation known as the British Pharmacopoeia. This gives an account of the drugs in general use amongst British medical men, including tests of their purity, standards of strength in active principles, methods of preparation, doses and so on. Unless there is a direction to the contrary the drugs ordered on a doctor's prescription must conform to the specifications of the current edition of the British Pharmacopoeia. The initials B.P.C. stand for British Pharmaceutical Codex, which includes drugs and preparations additional to those mentioned in the British Pharmacopoeia.

BRACHIAL. Derived from the Latin brachium, meaning arm, brachial is the name applied to various structures in this limb ; the chief artery of the arm is thus called the brachial artery, and the network of nerves which pass through the armpit is called the brachial plexus.

BRACHYCEPHALY. This word is the Greek equivalent for short-headedness. Certain races, such as the Germans, are naturally shorter-headed than others, but morbid short-headedness occurs in various kinds of idiocy.
See Skull.

BRADYCARDIA. This is the Greek equivalent for slowness of the heart. Exceptional slowness of the pulse is an uncommon symptom, and is of small importance as a rule. It is often noticed in jaundice. When the pulse is below 50 per minute the possibility of heart block has to be considered.

See Heart ; Pulse ; Tachycardia.

BRAIN. The large masses of nervous tissue forming the brain have an average weight of forty-nine ounces in a male adult. The structure of the brain shows extraordinary complexity. The larger

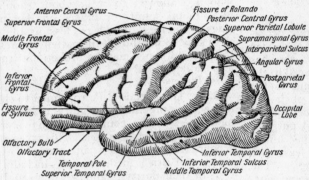

Anterior Central Gyrus
Superior Frontal Gyrus
Middle Frontal Gyrus
Inferior Frontal Gyrus
Fissure of Sylvius
Olfactory Bulb
Olfactory Tract
Temporal Pole
Superior Temporal Gyrus

Fissure of Rolando
Posterior Central Gyrus
Superior Parietal Lobule
Supramarginal Gyrus
Interparietal Sulcus
Angular Gyrus
Postparietal Gyrus
Occipital Lobe
Inferior Temporal Gyrus
Inferior Temporal Sulcus
Middle Temporal Gyrus

Left side of brain, showing how the fissures and sulci break up the grey matter on its surface into lobes and convolutions

part consists of the cerebrum in the form of two hemispheres, right and left, which are connected together by a broad band of fibres running transversely, and known as the corpus callosum. Below this come, in succession and on either side, masses of grey nervous matter, the optic thalamus and corpus striatum, and a stalk, the crus, literally a limb. Then there is the pons or bridge, and lastly the medulla oblongata or bulb which is continuous with the spinal cord (*q.v.*). Behind and below the cerebral hemispheres is the cerebellum, or little brain, which also consists of two hemispheres. These are connected with each other by a central part called the vermiform process and also through the pons.

Nervous matter is of two kinds, grey and white. The former consists of nerve cells and their processes, and the latter of medullated nerve fibres, that is to say. nerve fibres which have a protective white sheath Both the fibres and the cells are supported by a kind of connective tissue called neuroglia.

The outer surface of the cerebrum and of the cerebellum is composed of layers of grey matter, and this is infolded, forming convolutions, affording thereby an increase in the area of the brain surface. The optic thalamus, as stated, is composed of grey matter, and besides this there are other masses in the base of the brain, in the crus, the pons and the medulla. It is in the cells of the grey matter that nerve energy originates. The nerve fibres of the white matter merely transmit such energy.

Within the brain there is a series of cavities, known as ventricles, which communicate with each other and with a canal which runs down the centre of the spinal cord. These are filled with a watery fluid, called the cerebro-spinal fluid. The brain is covered by three membranes the pia mater, in close contact with the brain substance, the arachnoid and the dura mater. The last is in two layers, one lining the interior of the skull, and the other supporting the brain and sending folds into the deep fissures in the brain in order to accomplish this.

The space beneath the arachnoid is filled with cerebro-spinal fluid, which is in communication with the fluid in the ventricles of the brain through certain openings at the back of the medulla oblongata. This fact is of importance in connexion with the occurrence of hydrocephalus (*q.v.*). It will be appreciated also that, as a preventive against injury

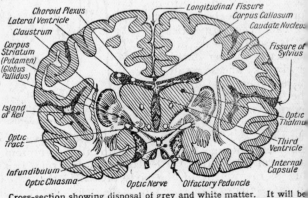

Choroid Plexus
Lateral Ventricle
Claustrum
Corpus Striatum (Putamen) (Globus Pallidus)
Island of Reil
Optic Tract
Infundibulum
Optic Chiasma

Longitudinal Fissure
Corpus Callosum
Caudate Nucleus
Fissure of Sylvius
Optic Thalmus
Third Ventricle
Internal Capsule
Optic Nerve
Olfactory Peduncle

Cross-section showing disposal of grey and white matter. It will be seen how the convolutions increase the surface area of the brain

the brain has the advantage of resting on a water cushion.

The deeper fissures seen on the surface of a cerebral hemisphere mark its division into lobes. The fissure of Rolando, which, beginning a little behind the top of the head, runs obliquely downwards and forwards, marks the boundary between the frontal lobe in front and the parietal lobe behind. The occipital lobe lies behind the parietal, and below these is the temporal lobe. The mention of these lobes simplifies reference to the functions of the brain. The grey matter on its surface contains millions of nerve cells, which are grouped according to the work they do. In front of the fissure of Rolando is the area concerned with initiating voluntary movements, subdivided into parts serving the leg, arm and face in this order from above downwards. The left side of the brain serves the right side of the body, however, and vice versa.

Sensation is to some extent served by this area, but more by the parietal lobe. Tactile sensations and those of pain and temperature are, however, appreciated by the optic thalamus, but this is under the control of the cerebral cortex or outer surface, and if this control is lost pleasing sensations become more pleasing and painful more painful. In the optic thalamus, also, it would appear that movements expressive of

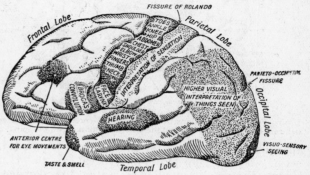

Brain. Control centres on the outer surface of the left side of the brain. The motor centres lie in front of the fissure of Rolando

emotion originate, smiling, for example, or grimacing from pain.

The centre for hearing is in the temporal lobe, and smell seems to be related to a part of the brain at the anterior extremity of this lobe. The centres for vision are in the occipital lobe. The speech centres appear to be in the lower frontal and parietal lobes on the left side for a right-handed person. The cerebellum is of importance in preserving equilibrium, and in co-ordinating the movements of muscles so as to permit of the performance of complicated actions.

From the brain come twelve pairs of nerves, whose names and actions are as follows : (1) olfactory, subserving smell ; (2) optic, nerve of vision ; (3) oculimotor, supplying most of the muscles which move the eyeball and the muscle which contracts the pupil ; (4) nerve supplying the muscle which turns the eyeball downwards and outwards ; (5) trigeminal, nerve supplying sensation to the face, etc., and to the muscles of mastication ; (6) nerve supplying the muscle which turns the eyeball outwards ; (7) facial, nerve supplying

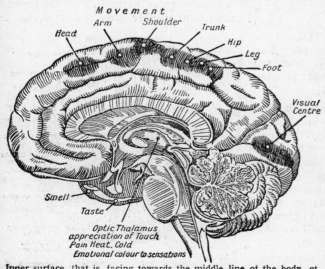

Inner surface, that is, facing towards the middle line of the body, of one cerebral hemisphere, showing situation of motor and other centres

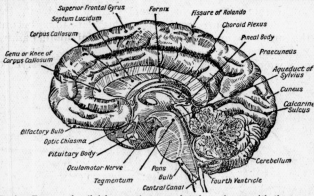

Brain. Four main divisions : the convoluted cerebrum with the cerebellum at its base, the pons, and the bulb, continuous with the spinal cord

the muscles of the face ; (8) auditory, subserving hearing ; (9) glosso-pharyngeal, a nerve of taste, also supplying sensation to the inside of the throat and activating some muscles there ; (10) vagus, or wandering nerve, supplying the heart, lungs, stomach and other viscera, etc. ; (11) spinal accessory, supplying muscles in the neck ; (12) hypoglossal, supplying the muscles moving the tongue.

The blood supply of the brain is derived from the internal carotid and the vertebral arteries. The venous blood and cerebrospinal fluid drain into the large venous channels, known as sinuses, which, in turn, pour their contents mainly into the internal jugular vein. At various points on the surface of the skull these sinuses are connected with external veins, which, if they become infected, may communicate infection to the veins within. One of the sinuses, the sigmoid, lies on the inner side of the mastoid process, and not infrequently becomes infected in suppurative disease of the middle ear.

Injuries and Diseases of the Brain. An injury to the head may cause stunning or concussion ; slight bleeding into the brain or on its surface, the pressure of a spicule of broken bone, meningitis or a commencing abscess following infection through a wound, may give rise to signs of serious irritation of the brain ; while considerable bleeding, a piece of depressed bone or a developed abscess, will result in signs of compression of the brain.

Concussion may give rise to nothing more than giddiness or slight headache of

short duration. Often, when recovering from stunning, the patient becomes sick and vomits. In worse degrees of concussion he is only semiconscious, and it may be difficult to rouse him. His skin feels cold and the pulse is weak. After a time he begins to come to, a reaction takes place, and he may develop some degree of fever. In other cases, however, signs of irritation or of compression appear.

Concussion which is supposed to be due to a shaking up of the brain tissues, without actual gross damage, is usually recovered from completely. In other cases it is followed by a weakness of memory and headaches when mental work is attempted.

The signs of irritation depend upon the amount and position of the brain tissue affected. If, for example, the centres for movement are irritated, convulsions occur which may be limited to a single limb, or be general, and then consciousness is lost.

A condition known as cerebral irritation sometimes follows concussion. It is due to laceration or tearing of the brain substance, probably of the frontal lobe. In this the patient is semi-conscious and manifests great irritability of body and mind, and usually after a few weeks he

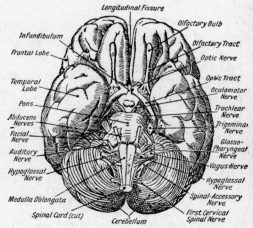

Lower surface of the brain showing the origin of the twelve pairs of cranial nerves

wakes up in a state of mental weakness or fatuity. In meningitis and abscess headache is marked, the temperature is raised and there may be rigors or severe shivering. There may be intense intolerance of light and noise of any kind, vomiting and so on. Compression of the brain results in the profound unconsciousness known as coma. The breathing is slow and stertorous, though later it may become rapid and irregular. Paralysis may affect the limbs on one side of the body, or in the later stages both sides may be powerless.

After concussion the patient should rest for some time, and in any but the slightest cases he should be put to bed. While awaiting the doctor, an attempt may be made to lessen the shock by putting hot-water bottles to his feet and by his sides. The room should be darkened and quiet. On no account, in any head injury, should alcoholic stimulants be given. When there are evidences of irritation or compression, an operation to remove the cause of either may be the treatment indicated. In other cases the conditions mentioned for concussion are continued, the bowels are kept open, the bladder is emptied, if necessary, by a catheter, and the patient is fed by the bowel.

Inflammation of the brain substance is called encephalitis (q.v.), and, when the grey matter is specially involved, polio-encephalitis. The latter condition is similar to the inflammation of the grey matter of the spinal cord, which results in infantile paralysis. It may be suspected when a child becomes suddenly ill and passes from one fit into another.

When the blood supply of a part of the brain is cut off, say, by an embolus, the part may die, and then it undergoes liquefaction or softening. Old people who exhibit mental deterioration are often said to have softening of the brain, and it may well be that, in consequence of a poor blood supply, there is degeneration of the brain substances.

Tumours of the brain include the glioma, the sarcoma and cancer, the last being almost always derived from cancer in other parts of the body, for example, the breast and the bowel. Tumours of any size usually produce certain classical symptoms, which are headache, vomiting, and optic neuritis, or, rather, a dropsical swelling of the optic nerve just as it enters the eyeball. Giddiness is another common symptom, and there may be mental changes. Tumours in the frontal lobe often produce a dreamy state. The position of the tumour may often be determined by observing alterations in the movements, sensations, etc., of various parts of the body and correlating the findings with what is known regarding the localisation of function in the brain. Some tumours can be removed successfully, and, where this is not possible, making an opening in the skull, an operation known as decompression, may do much to relieve symptoms.

Swellings due to tuberculosis or syphilis may act as tumours ; their treatment is that of the main disease, with operative interference in some cases.

See Apoplexy ; Disseminated Sclerosis ; Embolism ; Encephalitis ; Epilepsy ; General Paralysis ; Insanity ; Medulla ; Meninges ; Meningitis ; Nervous System ; Optic Thalamus ; Paralysis ; Spinal Cord, etc.

BRAIN FAG. An excess of mental work, of worry or of excitement, especially when combined with an insufficiency of sleep, is likely to be followed by signs of brain fatigue—restlessness, insomnia, inability to concentrate on intellectual work, and so on. Alcoholic and sexual excesses and the abuse of drugs like morphine and cocaine, or of tobacco, tea and coffee, precipitate the onset of brain fag ; while some people are born with brain tissues which are unable to withstand even a moderate strain. Rest and the adoption of sound hygienic habits form an essential part of any treatment.

See Fatigue ; Mental Hygiene ; Neurasthenia ; Weir Mitchell Treatment.

BRAIN FEVER. This is a term never used now by medical men. Apparently it was adopted to describe simple fever in which nervous symptoms were prominent, and also the fever associated with inflammation of the brain coverings.

See Meningitis.

BREAD. Ordinary bread made from wheat flour owes its sponginess to carbonic acid gas having been formed, along with alcohol, by the fermentation of sugar. Practically all the alcohol is driven off from the bread by the heat of the oven and is lost. Carbonic acid gas constitutes about two-thirds of the total bulk of a loaf ; its value consists in the fact that it allows the digestive juices readily to attack the bread. The formation of a sticky mass, or dough, when water is mixed with flour is due to the presence of a protein or flesh-forming substance known as gluten. Besides this, flour contains a large quantity of starch.

" Wholemeal " bread contains all parts of the grain, including the bran or grain covering. In " standard " bread part of the bran has been removed. In ordinary white flour all the bran has been removed, and also the germ of the grain. The loss of the bran and the germ implies the loss of vitamins, and also of the organic phosphorous compounds which these parts of the grain contain. This may not be of much consequence where a mixed diet is taken, but it is serious in the case of children who are fed almost entirely on bread. It interferes with their growth and is a factor in causing rickets.

White bread is more digestible than the others, and is to be preferred when there is any difficulty in digesting the latter ; but in this case milk, eggs or other

The Germ included in Standard Bread

All used for Whole Meal Bread

Bran. 15% to 20% added to flour for Brown Bread

Endosperm or Kernel used in White Bread

Proportion of Grain used in various Breads

Bread. Parts of wheat grain used in making several varieties

foodstuffs are imperative for the sake of vitamins, though bread of any sort requires the addition of fats to make it a sufficient diet.

Diabetic bread is supposed to contain little or no starch, so that it may make a suitable article of diet for people suffering from diabetes. It may be a gluten bread, which usually contains a varying propor-

tion of starch ; casein bread, made from the protein of milk ; or bread made with almonds or other nuts. It is necessary that supplies should always be obtained from a reliable maker.

See Diet ; Food ; Wheat.

BREAST. The female breast consists of a number of separate glands embedded in fat, the ducts of which converge to open on the nipple. The pink zone around the nipple is called the areola. After puberty the breasts grow rapidly, and in pregnancy the glands take on active development for the formation of milk, while the areola enlarges and becomes dark in colour. Sometimes supernumerary or extra breasts are found on various parts of the body.

Diseases of the Breast. Diseases of the female breast are mainly related to the changes which take place in the organ at puberty, in connexion with the function of suckling, and after the change of life. Acute inflammation of the breast, or mastitis, may occur in the first few days of life, due either to infection or to injury, such, for example, as is caused by people who ignorantly believe that the nipple strings have to be broken. All that is necessary for this condition is to ensure that the upper edge of the binder does not compress or rub on the inflamed breast, by placing a piece of gamgee or other dressing over the breast. Sometimes at puberty a similar thing occurs and a little fluid may discharge from the nipple. Here, again, all that is necessary is to protect the organ.

In women, apart from wounds and other injuries, mastitis generally occurs during the few days following labour. It is caused by infection through the nipple, owing to this being handled with dirty fingers or otherwise contaminated. Should the breast become engorged with milk, or " caked," the danger of mastitis is increased. The treatment for a " caked " breast is to give a dessertspoonful of Epsom salts or some other saline in a little water, and to massage the breast through flannels wrung out of hot water.

The movements are made from the base of the breast towards the nipple and continued till the organ is soft. The use of a breast-pump may help to reduce the engorgement. The breast should be supported by a bandage.

Should inflammation occur the breast becomes swollen and painful, or at any rate one part will be found to be tender, and the patient develops fever. In these circumstances, the breast should not be rubbed, but hot applications may be made and the organ supported. The bowels should be moved freely with salts. The child should be taken off the breast. Should the fever persist for longer than thirty-six hours it is probable that suppuration is occurring, and when an abscess has definitely formed it should be opened without delay. Sometimes when suppuration does not ensue the affected part of the breast may remain chronically inflamed ; or a similar thing may occur independently of acute inflammation or of pregnancy.

In women approaching the change of life chronic inflammation may affect smaller portions of the organ, being, however, much more diffused throughout it, and both breasts may be involved. Tiny cysts are formed in course of time, and one or more of these may swell sufficiently to give the feeling of a lump. In both forms of the disease there may be pain, which is often severe and tends to be worse at the menstrual periods. The first form may be sufficiently treated by supporting the breast and applying belladonna plasters for the pain. It may be said here that in order properly to rest the breast it is necessary to immobilise the muscle in which it lies. This is done by supporting the arm in a sling and binding it to the side. Similar treatment may help the diffuse inflammation, but more may be needed.

It will be evident, of course, that before starting treatment in these conditions the diagnosis must first be accurately made, as a lump in the breast may be one or more of a certain number of things.

Among these, in addition to chronic mastitis, are a chronic abscess, cysts, adenomata or glandular tumours, sar-

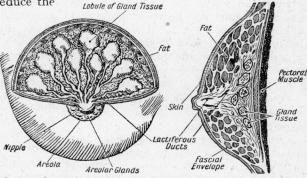

Breast. Internal structure, showing secreting and supporting tissues

coma and cancer. The existence of a lump in the breast inevitably gives rise to a suspicion of cancer in a woman's mind, and such is her dread of her suspicion being correct and of an operation being necessary that she often keeps her knowledge of the existence of the lump to herself. Anxiety preys on her mind and makes havoc of her health and happiness. This is quite wrong.

Immediately she becomes aware of the lump she should put herself in the hands of her doctor. She will either discover that simple treatment is all that is required, or if an operation is necessary and the lump proves to be cancer she will give the surgeon a fair chance to eradicate the disease.

A chronic abscess occurs usually in pregnant women, and is sometimes of a tuberculous nature. The treatment consists of evacuation of the pus and measures to improve the general health. Cysts, it has been noted, may occur in chronic mastitis. Other forms are the retention cyst, or galactocele, which contains milk and which occurs in women who are or have been nursing ; cysts due to irritation of the nipple, and so on. In some cases it suffices to lay the cyst open and pack it with gauze, but others should be removed.

Adenomata or glandular tumours are of several varieties. The commonest in younger women is the fibro-adenoma which appears as a small elastic lump with a fairly definite margin. It may be quite painless or, on the other hand, very painful. It should be removed. Sarcomata are found usually in women between thirty and forty years of age as roundish, somewhat elastic lumps, which rapidly increase in size. The glands in the armpit enlarge, and the growth is carried to other organs quite early in the course of the disease. It is not very common.

Possible Causes of Cancer in the Breast

Next to the womb, the breast is the most frequent site for cancer in women. It sometimes occurs in the male breast, but this is rare. It generally happens after forty years of age, but sometimes younger women are affected. The left breast seems to be more often involved than the right, and the disease usually begins in the outer half. Irritation of the breast by badly fitting corsets, changes induced by blows or squeezes, and chronic inflammation of the breast are among the causes noted as possibly having a share in originating the growth.

The disease is found in several forms, much the most frequent being that known as the scirrhus cancer. This is felt first as a hard lump, which may be painless or very painful. The skin at first moves over it quite freely. The glands in the armpit become enlarged and hard. If it is allowed to grow, sooner or later it becomes attached to the skin, which may be puckered in consequence, and the nipple also is drawn in. In later stages the skin may become ulcerated. This tumour grows rather slowly, and in old women sometimes very slowly indeed.

The encephaloid cancer grows more rapidly, and is felt as a rounded soft mass. The glands in the arm become enlarged very soon after the lump is noticed. Another kind is the duct cancer, which, if it forms near the skin, may appear as a rounded, dark red swelling.

Whenever cancer is present, or any condition which may justly be considered to be cancerous, the breast and the glands into which its lymphatics drain should be removed at the earliest possible moment. The X-rays and radium are sometimes used after the operation with a view to preventing recurrence, and they may be used when recurrence takes place,

and in cases which have been allowed to pass beyond the reach of operation.

Neuralgia of the breast, or mastodynia, specially affects young women who are anaemic and neurotic. The severe pain may arouse apprehensions of cancer, although pain in the breast is no more indicative of cancer than is the painlessness of a tumour evidence that it is not cancerous. The pain tends to increase in a marked way at the menstrual periods. Support to the breast and the use of belladonna plasters will be helpful, but earnest attention must be directed towards improvement of the general health.

Chronic eczema round the nipple will always give rise to the suspicion that it may be what is known as Paget's disease of the nipple, a condition in which eczema in this situation proves to be the forerunner of cancer in the underlying breast tissues. The suspicion will be justified if a thorough course of appropriate treatment fails to remove the eczema. The only prudent course, then, is to remove the breast, even although no definite tumour can be distinguished.

See Baby ; Cancer ; Fissure ; Pregnancy.

BREAST FEEDING. The natural and proper food for an infant is breast milk. This contains all the food materials necessary for growth in the proper proportions in the most digestible form, supplied at the proper temperature. Except in a few cases the mother's milk is free from infection with noxious germs, and the child is spared one of the undoubted risks of feeding with cow's milk. Only the gravest reasons can justify keeping or taking a child off the breast. The fact that the mother's milk does not appear to be sufficiently copious or to agree with the child is not a good reason, at any rate in the first place. An attempt should be made to improve the quantity and quality of the milk by giving plenty of nourishing food, and by ensuring that the mother takes sufficient exercise in the open air.

Details with regard to the frequency with which the child should be suckled will be found under the heading Baby. Should the mother's milk be insufficient to nourish the baby, it is better to give cow's milk or infant foods in place of some of the breast feeds rather than stop the latter altogether.

While suckling, a woman must be careful about taking purgative or other drugs, as some of these get into her milk and affect the baby. The doctor's advice should always be asked before doing anything of the kind. A child is weaned when nine or ten months old, but it may be kept at the breast longer if it is weakly, or if the time for weaning falls during hot summer weather, when the danger of polluted cow's milk is greatest, or if the child is sickly from teething or some other cause.

See Baby ; Childbirth ; Milk.

BREATH, BAD. A foul breath may be due to decaying teeth, constipation, indigestion, alcoholism, or enlarged tonsils with decaying matter in the small cavities or crypts on their surfaces. In a form of chronic catarrh of the nose known as ozoena, the breath has a very offensive odour, though the patient is himself quite unconscious of it. In bronchiectasis or dilatation of the bronchial tubes, the secretion of the tubes tends to accumulate and decompose. It is coughed up periodically, and the breath has a peculiarly offensive odour. Gangrene of the lung is among other causes of a bad breath, and this is so characteristically foul that the condition may be diagnosed from it. Mouth washes (*q.v.*) and scented pastilles may cover a bad breath, but the cause should be determined and remedied, if possible.

BREATHING EXERCISES. In breathing, air is drawn into the lungs by an increase in the capacity of the chest. This is brought about by a descent of the midriff or diaphragm and by the elevation of the ribs. In ordinary breathing the ribs are raised by the external intercostal muscles, the fibres of which pass from one rib forwards and downwards to the rib beneath. The air is forced out of the lungs by the elastic recoil of the ribs and of the abdominal wall, which has been forced forward by the diaphragm pressing on the abdominal contents.

It follows from these facts that breathing exercises, to be of any use, must consist in taking full breaths. Exercises such as swimming, which develops the muscles

passing from the chest wall to the arm, do not benefit breathing except in so far as they put one out of breath, and this, of course, can be done by running games, skipping and others equally well. A course of graduated hill climbing is about as good a breathing exercise as could be suggested.

It has been noted that the descent of the diaphragm pushes forward the abdominal wall. Therefore, when doing breathing exercises, not only should the chest clothing be slack but that covering the abdomen also. It must be further observed that these exercises, like all others, should be done either in the open air or in a well-ventilated room. Another most important point is that breathing should be performed through the nose and not by way of the mouth. The interior of the nose is so arranged that the air passing in is warmed, moistened and more or less filtered of injurious suspended matter. Air entering the air passages by the mouth is colder and dryer, and, far from being cleansed, it is actually polluted with the organisms which teem in what might be regarded as a clean mouth. It is not surprising, then, that "mouth-breathers" frequently suffer from catarrh of the air passages.

Young children with poorly developed chests should be subjected to a thorough and prolonged course of breathing exercises. If the opportunity is lost the ribs become rigid and much less improvement can be hoped for. When there is definite blocking of the nose from adenoids, or from any other cause, the obstruction should be removed by operation before beginning the exercises.

It is important that breathing exercises should not be practised by children with nasal obstruction without the advice and supervision of a doctor.

In performing breathing exercises of any kind, after the deep inspiration, it is an advantage to hold the breath for about ten seconds before breathing out. In the exercises which are done standing, the body should be held erect, though not in a stiff, strained attitude, and the shoulders should be thrown back. The following are a few typical exercises of this kind. Some are illustrated in Plate VIII.

Each exercise may be performed five, ten or more times.

(1) While standing erect with the arms hanging by the sides, breathe in deeply, hold the breath, and then breathe out.

(2) This time, while breathing in, raise the arms from the sides, above the head, and lower while breathing out.

(3) Repeat No. 2, but raise the arms in front.

(4) As in No. 1, but with the hands pressing on the lower parts of the ribs at the sides. After a few days the exercise is done with the hands about the middle of the side of the chest, and a few days later on the upper ribs.

(5) Stand erect with the arms above the head, take a long breath, stoop forward slowly as far as possible, and breathe out while doing so ; rise again slowly, at the same time breathing in deeply.

(6) Assume a sitting posture, with the legs stretched out in front and the knees slightly bent and turned outwards ; with the arms held above the head and the fingers clasped, take a deep inspiration : then stoop forward slowly as far as possible between the legs, bringing the hands to the lap, breathing out while doing so. Again, while breathing in, raise the body with the arms above the head. This exercise can be varied in the following way : while stooping forward take a deep breath, but so that the abdominal wall is pushed forward as far as possible—this means that the ribs are moved as little as possible— then breathe out slowly and repeat several times.

Breathing exercises are valuable not only for their effect upon the lungs ; they also improve the work of the heart and of the viscera.

See Adenoids ; Lung ; Respiration.

BREATHLESSNESS. *See* Shortness of Breath.

BRIGHT'S DISEASE. Nephritis or inflammation of the kidneys is commonly known as Bright's disease, after the doctor who first drew attention to the presence of albumin in the urine in this group of diseases. The varieties of Bright's disease may be classified as acute and chronic.

Acute Bright's disease usually occurs in the course of some acute disease, of which the most important is scarlet fever or scarlatina. It may occur also as a result of poisoning of the kidneys in diphtheria, typhoid fever, inflammation of the lungs (pneumonia), and in poisoning by mercury, Spanish fly and a large number of other irritant substances. It appears in some cases to follow exposure to cold, especially when this occurs in connexion with a drinking bout. It is a fairly common event in pregnancy.

In children the onset may be marked by the occurrence of convulsions ; the fact that fits in young children may be due to nephritis is not always remembered. The symptoms of the disease, however, may not be very pronounced ; the patient may complain of headache or of shortness of breath, or he may have a shivering fit and a small amount of fever. The pulse is rather more rapid than usual, the tongue is furred and the patient is generally constipated. There is usually very little pain, and, if present, it is seldom referred to the region of the kidneys.

Facial Swelling the Typical Symptom

The face is rather swollen, " pale, puffy, and pasty," and the ankles also may be swollen, but it is the swelling of the face that is typical of Bright's disease. The swelling is due to the accumulation of fluid, and this dropsy may proceed to any extent and ultimately may be the cause of death by interfering with the action of the heart. There is almost always some indigestion.

The most characteristic feature of acute Bright's disease is the diminution in amount of the secretion of the kidneys, and the fact that when chemically tested it is found to contain albumin ; it also contains blood and casts from the kidney tubules. As a rule, this disease runs a rapid course ; when properly treated, and especially when the treatment is commenced early, it is rarely fatal.

. The treatment of acute nephritis essentially consists in rest in bed and milk diet. The patient is put between blankets and is clothed in flannel. The amount of milk given depends on the degree of dropsy present. If this is very great, fluids of all kinds have to be given sparingly. In addition to plain water, home-made lemonade containing a teaspoonful of cream of tartar may be given to drink. This helps to keep the bowels active, but it is usually desirable to give also doses of Epsom salts, sodium sulphate or some other saline, dissolved in a little water only. This is to get rid of water and poisonous substances by the bowel and so relieve the kidneys.

For this reason it is necessary also to keep the skin active. This may be ac-

omplished by keeping hot-water bottles
a the bed and sponging the patient with
ot water, but hot baths may be necessary,
r hot packs or a hot-air bath. Min-
ererus solution and other diaphoretic
emedies are also sometimes used. Re-
overy is usually complete in about three
weeks. The return to solid food should be
radual. Alcohol is inadmissible. Anaemia
s generally a feature of the disease, and
s treated by iron preparations. Warm
lothing must be worn, and if the weather
s cold at home a change to a warmer
limate should, if possible, be made.

Chronic Bright's disease may succeed
he acute form, or may arise of itself.
n one form of the chronic disease, de-
cribed as the hydraemic type, resulting
rom what is called the large white kidney,
dropsy is present, and the urine may con-
ain a large amount of albumin. The
patient may note that his ankles and legs
are swollen after being about, and his face
puffy after the night's rest. The stomach is
asily upset, vomiting may be frequent,
and there may also be a tendency to
diarrhoea. When the symptoms are
pronounced the treatment must be similar
o that of the acute stage, and at all times
care must be taken to avoid chill by wear-
ng suitable clothing. The diet should be
plain and moderate. Where a large amount
of albumin is being lost in the urine
sufficient protein food, such as eggs, fish
and meat, are necessary to replace it.

Origin of the Azotaemic Form

In the other form of the chronic disease
known as the azotaemic, the urine is
abundant and watery, often containing
only a trace of albumin, and there may be
no dropsy, at any rate for a long time. It
may be a sequel to one of the forms already
described, or to arterio-sclerosis, a degeneration of the arteries. It may also
occur independently of these. Lead
poisoning, the abuse of alcohol, the im-
moderate use of rich food along with
sedentary habits, and syphilis, gout and
other diseases are amongst the underlying
causes. The disease may be present for a
long time without giving any plain hint
of its existence. Chronic dyspepsia,
possibly mistaken for bilious attacks, and
chronic bronchitis may, however, be
largely due to this form of kidney mischief.

The first knowledge some people have of
their kidneys being diseased is when they
consult an oculist for dimness of vision.
Inflammation at the back of the eye is
not uncommonly a result of nephritis.
Neuralgic pains and eczema are other
manifestations, though, of course, either
may be due to some other cause.

How the Blood Pressure is Affected

It has been stated above that kidney
disease may result from arterial disease,
and it must be added that chronic kidney
disease is followed by thickening and
hardening of the arteries, and the blood
pressure may be considerably raised.
One consequence of this is a liability to
rupture of a brain blood vessel with an
apoplectic seizure. Bleeding may take
place elsewhere in the body, and nose
bleeding is particularly common. The
heart becomes enlarged. This may be
attended by troublesome thumping or
even pain, while at some time evidences of
cardiac failure, breathlessness, dropsy, etc.,
may manifest themselves. In nephritis
there is always a possibility of fluid
accumulating in the pleural or peritoneal
cavity or in the pericardium.

It has been pointed out that the structural changes and symptoms of nephritis
are largely due to the retention of poisonous
substances in the blood. When these are
present in such quantities as to produce
clamant symptoms the condition is called
uraemia. The evidences of this condition
may be a tendency to drowsiness, headaches, nervous twitching, dimness of vision,
frequent vomiting, attacks of dyspnoea
or difficulty of breathing, and so on, but
sometimes convulsions resembling those
of epilepsy occur. These are followed
by a period of profound unconsciousness or coma, though this may happen
without the fits. Sometimes convulsions
of this kind are the first announcement
that the kidneys are diseased.

The treatment of chronic Bright's
disease in the earlier stages is not a matter
of drugs, though, of course, these may be
of value in relieving some of the symptoms
that are apt to occur when the disease is
further advanced. In general the treatment is a matter of diet and attention to
the sound rules of health. Constant attention to the diet is essential, especially

since indigestion is very frequent. It should be smaller than the average, but if there is no dropsy innocent fluids must be freely taken. Meat once a day is sufficient, and there may be a liberal allowance of farinaceous foods and, with the proviso just noted, of milk. Salt should be restricted in the hydraemic type. In the azotaemic a free supply of fresh vegetables is required.

The patient may carry on such work and recreations as he feels fitted for, but exposure to cold must be avoided. He must invariably wear wool next his skin and must encourage and facilitate the action of the skin by a regular use of baths. His danger is greatest during the cold weather ; when possible, therefore, he should spend the winter, if in Great Britain at all, in its warmest parts ; probably Bournemouth and Torquay are the most suitable places for patients suffering from this disease. The use of alcohol in any form is, in general, a danger. The lightest wines are allowed in some cases, but a doctor must take the responsibility of approving their safety in any particular case.

The treatment of Bright's disease can be much better controlled if tests of renal efficiency are carried out. That most often practised is to give the patient a dose of urea and determine how much of this is excreted within stated times.

See Albuminuria ; Arterio-sclerosis ; Dropsy ; Kidney ; Uraemia.

BROMIDE. There are several drugs of great use in medicine which owe their virtues to the possession of the chemical element called bromine. They are potassium bromide, sodium bromide, ammonium bromide and hydrobromic acid. They may be all considered together as their properties are almost identical ; the slight differences between them may, however, be noted.

It is usually considered that the salt containing ammonium has a slightly stimulant action and is therefore preferable for use where the patient is depressed or weak ; the salt containing sodium is neutral in this regard ; that containing potassium has a slightly depressant action. This is of practical importance only in a very few cases. Hydrobromic acid, the dose of which is 15 to 60 minims, is mor rarely used than the salts, but it is c value in the treatment of whooping cough, and is often combined wit quinine, since it tends to avert the un pleasant symptoms—such as headach and singing in the ears—which quinin sometimes causes.

The characteristic action of all thes drugs is upon the nervous system, whicl they depress uniformly throughout it whole extent ; they have no other action worthy of note. They are absorbed witl extreme rapidity and are removed from the body with equal rapidity by means o all the possible organs—the kidneys, the saliva, the skin, and the breasts, if these are acting.

Value of Bromides in Epilepsy

If a solution of a bromide be paintec on the throat the sensitiveness of the surface is reduced, but the effect can be better achieved by giving the drug in ternally for a day or two. This is often done prior to a thorough laryngoscopic examination, when the parts are unduly sensitive. If an immediate effect is necessary, cocaine or a similar drug would, of course, be used.

The disease in which bromides are of especial value is epilepsy. They may be administered in large doses, often amounting to 200–300 grains a day, and the administration has to be continued for long periods. The frequency and the severity of the fits are both, as a rule, markedly reduced, and, indeed, the symptoms of the disease may entirely disappear.

The bromides are also valuable in the treatment of sleeplessness, though, like all other drugs employed for this purpose, they are readily capable of abuse. They are of little value when the sleeplessness is due to pain or to other serious causes, but very successful when it is due merely to worry or overwork. The sleep produced is real sleep, which refreshes the patient. People who suffer from nightmare, and children who suffer from night terrors, are often benefited by bromides. The usual dose for such purposes as this is from 5 grains for a child up to 30 or more for an adult.

Much larger doses can be given in delirium tremens. Headache and many kinds of neuralgia are frequently relieved by bromides. These drugs are also given in various cases of spasm due to whatever cause—such as whooping-cough, lockjaw, poisoning by strychnine, and the curious symptoms often met with in rickety and weakly children which is usually called a "croupy cough." All forms of the drug are also extensively used in order to depress the sexual functions.

Full doses of bromides taken before going on board ship and during the voyage may help to prevent or lessen sea-sickness. The liquid preparations should be well diluted, and the best way to take one of the salts in powder is to dissolve it in half a glass of soda water. This applies to taking bromides for any purposes ; when taken with too little water they are apt to provoke sickness.

Poisoning by Bromides. In certain people bromides cause unpleasant symptoms of poisoning, the condition being known as bromism. When large quantities have been taken for a long period, the patient becomes depressed, stupid and unable to work. The sexual functions are abolished, the skin loses its sensitiveness and frequently displays a rash, which is very similar to acne and is sometimes called bromide-acne. The symptoms are easily removed by stopping or reducing the drug. By combining arsenic in a mixture with bromides the rash may be prevented in those who show an unusual susceptibility in this direction. It is undesirable to take bromides habitually, since in time it becomes impossible to sleep without them and the patient's intellect suffers.

BRINE BATH. A brine bath is often useful in chronic joint affections, and can be made at home by using coarse salt. The temperature of the water should be about 90° F., and the bath should last from 15 to 30 minutes.
See Baths.

BRONCHI. The air passages in the lungs are called bronchi, the word being the plural of bronchus. The trachea, popularly known as the windpipe, which leads from the larynx to the lungs, divides into two smaller tubes, one of which goes to each lung ; these are known as the right and left bronchus or bronchial tube. In

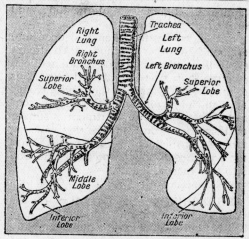

Bronchi : The system of air tubes in the lungs

the substance of the lung each of these divides and divides again, forming a sort of tree-like structure. When the bronchi become extremely small and lose their rigid character, owing to the absence of cartilage or gristle from their walls, they are known as bronchioles.

The bronchi are subject to various disorders, by far the most common of which is the inflammation of their lining membrane, or bronchitis. When the bronchioles are similarly affected the condition is much more serious, since the passage of the air to the air cells of the lung is seriously impeded. The bronchioles, which have a large quantity of muscular tissue in their walls, are very apt in certain people to be thrown into spasm, which naturally prejudices the act of breathing and which constitutes the basis of the symptoms of asthma.

See Asthma ; Bronchiectasis ; Bronchitis ; Broncho-pneumonia ; Lung.

BRONCHIECTASIS. When one or more of the bronchi become enlarged, forming cavities inside the chest, bronchiectasis is said to be present. Inside these cavities matter is apt to collect and has to be expelled by tremendous bursts of coughing. The contained matter commonly decomposes, and in consequence of this the breath and sputum have a highly offensive odour. This disease may be due to the presence of a foreign body in a bronchus or be a sequel to other diseases of the lungs, such as very severe and prolonged bronchitis, tuberculosis of the lung, and sometimes pneumonia.

Such a cavity has been laid open and drained. Another method of treatment especially useful is to produce an artificial pneumo-thorax on the affected side. This means injecting air into the pleural cavity so as to cause collapse of the lung. Apart from these measures, treatment is similar to that for chronic bronchitis, while an attempt is made to get antiseptics into the bronchus by inhalation or by injection into the trachea.

See Empyema.

BRONCHITIS. Inflammation of the bronchi takes various forms. It may be acute or chronic, and when acute may affect the larger tubes or the smaller, the latter being a very serious condition. An ordinary case of acute bronchitis is usually described as a bad cold in the chest. The inflammation affects the windpipe and the larger bronchi ; there is little or no interference with breathing, since the smaller tubes are not affected. It invariably attacks the bronchi of both lungs ; it may be brought on by exposure to cold, whether by a draught or by getting wet, or by the extension downwards of a cold in the head. Very often it is a symptom of another disease, such as influenza, measles, whooping-cough or typhoid fever.

The patient suffers from a distressing, racking cough ; often he has a sore throat and is hoarse, and there is some pain and sense of rawness behind the breast-bone ; he has scarcely any fever. At first the cough produces very little expectoration but is very painful. Later on expectoration is produced, and this becomes more and more abundant and the pain of the cough disappears. At first the sputum is tough, then white and frothy, but later it becomes mixed with yellow matter. The cough is usually worse at night and in the morning on waking up. When the doctor listens to the chest he hears little more than may often be heard by anyone who stands near the patient, that is, wheezing or whistling sounds, due to the passage of the air through the narrowed bronchial tubes.

There is no specific remedy for acute bronchitis. The disease runs its own course, lasting usually about a fortnight,

and all that can be done is to make the patient as comfortable as possible meanwhile. The first items of the treatment are bed and light, simple diet, such as gruel and slops. Some aperient medicine should be given, such as a dose of Epsom salts.

The pain of the cough and the rawness behind the breast-bone may be relieved by the use of drugs, such as ipecacuanha wine, in 10-minim doses three or four times a day, or one of the mild tinctures containing opium, such as paregoric ; but as useful a means as any is rubbing the chest with hartshorn and oil, turpentine liniment or the acetic liniment of turpentine. This draws a quantity of blood to the skin and relieves the congestion of the bronchi that lie underneath. For children, camphorated oil is very often employed. Grown-up people who can stand something more vigorous may employ a mustard plaster, or, if necessary, a linseed poultice or the kaolin poultice, B.P.C., on the front of the chest and another between the shoulders. A gamgee tissue jacket should be worn after this kind of treatment.

Relief from Steam Inhalation

The patient is much relieved by the breathing of warm and moist air. Dry, cold air irritates the bronchi and causes a great deal of painful and useless coughing, whereas he will cough very little if he is kept in a warm room, the air of which may be moistened by means of a steam kettle. A very useful measure also is the inhalation of steam containing Friar's balsam. In three or four days it becomes highly desirable to aid the patient in his efforts to cough up the secretion which is being produced in his bronchi. For this purpose the carbonate of ammonia is often given, usually in the form of sal volatile or the aromatic spirit of ammonia. This may be given in doses of half to one teaspoonful in a wineglass of water ; it is especially valuable in cases of bronchitis in children, in smaller doses, and old people.

The very serious and frequently fatal kind of bronchitis in which the smallest bronchial tubes are involved is usually met with in children as a consequence of measles and whooping-cough, and in adults as a result of influenza. The

PLATE VII

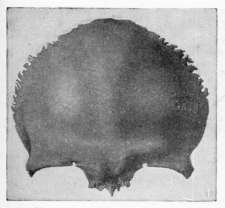

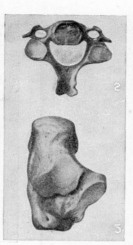

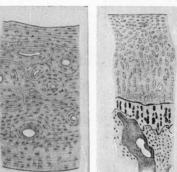

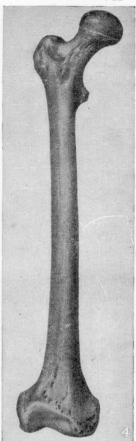

Bone : examples of the four types. 1. Flat
bone (frontal), 2. Irregular (vertebra).
3. Short bone (heel). 4. Long bone (thigh)

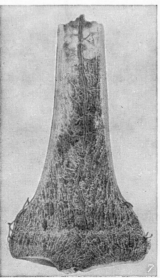

5. Bone sections showing Haversian canals for blood vessels and nerves
surrounded by bone cells in concentric rings. Right, section of cartilage

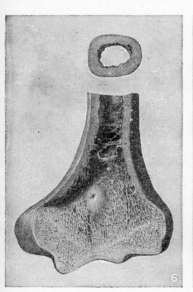

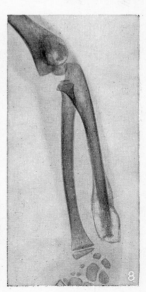

6. The shaft of a long bone is dense, while the extremity is of cancellous tissue, the open spaces containing
red marrow. 7. Details of blood supply. 8. Tuberculous disease of the ulna revealed by X-rays

PLATE VIII

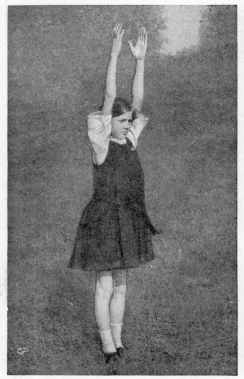

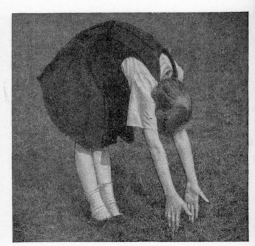

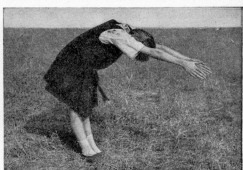

Breathing Exercises. 1. Stand erect, arms above head. 2. Stoop forward, exhaling through the nose. 3. Regain first position while inhaling

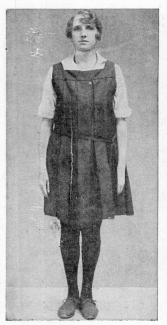

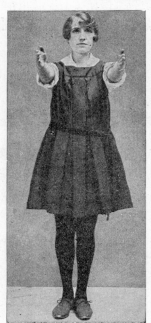

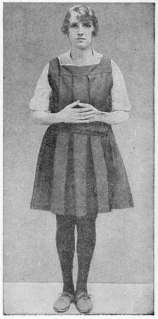

4. With arms hanging at the sides inhale deeply, hold the breath, then exhale. 5. While inhaling raise the arms in front and lower them while exhaling. 6. As in No. 4, but with hands pressing on the ribs

symptoms in general are not very different from those of pneumonia or inflammation of the lungs. There is extreme breathlessness and the breathing is very rapid ; the pulse is quick, there is a cough, the patient's face may become bluish, he is prostrated and has a dirty tongue. The temperature usually runs between 102° and 104° F. ; it may be lower, though a very low temperature is by no means a favourable sign.

Varied Duration of the Disease

The disease may run a rapid course. If it is fatal the patient usually dies within a week, probably from induced bronchopneumonia (*q.v.*) ; otherwise he may be convalescent in about a fortnight. There are other cases in which the disease drags on for weeks.

The treatment of this severe bronchitis is as follows : The patient must be put to bed in a warm room, the temperature of which should be from 60°–65° F. Although the air should be warm and moist, it must always be fresh. This is a most important point.

There can be little doubt that many children who suffer from this disease have been killed by neglect of the importance of ventilation.

The windows should be kept widely open, as there is less draught when they are so than when the opening merely consists of a narrow chink. It is very important to support the patient's strength, for the danger of this disease is that he might die of exhaustion. The diet must be very light, milk and soda-water being the staple. The patient's chest may be wrapped up in a flannel jacket or in what is known as gamgee tissue. Hot fomentations may be applied, consisting of flannel wrung out of very hot water and having perhaps a few drops of turpentine sprinkled upon it ; but the nurse must be very careful to see that the fomentations are light, so as not to interfere with the movements of the chest.

Various stimulants have to be given, such as sal volatile, whisky or brandy. Strychnine may also be employed, as well as digitalis and other heart stimulants.

It may be said that, despite all temptations, no form of opium or morphia should be employed in this disease. The patient's distress may be relieved in other ways which do not entail the serious weakening of his breathing powers which is caused by these drugs.

A most important matter is to attempt to clear out the patient's bronchial tubes, so as to enable him to breathe. When the act of vomiting occurs there also occurs a muscular contraction in the bronchi which causes them to empty themselves of their contents, and this contraction is more efficient than can be obtained in any other way. Hence emetics are constantly of value in the treatment of this disease, especially in the case of children, whose coughing powers are feeble. There is probably no better emetic than mustard, this being not only efficient as an emetic but also stimulating to the heart and to the breathing. A teaspoonful of alum, or a teaspoonful of ipecacuanha wine, repeated if necessary, may also be given, these doses being appropriate for a child.

If the breathing of a child should become suddenly very difficult and be accompanied by increased duskiness of the face, this may be due to collapse of portions of lung. While awaiting the doctor, place the child in a warm bath and sprinkle its body with cold water at short intervals. The object of this is to induce deep breaths.

Likely Victims of Chronic Bronchitis

Chronic bronchitis usually displays itself most markedly in the winter and is often called a winter cough ; it rarely undergoes complete cure, but tends to recur with the cold weather and finally to become permanent. It occurs most commonly in people who have abused alcohol, in the gouty, in cases of Bright's disease, heart disease, and in the very old. In consequence of the constant coughing and the strain on the lungs which it produces, the lungs actually become enlarged, many of the partitions between the little air cells breaking down and the natural elasticity of the lungs being thus reduced. The name emphysema is applied to this condition. The whole chest becomes enlarged and assumes the characteristic shape known as barrel-shaped chest.

It is the remoter consequence of the lung changes that leads usually in the course of years to the death of the patient, for the circulation of the blood through the lungs is interfered with, and this throws a great strain upon the right side of the heart, the business of which it is to force the blood through the lungs. Ultimately the heart breaks down.

The treatment of chronic bronchitis is, in the first place, the treatment of its cause if this is known, for example, alcoholism. If the patient can do so, he will benefit by emigrating to a drier climate such as Canada or Australia, or, if he can, to a warm island climate. He must persistently clothe himself in wool and must especially keep his feet warm. He will certainly prolong his life by breathing through his nose. Typical cough mixtures for chronic bronchitis are as follows :

Carbonate of ammonia ..	60 grains
Compound tincture of camphor	6 drachms
Syrup of Virginia prunes ..	4 ,,
Infusion of senega.. ..	to 6 ounces

A tablespoonful in water thrice daily after food.

Syrup of pix liquida ..	1½ ounces
Liquid extract of liquorice	2 drachms
Compound tincture of cardamom	3 ,,
Glycerin	4 ,,
Chloroform water ..	to 6 ounces

A tablespoonful in a wineglass of water three or four times daily.

These help to relieve cough, but there are two drugs which appear to help the underlying bronchitis ; these are potassium iodide and cod-liver oil.

See Bronchi ; Broncho-pneumonia ; Copaiba ; Dust Disease ; Emphysema ; Influenza ; Inhalation ; Laryngitis ; Lung.

BRONCHITIS KETTLE. In cases of irritability of the air passages, as in bronchitis, croup, and so on, it is advisable to moisten the air which the patient is breathing. For this purpose a bronchitis kettle may be used. It has a long spout somewhat expanded at its outer extremity. In emergencies an ordinary kettle may be used, to the spout of which a tube of cardboard, brown paper, or even ordinary newspaper is attached. This should

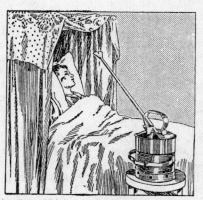

Bronchitis kettle for steam inhalation

be stiffened by having a piece of cane or a thin stick attached to its upper surface.

BRONCHOCELE. A goitre is sometimes spoken of as a bronchocele.

BRONCHO-PNEUMONIA. This disease is closely allied to acute bronchitis affecting the smaller bronchial tubes. Indeed this form of bronchitis usually causes death by means of inducing acute broncho-pneumonia. The compound name is meant to imply that not only the lung tissue but also the bronchi are affected in this disease. The disease must be distinguished from ordinary pneumonia, which usually starts directly in the lung tissues instead of spreading from the bronchi. Ordinary pneumonia is more common in adults ; broncho-pneumonia is the usual pneumonia of children and also of the aged.

The temperature may rise gradually instead of suddenly as in ordinary pneumonia, and the disease may run a longer and more irregular course. The symptoms, the dangers and the treatment are similar to those of acute bronchitis, but it may be noted that this disease may kill by causing a very high temperature. In such a case the fever must be attacked by applying an ice bag to the head and by cold sponging of the patient's skin, or even rubbing the skin gently with blocks of ice.

See Asthma ; Bronchitis ; Pneumonia.

BRONZING. A pigmented or bronzed condition of the skin is met with notably in Addison's disease, but it also occurs in exophthalmic goitre, diabetes, malaria, chronic arsenical poisoning, and other maladies. It occurs as a temporary annoyance in many cases of pregnancy.

BRUISE. Bruises are really wounds of the tissues underneath the skin. The characteristic colour of a bruise, as in a case of a black eye, is due to the blood which has been poured out into the tissues as a result of the injury. The changes in colour which a bruise undergoes are due to the changes in the red colouring matter of the blood as it is gradually absorbed and removed. The blue-black becomes brown and then green and yellow. The treatment consists in the application of cold and pressure at first and massage afterwards. The cold and pressure are of value only at the very first, before the bleeding inside the bruised tissues has stopped. If quickly applied they will often arrest the bleeding and thus limit the extent and duration of the bruise.

Pressure may be made through cloths wrung out of cold, perhaps iced, water, which are frequently changed. Cold should not, however, be long applied in the case of the aged or weakly. In the case of a black eye, care should be taken not to press on the eyeball but on the skin around it which has bone immediately beneath. Afterwards, gentle but firm massage is very useful, aiding in the removal of the blood and the waste products produced by the injury. Vaseline will facilitate the rubbing. At this stage bathing in hot water may relieve pain and reduce swelling. When the swelling has gone down, the disappearance of the discoloration may be hastened by applying compresses wrung out of a lotion composed of one part of surgical spirit to four parts of water, and covering with gutta-percha tissue.

Tincture of arnica has long enjoyed a quite undeserved reputation in the treatment of bruises. Any value it may have is due to the alcohol it contains. Moreover, it is a dangerous remedy if the skin is broken.

BRUIT. The term bruit, which is the French name for noise, is often applied to the abnormal sounds sometimes heard when the heart or a blood vessel is listened to with a stethoscope. The English equivalent of the word is murmur.

See Heart; Murmur.

BUBO. A swelling in the groin due to inflammation of the lymphatic glands is called a bubo. It usually occurs in gonorrhoea, syphilis or plague, but these glands may be inflamed and may suppurate when there is a septic sore anywhere in the region drained by the glands, from the foot upwards. The term is also sometimes applied to enlargements of other groups of lymphatic glands.

BUBONIC PLAGUE. *See* Plague.

BUNION. This very common deformity of the foot is the result of wearing boots or shoes which are too narrow, especially if they are also too short. As a consequence, a bursa forms over the great toe joint, which is liable to become swollen and inflamed. The treatment of bunions is dealt with under the heading Hallux Valgus.

See Bursitis ; Foot.

BURN. The distinction between burns and scalds is simply that the latter are caused by moist heat such as steam ; the injuries produced are the same whether the heat be moist or dry. Burning is a very common accident, and many cases could be prevented by the knowledge and avoidance of certain risks. Young children should never be left alone in a room with an open fireplace or a stove, unless there is an efficient fire guard.

Special care must be taken to keep from contact with naked lights flannelette clothing of any sort ; many children have been burnt from standing in front of a fire in a nightdress of this material.

The delicacy of a young child's skin is such that serious burning may be caused by applying an over-hot poultice. A hot-water bottle which is put into the bed of a patient who is unconscious—for example, one recovering from a general anaesthetic or who has a paralysed limb—should be well covered with flannel and, moreover, it should be placed so that it does not touch any part of the body.

A burn may only cause redness of the skin, or, in addition, blisters. If more severe, the skin may be destroyed partly or wholly ; the soft tissues may be damaged to a considerable depth ; or the bone may actually be charred. In addition, a burn of any severity is likely to be associated with the condition known as shock. It is important to remember that when this is so there may be no complaint of pain.

It is sometimes assumed that a child who has been severely burnt and who lies quiet and still cannot have suffered so much as might be expected. But the absence of crying has really a very grave significance.

Children are much more likely to be affected in this way than are adults, except that in old people the results resemble those seen in children. Burns of the trunk are more likely to be attended with shock than those of the limbs, and large superficial burns rather than deep burns of a smaller surface.

In burns of any severity a doctor should always be summoned. In the meantime, shock may be treated by putting the patient to bed and placing hot-water bottles near him. Stimulants should be given freely, spirits or sal volatile in water, or tea and coffee. Putting a child in a warm bath has at once the effect of relieving shock and of permitting easier removal of the clothing. Great gentleness should be exercised in taking away clothing from the burnt surface, and if, in spite of thorough soaking, it still adheres it is better to cut round the adherent piece. Pain will be much relieved by excluding the air from the burn by certain applications.

Where there is broken skin greasy applications should never be made.

The reason for this is that they may make the subsequent cleansing of the burn much more difficult, so that septic contamination results. The aim in all burns is to keep them free from suppuration. Where, however, there is merely reddening of the skin, carron oil, eucalyptus or zinc ointment, vaseline, cold cream or olive oil may be applied. Powders are also suitable, for example, boracic acid or oxide of zinc. Bicarbonate of soda is a good remedy when made into a thick paste with a little water and spread on thickly. Paraffin preparations of the type of ambrine (*q.v.*) are suitable for this and for severer degrees of burning.

An efficient treatment for burns is spraying with a $2\frac{1}{2}$ per cent. watery solution of tannic acid, or, for the face, an ointment of the same strength. Either preparation is used until the surface is tanned.

Large blisters should be pricked, the best way to do this being described under the heading Blister. The burns are then covered with cloths lightly wrung out of warm boracic solution, and this also applies to the severer degrees. In the case of a limb it may be immersed in a basin of water to which has been added a table-spoonful of boracic acid powder. When a burn has not gone beyond the stage of blistering, there is unlikely to be scarring, but in deeper burns scarring will follow.

If the burn affects surfaces which come into contact, for example, the under surface of the chin and the chest wall, or the back of the leg and of the thigh, these surfaces may adhere, or from the shrinkage of the scar may be drawn together. To defeat this it is necessary to exercise care as to the position of the parts during healing, and the instructions of the doctor in this respect must be scrupulously followed. When the raw surface is very large, healing may be much hastened by skin grafting.

Burns resulting from corrosive fluids are dealt with under the heading Poisoning.

See Ambrine ; Blister ; Carron Oil ; Graft ; Shock ; Skin.

BURSA. A late Latin word meaning purse, the name bursa is given to a little pocket, with a very smooth lining, which is usually closed, but which sometimes communicates with a joint cavity. Bursae occur in various parts of the body where it is necessary to avert the results of friction, and are thus found round most of the joints, such as the knee and elbow. They are liable to inflammation, the commonest cause of which is exposure to undue pressure.

BURSITIS. Inflammation of a bursa is called bursitis. The acute form is indicated by a hot, reddened and painful swelling, the pain being increased on movement of the neighbouring joint. The treatment consists in rest and hot fomentations. Sometimes matter forms within the bursa and must be let out. Chronic bursitis, of which the commonest example is housemaid's knee, results in the bursa becoming distended with fluid. This is also found in a bursa over the elbow in miners and others who lean on their elbows when at work ; and there are other situations.

The form of pressure which is the cause in any particular case must be avoided, and absorption of the fluid may be hastened by painting the skin over the bursa with the stronger tincture of iodine and by applying an elastic bandage. If the fluid persists it may be necessary to withdraw it. The condition may be prevented by using a hollow pad under the knee or the elbow, as the case may be, and varying the part which takes the pressure.

See Joint; Knee.

BUTTER. Containing, as it does, 74 to 90 per cent. of fat, butter is a very important article of diet. It ranks amongst the heat and energy producing foods; hence it is especially valuable in cold weather and in cold climates. Margarine has a composition very similar to that of butter, but that prepared from vegetable fats only does not contain the essential vitamin which is present in butter.

See Food; Vitamin.

BUTTER-MILK. This is the liquid residue formed during the process of butter-making. It is valuable in certain cases of gastritis and albuminuria.

See Lactic Acid; Milk.

BUTYRIC ACID. An acid with a very rancid smell which is formed in butter as it undergoes decomposition is called butyric acid. In certain kinds of indigestion this acid is also formed in the stomach and its presence may be recognized by the characteristic odour which it imparts to the patient's breath.

See Acidity.

CACHEXIA. Derived from Greek words meaning a bad habit, the term cachexia is applied to a condition, characterised by marked wasting and an unhealthy-looking grey or yellow skin, resulting from cancer, consumption, malaria and other diseases.

See Emaciation.

CAECUM. The first part of the large bowel is called the caecum, or literally the blind end. It is 2½ inches long and 3 inches broad, and forms a cul-de-sac below the entrance of the small bowel. The contents of the bowel may stagnate here and undergo marked putrefactive changes. The vermiform appendix leads off from the caecum.

See Appendicitis; Intestine.

CAESARIAN SECTION. The delivery of a child through the abdominal wall of the mother constitutes the operation known as Caesarian section. It becomes necessary when a child cannot be born in the natural way owing to deformity of the pelvis, obstruction of tumours and other causes. It should always be considered, however, in cases where birth by the natural route, although possible, is attended with serious risks to the mother or child, as the operation has a very small mortality when done either before or early in labour.

See Childbirth.

CAFFEINE. The alkaloid caffeine is the active ingredient of tea and coffee and is found in other vegetable preparations. It stimulates the nervous system, the heart and the kidneys. The mental faculties are freshened, and the sense of bodily fatigue is removed or prevented by its use. If taken in too large doses this stimulation expresses itself in nervous and muscular irritability, perhaps to the extent of convulsions and delirium. Caffeine increases the flow of urine, and it is therefore often combined with digitalis for the relief of dropsy.

For some purposes it can be used as it exists in tea or coffee, but the drug is also extracted. It is a crystalline substance with a dose of 1 to 5 grains. There are some preparations made from it, amongst them being caffeine citrate, dose 2 to 10 grains, and effervescing caffeine citrate, 60 to 120 grains. All of these are used for headaches, and a valuable powder for this purpose is one containing 10 grains of phenacetin with 2 grains of caffeine citrate. Caffeine is recommended also for asthma, and 2 to 5 grains of the citrate may be given at bedtime and again during the night.

See Coffee; Tea.

CAISSON DISEASE. This curious disorder may attack men employed in building foundations of bridges under water, or in other work which necessitates breathing an atmosphere of compressed air; hence it is sometimes called compressed air disease, or diver's paralysis. Severe pains may occur in the muscles of the limbs and trunk and are known as the bends. It has been shown that when the person who has been subjected to compressed air returns to an atmosphere of the usual pressure little bubbles of gas escape from their previous state of solution in the blood and so form obstacles to the passage of the blood through the smallest blood vessels, especially those of the nervous system;

hence the symptoms of paralysis and loss of consciousness.

The malady is very rarely fatal. In all probability it may always be avoided by making certain that the transition from the atmosphere of very high pressure to the atmosphere of the usual pressure is a very gradual one, thus allowing time for the excess of gas which, so to speak, has been squeezed into the blood to make a gradual and harmless escape. This is called decompression. When symptoms occur the patient is slowly put back under high pressure and then gradually " decompressed."

CAJUPUT OIL. A strong-smelling volatile or essential oil, cajuput is obtained from the leaves of a plant that grows in Singapore. Taken internally it acts as a carminative and antispasmodic, the dose being 1 to 3 minims. It is frequently used externally as a liniment mixed with two parts of olive oil, to relieve rheumatic and other pains.

See Oil.

CALABAR BEAN. The seeds of this tropical plant yield an active principle called physostigmine or eserine. This is a very powerful poison when administered in large doses, but in minute doses is of great value to the oculist. It contracts the pupil and lowers the tension within the eye : hence it is a valuable remedy in glaucoma (*q.v.*).

CALAMINE. The natural carbonate of zinc, known as calamine, after suitable preparation forms a smooth powder which is used in medicine as a local sedative and astringent. It may be used as an ointment, for example, 2 drachms of prepared calamine in an ounce of vaseline, or suspended in water as a lotion which is allowed to dry on.

See Zinc.

CALCIUM. The chloride of calcium, dose 5 to 15 grains, and the lactate, dose 10 to 30 grains, increase the coagulability of the blood and hence are often used for the arrest of bleeding. They are also good remedies for chilblains and for nettlerash. Calcium hypophosphate, dose 3 to 10 grains ; calcium phosphate, dose 5 to 15 grains ; and the syrup of calcium lactophosphate, dose ½ to 1 drachm, are used as tonics for general debility. Lime

is the oxide of calcium, and as slaked lime is used to prepare lime water. When this is added to milk it increases its digestibility. Lime water corrects acidity of the stomach and helps to check looseness of the bowels. It is often added to a baby's bottle feed. The dose for an adult is 1 to 4 ounces, and for an infant ½ to 1 teaspoonful. Outwardly it has an astringent action, and enters into lotions for eczema, etc. Mixed with equal parts of linseed or olive oil it is known as carron oil (*q.v.*), and is used as a remedy for burns. It is contained also in the black and the yellow mercurial washes.

See Chalk ; Chloride of Lime ; Mercury.

CALCULUS. The term calculus, literally a little stone, is applied to concretions of various kinds found in canals of the body. As might be expected, they tend to form specially in cavities which act as reservoirs, such as the gall bladder, the urinary bladder or the pelvis of the kidney. The materials of which they are composed come from the fluids in which they form, but usually there is a central nucleus consisting of dried mucus, blood clot or a small foreign body. A calculus may give rise to no symptoms till it begins to pass out from the cavity in which it has formed, when it may cause very severe pain, as in biliary and renal colic. Should the calculus become impacted or stuck in the tube down which it is passing there may be an accumulation of the secretion concerned behind the obstruction.

See Bladder ; Colic ; Gall-stone ; Kidney.

CALF'S FOOT JELLY. When an invalid is allowed an addition to milk diet, calf's foot jelly makes a pleasant change. It has only a partial food value, but is useful when taken as part of a mixed diet. It may be made as follows : Take two calf's feet, wash them thoroughly and divide into pieces. Put into a saucepan with 5 pints of cold water, bring to the boil and boil gently for six or seven hours. Strain into a basin, and when cold remove all fat from the top. The flavouring of calf's foot jelly must depend on the patient's taste, but a pleasant jelly, palatable to most, is made as follows : Take 1 quart of the jellied stock and put it into a deep saucepan with the grated rind of 3 lemons, 1 inch of cinnamon stick,

2 cloves, ½ pint of sherry, a small tea-cupful of lemon juice, 6 ounces of loaf sugar and the stiffly beaten whites and crushed shells of 2 eggs. Whisk vigorously until boiling, then simmer slowly for ten minutes. Strain through a jelly-bag and pour into moulds or glasses.

See Invalid Cookery.

CALLUS. During the process of the healing of a broken bone, new bone, or callus, is formed to repair the damage which has been caused. As a rule in a healthy person more callus than is neces-sary is formed, and after a few weeks the superfluous part is absorbed and dis-appears. But if the ends of the broken bone are not brought together, or if they are not kept at rest, a very considerable amount of callus is formed, and thick-ening at the site of the fracture may persist for a long time.

See Fracture.

CALOMEL. The subchloride of mer-cury, or calomel, is a white, almost taste-less powder which is taken most frequently as a purgative, though it has other im-portant uses.

See Mercury.

CALUMBA. The dried root of calumba is imported from East Africa in roughly disk-shaped pieces and is of value in medicine as a bitter (*q.v.*). It is used in the form of the infusion, which is made with cold water, dose ½ to 1 ounce, and the tincture, dose ½ to 1 drachm. Like quassia, it does not contain tannin, and thus does not become inky when mixed with preparations of iron. It stimulates the appetite and digestion, but its use must not be continued too long or a state of gastric irritation may result.

CAMOMILE. Tea made from the dried flowerheads of camomile is used as a remedy for coughs and for infantile colic. It also acts as a digestive tonic. A break-fastcupful of boiling water is poured over about a dozen of the flowerheads and set by the side of the fire to infuse for 10 or 15 minutes. The infusion is then strained, sweetened and served hot. The infusion of anthemis, obtained from a chemist, corresponds to this and has a dose of 1 to 4 ounces. The alleged virtues of a camomile poultice are probably to be ascribed entirely to the heat.

CAMPHOR. Camphor is obtained from the wood of an Asiatic tree and occurs as tough crystals with a pungent taste. Its common preparations are camphor water, dose ½ to 2 ounces ; spirit of camphor, dose 5 to 20 minims ; compound tincture of camphor (paregoric), dose ½ to 1 drachm ; liniment of camphor (camphor-ated oil) ; and the ammoniated liniment.

When rubbed on the skin it causes redness and so acts as a counter-irritant. The ammoniated camphor liniment is used for chronic rheumatism, sprains and similar conditions. Camphorated oil is a useful liniment for rubbing on the chest in the bronchial complaints of children. Chaps are often treated by rubbing the skin with a camphor ball. Equal parts of camphor and of chloral when ground up together form a liquid which may be rubbed over the painful spots in neuralgia. Camphor helps to relieve itching, and may be used in a lotion such as the following :

Prepared calamine	..	1 drachm
Glycerin ..	..	1 ,,
Camphor water	..	1 ounce

To be well shaken up before applying.

The following ointment acts similarly :

Zinc oxide powder ..	..	1 drachm
Camphor powder ..	..	1 ,,
Vaseline ..	..	1 ounce

A mixture of camphor and carbolic acid if applied to a decayed tooth may relieve toothache arising from it. Camphor is sometimes used to check an oncoming cold. An adult may take 10 minims of the spirit of camphor on a lump of sugar. Paregoric, which, it should be remembered, contains opium, is a common constituent of cough mixtures, and it is also useful for colic. Here the camphor acts as a carmina-tive, relieving flatulence.

In small doses camphor acts as a heart stimulant and is used in pneumonia, enteric fever and other diseases. A solu-tion in sterilised oil for hypodermic in-jection is the preparation usually employed in these cases. Camphorated chalk is a popular tooth powder. Camphor in vaseline is sometimes sniffed up the nose to clean it, but this should never be used for infants, as collapse may occur.

Poisoning by Camphor. In excessive doses camphor produces giddiness and a kind of intoxication. This may be followed by convulsions and unconsciousness. In cases of poisoning an emetic should be given and then strong tea or coffee, and water may be given freely. Hot fomentations should be applied over the heart, and hot-water bottles put at the feet and by the sides. If unconscious, half a pint of strong coffee may be injected into the bowel.

CANCER. Any malignant tumour may be described as cancer, whether it be a sarcoma or a carcinoma, but nowadays it is almost invariably the latter which is meant when the word cancer is used. In this sense cancer is a tumour beginning in, and consisting of, epithelial cells. These are cells which cover the skin and mucous membranes, form glands and occur in other situations in the body. The cancer cells resemble those from which they are derived ; on the skin, for example, they are flat, in the breast spheroidal and in the bowel columnar, being also arranged in imitation of the glandular structure of the bowel lining.

Cancer cells are altered somewhat in appearance and size from the original cells, however, and they have the further important peculiarity that they invade the normal tissues by which they are

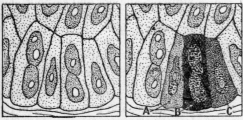

Cancer development. Left, diagram of normal epithelial cells. Right, same group : A and C, cells in precancerous state ; B, cancerous cell

surrounded and gradually replace them. This is one of the marks of malignancy distinguishing a cancer, say, from a simple fatty tumour. Another mark is that the cancer cells proceed along the lymphatics to lymphatic glands, and either from these, or through blood vessels in the tumour itself, make their way into the blood stream, reach in this way the liver or the heart, and from the heart may be sent to any part of the body. This dissemination of a malignant tumour to distant parts is known as metastasis.

The secondary growths are always composed of the same kind of cells as the original growth, so that if the latter is in the bowel and a secondary growth occurs in the liver this will have the appearances of a bowel cancer, whereas, if the original growth were in the skin the liver tumour would be a flat-celled epithelioma. Nor does the resemblance stop at the cancer cells, but even the stroma, or connective tissue framework in which the cells lie, is imitated.

Cancers vary very much in the amount of connective tissue which they contain. One which is found in the breast, the stomach and other organs contains a very considerable amount of connective tissue and is called a scirrhus, the literal meaning of this word being hard. The relative rate of growth of a scirrhus is slow. Where, on the other hand, the proportion of cells is very high, as in the soft or medullary cancer, growth is rapid. A form of skin epithelioma, known as a rodent ulcer, grows generally about the edge of the orbit and the side of the nose. It does not become disseminated, though, if untreated, it tends to eat deeply through the soft tissues and bone.

It has been pointed out that cancer cells resemble the epithelial cells among which they first begin to grow, and that this resemblance applies equally to secondary growths, perhaps far distant from the parent growth. As a fact, cancer cells are derived from, and pertain to, the epithelial cells, among which they grow, but they differ from normal cells in that they have acquired an independent existence. They have ceased to belong to the commonwealth of cells which constitutes the body, and now act as rebels or predatory aliens.

In producing this change in the nature of the cells there are probably two factors, whether the new growth be a sarcoma or a carcinoma. The first is the presence of some exciting agent, the nature of which is still under discussion.

The second factor is some change in the body cells which makes them susceptible to invasion by the virus. This may be induced in various ways ; in carcinoma it is due, in most cases, to chronic irritation. Chimney sweeps, working among soot, paraffin workers, and those who have to handle tar and pitch, often exhibit signs of irritation and often have cancer of the skin. A cancer of the tongue is often found associated with a jagged tooth or in men who smoke pipes with short, rough stems; in the latter circumstance the growth may be on the lip.

An epithelioma not infrequently forms on the site of old skin trouble due to syphilis and lupus. There is reason to believe that cancer of the breast and of the womb has followed chronic inflammation of these organs. There are grounds also for believing that cancer of the stomach may occur in those who take their food very hot, especially liquids. It is notoriously apt to occur on skin which has been badly burnt with X-rays or radium emanations.

Instances of the direct association of cancer with some irritant could be multiplied, and significance is impressed on such association by the fact that cancer may be artificially produced on mice by long-continued application of tar. These experiments have also shown that different species of animals vary in their susceptibility towards cancer produced by irritants, and that individuals belonging to the same species also vary. This is of importance in connexion with the question of cancer inheritance.

The disease is not inherited; though a susceptibility to develop it in certain circumstances may be transmitted. But such an inheritance must play a relatively small part in producing the disease and need not be seriously considered.

It has also been shown that young mice and old mice are equally susceptible, and it is suggested that the reason why cancer affects older people rather than younger is probably really a matter of the length of time during which irritation operates.

So much for the predisposing factor in the development of carcinoma. The rôle of a virus as the exciting factor has been enunciated by Dr. Gye as a result of his researches on a malignant tumour of fowls, the so-called Rous tumour, which is a sarcoma.

Gye's conclusions have been seriously shaken by Murphy, also working with the Rous sarcoma, who has produced cogent evidence of the exciting agent being of the nature of a ferment, formed within the body and not, like Gye's virus, introduced from without. It must be borne in mind, of course, that however this question is finally settled, it has still to be shown that what applies to these tumours in fowls is applicable to tumours in human beings.

In any case, it can be said that there is no reliable evidence of cancer being an infectious disease.

Cancer in human beings may manifest itself in various forms. It may be a lump felt in the breast or the stomach. It may appear on a skin or mucous surface as a wart, or as a thickening beneath and around a sore or fissure. When it is near the surface it readily ulcerates. Irregular bleeding occurring in a woman after the age of 40 or thereabouts, and notably the supposed irregular return of the courses after they have apparently ceased altogether, are extremely suspicious symptoms of the beginning of cancer of the womb, and a doctor should always be consulted at once.

Cancer sooner or later causes deterioration of the general health. At the beginning worry probably plays a part, but later on there are bleeding, pain and interference with the functions of important organs by the primary or the secondary growths.

It must be emphasised that while pain may be severe in the later stages, it is not a common early symptom, and it may be disastrous if, for example, a lump in the breast is assumed to be free from suspicion of cancer simply because it is painless.

Cancer is not common before 35 years of age, but it may occur. It is more common in women than in men on account of the frequency with which the womb and the breast are affected. In men the most common sites are the stomach, the lower lip and the rectum. The disease would appear to be on the increase, though allowance must always be made for increased accuracy of diagnosis and for the increased number who reach an age when cancer is likely to develop.

In dealing with the probable causes of the disease, the rôle played by some kind of irritation has been emphasised.

If people can be brought to realize the dangers lurking in certain substances with which they come into contact at work, and in certain personal habits, they at least know how a great deal of cancer could be avoided.

Chronic inflammation or irritation anywhere about the body should be cleared up if possible. If a lump, an ulcer, bleeding, or other possible signs of cancer develop, medical advice should be sought at once. An operation done in the early stages of the disease offers an excellent prospect of cure; an operation when the disease is thoroughly established, little or none.

Rodent ulcers can generally be cured by X-rays or radium, but in other forms of cancer this kind of treatment should be restricted to cases which have unfortunately passed beyond the reach of operation. In some of these cases treatment by rays may make an operation possible. In any case, much comfort may be derived in inoperable cases from their use. A considerable number of inoperable cases of cancer have been treated with injections of colloidal preparations of lead, and cures have been claimed.

See Dermatitis; Radium; Rodent Ulcer; Sarcoma; Tissue; Tumour.

CANCRUM ORIS. A very acute and dangerous affection of the cheek known as cancrum oris sometimes attacks very weak children as a complication of measles; it may also be witnessed in other people. Want and insanitary surroundings are contributory causes. Its essence is a form of mortification or local death which may attack the whole thickness of the cheek; it is due to some specially poisonous kind of microbe, and must be treated by the surgeon with the utmost promptness and energy. The only hope of saving the child's life is by early surgical operation.

CANNABIS INDICA. This is the name of a drug sometimes called Indian hemp. It is generally given in medicine in the form of an extract or of a tincture, and is used for neuralgia, menorrhagia, pruritis and other conditions. It is largely taken in India as an intoxicant, being made into preparations of various names, such as bhang, haschisch and ganga.

CANTHARIDES. A drug which consists of the dried and powdered bodies of a beetle known as the Spanish Fly is technically called cantharides. It contains a substance called cantharidin, which is a very powerful irritant. A large number of preparations of this drug are used for external application, and the tincture, which must be used with great caution and never in doses of more than 5 drops, is occasionally given internally. The chief use of the drug is to produce blisters for counter-irritation. Preparations for this purpose are cantharidin plaster, blistering fluid, cantharidin ointment and tincture of cantharidin. A pomade made up of 1 part of cantharidin ointment and 2 parts of soft paraffin is recommended for improving the growth of hair.

Poisoning by Cantharides. Poisoning may follow improper administration of the drug. The symptoms are those of intense irritation of the alimentary canal and the kidneys. Treatment demands medical aid, but may be begun before the doctor arrives by putting the patient to bed, keeping him warm, and giving him large quantities of simple soothing drinks such as water and barley water, in order to dilute the poison and thus weaken its irritant action. Since this drug has a special tendency to irritate the kidneys, it must never be given internally, save when those organs are known to be healthy; furthermore, since the drug is readily absorbed from the skin, it must never be used even externally without previous medical examination of the state of the kidneys. Nor must it be ever applied to a part of the body on which the patient lies, nor to paralysed limbs. In treating children, the aged and all weakly people, cantharides should not be used at all.

See Blister; Counter-irritation.

CAPILLARY. The minute blood vessels which continue the circulation between the smallest arteries and the smallest veins are called capillaries. The name is derived from a Latin word meaning a hair. They cannot be seen with the naked eye.

See Circulation of the Blood.

CAPSICUM. The pods of the capsicum plant are used to make cayenne pepper and certain medicinal preparations. When taken inwardly capsicum stimulates the flow of gastric juice and relieves flatulence; hence its use as a condiment, as a digestive stimulant in certain diseases, notably dipsomania, and its frequent inclusion in purgative pills where it is intended to prevent griping. When rubbed on the skin it has a stimulant effect, and so is used as a counter-irritant. Chilblains, provided that the skin is not broken, will benefit from being rubbed once daily with capsicum ointment or the B.P.C. stronger tincture. The ointment is popularly known as chilli paste and, with the liniment of capsicum, is a favourite remedy for lumbago and muscular pains elsewhere. Capsicum wool and capsicum gamgee tissue are used as applications for chest complaints and act like thermogene.

CARAWAY. This is the name of a very harmless drug with a pleasant odour, which is the fruit of the caraway plant. This yields an essential oil which is used for flavouring medicines, and as a means of soothing an irritable stomach or bowel. Caraway water may be taken in a mixture, or the oil of caraway, dose $\frac{1}{2}$ to 3 minims, on sugar.

CARBOHYDRATE. This large and very important group of substances owes its name to the fact that they consist of carbon and of hydrogen and oxygen, the last two being in the proportions in which they occur in water. Their importance lies in the fact that they are most valuable foodstuffs owing to the carbon they contain, which is capable of being burnt up in the body, thus producing heat and energy. It follows that the proportion of them in the food should vary, strictly speaking, with the temperature, much less being needed in summer than in winter, and with the amount of physical exertion undergone by the individual. But it may be stated that about a pound of carbohydrates each day represents a suitable average amount for an adult of average weight and energy.

The chief carbohydrate foods are all the forms of sugar (cane sugar, grape sugar, milk sugar) and starch. The substance called cellulose belongs to this class and can be digested by such animals as the ox, but is absolutely indigestible by man. This is a matter of practical importance; for example, a potato consists practically of an enormous number of minute cells of starch, each of these cells

30 Grams taken as equal to 1 ounce		Proportion of Carbohydrates in one ounce of food shown shaded 10 grams / 20 / 30	
Cereals	Wheat (flour)		20
	Oatmeal		18
	Barley (pearl)		21
	Maize		22
	Rice		22
Meats	Beef	Nil	
	Mutton	Nil	
	Bacon	Nil	
	Poultry	Nil	
Dairy Foods	Milk		1¼
	Cheese (cheddar)		1
	Butter	Nil	
	Eggs	Nil	
Vegetables	Potatoes (raw)		5
	Onions		3
	Dried Peas		3
	Green Peas		5
	Dried Beans		17
	Green Vegetables		1½
	Refined Sugar		
	Fish	Nil	

White Spaces represent Proteins & Fats and mineral matter

Carbohydrate value of certain foodstuffs

being enclosed in a wall of cellulose. Hence we cannot digest uncooked potatoes. The effect of the cooking is to burst the cellulose envelopes, and thus enable the digestive juices to reach the starch which is inside them.

While carbohydrates are capable of forming fat, they do not act otherwise as tissue builders. For this proteins are required. On the other hand, these can replace carbohydrates and fats as a source of heat and energy; but their use for these purposes is not economical.

See Diet; Food; Starch; Sugar.

CARBOLIC ACID. Phenol or carbolic acid is obtained from coal tar. The pure acid may be obtained in the form of crystals or as a thick liquid. This has a marked caustic action upon the tissues, and is only employed by the surgeon with the utmost caution when he desires completely to destroy the microbes in some small area of tissue. The common form in which the drug is employed is as a 5 per cent. solution in water. This is diluted in various degrees according to the purpose required.

For the treatment of wounds, ulcers or burns at home the 5 per cent. solution should have at least its own quantity of water added to it. This is used as a lotion, and then a piece of lint or gauze wrung out of the solution is applied as a dressing. If the dressing is covered with what is called oil-skin, or oil-silk, or gutta-percha tissue, or anything that can prevent the carbolic acid from travelling outwards, a weaker solution is used, say, 1 in 60. The oil-silk must be applied so as to overlap the dressing at all points.

A 1 in 100 solution is often used as a gargle for sore throat, and the same strength is a useful application for the relief of itching of the skin.

Poisoning by Carbolic Acid. It must never be forgotten that carbolic acid is highly poisonous ; there are several cases on record of its having caused death by absorption from a large surface of skin to which it had been applied as a surgical dressing. Thus the drug is a poison in quite a special sense as compared with ordinary corrosive acids. These kill by means of their local destructive action upon the tissues with which they come in contact ; but carbolic acid will readily kill by means of its action on the nervous system without having caused the slightest local injury or irritation anywhere. In this respect it resembles oxalic acid.

In poisoning by carbolic acid much may be done before the doctor arrives. When, as is usually the case, the acid has been swallowed in concentrated form, there are two distinct dangers to meet : first, the local action of the acid ; secondly, its effect upon the brain after it has been absorbed into the blood. Each of these dangers is to be met by corresponding treatment. The patient must be put to bed and kept warm. His stomach must be emptied, if possible, by means of a stomach tube or the application of a feather to the throat. White of egg may be swallowed in the hope that it will protect the surface of the stomach, but there are two proper antidotes. The first of these is chalk—plaster scraped off the walls may do—and the second is any kind of sulphate, such as Epsom salts. These substances combine with the carbolic acid and render it harmless.

The early signs of nervous poisoning by carbolic acid consist of deafness, noises in the ears, giddiness, stupidity and sickness. These symptoms will arouse the attention of anyone acquainted with them when they are exhibited by a patient who is being treated with carbolic acid either internally or externally. The urine becomes very dark, and any indication of this sort should be met by the instant administration of Epsom salts.

See Poisoning.

CARBONIC ACID. The commonest compound of carbon and oxygen, carbonic acid is formed during the process of breathing by combustion, fermentation and putrefaction. It must necessarily escape from the body if life is to go on. Living continuously in an atmosphere containing an excess of carbonic acid results in a greater or less degree of ill-health expressed by loss of appetite, headache, lack of energy or indigestion. The atmosphere constantly contains about 4 to 6 parts of carbonic acid in 10,000, and the second figure represents the proper limit, beyond which the proportion of carbonic acid should never go, if perfect health is to be expected.

It has been shown, however, that the importance of the carbonic acid gas index in air is ordinarily only as a measure of the efficiency of the ventilation, and that it is the loss of the stimulating effects of the circulating air that is responsible for the headache, malaise, etc., formerly attributed to poisoning by the gas. The deliberate increase of this gas in the inspired air is sometimes used to stimulate the respiratory centre, and opium poisoning and other conditions have been successfully treated in this way.

When taken by the mouth in a state of solution in aerated waters, carbonic acid increases the palatability of the waters and imparts a sharpness which has a stimulating effect. In a good many states of the stomach and bowel soda and potash waters, which owe most of their properties to carbonic acid, act as sedatives, relieving pain and irritation and promoting recovery.

Carbonic acid is a poison producing a loss of sensibility and asphyxia. Hence, when the vital powers are failing and death approaches, carbonic acid accumulates in the body. Thus it comes about that unconsciousness precedes death, and is ushered in by a drowsy state, in which the patient is quite peaceful. People who have gone to sleep near lime kilns or in rooms heated by charcoal braziers and not well ventilated, or having otherwise breathed air heavily charged with carbonic acid, suffer from asphyxia.

Carbonic acid solidified by cold and pressure is known as carbonic acid snow, and is used in the treatment of warts, birthmarks, lupus and other skin diseases. It acts by freezing and killing the tissues to which it is applied.

See Asphyxia ; Ventilation.

CARBON MONOXIDE. When combustion takes place in a limited supply of air, for example, in an anthracite stove, instead of carbonic acid there may be produced carbon monoxide. This gas, which is very poisonous, is also found in coal gas and in water gas. Its existence is one of the dangers attaching to the use of a geyser in a bathroom. It differs from carbonic acid in this way, that in poisoning by these gases the patient who has inhaled carbonic acid can generally have his blood easily cleared of the gas by artificial respiration, but when carbon monoxide has been inhaled it may be extremely difficult to do this on acount of the gas forming a compound with the colouring matter of the blood, from which it does not readily separate.

People who are inhaling carbon monoxide may suffer from headache, nausea, giddiness and a sense of profound weakness. Later there may be convulsions, followed by unconsciousness.

When it is discovered that a room occupied by any person contains coal gas, the window should be at once thrown up or have a pane knocked out, and the gas should be turned off. The person, if unconscious, is then carried or dragged into the fresh air, tight clothing is loosened, and, if breathing has ceased, the mouth and throat are examined to ensure their being clear, and artificial respiration is started forthwith. A doctor should be summoned without delay. Inhalation of oxygen gas is one of the best methods of treatment.

Those who carry out the rescue should cover their mouths and nostrils with damp towels to avoid inhalation of the fumes, or the breath must be held while in the room. On no account should a naked light be used.

See Artificial Respiration ; Asphyxia ; Oxygen.

CARBUNCLE. This is a name applied to a very painful and sometimes dangerous affection, which may best be described as a multiple or compound boil. As in the case of boils, carbuncles are most apt to occur in persons who suffer from some constitutional weakness, or in those who have actual disease, such as Bright's disease or diabetes. Its occurrence is usually later in life than that of boils.

The commonest site of the carbuncle is in the nape of the neck, after that the shoulders and the face. A painful, hard lump is felt beneath the skin, which becomes red or purple in colour. The lump soon softens and the skin gives way at several places, and through these openings the core of the carbuncle is seen as a greyish-white slough. The local inflammation of the skin and the structures immediately beneath it is accompanied by severe general disturbance, due to the absorption of poisons produced by the microbes in the carbuncle. The slough is gradually separated, but the process causes great exhaustion to the patient, and from this exhaustion, or more actual poisoning, death often follows.

The treatment of a carbuncle must be prompt and energetic. It must be freely excised to expose the slough. This may be treated with pure carbolic acid or another strong antiseptic. Afterwards antiseptic fomentations may be used to assist the separation of the slough. In addition to these vigorous local measures, it is necessary to take every step to support the strength of the patient by a generous diet, alcoholic stimulants and tonics such as, for example, Easton's syrup, in teaspoonful doses thrice daily. The bowels must be freely opened. The flowers of sulphur, 20 grains, given with marmalade, or sulphur lozenges, may be given thrice daily, as sulphur appears to be a good remedy.

See Boil.

CARCINOMA. *See* Cancer.

CARDAMOM. The seeds of the cardamom plant found in Malabar contain an essential oil, which has a very pleasant odour and taste. The compound tincture of cardamom is often used for flavouring other medicines and also as a carminative (*q.v*). The dose is $\frac{1}{2}$ to 1 drachm.

CARDIAC. This adjective describes anything that has to do with the heart, for instance, cardiac murmur, cardiac stimulant, and so on.

CARIES. The literal meaning of the term caries is decay, and it is used to describe a process which affects only bones or teeth, in which these structures are gradually destroyed. In bone the hard substance is replaced by granulation tissue (*q.v.*), and the cause may be inflammation due sometimes to septic microbes, to tuberculosis, or to syphilis. If due to septic microbes there is always a discharge of matter or pus.

Dental caries is different from that occurring in bone, and consists in the dissolving out of the earth salts in the tooth substance by acids formed in the mouth.

See Bone ; Necrosis ; Teeth.

CARMINATIVE. Drugs which dispel flatulence and relieve colic are carminatives. They act by stimulating and regulating the movements of the stomach and bowels. Alcohol, ether, and even water have this effect, but the principal remedies of this class are the aromatics, or substances which contain a fragrant or pungent volatile oil. Examples of these are allspice, cloves, cinnamon, cascarilla, bitter orange, dill, anise and peppermint. For babies a teaspoonful of dill water is often used, and for adults a wineglassful of peppermint water. In either case the addition of a little bicarbonate of soda is an advantage, and the combination is supplied in a convenient form in soda-mint tablets.

See Flatulence ; Indigestion ; Oil.

CAROTID. The great artery on each side of the neck is called the carotid. In the first part of its course upwards it is called the common carotid, but later, at about the level of the Adam's apple, it divides into two arteries, called the external and internal carotids, one of which supplies the scalp and the face and other structures outside the skull, whilst the other is the great artery which supplies the half of the brain on its own side of the body.

See Artery ; Circulation of the Blood.

CARRIER. It is often found that certain people have in their bodies virulent disease organisms which, if they are communicated to other people, produce their respective diseases. A person who harbours disease germs in this way is

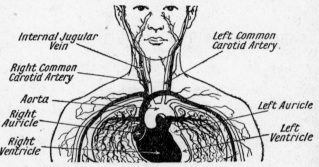

Internal Jugular Vein

Right Common Carotid Artery

Aorta

Right Auricle

Right Ventricle

Left Common Carotid Artery

Left Auricle

Left Ventricle

Carotid arteries, supplying blood to the face and to the brain

called a carrier of the particular disease. He may not himself have suffered from the disease ; on the other hand, he may have had either an unmistakable attack, or one so slight that its existence was not noticed. Some people harbour the germs of diphtheria or of cerebro-spinal fever in their throats ; others pass the germs of enteric fever or of dysentery in their stools. When these and other infectious disorders occur, the question of the existence of a carrier always arises and investigations are made accordingly.

See Contagion ; Infectious Disease.

CARRON OIL. This remedy, which owes its name to its having been introduced at the Carron Iron Works in Scotland, is still very popular in the treatment of burns. It consists of linseed or olive oil and lime water in equal parts. It is liable to become infected with germs, and therefore to be dangerous when the skin is broken. The addition of about 2 per cent. of carbolic acid, which also helps to relieve pain, or of eucalyptus oil, 1 part in 8, makes it more reliable, but even then it is only suitable if the skin is unbroken, as the application of any oily or greasy preparation to a raw surface caused by a burn interferes greatly with the cleansing of the wound.

See Burn.

CARTILAGE. This tissue, which is popularly known as gristle, is found in various parts of the body, such as the larynx, which consists entirely of a number of cartilages. The ends of the ribs next the breast-bone are also made of cartilage. The larger number of the bones of the body were originally cartilaginous, or gristly. But besides these instances of cartilage there is another kind, called articular cartilage, which is of the first importance in the formation of movable joints. Whereever a bone is jointed with another bone the surfaces of the two bones which are to move upon one another are covered with a smooth portion of articular cartilage.

In disease of joints due to tuberculosis the invasion of the articular cartilage by the microbes is usually signalised by the occurrence of what are called starting pains at night, the patient being roused by a pain in the joints just as he is dropping off to sleep. These cartilages are very sensitive, and when they become eroded in the course of the disease they greatly resent pressure; it is this which wakes the patient just when his limbs are moved by the complete relaxation which accompanies the beginning of sleep.

See Bone; Epiphysis; Joint; Ossification; Tissue.

CASCARA SAGRADA. The drug known as cascara sagrada, literally "sacred bark," is obtained from the bark of the Californian buckthorn. It is a bitter substance which stimulates the movements of the bowels and also removes flatulence. The common preparations are the dried extract, dose 2 to 8 grains, the liquid extract, ½ to 1 drachm, and the aromatic syrup of cascara, ½ to 2 drachms. It is one of the few purgative remedies which does not require to be given in increasing doses in order to maintain its effect, and so is eminently suitable in treating chronic constipation.

As the dose appropriate for different people varies somewhat, it should first be ascertained in an individual case how much is required to produce an easy action of the bowels. This is taken each day, either a single dose in the evening or a smaller dose thrice daily, for ten days or a fortnight, and then the dose is gradually diminished. The dried extract can be taken in pills or tablets. To cover the taste of the liquid extract it may be mixed with an equal part of liquid extract of liquorice, when it will often be found that half the ordinary dose of cascara will suffice; a little tincture of orange is then added and the whole is taken in a wineglassful of chloroform water. The aromatic syrup is a good preparation to use for children, 10 drops being usually enough for a baby.

See Aperient; Cathartic; Constipation.

CASCARILLA. From dried cascarilla bark two preparations are obtained: the infusion, dose ½ to 1 ounce; and the tincture, ½ to 1 drachm. The former has the drawback that it does not keep well, especially in warm weather. The drug is an aromatic bitter which has a deserved reputation as a means of promoting appetite and digestion, particularly during recovery from acute illnesses.

The following prescription will be found useful for these purposes:

Tincture of cascarilla	..	6 drachms
Tincture of orange	..	3 ,,
Glycerin ..	..	4 ,,
Orange-flower water		to 6 ounces

Take a tablespoonful thrice daily before food in a wineglass of water.

CASEATION. This term, from the Latin casea, meaning a cheese, is applied to the cheese-like change which occurs in many parts of the body when these are attacked by tuberculosis.

CASEIN. The most important protein constituent of milk is known as casein. In milk in its original state casein is not present as such, but occurs in a fluid form, caseinogen, which is transformed into a solid so soon as the milk is subjected to the action of the juices of the stomach. This is due to the action of hydrochloric acid or of rennet. Much depends upon the way in which the casein is formed in the stomach, since, if the curd be light, flaky and loose, it is easily digested, whereas if it is a solid, dense mass the digestive juices are scarcely able to attack it.

In the case of an adult with strong, healthy digestion this may matter little ; he may be quite well able to drink off a tumbler of milk and digest it successfully. But in the case of a child, or an adult with weak digestion, some sort of precaution must be taken in order to render the milk fit for treatment by the gastric juices. The proper way to take milk, however, is to sip it. One way of obtaining a light, flaky curd is to dilute milk with soda water. For a baby which is being fed on cow's milk the best substance for diluting milk is lime water.

See Milk ; Whey.

CASTOR OIL. The castor oil plant is a native of India, but is grown in many parts of the world. The oil is obtained from the seeds, and it is now usually extracted without the aid of heat ; when obtained by the latter method the oil is dark in colour and has a very disagreeable taste. Castor oil is a very efficient laxative : it does not cause griping, it is certain in its action, and it clears the whole length of the bowel. It is an old cure for diarrhoea due to the presence of irritating materials in the bowel. One or two tablespoonsful are given, and may be combined with 10 to 15 drops of laudanum.

It is, perhaps, the best opening medicine for pregnant women, and, if necessary, a teaspoonful or more may be taken each night. It is also the most reliable remedy for children ; 15 drops may be given to an infant, and larger doses for increasing ages. It is well suited to those who suffer from piles or other painful conditions in the lower part of the bowel. Its use, however, is mainly for temporary constipation, and when this condition is chronic cascara is preferable. The drug may be taken in the B.P. mixture of castor oil, the dose of which is 1 to 4 tablespoonsful.

There are several methods of taking castor oil so as to minimise its nauseousness. It may be taken with hot milk, or with an equal amount of glycerin, when half the intended dose of the oil will suffice, or it may be floated on peppermint water and then covered with a little brandy. It is also obtainable in capsules.

A drop of the warmed oil is a grateful application to the eye after the extraction of an irritating foreign body. Castor oil is often an ingredient of hair lotions, when it is mixed with spirit.

See Aperient ; Cathartic ; Constipation.

CATALEPSY. The extraordinary disorder of the nervous system known as catalepsy is very rarely witnessed, but is absolutely unmistakable to the expert eye. In catalepsy the patient—most frequently a young girl—is in a peculiar state of half-consciousness. She is quite unaffected by such things as a pinprick ; she has lost her identity. There are no convulsions of the usual kind, but, in whatever position the patient is placed, there she will remain ; the fingers may be placed at different angles, the arm held up in the air ; minutes pass before the limb, so placed, gradually sinks down under the action of gravitation.

Recognition of this disease is simple, the only exception being a very important one. It is a fact that severe and prolonged states of catalepsy have sometimes been mistaken for death. There are numerous differences, which can only be revealed by close examination. For instance, the breathing in catalepsy is so shallow, and the beating of the heart so weak, that evidence of the continuance of these functions has to be looked for with great care. At the same time, there is no doubt that the public mind has greatly exaggerated the risks of making this serious mistake.

A state similar to catalepsy may be produced by hypnotism, and, apart from this, the phenomena appear to be of a hysterical nature. The usual line of treatment is to put the patient to bed. The necessary functions must be performed for her, both as regards feeding and the evacuations, and if this be done she will not suffer the slightest harm, even though she may continue in the condition for weeks. On recovery from the attack treatment will be adopted for the hysteria. Amongst drugs used in this condition, valerian possesses some value.

See Death ; Hysteria ; Trance.

CATAPHORESIS. The process of passing drugs through the skin or any other tissue by means of an electric current is called cataphoresis. Of late years this method has been largely employed, and it doubtless possesses definite advantages in some conditions, such as painful affections of the joints.

See Ionisation.

CATARACT. A very common disease of the eye, which consists in the loss of transparency of its lens, is called a cataract. All light has to pass through the lens, and if this becomes opaque absolute blindness is the result. The

extracted when the cataract is ripe. When both eyes are affected, reading and other near work may be rendered easier by fitting a simple piece of apparatus to the better eye. It consists of a cone of cardboard of which the base is made to fit over the eye, while the other end is narrowed to form an opening of $\frac{1}{4}$-inch diameter or less. The inside is blackened. In consequence of the loss of the lens, the shape of which is indicated by the diagram, it is necessary to provide the

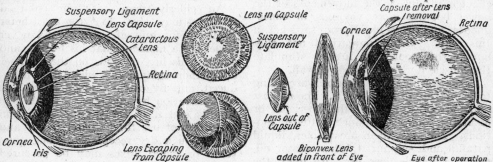

Cataract. How the diseased lens is removed and its function performed by a convex spectacle lens

condition sometimes occurs as the result of injury, and in such cases may be found in young people ; it may, in fact, be present at birth. Sometimes, also, the disease appears to be due to some constitutional malady, such as diabetes, but the vast majority of cases occur in elderly people, and seem to be simply due to a degeneration, or loss in vital power in the tissue of the lens. There is probably some hereditary tendency to the disease.

The opacity is usually very gradual, and not until the entire lens is opaque is the cataract said to be " ripe." It may begin in one eye only, but the second eye is almost invariably attacked sooner or later. An average period of ripening is about two years. The first sign of the presence of cataract may consist in persistent tiny specks before the eye. Vision is then noticed to become progressively worse. The patient usually sees better in a dim light, though there are cases where a bright light is preferred. For a time after objects cease to be visible there remains a perception of light.

No treatment other than operation seems to affect cataract, but this method is exceedingly satisfactory. The lens is

patient with an artificial lens, in other words, with spectacles having convex lenses like the natural lens.

See Eye.

CATARRH. Inflammation of a mucous surface of the body, such as that of the lining of the nose or the stomach, is known as catarrh. Thus a cold in the head might be described as acute nasal catarrh. The word implies a discharge from the inflamed surface such as is seen in the running nose, but when there is little or no discharge the name is sometimes retained, as in dry catarrh of the nose or of the bronchial tubes. It is also used for inflammation of the kidney tubules and the vesicles of the lung which are not lined with mucous membranes.

See Cold, Common ; Gastritis.

CATECHU. Obtained from a plant which grows in Southern Asia, catechu contains tannin and so has a powerful astringent action. The powdered drug, dose 5 to 15 grains ; the compound catechu powder, 10 to 60 grains; or tincture of catechu, 5 to 15 minims, may be given in the treatment of diarrhoea and other states of irritation of the bowel. Catechu lozenges are useful for a relaxed throat.

See Astringent.

CATGUT. In surgery, catgut is used for ligatures in tying blood vessels or for stitching tissues together. Since it is an animal tissue, it is readily absorbed so soon as its work is done.

CATHARTIC. This term, which literally means a cleansing agent, is used as a general name for purgative medicines. These act by stimulating the movements of the intestines or by making the intestinal contents more liquid. When the latter effect is produced, the movements of the bowel become more vigorous in consequence, and drugs like Epsom salts act in this way. Other purgatives not only liquefy the stools but directly stimulate the muscle fibres in the bowel wall.

Cathartics may be grouped according to the nature of their effects. The mildest remedies of this class, the aperients or laxatives, simply produce softened motions. Amongst them are prunes, liquid paraffin and sulphur. When castor oil, senna, calomel, aloes, etc., are used, the effect is greater, the stools being semi-liquid in character. When still more powerful drugs are used, for example, elaterium, croton oil, jalap, podophyllin or scammony, the stools are watery.

Whenever the bowels act very briskly there is always some degree of reaction in the form of constipation, so that the use of powerful cathartics is bad treatment for chronic constipation. The degree of action of these remedies, however, depends on their dosage, and aloes, which is not suitable for treating chronic constipation when given in moderate or large doses, is quite a proper remedy if the dose is small. Cathartics which act briskly are likely to cause griping, and to prevent this aromatics are usually given with them, such as ginger, cloves or capsicum. Powerful cathartics should not be given to children, old people or those who are weakly, except on medical advice ; they may easily depress the vitality to the verge of collapse.

See Aloes ; Aperient ; Colocynth ; Croton Oil ; Enema ; Epsom Salts ; Euonymin ; Jalap ; Podophyllum ; Rhubarb ; Scammony ; Senna.

CATHETER. In order to tap certain cavities of the body which are reached through narrow passages, tubes known as catheters are employed. What is called the Eustachian catheter is used for inflating the ear through the nose. It may be made of metal or of vulcanite. A catheter is often introduced into the urinary bladder, sometimes to carry antiseptic lotions within, but usually to drain off the urine. Such may be made of metal, of soft rubber, of silk web stiffened with varnish, or of some other material. A metal catheter should only be used by a doctor.

An elderly man with an enlarged prostate may have to pass a catheter regularly for himself. He should never forget for a moment that his health, and perhaps his life, depends on the catheter being thoroughly clean when it is introduced, and by clean is meant free from contamination by microbes. It will help to this end if in the intervals between the times of use the catheter is dry and is kept in a dry receptacle. Long glass tubes or metal boxes may be procured for this purpose.

To disinfect the instrument before use, a rubber or metal catheter should be boiled for a few minutes, but as gum elastic or silk web catheters would be spoilt by boiling, they are disinfected by letting them lie, preferably for an hour, in an antiseptic solution, such as lotion of perchloride of mercury, 1 in 2,000. Before handling the catheter the hands should be thoroughly washed with soap and water, and the end of the penis should be washed just before introducing the instrument. If lubrication is necessary, a little glycerin of borax may be used. After use the catheter should be well washed, inside and out, in running water. If there is difficulty in getting off grease a little methylated spirit will help. It is then thoroughly dried and put into its container. When a catheter becomes rough and worn it should be discarded.

See Prostate.

CAUL. This name is given to a cap formed on the head of a new-born child by a portion of the foetal membranes which cover it in the womb. As a rule the membranes are split during birth and the child's head passes through the gap, but sometimes the head carries the membranes forward and a piece is torn off circularly ;

or the child may be born within the intact membranes. It is an old superstition with sailors that if they take a dried caul to sea with them it will act as a charm against drowning.

CAUSTIC. Substances which have a destructive action upon the tissues to which they are applied are caustics. They may be solid or liquid. Typical caustics are nitrate of silver, usually called lunar caustic, caustic potash and caustic soda. In olden days before modern surgery, caustics were very largely used for the destruction of diseased tissues, ranging from cancer to warts and corns. It may be said that nowadays caustics have fallen out of use altogether, except in such cases as the application of lunar caustic, glacial acetic acid, or strong nitric acid to common warts.

Caustics cause great pain almost always. Their action is difficult to control and to limit ; furthermore, it is very difficult to secure healing after the use of a caustic, for it greatly weakens the vital powers, even of the tissues which it does not destroy. It is also known that the incautious and continuous application of caustics to various little growths—such as warts that may appear on the faces of elderly people—may cause them to become cancerous. Carbonic acid snow acts as a caustic, but the extent of its action may be fairly well regulated.

See Blue Stone ; Poisoning ; Silver ; Wart.

CAUTERY. The destruction of tissue, when necessary, is more satisfactorily accomplished by the cautery than by caustics, with the exception of corns or warts or such as can be dealt with by carbonic acid snow. There are many kinds of cautery, such, for instance, as the wire, or pair of wires, the tips of which are heated by passing electricity through them ; or the cautery which is heated in flame. But every kind of cautery owes its powers to its high temperature, and the especial value of this instrument is that its action can be exactly limited as the operator desires. An advantage of the cautery is that it absolutely prevents bleeding from any tissue which it touches, and it can very easily be used, just as a knife is used, for the division of tissues which contain a quantity of blood and would bleed profusely if otherwise cut.

See Thermo-cautery.

CELL. Every living thing consists either of cells—that is to say, minute bodies of various shapes each of which contains living matter, and is, up to a point, complete in itself—or else products of such

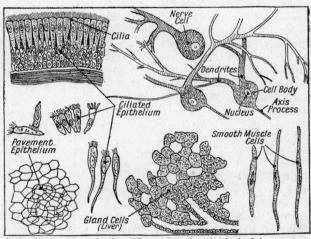

Cell, Various types having different functions in the body's structure. Ciliated epithelium is found, amongst other situations, in the windpipe, and pavement epithelium in the mouth and gullet

cells. These products are not themselves alive ; thus the enamel of the teeth is not alive, yet is formed by soft living cells.

Very many kinds of cells are found in the human body ; for example, the flat, horny cells of the skin ; the square or cubical cells that are found in glands and produce various secretions ; the rounded fat cells ; the elongated cells of muscle, which have the power of shortening and lengthening themselves ; the many kinds of nerve cells ; the cells of countless shapes which occur in various parts of the eye, the ear, and other organs of sensation ; and many more than have yet been named, notably the white and red cells of the blood. The body really consists of a vast commonwealth of cells.

Reference in this book is made to various types of cells under appropriate headings. Here it is necessary merely to note that the modern study of disease may be said to date from the time when the true relation of these cells to the life of the whole body began to be recognized ; in other words, modern pathology, or the study of disease, is " cellular pathology."

See Amoeba ; Blood ; Epithelium ; Lipoid ; Protoplasm ; Tissue.

CELLULITIS. Inflammation of the loose cellular tissue lying beneath the skin and between muscles is called cellulitis.

See Inflammation.

CEREAL. A very important class of foodstuffs, including wheat, oats, barley, maize and rice, constitute the cereals. These are, though in varied degree, rich in carbohydrates and proteins. Oats are the most nutritive of all cereals, a fact which bears on the value of porridge. Most biscuits are cereal products, so are semolina, vermicelli, macaroni and cornflour.

CEREBELLUM. This is the scientific name for what is called the small brain, that is, the part of the brain which lies behind and underneath the great brain or cerebrum.

See Brain ; Equilibrium.

CEREBRO-SPINAL FEVER. The acute, infectious disease which is more popularly known as " spotted fever " is called by doctors cerebro-spinal fever because, although like other specific fevers, it is a form of blood poisoning, yet the main brunt of the disease falls on the coverings or meninges of the brain and spinal cord. On this account it is also sometimes called epidemic cerebro-spinal meningitis.

The blood poisoning and the meningitis are caused by a germ known as the diplococcus intracellularis ; of this there are four types, any one of which may be present in an individual case, and which vary to some extent in their virulence. These germs invade the throat in the first place, and are often found in the throats of people who have had the disease and also of others who do not themselves suffer from it, but who can communicate it to others. A person who harbours disease-producing germs in his body, while enjoying ordinary health, is called a carrier (*q.v.*) of the particular disease and is capable of communicating it to others.

In any community there are always carriers of cerebro-spinal fever, and this danger increases in a marked degree when people are crowded together. Epidemics of the disease are therefore liable to break out in barracks, camps or elsewhere where overcrowding occurs, and for this reason they also occur most frequently during the cold months of the year. Doubtless dirt and bad sanitation of other sorts play a contributory part. In addition to these epidemic outbreaks, individual cases occur from time to time.

Children are most frequently affected, but people of any age may contract the disease. It is most fatal in the young and in the old. It usually begins suddenly, severe headaches and vomiting being common early symptoms and sometimes being wrongly ascribed to food poisoning. The patient becomes very irritable and cannot tolerate noises or bright light. Later he is semi-conscious and delirious.

Two symptoms make their appearance early, the first being a painful rigidity of the muscles at the back of the neck, so that the patient complains if any attempt be made to bend the head forward ; the other is what is called Kernig's sign. This means that when the patient lies on his back, if a thigh is bent to about a right angle with the body and an attempt made to straighten the leg at the knee, great pain is caused. It may also be noticed that the eyes are squinting, and other nervous symptoms may be present, for example, convulsions in young children.

So far all the symptoms described have been due to meningitis. The fever present is partly due to the same cause but also to the blood poisoning, and other effects of this may be reddish or purple spots on the skin (whence the name " spotted " fever), and inflammation of the joints, the lining and the covering of the heart, and other parts. Inflammation of the kidneys may be present, and in some cases has been the only symptom. Sometimes large patches of discoloured skin or purpura are found, these and the spots being due to bleeding under the skin.

Persons who contract this disease must be isolated, and all who have been in contact with them must have their throats examined to determine whether they harbour the germs ; meanwhile, they also are isolated. Treatment consists in tapping the spinal canal, described under the ading Lumbar Region, so as to permit the escape of the excess of cerebro-spinal uid, and the injection into the canal of e appropriate anti-meningococcic serum. his may also be injected into the ntricles of the brain and into a vein. At e same time vaccines, made from the rm, are generally used.

The patient may have to be fed through tube, and in cases which last any length time precautions must be taken against e occurrence of bed sores. Recovery ay be complete, but in some cases uinting, defective eyesight, deafness, aralysis of one or more limbs or mental npairment may be left. Patients may tain the germ of the disease in their roats for months after recovery, and it lps to remove them if a large amount time is spent in the open air.

See Carrier ; Meningitis.

CEREBRUM. This is the technical ame for what is called the great brain, hich in man is so enormously developed at it constitutes the greater part of the ntire brain, both by volume and by eight.

See Brain.

CERVICAL. Derived from the Latin ord meaning neck, cervical is an adjective hich describes anything that has to do ith the neck, as, for instance, the cervical lands, cervical nerves, or cervical verte- rae. The adjective is also applied to the ervix, or neck of the womb.

CHAFING. From the rubbing together f two skin surfaces of the body chafing ay result, that is to say, the skin becomes ed and painful, and perhaps raw. This ay also ensue from the rubbing of tight lothing. Common sites are the armpits nd the inside of the top of the thigh, and n both these instances the decomposition f sweat is doubtless a factor. Scrupulous leanliness will do much to prevent and ure this condition. The parts should be vashed daily with soap and water. Dusting powders are also useful, or zinc intment or cold cream.

See Eczema ; Erythema ; Intertrigo.

CHALK. Calcium carbonate or chalk as various uses in medicine. When round into powder it is called prepared halk, and in doses of 10 to 60 grains may e used for acidity of the stomach. Its

frequent use for this purpose, however, may lead to the formation of lumps or concretions in the bowel. For diarrhoea, chalk mixture, dose ½ to 1 ounce, aromatic chalk powder, 10 to 60 grains, or the aromatic chalk powder with opium, are useful remedies. Prepared chalk, either alone or mixed with other ingredients, is a common tooth powder.

See Calcium.

CHALK STONES. In people suffering from chronic gout, deposits are found in the ears, the eyelids, the knuckles and elsewhere, which are known as tophi or chalk stones, but which really consist of urate of soda.

See Gout.

CHALYBEATE. Waters which contain salts of iron, such as those at Tunbridge Wells and Harrogate, are called chaly- beate waters. People who suffer from bloodlessness can generally be treated properly with iron without resorting to spas. The main advantage of such places is that the patient is subjected to a regular and sensible life in healthy surroundings.

See Anaemia ; Health Resort.

CHANCRE. A venereal sore, which may be either of the hard or soft variety, may be described as a chancre, though usually nowadays the term means the hard sort, while the soft chancre is re- ferred to as a soft sore. The former is the primary lesion of syphilis and may appear from three to five weeks after contagion ; the latter appears, a day or two after the impure connexion, as a dirty yellow ulcer which discharges pus. This pus, if inoculated on other parts of the body, speedily reproduces the sore. The glands in the groin may become swollen and an abscess may form, par- ticularly if the person walks about. A soft sore can generally be cleared up quickly by antiseptics, but, as the infec- tion of syphilis may also be present, a doctor should always be consulted.

See Syphilis.

CHANGE OF LIFE. The period in a woman's life when the reproductive func- tions come to an end is popularly known as the change of life. Technical names for this time are the menopause and the climacteric. It usually occurs between the ages of 45 and 50 ; very rarely later than the latter date, but not infrequently earlier than the former. The child-bearing period lasts usually about 30 years. An artificial change of life may be produced by a surgical operation, which is sometimes found necessary for certain diseases of the pelvic organs.

The change is signalised by the cessation of the menstrual periods. This may happen all at once or the periods may occur irregularly for two or three years before disappearing altogether. The importance of the change of life from the point of view of the health of the individual lies in the fact that it is very often accompanied by various unpleasant nervous symptoms. The patient's temper may suffer, and so may her digestion and also her sleep ; she is very apt to have hot and cold turns and she flushes very readily. She very frequently tends to put on flesh ; but the tendency may be in the other direction. She may suffer from headache, though this may really indicate the need of glasses for reading and other near work. Amongst other disorders which may make their appearance at this time, mention may be made of inflammation of the joints or osteo-arthritis (*q.v.*)

It must be emphasised that irregular bleeding at or shortly after the menopause must be viewed with the strongest suspicion in view of the tendency to the development of cancer of the womb at this time. Therefore its occurrence should always be brought to the notice of a doctor.

The disagreeable incidents of this period may be diminished by regular, careful living : sufficient open-air exercise, sufficient sleep, a careful diet and attention to the bowels. A change of air from time to time is often of great service. Tea should be drunk in moderation and should not be strong, while alcohol is best avoided altogether.

The flushing may be relieved by the use of potassium bromide, 15 grains in half a glass of soda water from time to time. An effective remedy is sometimes found in ichthyol. A tablet of 2½ grains is taken thrice daily after food, and the number is gradually increased until in about three weeks' time four tablets are taken thrice daily. After a day or two the drug is dropped, and this should be

done if at any time during the course t patient has a persistent taste of the dr in her mouth. Flushing and other d agreeable incidents of the change of li are often successfully treated with ovari extracts.

See Menstruation ; Obesity.

CHAP. Chaps are due to a lack healthy elasticity of the skin induced l its exposure to cold. The effect of co is to prevent much blood from circulatir through the skin, that is to say, to mal the skin dry. If now the skin is put c the stretch it tends to crack. Though tl cause of chapping is thus mainly tl dryness of the skin, it must be remen bered that the worst thing for chappe hands is to leave them imperfectly dr after washing. This is by far the con monest way in which chaps are cause more particularly when the hands ar dried at the fire.

In washing, hard water should b avoided if possible, and if only such available it should be softened by tl addition of a little washing soda or bora: Towels must be perfectly dry, and may be advantageous to have a littl bowl of bran on the washstand into whic the hands may be plunged after drying Some people find that rubbing lanolir into the hands at bedtime is useful i cold weather. Others use glycerin an rose-water. Should chaps form, the must be protected from contaminatio like any other wound, or they may becom septic. They may be painted over wit flexible collodion or " new skin," c anointed with boracic ointment an covered by bandages or clean cotton glove

Chapped lips may be prevented b using a lip salve or rubbing on lanoline cold cream or a little vaseline befor going out into the cold. When they exis they are often aggravated by frequen moistening of the lips or by biting th lips or picking at them. They should b treated by putting on boracic ointment a night. Deep sores on the lips should no be allowed to persist ; they may lead t ugly scarring and they may be dangerous.

See Chilblain ; Skin.

CHARCOAL. Wood charcoal is o considerable use as a drug in some case of indigestion. It has the power of con trolling fermentation in the stomach, and, beyond this, also tends to absorb gases formed in indigestion. It must be taken dry in doses of 60 to 120 grains, either as lozenges or sprinkled on bread and butter. Its property of absorbing gases is utilised in the treatment of foul sores, to which it may be applied sprinkled on a poultice. By absorbing the gases it destroys the disagreeable odour attending such sores. Charcoal is often used as a tooth powder.

CHEST. The upper section of the trunk, the chest, is technically known as the thorax. The important organs it contains are the lungs, which take up the greater part of its space, and the heart. The chest has more or less the shape of a cone, expanding below and diminishing upwards. It is bounded below by the diaphragm, through various openings in which it communicates with the abdomen. The principal structural foundation of both chest and abdomen is furnished by the spine, but the chief difference between them is that, whilst the walls of the abdomen are entirely soft but for the spine, the part of the spine which helps to form the chest gives origin to 24 long curved bones called ribs, which help to form the wall of the chest. In front, the ribs, with the exception of the last two

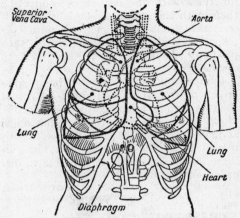

Chest : Its structure and principal contents

in girth during inspiration and expiration respectively, or, in other words, the range of movement. The phrase a weak chest is a vague one to which often very little meaning can be attached. It may mean that a person has a small chest, and if there is also a poor range of movement it is reasonable to suppose that such a chest implies, perhaps, some defect of vital power and an increased risk of pulmonary complaints, as may also the conjunction of a narrow chest with little flesh upon it, sloping shoulders and a long, thin neck. But the early stages of consumption may produce somewhat similar appearances. Any person whose chest exhibits any of these features should be much in the open air and should always sleep with his bedroom window open.

The barrel-shaped chest is frequently met with in elderly people, as a consequence of chronic bronchitis with much cough-

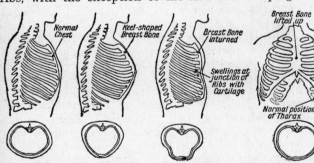

Normal chest and three types of deformity, namely, pigeon breast, rickety rosary and (right) barrel-shaped chest. Below, sectional aspects

pairs, are attached in some way to the sternum or breast bone. They are capable of movement by the muscles attached to them, and thus help in that process of breathing for the discharge of which the whole chest is designed.

The girth of the chest, which is usually measured about the level of the nipples, is in men usually from 33 to 40 inches, but the most important fact is the difference ing, which has caused the chest to become enlarged, in order to make space for the overstretched lungs. The range of movement may be very small, 1 inch or less, as the ribs occupy a nearly horizontal position. Two familiar deformities of the chest are due to rickets. Of these the most marked is what is called pigeon breast ; this is favoured by the existence of adenoids or by diseases, like whooping-cough, which interfere with breathing while the ribs are still soft and malleable. The other consists of a series of so-called "beads" upon the ribs, due to their being swollen at certain points of their junctions with the cartilages connecting them with the sternum. Usually there is one such swelling on each rib at a corresponding place. The deformity thus produced is often called the "rickety rosary."

Pain in the chest may be due to disorders of any of its contained organs or their coverings, reference to which will be found under their appropriate headings. It may be due to rheumatism of the intercostal muscles or pleurodynia. In some instances, however, it is due to disorders of the stomach.

See Breathing Exercises; Heart; Lung; Pleura; Pleurodynia; Poultice; Respiration; Shingles; Thorax.

CHEST PROTECTOR. Garments made of flannel and wool are often worn on the front and back of the chest. They may consist of a single layer, or, in front, in accordance with the universal delusion that the lungs are only to be found in that region, they may be double. It is probably safe to say that the chest protector is always undesirable; if it were sufficiently large and not too thick, and if it were regularly washed, and as absorbent as ordinary flannel underclothing, its use might possibly be justifiable on occasion, but it practically never answers to these conditions.

CHICKEN. Breast of chicken is the most easily digested meat known, and is thus of great value in invalid and convalescent cookery. A young bird should always be chosen, as the meat is more tender and of finer quality. Chicken broth is of value in fevers, chicken cream, mince, and fricassee are suitable for the early stages of convalescence, while roast chicken and other dishes may be given when the patient is put on a more substantial diet.

A good chicken broth suitable for invalid diet is made as follows. Half a chicken is used, the white meat from the breast being removed for serving separately or for adding later to the broth. The remainder is well washed, the fat and skin are removed, the meat cut into small pieces, and the bones broken. This is then covered with about two pints of water, to which a pinch of salt is added and allowed to simmer gently for four to five hours, water being added if the meat becomes uncovered. The broth should be skimmed at intervals. It is then strained through a fine sieve, left to get cold, and any fat then removed. If the breast is to be used, it is first pounded in a mortar and rubbed through a sieve, then added to the reheated broth with a teaspoonful of fine tapioca or barley and simmered until the latter is cooked.

See Invalid Cookery.

CHICKEN-POX. A very common infectious disease of childhood, chicken-pox is technically known as varicella, this word being really the diminutive of variola, which is the technical name for smallpox. The relation of the two names may be remembered, because it is noteworthy that smallpox, occurring in persons who have been very nearly but not entirely protected by vaccination, very often closely resembles chicken-pox; this may be a very serious matter, because the patient may not be isolated, and other people may catch the infection and die from it. The accident has frequently happened.

Chicken-pox is exceedingly infectious, and few children escape it. It is most common in children under six years, but older children and even adults may contract it. The microbe which causes it has not yet been identified. The disease usually shows itself about fourteen days (eleven to nineteen) after infection; in other words, the period of incubation is a fortnight. The rash, consisting of small red spots, appears on the first day of the symptoms, which are those of slight fever (q.v.). The chest, the back and the limbs are most affected. The rash may also occur on the face and scalp, and in the mouth, making swallowing painful. In a short time the spots turn into blisters (Plate XXXI, 3); soon these dry up and leave crusts which become detached. As a rule no permanent scarring results, except where the child has scratched the spots.

This is a mild disease; there are no complications except in the very rarest cases, when inflammation of the kidneys broncho-pneumonia may occur. The patient should not be allowed to mingle with his playmates until all the crusts have separated, including those amongst the hair; he should have a course of warm baths and a new outfit of clothes. Second attacks of the disease are not common. The treatment is that of a mild case of fever; warmth, slop food, and a mild laxative for the bowels if necessary. If any of the spots ulcerate, they should be smeared with an ointment consisting of equal parts

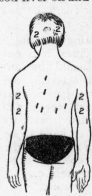

Chicken-pox rash: where and when it appears

of vaseline and white precipitate ointment. This or some zinc ointment may also relieve itching. Children who have been in contact with others suffering from the disease should not return to school till three weeks have elapsed since the last contact. From time to time chicken-pox is put on the list of notifiable diseases.

See Infectious Disease; Smallpox.

CHILBLAIN. Strictly speaking, a chilblain is a local inflammation of the skin and the tissues immediately under it, occurring on the toes, the fingers, the ears, and the nose, and due to the injury inflicted upon the tissue in question by cold. The first symptom of which the patient is aware is an itchiness or burning sensation. Soon the affected part swells and takes on a dark red colour, the skin being stretched and shiny. A blister may form, and this may burst, an event to be avoided, because the vitality of a part affected with chilblains is so low that the process of healing is exceedingly long and difficult.

Chilblains may be prevented by wearing warm clothes and stockings; by taking regular exercise of a vigorous kind, such as brisk walking, and skating when possible; and by daily rubbing of the parts most likely to be affected. Boots and gloves must be perfectly easy. It is better not to use a hot-water bottle in bed at night, but if one is used it should not be brought near to the feet. People who are prone to develop chilblains may derive benefit from taking cod-liver oil or cod-liver oil and malt during cold weather.

When chilblains threaten, the affected parts should be painted with the strong tincture of iodine, and the lactate of calcium may be taken in doses of 15 grains (5 grains for a child), thrice daily. The taste of this drug may be covered by taking with it as many drops of the liquid extract of liquorice. Should the parts still remain hot and irritable, zinc ointment or an ointment of ichthyol, 30 per cent. in soft paraffin, may be applied on lint. If the chilblains break, the ichthyol ointment may be continued, or a stimulating ointment such as the following may be used:

Birch tar	..	..	1 drachm
Zinc oxide powder ..	..	2½ drachms
Soft paraffin	..	..	5 ,,

A lotion of equal parts of hydrogen peroxide and warm water will make an excellent wash for the sores, especially if they are suppurating.

See Ambrine; Frost Bite; Skin.

CHILD. Infancy may be said to merge into childhood about the time when the infant is cutting the milk teeth, say in the 7th or 8th month, though others make childhood begin at the end of the first year. It may be said to merge into youth about the 6th or 7th year, when the permanent teeth appear and when the more formal education generally begins; or childhood may be considered as lasting on till adolescence ushers in the characteristics of maturity.

Childhood is marked by active bodily and mental development. The height at birth should be doubled in the first six years, and at 14 years is eleven-twelfths of the individual's adult height. The weight at the end of the sixth year is about double that at the end of the first year, and it doubles again at 14 years. Thus at six years a child will measure about 3 feet 6 inches and weigh about 3 stones, and at 14 the figures may be about 4 feet 9 inches and 6 stones respectively. A well-developed child walks as a rule at the end of the first year, or at any rate, at 15 months. Till about four years the gait is not very steady, however.

While strongly deprecating too much repression of childish activities, it is not intended that children should be uncontrolled. The more their activities can be engaged in wholesome games and occupations which interest them the better. When a child begins to walk its willingness to get about may have to be restrained. Heavy children may press too much on their legs, and in these cases a "baby walker," that is, a frame which allows the child to use its legs but takes some of the weight off, is often an advantage. Young children should not be taken long walks, otherwise the arches of the feet may be overstrained, and flat foot may develop.

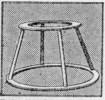
Baby "walker" in wood

It is necessary to ensure that children get a sufficiency of sleep, and up to the age of four a child should be encouraged to take a sleep in the afternoon. The hours of sleep generally required at various ages are as follows: four years, 13 hours; six years, 12 hours; eight to nine years, 11 hours; twelve to fifteen, 10 hours. Children vary, of course, as regards their need of sleep, but these figures afford some guidance. A good rule is to allow a child to sleep as long as it can; another is that a child should always go early to bed.

A close watch should be kept on children when they are attending school. Overstrain may be indicated by irritability of temper and a loss of appetite. In these circumstances, sufficient time for sleep must be insisted upon, and it may be necessary to diminish the child's work or even to take it from school altogether for a time. Children at school should not be allowed to spend too long over homework. Too much of this is often allotted to a child who, if he is conscientious, either overworks or is made unhappy by his inability to accomplish the task.

Attention must be paid to the posture assumed by children in school and at other times, as the habit of sitting or lounging with one shoulder higher than the other or with the shoulders stooped is a common cause of spinal curvature. It is now quite clearly recognized that a poor development of the skeleton in women is usually due to their being kept too much indoors in girlhood and their losing the benefits of the games which their brothers enjoyed.

A child should be brought up to enjoy the morning tub. When very young the water must, of course, be warm to tepid, but as they grow older they should wash in water from the tap. They must have a brisk rub down with a towel afterwards. If it is observed that they do not react well, the tub should be discontinued, but it will be beneficial to wash the neck and shoulders with cold water. These measures help to harden the child against catarrhal troubles, and prevent or diminish the skin troubles which are favoured by dirt.

A child should be much in the open air and sunlight, and should have its bedroom window open at night. A draught can easily be kept from the child's bed. The importance of sunlight is emphasised by its ability to prevent and cure rickets and its beneficial effects in surgical tuberculosis, and that of fresh air by its influence on consumption.

A close watch should be kept to see that a child is in the habit of breathing properly, and breathing exercises should be instituted if he does not do so. He ought to breathe deeply and through the

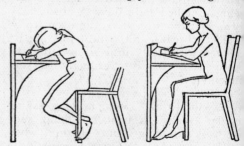
Child. Harmful and correct sitting postures
Courtesy of the Ling Association

nose. If he is a mouth-breather probably adenoids are present, and these will require to be dealt with before breathing exercises e undertaken. Clothing should be fficiently warm.

Children are often turned out in cold weather with bare feet and legs with a view to hardening them. Much trouble of the joints is caused in this way.
On the other hand, some children are verweighted with clothes. Boots should e broad at the toes and have low heels.
With regard to food, at one year a ild is having bread and other carbo-ydrate foodstuffs in addition to milk. hree or four months later it may have utter on the bread, and in a month or vo a thoroughly baked potato mashed ith a little butter may be added to the id-day meal. Crusts and rusks should e given for the child to exercise its teeth n. In the last quarter of the second ear eggs are added to the diet, though soft-boiled egg with breadcrumbs is ften enough given earlier. The pulp of baked apple may be given at the ourteenth or fifteenth month. Porridge vith milk should be given regularly from he eighteenth month.

Age at which Meat May be Given

After the age of two to two and a half ears the child should be trained to take ts food in three meals with only a little ailk or soup before bedtime. Meat is dded at the end of the third year, and s at first cut into small pieces. It is not ecessary to give meat oftener than once day, though it should be remembered hat as children grow older they require liberal allowance of meat, fish or eggs or the purpose of growth. The beverages t meals should be milk, cocoa and water ; ea and coffee should be withheld till about he tenth year, and with advantage onger if possible.

Fresh fruit and vegetables should lways be part of the diet, given in forms uited to the digestive powers. Pickles, ondiments, and highly seasoned foods hould not be given to children.

From the beginning a child should be trained to swallow its food without the help of any beverage to wash it down. Food should not be allowed between meals ; indulgence in this respect often enough ruins a child's digestion. The craving for sweets cannot be disregarded, but, if possible, these should be given with meals and not in any quantity before a meal, as they spoil the child's appetite for other food.

See Adenoids; Baby; Breathing Exercises; Clothing; Convulsion; Diet; Fire-guard; Growth; Nervousness; Rickets; Teeth.

CHILDBIRTH. As soon as a woman knows that she is pregnant she should engage a doctor and nurse and begin making other preparations for her confinement. When this is imminent the room in which it will take place should be prepared. Although childbirth differs usually from a surgical operation in that it is a natural physiological process, it resembles the latter in exposing the patient to the risk of infection with microbes. This fact must always be kept in mind in the preparation of the room, and in all handling of the patient during labour and subsequently.

If there is any choice in the matter, a large quiet room should be selected. The lying-in room should always have a fire-place. The carpet should be taken up and beaten, the floor and woodwork should be thoroughly washed with soap and water, and the walls gone over with a damp cloth. There should be no super-fluous furniture in the room, and the hangings should be few, washable and clean. The bedstead should be plain and clean. It should be placed so as to afford easy access from either side. It should have a spring mattress and hair mattress. Any tendency to sag should be prevented by placing boards across the frame. A waterproof sheet should be placed on the hair mattress or, if this is not available, several sheets of clean brown paper. Over this is put a blanket and then a sheet. The patient lies on a waterproof sheet covered by a draw sheet, made of a sheet folded to the width of a yard ; or in place of this a large sheet of gamgee may be used.

During labour the nightdress should be well tucked up to keep it clean, and a flannel or cotton petticoat should be worn. The advantage of this is that it avoids the necessity of changing the nightdress when the labour is over and the patient very tired. An ample supply of sanitary napkins should be available. The practice of keeping soiled sheets or clothing beneath the bed is thoroughly bad.

Labour takes place in three stages. In the first the womb is opening up to allow of the passage of the child ; in the second the child is being expelled ; and in the third the afterbirth comes away. The whole process takes about sixteen hours in the case of a first baby, though it may be much longer. It may be shorter, and generally is so at subsequent confinements.

The first stage is much the longest, and is marked by regularly recurring pains which increase in frequency and severity. The pain is felt first in the back and passes thence to the front of the body. These pains are characterised by their beginning in the back and by a discharge of blood-stained mucus, " the show," which accompanies them. If the patient walks about during this stage it helps to hasten the labour, but she must avoid tiring or chilling herself.

Second Stage of Labour

The second stage brings a difference in the character of the pains ; they are more grinding in character and the patient tends to " bear down." She should now be in bed and should not get out of bed for the relief of the bladder or bowels, but should use a bed pan. The neglect of this precaution has frequently led to the baby being born in circumstances which were awkward or dangerous for it. It may be said here that when the bowels move during or after labour the nurse in performing the toilet of the bowel should always wipe backwards, in order to avoid carrying infected matter towards the vagina, and should have some lysol in the water which she uses for the purpose. The nurse should have her hands scrupulously clean before changing diapers or washing the parts ; she should use hot water and soap with a nail brush, and should then soak the hands for a little in lysol solution, a teaspoonful to the pint.

When labour appears to have begun the doctor should be summoned. If labour is precipitate and it seems likely that the baby will be born before his arrival, the situation should be accepted with calmness. The patient should be made to lie on her left side, with the thighs bent and a pillow between the knees. She should be encouraged to cry out with her pains, as this will tend to diminish their force, and may prevent tearing of the passages.

When the child's head is born, it should be supported until the body is expelled, and meanwhile with a clean rag mucus may be cleaned off the mouth and nostrils. If the child is born with membrane over its face this should be cleared off, and if, as sometimes happens, it is born within the membranes these must be ruptured at once, or the child will be suffocated or drowned. If it should happen that the baby is born when the mother is standing an instant examination should be made as to whether the umbilical cord has been torn, and, if so, it should be tied about 2 inches from the infant's belly with a piece of tape or some strands of linen thread.

As soon as a child is born, after one or two gasping breaths, it usually cries lustily and vigorous breathing is established. If there is any delay in starting breathing, a smart smack on the buttock or sprinkling cold water on the face and chest may prove a sufficient stimulus. When the cord has been tied and divided the baby is wrapped in a warm flannel, care being taken to allow a sufficient air supply, and is placed near the fire. Details to be observed in giving the infant its first bath will be found under the heading Baby.

After the Baby is Born

In the absence of the doctor, the nurse standing on the mother's right side, should place her left hand on the patient's abdomen over the womb. This will be felt as a more or less distinct lump, upon which she will exercise gentle pressure. On no account should any attempt be made to hasten the expulsion of the afterbirth by pulling on the cord. When the afterbirth comes away the nurse will still keep up gentle pressure on the womb for a short time. Care should be taken not to expose the mother more than is necessary. If she feels chilly a hot diaper may be applied and a hot-water bottle may be placed at her feet.

After the expulsion of the afterbirth, attention is given to any injuries which the mother's parts may have received. She is then washed and made comfortable. Some doctors apply a binder, others do not. When labour is over the room should be darkened and the mother encouraged to sleep. When she has rested sufficiently, the baby is put to the breast.

It may be useful to state here the more necessary articles to be procured in anticipation of a confinement. One, preferably two, mackintosh or waterproof sheets; draw-sheets; at least three abdominal binders for the mother; two or three dozen sanitary napkins of the largest size; one or two pounds of absorbent cotton wool; some stout linen thread cut into lengths of about 10 inches, or strong narrow tape, for tying the umbilical cord; a bottle of lysol; large and small safety pins; a clean nail brush; antiseptic dusting powder; a pot of vaseline; clean scissors; and two basins.

Three or four lengths of the linen thread are tied together at each end to form a ligature, and two such are required. Before being used they should be boiled for half an hour, or in an emergency put in lysol solution. Lint and other dressings may be baked in a hot oven for half an hour, care being taken not to scorch them. This is best accomplished by placing them in a hot oven with a dying fire. Abdominal binders, towels, sheets, etc., should be freshly laundered and put away. The scissors should be left in lysol solution some time before being used to cut the cord. Bed pans should be rubbed over with lysol solution before use, and after use should be cleaned at once and rubbed over with lysol before being put away.

See Artificial Respiration; Baby; Flooding; Pregnancy; Presentation; Puerperium.

CHILL. A sensation of coldness, especially in the back, and attended by shivering, is spoken of as a chill. This may be followed by other symptoms of a common cold, but it may usher in influenza, pneumonia, or another acute disease. Chills are usual in malaria. The patient should be put to bed between blankets, with hot-water bottles at the feet and sides, and should be given hot drinks. It is often well to begin treatment with a hot mustard foot bath.

See Cold, Common.

CHILLI PASTE. *See* Capsicum.

CHLOASMA. Patches of discoloration of the skin, yellow, brown or black, occur in pregnancy, consumption and other conditions, and are known as chloasma. There is no special treatment for this beyond that for the underlying disorder.

See Pigmentation; Pityriasis; Skin.

CHLORAL. When reference is made to chloral, what is meant is chloral hydrate. It has long been regarded as an efficient hypnotic, as it quickly produces natural sleep from which one wakes properly refreshed. Like other similar drugs, it has, however, its dangers. If given in large doses it depresses the heart and respiration, and moderate doses may be dangerous to those who have fatty hearts or diseased blood vessels. It tends to lose its power if taken often, and, what is more, it develops a craving for itself.

Both mind and body are affected; a patient becomes excited and talkative; his digestion is upset; his sleep is at the mercy of the drug; his breathing is interfered with; he becomes liable to faint, and suffers from eruptions upon the skin; his mind may be so affected that it will never recover itself even though he give up the habit.

Chloral hydrate is given in doses of 5 to 20 grains, though 10 grains is usually sufficient. It may also be given as the syrup of chloral hydrate, dose $\frac{1}{2}$ to 2 drachms. Other conditions in which the drug is given include convulsions in children and sea-sickness.

Camphorated chloral B.P.C. is a useful preparation for rubbing over tender spots in neuralgia, or chloral menthol, which is similar, may be used.

Poisoning by Chloral Hydrate. Poisoning from an overdose of chloral hydrate is treated by giving an emetic and keeping the patient warm in bed with blankets and hot-water bottles. He should be roused and kept from going to sleep again, by slapping his chest with damp towels if necessary. Whisky, sal volatile and hot coffee are used as stimulants; if unconscious, a pint of warm coffee may be injected into the bowel.

CHLORALAMIDE. Derived from chloral, chloralamide acts also as a hypnotic and is safer. It is given in doses of 15 to 45 grains, 20 grains being usually a sufficient dose for a healthy adult. It may be dissolved in a wineglass of water containing a dessertspoonful of spirits. As a preventive of sea-sickness, 15 grains each of chloralamide and potassium bromide are recommended.

CHLORIDE OF LIME. By exposing slaked lime to the action of chlorine gas, a substance is obtained which is known as bleaching powder, chloride of lime or chlorinated lime. It acts as an antiseptic, disinfectant and deodoriser. For the latter two purposes it is frequently used in drains and privies. Clothing may be disinfected by soaking for 24 hours in water containing 2 ounces of chloride of lime to the gallon. By dissolving washing soda, with chloride of lime, in water, the solution of chlorinated soda is obtained, of which 2 tablespoonsful in 1 to 3 pints of water make a good antiseptic lotion. The weak solution can be used as a mouth wash. Eusol, Dakin's hypochlorite solution and similar preparations are made from chloride of lime and boracic acid, and are used as antiseptics.

See Disinfection.

CHLORODYNE. This name is given to a proprietary medicine used for relieving pain and promoting sleep. The compound tincture of chloroform and morphine is a similar preparation, and is given in doses of 5 to 15 minims. This is a very efficient remedy for many kinds of pain, and especially for colic. When this is apparently due to undigested or improper food, a dose of castor oil should be given at the same time. Another use for it is to allay a persistent dry cough.

The mixture is a very dangerous one to use for infants and children, and should not, indeed, be used by anyone except on the advice of a doctor.

An overdose produces the symptoms of opium poisoning, and the treatment is the same.

See Opium ; Poisoning.

CHLOROFORM. For the production of prolonged general anaesthesia chloroform or ether are the drugs employed, either singly or in combination with each other or with other drugs. Chloroform has the advantages of being more readily portable, of having a more agreeable odour than ether, and of acting more promptly. Ether would appear to be the safer, though it causes a free flow of the secretions of the mouth and bronchial tubes, and its use may be followed by bronchitis or even pneumonia. Chloroform should be used for the very young and for the old. As used at childbirth, it is a safe and valuable means of relieving the pangs of labour.

Chloroform is a colourless volatile liquid with a sweet pungent taste. It may be used to flavour mixtures and to exert a carminative effect, in the form of chloroform water or of the spirit of chloroform, the dose of the latter being 5 to 20 minims for repeated doses and 30 to 40 minims for a single dose. The compound tincture of chloroform and morphine, dose 5 to 15 minims, acts as an anodyne. Liniment of chloroform may be applied in muscular rheumatism or in neuralgia. It reddens the skin and relieves pain. It is a constituent of the A.B.C. liniment (*q.v.*), in which form it is generally used. A small piece of cotton wool soaked with chloroform and put into a cavity in a painful tooth often gives immediate relief.

See Anaesthetic ; Chlorodyne.

CHLOROSIS. *See* Anaemia.

CHOKING. There is a form of choking which is due to nervous disease affecting the functions of the muscles which open and shut the larynx. Choking may also be due to disease of the larynx. But the form of choking now to be considered is due to the presence of a foreign body in the upper part of the air passages.

When this is a piece of meat or of bone, or something similar, the finger, or the handle of a spoon (*see* Plate X, 1), should be passed to the back of the throat and the foreign body should be hooked forward. It is often a useful procedure to hold a child up by the feet and smack it once or twice between the shoulders and something of the same kind may be possible for adults. This should never be done, however, if there is any suspicion that the foreign body is in the windpipe. If, when the throat is clear, breathing is found to have ceased, artificial respiration (*q.v.*) should be started at once.

See Asphyxia ; Probang.

CHOLERA. Asiatic cholera, which at one time occurred periodically in Great Britain in epidemics, is now all but unknown, largely in consequence of the improved water supply of towns and especially of seaports. Cholera is due to a microbe, known, from its shape, as the comma bacillus, and, like enteric fever, is a water-borne disease. It gets into the body in drinking-water or in food which has been contaminated by infected water, for example, milk or salads.

Symptoms come on suddenly and severe diarrhoea is the chief of these. The motions of the bowels are profuse and watery, and from their appearance are sometimes spoken of as rice-water stools. The heavy drain of water from the body is shown by the shrinkage of the tissues. The face becomes pinched and the belly falls in. Severe cramps are felt in the limbs, and before long the patient is in a state of collapse.

Early and energetic medical treatment is necessary. Potassium permanganate is given in solution by the mouth and solutions of saline are injected into the tissues or veins. The patient should drink freely. Warmth and stimulants are needed for the collapse.

When cholera is prevalent all water used either for drinking or for washing food utensils should be boiled. Milk should also be boiled, and ice cream, salads and raw fruit, unless in perfect condition, should be eschewed. Before taking food the hands should be washed, and those in attendance on cases of the disease should also soak their hands in an antiseptic solution. Any tendency to diarrhoea should be arrested, a useful remedy being a tablespoonful of castor oil with 15 drops of laudanum. Vigilance should be exercised against contamination of food or food utensils by flies (*q.v.*). Cholera nostras or cholera morbus, due to eating over or under ripe fruit or tainted food, produces symptoms resembling those of Asiatic cholera, and is treated in the same way.

Infantile Cholera. The summer complaint of infants, or infantile cholera, is a very fatal form of diarrhoea which affects young children, principally those under two years of age. It occurs during hot weather, and is especially prevalent amongst hand-fed babies who live in dirty and insanitary surroundings. Infection reaches them through milk, and is either present when the milk is received from the dairy, or is introduced subsequently by dust, flies or dirty utensils.

Milk should be received in sealed bottles. It should be kept in a cool, clean spot in the house, and should be constantly covered. It should be sterilised, and bottles and teats, after being thoroughly washed, should be boiled before being again used. A dummy teat is a danger.

Should the disease occur, vomiting may be free, and the motions of the bowels are frequent, profuse, and watery. The face is pinched, and the belly feels hard and inelastic. The temperature is likely to be high. A doctor should be procured at once, and meanwhile the child may be put in a pack. A towel or piece of sheeting is wrung out of cold water and put round the body from the armpits to the feet. Over this a blanket is wrapped. Boiled water is all that is given till vomiting has ceased, when albumen water and whey may be given. Should the child show signs of collapse, that is, coldness, blueness and prostration, hot-water bottles should be put round it, and it should be given small quantities of weak spirits from time to time.

Soiled napkins should be placed in a solution of carbolic acid (1 in 20), or of lysol, before being washed. This precaution is very necessary, as flies may carry infection from soiled napkins to milk, and other children may be infected.

See Diarrhoea ; Normal Saline Solution.

CHOREA. *See* St. Vitus's Dance.

CHOROID. The middle layer of the eye is called the choroid. Inflammation of the choroid, or choroiditis, may assume various forms and have different causes. It may be disseminated or widely spread over the surface of the membrane, or it may be central, and when this is so vision is affected more or less seriously. This symptom may also be present in the other form, and then night blindness may be a prominent symptom. Old age accounts for some cases, others are of obscure origin, but a large number are due to syphilis, and should receive treatment for this disease.

In wounds of the eye, in purulent inflammation of the cornea (*q.v.*) and in other eye and general diseases, cerebro-spinal fever, measles, etc., a suppurative choroiditis may occur. This is an extremely serious disorder.

See Eye.

CHYLE. Chyle is the name applied to certain constituents of the food which are absorbed from the bowel, not by the blood as the other constituents are, but by means of a number of special channels called lymphatics. These particular lymphatics have the special name of lacteals (Latin lac, milk), because their contents during the process of digestion are very like milk in appearance. This appearance is chiefly due to the presence of a quantity of fat in the form of tiny little drops, which give it a white, opaque appearance. The chyle is carried by the thoracic duct to the left subclavian vein, where it is poured into the blood stream.

See Digestion.

CHYME. This is the name applied to the contents of the stomach when the process of digestion in the stomach is completed. When this stage is reached, the passage from the stomach opens, and the chyme passes through in small quantities at a time for further treatment by means of the digestive action of the bowel, and of the fluids which reach the bowel from the liver and the pancreas. The chyme is acid, and its entrance into the first part of the bowel leads to the formation of secretin, which is carried by the blood to the pancreas and excites it to activity.

See Digestion.

CICATRIX. *See* Scar.

CINCHONA BARK. This is also known as Peruvian bark or Jesuits' bark. The varieties of cinchona trees from which the bark is taken grow in South America, their original home in India, and elsewhere. These barks are the source of quinine and other similar alkaloids. Cinchona bark was introduced into Europe as a remedy for fevers, and is the specific for malaria. Formerly the powdered bark was taken when its remedial effects were called for, but it has two disadvantages. In the first place, samples of bark vary in the amount of the alkaloids which they contain, so that the resulting action cannot be precisely gauged ; in the second place powdered bark is apt to upset the stomach

Another of the alkaloids in cinchona bark, quinidine, has proved a useful remedy in some cases of auricular fibrillation, a form of heart failure, marked by a quickening and complete irregularity of the heart's action. The preparations of cinchona bark are the liquid extract of cinchona, dose 5 to 15 minims ; and the tincture and the compound tincture of cinchona, the dose of each being $\frac{1}{2}$ to 1 drachm. These may be used for fever or as tonics. The liquid extract of red bark is said to be of use in relieving the craving of dipsomania (*q.v.*).

See Quinine.

CINNAMON. The bark of the cinnamon tree, which grows in the tropics, contains a volatile oil, to which it owes its characteristic taste and smell. It is this which makes powdered cinnamon a useful condiment and aid to digestion. It relieves flatulence, and for this purpose either tablespoonful doses of cinnamon water or the compound cinnamon powder, in doses of 10 to 40 grains, may be taken.

Cinnamon oil is given in doses of $\frac{1}{2}$ to 3 minims, and may be conveniently taken on a lump of sugar. It may stop a common cold if taken early enough and frequently, and is also used in influenza. Applied to the cavity of a painful tooth, the oil acts as an anodyne ; it is also used as an application for warts.

See Cold, Common ; Oil.

CIRCULATION OF THE BLOOD. In the body the blood circulates continuously through a series of closed tubes, the arteries, capillaries and veins, in two circles, the heart being the starting point in each case. In the first or systemic circulation the blood is sent from the heart throughout the body, carrying food and oxygen to every organ and tissue and taking away their waste products, and in the second or pulmonary circulation the blood is sent from the heart through the lungs, where it gets rid of carbonic acid gas and receives oxygen.

In the first it is the left side of the heart, and in the second the right side, which pumps the blood onwards. From the head, trunk and limbs the blood finds its way through the veins to the right upper chamber (right auricle) of the heart. When the heart beats, the walls of this chamber contract, forcing the blood through a valve into the right lower chamber or right ventricle. The ventricle has thick muscular walls, and, when these in their turn contract, the blood is forced through the pulmonary artery and reaches an immense network of thin-walled little vessels, threaded amongst the air cells of the lungs.

Through the walls of these capillaries there is an interchange of gases between the blood and the air in the air cells of the lungs, carbonic acid passing out of the blood and oxygen passing in. The purified blood is collected into the pulmonary veins and carried to the left upper chamber of the heart (left auricle). Here, again, at the start of the heart beat, the blood passes through another valve, flowing into the left lower chamber or left ventricle of the heart. The walls of this chamber are very thick, and when they contract the blood is forced into the main distributing artery, the aorta, and reaches every portion of the body.

The farther it goes from the heart, the smaller become the branches of the arteries through which it passes, until finally it enters the minute capillaries. From the capillaries it passes into the veins, which progressively increase in size, and finally empty their contents into the right auricle of the heart, from which we have seen it start out in its course.

While the blood is in the capillaries of the body a free interchange takes place between the blood within them and the fluid which bathes the cells of the body, food and oxygen passing out of the blood and waste products passing in. It should be observed, however, that the blood which leaves a large number of glands, amongst them being the pancreas, the supra-renals, the thyroid and the pituitary, in addition to waste products, contains contributions from these glands,

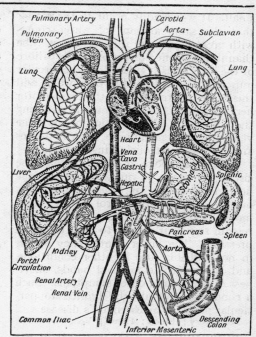

Circulation. Vessels carrying impure blood for cleansing, e.g., the pulmonary arteries running from heart to lung, are shown darker than those carrying pure blood to feed the tissues

known as internal secretions, which are of the greatest importance in the bodily economy.

A third circulation may be described, namely, the portal circulation. The blood coming from the walls of the stomach and intestines, where it has absorbed the products of digestion, etc., and from the spleen, is carried by the portal vein to the liver. Here it passes again through capillaries, giving up to the liver cells certain of its constituents, and being collected again into a large vein which carries it to the right auricle of the heart.

Reference has been made to the part played by the heart muscle in forcing the blood through the vessels, but it is essential to the maintenance of a sufficient blood pressure to carry on the circulation efficiently that the calibre of the medium sized arteries should be kept sufficiently

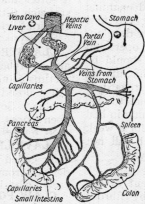

Portal vein that carries products of digestion to the liver

F

small. It will readily occur to the reader that the same amount of water comes with greater pressure from a narrow tube than it does from a larger one. The calibre of the arteries is regulated by the circular muscle fibres contained in their walls, and these are controlled by the vaso-motor nerves (q.v.). Another factor in assisting the circulation is the suction of the large veins by the right auricle when it dilates and by the chest during inspiration.

From the above it is clear that the circulation will be impaired when the heart is weakened by disease, and when, owing to defective control of the vaso-motor nerves, the blood vessels do not remain sufficiently tight to keep up blood pressure. The latter contingency occurs in neurasthenia and in other conditions, and is responsible for cold hands, shortness of breath and other symptoms. Such a condition may also be limited to particular parts, as in Raynaud's disease.

See Artery ; Blood ; Heart ; Vein.

CIRCUMCISION. The removal of the foreskin, which constitues the operation of circumcision, ought always to be performed in infancy when the part is long and cannot be retracted easily and thoroughly. It is a small operation and can be performed at home. If a tight foreskin is neglected, the secretions of the glands become foul and irritating, and there is difficulty in passing water, which leads to straining. Some of the consequences of neglect are bed-wetting, various nervous disorders and rupture.

As free bleeding occasionally follows the operation, the nurse should examine the dressing frequently during the first few hours. Owing to the greater development of the parts in an adult, the operation is not quite so simple, but it should be performed if there is much difficulty in washing the parts, a matter regarding which it is necessary to be punctilious. The operation will entail remaining in bed for, at any rate, 48 hours, and for a week after the operation the patient will not be able to get about very freely.

See Phimosis.

CIRRHOSIS. The replacement of the normal tissues of an organ by fibrous tissue is known as cirrhosis. The affected organ becomes hard and its power to carry on its functions is impaired to a degree corresponding with the extent of the replacement. The process may be observed in the liver, the kidney, the heart, the spleen and elsewhere in the body. The name is derived from a Greek word having reference to the yellowish colour assumed by a liver so affected. The small red kidney is the result of cirrhosis.

See Bright's Disease ; Fibrosis ; Heart ; Liver.

CITRATE OF MAGNESIA. The effervescent citrate of magnesia, dose 1 to 3 drachms, and solution of magnesium citrate, 5 to 10 fluid ounces, are used as laxative and refrigerant medicines.

See Aperient ; Fever.

CITRIC ACID. The juices of oranges, limes and lemons owe their tartness to citric acid, which is obtained from them in colourless crystals. The dose of the acid is 5 to 20 grains, and it is used to provide cooling drinks which are agreeable at any time, but specially so during fever. The acid may be used to make an effervescing drink, and this is often useful when the stomach is acutely irritated. It may be made by dissolving 20 grains of citric acid and 30 grains of bicarbonate of potash, each in half a glass of water, and then mixing the two in a large tumbler. It is drunk while effervescing.

The acid is used to form certain salts which have various uses in medicine, such as magnesium citrate, citrate of iron and quinine and sodium citrate. The last is often used in the strength of 1 grain to the ounce to render milk more digestible for an infant, which it does by producing a softer and looser curd in the infant's stomach. Citric acid is much used in making Imperial drink and home-made lemonade.

See Beverages.

CLAUSTROPHOBIA. The uneasiness and apprehension often manifested by the victims of neurasthenia when in rooms or other closed spaces is known as claustrophobia. Sometimes there is a dread of open spaces, and this is called agoraphobia.

See Neurosis ; Phobia ; Psycho-therapy.

CLAVICLE. The collar bone is technically called the clavicle, this name being derived from the Latin word for a key.

See Collar Bone.

CLAW FOOT. When the natural arch of the foot is exaggerated, the toes drawn backwards towards the instep, and the foot consequently shortened, the condition is described as claw foot or pes cavus. This may begin at an early age and although the appearance of the foot may

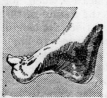
Claw Foot: exaggerated arch of the instep

not suggest it, it will be a suspicious circumstance if the child is rather awkward in running about and shows an unusual readiness to stumble. The suspicion will be confirmed if on attempting to bend up the foot towards the leg it is found that the angle in front of the ankle cannot be made less than a right angle, which ought to be possible for the normal foot.

At this stage an attempt may be made to rectify the condition by trying to bend up the foot several times each day. The boots worn should be sufficiently long, and it is recommended that a leather bar, half an inch in thickness, should be fixed across the sole of the boot beneath the tread in order to throw the fore part of the foot up. As the condition progresses the hollow beneath the sole becomes greater, callosities form, and at last, the foot is so deformed that the patient walks on the outer part of the upper surface of the foot. When the treatment first mentioned does not suffice, it is necessary to divide the Achilles tendon (*q.v.*) and in worse degrees, other structures also ; and bones may have to be removed.
See Foot.

CLEANLINESS. As dirt is notoriously either a direct or an indirect cause of disease, it follows that much disease can be prevented by cleanliness. The rôle played by dirt present in water and food, in the home and in the street, is explained when describing the origin of many diseases dealt with in this book. Here something may be said on the subject of personal cleanliness.

The surface of the skin is at all times exposed to contamination. Besides the sweating which is apparent, a large amount of sweat is poured out unconsciously. The watery part of this evaporates, but the substances dissolved in the sweat are deposited on the skin and with the secretion of the fat glands and with dust form a sort of varnish. Some of this is rubbed off by the friction of clothing and by rubbing with a towel, but in order to keep the skin clean it is necessary to have a hot bath and a thorough lathering with soap at least once a week. This applies even to those who take a daily cold bath ; the amount of dirt sometimes apparent when the skin is rubbed after a Turkish bath, shows that even regular hot baths may not succeed in removing all the dirt.

The neglect of sufficient washing is seen in inflammatory conditions of the skin, due either to the dirt or to parasites, bacterial and others, which are apt to infest a dirty skin or head. Workers who have to do with paraffin, tar, sugar and other substances are specially prone to dermatitis, and in some cases even to the development of malignant growths. In their case it is of extreme importance to be punctilious about personal cleanliness.

Besides washing the hair, it is necessary to brush it thoroughly and regularly, and to be careful that brushes and combs are kept clean, as otherwise dandruff and other contagious conditions may be spread. Neglect to clean the teeth regularly may result not only in their early decay, but in some general diseases which are apt to be associated with a dirty mouth. The teeth should be brushed at least twice daily, in the morning and again before going to bed. The nose acts as a filter of the air which is breathed in, and in certain circumstances a considerable amount of filth may accumulate in the passages. It is desirable, therefore, that children should be taught to use a handkerchief regularly and to keep their nostrils clean.
See Adenoids ; Antiseptic ; Baths ; Dermatitis ; Hair ; Mouth Wash ; Skin ; Soap ; Teeth.

CLEFT PALATE. Some children are born with a cleft or gap along the middle of the arch of the mouth, which may be limited to the soft palate or extend forwards to the hard or bony palate. It is often accompanied by hare-lip.

A baby which has a badly cleft palate cannot suck. When it attempts to swallow, much of its food passes through the cleft, and reappears at the nostrils ; this, of course, is very serious. Such a child has to be fed very carefully. Again, a child with cleft palate is much more liable than another to suffer from all sorts of inflammation of the throat, mouth and nose. Lastly, speech is very difficult to produce, and even more difficult to understand. Even a very small defect causes serious deterioration in the speech.

The treatment of cleft palate consists of a surgical operation, which may be performed between the third and sixth months, though some surgeons prefer to wait until between the second and third years. It essentially consists of loosening the membrane which covers the bony part of the palate on each side, and bringing the two portions of membrane together, so that they can be joined in the middle line.

See Hare-lip ; Mouth ; Palate.

CLERGYMAN'S THROAT. A chronic inflammation of the structures at the back of the throat is sometimes called clergyman's sore throat on account of its being caused to a large extent by an over use or improper use of the voice. The mucous membrane lining the back of the throat is dotted with little dark red elevations varying in size from a pinhead to a pea, or even larger in some cases. A dry cough and a tendency to hawking, which are important symptoms, aggravate the irritation, and the voice becomes weak and husky. The disorder may affect anyone who has to do much public speaking.

General treatment of some kind is usually necessary, and dyspepsia, constipation, anaemia, etc., should be remedied, if they exist. A visit to a spa possessing laxative waters is often beneficial. If there is any obstruction to nasal breathing it must be rectified. The granules at the back of the throat should be destroyed by the galvano-cautery or in some other way. The voice must be rested for as long as may be necessary. A correct method of voice production is of great importance in preventing the condition. Alcohol, tobacco and condiments should be avoided. As a temporary measure, the B.P. lozenge of benzoic acid, krameria or of red gum, or similar preparations, may be used.

See Larynx ; Pharynx.

CLIMACTERIC. *See* Change of Life.

CLIMATE. Here may be noted as briefly as possible the outstanding facts concerning climates of various kinds, in their relation to bodily health and to disease.

It is not sufficient to note the distance of a place from the equator, for many other factors also enter into the case, such, for instance, as the rainfall, the nature of the soil, the presence of vegetation, the height above sea level, and the nearness to large tracts of water. This last consideration is very important ; it does not do merely to divide climates into hot, temperate and cold, because an insular climate has its own characters, dependent not upon the distance of the place from the equator, but upon the influence of water in modifying the temperature of the air in its neighbourhood.

Hot climates are now frequently endured by Europeans, and especially by the Briton, but the measure of his adaptation to the new conditions is very small. He lives better in cold climates, yet here also his adaptation is imperfect, and though his mental activity is not so much diminished as it is in hot climates, his lungs and his kidneys are apt to suffer. The temperate climate is that to which the races of Europe are best fitted ; but it does not do to say that it is the climate which best suits the human race, because various races have undoubtedly undergone development under the influence of the climate to which they have been subjected.

Advantages of Living on an Island

The best variety of temperate climate is the temperate insular climate, such as that in which we live. The chief characters of an insular climate are the exceptional equableness of the seasons ; a summer only moderately hot, and a winter only moderately cold. The explanation of this fact is that during the summer the water surrounding the island tends to accumulate heat, thus largely sparing the land and air ; and during the winter the heat stored up in summer is given back to the air, thus moderating the cold which would otherwise be experienced. Furthermore, the dweller in an island such as ours is constantly undergoing change of air simply owing to the prevalence of winds ; and, lastly, his air is always a relatively moist air.

A cold, damp atmosphere is injurious to those suffering from rheumatism and chest affections, but a warm, moist atmosphere is beneficial to bronchitis with a dry, irritating cough. Very dry air, for example, desert air, which tends to deprive the lungs of their natural moisture, is very irritating. It may help bronchitis, however, when the expectoration is profuse. The insular climate is necessarily a rainy climate, but rain is a great purifier of the air, every shower of rain washing the air and removing dust and microbes from it. *See* Acclimatisation; Humidity.

CLINICAL. This term, from a Greek word meaning bed, is frequently used in medicine, together with its derivatives. A clinician, for instance, is a medical man who concerns himself entirely with the actual treatment of cases of disease, as distinguished from, say, a medical officer of health, or a bacteriologist. Again, clinic or clinique is the name of a lecture delivered at the bedside of a patient, or of a place where such instruction or treatment is given. A clinical thermometer is a thermometer (*q.v.*) used for estimating the temperature of a patient.

CLOT. *See* Coagulation.

CLOTHING. From the hygienic point of view, clothes are worn to afford protection against heat, cold, damp, wind and mechanical or other injuries. In hot climates, for instance, one must guard against the injurious rays in the strong sunlight, and also against the bites of such insects as the mosquito, which are capable of conveying disease infection. The body loses heat by radiation, conduction, and by the evaporation of sweat. In cold climates the clothing should therefore conduct heat badly, so as to retain it within the body, while in a hot climate the reverse is the case.

There is always a danger of chill if the clothing becomes damp with sweat, and to prevent this the clothing must absorb moisture well. Wool is a bad conductor of heat and is a good absorbent, and should be chosen for purposes of warmth, though silk, which also fulfils these requirements, may be preferred by those who can afford it. Cotton and linen, on the other hand, are good conductors of heat, and may be chosen for coolness, but as they do not absorb moisture well, they tend to become unpleasantly clammy, and

if one stands about after perspiring freely, a chill is likely to result. It is safer, even in hot weather, to have thin woollen or silk under-garments. For those whose skins do not tolerate pure wool, a mixture of wool and cotton or silk should be substituted.

Air is a bad conductor of heat and it is for this reason that fabrics which are loosely woven, and, therefore, have much air in their interstices, are warmer than those which have a dense texture. From this point of view cellular cotton is warmer than any other sort and may be warmer than some kinds of flannel. Also, several layers of thin clothing are warmer than a single thick layer, owing to the air between the layers.

The colour of the outer clothing is of some importance. Dark colours, such as black and dark blue, absorb heat, while lighter colours, for example, light grey and white, do this only slightly or not at all. Therefore black garments, by absorbing the heat of the sun, may be oppressive in the summer. Some dyes are capable of producing severe inflammation, so it is safer not to wear dyed fabrics next the skin.

Many people believe that by exposing the limbs of their children to all weathers, the children will be enabled better to withstand cold. This is a great mistake, and is the cause of much chest and joint trouble.

The exposure of the chest by women, either partially unclothed or covered only with thin cotton or linen, may expose them to chill, but tolerance is often acquired. All clothing should be loose enough to permit of the free play of the trunk and limb muscles. Young girls should not wear corsets as they tend to interfere with the development of the muscles of the spine. If they are allowed free, open-air exercise like their brothers, the need for corsets will probably never arise. Badly fitted corsets, sometimes worn to give a figure, do much harm. They press down the liver and other abdominal viscera, thus interfering with the digestive processes, and they press on the breasts and may give rise to trouble there. If a corset must be worn, it should support the breasts without compressing them.

Garters and other constricting bands about the clothing are harmful. Varicose veins are often due to constricting the legs with garters, and these should be replaced by suspenders. As far as possible all clothing should be hung from the shoulders.

Baldness in men has been attributed, and probably correctly, to wearing tight and badly ventilated hats. The tight brim certainly interferes with the circulation of blood in the scalp, and the moist warmth favours the growth of organisms.

Badly shaped boots are responsible for much suffering and disablement. A pointed toe on a boot is wrong, as it forces the great toe out of position and crowds all the toes together. Such a boot is modelled as if the axis of the foot ran down its middle, whereas in the normal foot the inner surface of the great toe and of the heel are in line. The boot should therefore have an almost straight inner border, and, moreover, the toe should be broad enough to allow free play for the toes, even when the boot is new. This point is illustrated under the heading Toe. In trying on a boot its fitness should be tested by standing up with it on, as in this position the foot always lengthens and broadens to some extent. A woman who walks on a high and narrow heel places her foot in an unnatural and unstable position. She therefore tires easily and is liable to sprain her ankle from trifling causes (*see* Plate II, 3).

Gloves should be sufficiently large to allow a proper circulation of blood in the fingers, or chilblains and chapping result.

CLOVE. Cloves, which are dried buds of an Eastern plant, eugenia caryophyllata, have important uses in medicine and in cooking. They owe their properties to a volatile aromatic oil which they contain. Applied outwardly, oil of cloves produces heat and redness of the skin, and may relieve muscular and other pain. If rubbed thoroughly over and into the hands it will disinfect them satisfactorily. It may be applied to a cavity of a tooth for the relief of toothache.

For internal use, oil of cloves may be given in doses of $\frac{1}{2}$ to 3 minims, and may be taken on a piece of lump sugar. By stimulating the flow of saliva and of gastric juice and increasing the movements of the stomach, it improves appetite and digestion. It is often prescribed in indigestion with flatulence. Oil of cloves also stimulates the movements of the muscles in the walls of the intestine and prevents irregular and colicky contractions. It is therefore frequently included in purgative pills in order to prevent griping, for example, in the B.P. colocynth pills.

CLUB FOOT. One or both feet may be deformed at birth, or may subsequently become so, as a result of paralysis of the muscles which move the foot, or from contraction of scar tissue following on disease or injury.

There are four main varieties of club foot. In the first, or talipes equinus, the heel does not reach the ground, the weight of the body falling on the ball of the foot. The opposite condition is found in talipes calcaneus, where the front of the foot is raised and the weight is taken on the heel. In talipes valgus and talipes varus the patient walks on the inner or outer border of the foot, respectively. Frequently the deformity consists of a combination of two of these types, that known as talipes equino-varus being the commonest.

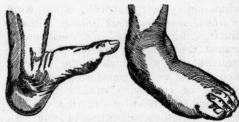

Club Foot. Left, variety termed talipes calcaneus ; right, talipes valgus, extreme flat foot

In congenital cases the mother or nurse may correct the deformity by manipulating the foot into the correct position several times a day. Such treatment, to be of any use, must be begun in the early weeks of life. Some form of apparatus must be applied to keep or bring the foot into a correct position. In other cases tendons and other structures have to be divided, and it may be also necessary to remove wedges of bone.

See Flat Foot ; Foot.

COAGULATION. Through the action of certain agents, such fluids as blood, milk and white of egg are clotted or coagulated, that is to say, they assume a more or less solid state.

The coagulation of milk is usually brought about by the ferment, rennet. In the presence of salts of lime, this ferment converts casein-ogen, a protein solution of milk, into the curd, which consists of casein and entangled fat. This process is a necessary preliminary to the digestion of milk and to the manufacture of cheese.

Blood coagulates when it is shed, the process usually beginning in from two to three minutes on the surface of the blood,

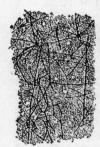

Coagulation. Left, network of fibrin threads shown on right filled with red blood cells

which becomes stiff and jelly-like. The whole mass of blood will be similarly altered in from 10 to 15 minutes. In a short time the clot begins to shrink and, in doing so, squeezes out a straw-coloured fluid, known as the blood serum. If the blood has been collected in a vessel, in an hour or two the clot will be found to be comparatively small and hard and floating in the serum.

The blood clot consists of a meshwork of fibrin filaments, imprisoning red and white blood corpuscles. The fibrin is produced from a substance known as fibrinogen, which is in solution in the blood plasma, the liquid part of blood. The change is brought about by the action of fibrin ferment, or thrombin, which is formed in the presence of lime salts from certain antecedent substances derived from injured white blood corpuscles and body cells, and probably also from the blood platelets.

The coagulation of blood is an important factor in the natural arrest of bleeding, as the clot which is formed blocks, more or less effectually, the opening of the cut blood vessel. It may be readily understood, therefore, that wounds must be handled very carefully as, in cleansing them, clots may easily be washed or rubbed away from the ends of the blood vessels, when bleeding will start afresh.

In some diseases, for example, haemophilia, haemorrhagic purpura, pernicious anaemia, and jaundice, there is an undue tendency to bleeding, either into the tissues or from slight wounds. This peculiarity is due to delay in blood coagulation depending upon a deficiency in some of the antecedents of fibrin ferment. In jaundice, it is the lime salts that are lacking, and so, when people suffering from jaundice must be operated upon, it is customary to administer the citrate or the chloride of calcium during the three days preceding the day of the operation.

When bleeding occurs in the tissues, as in a sprain, the clot may soften and disappear and the part recover perfectly ; but if the clot, or part of it, is not absorbed, it is gradually converted into fibrous or scar tissue, and this, by binding sinews and other parts together, is likely to cause subsequent pain and stiffness.

A thrombus is a clot which forms in the heart or blood vessels during life ; the process is called thrombosis. The expression " a clot of blood on the brain " may be taken to mean that clotting has taken place in a brain artery or that such an artery is blocked by a piece of thrombus detached from elsewhere.

See Bleeder ; Bleeding ; Blood ; Blood Vessel ; Embolism ; Milk ; Protein ; Thrombosis.

COAL GAS POISONING. *See* Carbon Monoxide.

COCAINE. The alkaloid cocaine is obtained from the leaves of the coca plant, which is found in South America, and which, it must be observed, has no connexion with cocoa.

It is largely used to produce local anaesthesia, and is of great value in the performance of operations on the eye, the nose and throat, and for tooth extraction. For most of these purposes it is combined with adrenalin, or extract of supra-renal gland, which helps to increase the anaesthetic effect. Sea-sickness and the vomiting of pregnancy are amongst other conditions which may be benefited by its use.

It is not a drug which can safely be taken often, as a habit is quickly formed.

The victim of cocainism, as the habit is called, rapidly loses all his moral sense; he usually suffers from sleeplessness, and may become clearly insane; his circulation, digestion and vision suffer greatly, the appetite is generally interfered with, and his body wastes.

An overdose of cocaine first excites and then depresses the brain, there is difficulty of breathing, and possibly convulsions. The treatment is to administer strong tea and coffee, sal volatile, and other stimulants. If the patient is unconscious a pint of warm coffee should be injected into the bowel. Chloroform may be necessary to stop the convulsions.

Eucaine, stovaine, butyn and other substances have been introduced at various times as substitutes for cocaine. The drug is one of those dealt with by the Dangerous Drugs Act.

See Drug Habits.

COCCUS. This name is applied to various kinds of microbes which are round in outline. The commonest of these are responsible for most cases of abscess, for many cases of blood poisoning and for erysipelas.

See Bacteria.

COCCYX. The lowest part of the spinal column is called the coccyx. It consists of four rudimentary vertebrae joined together, and is fixed to the lower end of the sacrum by a movable joint, but, as life advances, the union tends to become rigid. Should this occur prematurely in women it may give rise to difficulty in childbirth.

See Backbone.

COD-LIVER OIL. The value of cod-liver oil lies not only in the fact that it is a food and that, compared with other fats, it is very readily absorbed, but that it appears to have a powerfully stimulating effect on the general metabolism of the body. This is mainly due to its containing a plentiful supply of fat-soluble vitamins A and D. It is invaluable in rickets, in convalescence from acute diseases, in starvation, for people whose health is generally run down, as the saying is, for those constantly suffering from low spirits, in chronic diseases of the joints, and in chronic bronchitis, both in the young and the old; it is pre-eminently serviceable in every variety of tuberculosis.

The dose of cod-liver oil is generally stated to be from one to four teaspoonsful, but more can be taken if it is well digested. It should always be taken after a meal or at bedtime, and, when beginning a course of the oil, the first doses should be small. If the plain oil is taken the taste may be improved by adding a little pepper and salt or ketchup, or by taking it in milk or coffee. Most people find it easier to take an emulsion or a mixture of cod-liver oil and malt extract.

When there is great difficulty in taking the drug internally it may be rubbed into the skin. In a child a good site for this inunction is the abdomen; in adults it may be the skin under the armpits or on the inside of the thighs. These inunctions give rise to a disagreeable smell, but it is often well worth while to endure this.

COFFEE. The stimulating effects of coffee are due to it containing the alkaloid, caffeine, which is identical with theine, the active principle of tea. Coffee is a true stimulant, that is to say, it stimulates without producing subsequent depression, as occurs, for example, after the use of alcohol. It quickens the mental faculties and removes drowsiness, it temporarily increases the power of muscular endurance, it stimulates the heart, the kidneys, the bowels and the skin.

Its habitual use to stave off sleep to permit of brain work at night is dangerous, as it may lead to nervous exhaustion.

Muscular fatigue may be relieved or prevented, but, here again, it should not be used to allow of excessive strain. Coffee will be found to be a useful stimulant in heart disease and in prolonged fevers, such as pneumonia and enteric fever. In these cases also it affords a change of flavour for a patient on whom the monotony of milk diet is beginning to pall; and this is a matter of considerable importance. Coffee with breakfast is often an aid in securing a regular action of the bowels. Strong coffee may relieve a paroxysm of asthma. It may be used as a stimulant for the depression resulting from injuries, snake and insect bites, etc. It is an antidote in narcotic poisoning, and, if the patient is unconscious, a pint of strong, warm coffee may be injected into the bowel.

If coffee is drunk to excess it may cause indigestion, sleeplessness and various nervous symptoms.

See Caffeine; Tea.

COLCHICUM. Preparations of this drug have a remarkable power of relieving the most painful symptoms of gout, but they do not have any power in preventing the occurrence of gout, and do not affect its cause; they must only be looked upon as a mere means of relief. It is found that the drug must be used with care, since it is apt to cause irritation of the alimentary canal; it is therefore usually combined with alkalies. The commonest mode of administration is in the form of colchicum wine which is made with sherry. The active principle of the drug is colchicine.

See Gout.

COLD. The direct effects of cold in producing disease are seen in chilblains, frost bite, and some forms of rheumatism; indirectly it acts by lowering the resistance of the body and allowing scope for microbes. Cold may thus cause bronchitis, pneumonia, and a large number of other ailments. The effects of cold in causing disease are increased if it is combined with dampness; and a draught of cold air is more dangerous than still air at a much lower temperature.

As a remedy, cold is chiefly used in arresting bleeding, limiting inflammation and fever, and in relieving pain. Very cold water hastens coagulation of the blood and so arrests bleeding. It is chiefly useful where oozing is taking place; if blood is flowing freely the correct treatment is to put pressure on the bleeding spot. It arrests bleeding into the tissues, and relieves pain in sprains and other injuries. Iced cloths are applied, or what is known as an evaporating lotion. But cold should not be long continued for such purposes in the aged or infirm, or the tissues may possibly die.

An evaporating lotion or an ice-bag is often used to relieve neuralgia, and the latter also relieves the pain of pleurisy or of appendicitis and similar abdominal conditions. As the weight of an ice-bag might increase the pain, the bag is slung from a bed cradle (Plate IX, 1).

For the reduction of fever, cold may be applied by cold sponging, by a cold pack or a cold bath. Delirium and headache in fevers and in brain diseases may be diminished by applying cold to the head, either in some of the forms already mentioned or by the apparatus known as Leiter's tubes (Plate IX, 2).

See Baths; Bleeding; Cold Pack; Fever; Frost Bite; Leiter's Tubes.

COLD, COMMON. A common cold or, as it is technically named, coryza, is an acute infectious disorder due to a microorganism which has not yet been definitely identified, though there is good evidence to implicate the micrococcus catarrhalis. There is a great difference in the liability of different people to colds, some scarcely ever being affected. Others have a succession of them every winter, for the protection conferred by one attack may not last long; generally, however, it lasts for several months. Epidemics are common in the winter and spring.

Liability to infection does not appear to be diminished at all by vigorous general health; it is much increased by close contact with those suffering from colds, especially in rooms or other confined spaces; and the infection is widely disseminated by coughing and sneezing. A special tendency to take cold may depend on sources of irritation in the nose and throat, for example, enlarged tonsils or chronic irritation due to the excessive use of tobacco or alcohol. Chronic poisoning from pyorrhoea, constipation, etc., may also be a factor.

The gravity of a cold varies widely; it may not attack anything more than the lining of the nose and of the passages that communicate with the nose, such as the tear ducts, which carry the tears from the eyes to the nose, and the tubes which communicate between the ears and the back of the nose. Hence it is common to have some degree of deafness and unusual moistness in the eyes.

The throat may also be affected, though it very frequently escapes; sometimes the larynx may also be affected, or even the wind-pipe in the later stages of a bad cold.

At first the sneezing is accompanied by a thin, scanty secretion which is very irritating, and reddens the skin at the edges of the nose. Breathing through the nose is almost or quite impossible, because of the swelling of its lining ; and the speech is nasal. Later the swelling subsides, the secretion becomes abundant and thicker. Sometimes the lining of the eyelids is affected, and occasionally there may be some headache in the forehead owing to the swelling of a canal which leads from the nose up to the little cavities on the bone of the forehead, just above the nose and eyes.

The treatment of a cold depends on many circumstances. Most people take no notice of a slight cold, but if the temperature is definitely raised the patient should stay in the house, or even in bed. It should always be borne in mind that symptoms like those of a bad cold may inaugurate such diseases as measles and influenza.

How to Get Rid of the Germs

Further, it is necessary, as in every similar kind of disease, to get rid, as far as possible, of the poisons produced by the microbes that cause it, and to this end the patient must ensure free action of his skin by means of a hot bath, hot drinks, or some diaphoretic remedy such as Mindererus spirit, 2 to 6 drachms, or Dover's powder, 5 grains. An aperient should also be taken, a dose of castor oil or even something stronger, such as compound jalap powder, 10 to 60 grains.

Several remedies are used with the object of destroying the microbes concerned. These include ammoniated tincture of quinine, $\frac{1}{2}$ to 1 drachm, in a mixture or in tablets, and cinnamon essence or spirit of camphor, 15 drops of either on a piece of sugar. To have any effect, these remedies must be used at the very outset of the disease. A hot mustard foot bath may help to clear the head, and for this purpose also a variety of medicaments may be inhaled or sprayed into the nose, such as carbolised smelling salts, pinol, eucalyptus or menthol. These may be inhaled from the bottle, from a handkerchief or from steaming water. For spraying they are mixed with liquid paraffin in an appropriate spray apparatus. A sore throat may be treated by gargling with a weak solution of permanganate of potash.

The diet should be light and easily digested. If the cold leaves some general weakness behind it, a suitable tonic would be Easton's syrup, in $\frac{1}{2}$ teaspoonful doses, or the compound syrup of hypophosphites in teaspoonful doses thrice daily in a little water after food.

Liability to catch cold will be lessened by being as much as possible in the open air during epidemics of the disease.

Fresh air is also an important element in successful treatment, as there is nothing more calculated to increase the hold which the disease has on its victim than the plan of keeping to a hot room of which all the windows are closed.

The morning tub has the effect of increasing resistance to chills, and if for any reason it cannot be taken, some good accrues from douching the back of the neck and the shoulders with cold water every morning. A recurrence of colds may sometimes be prevented by the use of a vaccine.

See Bronchitis ; Cough ; Eucalyptus ; Eustachian Tube ; Influenza ; Lotion ; Nose.

COLD CREAM. The ointment of rosewater of the British Pharmacopeia is popularly known as cold cream. It may be used for inflamed or irritated states of the skin, sunburn, for example, or for any other purpose where an emollient is indicated.

COLD PACK. A high temperature—for example, in fevers or heat-stroke—may be lowered, and the highly nervous state often found in fevers may be soothed, by the use of a cold pack. It is applied as follows :

The bed is covered with a waterproof sheet over which a blanket is laid. A sheet is wrung out of cold water and spread out on the bed. On this the patient is laid, stripped, and it is then wrapped round him as high as the armpits, the legs being wrapped up separately. The patient is then covered with one or two blankets which are tucked well about him (*see* Plate IX, 3 and 4). He may be left in this from 15 minutes to half an hour, when he should be dried quickly.

See Delirium ; Fever.

COLIC. Pain due to irregular and violent contraction of various muscular tissues within the body is described as colic. According to the part affected we speak of intestinal colic, which is due to spasmodic contraction of the bowel ;

of biliary colic, due to irregular contractions of the bile ducts ; of renal colic, due to irregular contractions of the ureter—that is, the tube which passes downwards from the kidney to the bladder—and so on.

The cause of the spasmodic contractions is irritation of some kind ; for example, that due to a stone. All these muscular tissues are in regular action, but in health their work is entirely unnoticed by us. Their mode of contraction is wave-like, a sort of ripple of contraction runs along them, and this causes no sensation. But when their contraction becomes violently spasmodic extreme pain may be aroused.

Very often morphia must be employed, or a few whiffs of chloroform where this is available. Atropine, although it does not act so quickly as these others, has a remarkable power of relaxing muscular tissue of this kind and relieving the pain. It is injected beneath the skin by a doctor.

The commonest form of colic is that arising from irregular contraction of the bowel, and this may be due to a variety of causes, such as indigestible food, chill or constipation. In chronic lead poisoning intestinal colic is a prominent symptom. Severe griping pains are felt around the navel ; the abdomen may be distended, and there may be constipation or diarrhoea.

Difficulty of a Correct Diagnosis

It is sometimes very difficult to distinguish between pain due to inflammation, such as appendicitis, and that due to mere colic ; so that unless the colic is clearly due to indigestible food and responds quickly to simple remedies, it is well to call in a doctor at once.

The treatment alluded to consists in applying hot poultices or a hot water bag to the abdomen, and giving sips of hot water containing a little spirits, sal volatile, peppermint water or essence or the essences of ginger or cinnamon. Where irritating substances have been swallowed and the colic is accompanied by diarrhoea, a dose of castor oil may be given, and to this may be added 15 drops of laudanum. But if there is the slightest doubt as to the cause of the colic, a purgative should not be given. It will be safer, then, to try to move the bowels by an enema consisting of a pint of warm, soapy water containing a tablespoonful of oil of turpentine.

Colic in infants may be due to difficulties in digesting milk, but common causes are undue exposure during the bath and cold feet. Sips of warm water and of dill-water may be helpful, and also warmth applied to the abdomen by a fomentation or hot bag. It is necessary to emphasise the importance of precautions against burning the skin when making these hot applications.

After an attack of colic only milk food should be taken for a day, and for a few days longer the diet should be light, vegetables, fruit, or anything tough or stringy being studiously avoided.

See Carminative ; Constipation ; Diarrhoea ; Dill-water ; Indigestion, etc.

COLITIS. Inflammation of the colon or large intestine, technically known as colitis, may occur as a part of other diseases, for instance, the presence of a cancerous tumour in the bowel, appendicitis, tuberculosis, dysentery, etc., but it also occurs apart from other diseases and in several forms. These are simple catarrhal colitis, ulcerative colitis, and mucous or membranous colitis.

Acute simple catarrhal colitis begins suddenly with diarrhoea, pain in the abdomen and vomiting. The stools contain mucus or slime, and often bright blood. There may be cramps in the calves of the legs. Treatment for this and other forms of colitis should always be at the hands of a doctor, and in the present instance consists in putting the patient to bed, applying hot poultices to the abdomen and a hot-water bottle to the feet, and giving certain remedies, such as three minims of spirit of camphor every ten minutes for an hour, a starch and laudanum enema, etc. The diet should consist of such things as cold milk, to which may be added a tablespoonful of whisky or brandy to the glass, milk and lime-water, milk and isinglass, albumen water or barley water. The milk should be taken in sips.

Ulcerative colitis usually affects men who are past middle age. It is characterised by brownish liquid stools with a foul odour, and containing pus and blood, sometimes in the form of clots. The bowels are apt to move after food has been taken. Pain in the abdomen occurs in paroxysms, and may be of great severity. The disease may become chronic and leads to severe anaemia and prostration. The most successful treatment is by operation. The appendix is brought to the surface of the abdominal wall, cut off, and the bowel is then irrigated through the stump. This continues for many months.

Membranous colitis is so called because the patient passes from the bowel shreds of mucus, which sometimes may take the form of complete casts of segments of the bowel. This may be accompanied by great pain, and there may be considerable tenderness on pressing along the course of the large intestine. The patient is a chronic dyspeptic and usually presents symptoms of hysteria or neurasthenia. Women are much the most frequent victims, and the disease usually begins between the ages of twenty and forty. The course of the disease is very prolonged.

Dietetic treatment differs in the practice of various doctors, as some prescribe a light, easily-digested diet, consisting of pounded meat and fish, eggs lightly cooked, mashed potatoes, toast and similar foodstuffs, while others advise exactly the opposite, namely, plenty of cooked green food dressed with butter, wholemeal bread and other bulky foods. Chronic constipation is the rule, and may be corrected by daily enemata of warm water or daily doses of castor oil. The Plombières treatment of douching the lower bowel sometimes gives very good results when efficiently carried out.

The neurasthenic side of the symptoms must be met by appropriate treatment, rest, and interesting forms of light exercise, a change of environment, etc.

See Constipation; Diarrhoea; Dysentery; Intestine; Neurasthenia; Obstruction.

COLLAPSE. After profuse bleeding, in cholera, in severe poisoning, after serious burns, and in a large variety of other disorders, the patient may become collapsed. He is pale and cold, the pulse and breathing are feeble, and while in some cases the mind is quite clear, in others consciousness is more or less impaired. A doctor should be summoned at once, and in the meantime the patient is kept warm in bed with his head low. Hot-water bottles are placed at his feet and by his sides. It is not safe to give stimulants without medical advice, as, should the cause be, for instance, internal bleeding, this may be increased by stimulants.

See Bleeding; Burn; Fainting; Shock.

COLLAR BONE. The clavicle or collar bone is the curved bone which runs from the top of the breast bone outwards to the shoulder. It is a somewhat slender bone and is frequently broken, since in falls upon the shoulder, or upon the hand, the force is often transmitted through this bone. The consequence is that the shoulder falls forwards, downwards, and inwards, and, as one of the broken ends rides over the other, there is a lump on the course of the bone, easily detected by the finger. In order to make himself more comfortable, the patient usually supports the elbow on the injured side on the palm of his other hand.

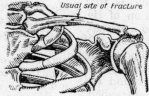

Usual site of fracture

Collar bone and its attachments

The first aid treatment is described under the heading Fracture and is illustrated in Plate X, 3–6. Generally a little deformity results if the patient walks about. Where, as in the case of a woman, it is desired to prevent any disfigurement, it can generally be achieved if the patient will agree to lie perfectly still on her back on a flat mattress and without a pillow until the broken ends have joined sufficiently firmly.

Either end of the bone may be dislocated, and in this case the limb is supported by a sling until a doctor can attend to the injury.

The subclavian artery runs beneath the collar bone, and about the middle of the bone is found to be lying on the top of the first rib. This is the site chosen to press on the artery for the arrest of bleeding. It is marked by a little depression or nest above and behind the collar bone (*see* Plate VI., 2 and 3).

See Bandage ; Bleeding ; First Aid ; Fracture.

COLLES' FRACTURE. A fracture of the lower end of the radius just above the wrist is known as a Colles' fracture. It is caused by a fall on the hand with the arm outstretched, and produces a characteristic deformity.

See Fracture ; Radius.

COLLODION. Flexible collodion is largely used as a means of protecting wounds. When it is painted on the skin it soon dries and forms a thin film, which protects the wound and, owing to contraction, tends to keep the edges of the wound together. It is absolutely airtight, is waterproof, and of course must only be applied to wounds which are perfectly sterile, that is to say, free from microbes and therefore yielding no dangerous products of inflammation. Collodium callosum and salicylic acid collodion are used to dissolve warts and corns.

COLLOID. If a vessel closed at one end with a parchment membrane and containing a solution of common salt be placed in another containing water, so that the salt solution is separated from the water by the membrane merely, salt will pass through the membrane into the water. If, however, a solution of gelatin or glue be substituted for the salt, none of the gelatin or glue will pass. For a substance that can pass through the membrane the name crystalloid was invented, and for a substance that cannot the name colloid.

It is now known, however, that a substance may be prepared in a colloid state although at other times acting as a crystalloid, and various metals and other substances are so prepared and used as drugs ; silver, sulphur and iodine, for example. In a colloid state these substances are practically harmless. It is also claimed that as the fluids of the body are, at least, mainly colloid solutions, colloid preparations are more readily effective in exerting the specific action of the drug.

See Drug.

COLLYRIUM. An eye lotion is sometimes called a collyrium, and the one most commonly used is made with boracic acid.

If as much boracic acid is added to hot water as can be dissolved, and this is allowed to cool, a saturated solution is obtained. Equal parts of this and of hot water can then be used to wash the eyes. This can be done by using an eye bath (*q.v.*) or by squeezing the lotion over the eye from a piece of absorbent cotton wool. The head is turned to one side so that the liquid can be received in a basin.

See Eye.

COLOCYNTH. The fruit of the bitter apple, or colocynth, acts as a drastic purgative. An extract of the pulp is used to prepare purgative pills, for example, a compound colocynth pill and pill of colocynth and hyoscyamus. The latter, which resembles Hamilton's pill, is less likely to gripe than the other. A medium dose of these pills for an adult is 5 grains.

See Cathartic.

COLON. The greater portion of the large bowel is called the colon.

See Intestine.

COLOUR BLINDNESS. This remarkable peculiarity of vision often goes by the name of Daltonism, since it was studied carefully by the great chemist, John Dalton, who himself was colour blind. Occasionally a person may become colour blind, but the disorder generally indicated by this term is a congenital affection.

The disease is hereditary, but in a very peculiar way. Like the bleeder's disease, it is practically confined to men. It often skips a generation, and is very frequently transmitted from a grandfather to his grandson by means of a mother who is herself free from any defect.

The most usual form is a difficulty in distinguishing red and green, these colours being confused with grey, blue and yellow. A violet-blind person confuses purple, red and orange. In some cases the defect is complete, and only black and white are distinguishable ; short of this the degree of difficulty varies, and sometimes merely consists of hesitation with regard to some colour combinations. The red-green defect is a bar to service on the sea or a railway when the duties include the recognition of these colours. There is no cure for the congenital defect.

Nor can anything be done when colour blindness is due to atrophy of the optic nerve, but where poisoning, as by alcohol, tobacco, diabetes, etc., is the cause, improvement usually follows the removal of the poison from the system. Alcohol and tobacco should be given up entirely. Colour blindness may be recognized by making a person match Holmgren's wools, which include many shades of colour; but the most reliable tests are those invented by Dr. Edridge-Green.

See Eye ; Tobacco.

COMA. The state of profound unconsciousness described as coma may be due to a large number of different causes ; for instance, pressure within or upon the brain, the production of various poisons inside the body, the introduction of various poisons into the body from without, such as alcohol, opium, prussic acid, and indeed the whole group of what are called nerve poisons.

The distinction between these various causes of coma may be immensely important, and may be difficult to detect, even for the trained doctor. Disastrous results only too frequently follow the inexpert opinion that a comatose person is drunk, when in reality he is suffering from some grave disease or form of poisoning which is threatening his life, and which might be controlled if it were recognized. Coma vigil is the name given to a condition which occurs in severe fevers and other diseases when the patient lies with the eyes open and mutters to himself, but is unconscious.

See Collapse ; Unconsciousness.

COMFORTER. The advantage of being able to pacify a baby by providing it with a comforter, or dummy teat, is heavily outweighed by the disadvantages. Its use may lead to deformity of the baby's jaws and palate, with narrowing of the nose passages and the institution of mouth breathing. In addition to this, it commonly introduces infection into the baby's mouth, thus leading to diarrhoea and other disorders. In no circumstances, therefore, should a comforter be used.

COMPLEXION. The skin of the face undergoes many important changes in disease, some of which enable the doctor to understand the nature of his case ; but in this article merely the conditions necessary for its health will be considered.

In the first place, it must be admitted that differences in complexion do not entirely depend upon health. The skin contains a certain amount of colouring matter, even in the white races, and the appearance of the complexion depends also upon the harmony between the tint of the skin and that of the eyebrows and hair. Pallor is dealt with under its own heading.

There is a common, popular belief that various kinds of rash or eruption upon the skin are due to bad matter making its escape in this fashion from the blood. In general this is a mistake. Spots and pimples, blotches and boils, are due in general to infection of the skin by microbes from without. If, therefore, the skin is to be kept clear, these microbes must be prevented from getting an entry.

As in the case of every other form of opposition to microbes, there are two courses to be pursued. First, there is the method of direct attack upon the microbes; second, that of rendering the soil unfit to support their life.

Cleanliness a Sine Quâ Non

With regard to the first method, in order to preserve the complexion it is first of all necessary to have the face clean, which is not always an easy matter for people who live in the filth-laden air of cities. Frequent washing with ordinary soap may, however, irritate the skin and produce blotches. If there is a tendency of this sort a change should be made to what is called a superfatted soap ; that is to say, one which has no free alkali. A delicate skin may sometimes be cleansed with cold cream.

To render the skin unsuitable for the growth of microbes, the most important means consists in a moderate massage of the skin every day with a rather rough towel immediately after it has been washed and thoroughly dried. A little friction and movement of the skin not only increases for the time being the amount of blood that nourishes it, but also tends to empty the little channels from the glands of the skin, and so promotes its general health.

A large number of the applications so frequently advertised for the care of the skin are of more than doubtful value.

Many of them interfere with the natural process by which the skin tries to keep itself clean. There is no form of application that has any title whatever to rank as a food for the skin. No tissue in the body is capable of utilising any kind of food until that food has been through a number of processes, and has passed into the blood, which distributes the food to every part in a fit state for immediate use. On the other hand, a good face cream may benefit a dry skin by increasing its softness and pliability.

A sallow, muddy complexion may be due to a septic mouth or pyorrhoea, to indigestion, constipation, and to neglect of various rules of healthy living, as, for example, a sufficiency of exercise in the open air, of sleep, and of fresh air in the bedroom at night. It would be necessary, therefore, to put such matters right in order to obtain benefit from care directed to the face itself.

See Breathing Exercises ; Cleanliness ; Constipation ; Cyanosis ; Exercise ; Freckles ; Indigestion ; Jaundice ; Pallor ; Skin ; Soap ; Sunburn ; Teeth.

COMPRESS. A compress is a folded cloth applied firmly to some part of the body to prevent haemorrhage or lessen inflammation. It may be wet or dry. A compress is often used to limit bleeding and thereby the subsequent disfigurement of a " black " eye. The application will be more successful if the cloth is wrung out of cold, and preferably iced, water. A sprain is another condition which may be benefited by a compress.

See Bruise ; Fomentation ; Poultice.

COMPRESSION. A state of the brain, termed compression, which depends upon the increase of pressure within the skull, may be due to pressure from outside, as when the skull is broken, or upon bleeding within the skull, upon inflammation of the brain or its coverings, or upon a brain tumour. The duty of distinguishing between compression and what is called concussion is one of the most important that the doctor has to discharge. The treatment of compression must plainly depend upon its cause.

See Brain.

CONCUSSION. Concussion of the brain is usually the result of accident, and consists of a violent shaking of the brain substance. It is most commonly due to a blow or fall upon the head, but sometimes may occur as a result of a fall upon the end of the spine, or even an unbroken fall upon the feet, the brain being very sensitive to mechanical shocks of this kind. Symptoms of concussion and details of treatment are given under the heading Brain (q.v.).

CONDENSED MILK. Condensed milk is cow's milk from which part of the water has been evaporated, and which has been sterilised by heat. The best is made from milk which is " whole," or to which cream has been added. Inferior condensed milk is made from skimmed milk and should only be used for cooking. A good deal of sugar is added to most kinds of condensed milk. When this is diluted sufficiently to make the proportion of sugar about right, the mixture is then deficient in cream. Unsweetened condensed milk, however, has not this defect, and on occasion it may be of use. It does not keep quite so well after the tin has been opened.

An infant's diet should not, as a rule, consist of condensed milk of any kind ; taken alone, such milk is a frequent cause of rickets. A restriction of the diet to condensed milk may also lead to the development of scurvy, as such milk does not contain the antiscorbutic vitamin. To remedy this defect the infant should be given a teaspoonful of orange-juice twice a day.

Dried milk, or milk in the form of a powder, is now made and is largely used in infant feeding. It avoids possibilities of infection inherent in fresh milk and, at least in the case of some brands, is said to be supplied with the necessary vitamins ; but even then orange-juice is advisable. Humanised dried milk is also obtainable, that is to say, cow's milk which has been so altered as to approximate in composition to human milk.

See Baby ; Milk.

CONFECTION. In pharmacy, drugs made into a mass with honey or moistened sugar are styled confections. Those contained in the British Pharmacopoeia are as follows : confection of pepper, a remedy for flatulence ; confection of roses, used for making pills ; confection of senna and confection of sulphur, purgatives. The dose in each case is 60 to 120 grains. Confections are comparatively agreeable preparations.

CONGENITAL. A disease or peculiarity which is present at birth, as, for instance, the possession of six fingers on each hand, or colour blindness, is said to be congenital. Much confusion still exists between the uses of the words congenital and hereditary. The terms are often used as if they were identical, but this is not so. Certainly everything which is truly inherited is present at birth, but there are many conditions present at birth which are in no sense inherited. For instance, a child may be born with a deformity of one of the limbs, due to an accident before birth ; this, of course, is not a case of heredity, but one of congenital deformity.

See Constitution ; Heredity.

CONGESTION. When any organ or tissue is too full of blood, that is to say, when the blood vessels in it are stretched and over-filled, it is said to be congested. There is no absolute line between the temporary congestion which is quite normal and the longer-continued congestion which is abnormal. Blushing, for instance, is a state of temporary congestion of the skin of the cheeks, and is not abnormal. But the cheeks may be similarly congested persistently, in consequence of disease of the tiny blood vessels in them, or some obstruction to the return of blood from them ; this would be a case of morbid congestion.

Congestion, also, is the first stage of the process which is called inflammation. It is not to be regarded as either bad or good in itself ; it may be either. Sometimes it is deliberately sought for its beneficial results, as when a mustard plaster is used, or in what is called Bier's treatment (*q.v.*) for joints affected by tuberculosis or other diseases. On the other hand, chronic congestion may be an annoyance, as, for instance, when it affects the womb, or the throat in people who have to use the voice extensively. Probably its most common causes are chronic irritation and over-use of the congested part ; and thus the treatment of congestion cannot be discussed as if this were a disease in itself, for it depends entirely upon the various causes which may lead up to the condition in any given case.

Congestion due to a sudden dilatation of the small arteries, such as occurs at the beginning of inflammation, is called acute congestion. When the blood vessels become over-filled from some kind of obstruction to the flow, passive congestion ensues. When this is due to gravity, it occurs in the parts of the body which happen to be lowest, and is then called hypostatic congestion. This may occur in the dependent parts of the lungs when old or debilitated people are left lying on their backs too long. It is desirable, therefore, that bedridden, helpless patients should have their position changed at fairly frequent intervals.

See Circulation of the Blood ; Hyperaemia ; Inflammation ; Liver ; Plethora, etc.

CONJUNCTIVITIS. The term conjunctivitis means inflammation of the conjunctiva, that is, the membrane that lines the eyelids and covers the white of the eye. This may arise from a large number of circumstances, and it is found in a variety of forms.

As there may be more or less serious damage to vision following in its wake, any but the slightest cases of conjunctivitis should have prompt medical care.

Simple catarrhal conjunctivitis may be caused by smoke, dust, the abuse of alcohol, the activity of microbes, and other causes. In the acute form the conjunctiva on the ball of the eye and that on the lids are both involved. The eye looks bloodshot, and the little fleshy mass at the inner corner of the lids is specially noticeable. There is itching, burning, and a sensation of grit under the eyelids. A sticky secretion is poured out from the conjunctiva, and through this it is often found that the edges of the eyelids and the lashes are glued together in the morning. Frequently the discharge contains pus or matter. Sometimes the eye becomes very painful and exposure to a bright light causes acute discomfort.

In treatment, the first thing to consider is the cause, since when this is removed, as, for example, a foreign body in the eye, simple measures usually bring about a quick cure. The eye should be washed frequently and freely with boracic acid lotion. A dropper may be used for applying certain medicaments, as shown in Plate X, 2. The edges of the eyelids should be anointed at night with an ointment consisting of vaseline, with 10 grains of boracic acid to the ounce, in order to keep them from adhering. If light is hurtful the eyes may be protected by wearing a wide brown paper shade, or one made of cardboard and covered with green fabric. As a rule, the eye should not be bandaged.

Chronic catarrhal conjunctivitis is usually limited to the conjunctiva of the eyelids, the edges of which may also show evidences of inflammation. The discharge may be slight and only show itself in little crusts at the inner corner of the eyelids and perhaps by sticking of the eyelids in the morning. The possibility of the inflammation being due to eye strain should be remembered, and the sight should be tested to determine whether or not glasses are necessary or, if already worn, whether they are suitable.

A useful lotion for this condition consists of 5 grains of boracic acid and 1 grain of zinc sulphate in an ounce of distilled water. If there is any deposit at the bottom of the bottle it should not be shaken up.

A very serious form of conjunctivitis is caused by the germ of gonorrhoea. Its importance may be estimated from the fact that it is responsible for a third of all cases of blindness. It should be noted also that nearly all the blindness due to this cause results from the occurrence of the disease in newly-born children, and that it is preventable.

Conjunctivitis in the Newly Born

In infants the first signs usually appear about the third day after birth. The eyelids become red and swollen, and there is a sticky discharge, clear or mixed with blood. A few days later the discharge consists of thick yellow matter. The cornea, or clear part of the eye, may become the site of a suppurating ulcer, and through this the whole eyeball may become inflamed and be destroyed; or, if the ulcer heals up, a white scar or leukoma remains, and this destroys vision according to its extent.

The treatment of this condition, which is known as ophthalmia neonatorum,

demands unremitting medical and nursing skill. The preventive measures which would almost invariably be successful are to wash the eyes with a clean rag first of all, when the baby has its first bath after birth, and the use by the doctor of drops containing some preparation of silver, such as colloidal silver.

Trachoma, which is also known as granular or Egyptian ophthalmia, is a

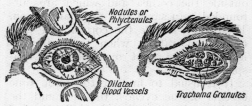

Conjunctivitis. Two forms of this inflammatory disease of the eye : left, phlyctenular type : right, trachoma, showing inner surface of eyelid

form of conjunctivitis in which granules appear on the inner surfaces of the eyelids. It is contagious, though the acute variety, in which there is more or less purulent secretion from the affected surfaces, is much more so than is the chronic form. The disease runs a long course.

There are two other forms of conjunctivitis which are sometimes confused with trachoma. One is the follicular conjunctivitis, which is usually found in young people, and which consists of pinkish-grey granules on the inner surface of the eyelids, chiefly the lower one. It is more tractable than is trachoma.

The other condition is known as spring catarrh. Here there are also granules on the inner surface of the lids, but these have a sort of tesselated or pavemented appearance. Besides this, the white of the eye on either side of the cornea may show a reddish-grey discoloration, and the surface of the conjunctiva may have an opaque, milky appearance.

Symptoms similar to those described for catarrhal conjunctivitis may be present, and there may be a mucous or a muco-purulent discharge. This disease occurs most often in young men, and hot weather seems to have much to do with bringing it on. The face is pale, and as the upper eyelid tends to droop the patient has a sleepy appearance. Treatment by radium seems to have some effect.

There is another form of conjunctivitis which is known as the phlyctenular, eczematous or scrofulous type. It is mainly found in children who are of a scrofulous habit or whose health has been reduced by an attack of measles, whooping-cough, scarlatina or something of the kind. It consists of minute pustules, or blisters filled with matter, which make their appearance on the white of the eye just outside the cornea and which are surrounded by a small area of inflammation. These may invade the cornea and give rise to ulceration, when the pain and intolerance of light may be very conspicuous.

It is usual to find at the same time eczema of the eyelids, the face and the head, and also chronic inflammation within the nose. Frequently the nose and upper lip are swollen. In addition to local treatment it is essential that the general health should be improved by fresh air, good feeding, cod-liver oil and perhaps syrup of the iodide of iron.

See Collyrium ; Copper ; Eye.

CONSTIPATION. The failure of the bowels to open easily and regularly, which is described as constipation or sometimes costiveness, is a very common complaint, probably more common nowadays and amongst civilized peoples than in the past and amongst savages. The reason for this is plain. The proper action of the bowels depends upon their due stimulation by their contents. This stimulation is always forthcoming when the food taken is coarse and contains an abundance of waste matter. The impulse to relieve the bowels is increased by the presence of liquid in the contents, and this is the reason why an enema is so speedily effective.

If the impulse is not followed up, it may pass away for the time being, and the bowel content becomes dried. The impulse may not return for several days, and the bowels may then be evacuated naturally and resume their regular action. But sometimes the hardened faeces irritate the delicate bowel lining and produce the painful affection known as fissure.

Some people allow their bowels to become bound up for several days and then seek relief by taking a brisk purge. This practice is wrong, because an action of the bowels caused in this way is followed by reaction in the shape of constipation, and thus a vicious circle is established. In the circumstances mentioned it is better to use an enema of soap and water, containing castor oil or olive oil. This also lessens the danger of a fissure.

Chronic constipation is liable to cause piles, and congestion also of neighbouring organs, as, for example, the womb in women. It may give rise to colicky pains in the abdomen and the digestion may be upset, the tongue being furred and the breath foul. The absorption of poisons produced by the stagnant bowel contents may cause very considerable depression of body and mind.

When it is asked what constitutes constipation, it must be allowed that what is normal for one person is not so for another. Undoubtedly the majority of people do rightly to observe the rule of " once a day "—a sort of natural rule which is convenient and safe. A regular time should be chosen, and the best is undoubtedly after breakfast, for the mere taking of breakfast helps to stimulate the bowel. Taking coffee with breakfast increases this stimulation, and many men find that a smoke does so also.

It follows from what has been said that the rational means of treating constipation is by a change in the diet, so that it comes to include more of those indigestible substances which are contained in the diet of natural man. For instance, the substitution of wholemeal bread for ordinary white bread may make the necessary difference, owing to the presence of the bran in the former.

Value of Fresh Fruit and Vegetables

Other foods that are desirable in this connexion may be noted : fruit in general, notably figs, raw apples, and prunes ; vegetables, especially those that have a large residue, such as cabbage, and also tomatoes ; honey and marmalade, which so many people use for this purpose ; and treacle and porridge. Many people might with advantage go the length of taking a course of vegetarianism.

Equally important to such modifications of the diet is the attempt to form a regular daily habit at a constant hour. There is no doubt that abdominal massage is often useful in restoring the tone of the bowel (Plate XXIV, 7 and 8). Much success has followed the device of filling a leather ball with swan shot and rolling it over the abdomen as one lies in bed in the morning. The ball should weigh about five pounds and, beginning above the right groin, should move round the abdomen in the direction of the hands of the clock. Short of this it is a useful measure to improve the tone of the muscles of the abdominal wall by bending the thighs up and down for a few minutes every morning in bed before getting up. Regular exercise in the open air i san important help.

But if all these measures have failed recourse must be had to the use of drugs, although full reliance must never be placed on them alone. A very large number of drugs which have an action upon the bowels either tend to lose their property in time, or they induce laziness on the part of the bowel itself, or they have a definite after-action, as explained above. These drugs have their uses at one time and another, but they are one and all condemned for cases of habitual constipation. In other words, the object of the drugs must be to give a tonic to the muscular wall of the bowel, so that by an improvement of its health it is enabled to do its own work for itself without artificial assistance.

Drugs that Have a Tonic Effect

Of drugs that answer to this description three may be noted. Aloes has long been popular, and is certainly the most widely used of all, since it is present so frequently in patent medicines. Nux vomica, containing the valuable tonic strychnine, is also widely employed.

Probably better than either of these in the majority of cases is cascara sagrada. It can conveniently be taken in the form of capsules, tablets or pills ; the liquid preparations have an intensely bitter taste, which may be corrected by flavouring agents, as in the aromatic syrup of cascara, and similar mixtures. Properly used, and accompanied by other measures, it is a means of curing, as distinguished from removing, the symptoms of chronic constipation. It may be given in small doses three or four times a day, or in a single dose at bedtime.

The doses usually taken are far too large for the best results. They should be just sufficient to produce one natural movement of the bowels each day. An adult might begin with 2 grains of the dry drug in pill or tablet, or 20 drops of the liquid extract, thrice daily, or 4 grains and half a drachm respectively at bedtime ; and either increase or diminish the dose until the correct one is discovered. This should be continued for about a fortnight and then be gradually reduced until in about two months' time the drug is discontinued altogether.

Amongst other drugs used for chronic constipation, mention may be made of sulphur and liquid paraffin. The habitual use of salts is decidedly not good treatment. Pregnant women appear to do best on a teaspoonful of castor oil at bedtime.

Treatment of the Condition in Children

With reference to constipation in children, it may be observed that during the first year of life the bowels usually move two or three times a day ; in the second year twice, and thereafter once daily. In the case of infants, constipation may be due to a deficiency of sugar or of fat in their diet, and an additional ration of either of these should be tried, fat being given in the form of fresh cream, a teaspoonful once or twice a day. When a child strains much at stool, better than opening medicine is a small enema of soap and water, or a glycerin or soap suppository.

It should be pointed out that much may be done in training even young infants to have regular habits in this respect. When constipation is habitual cascara is again probably the best remedy, and it should be used on the principles already laid down. The initial dose might be 5 drops of the liquid extract in simple syrup, or twice this amount of the aromatic syrup of cascara, once or twice daily. Olive oil, $\frac{1}{2}$ to 2 teaspoonsful, according to age, and given the last thing at night, is often successful in children.

Simple constipation only has been hitherto considered, but it must be noted that interference with the action of the bowels may be due to a large number of much more serious causes, such as the presence of various obstructions. The detection of the nature of such cases is a matter for the most expert skill.

See Aloes ; Cascara Sagrada ; Cathartic ; Grape Cure ; Intestine ; Intussusception ; Piles.

CONSTITUTION. It is well established that individuals inherit qualities of bodily structure and function from their forbears, and that in many cases these qualities may be of the nature of patent abnormalities ; in others, liability to certain diseases ; and in others, again, special powers of resistance to diseases.

Among abnormalities which may appear in successive generations may be included an excessive number of fingers or toes ; the peculiar skin disease known as ichthyosis or fish skin ; colour blindness, and haemophilia, or the bleeder's disease. An inherited proclivity may often exist to insanity, to epilepsy, migraine and other nervous diseases ; to gout and rheumatism, diabetes, psoriasis, asthma, tuberculosis, and other diseases.

In the same way an individual, in consequence of his descent, may not be prone to some diseases. The negro, for example, does not appear to contract yellow fever ; and malaria, which works havoc amongst white men in the tropics, is, in his case, a comparatively mild disease. A constitutional tendency to disease indicates a defect somewhere in the make-up of the individual, and this, under the ordinary wear and tear of life, comes into view in the form of some malady or other.

It is necessary to understand clearly, however, the precise rôle played by defects of this kind in the development, for example, of tuberculosis, a disease which is caused by a microbe, and which will not exist unless this microbe is able to invade the body. Inherited weakness here plays a relatively small part as compared with the opportunities for infection. If the children of a consumptive parent develop tuberculosis, it is almost certainly because they are too much exposed to infection. The sputum which a consumptive spits up is loaded with bacteria, and unless care is exercised in disposing of it, the consumptive's whole environment teems with infection.

Possibly a child could be born suffering from tuberculosis, just as many children are born suffering from syphilis ; but in both these instances the children suffer because germs have been transmitted to them by a parent, and so they may be said to inherit the disease from such parent. But if a person born with an inherited disease is cured of his disease and begets children while still free from the disease, these will not be affected by it.

It is otherwise with such a condition as epilepsy, for example. The disease is not due to anything extraneous, as in microbe infection, but to some defect in the nervous mechanism of the parent, and this defect he may pass on to his progeny. In them the defect may exhibit itself also as epilepsy, but not necessarily so ; the descendant may exhibit it, for example, in a tendency to migraine. It is to be noted, also, that the defect may not be passed on at all, but there is always a risk that it will be ; and if there are several children in the family, one or more is almost certain to have it.

If marriage takes place between members of a family in which such a proclivity exists, the defect is likely to show itself in an exaggerated form in their offspring. Consequently, those who marry in these circumstances may inflict a serious wrong on any children who may be born to them.

See Congenital ; Consumption ; Heredity.

CONSUMPTION. The disease which is best known as consumption or decline is sometimes also referred to as phthisis. All these names express the same thing, namely, the wasting away which occurs in this disease, and so long as the real nature of a disease is unknown, it is convenient to call it by the name of its prominent symptom ; but now that the nature of this disease is known, it is more accurately described as tuberculosis of the lung, which implies that it is a diseased process in the lung due to the presence and activities of a microbe known as the tubercle bacillus.

To say that a person is in a decline is to express, however, in a vivid way what is the most usual course of the disease. It consists of a gradual sapping of the strength and a gradual wasting of the body. Such things may be present before the development of a cough, though a short, dry cough is often the first thing that draws attention to the patient. It may be observed that when the patient attempts to go on with his work or exercise as usual, he is unduly fatigued and easily made short of breath. If his pulse is counted it may be found unduly quickened by exercise and slow to return to its ordinary rate when at rest, while the temperature, if taken for a number of successive evenings, may be above the normal.

The patient may also exhibit a pallor of the face which is shared by the lips and gums, and if his weight be taken at intervals of some days, a progressive fall may be evident. There may be a diminution of the appetite, and perhaps a complaint of dyspepsia. In the presence of circumstances such as these suspicion of tuberculosis of the lungs would arise, and the patient should be placed under medical observation.

Another suspicious symptom is spitting up blood. This may be the first sign of the disease, and occur in a person who is apparently quite well. Blood may be spat out in a number of other conditions— for example, unhealthy state of the gums— but when the amount approaches a teaspoonful it is safer to assume that it means tuberculosis of the lung, unless there is some other satisfactory explanation of its presence.

Symptoms of Advanced Consumption

However it begins, if the disease is allowed to progress the cough becomes worse, and some sputum is brought up. If this is examined it may be found to contain the tubercle bacillus. As time goes on the sputum becomes more purulent ; it may also become very offensive, due to the invasion of the lung by putrefactive bacteria. Signs of fever become more manifest : a constant elevation of the temperature with an additional rise at night, a hectic flush and drenching sweats at night or during the day if the patient goes to sleep. Loss of flesh continues till there is great emaciation, and the skin assumes a dirty grey appearance. Diarrhoea may be troublesome and with this may occur pain in the abdomen, these signs very often meaning an infection of the bowel from the sputum which has been swallowed. Sometimes the

larynx becomes infected, giving rise to huskiness, loss of voice, and, often, great pain in speaking and in swallowing.

Thus far chronic pulmonary tuberculosis has been described, but the disease may also occur in acute forms. These acute cases are popularly referred to as galloping consumption, and may either resemble lobar pneumonia (q.v.) or bronchopneumonia (q.v.). These almost always proceed rapidly to a fatal termination, though sometimes they settle down to the chronic form.

Carelessness of Germ Carriers

It has been already said that the direct cause of this disease is the tubercle bacillus, and that this germ may be present in the sputum of a person suffering from the disease ; it should be added that it may be present in enormous numbers. When the person coughs or talks loudly the germs are spread in the spray which comes from his mouth, and in this way they may be carried for a distance of many feet.

If the patient spits on the street, into a common spittoon, or into a handkerchief, the sputum may dry and the microbes be widely disseminated by the dust to which they become attached. There is thus a possibility that other people may inhale the infected air, when the microbes may be carried directly into the lungs. More frequently they adhere to the lining of the mouth or the throat through which they make their way, or they are swallowed and pass through the bowel lining. People who handle consumptive patients or their belongings may get the infection on their hands and convey it to their mouths.

The tubercle bacillus also occurs in cattle, and may be ingested in butcher's meat which has not been properly cooked. But this source of infection is insignificant as compared with the milk of tuberculous cows. The microbes are also found in butter and cheese made from tuberculous milk. Bovine tuberculosis is not common in adults, but is quite a frequent cause of enlarged glands and of acute tuberculous affections in children.

It is common knowledge that tuberculosis may occur as a family disease, the children of tuberculous parents very often becoming affected also. This has naturally given rise to an opinion that the disease may be inherited. There are undoubtedly instances where an unborn child is infected, but such are believed to be uncommon. It is considered also that in some families there may be inherent weakness of resistance to the activities of the tubercle bacillus.

Extreme Infectiousness of the Disease

In considering the chances of an individual becoming the subject of tuberculosis, this inherent susceptibility would appear, however, to be relatively unimportant as compared with his opportunities of becoming infected. Cogent evidence has been adduced for the proposition that infection with pulmonary tuberculosis always takes place in the first two years of life, and that whenever it occurs at a later age it is merely a recrudescence of the old disease. Sufficient has been said to show the imminent danger in a household, unless strict precautions are taken. The danger will be increased if the accommodation is restricted, and if the premises are dark and badly ventilated. It will be further increased if the inmates have an insufficient supply of food.

Damage to the lung by other diseases predisposes to tubercle, and thus the disease often attacks children who suffer from broncho-pneumonia, either in connexion with measles, whooping-cough or otherwise. The same liability is shown in the case of those whose occupations are carried on in an atmosphere charged with dust, such as steel grinders, quartz miners, potters and so on. It is quite a common thing for people who suffer from debilitating diseases, diabetes, for instance, to contract and die from tuberculosis of the lungs.

When tubercle bacilli invade the tissues of the body they are taken along lymphatic channels. They thus reach lymphatic glands where they may remain and multiply, or they may pass on to other glands. From these they pass out through the lymphatic vessels to different organs, and as the lungs contain an enormous number of such vessels it is natural that they should be such a common site of tubercular disease. From the glands they may make their way also into the blood stream and pass on till they reach the smallest blood vessels, the capillaries which also are found to an enormous extent in the lung tissue.

It is the habit of the white blood corpuscle to kill and devour microbes which it has taken into its substance, but this it has difficulty in doing in the case of the tubercle bacillus, because this organism has a protecting outer fatty envelope. It is thus the white blood corpuscle which is usually killed, while the microbe survives and multiplies. When this is going on the microbes become surrounded by a collection of cells forming tiny nodules, which are known as tubercles, whence the name tuberculosis is derived.

The tubercles may collect into masses and may infiltrate the lung tissue. This new material may degenerate into a cheesy mass, which may be softened and be coughed out, leaving a cavity; sometimes, however, it is converted into a hard mass through becoming permeated with lime salts.

For protection against the bacilli there tends to be produced round the tubercles new or scar tissue, and then the infection may be walled off. This process, which is known as fibrosis, may be very extensive, and as the scar tissue contracts, it may drag on the heart and displace it far from its normal position. Fibrosis is the natural process of cure. Sections of an infected lung are shown in Plate XI, 1-3.

The cavities which have been mentioned as having been produced in the lung have at first raw ulcerated walls. Vessels in their walls may become involved in the ulceration process and be opened, thus giving rise to more or less bleeding. These cavities also tend to be invaded by putrefactive organisms, and then their contents may become very offensive.

How Consumption Must Be Treated

The treatment of consumption requires the supervision of the doctor at every stage, and it will be sufficient here merely to outline the lines of treatment which are usually adopted. When the disease shows that it is active, for example, by a rise of temperature, loss of weight, and so on, the patient should rest in bed. It is a desirable thing that patients in whom the disease is even only suspected should rest until the true nature of their condition is cleared up.

In all cases where the existence of the disease in active form is established, rest in bed must be prolonged until it becomes quiescent, that is, for two months at least, though it may be four, six or more months.

As the object of rest in bed is to diminish as far as possible the movement of the damaged lung, it is necessary that the patient should do as little talking as possible so as to further this purpose.

The patient's bed should be placed either in a room close to a widely open window, one with the sashes taken out being the best, on a verandah or in a garden shelter. In certain circumstances it may be necessary to go to a hospital or to a sanatorium. Fresh air and sunlight are what principally matter in the choice of a sleeping apartment (*see* Plate XII).

If it is possible to have a shelter in the garden it is a decided gain (*see* Plate XII,1). This should preferably be a revolving one, but if not it should face south-west. It should have a shutter or a screen to let down quickly to keep off rain. The patient should begin sleeping in it in fine weather, and its benefits will be appreciable at once. The cough will be eased and the night sweats may cease.

The patient should be washed all over each day, and should have his teeth and mouth cleansed several times a day, using a weak antiseptic mouth wash (*q.v.*).

The diet must be as liberal as can be digested and assimilated, but the patient's powers in these directions will vary and must be studied. There is great scope in this connexion for skill and care in the choice, cooking and serving of food. An abundant supply of milk should be given, and when solid food appears to be digested with difficulty, recourse should be had to raw eggs and raw meat. The latter may be given in the form of meat juice or be pounded or minced, when it can be served in sandwiches, in milk, or in warm soup.

When the patient begins to get up he should be careful to rest for half an hour before, and the same time or longer after, his meals. While endeavouring to get him to take a sufficiency of food, care should be taken not to overdo it, other-wise his digestion may suffer or he may become obese and flabby. Cod-liver oil (*q.v.*) has long been known to have a favourable effect in tuberculosis. It acts both as a remedy and as a food, and should be taken whenever possible. It is best to begin with a small dose after a meal. The patient should not smoke, and should only take alcohol on the doctor's advice. Sometimes a little light beer or wine helps the appetite and digestion.

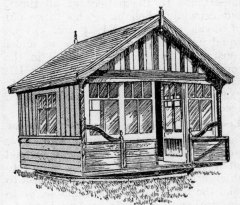

Consumption.   Open-air revolving shelter
Courtesy of Boulton & Paul, Ltd.

It may be necessary to do something for one or other of the symptoms on occasions when the doctor is not at hand. Thus, if the temperature runs up to the neighbourhood of 103° F., sponging with tepid water and vinegar will help to keep it within bounds. If there is pain in the chest or abdomen, it may be relieved by applying a hot-water bottle or a mustard plaster.

Bouts of prolonged coughing may be due to pharyngeal irritation, caused sometimes by cigarette smoking, and may be eased by gargling with warm water containing bicarbonate of soda or alum. A mixture of hot milk and soda water, half and half, containing a pinch of bicarbonate of soda is often useful, as are glycerin or liquorice pastilles. If the patient brings up a considerable amount of blood in coughing, he should rest quietly till the doctor sees him. Meanwhile, he can be reassured as to the outcome of the accident, as haemorrhage in consumption is rarely, in itself, fatal.

Night sweats may be lessened by sponging with tepid water and vinegar at bedtime. Sleeplessness is often cured by a glass of hot milk. If breathlessness occurs it may be relieved by giving a teaspoonful of sal volatile with the juice of half a lemon in a wineglass of water, mixed and taken quickly.

It is a great advantage to a patient to have a course of sanatorium treatment. Dryness and sunshine are the considerations leading to the choice of sites for these institutions, and this is of great importance to the patient at all times, but certainly when he is able to go out of doors (see Plate XI, 4 and 5). Of equal importance is it that he be under constant observation and trained in the routine necessary in treatment. His capacity for exercise can be accurately gauged, and exercise and work graduated accordingly.

Lessons to Learn from Sanatorium Treatment

The relapse of patients who have enjoyed sanatorium treatment would often appear to be due to a failure to observe the rules taught there, neglect to take the temperature, for example, or to exercise care when it is found to be going up regularly. People who have suffered from consumption require to take special care of themselves for the rest of their days.

After leaving a sanatorium it is an undoubted advantage to go to a farm colony. When the time comes to consider how a living is to be earned, a number of factors have to be duly weighed. *The mere fact that the occupation is carried on in the open air is no advantage if the work is too heavy and the emoluments insufficient.*

If an office or a factory is clean and well ventilated, the work not too hard, and the wage will provide a sufficiency of food and comfort, indoor employment may be quite a suitable choice.

Amongst the special forms of treatment which are practised and found to be of benefit in special cases, one or two may be mentioned. Injections of tuberculin are given in order to stimulate the natural resistance of the body to the disease. When the lung has become infected with other microbes in addition to the tubercle bacillus, marked benefit often occurs from measures dealing par-

ticularly with these. Thus, appropriate vaccine treatment may be instituted, or antiseptics may be introduced into the tubes and cavities either by using inhalers or by injecting the preparations into the trachea.

A very successful form of treatment in suitable cases is the production of what is called artificial pneumo-thorax. This means the introduction of sterilised air into the chest cavity on one side, thereby producing collapse of the lung and putting it at rest. Again, there are cases which benefit from an operation on the chest wall which allows of the ribs falling in and so diminishing the cavity of the chest on that side.

Two important questions are raised by a consideration of the means of preventing tuberculosis, namely, the supply of proper housing, and the supply of cheap good food, for the poorer classes of the community. Undoubtedly housing and food touch the problem very closely, and their provision is demanded for an adequate solution. A great deal could be done, however, in the houses we have if proper attention were paid to good ventilation and cleanliness. In one or both of these features, even many houses with ample space are more or less lacking. Their importance is increased when there is a patient suffering from tuberculosis in the house.

How to Clean a Consumptive's Room

In cleaning out the room occupied by a consumptive, care should be taken not to raise the dust. Tea-leaves should be sprinkled on carpets and rugs before sweeping, or a vacuum cleaner used, and dusting should be done with a damp cloth. Sweepings should be burnt at once, and dusters should be soaked in disinfectants after use. It is better, also, to dispense with a carpet and to lay down a few rugs which can be taken out and exposed to the sun, as sunlight has a powerful effect against the activities of the tubercle bacillus. For the same reason the rooms should, as far as possible, be kept flooded with light.

Turning to the question of food, it should be noted that growing children require a large amount of protein food and that this is most easily supplied in the form of meat. The cost of meat prohibits in very many cases the supply of an adequate amount of it for children, and so it should be remembered that oatmeal and fresh herrings are cheap and also valuable feeding stuff.

There has always been a difficulty in obtaining milk which can be guaranteed free from bovine tuberculosis. This is very important, in view of the fact that a very large number of children become infected with bovine tuberculosis. It is now possible, however, to obtain milk certified to be derived from cows which have successfully passed through a test with tuberculin, and which are presumably free from tuberculosis. A large amount of milk is, and probably will be, used which is not of this class. The tubercle bacilli may be killed by boiling milk for a few minutes, but if this be done it should be borne in mind that the milk has thereby been deprived of its supply of vitamin, so that this must be made up in other ways.

A consumptive mother should not nurse her baby, and should be careful about touching the baby's mouth or eyes, or the teats of feeding bottles, as she may readily convey infection on her fingers.

The bad habit of moistening the fingers when turning over the pages of a book is especially dangerous when employed by consumptives.

Those who have to handle consumptives, or even live with them, should be the last to forget the hygienic rule of washing the hands before handling food, whether at meals or otherwise.

The correct disposal of the patient's sputum is of the utmost importance in prevention of the disease. A patient who goes out of doors should always carry a sputum bottle or flask. This should contain a small quantity of some antiseptic solution, and care should be taken when spitting that all the sputum goes properly into the bottle. Pocket handkerchiefs should on no account be used for this purpose. When indoors, paper handker-

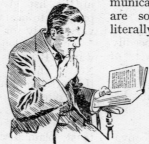
One way of spreading consumption

chiefs may be used, but should be burnt immediately. If jars or anything of the kind are used they should also contain an antiseptic solution.

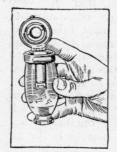
Sputum flask for consumptive patient

It is not safe to have children in a house with a patient who is expectorating tubercle bacilli. If the patient cannot be taken to a hospital, the utmost endeavour should be made to get the children away to a healthy environment. Bedclothes and other clothing used by the patient should be effectively disinfected by soaking in solutions of carbolic acid (1 in 20), or of lysol or some other disinfectant before being washed or sent to the laundry.

The possibility of pulmonary tuberculosis following whooping-cough, measles, influenza, broncho-pneumonia and other diseases should always be borne in mind. Convalescence from such affections should be carefully supervised, and every available means employed to restore the patient to vigorous health.

Tuberculosis is a notifiable disease, and in most places the sanitary authority will attend to the disinfection of clothing and of rooms. The existence of tuberculosis dispensaries and of health visitors is also of the greatest service in the treatment of the patient and in advising as regards preventive measures.

See Broncho-pneumonia ; Disinfectant ; Dust Disease ; Fibrosis ; Guaiacol ; Lung ; Pneumonia ; Sanatorium ; Tuberculosis ; Ventilation.

CONTAGION. Strictly speaking, a contagious disease is one which is communicated by touch or contact ; and there are some diseases of which this can literally be said, as, for example, syphilis, leprosy or ringworm. In such cases another person contracts the disease by coming into contact with a part of the patient's body which harbours the infective organism or with something which has done so.

The terms contagious and infectious are used, however, rather loosely as meaning the same thing and this association is easily explicable when it becomes apparent that in both cases an infective organism passes from one person to another, and that in every case, although it may be indirectly, contact of some kind must take place. A consumptive, for example, spits on the ground; the sputum dries and rises into the air as fine dust; the air is breathed by a second person, and he may contract the disease. A person suffering from influenza sneezes. The fine spray which he ejects carries infective organisms to a person who happens to breathe in the air charged with the spray.

Again, if the motions of a patient suffering from enteric fever are thrown into a river, people who are living miles away, and who drink the water, may become infected. Insects are often the agents which establish the contact. A mosquito drinks the blood of a person infected with malaria and injects the parasites into the body of a healthy person, who thereupon may show symptoms of the disease.

See Carrier; Flies; Infectious Disease.

CONTUSION. A bruise is technically known as a contusion. The injury consists of a crushing of the tissues without cutting or tearing. When, in addition to the bruise, the skin is broken, the result is a contused wound.

See Bruise; Wound.

CONVALESCENCE. The period which elapses between the end of an illness and the recovery of normal health is one of great importance. It may be prolonged by injudicious treatment, and out of it sometimes arise other and graver disorders, such, for instance, as tuberculosis. The gap between acute illness and the resumption of bodily health may be surprisingly short in such a disease as pneumonia, in which the patient may speedily acquire a good appetite and powers of digestion and assimilation. On the other hand, convalescence from influenza may be remarkably prolonged and unsatisfactory, even after apparently mild attacks.

The difficulty in dealing with convalescent patients is that often they insist upon overtaxing their strength, either from a mistaken optimism as to their capacity for exercise or work, or because they feel that it is their duty to shoulder the work and responsibilities of business. What a convalescent can do is always a matter for the doctor to decide, and patients and their friends will find it true economy to abide by his instructions in the matter.

Improving a Convalescent's Resistance

Fitness for getting up will be hastened by regular daily massage, and this may be begun early. Fitness for going into the open air will be furthered by keeping thoroughly well ventilated all rooms in which the patient may be. Draughts must, of course, be avoided, but this is best done by having a window widely open. Resistance to cold will also be improved by gradually cooling the water used for the daily sponge bath, but in this matter discretion will require to be exercised to keep within the patient's capacity to react to cold baths. When the patient sits up, and later gets out of bed, he should be kept warm by wearing sufficient clothing rather than by warming of the room. On the other hand, convalescents are often over-clothed, more particularly children.

Tact will be required with regard to the admission of visitors. At first few should be allowed into the sick-room and only for short visits, while later a discrimination must be exercised between those who help the patient and those who worry and bore him.

The subject of diet is very important at this period. The food must be such as is suited to the patient's powers of digestion, and items of diet will gradually become admissible in the stages roughly indicated in the list given below. The rate of progress from stage to stage will, however, vary widely for individual patients.

(1) Milk, alone or with soda or potash water, Benger's food, Allenbury's Diet No. 3, chicken soup, beef tea, egg flip, thin arrowroot made with milk, rusks, tea and coffee.

(2) Calf's foot jelly, chicken jelly, mutton broth, thin bread and butter, toast, plain biscuits, plain sponge cakes, milk jelly, junket.

(3) Oatmeal porridge, good milk puddings and custards, eggs poached or soft-boiled, steamed fish (whiting, sole, plaice or haddock) with milk sauce.

(4) Cauliflower with white sauce, spinach, tripe or sweetbreads, chicken or rabbit, baked apple, a little fresh fruit, roast mutton, or the eye of a tender mutton chop with a boiled mealy potato.

The nurse will herself make up the patient's menu. It is a great mistake to burden the patient with suggestions of this kind. If, however, he expresses a wish for any particular food, the propriety of letting him have it should be considered, and if there is any doubt about it the doctor should be consulted. Care and ingenuity expended in cooking and serving the invalid's food will be well repaid.

In many cases a tonic of some sort is an important aid to recovery. After fevers and other illnesses when the appetite is poor, it may be improved by giving a mixture like the following :

Tincture of cascarilla	..	3 drachms
Tincture of orange	..	2 ,,
Syrup of orange ..	..	4 ,,
Chloroform water ..	..	to 6 ounces

Take a tablespoonful thrice daily in a wineglass of water, after food.

Other useful tonics are the compound syrup of glycerophosphates, dose 1 to 2 drachms, and the compound syrup of hypophosphites, ½ to 2 drachms, the dose of either of these being taken thrice daily in a little water after food.

Children may be given the compound syrup of iron phosphate B.P.C. (chemical food), 10 to 30 drops or more, or syrup of the iodide of iron, 10 to 20 drops.

Value of Cod-liver Oil

In many cases it proves of immense advantage to give cod-liver oil in some form. It is better to begin with a small dose once daily after food. The pure oil may be taken in doses of 1 to 3 teaspoonful or more, though generally an emulsion or a mixture of the oil and malt is better tolerated.

Cod-liver oil may also be administered to infants and children who are unable to take it otherwise, by rubbing it on the belly and applying a flannel binder. The smell is somewhat unpleasant, but the improvement produced is often astonish-ing. When convalescence is slow an attempt should be made to secure a change of air, if the weather and other circumstances are suitable.

See Diet ; Health Resort ; Invalid Cookery; Massage ; Nursing.

CONVULSIONS. Involuntary paroxysmal movements of certain of the muscles of the body, or convulsions, are due to some disorder of the nervous system, which controls them all. Convulsions may be local or general, and their causes are very numerous. This article will be confined to the convulsions of children, usually known as infantile convulsions.

These occur, it is said, amongst children because their nervous systems are more sensitive than those of grown-up people, and this is true so far as it goes. Again, it seems certain that convulsions are more likely to occur in children who inherit a certain unsteadiness of the nervous system, children who come of what is called a neurotic stock.

The great majority of children who suffer from infantile convulsions, however, show clear evidence of the existence of rickets.

Given these conditions, and especially the last, very trivial causes will set up convulsions, chief amongst them, without a doubt, being a disturbance of the alimentary canal. Convulsions often usher in acute infectious diseases in children.

The child is seen to become pale and unaware of its immediate surroundings, then it becomes unconscious and the convulsions begin. Afterwards the child is very sleepy. It is almost always noticed that its fingers are tightly clenched upon its inturned thumbs.

The large majority of cases of convulsions do not indicate immediate danger. If the child is put in a comfortable position in bed, with its clothes quite loose, it will soon pass into a state of more or less natural sleep. There is no need to apply cold water to its head unless high fever is present. There seems to be no question that the placing of a child in a warm bath has a wonderfully soothing effect upon the nervous system ; if the water is very hot the opposite effect may result. It is often beneficial also to clear the bowel by an enema of soap and water. Great care must be exercised in giving this.

But it is less important to interfere with the convulsions themselves than to remove the cause which produces them; and this is not done by drugs, save in a very small degree.

In all cases evidence of the presence of rickets should be sought for and, if found, appropriate treatment should be adopted.

See Eclampsia; Epilepsy; Fit; Hysteria; Rickets; Strychnine; Teeth.

COPAIBA. Obtained from trees which grow in South America, copaiba belongs to the class of substances known as oleo-resins, that is to say, mixtures of essential or volatile oils and a resin. It is chiefly used in medicine for the treatment of gonorrhoea; but it has other uses, as, for example, in chronic bronchitis, where it acts as a stimulating expectorant. The dose of copaiba is ½ to 1 drachm, and that of the oil extracted from it 5 to 20 minims. It may be given with water, but is better taken in an emulsion, in a paste, or in capsules. Sometimes a rash, which resembles measles, comes out on the skin of a person taking the drug.

COPPER. Salts of copper are used in medicine. Blue stone or copper sulphate is sometimes given as an astringent to check chronic diarrhoea, but the chief purpose for which it is used internally is as an emetic, when it is given in doses of 5 to 10 grains. Its action is rapid, and it is especially valuable in poisoning by narcotics and in acute phosphorus poisoning. It should only be used under medical supervision, however.

Blue stone is often used to reduce what is known as exuberant granulations or proud flesh. Solutions of the drug are antiseptic, and a 1 per cent. solution is sometimes painted over a stye after the lash in the centre has been pulled out. The application is made every hour.

Cuprol or copper nucleinate is made from copper oxide and nucleol, a substance obtained from yeast. It is a fine powder, and 5 to 10 per cent. solutions have been used for chronic forms of conjunctivitis (*q.v.*), as, for example, trachoma.

Poisoning by Copper. Verdigris is acetate of copper, and its accidental ingestion may cause symptoms of acute

irritant poisoning, vomiting and so on. The treatment is to wash out the stomach by copious draughts of tepid water and to give white of egg. A greenish line is said to form along the gums in chronic poisoning by copper.

See Poisoning.

CORN. It is a general rule that pressure upon any part of the body, provided that it be not continuous but intermittent, tends to cause overgrowth. According to our present customs, our toes and also the soles of the feet are exposed to this intermittent pressure, and the result very frequently is overgrowth of the part most exposed to it. The overgrowth, in the case of a corn, mainly consists of the outermost layer of skin. This in itself is quite insensitive, and the pain of the corn is entirely due to the pressure which the thickened outer skin transmits to the sensitive tissues beneath.

This pressure not only causes pain, but it brings an increased supply of blood to these tissues, thus leading them to produce more of the outer skin than ever. In other words, the corn will grow more quickly the less frequently it is pared. The paring of a corn has in itself no action tending to make the corn grow, provided it be done carefully and not carried too deep.

The obvious means to prevent corns is to have the footwear sufficiently roomy, but not too much so, otherwise the foot will move about too much within the boot and cause rubbing. If there are ridges, creases, or lumps in boots or shoes, they should be removed by a shoemaker.

The proper way in which to dispose of the corn is first of all to pare it down and then to paint it night and morning with some such substance as salicylic collodium or collodium collosum. Afterwards, in addition to wearing proper boots, pressure may be taken off the site of the corn by means of a corn plaster, which is a pad with a hole in the middle. If this be done the whole corn will disappear and will remain away so long as the cause which originally produced it is not applied again (*see* Plate X, 7 and 8).

Soft corns require rather different treatment, because it is impossible to dispose of them until they are made dry. This is to be done by separating the toes with cotton wool and covering the corn with some boracic acid or some other dry antiseptic powder ; and then, when the corn becomes quite dry, it can be disposed of in the same way as the others.

It is to be noted that in very old people, whose blood vessels are diseased, there is some risk of causing mortification if a corn is pared so closely as to admit germs into the living layer of the skin.

CORNEA. By the cornea is meant the transparent part of the eye, through which are seen, when looking at an eye, the coloured ring of muscle, the iris, which lies behind, and the pupil, the dark hole in the middle of that ring. The cornea is

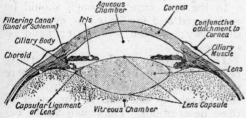

Cornea and parts of the eye lying behind it

plentifully supplied with nerves, and is very sensitive. A foreign body in this situation, therefore, causes considerable discomfort, and may be very painful. Frequently by the closure of the lids and the free flow of tears the foreign body is whisked or washed off, but it often adheres to the surface, and may be embedded in the cornea. If it is a chip of hot steel or a piece of cinder, the cornea is also burned.

Unskilled efforts to remove the foreign body may result in its being pushed farther into the cornea, and the same may happen from rubbing the eye. Beyond putting a little clean castor oil or vaseline or, at factories where it is provided, weak cocaine ointment into the eye, nothing should be done pending the attention of a doctor. After injuries of this kind the eye must be protected for a few days and washed frequently with boracic acid lotion.

Inflammation of the cornea, which is known as keratitis, may result from various causes, and leads to a clouding of its transparency, either gradually or in spots. Ulceration of the cornea may follow

on injury or disease, and usually causes severe pain, a free flow of tears and intolerance of light, so that the patient must keep his eye shut. Some ulcers tend to sink deeply into the cornea, and may bring about perforation, opening into the anterior chamber of the eye, which lies just behind the cornea. Other ulcers show a tendency rather to spread, and sometimes are not very painful, but they may seriously and permanently affect vision.

After ulceration or inflammation scars may be left in the cornea, and if near the middle of the structure may interfere with vision. The smaller type is known as a nebula, the larger as a macula.

Very frequently the cornea is not perfectly shaped ; it is curved too much when looked at from above downwards, as compared with its contour from side to side ; or vice versa. This is the cause of the very common defect of vision known as astigmatism (q.v.), which may require specially ground glasses for its correction.
See Collyrium ; Conjunctivitis ; Eye ; Keratitis ; Pterygium ; Spectacles.

CORPULENCE. See Obesity.

CORPUSCLE. Meaning literally a little body, corpuscle is the name applied to the cells of the blood.
See Blood.

CORROSIVE. Substances which destroy tissues with which they come into contact are called corrosives. Oil of vitriol is an example.
See Caustic ; Poisoning.

CORROSIVE SUBLIMATE. This is the name of a compound of mercury, technically known as perchloride of mercury. It is of very great importance, since it is an exceedingly powerful antiseptic, and very cheap. A solution of it in water to an extent of one part in 4,000 is a thoroughly trustworthy antiseptic for almost all purposes. It possesses the disadvantage that it spoils steel instruments if used to disinfect them.

It is also used internally in exceedingly minute doses for the general purposes of mercury ; in large doses it is a most dangerous poison, producing intense irritation of the alimentary canal, severe pain, vomiting and diarrhoea. The symptoms have a considerable resemblance to those of cholera. The treatment is not very satisfactory except when it is undertaken very soon. If a quantity of a solution of this salt is swallowed by mistake, for instance, the best antidote is white of egg, which, if swallowed immediately and then followed by an emetic, may avert ill consequences. The white of egg combines with the poison and renders it harmless.

See Antiseptic ; Mercury ; Poisoning.

COTTON WOOL. The soft substance known as cotton wool is made from the hairs surrounding the seeds of the cotton plant, and contains no wool whatever in the ordinary sense of the word. When the oil which is naturally present is removed, the cotton wool becomes very absorbent, and is capable of picking up a large quantity of fluid. Owing to its texture, this substance is very much warmer, that is to say, a very much worse conductor of heat, than is an ordinary cotton fabric.

Absorbent cotton wool is used largely in surgery. It is an important dressing, as it readily absorbs discharges of all sorts, and it protects injured parts from cold or pressure. It affords a much cleaner and safer means of cleansing wounds than sponges. When buying cotton wool for these purposes it is important to get the absorbent material, as a variety is sold which, although useful enough to apply to the chest, for example, is not absorbent, and so is useless as a dressing.

See Dressing ; Gamgee Tissue.

COUGH. A cough may have a large variety of origins ; it may indicate grave disease of the lungs, for example, or be due to the pressure of wax in the ear, or to irritation elsewhere outside the breathing apparatus. Nor is it safe to interpret a cough according to its character except with very great care. For instance, there is no kind of cough characteristic of advanced tuberculosis of the lungs. The hollowest kind of cough known, a loud, rich, resonant, penetrating cough, is usually associated with hysteria. The most serious cough of all—that is to say, a cough indicating the most serious disease—is the short, suppressed, almost inaudible cough of the patient who is dying of pneumonia, or the voiceless cough of the patient who has tuberculosis of the larynx.

A cough is not necessarily to be regarded as an evil thing in itself. The cough of a person who has nearly choked will save his life by expelling the cause of the obstruction. The cough of bronchitis in its later stages is of the utmost importance as a means of draining the air passages ; so far as nature is concerned, it must be regarded as a proper and effective means of removing objectionable matter from the air passages.

It is important to be able to distinguish, in any particular case of coughing, between a desirable and beneficial response of nature to a particular emergency, and a painful, exhausting and useless symptom.

In the first case the cough should be encouraged and facilitated in every possible way ; in the second, it should be suppressed.

The question needs careful study, because in one and the same disease there may be periods when the cough answers respectively to one and to the other of these descriptions. The cough at the beginning of bronchitis, for instance, is due to the irritation of the air passages ; there is nothing to remove, and the cough merely induces more irritation, pain and swelling. The patient must, therefore, be persuaded to control his coughing as much as possible, and must be given drugs which will tend to deaden the sensitiveness of the nerves that run to the brain from the air passages.

At a later stage, in the same case, quantities of fluid and semi-fluid are poured into his air passages from their walls, and it is imperative that these be disposed of. Hence he must be given drugs which add to the vigour of his coughing instead of relieving it. In many cases it is probably only too true that the patient has been choked in consequence of the reckless administration of drugs which have effectively relieved his cough.

The parts of the body in which the irritation may arise that expresses itself as a cough are as follows : the nose, ear, throat, gullet, larynx, windpipe, bronchi, lungs, the covering of the lung (which is called the pleura), the liver, spleen and stomach. In addition, there are certain areas of the skin, especially upon the throat and chest, irritation of which may lead to coughing. A cough may also be of purely nervous origin, as in hysteria, and also, as everyone knows, may be due to suggestion, as when a person coughs in church and other people who have no reason for coughing do likewise.

The so-called stomach cough does not occur in one per cent. of the cases that usually go by that name. It is an improper thing to come to the conclusion that a cough for which no particular reason can be discovered is a stomach cough ; the name is an excuse for convenience and laziness. Only too frequently it is found on examination that there are early stages of tuberculosis. A true stomach cough may be at once relieved by giving half-teaspoonful doses of bicarbonate of soda. In other cases, when the throat is attended to, the so-called stomach cough disappears, and in yet others, it is a symptom of hysteria. The term winter cough is often applied to the exacerbations of chronic bronchitis during cold, damp, wintry weather.

Drugs and Other Modes of Treatment

The treatment of a cough depends upon the discovery of its cause. Paregoric will obviously not do much good to a cough which depends upon the presence of a plug of wax in the ear ; nor is it likely to be of benefit to a hysterical cough. Once the cause is discovered, the treatment is usually simple enough, if the cause be in any part of the breathing apparatus. The essential thing is to ascertain whether the cough is a beneficial one, or is harmful.

A large number of drugs are employed for the treatment of various kinds of cough. Those which soothe the cough contain either opium or some of its constituents, such as morphia and codeine. Those which are intended to strengthen a weak cough, such as too frequently occurs in children and the aged, almost invariably contain some form of ammonia, this being by far the most powerful and rapid stimulant of the act of coughing that is known.

It must be remembered that drugs are not the only means of treatment of a cough which must be soothed. Very often the cough will cease if the air that the patient breathes be made warmer and moister than usual. In cases of cough due to the early stages of bronchitis, or of inflammation of the larynx, much benefit follows the inhalation of steam from a special inhaler, or from a kettle or teapot. To the hot water which produces the steam, may be added many soothing and antiseptic drugs. One of the best, and perhaps the most popular of these is Friar's balsam. A cough may sometimes be relieved by sucking demulcent lozenges, for example, glycerin or liquorice pastilles, or lozenges which contain menthol. Again, it may be relieved by gargling with a pinch of common salt or alum in a half glass of water. Coughing is often due to excessive cigarette smoking, and ceases when cigarettes are given up or much reduced.

In the case of children suffering from very grave bronchitis, where so much foreign matter is poured into the air passages, that death by suffocation is threatened, relief may often be obtained by administering drugs which do not directly affect the act of coughing but which produce vomiting, such as a teaspoonful of ipecacuanha wine, repeated if necessary. This is usually accompanied by coughing, and in addition, is probably also accompanied by movements of the muscular tissue that surrounds the air passages, in such a fashion as to empty them.

The cough in elderly people due to a slight defect in the circulation through the lungs, caused by weakness of the heart, will fail to respond to a host of remedies, so long as attention is not directed to the cause of the trouble. As soon as a heart tonic is administered the cough will disappear.

The application of poultices, mustard plasters, or other counter-irritants to the lungs is another method of relieving cough due to chest affections.

See Atomiser ; Balsam ; Barking Cough ; Bronchitis ; Consumption ; Counter-irritation ; Croup ; Expectoration ; Hysteria ; Whooping-cough, etc.

COUGH MIXTURE. It is always necessary to understand the exact cause of a cough and to appreciate whether it is beneficial or not, before prescribing or taking a cough mixture. It would be a disastrous mistake, for example, to go on with one cough mixture after another in an attempt to cure a cough which is due to the presence of consumption. For winter cough, the cough which troubles elderly people in cold and damp weather, the following is often of service :

Ammonium chloride	120 grains
Compound tincture of camphor	4 drachms
Liquid extract of liquorice	2 ,,
Glycerin	4 ,,
Chloroform water	to 6 ounces

A tablespoonful every four hours in a wine-glass of water.

See Anise ; Balsam ; Cough.

COUNTER-IRRITATION. Deliberate irritation of the skin in order to produce an effect upon some organ that lies beneath it is known as counter-irritation. The familiar instance is rubbing the chest of a child with camphorated oil in order to relieve a slight cold. There is here a condition of deep-seated congestion, and by way of curing it, an application is made to the skin over the part involved irritating enough to redden it. Severe counter-irritation may cause actual blistering or destruction of the skin.

Counter-irritation is of marked value in very many cases. It is applicable to all parts of the body, to acute and to chronic cases, and to diseased conditions of most various kinds. Whilst so widely useful, counter-irritation has the advantage of being almost always harmless in itself. It is probable that massage is responsible for a certain amount of the benefit derived. It is better to rub in a liniment than merely to apply it ; both the rubbing and the counter-irritation of the skin result in improving the circulation throughout the underlying structures, and so helping them to recover.

See Blister ; Cantharides ; Cautery ; Liniment ; Mustard.

COURT PLASTER. Small wounds may be covered over, or the edges of cuts brought together, by court plaster. It consists of a mixture of isinglass, glycerin and alcohol spread on silk.

COWPOX. There is reason to believe that the disease known as cowpox or vaccinia, in which vesicles or blisters appear on the udder and teats of the animal, is essentially the same disease as smallpox. Cowpox is a relatively mild disease, however. It is contagious amongst cows and is also communicable to man. It was an observation made to Jenner, that milkmaids who contracted cowpox did not afterwards take smallpox, that induced him to pursue the investigations which resulted in the system of vaccination. The lymph used to communicate the disease to human subjects is taken from vesicles on calves, and is treated with glycerin before being put up for use.

See Vaccination.

CRAMP. An involuntary contraction or spasm of a muscular tissue in any part of the body is known as cramp. Sometimes the name is confined to the muscles over which we usually have control, such as the ordinary muscles of the limbs : whilst the term colic is applied to spasms of the muscles in the interior of the body, over which we have no control, and of the action of which we are usually unconscious. The commonest instance of cramp is that which occurs in the calf of the leg, particularly when one is asleep in bed.

The patient can almost always be relieved very quickly if the proper measures are taken. As a general rule, a muscle which is in a state of uncontrollable spasm will relax if the part of the body is so bent that the muscle has not to be on the stretch, for it is the stretched muscle that is the most irritated muscle. Therefore the first thing to do in cramp of the calf is forcibly to bend the knee to its utmost, so that the muscles are relaxed as far as possible. When this has been done, rub the part vigorously, and more in an upward than in a downward direction.

A tendency to cramp at night is associated with flatulent indigestion, and it may be found of some use to take a teaspoonful of sal volatile in a little water before going to bed. Other measures should be adopted at the same time to cure the dyspepsia.

On the other hand, cramps sometimes occur in muscles that are not sufficiently nourished with blood. They are very common in the legs of bloodless girls at night, and in this case the treatment is to increase the amount of blood that goes to the limbs. This can be done by getting out of bed and standing up, not forgetting to keep the feet warm.

Cramp in the stomach gives rise to very intense pain. A hot-water bottle, a mustard

PLATE IX

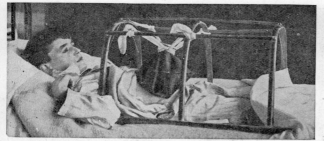

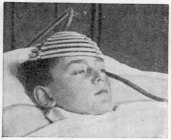

Cold Applications. 1. Ice bag used to relieve abdominal pain.
By suspending it from a bed cradle pressure is avoided

2. Leiter's tubes in cap form
to relieve headache in fever

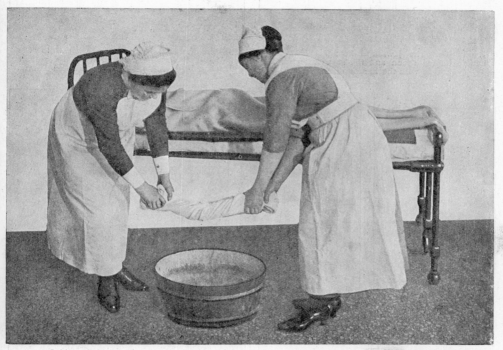

3. Cold pack for treating febrile disorders. A sheet is wrung out of cold water at tap temperature

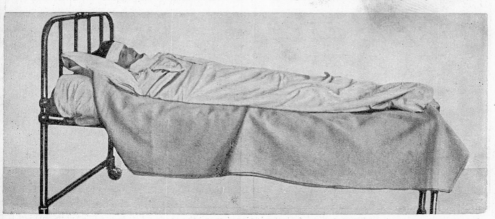

4. The wet sheet is wrapped round the patient, who is then covered with the turned-up blanket

PLATE X

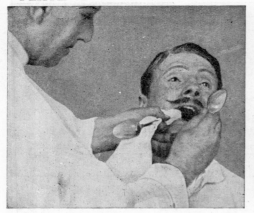

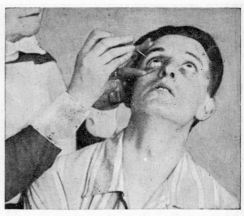

1. Choking. The jaws are kept apart by the handle of one spoon and the obstruction raked forward with the handle of another

2. Conjunctivitis. Drugs are applied to the inflamed membrane by a dropper, the patient looking up while the lower lid is drawn down

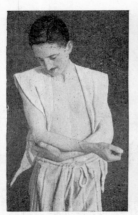
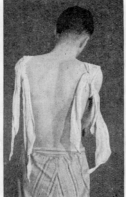
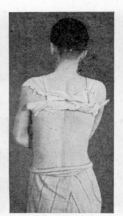
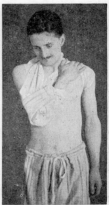

Collar Bone : first-aid treatment of a fracture. 3. Two triangular bandages are folded and laid over the shoulders. 4. Each is tied behind the shoulder and then (5) knotted across the back as shown. 6. Another triangular bandage is applied as a sling, the hand being placed on the sound shoulder

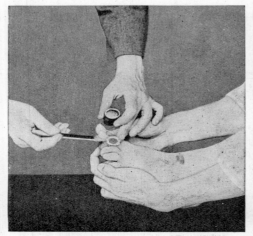
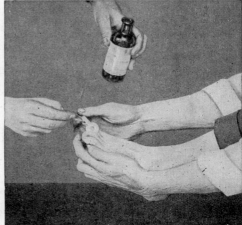

Corn : treatment of the soft variety. 7. A plaster is placed round the corn and its cavity filled with powdered salicylic acid. 8. Plaster and contained salicylic powder are then covered with collodion

plaster or a poultice should be applied over the stomach, and half a teaspoonful of bicarbonate of soda should be given in a little soda water, or in peppermint water if this is at hand. Ginger or any other carminative (*q.v.*) would also be useful.

Cramp in the legs is often troublesome to women in childbirth, and is caused by the pressure of the child's head on the large nerves which supply the lower limbs. The affected parts should be rubbed briskly.

See Colic ; Muscle ; Writer's Cramp.

CRANIAL NERVES. The twelve pairs of nerves which come from the brain and serve the purposes of the special senses and of movements and sensation about the head and neck are called the cranial nerves.

See Brain ; Nervous System.

CRANIUM. The term cranium may be applied to the skull as a whole, though properly it means only the part which contains the brain. The skull would thus consist of the cranium and the bones which form the face.

See Skull.

CRAPULENCE. The state of body which results from over-indulgence in food and drink is denoted by the term crapulence. It means either ordinary alcoholic drunkenness, in which the stomach is upset, or a similar condition consequent to gluttony.

CREAM OF TARTAR. The bitartrate of potassium, commonly known as cream of tartar, is given in doses up to half an ounce as a purgative. It may be taken dissolved with water or mixed with marmalade. A form of Imperial drink can be made by adding cream of tartar, in the proportion of a teaspoonful to the pint, to home-made lemonade. This is used as a beverage in fevers.

See Beverages.

CREMATION. The practice of burning the dead has much to commend it. It is essentially cleanly and decent ; it economises space ; and although, by a proper use of disinfectants, the bodies of those dying from virulent infectious diseases can probably be rendered innocuous, still cremation definitely disposes of all possibilities of infection. The stringent regulations regarding death certification do away with the possibility of crime being concealed, and, in conjunction with the time which must elapse before cremation, of the possibility of people being cremated while in a trance. The cremation companies give every assistance in carrying out the procedure required.

See Death.

CREOSOTE. Creosote is a colourless or pale yellow liquid, with a penetrating odour, which is obtained from wood-tar. It is a powerful antiseptic and has been much used in the treatment of pulmonary tuberculosis. The dose is 1 to 5 minims, and it is given in capsules, in a mixture, or in cod-liver oil. It is also administered by sprinkling it on the sponge of an inhaler, and when thus used may relieve an irritating cough. It corrects gastric fermentation. It may be applied on cotton wool to the cavity of a carious tooth for the relief of pain. From creosote may be obtained guaiacol (*q.v.*), which is also used for tuberculosis. Guaiacol carbonate is valuable in the treatment of rheumatoid arthritis if given for many months.

CRESOL. Obtained from coal tar, cresol is a light brown liquid which is much used as an antiseptic and disinfectant. It is used to prepare the liquor cresolis saponatus which resembles lysol and is used in the same way. To make an antiseptic solution, add one or two teaspoonsful of either of these to a pint of hot water and mix thoroughly. Vaporised cresol is sometimes used to lessen the severity of whooping-cough, by impregnating the air with the drug. This can be done by heating a large metal spoon, or something of the kind, in the fire and then pouring on a teaspoonful of cresol ; or a vaporiser for the purpose may be bought. In poisoning by cresol water should not be given, but white of egg, oil or butter.

CRETINISM. A number of glands in the body have no duct whereby they can get rid of the substances they manufacture and these are clearly poured directly into the blood stream. The thyroid gland, which is situated in the neck below the Adam's apple, is one of those glands, and its secretion has a marked influence upon growth. This was observed by noting the relation between the gland and the diseases known as cretinism and myxoedema.

If a child is born with the gland undeveloped, or if it degenerates before the period of puberty, cretinism results ; if, after growth has taken place, the gland becomes ineffective, there occur mental and bodily degenerative changes to which the name myxoedema has been applied. A cretin child is distinguished by the fact that it does not grow ; before the nature of the disease and its treatment were discovered, cretins who reached adult life would average only about three feet in height. The cretin child has a protuberant belly ; the face is large, the lips are thick, and the tongue appears too large for the mouth and may protrude between the lips. The hair is coarse and scanty. As for mental development, such children are imbecile or idiots.

If, however, the defect of thyroid secretion is made good by feeding the child with thyroid glands from the lower animals, say, the sheep, or with extracts of these glands, a wonderful change takes place. Growth begins and proceeds briskly ; in five or six months the child may add as many inches to its stature ; the other physical abnormalities disappear, the hair grows normally, and the child assumes ordinary mental capacity, except that, of course, it is backward for its age. But it is now capable of education. Treatment of this kind must be commenced early, however, to get the best results, for if the child has been allowed to remain untreated for some time, although good bodily development may be achieved, it may not be possible to reach the proper standard of mental capacity. As thyroid substance is such a powerful remedy, it is necessary that the treatment should be controlled by a doctor. The extract may be given in liquid form or in tablets, and the commencing doses must be small. An excessive amount of thyroid activity causes Grave's disease or exophthalmic goitre.

See Endocrine ; Exophthalmic Goitre ; Myxoedema ; Thyroid Gland.

CRICK. A sudden painful stiffness somewhere in the neck or back is popularly described as a crick. It is probably due in most instances to muscular spasm, though an alternative explanation is that it is caused by the tearing of a few muscular or tendinous fibres. Relief will be obtained by gently rubbing the part with the tips of the fingers, using some warm oil or a liniment.

CRIPPLE. *See* Deformity.

CRISIS. This is the name applied to the manner in which certain fevers come to a termination. In popular language it is supposed that there is a crisis in every illness, but that is not really a proper use of the word. In general there are two ways in which fevers terminate, either by crisis or by lysis. Typhoid fever is an example of the latter : the patient's temperature comes down gradually, each day it is a little lower than it was the day before, and so at last it reaches the normal.

Pneumonia is an excellent example of the fever which terminates by crisis. The patient's temperature is very likely as high as 104° F. and has been so for some days, then quite suddenly it falls in a few hours ; it may fall actually 6 degrees or more, that is to say, to a point much below normal, and then rise again to the proper height. It is to this very sudden fall in the temperature that the term crisis is properly applied.

So rapid and so great a change of temperature naturally denotes profound changes in the working of the body ; hence there are certain dangers and symptoms peculiar to crisis, and these are commonly known as critical symptoms. Just before the crisis the temperature may rise higher than it was before, and there may be delirium. The fall of temperature may be accompanied by profuse sweating, the passage of a large quantity of urine, and sometimes by diarrhoea.

The term crisis is also applied to the sudden attacks of pain which occur in various parts of the body in locomotor ataxia.

See Fever.

CROTON OIL. Croton oil is an exceedingly powerful drug which is occasionally used when a very active purgative is required. It is far too powerful for ordinary use, and must be very carefully distinguished from castor oil, for the seeds that yield the oil in the two cases are very similar and have occasionally been mistaken for one another, with disastrous results.

Whereas the dose of castor oil is almost indefinite, one ounce, for instance, being a quite sufficient and harmless dose, the utmost quantity of croton oil that should ever be given at one time is one drop.

Obviously, this drug has the advantage that since its effective dose is so small in bulk it can easily be administered to unconscious or insane patients; for if the drop is placed on the back of the tongue it has to be swallowed. A dose of croton oil should never be repeated; the drug is exceedingly irritant, and must never on any account be administered when there is any kind of disease of any part of the bowel, but only in cases of simple obstinate constipation.

Croton oil exerts its irritating properties upon the skin as elsewhere, and it is used in a liniment which is sometimes employed for purposes of counter-irritation. The same liniment, carefully diluted, is sometimes used in order to stimulate the scalp in cases of baldness.
See Cathartic.

CROSS-EYED. *See* Squint.

CROUP. The term croup has the same significance as croak, and has been applied to conditions characterised by a cough with a croaking quality about it. Associated with such a cough there may be huskiness or even loss of voice, and perhaps stridor or crowing, which is a peculiar, sharp vibratory sound heard when the patient inhales. As in these circumstances there is obviously interference with the free supply of air to the lungs, the face becomes dusky.

Attacks of croup may affect children suddenly during the night. They start up in bed and present symptoms such as have been described. Under treatment the difficulty of breathing passes off and they fall asleep, to awake perhaps well, or perhaps still somewhat hoarse and with a croupy cough. The attacks of difficulty of breathing may recur on one or more successive nights before finally disappearing. Such a condition of things occurs when there is inflammation in the larynx and voice-box, and in addition some spasm of the vocal cords. Very frequently the child suffers from adenoids and enlarged tonsils, and these must be got rid of when there is a tendency to croup of this kind.

There is another condition in which sudden difficulty of breathing may cause children to start up in bed. It usually affects those who suffer from rickets. It is due simply to spasm of the vocal cords, and commonly spasms occur elsewhere as, for example, at the wrists. The child holds its breath to such an extent that it tends to become black in the face; then it takes a breath accompanied by the peculiar sound known as stridor. The attack then passes off, as a rule, and the child goes to sleep.

But while difficulty in breathing, a croupy cough and stridor may be due to the foregoing causes, the first thing that should be thought of is diphtheria, in which the symptoms are caused not only by inflammation and perhaps spasm, but by the presence of membrane in the larynx which may block the air passage mechanically, and quickly suffocate the patient. In cases of croup the doctor should therefore be summoned immediately, and, in sending for him, it would be wise to let him know the nature of the emergency.

Meanwhile, a tent should be rigged up over the patient's bed with sheets on a clothes'-horse or over ropes, and steam from a bronchitis kettle should be let into the tent. While these arrangements are being made the child should be put into a hot bath to which two tablespoonsful of mustard have been added and kept there for a few minutes. It is then taken out, put to bed, and a hot fomentation applied to the throat. Care should be taken that the steam from the kettle is not delivered too near to the child's face. If the difficulty of breathing persists, vomiting should be induced by giving a teaspoonful of ipecacuanha wine, if this can be got quickly.
See Bronchitis Kettle; Diphtheria; Rickets.

CROWING. *See* Stridor.

CRUTCH. A crutch used to assist an invalid in walking should be as light as possible consistent with strength. Care must be taken that the head of the crutch does not press too much, or for too long a time, on the armpit, otherwise the nerves going to the upper limb may be damaged, and cause what is called crutch paralysis (*see* illus. in page 45). The nerve most frequently injured is the musculo-spiral, and one of the effects is wrist drop.

The pressure may be taken off to some extent by having a bifurcated crutch with a cross-piece for the hand grip, or a spring apparatus may be fixed to the head of the crutch. A modified crutch is made which does not come higher than the middle of the upper arm, where it is fixed by a horseshoe-shaped metal spring. A pair of these is generally used.

Crutch : four different shapes

CUBEBS. The dried unripe fruit of the piper cubeba, which grows in Java, is used in medicine in the treatment of gonorrhoea, when it is generally given in combination with copaiba or with sandal-wood oil. It is also valuable in bronchitis when there is profuse expectoration. The dose of the powdered fruits is 30 to 60 grains, and in this form the drug is usually made into an electuary with glycerin or something similar, wrapped in a piece of wafer paper and swallowed. The oil, extracted from the fruits, the dose of which is 5 to 20 minims, may be taken in capsules. The tincture of cubebs, dose $\frac{1}{2}$ to 1 drachm, may be taken in linseed tea. The drug is also made into cigarettes for smoking in the type of bronchitis above mentioned.

CUPPING. In congestive disorders of the lungs, the kidneys or other parts, much relief may be obtained by the operation of cupping. The cups are made of thick glass, and when applied to the skin the air within them is reduced, so that the skin swells up within the glass and becomes dark in colour from the blood with which it becomes engorged.

The glass may be capable of being attached to an air pump and of being exhausted in this way, but the method almost universally carried out is to moisten the inside of the cup with methylated spirits and to set this alight. The cup is immediately and accurately applied to the skin. The flame is thus at once extinguished and a partial vacuum is created. Six or eight cups may be applied.

This is called dry cupping because the blood is only drawn to the surface, but if it is desired to draw off blood by wet cupping, as soon as the skin has been properly drawn up into the cup, the latter is removed, and a number of small incisions are made on the skin by an instrument known as a scarificator. The cups are then reapplied as before and soon become filled with blood. Wet cupping may be used instead of bleeding by venesection, and when the heart is finding difficulty in pumping the volume of blood along, its work may be lessened for it in this way.

See Bleeding.

CURD. *See* Casein.

CURETTAGE. The operation in which diseased tissues are scraped away by an instrument known as the curette, is technically known as curettage. It is employed in diseases of the womb and other disorders.

CURVATURE OF THE SPINE. The spine normally presents curves in a forward and backward direction. Pathological curvatures may consist in an exaggeration of these or in lateral curvature.

See Backbone ; Pott's Disease ; Spinal Curvature.

CUSPARIA. The bark of the cusparia febrifuga, also known as angostura bark, acts as a bitter tonic. The infusion of cusparia is given in doses of 1 to 2 ounces.

CUT. Small simple cuts are best treated by dabbing tincture of iodine over them. There is some smarting, but this is momentary, and the iodine helps in arresting bleeding, and is also a powerful antiseptic. The wound is then dressed with boracic lint or a clean cotton or linen rag.

When a cut is larger and deeper, bleeding may be considerable, and the first thing to do is to arrest this, a finger being pressed on the bleeding point while a pad of some clean material is being prepared. The wound may then be washed gently with water which has been boiled and then cooled, or with boracic or some other antiseptic lotion. In the case of a severe cut a doctor may stitch the skin edges together or use strips of plaster for this purpose.

See Adhesive Plaster; Antiseptic; Bleeding; Collodion; Court Plaster; Wound.

CUTANEOUS. This is an adjective derived from the Latin word cutis, the skin, and applied to anything that has to do with the skin. From it, in turn, is derived the word subcutaneous, denoting anything administered or that occurs just under the skin; and also percutaneous, anything administered through the skin.

CUTICLE. Practically a Latin word meaning the little skin, the term cuticle is sometimes applied to the surface layer of the skin or the epidermis, of which we rub off quantities every time we wash our hands.

CYANOSIS. The literal meaning of cyanosis is blueness, and the term is applied to the blue or purple discoloration of the skin and mucous membranes which is due to defective aeration of the blood. The whole surface of the body may be affected, but the word may also be applied to a state of affairs sometimes seen in the fingers and ear tips, and elsewhere, as the result of interference of the circulation by cold. Where there is general cyanosis of a slight degree the condition is most easily observed on the finger nails and lips, but when of greater degree it is plainly visible on the face and elsewhere.

Such general discoloration may occur in many disorders. It is common, of course, in respiratory and heart diseases. It may exist from birth in congenital heart disease, and is then due to a mixing of the venous and arterial blood at the heart. It may occur in emphysema, apparently from a similar mixing of blood in the

vessels of the lungs. In both of these cases, although the patient looks very blue, he may be able to get about quite well.

The condition may be met with in poisoning by benzol, nitro-benzol, opium and other drugs; and apparently poisons capable of producing it can be manufactured in the intestinal canal of the patient himself. Treatment must be directed to the underlying cause. In some cases oxygen may be administered with benefit.

See Asphyxia; Raynaud's Disease.

CYCLITIS. The ciliary body of the eye lies behind the iris or movable curtain at its outer circumference, the two structures being continuous. Inflammation of the ciliary body, known as cyclitis, is usually associated, therefore, with that of the iris also, when the condition is called irido-cyclitis.

Cyclitis is a very serious malady, and if it persists blindness in the eye will probably result. In addition to this, its existence in one eye may lead to its appearance in the other also, more especially if the cyclitis is due to a penetrating wound of the eye, and if a foreign body is retained in the eye. The affection in the second eye tends to lead to widespread trouble there and is known as sympathetic ophthalmitis.

Among the symptoms of cyclitis is a pink zone of congestion just outside, and all round the cornea or clear part of the eye. There is pain in the eye which is also tender to pressure. Pain may be felt in the forehead. Vision is more or less dimmed.

See Eye; Iritis; Ophthalmia.

CYST. The term cyst is derived from a Greek word meaning a pouch, and is applied to swellings which may occur in many parts of the body, and which are essentially bags with more or less fluid contents. They may be quite minute, or, on the other hand, may grow to an enormous size, as in the case of ovarian cysts. They may form in pre-existing spaces, or, again, where there is no such space.

To the first type belong what are known as retention cysts. When the duct of a secreting gland is blocked, the secretion may accumulate behind the obstruction and give rise to a retention cyst. The common wen or sebaceous cyst which is often seen on the scalp is an instance of this. Here the duct of one of the sebaceous glands is blocked, and the cyst is found to contain soft cheesy material, which represents the oily secretion of the gland in a concentrated state. A ranula, which forms usually in connexion with the sublingual gland, the salivary gland situated beneath the tip of the tongue, is another instance.

A cyst which forms at the site of a bleeding into the tissues or round a foreign body, is an instance of one forming apart from a pre-existing space. Dermoid cysts are curious structures which often contain hairs, teeth, nails and the like. They arise from cells similar to those which produce such structures, but which, having been misplaced in the developing embryo, grow out of place and out of season. Other cysts also arise from embryonic structures. Cysts are often found in the liver and elsewhere in the body which are produced by the hydatid worm, which lives in the intestine of dogs, and these may be of large size.

The treatment of a cyst depends upon its nature, its size, its position and other considerations. Many may be left alone, but others must be removed, and it is usually necessary when doing this, to take away all or, at any rate, most of the cyst wall in order to prevent a recurrence of the cyst.
See Wen.

CYSTITIS. This is the technical name for inflammation of the bladder (*q.v.*).

DACTYLITIS. This name is sometimes applied to inflammation of a finger, the Greek word for a finger being dactyl.

DALTONISM. *See* Colour Blindness.

DAMP. Damp is accused of causing many illnesses, and there is no doubt that in certain people it is capable indirectly of causing disease. How it acts no one knows, but it must be remembered that the skin is constantly losing moisture to the atmosphere, as also are the lungs in the act of breathing. This is a necessary function of the body, enabling a quantity of water constantly to circulate through it, so as to keep it clean and free from impurities, in addition to the heat-regulating function of perspiration.

The presence of much damp in the atmosphere very much reduces the speed at which the skin and lungs are able to rid themselves of water vapour, and the interference with this function may particularly account for the bad influence of damp on certain people. Further, it is to be noted that damp probably favours the growth of microbes. But it is probable that most of the harm done by damp is due rather to cold than to the moisture itself. Rheumatism and chest complaints are notably affected by cold and damp.

The damp heat which may occur in certain states of the weather must also be remembered, since it gives rise to oppression or even heat stroke. In selecting a climate for those with chronic bronchial complaints it will generally be found that if the cough is dry or accompanied only by a scanty sputum, residence in a moist warm climate such as one finds at Torquay,

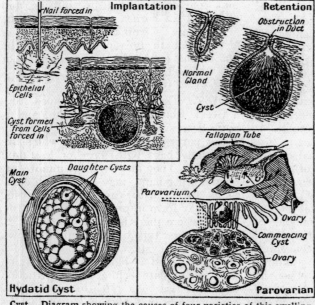

Cyst. Diagram showing the causes of four varieties of this swelling

Madeira or Algiers, is likely to be suitable, whereas if the sputum is profuse, a dry, warm climate should be chosen.

See Climate ; Cold ; Fog ; Humidity.

DANDRUFF. Scurf or dandruff consists of a great accumulation of dead matter, once living cells, which has been cast off from the surface of the scalp. It is an exceedingly common symptom of defect of health in the scalp, the defect being of the nature of a very mild and chronic inflammation of certain parts of the scalp, and this it is which gives rise to the excessive casting of the cells that constitutes dandruff. The technical name for this condition is pityriasis simplex, or alba capitis.

Occasionally the disorder may go considerably further, and pass into an unmistakable inflammation of the scalp, and perhaps there may also be red, scaly patches on the forehead and face ; but as a rule the production of dandruff continues in its slow and inconspicuous fashion for months and often for years, without any further change, except, and the exception is very important, that the hair gradually becomes thinner.

There is no doubt at all that microbes are involved, and it is evident also that it is difficult to keep the scalp clear of microbes. These may be transferred from one person to another by hair brushes and in other ways. There is also some difficulty in thoroughly applying remedies to the scalp, especially in the case of women with long hair, but it is nevertheless true that dandruff can be got rid of if people will take sufficient trouble.

The best remedy would appear to be sulphur, and this can be applied in several ways. It may be used in a sulphur soap, made by a reputable maker, with which the scalp is washed two or three times a week. Instead of this an ointment may be used, of which the following is a good example :

Precipitated sulphur	30 grains
Salicylic acid	10 grains
Soft paraffin	1 ounce

This must be rubbed into the roots of the hair, as thoroughly as possible, with the tips of the fingers. In order to go properly over the scalp it has been suggested that a quarter of the area should be covered each day, and that the head should be washed on the evening of the fifth day. The ointment is then resumed and the routine followed for as long as may be necessary. Those who object to greasy applications might ask their chemist for one of the colloidal preparations of sulphur which are sold for this purpose.

If there is any difficulty in removing the scales, the head should be thoroughly shampooed with tincture of green soap, after which it must be rinsed with several changes of water.

It is important to remember that the dandruff scales falling on other parts may give rise to inflammation there. Acne of the back, for instance, is often associated with dandruff of the scalp, and treatment, to be successful, must deal also with the latter.

See Acne ; Baldness ; Dermatitis ; Seborrhoea.

DEAD FINGERS AND TOES. The blanching and coldness of the fingers or toes due to disturbance of the nervous control of blood vessels, is often popularly referred to as dead fingers or toes. The condition is an example of what is described as Raynaud's phenomena.

See Circulation of the Blood ; Raynaud's Disease.

DEAF-MUTISM. Persons who are deaf and dumb are commonly referred to in scientific works as deaf-mutes. The subject of deaf-mutism is one of very great importance for the reason that so much can be done for the relief of these unfortunate persons if sufficient skill and sympathy are engaged in their behalf.

In the first place, distinction must be made between the cases of deaf-mutism which are due entirely to deafness, the inability to articulate being the direct consequence of the inability to hear, and those cases in which the dumbness is a consequence of defective mental development. Here only the first class of cases will be considered.

It would appear that about one-half of the total number of these patients are deaf from birth, whilst the remainder acquire their deafness in consequence of certain diseases. Of these the chief are inflammation of the covering of the brain, scarlet fever and measles. A very large number of cases of deaf-mutism due to the two latter diseases might have been entirely prevented. If a child born with good hearing becomes deaf before the age of four it will be a deaf-mute, and there is a danger of this happening to any child becoming deaf before the age of eight unless painstaking efforts are made to keep it talking.

The other most important aspect of this question, in relation to the prevention of deaf-mutism, is concerned with the inheritance of congenital deafness, that is to say, deafness from birth.

It must most positively be laid down that it is an improper thing for persons afflicted with congenital deafness to marry.

Prevention of deaf-mutism is thus of paramount importance, but there remains to be considered the mitigation of the lot of patients in whom this defect is already present. Very little can be done by way of absolutely curing these cases; surgical treatment of the ear and of the throat may be of some service, but it does not count for much. These children, however, can be taught to understand a spoken language and, although there is much more difficulty about this, to reproduce it in a curious monotonous speech by means of lip-reading (Plate XIII, 5). Taught by a careful and patient teacher, they learn to recognize much of what he is saying, by simply observing the movements he makes in speaking, and afterwards they are able to imitate these movements.

This method of enabling deaf-mutes to communicate with their neighbours is called the oral method, and in those cases where it succeeds it is of far more use to the patient than what may be called the finger method. If it fails, however, there always remains what is called the deaf and dumb alphabet, which is easy to learn and understand, and which is of avail in every case where the deaf-mutism is not due to mental defect. It is well to note in connexion with this last class of case, that very often cretinism is involved, and remarkable success may follow the administration of thyroid substance.

DEAFNESS. Deafness may be due to many different causes, but, in general, there are two kinds of deafness, which are fundamentally distinct in their cause, their character and their possibilities of treatment. One kind is what is called nerve-deafness and is due to some defect in the nerve of hearing or in the brain. In general these cases derive very little benefit from treatment; no artificial drum or application of lotions or any measures of that kind avail in nerve deafness.

In contra-distinction to these cases are those of what is called obstructive deafness. Here the whole nerve apparatus of hearing is intact, and the difficulty lies in the fact that the sound is imperfectly conveyed to it. A large number of different disorders causing deafness may be found in the extremely complicated apparatus designed for conducting sound from without to the nerve of hearing; but nevertheless these cases are distinguished from the others by the fact that in very many instances they are capable of successful treatment.

Temporary Deafness and Its Cure

Sometimes this may be simply treatment for the relief of a mild inflammation, such as applying counter-irritation in the form of a blister behind the ear, or the use of antiseptic washes; in other cases it may be necessary to perform a surgical operation, which may vary in degree from the simple removal of a small portion of dead bone to an extensive operation involving the whole of what is called the middle ear. Merely temporary deafness may be due to wax in the ear, and this can be cured by syringing (*see* Plate XV, 1).

It is well to note here also that certain cases of deafness are due to hysteria, and must be treated not as a disorder in themselves, but merely as symptoms of that malady.

The all-important thing upon which to insist is that no real progress can be made in the treatment of any case of deafness until its true nature has been discovered.

There are many different aids to hearing, some of which are of considerable use, others of doubtful utility. Among them may be mentioned: (1) Artificial ear drums; a patient can provide these for himself by making a little ball of cotton wool, tying a thread firmly to it, dipping it into collodion and, when this is dry, putting it into the ear in the position in which he hears best. (2) An apparatus for conveying sounds through the bone, for example, by grasping part of the apparatus with the teeth. (3) Electrical apparatus on the principle of the telephone. (4) Ear trumpets and tubes (*see* Plate XIII, 1–4).

It may be that hearing is improved by aids such as these, but even then, and certainly in cases where hearing will progressively become worse, the patient should seek out a teacher of lip-reading and earnestly endeavour to acquire the art. Much might be done for the child who is hard of hearing if the mother will find time to take it aside often and converse to it on the topics which interest the family, bringing her mouth sufficiently near to the child's ear to allow of it hearing. It has been suggested that if this were done in front of a mirror (*see* Plate XIII, 5) the child would at the same time acquire ability in lip-reading, thus mitigating the hearing defect, while the conversations would keep the mind alert.

Tests for deafness are considered under the heading Hearing.

See Ear; Eustachian Tube; Hearing; Noises in the Ear.

Deafness. Artificial ear drum consisting of a small ball of cotton wool

DEATH. The signs of death constitute a subject of great importance, to which a great deal of attention has been paid, especially from the medico-legal point of view. It is only in a very small percentage of cases of death that any difficulty or doubt is likely to arise; but nevertheless cases of this kind are quite frequent enough to demand very careful enquiry. The bodily states which most closely resemble death are extreme cases of what we call fainting, cases of asphyxia and cases of trance or catalepsy.

The following are the principal signs of death:

(1) The action of the heart and the breathing must have absolutely ceased; it is not sufficient that there is no pulse to be felt at the wrist, or that the chest becomes motionless. The heart itself must be listened to by a skilled ear for a few minutes in absolute quietness so as to make certain that it is motionless; similarly, the faintest signs of breathing must be tested by noting whether a cold mirror held before the face is dimmed, or whether a piece of cotton fluff is moved to and fro. A further test for the cessation of the circulation consists in tying a tight band round one of the limbs and noting whether the part beyond the band gradually becomes swollen as it always would during life. If doubt remained as to whether the heart was beating, the fact could be demonstrated by an electrical cardiograph.

(2) A short time after death the muscles of the body undergo a curious change; they become stiff, owing to the solidifying of the fluids within them. This change is known as rigor mortis, that is to say, rigidity of death. The time at which it comes on and during which it lasts varies very much in different cases; on the average it begins in about six hours and lasts for twenty-four.

(3) After death the body begins to cool and is usually quite cold in less than twenty hours; though it may not reach air temperature for four days.

(4) The eyes very quickly lose their brightness after death.

(5) The skin undergoes changes after death. It ceases to be elastic. First of all very pale, it afterwards becomes discoloured in its lowest parts, varying according to the position in which the body lies. This is due to the fact that the blood, under the action of gravitation, naturally sinks to the lowest possible points, and so these points are stained with blood. This discoloration appears usually in from eight to twelve hours.

(6) Finally, and most important of all, the body undergoes changes of putrefaction. This is an absolutely infallible test; those, however, who assert that it should always be waited for before the fact of death is taken as proved are quite

unjustified in their opinion. Certainly neither burial nor cremation should be undertaken until the fact of death is beyond all dispute whatever ; but not in one case in millions is there the slightest need to wait for changes due to putrefaction.

See Auscultation ; Cremation ; Unconsciousness.

DEATH AGONY. During the few moments of the process of death, there are frequently observed certain spasmodic movements of the body, and these have given rise to the idea that the moment of death is preceded by great agony of mind, or body, or both. This is not correct, as consciousness has already ceased and the movements belong to the phenomena of asphyxia.

See Carbonic Acid.

DEATH RATE. The study of the death rate from all causes, and of the special death rates, must be pursued in full knowledge of the manner in which the figures are arrived at. They are the product of death certificates. These are furnished by the doctor in attendance at the time of death, and he only states the best opinion that he is able to form under the circumstances ; where he is in doubt, he often has to describe as the cause of death some immediate cause, which throws no light upon the underlying disease.

An apparently rising death rate in any particular disease may be due to increasing accuracy of diagnosis, as was shown in the article on cancer (*q.v.*). Another most important point as to the accuracy of asserted death rates from various diseases is that in Great Britain there is no secrecy as regards the contents of the certificate, one consequence being that the part played by alcohol in causing death is not always or even often disclosed. Chronic alcoholics are more likely to succumb to pneumonia and other diseases than are others, but the death may be shown as simply due to pneumonia or some other acute or chronic ailment. Hence, it actually arises that according to the official figures the proportion of deaths due to alcoholism is small.

The death rate in England and Wales, that is to say, the number of deaths in every thousand of the population, was 12·3 for males in 1927. At all ages the female death rate is lower than the male death rate. It is frequently held that a high birth rate is a cause of a high death rate because of the large number of infants who die, the rate in 1927 being 69 for England and Wales. This, however, is an error, because if the high birth rate continues there will be a large proportion of young adults in the population ; moreover, a high birth rate implies the existence of a large number of people at the child-producing age, which is a healthy one.

At present in Great Britain, as in almost all civilized countries, both the death rate and the birth rate are falling. The general death rate is influenced by certain conditions, and is usually highest in the first quarter of the year ; it is lowered by a cool summer or a mild winter despite the nonsense talked about " unseasonable weather." A severe winter kills off many of the young and many of the old who would have otherwise survived ; a hot summer, as a general rule, enormously increases the infantile death rate, though to this there have been striking exceptions.

Vital Dangers of Overcrowding

Overcrowding and the death rate increase and decrease in proportion to one another. The most important fact about overcrowding, in relation to the death rate, is not the number of people in a given area, but the number of people that inhabit a single room. Overcrowding increases the death rate because it means bad ventilation ; this is an all-important fact which cannot be over-estimated. Overcrowding also means increased liability to contract infectious diseases, and it implies poverty ; people living in such conditions are insufficiently fed and clothed.

It is, of course, evident that there are certain ages at which death is more likely to occur than at others ; as, for instance, infancy and extreme old age. Hence, in comparing one year or one country or one place with another, it is necessary to ascertain the ages of the population. For instance, in a district containing a number of almshouses, or a very large number of children, there will be a much higher death rate than in a district which is mainly inhabited by people of the robust ages. It would be absurd to argue from the comparison of the two death rates that the second district was healthier than the first.

Incorrect interpretation of death rates is especially conspicuous in relation to the familiar question as to the relative healthiness of town and country. People who desire to support the reputation for health of cities, and notably of London— the low death rate of which is so often quoted—imagine that because the death rates of so many towns compare favourably with those of the country, towns in general are as healthy as the country. This is quite wrong. Directly the figures are corrected in accordance with the age distribution of the population, and in respect of many other factors, the superior healthiness of the country becomes apparent.

The question may arise in the mind of the thoughtful reader, how much further is the death rate likely to fall ? Occasionally we hear in isolated parts of death rates that may be represented in a single figure. Now, it may be said that at least one half of the total death rate is due to preventable disease of infectious character. When the conditions which favour the spread of these diseases are removed, and when the dangers of alcohol are met, the death rate will fall, without any doubt, to a figure ranging somewhere between five and eight per thousand per year.

See Birth Rate ; Expectation of Life.

DEBILITY. There are so many and such varied causes for the sense of weakness sometimes referred to as debility, that it is a mistake, and sometimes a dangerous one, to label such symptoms as debility without consulting a doctor as to the probable cause. In different individuals, who find themselves debilitated, the cause may be anaemia, indigestion, constipation, chronic kidney disease, or a malignant growth, to mention only a few of the possibilities. It is obviously wrong, therefore, for a person to make prolonged attempts to pull up his strength by taking tonics, stimulants, extra feeding, changes of air and so on, until the real nature of his condition is understood. Apart from such definite causes, it is certainly the case that large numbers of people are kept in a more or less debilitated state by bad ventilation, insufficient exercise in the open air, improper and insufficient feeding, and the abuse of tea, alcohol and tobacco.

See Anaemia ; Consumption ; Diet ; Exercise ; Food ; Health ; Indigestion ; Ventilation.

DECLINE. *See* Consumption.

DECOCTION. A preparation of a drug made by boiling it in a covered vessel for a few minutes and then straining, is called a decoction. The difference between a decoction and an infusion is very small, the latter being made, as everyone knows in the case of tea, by pouring boiling water upon the material that is used. In the British Pharmacopoeia the following decoctions are given, the dose in each case being $\frac{1}{2}$ to 2 ounces : decoction of acacia bark, astringent, used as a gargle for relaxed throat ; of couch grass or agropyrum, diuretic and aperient ; of logwood or haematoxylin and of sappan wood, both astringent and used for diarrhoea ; and of ispaghula, demulcent, like barley water.

DEFORMITY. A lack of the normal shapeliness of the body or its members may exist at birth, and may then represent some inherited peculiarity or be due to some accidental occurrences affecting the development of the child. An excessive number of fingers or toes is an example of the former, and to the latter class belong those errors of development like hare-lip or spina bifida, and also deformities resulting from injuries received within the womb, as, for example, the amputation of a limb.

Congenital club foot may be due to the foot having been crushed into and retained in a bad position before birth. Deformities arising after birth may be the results of injuries, as, for example, when a fractured bone has united in a bad position, or when the parts are dragged on by extensive scarring following burns ; or they may be due to disease in the deformed part, as where angular curvature follows tubercular disease of the spine.

Deformities quite frequently result from nervous diseases, in which, owing to paralysis of one set of muscles, the influence of gravity and the action of the opposing set of muscles drag the part into an abnormal position. Instances of this occur in infantile paralysis and other nervous disorders. References to deformities of various parts of the body will be found under the appropriate headings. The branch of surgery specially concerned with the correction of deformities is known as orthopaedic surgery.

DEGENERACY. In contrast to the great mass of people who are sufficiently suited for a social existence to be regarded as normal types, here and there one can recognize in individuals the marks, or, as they are called, the stigmata of degeneracy. In the presence of notable weakness of mind there is, of course, no difficulty, but there are degenerates whose mental powers, on a casual examination, appear to be quite up to the ordinary standard, or in fact they may notably transcend this, especially in the direction of artistic capacity. A more intimate knowledge of such people would bring to light, however, qualities which separated them from the average man : an inordinate egotism, a weakness or even an entire lack of will power, inability to control their instincts and their emotions, eccentricity of conduct, and perhaps sexual perversions. Habitual criminals are often drawn from this class.

Frequently in persons who show the mental and moral stigmata of degeneracy there are physical peculiarities, such, for example, as a misshapen head, misshapen or badly placed ears, a high arched palate, and so on ; and, sometimes, a functional defect such as a high degree of impairment of vision or impairment of speech. Not every person who presents one or other of these physical stigmata is a degenerate, of course, but this is likely to be the case if there are several of such marks together ; it may also be found that the person is an epileptic.

See Feeble-minded.

DEGENERATION. In connexion with the various organs and tissues of the body, fatty, amyloid, hyaline, or some other form of degeneration may occur. What is meant by this is that the living, functioning substance of the tissues becomes replaced by a new material which is quite inert, the result being that the tissue ceases to perform its duties according to the extent to which the change has taken

place. A liver cell, for example, which in the ordinary course stores up sugar, manufactures bile, destroys poisonous substances coming to it in the blood, and so on, can do none of these things if its protoplasm is replaced by fat or by amyloid substance.

There are numerous causes of such degeneration. A general fatty degeneration throughout the body may occur in certain fevers, in poisoning by phosphorus or arsenic, or other poisons, and in the disease known as acute yellow atrophy of the liver. The liver, the kidneys and the heart muscle are the parts more particularly affected. That is an instance of degeneration from toxic or poisonous influences.

To deprive a tissue of its nourishment by cutting off the blood supply is another way in which degeneration may be brought about. The softening of the brain which occurs when one of the brain arteries is blocked is an instance of fatty degeneration, and this may occur also in tumours which grow too fast to provide themselves with a sufficiency of blood vessels to carry on the circulation within them. In amyloid, also known as waxy and lardaceous degeneration, a heavy, translucent material replaces the normal tissue. This is easily permeable by water ; hence when it occurs in the kidneys there is a free flow of watery urine, and when in the bowel, diarrhoea.

Mucin, which is found normally in the secretion of mucous glands, in the saliva and elsewhere, may also occur as a degeneration in tumours of the ovary, some cancers, etc.

When a nerve is divided, degeneration takes place in the part which is cut off from connexion with the nerve cell. This is because the nourishment of the nerve fibre is controlled by the cell. In the case of a nerve outside the brain or spinal cord, regeneration takes place and a new nerve fibre grows down to take the place of the former one, but inside these masses of nervous matter nothing of the kind happens, and function which is lost through injury or disease breaking into the continuity of nerve fibres there is lost beyond recall.

See Kidney ; Liver ; Nervous System, etc.

DELIRIUM. The mental excitement and disorder which may occur in the course of high fevers, certain brain diseases and in a variety of other circumstances, is spoken of as delirium. A delirious person may be living a vivid waking dream, in which all sorts of extraordinary and perhaps terrifying things occur. He may see people, animals or things which have no existence, or his imagination may distort objects within his view into something quite different, and confuse the identity of people. He may imagine voices or other sounds, and he may misinterpret those which are real. He may entertain suspicions of someone in attendance on him of poisoning his food, of being in league with his enemies, or of something else of the kind, and in consequence of this he may attempt violence or may try to make his escape from the room. Delirious patients have sometimes sustained serious, and even fatal injuries, by falling from windows or downstairs.

Onset and Control of Delirium

The onset of delirium in feverish disorders may be preceded by a certain amount of confusion of ideas, shown when the patient first wakens out of sleep; it may, however, come on quite suddenly. It therefore behoves all those in charge of cases of pneumonia, of enteric fever, or of any other high fever, to mark well any indications pointing to mental confusion; and when active delirium has developed, the patient should never be left for a moment unobserved. The treatment of delirium will be controlled, of course, by the doctor, but it may be said that the application of an ice-bag or of iced cloths to the head, sponging the body and limbs with cold water, or the application of a cold pack, are measures which may prove very useful. The patient must also be humoured as far as possible, and will be quieter when in charge of someone whom he trusts.

There is another sort of delirium which sometimes occurs towards the end of fevers or other serious illnesses. It is what is called low, muttering delirium. The patient lies with his eyes half open, but is unconscious. He keeps on muttering to himself, and his hands may be active, picking at the bedclothes, or as if catching flies in the air. In this condition the fires of life and energy are burning very low. Care must be taken to maintain warmth as far as possible by watching the temperature of the room, and by the use of hot-water bottles in the bed. A little whisky or brandy, if the doctor so orders, is often of great use at this time. *See* Fever.

DELIRIUM TREMENS. Delirium tremens, which literally means trembling delirium, is a name given to a very distinct form of alcoholism. Sometimes it is described as acute alcoholism, but that term is misleading, since any case of drunkenness might be so described. Delirium tremens is a quite distinct affection; it is so common and important that it must be carefully considered.

For the time being the patient is undoubtedly insane; this condition is not due to the direct action of alcohol, otherwise, of course, it would be far more common even than it is, but to changes in the brain produced by the prolonged abuse of alcohol. It may occur in a patient who has never been drunk; this is often the case with women. The attack comes on often in consequence of some extra strain thrown upon the brain, such as an accident, some acute illness, or an exceptional amount of drinking.

As the name implies, trembling (especially of the limbs and fingers) is a marked symptom; the patient becomes sleepless and loses his appetite, then his mind goes, he becomes the subject of all sorts of baseless suspicions, and is in constant terror, partly on that account, and partly because he imagines that he sees all sorts of insects and horrible creatures on his bed and all around him. The patient usually has some fever. According to circumstances, he may recover altogether, or he may die during the attack, or he may recover physically but sink into a state of permanent insanity. The kind of insanity called dementia is the natural sequel to a succession of attacks of delirium tremens.

The treatment of this disease consists mainly in attempting to support the patient's strength. This is to be done by keeping him in bed, if possible by mere persuasion, but if necessary, by force, in feeding him on a simple, digestible and nourishing diet, and in compelling him to sleep, by hypnotics if necessary; no alcohol must be used.

It may be noted that shortly before an attack of this disease the patient very frequently not only loses his appetite for food, as already noted, but also his appetite for alcohol. Hence his relatives are often apt to say that it is the cessation of alcohol that has produced the acute symptoms, and they demand that the poisonous drug be resumed. But, of course, it is not the cessation of alcohol that has produced the delirium, and it is absolutely necessary to prohibit the use of this drug, whether or not the patient has already discontinued it for the few preceding days.

See Alcohol; Delirium; Dementia; Insanity.

DELUSIONS. It is rather difficult to define a delusion because it is almost impossible to make a definition which cannot be applied to certain of the beliefs of apparently sane people. So far as a definition can be made, a delusion is a false belief directly opposed to the evidence and incapable of being affected by any kind of argument or proof. The presence of such a delusion must certainly be regarded as a sign of insanity, but obviously it is very difficult in many cases to say whether the belief in question really answers to the definition given.

The commonest kinds of delusions are those in which the patient wrongly imagines that he suffers from some bodily disease or that he has lost his memory, or that he cannot walk, or that he is the special object of the wrath of the Deity, or that he has been poisoned, or has come into a great fortune. In a great many cases there may be only one particular delusion or group of delusions; two of the commonest are the " delusions of grandeur," as when a patient thinks that he is a millionaire or is the Deity, and " delusions of persecution," when the patient is in the constant belief that some person or body of persons is threatening his life or fortune or happiness.

See Delirium; Hallucination; Illusion; Mental Disease; Will Making.

DEMENTIA. Dementia is the general name applied to all those forms of insanity of which the chief characteristic is not perversion of the mind or alteration of it in any particular direction, but simply loss of mind. The exact English equivalent for this Latin word is mindlessness, and that is precisely what it means.

A progressive mindlessness, or dementia, is, so to speak, a normal symptom of extreme old age, but often occurs far sooner than it should, and often apparently as simply an effect of decay. In other cases, however, there is some brain disorder to account for it, a haemorrhage or a tumour, for example; or the brain disorder may follow on abuse of alcohol or other drugs, or occur as part of the general defect in cretinism or myxoedema. Other forms of insanity, whether there is excitement or depression, are apt to end in dementia.

People suffering from dementia will require care and control according to the degree of mental enfeeblement. Special causes may benefit from appropriate treatment; much benefit will be produced in cretinism and myxoedema by the administration of thyroid extract.

Dementia praecox is a name which is given to certain cases in which, perhaps after delirium with hallucinations, there is a rapid loss of mental capacity. There is some difference of opinion as to its nature, some authorities ascribing the mental symptoms to degenerative changes in the brain and elsewhere; while others think that the degeneration begins in the thinking processes themselves. Its onset has reference to the development which takes place during the periods of puberty and adolescence. Amongst other methods of treatment suggested for this condition is a systematic re-education of the patient.

See Insanity; Mental Disease.

DEMULCENT. Drugs or other substances which have a soothing action upon surfaces of the body, and especially mucous surfaces, are demulcents. A soothing ointment, for instance, is a demulcent to the skin, and white of egg is demulcent to the stomach.

DENTIFRICE. A substance used for cleaning the teeth is a dentifrice; it may be a liquid, a paste or a powder. Powders and pastes by their physical nature help to rub away deposits on the teeth, but they should not be too gritty or they may injure the enamel. Camphorated chalk is a useful and inexpensive dentifrice.

DENTINE. The hard, ivory-like substance which forms the main bulk of a tooth is known as dentine. The chemical

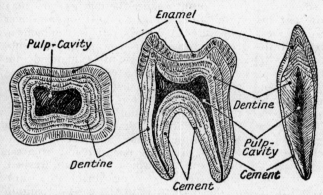

Dentine. Sections of teeth showing the structure of dentine, covered with enamel over the crown of the tooth and with cement in the socket

composition resembles that of bone, but its minute structure is different. It contains a large number of very minute branching tubes, which pass out from the pulp cavity towards the surface of the dentine. These tubes contain prolongations of the tooth pulp. The dentine may be sensitive when it is exposed.

See Bone ; Caries ; Teeth.

DEODORANT. Substances which mask or destroy foul odours are called deodorants. The smoke of tobacco, of brown paper, or of other materials is sometimes used for this purpose, as are eau de Cologne and other perfumes. It must always be remembered that merely to cover a bad smell may in no way dispose of dangers of disease contamination from the cause of the smell, whatever that may be. A solution of permanganate of potash or some chloride of lime, if properly used, will act both as a deodorant and disinfectant.

See Antiseptic ; Disinfectant.

DEPILATORY. This is the technical name applied to any drug or measure which removes hair. A depilatory paste will remove hairs if properly used, but they will grow again in the course of a few weeks. The active drug in most of these pastes is the sulphide of barium.

The following is a formula for such a paste :

Barium sulphide	..	..	..	2	drachms
Orris root powder	..	..	..	2	drachms
Starch	..	..	..	..	4	drachms

A small quantity of the powder is made into a stiff paste with a little water, and is applied to the skin from which the hairs are to be removed. It is left on about 5 minutes, and is then scraped off with a blunt knife. The hairs come away with the paste. As a rule there is no pain or irritation, but it is well not to leave the paste on longer than for five minutes, or it might cause irritation. The skin is washed after the paste is removed, and a little cold cream is then applied.

It is possible that a depilatory, like shaving, might cause the hairs to have a stronger growth in course of time. There are two depilatory measures, however, which are quite effective, though far from being perfect. In the case of small, delicate hairs, the strength of which has not been increased by shaving, the method known as electrolysis is quite effective ; it consists in passing an electric current through the root of each hair, one by one, and so destroying it. In the case of hairs placed closely together and having considerable thickness, even this method will not succeed in destroying hair without leaving permanent marks upon the skin. Another depilatory measure which may be used consists in the employment—under very careful supervision—of the Röntgen Rays.

See Barium ; Electrolysis ; Hair ; Skin ; X-Rays.

DEPRESSION. The subject of depression is one of great difficulty and importance. The depression of mind which is due to some sufficient cause, such as a great misfortune, is hardly a matter for medical enquiry, but there is a large amount of depression which is not due to any such sufficient cause. Sometimes it occurs in cases of insanity, but depression of mind also occurs very frequently amongst persons who are not insane, and who have had no misfortune, or only such as other people would bear without difficulty.

As a rule there is some bodily reason for these cases of depression. Sometimes there is positive disease; but more frequently it will be found that the patient has been abusing his body in some way, or that he has indigestion, or that his nervous system has been strained by over-work, or that he suffers from that disturbance of ideas which is called a complex.

A constant resort to stimulants such as tea and coffee, and more especially alcohol, in order to dispel depression, is greatly to be deprecated, as this will probably only aggravate the condition. The cause must be investigated. If it is overwork the patient should rest or have a change; in some cases more open-air life is needed, and so on. People who suffer from depression which their own minds tell them has no really sufficient cause, should be aware that their condition demands serious attention, for otherwise it may lead, in a certain number of cases, to permanent disorder of the mind. Psychotherapy is often of benefit in these cases.

See Change of Life; Neurasthenia.

DERBYSHIRE NECK. Certain localities have been notoriously associated with forms of goitre, and amongst them, Derbyshire; a popular name for the disease is therefore Derbyshire neck.

See Goitre.

DERMATITIS. Inflammation of the skin is technically called dermatitis. The area of skin inflamed may be uniformly affected, or there may be larger or smaller patches scattered over it with sound skin intervening. The signs are those which one is accustomed to associate with inflammation, that is to say, redness, swelling, heat and pain. After exposure to the sun, for instance, the face may become red and swollen, so much so, perhaps, that the eyes almost disappear. The face feels hot and burning, and perhaps itchy. Afterwards the skin may peel and some brown pigmentation may be left.

In some cases blisters are formed; if small, these are known as vesicles, if large, as bullae. If a vesicle becomes filled with pus or matter, it is a pustule. Should any of these burst, an ulcerating surface may be left which may continue to discharge, or the discharge may dry up and form a crust or a scab. In some cases of dermatitis, papules or pimples make their appearance and may give rise to intense itching.

External irritants other than sunlight may also produce dermatitis. It may result from cold, from heat, or from over exposure to X-rays. It is common in certain occupations owing to the substances which have to be handled; for example, paraffin workers; workers amongst tar; cabinet makers; grocers, in whom it appears as grocers' itch, apparently from handling sugar; gardeners, from handling certain plants, notably some primulas and poison ivy; steel-workers, from the fine grit and from the dirty tubs in which tools are washed. The importance of recognizing the cause of the dermatitis in the case of paraffin and tar workers is that if the irritation be allowed to operate for a long time, cancerous disease of the skin may be produced.

Drugs that Produce a Rash

Poisonous substances in the blood may also cause dermatitis. The nature of some of these poisons is obscure, but often a clear connexion can be shown between dermatitis and some drug which has been introduced into the body. Arsenic, bromides and iodides are instances of such.

The prevention of what are called the occupational forms of dermatitis is clearly a matter of great importance. In every case scrupulous cleanliness should be practised, and this would do much towards prevention. In some cases it may be possible to use gloves or something of the kind when handling irritating substances. There will always be certain persons whose skins show an undue readiness to irritation by particular things. The only feasible plan in this case may be a change of occupation.

The treatment adopted for dermatitis will vary according to its severity and its cause. In some cases, as where the cause is a drug, merely to discontinue this may be quite sufficient. Where there is heat and itching a sedative may be applied. This may take the form of a lotion, for example, calamine lotion; of a dusting powder, such as one made up of 1 part of zinc oxide, 1 part of boracic acid, and 8 parts of starch powder ; or of some emollient, like vaseline, lanoline, cold cream or zinc ointment.

The reddish or salmon-pink scaly patches which sometimes appear on the back, the chest, the brow or elsewhere, and usually when the patient is subject to dandruff, are sometimes called seborrhoeic dermatitis, and are due to a microbe. Such patches will disappear quickly, as a rule, under an ointment such as this :

Salicylic acid	10 grains
Precipitated sulphur	10 grains
Powdered zinc oxide	1 drachm
White vaseline ..	to make 1 ounce

The dandruff (q.v.) should always be attended to.

The name exfoliative dermatitis is given to cases where the signs of inflammation of the skin are followed by the profuse formation of scales which continue to be shed for a longer or shorter period. This condition may occur at any age and under a variety of circumstances ; it may, for instance, occur as an epidemic.

The herpetiform dermatitis is one in which the signs of inflammation, whether papules, vesicles or bullae, occur together, and vesicles are often grouped as one finds them in herpes (q.v.) This disease, which usually affects adults, appears often to have a definite association with some nervous disorder which may contribute to its origin. Dermatitis occurs of course in most skin diseases, but where there are special features the disease is given a special name as, for example, eczema, erysipelas, psoriasis, herpes, and so on.

See Lotion ; Occupational Disease ; Ointment ; Pemphigus ; Skin.

DERMOID. This name is applied to certain growths which are occasionally found in the body, and which, when removed, are seen to contain structures that really belong to the skin. Often, for instance, a dermoid tumour is found to contain a quantity of hair that has grown within it.

See Cyst.

DESQUAMATION. Derived from the Latin word squama, a scale, desquamation is a word used to describe a condition that follows some diseases, the most striking of which is scarlet fever. The outer skin is more rapidly shed than at other times, and comes off in the form of a multitude of tiny scales. In scarlet fever large flakes may peel off, perhaps even like a glove or slipper. A great deal of importance has been attached to this process because it was once thought that the scales contained the infectious microbes of the disease, and therefore the patient was an object of danger to his neighbours until the peeling had ceased. It is now held by authorities that desquamation is relatively unimportant,

See Scarlatina.

DETERGENT. A detergent is simply a cleansing agent, for example, soap and water, turpentine, olive oil, and so on.

DEVONSHIRE COLIC. At one time colic due to lead poisoning was frequently caused by drinking cider. From this arose a custom of calling chronic lead poisoning Devonshire colic. It is possible that lead was added to reduce the acidity of the cider, but the more likely explanation of its presence in the beverage is that there were lead parts used in the construction of the cider presses. Nothing of the kind need be anticipated from cider nowadays.

See Lead.

DIABETES INSIPIDUS. This is a rare and very peculiar disease, the one distinctive symptom of which is the persistent production of an extremely excessive quantity of urine. Naturally accompanying this symptom is a persistent and excessive thirst. The precise cause of the disease is unknown, though it is perhaps due to some peculiarity in the neighbourhood of the pituitary gland.

The disease is not in itself fatal, but may be accompanied by damage to the kidneys, and there is a tendency to contract disease of the lungs sooner or later. Treatment by injections of pituitary extract usually produces at least temporary release from symptoms, and the withdrawal of cerebro-spinal fluid by lumbar puncture has been beneficial occasionally. The patient must be kept warm and should avoid fatigue. He should restrict the fluids taken so far as this can be done comfortably.

DIABETES MELLITUS. Generally referred to simply as diabetes, this disease is quite distinct from diabetes insipidus described above, is far commoner and of much greater importance. In this, as in the other form, there is a great excess in the amount of urine passed, but here the resemblance between the two diseases ends   In diabetes mellitus, or true diabetes, the almost constant fact is that, apart from treatment, the urine contains a certain amount of sugar ; whereas there is no sugar in normal urine.

It must not be supposed, on the other hand, that whenever there is sugar in the urine there is diabetes.   There are conditions in which there is a temporary glycosuria, this being the term used for the presence of sugar in the urine.   But when it is found that the urine constantly

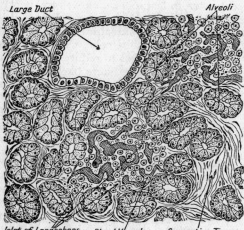

Large Duct   Alveoli

Islet of Langerhans   Blood Vessels   Connective Tissue

Section of the pancreas showing the islets of Langerhans, disease of which causes diabetes

contains sugar, and that the amount of sugar in the blood is increased, then diabetes mellitus is present.

It is believed that the disease, at any rate in a large number of cases, is due to damage affecting the pancreas, the gland which lies near the stomach and which is so important in digestion (q.v.) ; but it is not the part of the pancreas concerned with digestion which has to do with diabetes, but rather the little collections of cells which are embedded in the gland proper.   These are known as the insulae or islets of Langerhans, and they appear to produce a secretion which they pour into the blood, and which has the effect of ensuring that the sugar in the body will be burnt up and utilised.

In disease of the pancreas, affecting these islets and leading to a failure of their secretion, it is not surprising, therefore, that diabetes should occur.   The truth of this view of the part played by the islets in causing diabetes is borne out by the fact that an extract made from the islets, which is well known as insulin, has the effect, if injected into the body, of removing the symptoms of diabetes.

Normally, carbohydrate food is converted into grape sugar in the intestine, absorbed as such and carried to the liver, where it is converted into and stored up as glycogen, a starch-like substance.   Glycogen is stored in the muscles also.   From time to time, as sugar is required in the blood, glycogen is re-converted into sugar and is passed into the blood stream.   But in diabetes mellitus this scheme is upset, and carbohydrate food, and in some cases even protein food, is converted into grape sugar which is not stored up but accumulates in the blood, and is forthwith discharged into the urine.

The damage to the pancreas may arise from infection of some kind.   In considering the causation of this disease, other facts must, however, be noted.   It appears to be a family disease in a large number of cases.   In others the symptoms have followed an injury about the base of the skull ;   or excessive eating, especially of carbohydrates. over a prolonged period ; or severe grief or worry, or a nervous shock of some kind.

In consequence of the changes in the body chemistry the patient loses flesh and strength, despite his large appetite and great thirst ; he becomes thinner and thinner, and various complications may supervene.   When the disease occurs in the young it is much more acute, and also more rapidly fatal.   Occurring in the elderly, it is often very mild, not very much sugar being lost, and it may last for years without very markedly affecting the health of the patient.

People who suffer from diabetes are specially liable to the infection from tuberculosis, and not infrequently they are carried off by tuberculosis of the lungs. The most characteristic end of the disease, however, is by coma, by which is meant profound unconsciousness.   This is brought about by a poisoning of the blood, commonly called acidosis (*q.v.*), which results from the perverted body chemistry.

Even prior to the introduction of insulin treatment, glycosuria in elderly people could generally be controlled by a properly adjusted diet, and this was accomplished also in many instances of diabetes occurring in younger people, but here the benefits of dietetic treatment were only temporary, as the disease reasserted itself after a year or two. The diet must contain some carbohydrate, as, if it is withheld, fats are not properly metabolised, and acidosis results ; and, on the other hand, if too much carbohydrate is taken, sugar appears in the urine. The first thing to be done, therefore, is to find out the extent of the sugar tolerance of the patient, that is, the amount of carbohydrate which he can take without unduly raising the amount of sugar in the blood.

This may be done by putting the patient on a diet of meat, eggs, green vegetables, and a limited amount of carbohydrate, for example, 4 ounces of bread daily. The amount of sugar represented in the carbohydrate given is known, and it can be judged by an examination of the urine whether it is necessary further to reduce carbohydrates or possible to increase them.

When and How Insulin is Given

It must next be considered whether the diet reached in this way satisfies the patient's demands as laid down under the heading Diet, due regard being paid to the amount of the daily work. For many elderly people it may be found sufficient, but it is very unlikely that younger patients will be able to get on without an increase of carbohydrate. This will be made possible, however, by the daily use of insulin, the requisite number of units being injected under the skin, twice as a rule, once before the morning meal and again before the evening meal. More frequent dosage can rarely be tolerated. Should the patient become affected with an infectious disorder, influenza or pneumonia, for example, the amount of each dose must be increased three or four times at least.

Care should be taken to avoid overdosage with insulin, otherwise there occurs an undue diminution of the sugar in the blood, or hypoglycaemia. This is signalised by such symptoms as faintness, giddiness, trembling of the hands, sweating and drowsiness. These symptoms will be relieved by taking cane-sugar or glucose, and it is a useful precaution for a patient who is taking insulin to carry around with him a stick of barley-sugar.

Insulin has proved of immense value in cases of diabetic coma, in which formerly the outlook was of the blackest.

What a Diabetic May Eat

For purposes of reference it may be useful to mention some of the things which may be taken by a diabetic and others which are forbidden, unless ordered by the physician. He would do so when the patient was allowed a certain amount of carbohydrate. The following may be given : clear soup, tea and coffee (without milk or sugar), soda water, unsweetened lemon drinks, bread and biscuits made with almond, gluten or bran, cucumbers, celery (sparingly), tomatoes, asparagus (the green part), and all green vegetables, all kinds of fish and shellfish (except cod's liver), fresh meat (except liver), poultry, eggs and butter, and all acid fruits, particularly oranges, currants and sour berries.

Diabetic bread and biscuit must be obtained from a reputable firm, and a doctor's advice should be asked with regard to any food of the kind which it is proposed to take. Saccharin may be employed in powder or tablets to sweeten tea, coffee and other beverages, and fruit or other foods which may be taken.

The following are forbidden : bread of all kinds (except such as is made for diabetics), rice, tapioca, potatoes, beets, turnips, vegetable marrows, parsnips, artichokes, all malted liquors, sweet wines, and any beverage sweetened with sugar. Milk should not be given without the doctor's sanction ; it is sometimes submitted to treatment which fits it for diabetics on a carbohydrate-free diet.

See Acidosis ; Bread ; Diet ; Food ; Pancreas ; Urine.

DIACHYLON PLASTER. *See* Lead.

DIAGNOSIS. The process by which the doctor attempts to discover the nature of the disease from which his patient is suffering is called the **diagnosis**. Important help in recognizing the **nature**

of a complaint may be derived from a knowledge of illnesses which have occurred to the patient's forbears or other blood relations, or in his own life. In addition to this, there are two leading methods by which the doctor attempts to discover the nature of a disease, and sometimes the words symptoms and signs are used to distinguish the two methods.

In general the word symptoms indicates the facts of the disease which the patient feels for himself. Pain, for instance, is a symptom which the doctor cannot discover directly, but of which the patient informs him. Naturally, in attempting to make a diagnosis, the doctor first learns all he can about the patient's symptoms, and after that he examines the patient's body so as to discover, if possible, the state of affairs which has led to these symptoms. Thus he finds the physical signs.

Modern Methods of Diagnosis

This, however, is not all. Even when he has examined the patient's body in every available way, by looking at it, by feeling it, by tapping it, so as to observe the condition of the organs that lie underneath the points where he taps, by listening to it, so as to hear the sounds made by the heart and the lungs, by examining the back of the eye with a special mirror invented for the purpose, and by other means of the same kind—even then modern means of diagnosis are not exhausted.

The whole elucidation of the case may depend upon chemical examination of the urine, and in other cases the diagnosis may entirely depend upon examination of the blood, as, for instance, in suspected cases of typhoid fever. Again, certain minute portions of the body may actually be removed for the special purpose of examination, as, for instance, when a surgeon removes a minute portion of a tumour which may prove to be cancer, and examines it under the microscope to see whether it contains structures characteristic of that disease.

Since surgical operations have become so safe, in cases of obscure disease of the brain or of the abdomen, the surgeon very often undertakes what is called a diagnostic operation for the purpose of finding out exactly what the condition is,

and then dealing with it to the best of his power. The X-rays are an indispensable aid to diagnosis in many cases.

See Constitution ; Disease ; Heredity ; Pain ; Prognosis ; Wassermann Reaction ; X-Rays.

DIAPHORETIC. This is the name applied to any drug or other means of treatment which causes the skin to produce a quantity of sweat or perspiration ; exposure to hot air, as in a Turkish bath, is a typically diaphoretic measure, and many drugs have a similar action.

The skin is one of the organs by which the body gets rid of poisons that may have gained admission to it, or that may have been produced within it. Hence it is often desirable, for example, in cases of fever and Bright's disease, to employ some kind of diaphoretic to urge the skin to greater activity. Moreover, free perspiration helps to lower the temperature in fevers.

Sweating can sometimes be quickly induced, for example, in malaria, by wrapping the patient in a blanket, surrounding him with hot-water bottles, and giving him hot drinks. By the use of a large bed cradle and lamps, a patient may be given a hot-air bath or a vapour bath in bed.

Amongst the drugs which have this effect the most commonly used are probably the solution of acetate of ammonium or mindererus solution, the dose of which is 2 to 6 drachms ; sweet spirits of nitre, dose 15 to 60 minims ; and Dover's powder (*q.v.*) which contains opium and ipecacuanha and is given in doses of 5 to 15 grains. The last named is often taken at the commencement of a cold, if the patient can go to bed. A simple diaphoretic mixture for an adult would be as follows :

Spirit of nitrous ether	3 drachms
Solution of acetate of ammonium	2 ounces
Syrup of oranges	4 drachms
Camphor water ..	to make 8 ounces
Dose : Two tablespoonsful every 4 hours.	

When a very rapid and powerful effect is wanted pilocarpine is generally used, but this should only be under medical supervision. Care has to be taken, after the use of any of these diaphoretic remedies, against exposure and chilling.

See Baths ; Fever ; Sweat ; Warburg's Tincture.

DIAPHRAGM. The dome-shaped partition between the cavities of the chest and abdomen is known as the diaphragm or midriff, the latter being an old English word meaning the middle of the belly. It consists of flat muscles at the sides and of tough membrane at the centre, and is attached to the six lower ribs, the backbone, and the lowest part of the breast bone.

It is perforated by several openings for the passage of the oesophagus or gullet, the abdominal aorta or large artery supplying the lower part of the trunk and the lower limbs, the inferior vena cava or large vein returning the blood from these parts, and of other structures. It is supplied by the phrenic nerves. The descent or flattening of the diaphragm increases the height and therefore the capacity of the chest cavity, and air is thus drawn into the lungs.

See Abdomen ; Respiration.

DIARRHOEA. The frequent passage of softened motions by the bowels, which is what is meant by the term diarrhoea, should always be looked upon as a symptom, and not a disease in itself. Along with diarrhoea there may be the rumbling of gas in the bowel, and colicky pain. In some cases there is frequent and useless painful straining ; this symptom is commonly referred to as tenesmus. If diarrhoea is at all sharp the patient may be more or less collapsed.

The most common cause of diarrhoea is the presence in the bowel of some irritating substance. In such a case the first business of the doctor is to get rid of that substance, and therefore he gives some drug which makes the bowels act more vigorously than ever ; then, when the cause of irritation is removed, the diarrhoea ceases. On the other hand, there are many cases of diarrhoea which depend upon a diseased condition of the wall of the bowel itself. In such cases a purgative drug would make the condition worse in every way.

Thus, it is clear that no one should attempt to treat any case of diarrhoea until the cause of the condition has been ascertained.

Acute diarrhoea is exceedingly common and is most frequently caused by irritation, though in other cases it is due to chill, and, in the peculiar condition known as examination diarrhoea because it is apt to affect students who are facing an examination, it is due to nervous influences accompanying excitement. There is another type of diarrhoea which tends to occur whenever a meal is taken. It should not be forgotten also that diarrhoea may usher in enteric fever, dysentery, or some such disease. Occurring in a young child in hot weather, it may constitute the exceedingly fatal malady known as summer diarrhoea or infantile cholera, which is described under the heading Cholera.

When diarrhoea is due to something indigestible having been taken, it is best treated by giving about an ounce of castor oil to which a few drops of tincture of opium or laudanum have been added. The castor oil removes the irritating substance, and the opium soothes the angry bowel. When the diarrhoea is at all serious, the food should be confined to liquids, milk, of course, being its best ingredient. Milk should be sipped, and it may well be mixed with an equal part of warm water, soda water, or of lime water. In hot weather the milk should be boiled, and it may be an advantage to do this at any time.

Value of Warmth and Rest

Warmth to the belly not only eases any pain there may be, but tends to diminish the diarrhoea. Another means of doing this is to rest in bed, or at any rate to lie down. If there is faintness a little spirit of sal volatile may be given in some water ; but if diarrhoea is as severe as this, or if it does not respond quickly to simple remedies, a doctor should be called in.

If looseness of the bowels persists after the irritating substances have been cleared away, doses of salicylate of bismuth, 10 grains, of chalk mixture, $\frac{1}{2}$ to 1 ounce, or of vegetable astringents like catechu or kino, may be given every three or four hours.

After an attack of diarrhoea, the diet should be light and bland for a few days. Of this description would be milk puddings, steamed white fish, sweetbreads and chicken jelly. Stringy meat or vegetables and fruit skins must be avoided. It is a great mistake for a patient with chronic diarrhoea to go on treating himself with diarrhoea mixtures without reference to a doctor. A very careful expert examination is required in these circumstances to determine the nature and cause of the diarrhoea, and the sooner this is done the better.

See Astringent ; Cholera ; Collapse; Indigestion ; Intestine ; Lianteric Diarrhoea.

DIET. For a healthy person who has an ample supply of fresh food and leads an active life out of doors, the principles of diet are likely to have a merely academic interest. A proper understanding of these principles is of the utmost importance, however, for those whose food supply, from reasons of expense or otherwise, is limited, for those dependent largely on artificial or preserved foods and for those in poor health.

The essentials of a proper diet are that it should provide for growth and for the replacement of waste, that it should furnish the heat and energy required by the body, and that it should furnish also a measure of stimulation to metabolism and to the functions of the alimentary tract. An analysis of foodstuffs shows that they are made up of certain constituents, namely, proteins or nitrogenous substances, carbohydrates, fats, salts, vitamins and water.

Dual Function of the Proteins

The proteins, of which white of egg and lean meat are examples, are the tissue-builders and make good the loss of tissue due to the wear and tear of living ; they also go to the making of the secretions of the body. The daily amount of tissue waste in an adult person is not very great, and hard work makes no appreciable difference, because the energy expended is derived from other kinds of foodstuffs. An increased consumption of meat, therefore, on account of harder work has no physiological justification. A growing person, on the other hand, requires a liberal allowance of proteins.

These substances are contained in flesh, fish and fowl and also in wheat and other vegetable foods, but those of animal origin have in addition a certain dynamic quality which explains the craving for animal food in cold climates and the lessened inclination for it among dwellers in temperate climes during the hotter weather. Another advantage of flesh foods is that they present their proteins in a concentrated and easily digested form.

Proteins also furnish a certain amount of heat and energy, but the proper sources of most of our requirements of these are carbohydrates and fats. If more protein is taken than is required for growth and repair, more energy will certainly be provided, but the body will be taxed to dispose of much that is not otherwise utilised ; there will be an excess of ash, as it were, for the fuel consumed, whereas fats and carbohydrates produce no ash.

The Calorie as Unit of Energy

The amount of heat, and incidentally of energy, as heat and energy are convertible into one another, furnished to the body by fixed amounts of protein, fat and carbohydrate, can be estimated by burning them outside the body. The amount of heat is calculated according to a unit known as a calorie or, as is usual when dealing with foodstuffs, a large, or kilogramme, calorie.

A calorie, or small calorie, is the quantity of heat required to raise the temperature of 1 gramme of water through 1° C. ; a large calorie, that required to raise the temperature of 1 kilogramme, or 1 litre, of water also through 1° C. In what follows, and elsewhere in this book, when the term calorie is used it is the large calorie that is meant.

It has been found, then, that 1 gramme of either protein or carbohydrate produces 4 calories, while the same amount of fat produces 9 calories. The excellence of fat as a source of heat is apparent, and, for a reason to be mentioned hereafter when treating of vitamins, fat is an essential part of any diet. It might appear, then, that fat might be used altogether in place of carbohydrate, but this is not so ; the body cannot burn up fat properly unless in the presence of a relatively large amount of carbohydrate. Otherwise poisonous substances accumulate in the blood, as described under the heading Acidosis.

From experiments it has been found that the number of calories expended and required in the 24 hours by various classes of persons are as follows :

Man doing hard muscular work	4,000 calories
Man doing moderate muscular work	3,500 ,,
Man doing light muscular work	3,000 ,,
Man doing sedentary work	2,500 ,,
Average woman	2,500 ,,
Man in bed, feeding	1,850 ,,
Man in bed, fasting	1,700 ,,

Different opinions have been expressed regarding the relative proportions of the three food constituents which should be represented in the diet. Two scales which have been suggested as suitable for a man doing light work, that is, requiring 3,000 calories, are as follows :

Protein	Carbo-hydrate	Fat	Actual Calorie value
120 grammes	500 grammes	50 grammes	3,007
100 ,,	350 ,,	100 ,,	3,090

As regards the differences, it may be said that most people could do with less protein than is commonly taken, that is, with the second scale as stated above, while with regard to the proportions of carbohydrate and fat, the former should bulk more largely as compared with fat when a rapid output of energy is required.

Under the heading Food, tables of the principal articles of diet are given, from which, by the application of the facts mentioned above, an intelligent scheme of dieting can be produced.

The salts in foodstuffs include those of iron, calcium, magnesium, sodium and potassium, and are necessary in tissue building or, in various ways, in the chemical processes which go on in the body ; iron is a necessary constituent of the red blood corpuscles, for example, and calcium of bone, while sodium chloride is a constituent of blood, etc., and the source of hydrochloric acid in the gastric juice.

Even should a diet be corrected, however, in all the particulars which have been mentioned up to this point, it will not be a good diet unless the foods included contain certain substances known as accessory food factors or vitamins. Several of these vitamins have been recognized, namely, three which are soluble in fat, but not in water, and known respectively as A, D and E, and three which are soluble in water and known as B, B2 and C.

Fat soluble A prevents xerophthalmia, D prevents rickets, and E has been shown to be necessary to reproduction in rats fed on an artificial diet in which A and D were present ; the absence of water-soluble B leads to beri-beri, and it is therefore also known as the anti-neuritic vitamin ; B2 prevents pellagra ; while the absence of water-soluble C leads to scurvy and it is therefore called the anti-scorbutic vitamin. It is probable that ill-defined diseases occurring in those who feed on artificial foods is explained by vitamin starvation.

In the following table the vitamin content of various foods is set out :

Foodstuff	Fat Soluble A	Water Soluble B	Water Soluble C
Milk	+ +	—	+
Butter	+ + +	—	—
Cream	+ +	—	+ ?
Egg yolk ..	+ +	+ +	—
Beef fat.. ..	+	—	—
Mutton fat ..	+	—	—
Lard	—	—	—
Pork	—	—	—
White fish ..	—	—	—
Herring ..	—	—	—
Cod-liver oil ..	+ + +	—	—
Margarine (containing animal fat) ..	+	—	—
Vegetable oils	—	—	—
Wheat (whole grain) ..	+	+ +	—
White flour ..	—	—	—
Polished rice..	—	—	—
Fresh fruit (especially orange, lemon, grape fruit, tomato) ..	—	—	+ + +
Nuts	—	+ + +	—
Green vegetables (raw) ..	+ +	—	+ + +
Green vegetables (cooked for a short time)	+ +	—	+
Potato	—	+	+
Swede turnip	—	+	+ +
Yeast	—	+ + +	—

+ + + = abundant supply ; + + = moderate supply ; + = fair supply ; — = none.

Foods which contain vitamin A generally contain D also, and the statements in the first column above, regarding the presence and richness of vitamin A, may be taken as applying equally to vitamin D. There is very little vitamin D in green vegetables, however, and conversely the body fat of fish contains no vitamin A but a fair proportion of vitamin D, so that herrings, for example, may be used as a source of the latter. What is said about vitamin B above applies more or less to vitamin B2, but milk, which does not contain the former contains the latter and this also occurs in lean meat, fish, cheese and eggs.

Other characteristics of a good diet remain to be considered. It must excite the digestive functions and must contain a sufficient amount of indigestible material, or, as it is called, roughage, to stimulate the muscular movements of the gut and so promote regularity in the action of the bowels.

Preserving the Teeth by Eating Apples

Appetite and digestion are improved by variety in the diet and by good cooking. Foods which require chewing are helpful because they allow time for the action of saliva, and the act of chewing stimulates the flow of gastric juice. Moreover, it should be recognized that chewing crisp food, such as an apple, is a natural method of cleansing the teeth, and if young children were given such foods regularly there would be much less dental caries than is encountered at present. Roughage is supplied chiefly by the cellulose contained in vegetables and fruits and stimulates the bowel mechanically. Constipation may be cured simply by taking more of such foods ; on the other hand, when there is diarrhoea, foods providing roughage should be discontinued for the time being.

Reference has been made to diseases ensuing on a partial or total lack of vitamins or of carbohydrates. It may be noted also that anaemia may result from iron starvation, as when a patient is kept on a purely milk diet for a long period, and goitre from iodine starvation, the thyroid gland enlarging in the effort to make good such deficiency.

An excessive diet strains the digestive and excretory apparatus of the body, leading to indigestion and auto-intoxication (q.v.). Some of the excess is laid down as fat, and a flabby obesity is also the common result of an excessive consump-

tion of carbohydrates, another result being flatulent indigestion.

Babies, up to about the age of six months, are unable to digest starch, as they lack the necessary ferments ; in the permissible types of the infant foods which are prepared from wheat, the starch has been converted into the sugar known as maltose.

In some diseases adjustment of the diet is the most important part of the treatment. In diabetes mellitus, for example, the supply of carbohydrates must be strictly controlled, and in gout the supply of proteins. In nephritis the protein supply must also be diminished as a rule, though in chronic cases, where the loss of protein in the urine is very considerable, it may be necessary to make good this loss. In asthma and eczema it may be found that attacks are precipitated by some protein, that of eggs, for instance, and such must therefore be avoided.

A sharp difference of opinion exists on the subject of the correct diet for acute febrile diseases. The traditional method is to " starve a fever," and is dictated by the impairment in the digestive and excretory powers of the patient. The question is dealt with in the article on fever (q.v.).

The diet in chronic diseases varies considerably according to the nature of the disease, but one observation should be made, namely, that often the diet is not sufficiently varied ; this, perhaps, applies particularly to dyspepsia, as the patient often subjects himself to vitamin starvation by too narrow a selection of foods.

Elderly People Should Eat Less

After a person has passed middle age his dietary should be reviewed frequently and the quantity should diminish pari-passu with his output of work as the years go on. Possibly, as he gets older, he may become more inclined to constipation and it will be important to have plenty of roughage in his food. For old age food must be simple and easily digested, and, as the body heat is less easily maintained, it should contain an adequate amount of fats and carbohydrates.

See Banting ; Carbohydrate ; Digestion ; Fat ; Food ; Invalid Cookery ; Protein ; Salisbury Diet ; Tuffnell's Diet ; Vegetable Foods ; Vegetarianism ; Vitamin.

DIGESTION Digestion is the name of the process by which the food, after it has been dealt with by the teeth, is changed in such a fashion that it can be absorbed from various points in the alimentary canal, and in this way reach the body in general.

It is a useful thing to think of the alimentary canal as a long tube that runs down the middle of the body. In a sense, therefore, anything inside that tube is not really inside the body; it must get through the walls of the tube before it is really made part of the body itself. This is an important idea, for it leads us to understand that we live, not by what we eat, but by what we digest and absorb and assimilate.

Another note must be made as to the meaning of the word indigestible. This is used in two senses. Sometimes it is used to describe substances which in the nature of the case cannot be digested; paper, for instance, is indigestible, and coal, and the fibres in cabbage stalk. There is no apparatus within the human body for reducing these things and many others to a form in which they can be absorbed; they cannot be digested, and therefore they are properly described as indigestible.

But the word is often used also to describe substances which get digested by the healthy body, but which tend to upset the digestion, as the saying goes. In certain cases this is a useful meaning of the word, but the first meaning must never be forgotten. It must always be remembered that the natural digestive powers of the body have a certain limit, and, further, that a certain proportion of most of the foods consumed lies outside those limits, and is therefore properly called indigestible.

There appears to be a common belief that the digestion is performed exclusively in the stomach, but this is quite wrong.

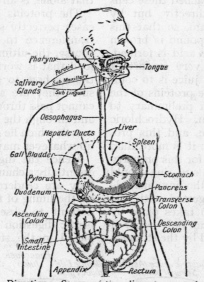

Digestion. Course of the alimentary canal with some of the principal accessory organs

Labels: Pharynx, Parotid, Salivary Glands, Sub Maxillary, Sub Lingual, Tongue, Oesophagus, Hepatic Ducts, Liver, Spleen, Gall Bladder, Pylorus, Stomach, Duodenum, Pancreas, Transverse Colon, Ascending Colon, Descending Colon, Small Intestine, Appendix, Rectum

The digestion performed in the stomach is of very much less importance, is very much less complete and very much less comprehensive and versatile, than the digestion which is performed in the bowel. In addition to its services to digestion, the stomach acts as a receptacle in which it is possible to put a quantity of food at a time, a convenient arrangement for enabling us to take a meal and then go about our business.

The first stage of digestion begins in the mouth. The saliva which is poured out into the mouth during the act of chewing helps not only to put the food into a convenient form for swallowing, but also contains a digestive ferment known as ptyalin, which gets thoroughly mixed up with the food if the act of chewing is properly performed and not scamped. What enters the stomach, then, consists of thoroughly chewed food mixed with saliva. Saliva is alkaline, and the juices of the stomach are acid, but it takes some time for the gastric secretion to penetrate the masses of food, and until this happens salivary digestion goes on.

The gastric juice has no power of dealing with the starchy elements of the food, and has only a slight action on oils and fats, except in so far as the movements of the walls of the stomach tend to mix them thoroughly with other constituents of the food and so render them more fit for treatment further on. It has, however, on proteins, which it owes to certain of its contents. This juice, which is a complicated secretion produced by the innumerable tiny glands lying in the lining of the stomach, is found, when analysed, to be a watery substance, having no colour or odour, and consisting to the extent of more than 99 per cent. of water. The remainder, however, has some important constituents, especially the acid called hydrochloric acid.

In some inexplicable way the living cells in the glands of the walls of the stomach are able to affect the common salt which is an indispensable ingredient of food, and which has reached these cells not from the stomach directly, but by means of the blood stream, so that this very firm and stable compound is broken up and free hydrochloric acid is formed.

The function of this very important constituent of the gastric juice is to combine with and dissolve the proteins of the food, this process being a preliminary to their satisfactory digestion. Hydrochloric acid is also an antiseptic, and this property is of extreme value ; it is more than probable that, were it not for this property of the gastric juice, much suffering would result from swallowing the innumerable varieties of microbes ingested with the food. So far as infection takes place by way of the stomach, it can only occur if the production of this acid by the stomach

combines with and dissolves the proteins of the food, and then the pepsin proceeds to digest them, that is to say, to produce chemical changes of such a character that they are able to be absorbed by the wall of the bowel at a later stage ; that, and that alone, is all that digestion means.

The proteins of the food are in some cases perfectly suitable for almost direct transference to the blood, which is, of course, the ultimate destination of all the food that is worth taking. But the question is how to get these proteins there, since they are so constituted that they cannot pass through the wall of the bowel and through the walls of the minute blood vessels which lie in its lining, ready to take up whatever may be worth having.

Hence the digestion of the proteins is essentially a change due to pepsin, whereby they are rendered capable of absorption by the lining of the bowel. It is most important to observe that the process of peptic digestion is practically never completed in the stomach ; as a matter of

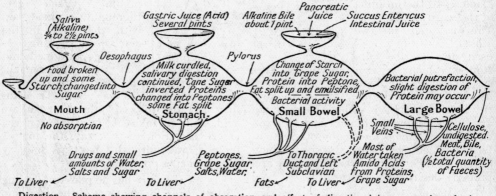

Digestion. Scheme showing channels of absorption and effect of digestive juices on various foods

wall is defective, or if the microbes are exceptionally resistant, or reach the stomach just when the gastric juice is very much diluted by the food, and therefore unable to exert its full antiseptic powers.

The other most important constituent of the juice is a ferment called pepsin ; it can easily be obtained by itself, and is found to be a pale yellow powdery substance. There is also a small quantity of another ferment called rennin, which curdles or coagulates milk.

After the first stage of gastric digestion, already described, the hydrochloric acid

fact, it usually stops about half-way. The soluble form of protein which is the product of this digestion is known as peptone.

What happens during the gastric digestion of certain common articles of diet may be briefly noted. The protein substance which is the chief constituent of milk is first of all solidified or coagulated by the rennin (the size and density of the clot that is formed markedly affects its ease of digestion) ; thereafter the clot is first of all dissolved by the hydrochloric acid and then half digested by the pepsin.

If milk were not so coagulated it would run straight through the stomach into the bowel.

In the case of the fat cells, such as those that constitute the ordinary fat of meat, all that gastric digestion accomplishes is to dissolve the envelopes of the cells and liberate the fat, or rather the oil, which they contain. It is important to remember that fat and oil really undergo only an insignificant amount of digestion in the stomach ; such substances, in fact, tend to lessen the secretion of gastric juice.

If the gastric juice is to do its work properly certain conditions must be established. The food must be palatable, it must be well masticated, it must obviously be capable of digestion by the juices of the stomach (as a great many articles of diet are not), and it must be taken at regular intervals. For successful gastric digestion there must also be absence of severe mental and muscular effort. While laying down these rules, it must freely be admitted that certain people are able practically to defy them all ; but these are the rules that apply to the great majority of people.

Propulsive Function of the Stomach

But this account of gastric digestion would be very incomplete if no mention were made of another function of the stomach, not a digestive function in one sense, but nevertheless a most important aid to digestion. Very soon after a meal is swallowed the wall of the healthy stomach begins to throw itself into waves of movement ; at first these are very slight, but the more acid the contents of the stomach become the more vigorous are the movements. They consist of regular waves travelling down the pyloric portion of the stomach to the valve which opens into the bowel. They go on steadily during the whole period of digestion, lasting on the average from three to five hours.

During this period, when a portion of the stomach contents is sufficiently acid and has been reduced to what is called chyme, small quantities of this semi-fluid material are expelled into the bowel at intervals of from two to five minutes. The advantage of this process is obvious, and exactly corresponds to the advantage of masticating one's food properly and not bolting it. As each little dose of chyme enters the bowel, it can be thoroughly mixed with the juices which it meets there, and which, as we shall see, are really more important than the gastric juice itself.

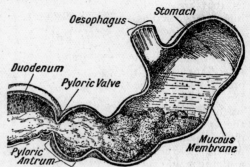

Passage of chyme from stomach to intestine

It has long been taken for granted that a quantity of food, after digestion, is absorbed into the blood through the walls of the stomach ; that is now known, however, to be quite a mistake. Apart from alcohol and other drugs and salts, absorption from the stomach does not take place. This has been proved by actual observation. The stomach, then, serves as a receptacle for a considerable quantity of food taken at one time ; it is the site of a certain stage of digestion which depends upon the activity of the saliva ; by its own juice it prepares the food for entering the bowel, by rendering soluble and half digesting the proteins, and kills microbes ; it guards the bowel by injecting into it small portions of chyme at suitable intervals, so that each portion may be well mixed up with very important juices ; and, finally, it may perform a very important function for which it never gets any credit, that of protecting the bowel and the body in general from all sorts of unsuitable substances which are often offered to it and which it rejects.

Next there follows the all-important process which is so often forgotten, and which is called intestinal digestion. The most important part of this process is not performed by the activity of the intestine or bowel itself, but by that of certain fluids which are poured into it from without ; of these, one is the bile, which needs no further discussion beyond noting that it helps absorption of fats by forming soaps and further assists the action of the pancreatic ferments.

Of greater importance is the fluid which is formed by the pancreas, and which is poured into the bowel at the same point as that where the bile enters, that is, at a distance of about 4 inches beyond the point where the stomach opens into the bowel. This juice resembles saliva to the eye, but is far more important and potent ; it contains a number of very active ferments, and is conspicuously contrasted with the gastric juice in that it is markedly alkaline. The fluid is poured into the bowel by a remarkable mechanism which ensures its coming just exactly when it is wanted.

For long it has been known that there is a nervous connexion which, so to speak, tells the pancreas when to send its juice to the bowel. It has now been discovered that there is, in addition, a remarkable chemical substance, known as secretin, the production of which by the lining of the duodenum, or first part of the bowel, is provoked by the acid chyme coming from the stomach. This is absorbed into the blood, and when it reaches the pancreas acts as a stimulant to it. The pancreatic juice is an extremely powerful digestive ; it can completely digest a number of substances which are entirely unaffected by the saliva or the gastric juice.

The pancreas is by far the most important organ of digestion. In the first place, its juice contains a ferment,

trypsinogen, which, by means of another ferment secreted by the small intestine, and known as enterokinase, is converted into an active form as trypsin. The function of this ferment is to convert into peptone any protein that has escaped the action of the gastric juice, and to carry the digestion of peptone a stage farther. Proteins cannot be absorbed from the bowel except in the form of what are called amino-acids, and, to arrive at this last stage of protein digestion, the aid of still another ferment is called in, namely, erepsin, which, like enterokinase, is secreted by the lining of the small intestine.

The digestion of fat is also accomplished by the pancreatic juice ; this is done by another ferment which has the power of splitting fats or oils into soap and glycerin which can be readily absorbed by the lining of the bowel. Thus, it is noticed that when the pancreas is diseased, or when, for any reason, its juice is prevented from entering the bowel, the greater part of the fat which is taken in the food leaves the bowel unchanged and unutilised.

So powerful is the pancreatic juice in this respect that it can digest a considerable amount of fat or oil, even if this be not emulsified, that is to say, broken up into a number of tiny little droplets. But it is well to remember that the digestion of all oils is far easier and more complete when they are made into emulsions ; and, in fact, the bile and the pancreatic juice do their best to convert

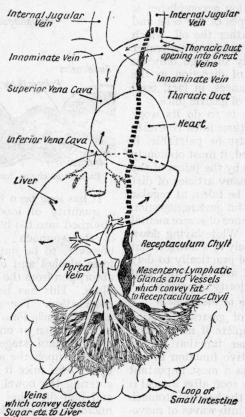

Internal Jugular Vein

Internal Jugular Vein

Innominate Vein

Thoracic Duct opening into Great Veins

Superior Vena Cava

Innominate Vein

Thoracic Duct

Inferior Vena Cava

Heart

Liver

Receptaculum Chyli

Portal Vein

Mesenteric Lymphatic Glands and Vessels which convey Fat to Receptaculum Chyli

Veins which convey digested Sugar ets. to Liver

Loop of Small Intestine

Digested fats pass upward through the thoracic duct, in order to reach the great veins at the neck

all the oil that reaches them into an emulsion prior to digesting it.

But the power of the pancreatic juice is not yet exhausted ; it contains a third ferment which exercises the same action as the ferment contained in the saliva, but in a far more marked degree. Hence the process which went on in the stomach for a short time under the action of the saliva is resumed, and much more vigorously, in the bowel. The result is that all the starch and starchy elements of the food are converted into a particular kind of sugar, the name of which, glucose, is quite familiar in commerce, and which has the form perfectly adapted for absorption into the blood.

In addition to the actions of the intestinal juice already mentioned, it should be added that certain digestive actions are carried out by the bacteria which normally inhabit the bowel.

Finally must be considered the absorption of the food thus digested. It has been seen that the stomach may practically be ignored as an organ of absorption ; on the contrary, the lining of the bowel is perfectly adapted for this purpose. The large and highly developed cells which lie on the surface of this lining are really the active agents of absorption. From the bowel they take up water, the various desirable salts of the food, the sugar and the broken-up proteins, now in the form of amino-acids ; and each of these passes into the tiny blood vessels which lie immediately underneath the cells.

How Fat is Absorbed by the Blood

The only other substance to account for is the fat or oil of the food. It has been shown that fat has been split up by the pancreatic juice, and the substances into which it has been split are taken up by the absorbing cells which, in some marvellous way, have the power of putting them together again so that tiny drops of oil soon begin to appear in the cells. These do not pass into the blood vessels that lie just beneath them, but into what are called the lymph vessels. These particular vessels, however, are usually called lacteals (from the Latin word for milk), because when they are looked at after the process of digestion they are seen to be filled with a fluid that has a milky appearance.

This fluid is simply ordinary lymph with the addition of the oil globules that have been passed into it through the absorbing cells of the bowel, and is often known by the special name of chyle. The chyle passes upwards, the lacteals gradually uniting with one another and forming larger but fewer tubes, until at last it finds itself in a long, slender, single vessel called the thoracic duct, by means of which it is poured into one of the large veins at the root of the neck. Thus, at last, after all these wanderings, the fat which has been taken by the mouth enters the blood, which distributes it to every part of the body.

The large intestine absorbs water, so that the bowel contents become more and more solid. It would also appear that it can absorb the products of peptic digestion, if this is prolonged, and glucose, as in rectal feeding.

Secondary or Essential Digestion

This completes the description of the essentials of digestion, but lately it has become common to apply a somewhat wider meaning to the word. This is done by drawing a distinction between primary digestion and secondary digestion. The long and complicated series of changes which have been described, resulting in the absorption of the nutritious elements of the food by the wall of the bowel, are all included under the term primary digestion.

The term secondary digestion may very properly be applied to the process by which the living cells of every tissue and organ of the body are able to take up the various substances they require from the blood, and utilise them for the purposes of their own life. Obviously it is correct to recognize this as the essential digestion. Hence all the processes of what is commonly called digestion should be regarded as mere preliminaries, necessitated by the vast complexity of the human organization, and essential digestion would consist in the process by which the tissues utilise and build up into themselves the food substances which the blood distributes to them.

A true conception of these facts is very useful to the student of disease, for he is able to distinguish between states of improper nutrition that depend upon some disorder of the primary digestion and those which depend upon far more subtle and mysterious disorders of the living tissues of the body, interfering with that process of secondary digestion—the essential digestion—upon which their life depends.

See Appetite ; Bile ; Chyme ; Eating ; Indigestion ; Intestine ; Pancreas ; Saliva ; Stomach.

DIGESTIVE. Food is digested within our bodies by the action of certain ferments, and in cases of dyspepsia it is often found useful to reinforce the natural supply of these ferments by giving those obtained from animals, or similar substances, or, as in peptonising milk, by adding these to food and partially digesting it before it is consumed.

The stomach ferment, pepsin, the dose of which is 5 to 10 grains, may be given as a powder, a pill, a cachet or a tablet ; or it may be given as the glycerin of pepsin, dose 1 to 2 drachms, when it is usually combined with 10 or 15 minims of dilute hydrochloric acid. Pancreatic solution contains a ferment which, like pepsin, digests protein foods, of which lean meat and white of egg are examples, and another which digests starch. It is given in doses of 1 to 2 drachms.

In peptonising milk and other foods to be taken by the mouth, the pancreatic ferments, in the form of solution, tablets or powders, are used, because pepsin, when employed for this purpose, produces bitter substances which are very unpalatable. Benger's food, which contains wheaten flour and is given made up with milk, has also an admixture of pancreatic ferments. When the prepared food is warmed the ferments act upon it, starch being converted into sugar, and the proteins, of both flour and milk, peptonised.

The longer the process goes on the more thorough is this predigestion, so that patients can get the food in the precise stage suited to their digestive capacities. If this is very weak, the ferments are allowed to act for a considerable time, but as the digestion improves the period is shortened until finally the patient is able to take ordinary food.

Amongst other digestives of starch are taka-diastase, dose 1 to 5 grains, in cap-

sules, and extract of malt, dose 1 to 4 drachms. Malt is an excellent digestive for children suffering from dyspepsia, who may be given a teaspoonful thrice daily.

DIGITALIS. The leaves of the purple foxglove, Digitalis purpurea, furnish one of the most valuable of all known drugs in its action on the heart. As a stimulant and tonic for the heart it is much more widely used than any other substance.

It is a very powerful drug and must never be used except under medical supervision.

Though digitalis certainly slows the pulse, yet it greatly increases the force of every beat of the heart, not only by slowing the pulse, but also by prolonging the period during which the heart muscle rests, that is to say, during the period between two beats. A further service done by this drug is that in lengthening the period of rest it lengthens the period during which the blood that nourishes the heart itself is able to flow through the two small arteries which pass into the substance of the heart muscle. At the time when the heart muscle is actually contracted the blood vessels in its substance are naturally squeezed ; hence it is only when the muscle relaxes its efforts for the rest of the body that it is able to receive its own nourishment. Probably the value of the drug is that it thus aids the nutrition of the heart.

Poisoning by Digitalis. Digitalis is one of the drugs which have a cumulative action, that is to say, after being taken regularly for some time there may be a sufficient amount of the drug in the system to give rise to symptoms of poisoning. It may be that the patient simply suffers from palpitation, but in severe cases his lips and finger-nails, or perhaps the face, become blue, and he is very breathless.

In these circumstances the patient should be made to lie down in bed, in the position which is easiest for him, and, while awaiting the doctor, hot coffee or spirits or sal volatile in water should be given. When a poisonous dose of digitalis has been taken an emetic should be given, and thereafter draughts of tepid water in order to encourage vomiting.

See Heart ; Poisoning.

DILL-WATER. This is a favourite and harmless drug for administration to children. It has a very similar action to other drugs that contain volatile or essential oils. Dill-water is very dilute, and a teaspoonful of it may be given to the smallest baby and freely repeated ; when given to a baby it should, of course, be warmed. Its value lies in the fact that it is able to relieve colicky pains in the stomach or bowel such as very often trouble young children. If the dill-water be given cold to a baby, the cold itself is apt to set up the very same disturbances as those which the drug is supposed to relieve.

It is very important to remember that dill-water is only a means of relieving symptoms ; it does nothing whatever to remove the cause of those symptoms, namely, improper diet.

Certainly let the child have dill-water when colic keeps it awake at night, but begin to reform its diet in the morning.
See Baby ; Colic.

DINNER PILL. The practice, and it is an old one, of taking a laxative pill regularly just before or after dinner is objectionable for two reasons. The first is that anyone who actually suffers from chronic constipation should attempt to cure himself of this condition so that he becomes independent of drugs, and the second is that the use of such pills permits a risk of overmuch and over-rich feeding. It must be pointed out that while, by the use of dinner pills, the consequences of high living may be postponed, they are not at all likely to be averted.
See Constipation ; Diet.

DIPHTHERIA. Diphtheria is a very infectious disease which is caused by a particular microbe called the diphtheria or Klebs-Loeffler bacillus. In the later stages of the disease, this bacillus is greatly aided in its inroads upon the body by a number of other microbes for which it has prepared the way.

The infection is usually direct from person to person, that is to say, from throat to throat, but it may be carried by milk, particles of dirt, slate-pencils, handkerchiefs, towels, etc. The disease is most common in youth, in cold climates,

and in cold weather ; it definitely has what is called a seasonal incidence, causing most deaths in the last four months of the year. About two-thirds of all the cases of diphtheria occur under the age of ten years.

The introduction of the antitoxin treatment has completely revolutionised the whole aspect of the disease, and the mortality, which at one time depended on the age of the patient, nowadays depends far less upon age or any other condition whatever than upon the treatment, or want of treatment, by antitoxin and the date in the history of the case at which such treatment was begun.

Diphtheria is known to attack the lower animals, and definite instances are on record of its communication from cats to man, and vice versa, though the view is taken amongst veterinary surgeons that diphtheria, at any rate in the large proportion of cases, is a somewhat different disease from that occurring in human beings.

The bacillus of diphtheria may attack any part of the body to which it can gain access except the unbroken skin ; but by far the most common site of its attack is the throat, the nose and the larynx being next in frequency. The incubation period of the disease, that is to say, the time that elapses between infection and the appearance of the first symptoms, is short, being very rarely prolonged beyond four days ; it is generally understood to range from two to ten days.

It is most important to remember that the symptoms of this disease show themselves very gradually and insidiously.

At the very beginning of the illness there is, unfortunately, nothing that is really characteristic. The child is obviously unwell, refuses food and is restless at night. The throat may be complained of, though this does not always happen ; but when it is examined it does not at first exhibit anything characteristic, even to the expert eye. Obviously this difficulty is still greater in the few cases of laryngeal or nasal diphtheria which have begun in those sites and have not spread from the throat.

When the false membrane, as it is called, appears in the throat, the diagnosis is usually made plain. The appearance of the false membrane varies. Sometimes it is thin and of a bluish-grey colour, when it will be found that only the diphtheria bacillus is present. But in other cases it is thick and leathery and of a yellowish-white colour, showing that there is a mixed infection, the diphtheria bacillus being accompanied by several other microbes. In a pure case there is very little swelling, redness or pain, so that, as stated above, the child may never mention the throat. The membrane adheres firmly as a rule, and leaves a bleeding surface if it is detached. Under the influence of the modern treatment, however, it loosens and may disappear gradually or be detached in shreds.

The little glands in the neck are usually enlarged, the pulse is at first rapid but may become slow and irregular, and as a rule the patient is prostrated. The temperature is rarely high, and after the first two or three days it is apt to fall below the normal ; this fact and the prostration and the state of the pulse all indicate that the danger to be feared in diphtheria is poisoning of the nervous system and of the heart. It is from failure of the heart that death is apt to occur, and this may be in the third or often in the fourth week of the illness.

Convalescence is very prolonged, and exceedingly apt to be interfered with by complications. The patient must be regarded as in danger of cardiac failure for no less than four weeks after the beginning of his symptoms. Thus in many fever hospitals it is the rule that diphtheria patients are to be kept in bed for at least three weeks and are not even to be allowed to sit up in bed in order to be examined.

The complications of this disease now comparatively rarely witnessed consist of trouble with the ears, the spread of inflammation to the lungs, interference with the action of the kidneys, and, most especially, diphtheritic paralysis, due to the action upon the nerves of the poison produced by the bacilli. This is most commonly witnessed in the soft palate, the paralysis of which causes difficulty of speaking and swallowing. The muscles in the eye which adjust the lens for reading and other near work may be paralysed, and it has happened not infrequently that the loss of power to see print distinctly has provided the first hint that the person had been suffering from diphtheria.

This disease must always be regarded as extremely grave, the most urgent and immediate treatment being demanded. What appears to be the mildest case may die of heart failure or of suffocation due to the spread of the false membrane to the larynx.

The treatment of diphtheria is one of the greatest triumphs of modern medicine. It consists of the injection under the skin of a substance called the diphtheria antitoxin or the antidiphtheritic serum. This is obtained by injecting the poisons produced by the bacilli, when they are grown in the laboratory, into the blood of horses kept for the purpose ; in the blood of these animals there appears, after a time, the antitoxic substance.

The results of this treatment are extremely striking. The membrane ceases

Diphtheria. Chart showing how an increased death rate follows delay in administering antitoxin

PLATE XI

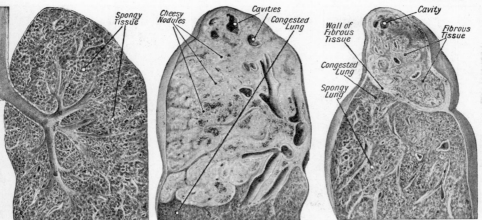

Consumption. 1. Normal lung. 2. Caseation by tubercles. 3. Patches walled off by fibrous tissue

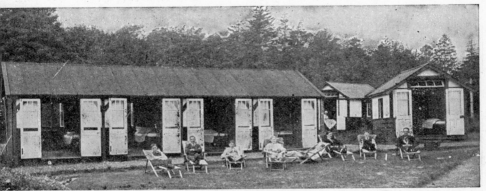

4. Garden shelters for sanatorium patients, enabling even bed cases to be virtually in the open air
Courtesy of Boulton & Paul, Ltd.

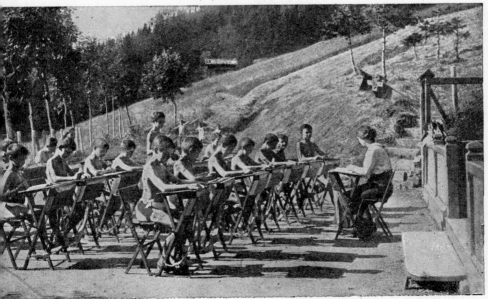

5. Fighting consumption at Leysin, young patients being continually exposed to sunlight and fresh air

PLATE XII

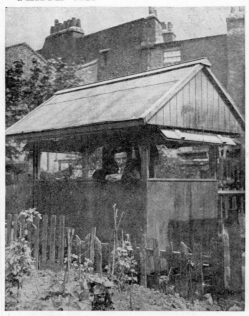

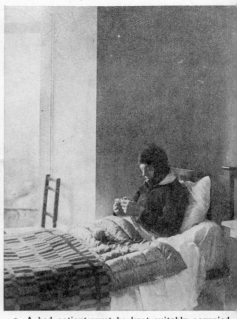

Consumption.   1. Outdoor sleeping shelter for patient unable to take sanatorium treatment

2. A bed patient must be kept suitably occupied during the daytime and not allowed to sleep

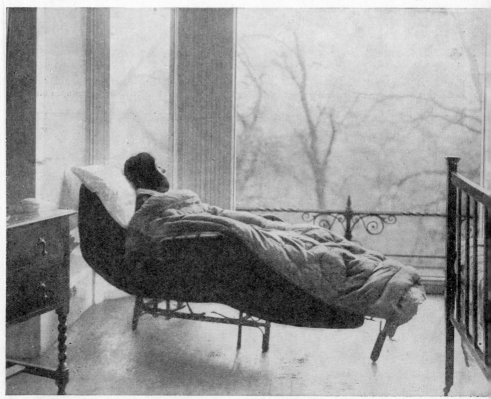

3. First stage in convalescent treatment.   When the patient is allowed out of bed he spends gradually extended periods on a couch, until he is allowed to walk about the room and to be up most of the day

to spread or to reappear if removed ; that which is present soon vanishes ; the foul discharge from the nose disappears, and with it the difficulty in breathing and swallowing ; the inflammation in the neck subsides ; the temperature and pulse rate approach the normal ; and the complications are practically unknown. This is the all-important item of the treatment ; it has really robbed diphtheria of its terrors.

If antitoxin be given on the first day, the disease is almost always cut short. The prospects become rapidly worse, however, the longer serum treatment is delayed.

In addition to this essential treatment, it must be remembered that the patient's heart is in danger. Therefore he must be permitted to make no exertion whatever, and must be protected from any kind of shock. In many cases the patient cannot be allowed to sit up, and a bed-pan must be used. The patient must be liberally fed, milk and strong broths being given in small quantities frequently, or other food if the digestive powers appear to warrant it.

Various antiseptics and soothing applications may be used for the throat, but they are really of secondary importance unless the throat is very foul. In making applications to the throat the nurse should protect her eyes with goggles, and if anything is spluttered on to her face it should be wiped off with a piece of cotton wool dipped in an antiseptic.

Cases are still occasionally seen which may present the grave complication which used to be so familiar, the child being threatened with death by suffocation. The antitoxin must, of course, be immediately employed ; but if the child threatens to die on the spot more must be done, and the choice lies between two operations. The first is sometimes practised, especially in fever hospitals. It consists in inserting a rigid tube within the child's larynx so that, no matter how much the membrane grows, there is still a passage left for the air. This operation of intubation, as it is called, has often proved very successful. The other operation is what is known as tracheotomy.

Finally, it is to be remembered that the disease is extremely infectious. Whenever, therefore, there is the least suspicion that anyone is suffering from diphtheria, he should be at once isolated. No one should be allowed to enter the sick-room except the persons in attendance. Discharges from the nose or mouth should be wiped off with cotton wool or with rags, and these should be burnt immediately. Clothing and bed or personal linen should be put to soak in a disinfectant before being taken from the sick-room.

By a method known as the Schick test, which is carried out by inoculations on the skin, it can be determined whether anyone is particularly prone to contract diphtheria, and protective inoculations of what is known as a toxoid-antitoxin mixture can be made. This is a great gain in dealing with outbreaks of diphtheria in schools, institutions and elsewhere.

A very important agent in spreading the disease is a person known as a carrier. The germs of diphtheria occur frequently in the throats of people who are not suffering from the disease, and sometimes the germs are active and capable of communicating the disease to susceptible people. In all outbreaks it is of supreme importance, therefore, to discover such carriers, and to disinfect their throats.

A person who has been suffering from diphtheria is a danger to others for at least three weeks from the disappearance of the membrane, and until two swab tests have proved negative. Anyone who has been in contact with a person suffering from diphtheria must be kept in quarantine till by sufficient swab tests the throat has been shown to be free from the germs.

See Antidiphtheritic Serum ; Croup ; Disinfection ; Infectious Disease.

DIPSOMANIA. The craving for alcohol which comes from habitual tippling is not properly what is meant by dipsomania. By this term is understood an uncontrollable craving which descends on its victim at intervals, sometimes of weeks, but in other cases after longer periods. The craving is constitutional, a legacy from ancestors. During the intervals the individual is not addicted to alcohol, and may, in fact, have a pronounced distaste for it.

H

There are certain indications which may give warning of the approach of an attack. The behaviour may be different, there may be marked restlessness and the appetite may fail. If an outburst cannot be averted, the individual begins to drink and goes on till he is pulled up, perhaps by developing a disgust for liquor, by severe vomiting and retching, or by an attack of delirium tremens. The friends of a victim of dipsomania should be alive to the portents of the approaching storm, and when they think that such is imminent a doctor should be called in.

The use of apomorphine, by inducing sickness and vomiting, may ward off or cut short an attack. Sometimes drugs are successful in taking the place of alcohol and in relieving the craving, and the following combination is well worth trying :

Tincture of capsicum .. .. 1½ drachms
Liquid extract of red cinchona 2   ,,
Syrup of ginger 4   ,,
Chloroform water .. to make 6 ounces
  A tablespoonful of this to be taken in a wineglass of water whenever it may be necessary.

In some cases hypnotism, as practised by doctors who possess the necessary skill and experience, appears to have been effectual in abating the craving.

See Alcoholism ; Delirium Tremens.

DIRT. Dirt has been defined as " matter in the wrong place " ; but the word is used in special senses, some of which are so important that they must be mentioned here. The chemist has a special meaning for dirt ; when he talks of a dirty vessel he means one that contains even the smallest quantity of some chemical substance of which it has been supposed to be rid. Nowadays, when a medical man says that anything is dirty he means that it contains microbes which are to be feared. Similarly, when he says that a thing is clean he usually means, not that it is clean in the ordinary sense, but that it is free from microbes ; or, to use his own special language, that it is sterile or antiseptic. This new standard of what constitutes dirt and what constitutes cleanliness is all-important, for it transfers the attention from mere appearances to essentials.

See Antiseptic ; Sterilisation.

DISEASE. It can be readily understood that the earliest notions of mankind regarding the ills which affect the body should have given greater prominence to the symptoms of disease than to its causes. It has thus come about that the general name applied to such ills is one expressive of the interference with the sense of comfort or well-being, for these are the original meanings of the term disease.

The progress of medicine has largely consisted in the discovery of the essential nature and causes of disease, thus relegating to their true position such symptoms as jaundice, fever, pain, diarrhoea, and the like. Owing to the imperfection of medical science, however, it is still often necessary to be content with treating symptoms of which we do not know the cause ; and even when this is known it is sometimes necessary to give treatment for the relief of symptoms which are particularly troublesome to the patient.

Interdependence of Body Tissues

A clear conception of the nature of disease is only possible if we bear in mind that our bodies are built up of millions of minute living particles or cells combined to form various tissues and systems, as they are called, which are more or less interdependent. Thus there is the digestive system, furnishing food for the body ; the circulating system, forming and distributing blood ; the nervous system, stimulating the other systems to action and controlling and co-ordinating their activities, and so on.

If disease affects one system, the others suffer in greater or less degree much in the same way as a community is affected when one or more of its industrial sections, for example, its coal-miners or its transport workers, go on strike. And just as such an industrial section consists of a large number of individual human beings, upon whose health and vigour the productiveness of the section depends, so with the systems of the body and the cells of which they are composed. These cells may be damaged by heat and cold, by starvation, by poisons, especially those produced by bacteria, and by other agents.

One does not wish to push the analogy too far, but it is true to say that, just as the efficiency of an industrial section of the community does not wholly depend on the mass sentiment and activities, but largely also on the care which the individual workers take of their health and energy, so each tiny body cell will make an effort to maintain its life and health. This is the basis of what is termed the healing power of Nature.

It should be noticed, finally, that there clearly is a possibility of the body affecting what we call the mind, and vice versa. Just as soundness and vigour of our bodily tissues can maintain and elevate mental vigour and the spirits, and bodily ill-health depress them, so does the mind react on the health of the body.

The department of medical science which deals with disease processes and their effects on the tissues of the body is known as pathology.

See Constitution ; Diagnosis ; Functional Disease ; Health ; Heredity.

DISINFECTANT. Any agent which kills the germs responsible for causing infectious diseases may be classed as a disinfectant. There is an important distinction between such an agent and an antiseptic. The latter does not necessarily kill germs, though it prevents their multiplication. In the case of wounds, to accomplish this much is enough, because the living tissues then dispose of the comparatively few microbes which exist in their midst. But in dealing with the infectious discharges of patients, their linen, and the rooms in which they have lain, something more is necessary : the microbes must be killed outright.

Heat of sufficient intensity is a thorough disinfectant and can be readily utilised. Thus, combustible articles from infected surroundings, and of no particular value, should be promptly burnt. For some articles of value, dry heat in the form of hot air is effective, and it is utilised for disinfecting books, etc. This must be done, however, in an apparatus under expert supervision. Articles which can be kept boiling for half an hour or longer are efficiently disinfected.

The best way to disinfect bedding, clothing, and other fabrics is by exposing them to steam at a high pressure in a special disinfector, the method adopted for such things by the sanitary authorities. The steam penetrates to all parts of the articles submitted to its action, and disinfection is quick and thorough.

There are many reliable chemical disinfectants, including corrosive sublimate (perchloride of mercury) biniodide of mercury, carbolic acid, lysol, and other substances derived from coal tar, bleaching powder, formaldehyde, the vapour of burning sulphur, permanganate of potash, iodine, hydrogen peroxide, and numerous other substances. There are many good proprietary disinfectants on the market, most of which owe their value to substances similar to those found in lysol.

It must always be borne in mind that the substances above mentioned only disinfect when they are used in sufficient strength and for a sufficient time. Weak solutions of permanganate of potash, for example, cannot be depended on to disinfect thoroughly, though they will remove disagreeable odours.

Substances which either remove or cover bad odours are classed as deodorants. The smoke of tobacco or of brown paper and eau-de-Cologne are used for this purpose, but they do nothing to interfere with the danger lurking in the substance which causes the smell. Permanganate of potash and chloride of lime deodorise, and in strong solutions also disinfect.

Scrubbing woodwork, etc., with soap has some value in disinfection, and so has exposure to sunlight and fresh air, especially after articles have been properly washed ; but the exposure to sunlight should extend over several days.

See Antiseptic ; Cresol ; Eusol ; Formalin ; Hydrogen Peroxide ; Infectious Disease ; Sulphur.

DISINFECTION. The problem of the disinfection of a room which has been occupied by a patient suffering from an infectious disease is much simplified if the room has been previously prepared for the reception of such a patient. The carpet will have been taken up and replaced by one or two light rugs, heavy hangings will have been replaced by light, washable curtains, unnecessary furniture will have been taken from the room and stuffed chairs and couches replaced by plain washable furniture. Books, pictures and things of the kind will also have gone. The only books allowed in the sick-room should be such as can afterwards be burnt.

Where, however, a patient has sickened with an infectious disorder in a room containing articles of the kind mentioned, nothing should be taken from the room without first consulting the doctor or the sanitary inspector. In most instances the disinfection of rooms, bedding and clothing is undertaken by the sanitary authority, with a minimum of trouble to the householder. It may happen, however, that the latter has to carry out disinfection himself.

While the patient is still in the sick-room disinfection will have to be done. In most cases of infectious disease paper handkerchiefs should be used for nasal discharges and sputum, and should be burnt immediately. When the discharges of the bladder and bowels may be infectious they should be received into a vessel containing some disinfectant. For this and other purposes a useful disinfectant consists of a solution of lysol in the strength of a teaspoonful to the pint When a motion has been passed, more of the antiseptic solution will be poured over it and the motion will be thoroughly broken up with a piece of stick and mixed with the solution. The motion should then be allowed to stand for two hours before being put down the privy stool or buried.

How to Deal with Fabrics

The patient's discarded clothing, bedclothes, etc., should be put in the antiseptic solution and left to soak in it for twenty-four hours before being taken out to wash. The washing should be thorough, and blankets and other heavy fabrics should be put out to the fresh air for three or four consecutive days. If they can have the benefit of sunshine so much the better.

After handling the patient, and always before taking food, the nurse should immerse her hands in the antiseptic solution for a minute or two. If the sanitary arrangements of the house include sinks and a water closet, strong solutions of soda in boiling water should be put down the pipes at frequent intervals. A pint of the antiseptic solution should then be allowed to remain in the stool or pipes for half an hour, that is to say, the plug will not be pulled nor water run through the sinks during that time. Bad smells may be removed by pouring a solution of permanganate of potash, chloride of lime or formalin down the pipes.

With regard to the disinfection of the air in the room, the only thing that matters, and it matters a great deal, is to have free ventilation. Saucers of solutions of permanganate of potash, carbolic acid or anything else, placed about the room are perfectly useless.

When the time comes to disinfect the sick-room the best agent for the ordinary person is probably sulphur. It must be remembered, however, that sulphur vapour is not active except in the presence of moisture. It is necessary, therefore, to moisten thoroughly the walls of the room. Metallic articles should be washed with the disinfectant solution and taken from the room. Cupboards should be opened and drawers pulled out. A deal table should be stood in the centre of the floor, and on this a large basin or a shallow bath containing a little water. The chimney is stopped by newspapers and the seams of the window-sashes by gummed paper (see Plate XIV, 1 and 2). Water is freely sprinkled over the floor and the table.

Roll sulphur may be used, 4 lb. for each 1,000 cubic feet of space, or sulphur candles may be obtained of an appropriate strength. The sulphur is placed in a small basin or plate which is put on the water in the large basin, and if roll sulphur is being used it should be moistened with methylated spirit. The sulphur is now lit and the seams in the door are closed with gum paper. After twenty-four hours the room may be opened, and when it becomes possible the windows are thrown widely open and the chimney cleared ; for a day or two doors and windows should be left open so that there will be a through draught. The paper should be stripped from the walls and burned, the ceiling limewashed and the floor and other woodwork thoroughly scrubbed with soap and warm water.

See Infectious Disease; Ventilation.

DISLOCATION. A dislocation is an injury to a joint in which the bones that form the joint are displaced from their normal relationship (Plate XIV, 3–6). For this to happen, the strong, fibrous textures called ligaments, that enclose the joint and keep the bones in their places, must be torn. The position of the tear, and the principal direction in which the bones depart from their proper position, will depend upon the direction of the force that has caused the injury.

Occasionally dislocations occur from causes less obvious. For instance, there may be a progressive disease of a joint, especially tuberculosis, which gradually destroys the ligaments or wears away the bones, and thus gives rise to a dislocation. And in other cases, such as in the very common condition known as congenital dislocation of the hip joint,

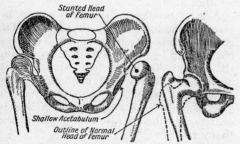

Stunted Head of Femur

Shallow Acetabulum

Outline of Normal Head of Femur

Examples of congenital dislocation of the hip. That on the right is termed coxa vara

the bones that enter into the joint have never properly developed, and thus, when strain is put upon it, dislocation ensues.

Dislocations are usually divided by surgeons into three kinds : simple, compound and complicated. In the first there is nothing but the dislocation ; in the second the skin is broken and there is a track leading from the exterior down to the dislocated joint ; in the third the dislocation is complicated by fracture of one or more of the bones that enter into the joint.

The violence that causes the ordinary kind of dislocation may be external violence, as in the case of a fall, or a blow upon the back of a stooping person, such as often causes dislocation of the hip joint ; or it may be due to too violent muscular action, as in the case of an extreme yawn, which occasionally causes a dislocation of the lower jaw (Plate XIV, 3 and 4). Dislocation is commonest in adult life ; in the young and in the elderly the bones, rather than the joints, give way.

The symptoms of dislocation are what might be expected : the movements of

the joint are restricted, and there may be kinds of movement which are not possible in a normal joint. In a dislocated shoulder or hip joint, it will be found, when the injured limb is compared with its fellow, that they are not of the same length ; in some cases the dislocation causes lengthening, in others shortening, of the limb. In addition, there are numbness and pain due to unusual pressure upon the nerves, and the limb usually swells, since the veins that bring the blood back from it are commonly pressed upon.

If a dislocated joint is allowed to remain unreduced, various changes occur which make subsequent reduction difficult. In certain cases, when dislocation has been thus neglected, it is necessary to perform a surgical operation. But when a dislocation is seen at once by the surgeon he is able to manipulate the displaced bone back into position and bind the part up so that it stays there.

Every kind of dislocation needs expert surgical treatment. The injury that has been done to the joint may be much increased by the efforts of incompetent people to reduce the deformity. First-aid treatment consists in resting the part, for example, putting the upper limb in a sling, and applying cold cloths to relieve pain. Shock is treated by keeping the patient warm.

See Ankle ; Joint ; Knee, etc.

DISSEMINATED SCLEROSIS. Disseminated, multiple or insular sclerosis is a chronic disease of the brain and spinal cord. By sclerosis is meant the replacement of nervous tissue by fibrous or scar tissue, entailing the destruction of nerve cells and the interruption of nerve fibres. The scar tissue occurs in plaques of varying size disseminated through the brain and cord, and the symptoms of the disease depend upon the precise situation of these plaques. They begin as areas of inflammation, and, although there is a strong suspicion that this inflammation is wrought by microbes, it cannot yet be proved.

The disease affects young people chiefly, and the first symptoms noticed may be stiffness and weakness in the legs. Perhaps before this is definite the patient may have observed a tendency to stumble. A notable symptom is what is called "intention" tremor. This means that when the patient puts his mind to do something, for instance, lift a glass of water to the mouth, the hand and arm shake, perhaps so violently as to spill the water. This is first noticed, as a rule, in the upper limbs, but later on may extend to the head and lower limbs.

Another notable symptom is a peculiar oscillation of the eyeballs known as nystagmus ; the vision may also become affected. There may be areas of anaesthesia or insensitiveness to touch, perhaps of one side of the body. Mental symptoms, such as weakness of memory and emotional excitability, may also appear. A peculiar sort of speech is found in many cases ; in pronouncing words the syllables are more or less separated, so that a staccato effect is produced.

A noticeable feature of disseminated sclerosis, and one which must be borne in mind, is that improvement may set in and last for a long time, so that false hopes of cure may be aroused. This is not infrequent in inflammatory nervous diseases. Another thing to remember is that early cases of this disease are sometimes mistaken for hysteria.

The treatment of the disease is not very satisfactory, though some benefit seems to accrue from large doses of arsenic. The patient should be kept warm, and should avoid either mental or bodily strain. In the later stages of the disease, when the patient is bedridden, care must be taken to prevent bed sores (*q.v.*).
See Nervous System.

DIURETIC. A diuretic is a drug, or indeed any measure, which aids the flow of the secretion of the kidneys. Diuretics are very numerous and various, and their action is so valuable that they are very frequently employed.

It is well to remember that by far the best of all diuretics, as well as the safest and the most widely useful, is water. There are a number of people who do not drink sufficient water and whose urine is therefore apt to be too concentrated ; but there are a number of cases in which the object of stimulating the kidneys is to aid in the removal of excess of water present in the body. In such cases, of course, other diuretics than water must be used.

Another consideration is that the urine is a very complicated product ; it largely consists of water, but contains also a quantity of solids in solution. Properly speaking, distinction should be made between drugs that increase the amount of water and those that increase the amount of solids, and it is very often important to know which solids are increased and to what extent. Hence it is a common device, in the absence of a more exact knowledge of this subject, to give a number of diuretics in combination, hoping that one will perform one service and another another.

A large number of diuretics act by increasing the force of the circulation. The result of their action is mainly to increase the amount of water that is removed from the body. Amongst them are digitalis, alcohol and coffee. The other great group of diuretics are simply salines, or mineral salts, such as the acetate and citrate of potassium, the citrate of sodium and many more.

It is a general rule in the case of salts that if they are given in small doses they pass into the blood and stimulate the kidneys, and therefore are diuretics ; whereas if they are given in much larger doses they do not pass into the blood at all, but stimulate the bowel by their contact with it and so act as purgatives.

The spirit of nitrous ether, dose 15 to 60 minims, and the solution of ammonium acetate, otherwise Mindererus solution, 2 to 6 drachms, are useful diuretics, and are much given in fever cases. Another simple diuretic in such cases is Imperial drink, that is, home-made lemonade containing a teaspoonful of cream of tartar to the pint. This may be taken freely. Other diuretic remedies are squill, calomel, broom, turpentine, copaiba, etc.

Cold applied to the body has a diuretic effect, and most people have noticed how the outflow of urine is increased in cold weather. This is a normal occurrence and need occasion no alarm.
See Kidney ; Urine.

DIZZINESS. When a person is dizzy he may feel himself whirling round or up and down ; on the other hand, he may appear himself to be steady while the objects around him are whirling. If the dizziness is severe he may fall to the ground, and he may become sick and vomit.

A slight more or less constant giddiness is common in neurasthenia, in chronic gastritis, in that loss of elasticity of the arteries in elderly people which is known as arterio-sclerosis, and in those who use tea, coffee, alcohol or tobacco immoderately. It is found also in those whose vision is defective, more particularly when there is a tendency to squint ; in such cases the provision of properly fitting glasses may completely remove the giddiness.

Balance Affected by Digestive Disorders

People who have thickened arteries very often feel giddy when they look upwards and in assuming the erect position quickly, for example, in getting out of bed. A sudden severe attack of dizziness may be one of the symptoms of acute indigestion, when it is likely to be associated with headache, blurring of vision, sickness and vomiting. There may even be some mental confusion. Here the giddiness as well as the other symptoms may be greatly relieved by free vomiting, and an attempt should be made to induce this by an emetic or by tickling the back of the throat. The stomach will be more effectually cleared if the patient takes large draughts of tepid water.

Another cause of sudden dizziness is epilepsy, when the symptoms may occur either as part of the aura which precedes a fit, or as an attack of petit mal, the form of epilepsy in which the patient is not convulsed and the loss of consciousness is only momentary.

Dizziness may be connected with the ears ; a plug of impacted wax, for instance, or even syringing may bring on giddiness and sickness. Disorders of the inner ear or labyrinth may bring on what are called Ménière's symptoms. There the giddiness is sudden and severe ; the patient may fall and may lose consciousness for a moment. There are noises in the head, hissing, blowing or banging, and more or less deafness.

Attacks such as this are likely to recur at longer or shorter intervals, and meanwhile there may be a persistent slight giddiness.

Disease of the brain, and of the cerebellum in particular, is another of the many causes of giddiness.

Treatment of dizziness obviously depends upon the cause in each case.

See Dyspepsia ; Ear ; Epilepsy ; Equilibrium ; Neurasthenia.

DOGS. Dogs are of some medical importance since they are subject to certain diseases which may affect man, and which may be transmitted to man under certain conditions. Of these, the most important is hydatid disease, of which the dog is the sole source of infection. It is due to a worm which lives in the bowel of the dog, and may be communicated to man by licking or in other ways. Women who kiss their dogs run a risk of contracting the disease

See Bite ; Hydatid Disease ; Hydrophobia.

DOMESTIC MEASURES. It has been customary to use spoons and other domestic utensils as measures for drugs when they are being given to a patient, the capacity of those commonly used being as follows :

One teaspoonful	1 drachm
One dessertspoonful	2 drachms
One tablespoonful	½ ounce
One wineglassful	2 ounces
One teacupful	5 ,,
One breakfastcupful	10 ,,
One tumblerful	10 ,,

It should be borne in mind, however, that the capacity of such things varies considerably, so that when accuracy is necessary a properly graduated glass must be used to measure out a dose. Though a doctor's instructions on a prescription generally state the dose in spoonsful, it is intended that one or more drachms, as the case may be, should be measured.

See Apothecaries' Weights and Measures ; Dose ; Drug ; Medicines ; Prescription.

DORSAL. Dorsal, derived from the Latin word dorsum, meaning the back, is the term applied to anything that has to do with the back ; for instance, the bones of the spinal column that lie below the neck and above the small of the back are called the dorsal vertebrae. The name is also applied to the back of the hand and that part of the foot for which there is no popular name but the top of the foot.

DOSE. The whole subject of dosage is both difficult and important, not only because drugs differ in their action according to the dose in which they are given, but because there are so many individual variations in different people. Other things being equal, it should always be remembered that the action of any drug must depend on the proportion between the amount of it that is given and the total mass of the body in which it acts.

Thus the really scientific method of giving drugs would be to calculate the dose in proportion to the patient's weight, and this is now often done, especially in scientific study of the action of microbes and the poisons which they produce. It is now the regular thing to speak not of doses employed in the ordinary way at all, but of the dose per ounce, per pound or per kilogramme of the body weight.

Another most important point in dosage is that the age of the patient has an important influence, quite apart from the weight. In the case of some drugs, such as arsenic, it is often possible and desirable to give larger doses to a child of twelve than many adults can tolerate. On the other hand, it would not do at all to calculate the dose of opium to be given to a baby merely by estimating its weight, for babies are very susceptible to this drug, and indeed it is only in the very rarest cases that any dose of opium should be given to a baby under one year old. In the case of old people similar differences in response to drugs are found, independently of the body weight.

Estimating the Dose for a Child

A rough rule for determining the dose suitable for a child is to give a fraction of the adult dose calculated by taking the child's age as the numerator and the age plus 12 as the denominator. Thus, the fraction of an adult dose of, say, 20 minims for a child of 8 would be $\frac{8}{8+12}$ or $\frac{2}{5}$ of 20, that is, 8 minims.

The doses of drugs in the British Pharmacopoeia are stated as being from so much to so much, for example, 5 to 15 minims, a dose between these limits being supposed to represent what should be efficient in most cases and what is safe. In the case of powerful drugs, mercury, for example, it is usually advisable to begin with the minimum dose or even less, for some people have an idiosyncrasy for certain drugs, and alarming or unpleasant symptoms may follow quite small doses.

When a single dose is to be given, it is often larger than what is expedient for repeated doses. Epsom salts may be given in a dose of $\frac{1}{2}$ to 1 ounce for a single dose, but repeated doses only amount to 30 to 90 grains. Compared with the dose of a drug given by the mouth, the dose when it is injected under the skin is about a half only, but when given by the bowel it is, with a few exceptions, twice as much.

The effect of drugs is sometimes much modified by disease. In fevers, for example, large quantities of alcohol may sometimes be given without producing effects which would be expected in an ordinary person ; on the other hand, repeated small doses of mercury would be disastrous to a person suffering from Bright's disease.

See Apothecaries' Weights and Measures ; Drug ; Medicines ; Prescription.

DOUBLE CONSCIOUSNESS. A remarkable disorder of the mind is sometimes met with, the feature of which is that the individual seems to have two personalities. At one time, for instance, he may be quiet, religiously inclined, familiar with foreign languages, and a student ; at another time he may be noisy, blasphemous, unable to understand any language but his own, but perhaps clever at music or something else for which his other personality does not care.

This extraordinary malady does not confine itself to mere doubling of the personality. There are cases on record where as many as nine, ten and eleven distinct personalities may have been recognized in one individual. One personality may have some knowledge of the others, but there may be no such knowledge, and then there may be intervals of life of which the patient can give no account. By hypnotism the new personalities may be discovered, and by their revelation to the patient mental unity is obtained.

See Epilepsy ; Hypnotism ; Pyscho-therapy.

DOUBLE VISION. This disorder has a technical name, diplopia. It may be due to various causes, but by far the commonest is a defect in the very delicate arrangement by means of which the two eyeballs have their movements adjusted to one another, so that the images of any external objects that are formed upon the membrane at the back of each eye lie in exactly corresponding positions.

A simple experiment will show how ordinary vision with two eyes depends upon the delicacy of this adjustment. If we look at any object and then press one eyeball firmly with the finger, we see two images of it, this being due to the fact that the images formed in the two eyes lie no longer in exact correspondence to one another, and so the seeing centre in the brain recognizes two images independently. The interference of alcohol with the delicate adjustment of the eyes, with consequent double vision, is a familiar occurrence.

See Binocular ; Eye ; Squint.

DOUCHE. This is the name given to treatment of any part of the body by means of a stream of water. It is a very valuable measure, and its value is simply the same as that of the application of water to the skin. It washes and cleans the part to which it is applied. The most frequently used form of douche is that employed by women. A douche may also be applied to the nose (*q.v.*).

Two precautions should be taken regarding the water that is used. As the risk from microbes is greater in the case of water that is used for washing the interior of the body than when it is applied to the very resistant skin, all water used for douching purposes should be first boiled ; secondly, it must be raised, or rather allowed to cool after boiling, to the temperature of the blood, that is to say, about 100° F.

The application of a cold douche to any part of the interior of the body is injurious, and is apt to cause congestion afterwards.

The word douche is sometimes applied to the application of water to the exterior of the body, and in such cases a cold douche is sometimes desirable ; not, in this instance, for its cleansing action, which is much less than that of warmer water, but as a stimulant to the nervous system.

For a vaginal douche one may use an apparatus consisting of a container from which a rubber tube about six feet long

is led, having at its other end a tube for introduction into the vagina. The container may be made of tin or of glass, or may take the form of a rubber bag ; the vaginal tube may be of vulcanite or glass. The latter form has the advantage of being sterilisable by boiling. Such an apparatus must be kept scrupulously clean. The force with which the lotion used for the douche flows through the tube will vary, of course, with the height at which the container is placed. If at the full length of the tube the force will be considerable, and might be dangerous owing to the fluid reaching further than it should ; but when the container is only raised two or three feet the flow will be gentle, though generally sufficient for the purpose.

The vaginal tube may be smeared with clean vaseline or boracic vaseline, if desired, and before introducing it the fluid ought to be allowed to run until all the air has been driven from the rubber tube. The vaginal tube should not be introduced for more than three inches. The returned fluid may be received into a bedpan, or the patient may squat over some other receptacle.

The lotion used will depend upon the condition for which douching is required. A good antiseptic lotion consists of a tablespoonful of lysol in five pints of water. A deep pink solution of permanganate of potash is also useful, and will help to remove any disagreeable odour. To get rid of discharge the addition of a tablespoonful of common salt or of bicarbonate of soda to a quart of water will generally suffice. Astringents, such as zinc sulphate, alum, etc., may be ordered by a doctor.

See Baths ; Ear ; Enema ; Nose ; Rectal Douche ; Vagina.

DOVER'S POWDER. The compound ipecacuanha powder, the essential ingredient of which is opium, is popularly known as Dover's powder, and it contains one grain of opium in ten grains. This is a considerable proportion, and the powder should not be used except on a doctor's prescription. At the beginning of a severe cold the drug is very valuable, as also at the very beginning of bronchitis. It soothes the air passages and usually ensures sleep, these actions being due to the opium ; whilst both the opium and the ipecacuanha cause the skin to act freely, and so tend to control the temperature and to help the patient to get rid of the poisonous matter by perspiration.

DRAINS. It is the duty and interest of a householder to ensure that the drains, or pipes which carry sewage from his dwelling to the common sewer, are efficient and in good repair. The pipes may be blocked, they may leak or they may bring sewer gas into the house.

A waste pipe from a sink may be blocked by parings of potatoes or other vegetable refuse, perhaps in conjunction with an excess of grease. Such things should be strained from water before it is allowed to pass down the waste pipe. Soil pipes from water-closets may be blocked by an over abundance of coarse ordinary paper, rags or something of the kind. The waste pipe of a wash-hand basin may be blocked by loose hairs when the women of the family use the basin for hair-washing.

Blocking of pipes will be indicated by delay in water flowing away, or the flow may cease altogether. Pouring boiling water, in which a considerable amount of washing soda is dissolved, down the pipes may affect a clearance, or this may be accomplished by pushing a long, stout wire, hooked at the end, up and down the pipe. The trap or bent pipe below a sink generally has an opening closed by a screw stopper, which can be removed for clearing the pipe. A rod and plunger is another method which can be adopted.

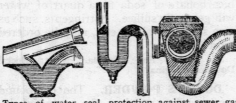

Types of water seal, protection against sewer gas

The condition of a soil pipe can be tested by pouring water coloured by lime into the stool and letting it into the soil pipe. The character of the flow may be observed at the lower end, at the manhole, or observation pit, into which the pipe opens. If the flow is very slow the pipe is choked, if the lime-water is discoloured the pipe is dirty.

Pipes of one kind and another may leak and cause dampness of the walls or foundations of a house ; should it be a soil pipe that leaks, the decomposing sewage will be at once unpleasant and a menace to health. This menace will be increased if the sewage can make its way into a well from which drinking water is taken, or occurs in any other situation where it can contaminate food.

A leak can be tested for in various ways. One is to pour an ounce of oil of peppermint, or some other pungent substance, into the topmost water-closet, sink or bath, as the case may be, and observe whether the substance can be smelled at any point below other than a normal opening of the pipe. Other methods are to pump air under pressure, or smoke, into the suspected pipe, the other opening of the pipe having been closed. An escape of air or smoke at a joint or elsewhere would locate a leak.

Danger from the Scullery Sink

The entrance of sewer gas to a house is a cause of annoyance or danger. This gas is capable of causing sore throat and debility, and while it probably does not directly cause such diseases as diphtheria or scarlet fever, by interfering with the health of the throat and of the body generally, it may predispose to these and other diseases. The people who are most likely to be affected by sewer gas are those who stand for prolonged periods over a sink, particularly in a badly ventilated and small scullery.

The entrance of sewer gas would ordinarily be favoured by the warmth in the house and by the rush of water in sewers. It is sought to prevent this danger by having traps on the pipes of the drainage system and especially by thorough ventilation of the system. A trap is an arrangement which allows water to flow freely down the pipe, but which prevents the return of air or gas through the pipe. The only efficient trap is one which has a water-seal and which is self-cleansing.

A water-seal is secured by bending the pipe so that a sufficient depth of water will always lie at the bottom of the bend to close the pipe against gas. This is found in the modern stool of a water-closet, and a similar arrangement occurs at lower levels on the various pipes. This type is known as a siphon trap. When the plug is drawn, the stool fills with water till the flow fills the thickness of the soil pipe, and the contents of the stool are sucked or siphoned out. This is what is called self-cleansing.

The pipe from the stool should enter the soil pipe at an acute angle so that the flow will be quick and easy. The soil

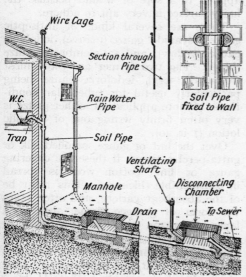

Drains. Soil pipe and its connexions above and below

pipe should be continued upwards for three or four feet above the eaves of the house, the upper end being open or protected by a wire cage to keep out birds or leaves. There is thus free air communication between the manhole and the upper air, and a current of air passes upwards. A soil pipe from a water-closet on an upper floor should run on the outside of the house-wall.

When entering a new house it is desirable to have the drains tested. When building a house the passage of drains beneath the house should, if possible, be avoided. If they must so pass, then it is necessary to embed them in cement, at least six inches thick, and there should be an inspection pipe at either end. The soil pipes of a new house must be passed by the local authority before being covered in.

See Dysentery; Grease Trap; Housing; Sewage; Ventilation.

DREAMS. It is doubtful whether there is any such thing as dreamless slumber, but, without expressing a dogmatic opinion on the subject, it can at any rate be said that people dream a great deal more than they imagine.

The dream state probably begins with events of the day which has passed, but the mind may wander on to scenes and experiences that are remote and which, in his conscious state, the individual may imagine that he has quite forgotten. Persons who have died, or otherwise gone out of one's life for many years, may be seen and conversed with.

Those inner conflicts of the mind which may be unknown to a patient, but which are recognized as capable of affecting his health, may come into dreams, and, in fact, are likely to do so. These may belong to the early years of life and may have the sexual character ascribed to them by Freudians, or they may be the problems arising in present activities. In either case they may surge towards a solution in dreams, and thus pent-up emotion may be able to express itself. The nature of a person's dreams can be found out, possibly by tracing backward from remembered dreams, or at any rate by hypnotism, but their interpretation is not usually easy.

The waking thoughts are modified by those standards of conduct and propriety derived from training and connoted by the word conscience. In dream-thought there is control of a similar kind, the controlling influence being described as the censor, and the modifications of thinking due to the censor must always be reckoned with.

People sometimes say that sleep has not been refreshing because it was disturbed by dreams, but the truth about this would appear to be that sleep was not refreshing because it was not sound. Throughout the night, or for large portions of it, the person has been on the threshold of consciousness. This state of affairs may be due to a close, badly ventilated bedroom, an uncomfortable bed, noisy surroundings, a heavy meal before going to bed, or the reverse, the need of a little food at bedtime. It occurs in many feverish disorders. Many people, also, seem to have dreams of this sort when they lie on the back. Attention to these and other details may secure sound sleep, and the dreams which then occur seem to be consistent with perfect physical rest.

See Freudism ; Nightmare ; Psycho-therapy ; Sleep.

DRESSING. In surgery the materials used for the protection of parts, or to favour healing, are described as dressings. In some instances protection may be needed against cold or rubbing or other kinds of mechanical injury ; more often it is against infection by the microbes which cause inflammation and suppuration. Instances of protective dressings are covering a burn with a waxy film like that of ambrine, or an abrasion with new skin or with collodion. Fabrics used for this purpose must either be sterilised by heat or be charged with chemical antiseptics.

In other instances a stimulating effect is wanted, when an ulcer may be dressed with, say, red lotion ; or a soothing effect is needed, so it is dressed with lead lotion, zinc ointment or something similar.

When a wound or ulcer is discharging it is all-important that the dressing should be able to absorb the discharge. When possible, a dry dressing is used for a wound because the heat and moisture of a wet dressing may favour the growth of germs ; but when a wound or ulcer is inflamed or covered with crusts a wet dressing is better suited for cleansing the parts, and the fabric used is lightly wrung out of an antiseptic lotion and generally also covered with gutta-percha tissue or oiled silk, so that it acts as a fomentation.

When the surface of an ulcer is covered with delicate granulations, which bleed easily and adhere to gauze or lint dressings, a layer of oiled silk, which has been dipped in an antiseptic lotion, is often applied to the surface of the ulcer before anything else is put on. A number of buttonhole openings are made in the silk to permit discharge to escape.

Otherwise, the first dressing applied is either lint or gauze. Plain white or surgeon's lint and plain gauze may be sterilised by heat, and packages containing these sterilised dressings can be bought ; for emergencies unsterilised gauze and lint are more commonly used, and before applying are firmly wrung out of carbolic, lysol or another antiseptic lotion. Boric or pink lint is ordinary lint which has been soaked in a saturated solution of boracic acid and allowed to dry. It may be put on dry or may be wrung out of boiled water.

Lint, it will be observed, has a smooth and a hairy side ; the former should be applied to a sore or wound because the hairy surface is very apt to adhere.

There are several kinds of antiseptic gauze : cyanide gauze (mauve), iodoform gauze (yellow), and sal-alembroth gauze (blue). The two former are those most frequently used, iodoform gauze being particularly useful for tubercular conditions. Before application, either gauze is very often firmly wrung out of carbolic lotion (1 in 40).

Over the lint or gauze, or oiled silk or gutta-percha tissue, if these are covering gauze or lint, cotton wool is spread in considerable thickness. This must be of the absorbent variety, and often takes the form of gamgee tissue, that is, a layer of cotton wool with a layer of gauze on either side of it. Cotton wool charged with some antiseptic, and also sterilised by heat, can be obtained. Last of all a bandage is applied (Plate II, 6).

Careful Handling of Sterilised Dressings

Dressings which have been sterilised by heat cease to be aseptic when they are opened out and handled in circumstances which permit of microbic contamination. This happens, for instance, if the hands of the person dealing with them are not covered with sterilised rubber gloves or otherwise sterilised, or if the dressings are laid down on a bed-cover or anything else which has not been sterilised. For dressings done at home it is safer, therefore, to use those charged with some antiseptic. Even these are not safe unless they are kept clean, and it is recommended that in storing them at home the dressings should be kept in clean paper packages which are put into a tin box with a tight cover.

See Ambrine ; Antiseptic ; Collodion ; Cotton Wool ; Fomentation ; Gamgee Tissue ; Iodoform ; Jaconet ; Sterilisation ; Wound.

DROPSY. An accumulation of watery fluid in the tissues and serous cavities of the body is described as dropsy or oedema.

This fluid is always present in tissues, filling up the interstices between the component cells, and is derived from the blood. In dropsy it is greatly increased ; the tissues are, as it were, water-logged and they become swollen.

When it affects the skin the existence of dropsy is shown by what is called pitting ; when the skin is pressed firmly with the finger a depression is left which takes some time to fill up again. Pitting is caused most easily when pressure is made on skin overlying bone or tendon, and when a slight degree of dropsy is suspected in the leg pressure is generally made on the inner surface of the shin bone, over one of the prominences of the ankle or over the Achilles tendon ; on the face, pressure is made on the bone below the lower eyelid.

Dropsical fluid in a serous cavity may accompany dropsy of the skin or occur independently ; when it occurs in the peritoneal cavity, that is, the space between the abdominal viscera and the abdominal wall, the condition is usually referred to as ascites ; when in the pleural cavity it may be called hydrothorax, and in the pericardial, hydropericardium.

Dropsy a Symptom, not a Disease

Dropsy may occur from many and various causes ; it is not a disease in itself, but merely a symptom. A common cause is obstruction of the veins, and the dropsy is then due to back-pressure. A tight garter, for example, may cause dropsy in the limb below it ; or varicose veins may result from blocking of a vein by a clot, or thrombus, or from the pressure of a tumour. In cirrhosis of the liver the flow of blood in the portal vein is obstructed by scar tissue pressing on the veins within the liver and ascites is likely to result. When the heart is weak and the circulation feeble, dropsy may appear in the legs after the patient has been walking about, or in advanced cases there may be dropsy all over the body, including the serous cavities.

Poverty of the blood, as in anaemia, may also cause dropsy. During the great war, in communities which had not sufficient food, many cases of what was called war oedema occurred. It is a common symptom of beri-beri, a disease caused by vitamin starvation. Oedema about the face and neck may occur from shellfish poisoning, and localised or general oedema results from nervous disturbance in the disease known as angioneurotic oedema. More or less oedema tends to accompany inflammatory disturbance, particularly when it occurs in the loose tissue beneath the skin, as in cellulitis.

The most common cause of general dropsy is acute nephritis or Bright's disease, and here the earliest site is usually about the eyes. Swelling is seen in the morning ; if the patient gets up it may disappear as the day wears on.

The treatment of dropsy depends on the cause. Unless it is due to such an obvious thing as a tight garter, a doctor should be consulted without delay.

See Ascites ; Bright's Disease.

DROWNING. * A person taken from water in an unconscious condition may be suffering from syncope, or more or less complete arrest of the heart's action, induced by impact with the water, fright or fatigue, or from asphyxia, due to the filling of the air passages with water. The first thing to do is to open the mouth and clear the throat of any gravel, sand or weeds which may have been sucked in by convulsive attempts at breathing. The patient should then be turned on his face and artificial respiration (*q.v.*) commenced without delay. The compression of the chest which forms part of this procedure will force water from the lungs and air passages. Artificial respiration should be continued until a doctor arrives. or for an hour at least.

Meanwhile, dry blankets and clothing, hot-water bottles, stimulants and a stretcher may be procured, and, if it can be done without interfering with the movements of the operator, wet clothing may be taken from the lower limbs and dry put on. When the patient starts natural breathing, but not before, brisk efforts should be made to improve the circulation by putting hot-water bottles between the legs and chafing the limbs, the patient being covered with blankets or dry clothing. When he can swallow, he may be given a little diluted spirits or sal volatile, or tea or coffee.

In handling the patient it should be borne in mind that he may have broken a bone by striking against something in falling into the water or by his struggles.

The patient should not be allowed to walk home but should be carried, preferably on a stretcher of some kind. He should be kept lying down, and, in the course of his removal and for an hour or two after he has been put to bed, a close watch must be kept on him, lest breathing should again stop; if it does, artificial respiration should be resumed at once.

See Artificial Respiration; Asphyxia.

DRUG. Substances, other than foods, which are used in medicine to modify the activities of the body are described as drugs. Some are vegetable products; some, minerals; some are of animal origin and the others are synthetic, that is, built up in the laboratory.

The medicinal virtues of a plant usually reside particularly, or even exclusively, in one of its parts: the leaf, the root, the wood, a gummy or resinous exudation, or some other part. Such are supplied to the pharmacist in a crude state, and, by a variety of processes, such as pulverisation, infusion, distillation or maceration, he makes from them powders, infusions, essential oils, tinctures, pills, ointments and other preparations, an account of which will be found under appropriate headings in this volume.

Active Principle of a Drug

In such preparations many of the constituents of the crude drug may be included; but one or more of these is the actual agent in producing the effects of the drug on the body, and so is described as the active principle; it may be an alkaloid like morphine, a glucoside like digitalin, a tannin or something else.

Samples of crude drugs are found to contain very varying amounts of active principle. The treatment of disease by drugs can only be safe and efficient, however, if equal doses of the same preparation of a drug always contain the same amount of active principle, and in compilations like the British Pharmacopoeia the amount which must be present in each preparation mentioned is laid down.

Crude mineral drugs usually require to be purified as, in natural deposits, they may be associated with other chemicals; from the purified drug salts and other preparations are then made. Animal products which have long been used in medicine include Spanish fly, spermaceti, lard, pepsin and pancreatic extract. More recently the extracts of the thyroid and pituitary glands, of the supra-renal bodies and of the islets of Langerhans in the pancreas, or insulin, have come into use and have proved of such signal value that the extracts of other animal glands and tissues have been introduced; the claims made for some of these, however, are not yet sufficiently substantiated.

Synthetic drugs are very numerous, and new ones are constantly making their appearance. Many, including antifebrin and similar drugs, are coal-tar derivatives. Aspirin is another example of a synthetic drug, and salvarsan, an organic preparation of arsenic, has proved of the utmost value in treating syphilis and other diseases.

Varied Action on Body Tissues

Besides classifying drugs according to their source, they may be classified according to their main action on the body, as antacids, depressants, stimulants, tonics and so on. Some, such as iron, lime, sodium or iodine, which are normal constituents of the body, may be administered when it is thought that there is a deficiency in the body, and then would act rather as foods than as drugs. Other drugs, such as alcohol, of which a certain amount may be burnt up in the body and furnish heat and energy, act as foods in so far as that happens.

Most drugs are given either to increase or depress the functions of one or more of the organs or tissues of the body, according as it is imagined that this is sluggish or over-active in the circumstances of the case. Other drugs, such as mercury, quinine and organic compounds of arsenic, are given to kill parasites within or on the body. As regards parasites in the blood and tissues, such drugs act, not directly, but by increasing the antiparasitic powers of the body itself; within the alimentary canal or on the body surface they can act directly.

Vaccines and sera, which are described under their respective headings, may be considered as drugs of very complex composition, and are intended to increase the resistance of the body to infection.

See B.P.; Colloid; Dose; Extract; Infusion; Inunction; Ionisation; Liniment; Lotion; Lozenge; Medicines; Mixture; Mucilage; Pill; Prescription; Serum-therapy; Suppository; Tincture; Vaccine.

DRUG HABITS. Many useful drugs are saddled with the heavy disadvantage that they possess seductive qualities and tend to create a craving in any person who employs them habitually, perhaps even for a short time. This craving may become nearly irresistible, so that addicts reach a point when they will readily lie or even steal in order to obtain a supply of the drug which they are in the habit of using.

Drugs of this sort produce a temporary sense of well-being through their action on the nervous system, but this is followed by reaction in the form of depression or discomfort, to relieve which further dosing is resorted to and a vicious chain is forged. Sooner or later ill effects become apparent; digestion and sleep are impaired, there is nervous irritability, sanity may be lost and the patient may die from poisoning or take his or her own life.

Prevention of the Evil

A drug habit is very difficult to eradicate, and the only really hopeful way of dealing with the problem is to prevent the habit being formed. Legislature has helped in this direction by enacting strict regulations for the supply to the public of opium, its derivatives, cocaine and preparations containing more than a certain small percentage of any of these. Except in so far as those drugs are used by qualified dentists and veterinary surgeons, they can only be supplied on a medical prescription. The chemist who dispenses the medicine must retain the prescription, so that a patient cannot procure further supplies than those stated on the prescription without consulting a doctor.

A further means of preventing the evil is to replace dangerous drugs in treatment by others whenever possible, as the use of a drug for some chronic or recurring ailment often starts a drug habit.

When a drug habit has been formed the only satisfactory method of treatment is to get the patient into an institution where it will be impossible to obtain the drug. Tonic medicinal treatment may form part of the cure, to relieve depression following the discontinuance of the drug, but moral treatment is what is really valuable, in the form of helpful advice and encouragement. The patient must therefore remain sufficiently long in the institution to recover from the physical effects of the drug, in so far as this is possible, and acquire sufficient control and self-respect to renounce its fascination. If he leaves the institution with the mental attitude of a discharged prisoner, treatment cannot have been particularly efficacious.

All this applies to alcohol equally with other drugs. Little or nothing can be expected from nostrums exploited as " drink-cures "; some of these aim at their effect by inducing nausea, others by suggestion, but all are broken reeds if a drink habit has really been established.

It is sometimes forgotten that tobacco, tea and coffee or similar beverages are also drugs. While it is true that their use in moderation is not only harmless to the great majority of people, but probably actually beneficial, it is no less true that over-indulgence in any one of them may have a very injurious effect on health. Further information on these and on other drugs for which a habit might be formed is given under appropriate headings.

See Alcohol; Cocaine; Opium; Poison.

DUCT. Derived from a Latin word meaning to lead, the term duct is used for some of the tubes in the body which act as conduits for liquids, most of them being main tubes through which a gland pours out its secretion. Examples are the ducts of the sweat glands, the bile ducts, the salivary ducts, and so on.

See Gland.

DUODENUM. So called because its length was estimated at twelve finger-breadths, the duodenum, which is the first part of the small intestine, is actually about eleven inches long in the average adult. At its commencement it is continuous with the pyloric end of the stomach, and, at its termination, with the jejunum or next part of the small gut. It is disposed somewhat in the shape of a horseshoe, the ends of the limbs being about two inches apart. In the hollow lies the head of the pancreas. The duodenum comes into contact also with the lower surface of the liver, the gall bladder and the right kidney.

The cavity of the duodenum is separated from that of the stomach by the pyloric valve, and about three or four inches below the valve there is a little projection, a papilla, on the lining membrane of the gut which marks the common entrance of the bile and pancreatic ducts. While digestion is going on in the stomach the pyloric valve opens periodically, and some of the acid contents of the stomach, the chyme, is discharged into the duodenum and by its contact with the lining of the latter stimulates closure of the valve. It mixes with the alkaline pancreatic juice and bile, however, and the acidity is neutralised; when this happens the valve again opens and lets in more chyme.

It is noteworthy that a duodenal ulcer almost always forms above the point of entry of the alkaline juices, and, therefore, where the lining is exposed to the action of the acid chyme. It is thought, however, that an important factor in causing such ulcers is sepsis, either swallowed from an infected mouth, nose or throat, or coming from a diseased appendix or gall bladder. An extensive burn is not infrequently followed by a duodenal ulcer. Inflammation of the bowel wall from sepsis, followed by a minute abscess or death of a small portion of the lining, makes the first breach, and this is extended and deepened by the erosive power of the gastric juice. The ulcerative process may open into a considerable artery and cause dangerous bleeding, or it may perforate the gut and cause peritonitis.

A duodenal ulcer is more common in males. It usually causes pain, the common site of which is to the right of the middle line in the upper half of the abdomen. It comes on generally from two to three hours after a meal, and its ap-

A duodenal ulcer is apt to form near the pyloric valve, where the acidity is greatest

pearance often coincides with the patient becoming hungry for his next meal; this is called hunger pain, and may occur in the early hours of the morning. The pain is relieved by taking some food or by a large dose of bicarbonate of soda.

More or less bleeding takes place from the ulcer; if very slight it can only be detected in the stools by careful examination by special methods; if in large quantity it may cause black motions, or melaena, or even appear as red blood. Sometimes blood is vomited.

If there are definite signs of a duodenal ulcer, medical treatment, such as rest, diet and alkaline drugs, may be tried, but the desirability of early operative treatment is founded on the risk of serious haemorrhage or a perforation, and on the likelihood of an ulcer which has healed under medical treatment breaking down again. There is little or no risk of cancer, however, which is such a common sequel to a chronic gastric ulcer.

The operation which is done is called gastro-jejunostomy; the stomach is connected to the jejunum and its contents do not then pass through the duodenum, thus allowing the ulcer to heal soundly. A diseased appendix or gall bladder should be dealt with at the same time.

See Digestion; Gastric Ulcer; Indigestion; Intestine; Stomach.

DUPUYTREN'S CONTRACTION. In middle-aged people, especially men, the ring finger, perhaps also the little finger and less frequently the middle and index fingers, may be bent into the palm at the knuckle joint. This deformity is known as Dupuytren's contraction. The affected fingers may also be bent to some extent at the middle joint, but at the end joint they are extended, or straightened out.

The condition is due to thickening and shortening of the palmar fascia, which sends down processes to be inserted into the fingers. At the beginning hard nodules will be felt in the palm of the hand.

Irritation by the pressure of some implement or tool has been blamed for starting the thickening of the fascia, but this is hardly likely, as both hands may be affected, although the hard use of a tool is confined to one hand. Heredity seems to play a part in causation. The treatment is to remove the fascia.

A congenital form of contracted fingers should be distinguished from Dupuytren's. There the fingers are extended at the knuckle joint, probably even bent towards the back of the hand, while at the other joints the fingers are flexed.
See Finger.

DURA MATER. The tough fibrous membrane which is the outermost of the three coverings of the brain and spinal cord is called the dura mater. These are Latin words meaning the hard mother. The name given to the innermost layer, a delicate membrane, is pia mater or the tender mother. The dura forms the inner lining of the skull bones, and along certain directions the two layers of which it consists are separated to form the larger venous sinuses, or channels of the skull which carry off blood from the brain. In fracture of the bones of the skull the dura may be torn and infection may thus be able to reach the brain.
See Brain; Meninges.

DUST. Except, perhaps, on the tops of mountains and out at sea, there is always a certain amount of suspended matter in the air. It may not be visible until a beam of light throws its particles into view, but in towns and at industrial centres much grosser particles are added in the form of soot and other pollutions. Sometimes droplets of moisture adhere to the soot particles and occasion a town fog, but even in the absence of fog a large amount of sunshine is shut out by a smoky atmosphere. Domestic fires, it must be said, are considerably to blame for this loss of health-giving light rays.

A dusty atmosphere provokes catarrh of the air passages by the mechanical or chemical irritation of its dust, but, in addition to this, bacteria of all kinds may adhere to dust particles and be inhaled, or may fall on food, in either case possibly causing some disease. It is for this reason that dusting with a dry duster and dry sweeping are unhygienic. The most satisfactory way to get rid of dust is by using a vacuum cleaner, but, failing this, wet tea leaves should be sprinkled on floors when sweeping them out, and dusters should be damped.

Spitting on the street or on the floor of a vehicle or elsewhere is highly dangerous, because the sputum dries into dust. In certain employments, as explained under the heading Dust Disease, lung disorders are caused by dust. Silica dust also appears to be responsible for some cases of Bright's disease. Chemical dust, such as lead, may cause poisoning.
See Air; Cleanliness; Fog.

DUST DISEASE. The excessive inhalation of dust, which is incidental to many occupations, is liable to set up morbid changes in the lungs, known as pneumokoniosis, or dust disease. The dust particles are deposited in the lungs and cause irritation and inflammation, followed by fibrosis, or scar formation, which is Nature's method of sequestering the irritating substance. The scar tissue takes the place of spongy lung, however, and to the extent to which this happens there is subtraction from the functional activity of the organ.

There are catarrhal processes in the air cells and in the bronchial tubes, the symptoms of the disorder when established being those of chronic bronchitis. There is cough and more or less profuse sputum, often coloured by the inhaled dust, shortness of breath and some degree of general debility.

Many sufferers contract tuberculosis of the lungs, though the liability to this is very much greater when the dust includes particles of silica, as in that inhaled by stonemasons, potters, printers, those employed in quartz mines and others. Silica has a poisonous action on the lung tissue which makes the latter much less resistant to the attack of the tubercle bacillus. Disease caused by mineral dust containing silica is called silicosis, by iron dust siderosis, and by coal dust anthracosis. The inhalation of coal dust does not predispose to tuberculosis of the lungs.

In occupations in which workers are exposed to the risk of dust disease, an effort to remove the risk should be made by good ventilation, by the use of exhaust fans, by moistening the substance creating the dust, by spraying the air and by the use of respirators.

When the signs of bronchial irritation first appear it may be possible by treatment and by a change of occupation to arrest the disease, but when the morbid process has become established, beyond relieving the cough and improving the general health by cod-liver oil and other tonics, little can be done.

As regards occupations involving a risk of silicosis, a medical inspector may suspend a workman from following the occupation if when the workman is first examined his physique does not appear to be satisfactory.

See Bronchitis; Consumption; Silica.

DYSENTERY. An infectious disease, characterised by inflammation and ulceration of the bowel, dysentery is mainly a disease of warm climates, though sporadic cases occur elsewhere and occasionally even epidemics in institutions such as asylums. Mostly the disease is caused by a bacillus, Shiga's or Flexner's, or by a minute animal parasite, or protozoon, the entamoeba histolytica; in the latter event the disease is also known as amoebic or tropical dysentery. Occasionally the disease is caused by another protozoon, balantidium coli, or by parasitic intestinal worms, and dysenteric symptoms may occur in malaria.

Infection occurs through food or beverages which have been contaminated by infected faeces. It may be by drainage into shallow wells or streams from which the water supply is drawn, by flies, or by persons who carry the infection being allowed to handle food. Uncooked fruits or vegetables which have been washed with polluted water or have not been thoroughly washed with clean water may introduce the infection. The risk of dysentery becomes very considerable when the superficial ground temperature rises to a certain point.

The disease commonly begins like a sharp attack of diarrhoea, but the calls to empty the bowel become very frequent, and the patient may be allowed very little rest. The first evacuations may consist of thin faeces, but blood and mucus, or slime, appear very soon and ultimately the motions consist of little else. They have an intensely disagreeable odour. There is much painful straining when the bowels move and probably also in emptying the bladder.

There is pain in the abdomen, often fever, and the patient is very thirsty. Pain and lack of rest lead to much exhaustion and possibly collapse and death, though bacterial poisoning or some complication may largely contribute to such an end. There are numerous cases, however, in which the disease occurs in a slighter form.

An acute attack of dysentery may terminate spontaneously but usually tends to become chronic; the patient may have recurring bouts of diarrhoea, with the passage of slime and mucus, and be either apparently normal in the intervals or subject to constipation. Efficient treatment during the initial attack may cure the disorder, but sometimes recurrences take place even after such treatment; or a patient, although he presents no symptoms of the disease, may still have the parasite in his body and thus be a danger to others.

Various complications may occur. The bowel may be perforated by ulceration and acute peritonitis ensue. In the bacillary form there may be inflammation of joints (arthritis) or of nerves (neuritis), and in the amoebic form inflammation or an abscess in the liver or in the brain. Such abscesses may occur long after an attack of dysentery.

How to Prevent the Disease

Preventive treatment consists in destroying flies and preventing their access to food, using only boiled water for drinking and for washing food and food utensils, washing the hands scrupulously before taking food and preventing " carriers " from handling food intended for others. The motions of a person suffering from dysentery should be burnt.

During an attack of dysentery the patient should rest in bed and the diet to begin with should consist of albumen water, rice water and then arrowroot or cornflour. Milk should be withheld until the symptoms have abated. Abdominal pain is treated by hot poultices or fomentations. Medical treatment depends upon which parasite is responsible. For the amoebic form emetine hydrochloride or emetine bismuthous iodide is usually given, the former hypodermically, in doses of $\frac{1}{2}$ grain twice daily, and the latter by the mouth, in doses of 1 grain twice daily, treatment in each instance lasting for about twelve days. The old treatment was to give powdered ipecacuanha, of which emetine is an active principle.

Bacillary dysentery is treated with magnesium sulphate, 60 to 120 grains, in water, every hour until the stools resume a faecal character, say for eight doses, and then at less frequent intervals. An antidysenteric serum, appropriate to the bacillus found to be present, or a mixed serum, is also used.

When there is no immediate means of finding out which type of dysentery is present, treatment by magnesium sulphate should be tried and a few doses of one of the emetine preparations, but the earliest opportunity of having the stools bacteriologically examined should be taken, even should the disease appear to be cured.

See Beverages; Colitis; Drains; Flies; Ipecacuanha; Liver; Peritonitis.

DYSMENORRHOEA. The onset of the menstrual flow is preceded in some women by a sense of weight in the pelvis, perhaps to an uncomfortable extent, which disappears, however, as the flow becomes established. Some women, on the other hand, experience a considerable degree of pain in the back and lower abdomen, preceding and accompanying the flow, and are then said to suffer from dysmenorrhoea. Mostly the pain takes the form of a dull ache, but along with this or independently there may be sharp, colicky pains. The aching is due to congestion of the internal genital organs, the colic to irregular spasmodic contractions of the womb in expelling the discharge.

Regular and painless contractions take place, of course, in normal menstruation, but these may be interfered with by the womb being somewhat underdeveloped, by its being tethered, as it were, by adhesions resulting from previous inflammation, by narrowness of the inner opening of the neck of the womb, by some displacement of the womb, by copiousness of the discharge, particularly when

there are clots, or by reflex nervous disturbance. Congestion is liable to occur in full-blooded women, especially when they suffer from chronic constipation, and in those who have had, or suffer from, inflammation in the pelvis or some other abnormality.

The tendency to dysmenorrhoea will be lessened if girls and women exercise freely in the open air and take reasonable exercise during the periods. The bowels should be kept open and it may be desirable to take $\frac{1}{4}$ to $\frac{1}{2}$ ounce of Epsom salts at the beginning of the period. If, however, the pain is very severe, rest is indicated. A hot bath often does good. Bromides, liquid extract of viburnum, aspirin and other drugs are sometimes required, but alcohol or opiates should not be taken as a habit may easily be induced. Organo-therapy may prove of great service. Something may require to be done to correct a displacement or some other abnormality.

See Amenorrhoea; Guaiacum; Menstruation; Womb.

DYSPEPSIA. *See* Indigestion.

DYSPHAGIA. Derived from Greek words meaning difficult and to eat, the term dysphagia means difficulty in swallowing (*q.v.*).

DYSPNOEA. *See* Shortness of Breath.

EAR. The hearing organ, or ear, is a mechanism by which air waves produced by vibrating bodies are communicated to the ends of a special nerve, the auditory, thus giving rise to impulses in the latter which are carried to the brain and there appreciated as sounds. It is customary to describe this mechanism as consisting of three parts, the external, the middle and the internal ear, though it must be understood that all these are continuous parts of the apparatus.

The external ear comprises the auricle, or pinna, the ear in the popular sense, and a passage, the external auditory meatus, leading inwards from this and ending at the ear drum or tympanic membrane. The auricle consists of a thin plate of cartilage thrown into folds and covered with skin; in the lowest part, however, there is no cartilage. There are some tiny muscles in the auricle and others which connect it with the skull; in the lower animals these actually move the auricle in various directions so as to assist listen-

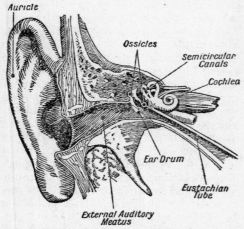

Ear. Sound waves pass along the external auditory meatus, reach the drum and set the ossicles in motion

ing, but in man they are merely vestigeal and the auricle only serves to a slight extent as a sound collector.

The external auditory meatus, about an inch long, is not a straight tube; about its middle it makes an upwards and also a backwards bend. Hence when syringing an ear the auricle must be pulled upwards and backwards in order to straighten the passage. This is rendered possible by the outer portion of the tube having cartilaginous walls; those of the inner portion are bony. In the skin lining the outer part there are modified sweat glands, secreting a thick yellowish waxy substance, known as cerumen.

The ear drum is firmly attached to the bony tube all round its circumference and has rather a slanting position, its lower margin being further in than the upper. Within the membrane is the middle ear, or tympanum, a cavity which is only $\frac{1}{12}$-inch across at its narrowest part and $\frac{1}{6}$-inch at the broadest; its height is about $\frac{1}{2}$-inch and the distance from before backwards rather more. Its principal contents are three tiny bones, or ossicles, namely, the malleus, or hammer;

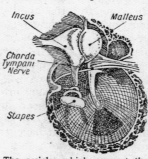

The ossicles which connect the drum with the internal ear

the incus, or anvil; and the stapes, or stirrup. The first is attached to the ear drum and is jointed to the incus, which, in turn, is attached to the stapes. The "foot-piece" of the last is fitted over a membrane which covers an opening in the inner, and bony, wall of the middle ear, known as the fenestra ovalis, or oval window. In front of this opening is the fenestra rotunda, or round window.

Into the front part of the cavity opens the Eustachian tube, coming from the throat just behind the back opening of the nose. When the lips are closed and the cheeks puffed out there is a sensation of pressure on the ear drums. This is due to air being forced up the Eustachian tubes into the middle ears; the function of the tube, in fact, is to maintain a constant quantity of air in the middle ear, and if, through the tube becoming blocked by catarrh, air is prevented from passing, deafness results from the air already in the middle ear becoming absorbed so that the ear drum is forced inwards by atmospheric pressure.

The uppermost part of the middle ear, known as the attic, presents at its back part the opening of a narrow canal leading into the mastoid antrum, a cavity in the upper part of the mastoid process, the nipple-shaped piece of bone at the back of the ear. Through this opening infection may spread into the antrum from the middle ear; also, the facial nerve passes outwards beneath the floor of this opening, and from septic mischief destroying its bony covering the nerve may be exposed and injured so that the face on the same side becomes paralysed.

Another danger of sepsis is that it may spread from the antrum to small spaces in the mastoid process, known as the mastoid cells, from which it is difficult to dislodge, and that it may spread into the lateral sinus, a large venous sinus within the skull, or even to the brain itself.

The internal ear or labyrinth consists of three parts: the cochlea, or hearing portion in front; the semicircular canals, which are concerned in preserving the balance of the body ; a space behind and between these known as the vestibule. All of these are hollowed out in the petrous portion of the temporal bone, but inside the bony semicircular canals there are closed membranous tubes of the same shape, and inside the vestibule are little membranous bags communicating with the membranous canals and with the canal of the cochlea.

The cochlea, literally a snail shell, has its apex towards the inner wall of the middle ear and its base towards the inside of the skull. It consists of a passage comprising two and a half turns round a central pyramidal pillar, the modiolus. Projecting into the passage from the modiolus, all round the turns, is a little ledge of bone, the lamina spiralis, and this and a membrane, the basilar membrane, from its edge to the wall of the passage divides the latter into two divisions, one towards the apex, known as the scala vestibuli, and the other towards the base, the scala tympani.

Another membrane from the bony ledge cuts off a part of the scala vestibuli in order to form the canal of the cochlea ; this is quite separate from the scalae but these communicate with each other at the apex of the cochlea. There is fluid in the scalae, the perilymph, which is continuous with fluid in the vestibule and around the membranous semicircular canals. Fluid in the canal of the cochlea, the endolymph, on the other hand, is continuous with fluid within the membranous semicircular canals. The lower end of the scala vestibuli is at the fenestra ovalis and of the scala tympani at the fenestra rotunda, which, it has been pointed out, are on the inner wall of the middle ear.

Along the canal of the cochlea, situated on the basilar membrane, there is a structure, known as the organ of Corti, which is the essential organ of hearing. This is made up of several kinds of cells, including some which terminate in hairs projecting into the endolymph while their other ends come into relation with the ends of the cochlear nerve, which,

passing up the centre of the modiolus, sends out branches all along the lamina spiralis.

When sound waves fall on the ear drum this is set vibrating, and with it the ossicles. The foot-piece of the stapes moves in and out of the fenestra ovalis, so altering the pressure of the perilymph in the vestibule ; this alteration is communicated along the scala vestibuli and back along the scala tympani till it impacts on the elastic membrane covering the fenestra rotunda.

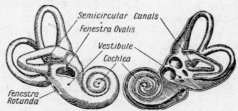

Labyrinth of the ear (shown in section on right), the functions of which are concerned both with balance and with hearing

The changes in the scalae are communicated to the endolymph in the canal of the cochlea, so stimulating the hair cells, from which impulses are passed along the branches of the cochlear nerve. This nerve joins with the vestibular nerve from the semicircular canals to form the eighth cranial or auditory nerve, and impulses are thus carried to the bulb, or medulla, of the brain and thence to the transverse and superior temporal gyri of the large brain, a gyrus being one of the folds or convolutions into which the surface of the brain is folded.

Diseases of the Ear. Congenital deformity may affect the auricle ; this may be misshapen or, in rare instances, missing altogether. It may be the seat of eczema or some other skin disease, and is particularly liable to frost bite. Gouty stones, or tophi, may form on it. A blow on the ear may occasion a swelling from the effusion of blood. This is called a haematoma auris, and sometimes occurs in the insane, apart from any injury.

As regards the external auditory meatus, the commonest abnormality is the accumulation of wax, which may cause itching, irritation

Sectional view of the cochlea, the internal organ of hearing

or pain in the passage, cough, giddiness or deafness. Sometimes, from water being admitted and causing the wax to swell, symptoms may come on suddenly.

No attempt should be made to dig out the wax with a hairpin or any other instrument, for fear of injuring the ear drum ; but, after dropping in some warm almond or olive oil or solution of bi-carbonate of soda and waiting for a little, a cautious attempt may be made to dislodge the wax by syringing. Ordinary warm water should be used and a small glass syringe ; the larger brass syringe is too powerful to be used except by the experienced (*see* Plate XV, 1).

How to Syringe the Ear

A large soft towel is placed about the patient's shoulders, and a bowl is held beneath the ear and in contact with the cheek to catch the water as it runs away. The auricle is drawn upwards and backwards, and the jet of water is directed from the nozzle of the syringe, which is held at the earhole but not actually in it, against the back wall of the passage. This is continued until all the wax appears to have been dislodged, but if there is difficulty in stirring the plug it is safer to put in more oil and, after some hours, syringe again ; if this fails a doctor should be consulted.

Children sometimes put beads or other objects into their ears, and here again syringing is the correct treatment, but should, if possible, be done by a doctor.

If the foreign body is a pea, or anything else likely to swell from contact with water, no water should be admitted to the ear by syringing or otherwise, but a little oil may be dropped in pending the services of a doctor.

The meatus may be the site of eczema, and the cause of this may be a purulent discharge from the middle ear, though poking in the ear with pins is one of the possible causes. There is heat, itching and more or less of a sticky discharge, and scratching aggravates the condition. Sometimes crusts or scales accumulate and block the meatus, an event which is made easier by the swelling of the lining of the passage, which may be considerable.

Again, a boil or furuncle may form in the passage, and may cause great pain and constitutional symptoms, suggesting perhaps the possibility of mastoid disease. Another painful complaint is myringitis, or inflammation of the ear drum. The drum may be ruptured by violence ; by diving, for example, by a box on the ear or by an instrument driven along the meatus. There is pain accompanying and following the accident, and the discharge of a little blood. All these conditions require immediate treatment.

On the wall of the external auditory meatus a hard, bony tumour may form. It may not always occasion discomfort, but, on the other hand, may cause great pain and may block the passage In the first instance the treatment is to keep the passage clean, but if urgent symptoms occur removal of the growth by operation may be necessary.

It has already been pointed out, in the account of the ear, that catarrh in the Eustachian tube may block this passage and cause deafness by preventing the admission of air into the middle ear ; but the catarrh may also spread right up the tube into the ear itself. This may cause acute pain and more or less fever. The middle ear, which, it has been noted, is a very small cavity with rigid walls except for the ear drum, becomes occupied by inflammatory discharge. This may actually be pus, a likely contingency when the ear trouble occurs as a complication of measles, scarlet fever, influenza and other diseases. In these circumstances it should be remembered also that adenoids, unhealthy tonsils and septic conditions about the nose and mouth generally, predispose to ear complications, and may themselves be responsible for recurring septic catarrh in the Eustachian tube and middle ear.

Hot Applications to Relieve Pain

When acute catarrh has invaded the ear some relief from pain may be secured by hot applications over the ear, or by dropping some warm water or some medicated liquid into the ear. The hot application may be a linseed poultice, a hot-water bag, common salt heated on a shovel and put into a flannel bag (*see* Plate XV, 2), or a big potato boiled in its jacket and wrapped in flannel. When the drum ruptures, allowing the escape of the imprisoned discharge, there is usually immediate relief from pain ; but it is dangerous to wait for this, because the pent-up infection may spread.

Persons suffering from pain in the ear, either in connexion with the diseases mentioned or otherwise, which does not quickly disappear when treated with warmth, should be under expert care, so that, if necessary, an opening may be made in the ear drum to allow the discharge to escape.

Besides minimising the risk of extension of the infection to the mastoid antrum and other surrounding parts, prompt interference of this kind will lessen the risk of the disease assuming a chronic form, either as a catarrhal or a suppurative otitis media. In the latter condition the continuance of the suppurative process entails certain consequences and risks. The drum and the ossicles may be destroyed ; the openings into the internal ear may be blocked by inflammatory thickening, and hearing impaired ; granulation tissue may enlarge to form a polypus blocking the ear passage ; cholesteatomatous masses may form and block the cavity of the middle ear.

Dangers of a Chronic Discharge

The general health may be affected by the absorption of toxins into the blood. The constant flow of purulent discharge may occasion eczema or boils in the ear passage. There is an ever-present risk of acute suppurative mischief in the mastoid antrum and in the cells, or tiny spaces, in the mastoid process ; thence there may be extension outwards, forming an abscess over the mastoid process or in the neck, or there may be an extension inwards destroying the internal ear, causing infective thrombosis in the lateral sinus, meningitis or a brain abscess.

An earnest endeavour must therefore be made to prevent the discharge from becoming chronic, and to cleanse the ear should a chronic discharge exist.

Either aspect of the case requires expert advice and supervision. For cleansing, a common method is as follows : The ear is syringed gently with a warm boracic solution, at least once a day, and when the outflow is clear the ear is drained by bending over the head on the affected side, and then dried by means of a tiny mop of cotton wool on a splinter of wood. The cotton wool must project well beyond the end of the splinter. A few drops of a solution of boracic acid powder in rectified spirits, 10 grains to the ounce, are then instilled into the ear, or some of the powder is blown in by insufflation (*q.v.*). A small pad of cotton wool may be applied over the earhole, but on no account should this be blocked by a plug of cotton wool ; such would simply dam up the discharge and probably precipitate an extension of the sepsis.

In all cases of chronic suppuration in the ear it is necessary to make sure that there is no obstruction in the nose or pharynx, and no lurking sepsis there or in the mouth ; the possibility of sepsis about the teeth, for example, should be investigated.

Insidious Menace to Hearing

The middle ear may be the site of chronic non-suppurative inflammatory processes which, while they do not menace life as does the suppurative form, yet are very serious because of their lessening or even destroying the hearing. In one form there is exudation into the ear. The beginnings may date back to scarlet fever or measles in childhood, or to some other circumstances leading to sepsis in the nose and throat. Although the fluid in the ear is not pus, there is likely to be some degree of sepsis associated with the disorder ; this leads to persistence of the fluid and to thickening of the membranes over the openings into the internal ear ; also to adhesions which limit the movements of the ossicles or, what has the same effect, to stiffening of the joints between the latter. If this disorder persists there is a progressive loss of hearing.

The most important item of treatment is opening the drum so as to allow the exudation to run off, and this should be done by an expert whenever there is reason to believe that exudation is present. The patency of the Eustachian tube must also be ensured by inflating it with a Politzer bag. The nose and throat must be cleaned up if necessary, and this is also important in prevention.

In middle-aged people a type of otitis media in which there is no exudation is more common; this is sometimes called otosclerosis, and the main feature of it is thickening of the bony walls of the middle ear. Heredity seems to play a part in its induction, but the nasal and throat conditions which have been mentioned as important in connexion with the exudative type of otitis media, whether suppurative or otherwise, also have to be taken into account here both as regards prevention and treatment.

In some cases of ear trouble the underlying cause is tuberculosis or syphilis, and in other instances general diseases like anaemia may aggravate a local disorder; in all such cases appropriate general treatment is also required.

See Deafness; Dizziness; Equilibrium; Eustachian Tube; Hearing; Mastoid; Noises in the Ear; Sound.

EAR-ACHE. Pain in the ear may be due to the pressure of foreign bodies in the passage, or to inflammation there or in the middle ear. Children with earache should have immediate medical care, as timely interference may prevent possible extension of septic mischief to the mastoid region and would often prevent serious loss of hearing in later life. Ear-ache is sometimes due to the presence of decay in the back teeth. Treatment depends on the cause, but hot applications are useful in relieving pain temporarily.

See Ear.

EARTH - TEMPERATURE. It has been noted that when the temperature of the earth, taken at a depth of 4 feet, falls to 47° F. or less there is an increased tendency to respiratory disorders, and when it is over 56° F. infantile diarrhoea will almost certainly become epidemic. When the surface of the ground attains a certain warmth there is also a tendency to epidemic dysentery.

EASTON'S SYRUP. Syrup of iron phosphate with quinine and strychnine, or Easton's syrup, is well known as a nervine and general tonic. It is often of use in carrying one through a period of physical or mental strain, such as during the last weeks before an examination, and in convalescence from debilitating diseases. The dose is ½ to 1 drachm. Those who object to the bitter taste of the syrup can obtain its equivalents in tablet form.

These tablets should never be left within reach of children, as fatal strychnine poisoning has occurred from neglect of this precaution.

See Strychnine; Tonic.

EATING. While it may be correct to say that one should eat when hungry, this does not mean that there should be anything haphazard about the choice of meal times. The digestive apparatus, like most things in nature, is subject to habit, and irregularity as regards meals is likely to upset its function. Meal times should be spaced out through the day, however, so that there is a call for food when the meal time arrives.

The principal meal of the day should be taken when circumstances favour its digestion, and this for hard-working people is usually at the end of the day. A short rest after hard work and before taking a meal helps to encourage appetite, and there is also some truth in the saying that " appetite comes while eating "; merely to begin a meal may create a possibility of enjoying it. Should there be a positive distaste for food, however, it will, as a rule, be well to take Nature's hint and abstain for a short time; appetite will return when the digestive and assimilative apparatus are ready for it.

It should be clearly understood that what matters at a meal is whether eating is properly performed. Sprightly conversation, the newspaper or a book may make a meal more enjoyable and by mental action favour its digestion, but if one or other interferes with the thorough mastication of food it is entirely harmful.

Satisfactory mastication requires, first, a sufficiency of teeth and, second, sufficient time devoted to chewing; it can hardly be satisfactory if liquids are taken while food is in the mouth, as much half-chewed food is thus washed down. In Fletcherism, an American body of doctrine relating to eating, the principles are that food should be retained in the mouth until it is liquid, no liquids being taken into the mouth meanwhile. To encourage a correct habit of chewing it is directed that the food taken at the beginning of the course of treatment should be firm and restricted to one dish. When the patient has formed the habit of thorough mastication more variety may be allowed, however. Restriction to a single dish means that the patient takes less food, and thorough mastication also helps in this direction, and the adoption of such methods is of very great use to those who have been in the habit of taking too much food.

The inclusion of firm food in the meal has the further advantage that it helps to keep the teeth clean, and an apple at the end of a meal is excellent on this account.

Thirst may be relieved by taking liquids at the end of a meal, though the best time is between meals, as the addition of much liquid during the digestion of a meal may be harmful by diluting the gastric juice.

The most important precaution with regard to liquids is to keep them out of the mouth while chewing food.

It is often said that one should rise from a meal with an appetite, and certainly no meal should be continued until no more can be taken. When one must share in a meal consisting of numerous courses, there is a danger of over-eating unless the earlier courses are partaken of sparingly. Strenuous physical or intellectual work should not be undertaken just after a meal; a half-hour's rest will help digestion by preventing blood necessary for that purpose from being withdrawn for the exercise of brain or brawn.

See Appetite; Diet; Digestion; Indigestion; Overfeeding.

EAU-DE-COLOGNE. A spiritous preparation containing oil of rosemary and other essential oils, eau-de-Cologne is very useful in the sick-room. Its addition to the water used for washing or sponging a patient makes this more cooling and refreshing. With a little water it may also be used to make an evaporating lotion out of which one or two layers of gauze are wrung and applied to the forehead, or inflamed joint, or wherever cooling is required. In virtue of its spirit it removes grease from the skin and has a tonic, astringent effect; so it is much used in cosmetics. A solid preparation of eau-de-Cologne is sold and imparts freshness to skin over which it is rubbed.

See Nursing.

ECLAMPSIA. Sometimes the ordinary course of pregnancy, especially the first, is interrupted by eclampsia, or the occurrence of fits which resemble those of epilepsy. These never occur during the early months and are most common in the last three months; they may not begin till the woman is actually in labour or even until labour is over, when the condition is called puerperal eclampsia. They are most dangerous when they occur before labour has begun and next when they begin during labour; they generally cease when the child has been delivered.

Eclampsia is due to poisoning consequent on the presence of the child in the womb; but the only thing that is definitely known about the nature of this poisoning is that the kidneys do not function properly, and that albumin is present in the urine. Very often there are symptoms pointing to the possibility of eclampsia, such as flashes of light before the eyes, dimness of vision or even temporary blindness, persistent headache, persistent indigestion, or diminution of the amount of urine passed in the 24 hours. A pregnant woman should keep in touch with her medical attendant and should report abnormal circumstances to him.

Alarming Onset of the Convulsions

A fit is ushered in with a cry and the face begins to twitch. Soon the whole body becomes rigid and, from interference with breathing, the face becomes dusky; the teeth are tightly clenched and the tongue may be caught between them. After about 1½ minutes rapid spasmodic movements begin, and these last for 2 or 3 minutes, and when they cease the patient lies in a comatose state.

Medical assistance should be summoned at once. Meanwhile, the patient should be extended at full length on the ground or in bed, if she happens to be there, and turned on one side. This is very important indeed, for if she lies on her back saliva may be drawn into the windpipe and may choke her. A piece of wood or the handle of a spoon wrapped in a handkerchief should be inserted between the back teeth on one side to prevent biting of the tongue. Clothing about the neck, chest and waist should be loosened in order to allow free breathing. The movements should be restrained sufficiently to prevent the patient from hurting herself, but no forcible attempt should be made to suppress them entirely. There may be only one fit or very many, and they may occur in rapid succession.

If medical help is delayed, an attempt may be made to prevent the recurrence of the fits by putting an ice-bag at the back of the head and neck and by fomentations or poultices over the kidneys, and the patient should be kept warm with hot water bottles and blankets in order to encourage sweating. If the patient is conscious, half an ounce of Epsom salts should be given dissolved in a little water, and this dose may be repeated in an hour.

See Childbirth ; Pregnancy.

ECSTASY. In rare instances some individual may have visions of such transcendent splendour as to make him, or her, oblivious to external surroundings. He may stand still in rapt contemplation and adoration of the vision or may express his excitement in appropriate movements, and in either case may give utterance to his sense of the wonder and beauty of the glories he beholds. Usually such visions are of a religious nature. This state is described as ecstasy and is a manifestation of hysteria. Apparently it was once of commoner occurrence than it is now. A state of ecstasy may follow an epileptic convulsion.

See Hysteria.

ECTOPIC GESTATION. The development of a fertilised ovum outside the womb is described as ectopic gestation. Its site is almost always in the outer part of the Fallopian tube. The ovum is usually fertilised in the tube and then moves on into the cavity of the womb, but in the cases under consideration something prevents it from doing so ; most frequently it is narrowing of the tube from antecedent inflammation. The ovum develops for a time but eventually, at some time between the 6th and 12th weeks of pregnancy as a rule, there is abortion or a rupture of the tube. There is usually then such considerable bleeding as to constitute an immediate threat to the life of the woman.

When ectopic gestation takes place there are the usual general signs of pregnancy, though they may be overlooked. A common history is that a woman, having missed one period, begins to have recurring small bleedings from the womb. Also, colicky pains occur in the lower part of the abdomen, and when such is the case in a woman who may possibly be pregnant, she should at once consult a doctor, whether or not she has a bloody discharge.

The only treatment is by operation, but if this is timely the woman's life will almost certainly be saved ; if rupture or bleeding has been allowed to occur, however, the prospects of success are very uncertain.

See Pregnancy.

ECTROPION. Turning outwards of the margin of the lower eyelid, a condition called ectropion, may be due to the contraction of scars following burns, ulceration, etc., or to chronic eczema of the lid-margin. It may be due to facial paralysis, and sometimes occurs in old people merely from relaxation of the tissues. It causes inability to close the eye properly, in consequence of which the conjunctiva of the cornea may suffer from irritation. Treatment is by operation.

See Entropion ; Eye.

ECZEMA. A large number and variety of substances, if long enough in contact with the skin, cause inflammation, or dermatitis, but if the skin is protected from the irritating substance and treated with soothing remedies it quickly recovers and remains well without any tendency to relapse. Eczema is also an imflammation of the skin, but it is a capricious disorder compared with the simple dermatitis just described ; it may come into existence for no obvious reason, and in the course of treatment may relapse on slight, or even no apparent, provocation.

It is thought that the explanation of this state of affairs is that the skin is sensitised to some substance which may reach it by the blood or come into contact with it, and that the manifestations of eczema are, as it were, explosive phenomena comparable to those of an attack of asthma, the kind of reaction which occurs in anaphylaxis (*q.v.*), etc. Sometimes attacks of asthma and eczema alternate, or they may occur together.

In asthma it is recognized that an attack is often precipitated by the patient swallowing some food, such as an egg, or inhaling horse-dandruff or some other substance, and the same may apply to an outbreak of eczema. In both cases also the liability to the disease may be inherited. In creating this tendency to eczema or in provoking an attack, it is thought that the poisons manufactured in the patient's alimentary tract, or toxins coming from some focus of infection somewhere in his body, may sometimes play a part. Local irritation may also be of importance in precipitating an attack in some people ; in others sunlight, coarse soap, sugar and so on.

Acute eczema oftenest appears first on the face. The skin becomes reddened, swollen and itchy, and then hot and tense. Blisters then appear, tiny at first, but perhaps coalescing to form larger ones. Itching is a prominent symptom in most cases of eczema, and either by scratching, or spontaneously, the blisters rupture and pour out a clear sticky discharge which is characterised by the fact that it stiffens linen like starch.

Later the discharge dries into yellow crusts, or, if blood has been drawn by scratching, the crusts are brown. After a few days the swelling abates, the crusts drop off, and there remains a reddened and scaly surface. Scaling goes on for a few days or even weeks, and the skin then resumes its normal appearance. But during this time some article of food or some application may cause a relapse, and the various stages are repeated.

The disease may spread from the face, or wherever it begins first, to other parts, and, especially in children, may cover the whole body. If much skin is involved there may be fever and loss of appetite. While the skin is inflamed it is readily invaded by microbes which may cause pustules like those of impetigo, crops of boils, or perhaps erysipelas.

Rôle of Diet in Treating Eczema

The general treatment should include a scrutiny of the diet, and, if there are successive attacks, it may be possible to fix responsibility on some particular item. In severe cases a light milk diet with vegetable soups is usually given, though it should be remembered that there are some people with whom milk does not agree. Water, barley water, or a natural alkaline water should be given very freely. When the disease is more localised, a grilled mutton chop and vegetables are usually safe. Alcohol, tea and coffee are not allowed. Clothing next to the skin should be of the cellular cotton type, with only sufficient bed and personal clothing to keep the patient comfortably warm. The bowels should be kept freely open by giving salines.

The kind of local treatment depends on the stage of the disease. In the weeping stage, that is, when there is discharge, some doctors use drying pastes or powder, but most use lotions. A good one consists of the dilute liquor of lead acetate, B.P., or one made by shaking up ½ ounce each of powdered zinc oxide and prepared calamine, and ½ ounce of glycerin with a pint of distilled water. Glycerin irritates some skins, however, and if this is so in the particular instance, it should be left out of the lotion.

How to Remove the Crusts

These lotions are applied on strips of butter-cloth or linen which should not be allowed to become dry, though it is better not to cover them over with any impermeable protective. Greasy applications are harmful at this stage as a rule, especially if there is any pus in the discharge. If there is much crusting, this can be removed by applying a starch poultice ; this is made by mixing a tablespoonful of wheat starch into a paste with a little cold water, pouring it into a pint of boiling water, and stirring briskly to mix thoroughly. The starch, when cool, is applied on pieces of linen, the surface having first been sprinkled with boracic acid powder.

Throughout the treatment plain water should not be used for cleansing, the lotion or a starch poultice sufficing in the early stages ; later, when ointments or pastes are being used, cold cream or oil of sweet almonds will be suitable cleansing agents. In a type of disease known as seborrhoeic eczema, thorough washing of the skin, on the contrary, is of the utmost importance. A change is made to creams, ointments or pastes when the weeping stage is over, Lassar's paste (q.v.) often being used at this stage.

Chronic eczema may follow an acute attack, but most frequently begins as such, that is to say, the lesions on the skin appear without the dramatic suddenness of the acute type. In one case the disease may mainly be of the weeping form, in another dry and scaly, while in a third the chief tendency is towards what is called lichenisation, that is, to the development of groups of papules, or pimples, such as occur in lichen (*q.v.*). In all cases, however, there is more or less thickening of the skin, and often fissures or cracks are present. ⌐ There is usually intense itching, increased by warmth, so that it may become intolerable when in bed at night. In this connexion it may be said that sometimes eczema spread over the limbs and trunk, which resists ordinary treatment, may be due to the itch-mite of scabies (*q.v.*).

How to Treat Weeping Eczema

For the weeping type the lotions already mentioned may be tried, with the addition of 2 drachms of liquor carbonis detergens to the ½ pint. When there are cracks, painting with a solution of 15 grains of silver nitrate in 1 ounce of sweet spirit of nitre is very effective, care being taken to avoid the sound skin, which would be blackened. In any case it is desirable to protect the sound skin around the patches with Lassar's paste, whatever the treatment used for the patches. It is often sound treatment to paint the patches (and this applies also to other types of chronic eczema) with pure tar, pix carbonis praeparata B.P.; itching may be wonderfully relieved by this application.

In the treatment of dry and papular eczema, ointments or pastes containing tar, ichthyol, juniper tar oil or something similar may be used. The following is an example of a suitable formula :

Liquor carbonis detergens	..	1 drachm
Zinc oxide powder	.. ..	120 grains
Powdered starch	.. .. ..	120 ,,
Vaseline and lanolin equally to make 1 ounce		

Other formulae are given under the headings of the drugs above-mentioned. Radium, X-rays and ultra-violet rays, when used by experts, are often of much service in obstinate cases of chronic eczema. The papular form tends to occur on parts of the skin exposed to friction, such as the neck, the shoulder and the front of the forearm, and means should be taken to eliminate this as far as possible.

See Bakers' Itch ; Dermatitis ; Seborrhoea ; Skin.

EFFERENT. This term is used to describe motion away from a particular centre, a blood vessel from an organ, for example, a duct from a gland or a nerve impulse from a centre.

See Afferent.

EFFERVESCENCE. A brisk escape of carbonic acid gas bubbles, or effervescence, by its sharp effect on the lining of the back of the throat, produces general stimulation reflexly, and for this reason soda water is more refreshing than still water. On the stomach lining the effect of effervescence is to cause a free flow of gastric juice, but the carbonic acid gas also appears to act as a sedative, and soda water or an effervescent mixture often relieves nausea and sickness. Nauseous drugs are somewhat more tolerable if the medicine is taken while effervescing.

An effervescent mixture is made by combining citric or tartaric acid, or both, with the carbonate or bicarbonate of sodium or some other base. The acids and carbonates may be dissolved in separate bottles, and a certain quantity of each is to be mixed just before taking; or, like a Seidlitz powder, the dry ingredients may be in separate packages to be separately dissolved and then mixed, or the acid may be made up with the carbonate in a single powder.

Some of the saline cathartics can be obtained as effervescent powders, for example, Epsom salt and sodium sulphate. Citrate of caffeine can also be obtained in this form.

See Beverages ; Cathartic.

EFFUSION. The escape of blood or serous fluid into the tissues or serous cavities of the body is described as effusion, though the collection of fluid thus poured out may also be described as the effusion. Thus there is an effusion of blood beneath the skin after bruising, and the fluid between the lung and the chest wall which may occur in pleurisy is called a pleural effusion.

See Bruise ; Pleura.

EGG. The contents of an egg form a complete diet for a developing chick, just as milk does for a young mammal. There are differences between the two, however, as an egg contains only an insignificant amount of carbohydrates, so little that eggs are allowable for diabetics on a strict diet ; on the other hand, an egg is relatively rich in iron and in lecithin, a phosphorised fat, which is found in large quantity in nervous tissues. It has a liberal content of lime also. It is thus a good food for the growing person and in anaemia ; it is useful also in tuberculosis and in convalescence from acute diseases. The white of the egg, or egg-albumin, is almost a pure solution of proteins, chiefly albumin ; fat, lecithin, cholesterol, a protein called vitellin, vitamin and mineral salts are contained in the yolk.

The digestibility of white of egg is increased by whisking it. A hard-boiled egg takes about twice as long to digest as a lightly boiled one, but its digestibility can be increased by mincing finely. Eggs may have a constipating effect, possibly because they leave hardly any residue in the bowel and contain lime. Some have difficulty in taking eggs in any form ; they may induce biliousness or provoke outbreaks of asthma or eczema. Such people are apparently sensitised to eggs, probably to the white.

See Albumin ; Anaphylaxis ; Beverages ; Food ; Invalid Cookery.

ELASTIC BANDAGE.

Included in this description are the pure rubber, or Martin's bandage, the woven elastic and the crêpe bandage. Any of these may be used to support varicose veins, but the pure rubber has the disadvantage that it imprisons the sweat and so may cause much irritation. To lessen this risk perforated pure rubber bandages are sold, but even these are not very satisfactory from this point of view. It is safer, therefore, to rely on one of the others. A bandage is a better support for varicose veins than an elastic stocking, but should be put on evenly from the foot upwards and before getting out of bed in the morning ; nor should it be removed until in bed again.

Another use for an elastic bandage is to support and exercise pressure on an injured joint ; it should be put on as a figure-of-eight. Woven elastic caps for a joint can be procured for use instead of a bandage. Although not quite so firm as the others, a flannel bandage possesses a certain amount of elasticity and is comfortable for a joint.

The pure rubber or woven elastic bandage is often used to compress the blood vessels and control bleeding during an operation, and in delayed union of bones, after a fracture or other affections of a limb. It is often beneficial if an elastic bandage is put on the lint above the disordered part sufficiently tightly to retard the return of the venous blood, but no more. This seems to improve the nutrition of the part and favours healing.

See Bandage ; Bier's Method.

ELBOW.

On the front of the elbow there are several large veins just beneath the skin. One, the basilic, runs upwards in the groove on the inner side of the biceps muscle, and another, the cephalic, occupies the groove on the outer side of the muscle. Crossing the front of the elbow, running obliquely upwards and inwards from the cephalic to the basilic, is the median vein, which lies in front of the brachial artery but separated by a strong strip of fascia, the bicipital fascia.

Elbow. Veins of the arm that cross the front of this region

These are the veins almost always used for blood-letting and for intravenous injections, and usually the median, the risk of wounding the underlying artery being minimised by the presence of the bicipital fascia. The brachial artery divides into the radial and ulnar arteries about a finger-breadth below the bend of the elbow.

The bones forming the elbow joint are the humerus above and the radius and ulna below. The upper end of the ulna possesses a notch which grasps the lower end of the humerus, the upper, or back, part of the notch being formed by the olecranon process, and the lower, or front, part by the coronoid process. The olecranon process forms the point of the elbow.

The upper end of the radius is in the form of a broad-rimmed disk, the upper surface of which articulates with the humerus, while the rim is applied to a depression on the side of the ulna. A strong ligament, the orbicular, passes from the ends of this depression round the neck of the radius, completing a ring within which the head of the radius revolves when the forearm is turned so as to bring the palm of the hand uppermost or downmost.

The elbow is a good example of a simple hinge joint, possessing only the move-

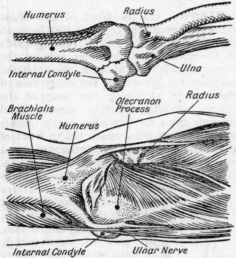

Above, fracture of humerus involving elbow joint
Below, muscles on outer side of right elbow, showing also position of the ulnar nerve or "funny bone"

ments of flexion, or bending the arm, and extension, or straightening it out. It does not move from side to side. When the forearm has been straightened out till it is in line with the arm, it is prevented from going any further by the olecranon process fitting into a depression on the back of the lower end of the humerus known as the olecranon fossa.

The elbow joint may be sprained or dislocated, or the bones may be broken in its neighbourhood. A dislocation of both bones is usually backwards, the elbow being more or less fixed with the olecranon process very prominent; sometimes the radius only is dislocated, and this is generally forwards. A fracture of the bones near the joint may extend into the latter, or otherwise threaten its future mobility. The first-aid treatment of these accidents is described under the headings

Dislocation, Fracture and Sprain, and diseases under the heading Joint.

What is called a tennis elbow is usually either a strain of the muscle on the outer side of the elbow in front or inflammation of a bursa (*q.v.*) which lies beneath those muscles. It may be caused by an over-powerful backhand stroke or by continuous overstrain of the muscles in such strokes. A tennis elbow is sometimes a strain of the muscles on the inner side of the front of the elbow, and this also is what constitutes a golf elbow. The usual treatment is to fix the elbow with strips of adhesive plaster, but if there is an inflamed bursa it may require operation.

There is also a bursa between the olecranon process and the skin to relieve pressure on the former when the elbow is rested on a hard surface. Swelling of this bursa is described as student's elbow or miner's elbow, and is similar to a house-maid's knee.

The ulnar nerve runs at the back of the elbow between the olecranon process and the inner prominence, or condylar process of the lower end of the humerus. It lies close to the skin and may readily be jarred by knocking this part of the arm against some hard corner, when a peculiar sensation runs down the forearm. Hence the name funny-bone applied to this part of the elbow. The nerve may be dislodged from its position and cause sufficient trouble to require an operation to replace it. Sometimes workmen who use the elbow vigorously, as in wielding a sledge-hammer, irritate the nerve so that it becomes thickened and more or less paralysed.

Just above the inner condylar process there is a lymphatic gland, the lowest on the limb, which may be enlarged and painful when there is septic mischief further down the arm.

See Dislocation; Fracture; Joint; Sprain

ELECTRIC BELT. If a so-called electric belt ever does any good it is not through any electricity it may produce, but purely and simply by suggestion. A sufficient current of electricity can only be procured from other kinds of apparatus, some of which, however are quite cheap. But the correct application of electricity for any purpose requires skill and judgement

ELECTRICITY IN MEDICINE. Treatment by electricity may be employed in various forms of disease ; in some it is an alternative which may be used if convenient, but in others it is necessary that it should be procured.

The best-known forms of electricity used in medicine are those of galvanism and faradism. The former is constant current electricity ; the latter is an induced current of an alternating nature. An alternating current in which the alternations take place very smoothly is known as the sinusoidal current. A high-frequency current is one which reverses the direction of its flow so rapidly that there may be as many as two million alternations per second. Diathermy, which is a heat-producing agent, is carried out by an intense current of this description.

It is not possible in a work of this kind to enter into technical details regarding the sources and methods of applying these currents, but their uses will be indicated.

The galvanic current is used in ionisation (*q.v.*) ; for treating neurasthenia and other constitutional diseases ; to stimulate paralysed muscles ; for nerve and muscle testing ; in electrolysis for the removal of birth marks and superfluous hairs.

The faradic current is of value in the regeneration of wasted muscles ; in obesity, this form of electricity being used in the Bergonié method ; and in certain gynaecological conditions.

The sinusoidal current is used for prolapse of the abdominal viscera ; in constipation ; for threatened curvature of the spine in growing children ; for difficult and painful menstruation.

High frequency is especially valuable in conditions of pain and congestion, and in treating skin lesions such as boils and ulcers. Diathermy is used to destroy piles and various kinds of tumours ; to increase metabolism ; to relieve neuritis ; in pneumonia, and for other purposes. Diathermy is much superior to poultices and similar hot applications, because the heat is produced in the tissues themselves.

What is called the electric breeze, which can be produced by high-frequency apparatus, is often effective in soothing headache or neuralgia, and in stimulating recovery in chronic eczema and other skin diseases.

Static or frictional electricity is especially useful where a constitutional sedative is required, and for its action on the circulation in the deeper structures.

The application of electricity to the diagnosis and treatment of disease can only be carried out properly by a doctor or under his immediate supervision ; much of the work is done by specialists.

Indirectly, electricity is used in medicine to operate the electro-magnet, used for removing metallic foreign bodies from the eye ; burrs, used in operations on bone and on the teeth ; and vibratory machines for massage. Instruments on the principle of the telephone are used as aids to the deaf. Electric lamps are used for radiant heat baths, and electric currents, with suitable apparatus, are necessary for the production of artificial sunlight and of X-rays.

See Ionisation ; Radiant Heat ; X-Rays.

ELECTRIC SHOCK. A severe electric shock causes a person to cry out, and he may fall to the ground and stop breathing. If he remains in contact with a live wire the current should be turned off. If this cannot be done at once, his connexion with the wire should be broken ; but proper precautions must be taken in doing so. The rescuer should stand on a pile of dry clothing, if a dry rubber mat is not available, and his hands should be covered with rubber gloves, tobacco pouches or dry woollen clothing. A dry stick, if at hand, may be used to push the wire off the body. It will be noted that emphasis is laid on everything used in connexion with the rescue being dry ; moisture conducts electricity very readily (*see* Plate XV, 6).

If the patient has stopped breathing, artificial respiration (*q.v.*) should be carried out. Probably a person who has ceased breathing after an electric shock has been killed by stoppage of the heart, but a decision as to this should be left to a doctor, who will have been summoned.

Smelling salts may be held to the nose, or if the patient can swallow he may be given diluted spirits of sal-volatile. He should be kept as warm as possible.

ELECTROLYSIS. When an electric current is passed through certain solutions decomposition takes place, some constituents moving towards the positive electrode and others to the negative. Electrolysis is made use of in medicine because, as the body fluids contain, in addition to other things, a considerable quantity of common salt, it means that if a current is passed through body tissues caustic soda is formed at the negative pole and hydrochloric acid at the positive, either of these substances having a caustic effect.

If, therefore, a current is passed through a naevus, a form of birth mark (*q.v.*), or a wart, there is coagulation of the blood and the growth atrophies and disappears. Similarly, when a platinum needle attached to the negative pole is pushed into a hair follicle, while the positive electrode is placed somewhere else on the body and an electric current passed through, the root of the hair is destroyed and superfluous hairs can be thus removed. Only large, coarse hairs are dealt with by electrolysis. This method of treatment should be done by an expert. The inexperienced may either fail to remove the blemish or may cause excessive destruction which is followed by disfiguring scars.

ELEPHANTIASIS. The tropical disease known as elephantiasis, or Barbados leg, owes its name to the enormous swelling which may affect the legs, the scrotum, the vulva, or, more rarely, the breasts, face or arms of those who are its victims. The swelling is the result of inflammatory

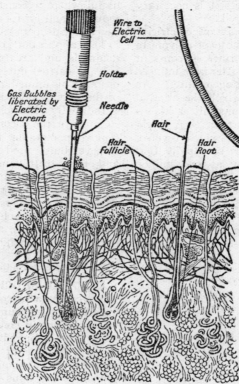

Electrolysis : removing hairs by destroying their roots

overgrowth and obstruction to drainage through the lymphatic channels, caused by a parasitic worm, filaria bancrofti, the adults of which, from 3 to 4 inches long, inhabit the lymphatics.

The embryos of these worms are introduced into the body by the bite of a mosquito ; here, having attained maturity, they breed and produce swarms of fresh embryos, which pass into the blood stream. They do not, however, appear in the peripheral vessels except at night.

The production of swelling in any part of the body is preceded by inflammation there and by bouts of feverishness. The increase in size is accompanied by coarsening of the skin, which also forms more or less massive folds at the joints of an affected limb, especially at the ankle. Very great deformity and incapacitation often occurs.

While the progress of the disease can be delayed, perhaps, by resting with the limb elevated and by the use of an elastic bandage, surgical treatment is usually required sooner or later and this may mean an amputation. Success in diminishing the number of the parasites and lessening the swelling has been claimed for treatment by intravenous injections of tartar emetic.

In temperate climates considerable swellings, sometimes referred to as pseudo-elephantiasis and due to lymphatic obstruction, may occur in different parts from pressure by tumours, scar tissue, etc. The lymphatic circulation is also at fault in Meige's or Milroy's disease, an uncommon hereditary affection, in which there

PLATE XIII

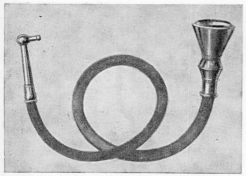

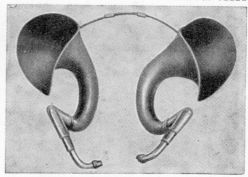

Deafness. 1. Conversation tube : the voice is directed across, not down, the mouthpiece

2. Head auricles ; if the wearer is a woman the hair can be so dressed that they are hidden

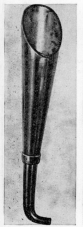

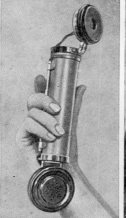

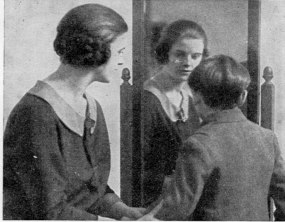

3. Tortoiseshell ear trumpet. 4. The uniphone, an electrical instrument

5. In chronic deafness lip-reading should be taught as soon as possible. One way is with a mirror

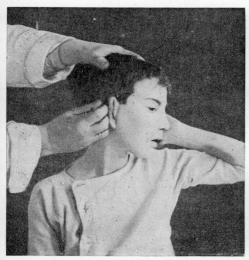

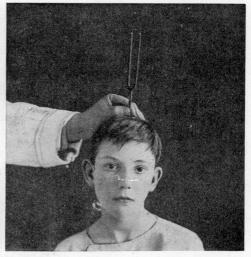

6. Test of hearing by conduction through the mastoid bone. A tuning-fork is placed on the bone and the length of time noted during which the sound is heard. 7. Weber's test : a tuning-fork placed on the head of a patient with obstructive deafness in one ear is heard better in that ear than in the sound one

1, 2 and 4 *courtesy of Hawksley & Sons*

PLATE XIV

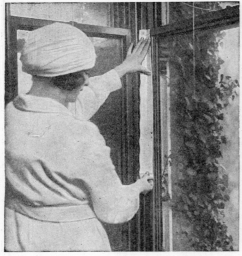

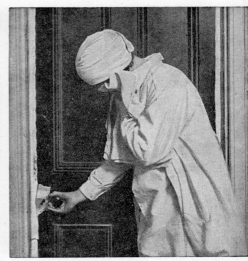

Disinfection. 1. Before lighting a fumigant the windows are sealed with strips of gummed paper

2. When the fumigant is lit, door and keyhole are sealed. The face must be protected

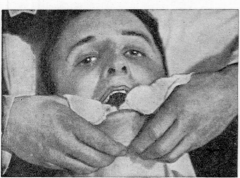

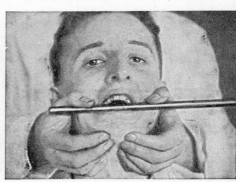

Dislocation. 3. A dislocated jaw can be reduced by pressing with the thumbs back and down

4. A thin walking-stick used instead. Either should be placed as far back as possible

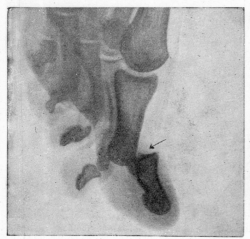

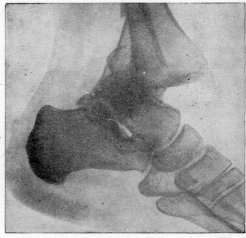

5. Dislocation of the great toe; this might occur from kicking hard with unprotected toes

6. Dislocation at the ankle joint; the foot is here seen to be displaced backward

To face page 249

is very considerable swelling, suggesting that of Barbados leg. Marked swelling may also happen in a limb from thrombosis of the deep veins.

See Dropsy ; Filaria ; Lymphatic System.

ELIXIR. Some sweetened and aromatic spiritous preparations are known as elixirs. An elixir may contain an active drug and be used itself as a medicine ; others are used to cover the taste of nauseous drugs, for example, the aromatic elixir, U.S.P. The following are some of the elixirs with their doses and uses : elixir of cascara, ½ to 2 drachms, laxative ; elixir of glycerophosphates, 1 to 4 drachms, tonic ; peptic elixir, ½ ounce after each meal, digestive. There is a long list of elixirs, however, some of which are proprietary preparations.

EMACIATION. Severe general wasting of the body, or emaciation, may occur from a variety of causes. It may happen quickly from a large loss of liquid by watery motions, as in cholera and the summer diarrhoea of infants, a loss, however, which is quickly made up if the patient recovers. It may happen fairly quickly also from the burning up of the tissues in fevers, or from the active chemical changes going on in the body in exophthalmic goitre. In infantile atrophy or marasmus, which occurs chiefly during the first six months of life, there is often no abnormal change in the organs to account for the wasting, and the adoption of a suitable diet produces a striking improvement.

There may be much emaciation in diabetes. Malignant tumours are another cause, more especially when one obstructs the gullet and prevents food being taken, or when a tumour otherwise interferes with the digestion or absorption of food. Tuberculosis of the lungs owes its other names, consumption and phthisis, to the emaciation which it causes, though tuberculosis elsewhere in the body will have the same result if it persists in an active state sufficiently long. Syphilis may have the same effect, and emaciation in young children is a common symptom of the inherited disease.

A person suffering from melancholia may be very much wasted, also one in the later stages of locomotor ataxia, and the instances of emaciation exhibited to the public as living skeletons are victims of a degenerative disease of the muscles.

See Atrophy : Starvation.

EMBOLISM. Sometimes there are particles floating in the blood which are able to block blood vessels, or, to use the scientific name for this occurrence, to cause embolism, the plug itself being called an embolus. With the exception of the branches of the portal vein, which in the liver become smaller and smaller and end in capillaries, it is always an artery that is blocked, and generally one of the smaller of these.

Most commonly the embolus is a piece of thrombus, by which is meant a clot formed in a vein or in the heart, or it may be a vegetation, a small fibrous mass, which has been detached from a diseased heart valve. Clotting, or thrombosis, is not uncommon in a varicose vein and it always takes place extensively in the veins of the womb after childbirth, and it sometimes happens that a portion of the thrombus breaks off, floats up through the great veins, through the right side of the heart, and lodges in one of the branches of the pulmonary artery. Similarly a thrombus from one of the tributaries of the portal vein may lodge in the liver.

After a fracture fat globules may occur in the blood, as they may in other conditions, and after a wound in a large vein, especially of the neck, or after labour, air may make its way into a vein. Either the fat or the air may act as an embolus. Other emboli consist of parasitic worms or portions of malignant tumours, and wherever the embolus of tumour tissue lodges a fresh growth begins.

Sometimes an embolus is infected with bacteria ; it may be a portion of a thrombus from an infected source or a mass of bacteria which have multiplied and remained clumped together somewhere in the heart or a blood vessel. It is then likely that an abscess will form at the site of the embolism and that further particles will be detached from the abscess and spread widely over the body, each giving rise to an abscess where it comes to rest.

Apart from this possibility of infection, the consequences of embolism depend upon its situation, the organ in which it occurs, and the size of the artery which is blocked. Where there is free anastomosis of the arteries, that is, where their branches intercommunicate freely, the stopping of the circulation beyond the plug is very short, because blood flows in from neighbouring blood vessels.

But in certain situations there is so little anastomosis that the arteries may be termed end arteries ; they are like a branch of a tree and its twigs, which can only obtain their sap through the branch. The coronary arteries which supply the heart are of this description, and embolism of one of these means sudden death. This might also occur were a considerable branch of the pulmonary artery in a lung the site of embolism. If not immediately fatal, a pulmonary embolism is accompanied by a sudden sharp pain in the chest and breathlessness, followed by the spitting up of blood.

What happens here is that in a wedge-shaped portion of lung the temporary anaemia is followed by a back flow of blood from the veins, so that the wedge becomes engorged with blood, or, in scientific language, it becomes the site of a haemorrhagic infarction. This portion of lung may die and be cast off, leaving a cavity, or it may be converted into scar tissue.

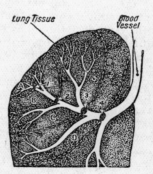

In the eye embolism causes sudden and permanent blindness, and in the brain the commonest result is sudden paralysis of one side of the body ; sudden death might occur if the part of the brain containing the centres for the heart and lungs were affected.

Emboli, numbered 1–4, are shown blocking blood vessels which serve the lung areas A–D

Other end arteries occur in the spleen and the kidney, and embolism causes pain over the organ involved ; there is not usually engorgement of the area supplied by the occluded artery, but what is called a pale infarction is formed by coagulation of the tissues, and this is later replaced by a scar.

The recognition of the occurrence of an embolism is not likely to be possible for any but a doctor. The possibility of its occurrence in connexion with heart disease or venous thrombosis and after labour should be borne in mind ; a person with heart disease should abstain from violent, or even much, effort, and in the other cases mentioned strict rest should be enjoined as long as the danger lasts.

See Apoplexy ; Infarction ; Pyaemia ; Thrombosis ; Varicose Vein.

EMBROCATION. *See* Liniment.

EMBRYO. A new creature comes into existence when the female cell, or ovum, has been fertilised by a male cell, or spermatozoon. Immediately thereafter cell division begins, one becoming two, two becoming four, and so on until a globular mass of cells is produced. On the surface of this some of the cells are differentiated to form the embryonic area, which has a length of 0·0076 inch and from which the embryo develops.

At the end of the second month of development, when the young creature has acquired a definitely human form, it ceases to be called an embryo and is known from then onwards till birth as a foetus. Of the other parts of the ovum, a portion is utilised for nourishing the young creature until it can be nourished from the blood vessels of the mother, and the remainder, with the lining membranes of the womb, form membranes for the protection of the creature, and also the placenta, through which a communication takes place between the blood circulations in the mother and her progeny.

For the first three months the mass, containing the embryo, or foetus, and situated on the inner wall of the womb, is still called the ovum, and it is customary to say that at the end of the first month it has the size of a pigeon's egg ; at the end of the second month, of a hen's egg ; and at the end of the third, of a goose's egg.

The foetus is 3 inches long at the end of the fourth month, or sixteenth week, and the sex is clearly defined ; by the end of the fifth month it is 4½ inches long ; by the end of the sixth, rather over 6 inches long; and by the end of the seventh, 8 inches long. If the child were born at this stage special efforts might be successful in making it survive.

See Abortion; Ovum; Pregnancy.

EMETIC. A substance which causes emesis, or vomiting, is described as an emetic. The stomach should be emptied at once when an irritant or narcotic poison has been taken, and it devolves on those who are at hand to give an emetic, which should be the first procurable.

An emetic should not be given, however, if there are stains or other evidences pointing to the poison as belonging to the corrosive group.

It is often desirable also to induce vomiting in cases of gastritis and thus get rid of irritating substances. Another circumstance in which vomiting may be useful is in bronchitis, when the bronchial tubes are filled with secretion, which may be cleared in this way.

The handiest emetics are common salt, two tablespoonsful in sufficient water just to dissolve it, and mustard, a tablespoonful in half a tumbler of water. A tablespoonful of alum in half a glass of water would also act. Zinc sulphate, 10 to 30 grains, and copper sulphate, 5 to 10 grains, dissolved in water are rapid emetics. Ipecacuanha wine is somewhat slow in its action; the doses are two tablespoonsful for an adult and a small teaspoonful for a child. Apomorphine, which is derived from morphine, is a rapid and reliable emetic; it is given hypodermically. For elderly people suffering from bronchitis, ammonium carbonate, in a dose of 10 grains in water, is a good emetic for clearing the tubes, as it does not cause the depression which follows most other emetics and which would be dangerous to one in an enfeebled state.

If one emetic fails to act another may be tried, but common salt must not be used with zinc sulphate. It will probably be found that tickling the back of the throat with a feather, the finger or a paper spill will succeed in bringing an emetic into action. When vomiting begins it should be encouraged by giving large draughts of tepid water, and this will further benefit by washing out the stomach.

See Apomorphine; Copper; Poisoning; Stomach Pump; Vomiting.

EMOLLIENT. External applications which protect, soothe or soften the tissues are described as emollients and include such substances as oil, soft paraffin, vaseline, cold cream, starch powder or chalk powder, and also poultices and fomentations. An internal remedy with the same actions is called a demulcent.

EMPHYSEMA. The tiny air vesicles of the lung and the passages leading into them have elastic walls, so that, while they expand when air is drawn into the chest, they shrink again when air is expelled. Should they remain more or less dilated, however, the affected part of the lung is said to be in a state of emphysema. If such a condition is widespread throughout a lung, this differs from a normal one in being larger and in the fact that if the chest were opened it would not collapse as the normal one does. As the disease advances the vesicles become more and more dilated, their walls atrophy and give way, so that large air spaces form, sometimes as large as a hen's egg (Plate XV, 7).

The subdivision of the normal lung into minute air cells provides an increased surface in which blood capillaries may run and so increases the opportunity for aeration of the blood; their destruction in emphysema results, therefore, in insufficient aeration of blood. Two consequences of this are that the patient is short of breath and cyanosed, though in some instances he may be very dusky but not so short of breath as would be expected from his appearance.

The enlargement of the lung pushes up the ribs so that the chest tends to be round or barrel-shaped, and there is also a tendency to be round-shouldered.

The subjects of emphysema suffer from chronic bronchitis, more particularly in the winter. The diminution of the available capillary blood vessels in the lungs means that the right heart has to work harder in order to push the blood through. In order to overcome its difficulties it hypertrophies, but as years go on it tires, becomes dilated and inefficient, so that dropsy and other signs of heart failure appear. People with emphysema are ill-prepared to resist pneumonia.

Anything that raises the pressure within the lungs tends to produce emphysema.

Hard physical toil, involving much holding of the breath, will do it, and occupations such as glass-blowing and playing on wind instruments. In asthma forcible efforts have to be made to expel air from the lungs, and in chronic bronchitis the stress of cough strains the lungs, though both of these conditions may also be effects of emphysema as well as causes. It is thought that some people are born with deficient elasticity in their lungs so that they develop emphysema very readily and even in childhood

An emphysematous state of the lung cannot be removed, but something can be done to prevent it from getting worse. If at all possible a change should be made from an occupation involving straining efforts to one which does not ; much stair climbing should be avoided and also exercises which put one out of breath. Dusty occupations should be eschewed, as they are provocative of bronchitis and fibrosis of the lung, and for the same reason it is desirable to winter somewhere away from the cold and damp and the fog of cities. Asthmatics, however, may have to stay where they are least liable to attacks ; this is often in a town.

The risk of bronchitis will be lessened by keeping the chest well covered, front and back, by avoiding quick changes from a hot to a cold atmosphere, by simple food in a moderate quantity and by strict moderation in the use of alcohol. Bronchitis should be treated as described under that heading.

See Bronchitis ; Cyanosis ; Health Resort ; Lung.

EMPYEMA. Although the term empyema, meaning a gathering, is sometimes applied to a collection of pus, or matter, in the maxillary antrum (*q.v.*) or a frontal sinus (*q.v.*), it usually signifies such a collection in a pleural cavity, that is, in the space between the lung and the chest wall. This may happen with or following pneumonia, or from tuberculous

infection, or in connexion with a specific fever, especially scarlet fever. Amongst other causes are a wound of the chest wall or the extension into the chest of a suppurating process in the abdomen, for example, from a liver or kidney abscess.

There is first a pleurisy with effusion, or wet pleurisy, but the effused fluid speedily becomes loaded with pus cells, though sometimes it may be a considerable time before this happens, and often enough a wet pleurisy does not go on to the stage of empyema at all. When it occurs with scarlet fever an empyema may not at first cause symptoms pointing to the chest, but the patient does not recover properly from the fever.

Similarly, when it follows pneumonia, the temperature does not become normal when it might be expected to do so, though it becomes remittent or intermittent ; or having become normal it recurs. Severe delirium in a child with pneumonia would be suggestive of a coexisting empyema. When a child is wasting and has symptoms suggestive of consumption, an empyema should be thought of as a possibility.

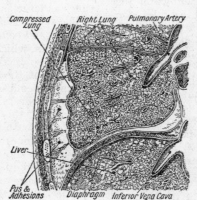

Compressed Lung   Right Lung   Pulmonary Artery

Liver

Pus & Adhesions   Diaphragm   Inferior Vena Cava

Empyema : pus in the pleural cavity, the space between the lung and chest wall

An empyema may cause sharp pain in the side and there may be a short, dry cough, but, in any case, whenever a doctor suspects the existence of empyema he tests his suspicion by drawing off some of the fluid for examination. It is sometimes difficult to locate an empyema, however, as it may be of small quantity and situated between the lobes of the lung, or be shut up towards the apex of the lung by adhesion of the two layers of the pleura.

To the extent to which it occupies the pleural cavity an empyema compresses the lung, and, if this persists for some time, the pleura covering the lung becomes thickened and contracted so that even when the fluid is withdrawn the lung is unable to expand. Inflammatory processes also invade the lung itself, which becomes firm and contracted from the rmation of scar tissue, while dilatations rm on the bronchial tubes, a condition nown as bronchiectasis.

It is therefore desirable to evacuate an mpyema as soon as possible after its iscovery. This is done by naking an opening in the hest wall at the side, a ortion of a rib usually being aken away, and inserting a rainage tube. The patient , thereafter, encouraged to reathe freely in order to romote expansion of the ing. Should this not be omplete a cavity will re- aain which will continue to uppurate unless the chest all falls in and closes it.

Sometimes the collapse f the chest wall is very onsiderable and causes a ateral curvature of the spine, he hollow of the curve being towards the ffected side. If healing does not take lace in this way, it becomes necessary to emove portions of a sufficient number of ibs to allow the chest wall to fall in.

See Bronchiectasis ; Consumption ; Lung ; Pleurisy ; Pneumonia.

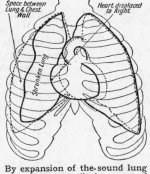

Space between Lung & Chest Wall

Heart displaced to Right

Shrunken Lung

By expansion of the sound lung and consequent displacement of the heart, the cavity resulting from empyema may be obliterated

EMULSION. In the ordinary way an il or a resin will not mix with water pro- erly, but if a little gum acacia or gum ragacanth be added, and the substances ubbed up together in a mortar, a good nixture is got in the form of a milky- ooking liquid. This is called an emulsion, nd in it the fat or oil is present in very mall droplets, which are prevented from unning together by the coating of gum vhich each has received.

Milk and yolk of egg are natural mulsions, and gum-resins, such as am- noniacum or asafoetida, form natural mulsions, a substance of this kind only requiring to be rubbed up with water. Yolk of egg is often used in making cod- iver oil emulsion. Other agents frequently ised are alkalies, usually a solution of ootash ; soap ; tincture of quillaia and incture of senega. The active constituent n these tinctures is a glucoside called saponin. Shampoos are generally made with tincture of quillaia.

See Cod-liver Oil ; Quillaia.

ENCEPHALITIS. Inflammation of the brain, or encephalitis, chiefly affects the grey matter, and may occur from extension of sepsis from a wound on the head or a suppurating middle ear, from the attack of microbes circulating in the blood, or from alcoholic or other poisoning. It frequently accompanies meningitis, but may occur independently, though sometimes it is difficult to distinguish it even then from meningitis. It may be associated with one of the infectious diseases, for example, measles, scarlet fever, whooping-cough or influenza.

The onset of encephalitis may cause irritability, drow- siness and perhaps vomiting, ensuing upon which there is progressive clouding of the faculties, per- haps passing into deep unconsciousness, or coma ; sometimes there are convulsions. The temperature may be high. Conscious- ness may not be regained, but, on the other hand, after the lapse of some days or weeks, there may be decline of the fever and awakening to consciousness, though mental dullness and paralytic symptoms may persist for some time.

Acute polio-encephalitis, so called because the grey matter is the site of the disease, is infectious, and presumably due to the virus which causes acute polio-myelitis, or infantile paralysis ; in fact, it may occur with the latter. It affects young people especially. It may be ushered in by a succession of severe convulsions, the child passing from one into another. There is irritability with vomiting, and more or less loss of con- sciousness. There is fever to begin with, but this disappears. Paralysis of eye, face, swallowing or trunk and limb muscles may be present, or blindness or other sensory paralysis. Often such paralysis disappears as the patient recovers. Death may occur during convulsions or after coma has lasted for a time.

Encephalitis lethargica. This form of encephalitis is popularly known as sleepy sickness because a striking feature of many cases has been drowsiness, from which, however, the patient could be aroused to give intelligent answers to questions. There are, however, frequent instances of the disease without drowsiness, and, indeed, the patient may be restless and sleepless. There is more or less fever and perhaps vomiting. Squint and double vision from paralysis of eye muscles is common, and a notable symptom which is sometimes present is persistent hiccough.

The patient may become profoundly unconscious and may die. If he recovers it may be completely; on the other hand, there may be serious sequelae. Some patients are left with symptoms resembing those of paralysis agitans, or Parkinson's disease (*q.v.*); others those of St. Vitus's dance (*q.v.*); others suffer from severe ataxia, their movements resembling those of a drunken person. Still others exhibit mental and moral defects; they are unclean, lying or thievish in their habits, and so on. Sometimes there is a constant free flow of saliva which is very disagreeable.

Rest a Vital Necessity

It should always be remembered that this disease may occur in slight degree, so slight indeed that it may be overlooked altogether, and nevertheless be followed by one or more of these sequelae. Whatever the cause or the extent of encephalitis, its treatment must include rest in bed in a quiet room.

Neglect of rest, even in very mild cases of encephalitis lethargica, may have very serious consequences, and during epidemics of the disease apparently trifling indisposition of a vague character should be reported to a doctor.

Although another explanation will usually be found for the symptoms, the benefit accruing in the exceptional cases will amply compensate for what in others would ordinarily be unnecessary fuss. Prolonged headache, sudden visual disorders, forgetfulness about the small matters of daily life, are examples of the symptoms alluded to above.

The diet should be light, and the bowels must be kept freely open. Headache may be relieved by cold applications to the head. Further treatment depends on the precise cause at work. A septic wound or suppurating middle ear, or a brain abscess will necessitate an operation.

Acute polio-encephalitis and encephalitis lethargica are notifiable diseases.

See Brain; Fever; Infantile Paralysis; Meningitis; Paralysis.

ENDARTERITIS. Inflammation of the internal coat of an artery is described as endarteritis. Acute inflammation which, however, probably involves all the coats of the artery, may occur from sepsis and, rarely, from other causes, its interest and importance mostly merging in the septic condition of which it is a part. Chronic endarteritis may occur in several forms, but in all there is a thickening of the internal coat caused by the growth of new cells. When widespread this constitutes the condition known as arterio-sclerosis (*q.v.*).

A patchy endarteritis, or atheroma, usually affects the aorta or some other large artery. The thickened patches project into the lumen of the vessel as flattened nodules. Fatty degeneration may occur in the interior of a nodule forming a soft mass called an atheromatous abscess, and if this bursts through its containing wall a so-called atheromatous ulcer is left.

Frequently there is a deposition of lime salts in the deeper parts of the nodule, a process described as calcification, and hard plates may be formed. Calcification may also occur in the middle, or muscle coat of the vessel beneath the atheromatous patch or in this coat in other parts of the same vessel, or this may occur independently of any atheroma. Arterio-sclerosis and atheroma, generally speaking, are diseases of middle or later life.

In one form of endarteritis the disease tends to block or occlude the vessel, and hence is called the obliterative or plastic type. This may occur in arteries in the neighbourhood of chronic ulcers, and then has the salutary effect of lessening the risk of bleeding. Syphilis is a common cause, and tuberculosis. The condition also occurs in silicosis of the lungs, the disease caused by the inhalation of rock-dust, and in chronic nephritis.

It sometimes occurs in the arteries of the lower limbs, causing the disorder known as intermittent claudication, in which, after walking for a short distance, the patient is pulled up by an acute burning pain in the limb. This passes off after resting for a short time, but recurs after another short walk. In course of time there is likely to be gangrene of the toes, the foot or even a larger portion of the limb. Syphilis or the abuse of tobacco appears to be the usual cause, and treatment should be directed appropriately.

See Arterio-sclerosis; Artery; Intermittent Claudication.

ENDEMIC. A disease is said to be endemic in any place where instances of it are always occurring. Thus, cholera and plague are endemic in parts of India and elsewhere in the Far East. When circumstances become favourable the disease is apt to assume an epidemic form and spread. Solitary cases of an infectious disease are said to be sporadic.

See Epidemic

ENDOCARDITIS. Inflammation of the lining of the heart is known as endocarditis. The valves are mainly affected and almost always those of the left side. Along the lines where the flaps come into contact during the closure of the valve fibrinous deposits take place, which may prevent the valve from closing or obstruct its orifice. Very occasionally part of the fibrin is broken off and gives rise to embolism (*q.v.*).

When the inflammation abates the deposits are invaded by tissue cells and absorbed, but the parts on which they have rested are changed into scar tissue, more or less, and by subsequent contraction of this the valve may become either incompetent or stenosed, or both. Should inflammatory processes persist, the valve flaps become thickened and deformed, and lime may be deposited in their substance, making them rigid and brittle.

The most common cause of this type of endocarditis is acute rheumatism in one of its forms, or St. Vitus's dance, but it may occur in connexion with one of the infectious fevers. The heart condition usually supervenes without any warning, and may, in fact, only be discovered when valvular mischief is considerable enough to cause disturbance of the circulation. Congenital malformation of a valve predisposes to endocarditis there.

Following on infected wounds, pneumonia and other conditions in which the blood stream may be invaded by swarms of bacteria, acute endocarditis of the ulcerative, or malignant, type may develop. The vegetations on the valves are not confined to the lines of contact of the flaps, and ulceration occurs. From the heart, emboli, containing bacteria, are distributed all over the body.

The disease may be ushered in by a feeling of chilliness, perhaps severe enough to constitute a rigor, and there is high fever and prostration. Bleeding may take place from the nose, the bowel, into the skin and elsewhere. The temperature may tend to go up and down irregularly, and there may be profuse sweating. Abscesses may form in many parts of the body. There may be diarrhoea. The patient may be drowsy and may sink into deep unconsciousness. The disease is very fatal, death usually occurring in from a few days to three or four weeks.

There is a type known as sub-acute bacterial endocarditis which usually occurs in hearts damaged by previous disease. Here again small emboli are distributed throughout the body, though they do not give rise to abscesses. There is progressive anaemia with pallor, or the skin may assume what has been called a café-au-lait tint, or a dark brown one. Scattered here and there, small bluish spots, or petechiae, may mark the sites of minute haemorrhages, and tender pink nodules may form on the pads of the fingers and toes.

Characteristic Clubbing of Fingers

Fever is rather irregular and may disappear for considerable periods. The spleen is found to be enlarged. The fingers become clubbed or swollen at their extremities. Minute bleedings occur in the retina of the eye, and embolism there may cause sudden blindness.

The duration of the disease may be anything from about three months to two years.

The recognition and treatment of endocarditis can only be undertaken by a doctor. It may be said, however, that in the acute rheumatic type salicylate of soda is given, and in the infective variety injections of sodium cacodylate, an organic preparation of arsenic, may do good. A person whose heart has been damaged should live carefully and should get rid of sepsis about his teeth or anywhere else.

See Heart; Rheumatism.

ENDOCRINE. The processes concerned in the development and functioning of the body are very complex and require some sort of control to ensure harmonious activity. Much of this control is exercised by the nervous system, but a large amount is accomplished by substances known as hormones or chemical messengers. Body cells, whatever their function, whether, for example, they are muscle fibres, secrete useful ferments or perform some other kind of service, can be whipped into activity, or restrained by an impulse coming along a nerve fibre; similar effects may be caused by substances reaching the cells in the blood.

An important group of hormones comprises the secretions of various glands which are poured direct into the blood and not out through a duct. Such a secretion is called an internal secretion, or endocrine, and the gland a ductless or endocrine gland. Some glands which have ducts for one secretion also contain within their substance groups of cells which furnish an internal secretion.

The endocrine glands include the thyroid, parathyroid, supra-renal, pituitary, the interstitial cells of the ovary and the testis, the thymus, the pineal, the islets of Langerhans in the pancreas, and scattered masses of cells here and there in the body, which resemble those of the supra-renal medulla. Other glands are

credited with an internal secretion, th mammary, for example, but the evidenc for this is not so definite.

Some even of the ductless glands furnish more than one secretion. Thus, th pituitary has two lobes with differen functions, and the same applies to the inter nal part, or medulla, of the supra-rena and its external, o cortical, part.

The fact that gland has no duc raises the presump tion that it has ar internal secretion but it must also be shown that its ex tract contains a de finite chemical sub stance and that i has a physiologica action of some kind when injected into the body. Evidence is also furnished by disease.

It has been shown that disorders with well-defined fea tures depend upon changes in particu lar endocrine glands changes resulting either in a deficiency or an excess of the inter nal secretion. Thus, cre tinism and myxoedema are caused by deficient thyroid secretion, while an excess of this causes exophthalmic goitre. In Addison's disease there is a deficiency of the secretion of the medulla of the supra-renal, in acromegaly an excess of that of the anterior lobe of the pituitary. Diabetes insipidus depends on some alteration of the posterior lobe of the pituitary, and diabetes mellitus on a deficiency of the secretion of the pancreatic islets. Deficiency of parathyroid secretion causes the nervous affection known as tetany.

Overgrowth of the cortical part of the supra-renal in the female invests her with male characteristics, a growth of hair on the face, deepening of the voice,

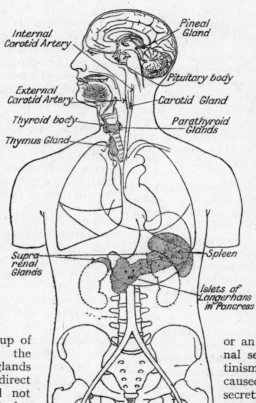

Internal Carotid Artery

External Carotid Artery

Thyroid body

Thymus Gland

Supra-renal Glands

Pineal Gland

Pituitary body

Carotid Gland

Parathyroid Glands

Spleen

Islets of Langerhans in Pancreas

Coccygeal Gland

Sites of the principal endocrine glands

iminution of the breasts, and alteration of even the general shape of the body and of mental qualities. Overgrowth of the pineal causes mental and sexual precocity. Besides such well-defined results of glandular defects, there may well be others less definite when the interference with the secretion is of lesser degree.

Extracts of endocrine glands are made and have been extensively used in laboratory experiments and in the treatment of disease. The administration of such may completely remove the symptoms, as thyroid extract may do in myxoedema, though the administration must continue throughout life ; on the other hand, as when adrenalin is given for Addison's disease, although the symptoms are improved the disease persists. Treatment by such extracts is commonly referred to as organo-therapy.

The active principle of extract of supra-renal medulla is adrenalin, a substance which may now be built up artificially by a chemist ; that of extract of the pancreatic islets is insulin, and this can be prepared in a crystalline form ; and that of thyroid extract is thyroxin, an organic preparation of iodine. Extract of the posterior lobe of the pituitary is called pituitrin, but its exact constituents are still uncertain.

The isolation of the active principles of internal secretions clinches the evidence of their existence, and the part which they play in disease gives some idea of the scope and variety of their activities in ordinary physiological operations, such as growth and metabolism. They are important factors also in combating bacterial or other poisons in the body. Some doctors distinguish adrenal, pituitary and thyroid types of bodily development with corresponding mental characteristics, and, indeed, it is generally recognized that psychological processes cannot be properly considered without reference to the activities of the endocrine glands and their relative preponderance.

The reader is referred to articles under the headings of the various glands and diseases mentioned.

ENDOMETRITIS. Inflammation of the lining membrane of the womb is called endometritis and may occur in acute and chronic forms. When acute, the inflammation almost always occurs in the wall of the organ as well as the lining, and should chronic endometritis last for a considerable time the morbid processes will probably extend into the wall.

Acute endometritis is mostly due to the extension of infection up the genital passages into the womb, either when portions of after-birth or membrane remain in the cavity, after labour or abortion, or as a result of gonorrhoea. The former event constitutes a type of puerperal fever. In acute endometritis there is a risk of blood poisoning and of inflammation spreading to structures surrounding the womb.

Signs of the Acute Form

There may not be much pain in puerperal cases, though the womb is very tender. In gonorrhoeal cases pain may be very severe and, as in puerperal cases, there may be considerable fever. A free purulent discharge from the vagina makes its appearance, and if the onset is during a monthly period the menstrual flow is arrested. Immediate medical care is required. Pain may be relieved by applying an ice-bag or hot fomentations to the abdomen. In puerperal cases the womb must be cleared of anything that may have been retained.

Chronic endometritis may follow the acute form or occur independently. It is always due to bacterial infection, but displacements of the womb, the presence of growths, excessive coitus, constipation or any other circumstance that causes congestion of the organ predisposes to such infection. A more or less profuse discharge is present, consisting of pus and mucus, and, from its appearance, described as leucorrhoea or the whites. There may be a sense of weight in the pelvis, and at the menstrual periods the discharge may be excessive or be accompanied by pain. Signs of nervous fatigue are often manifest in patients in whom the condition has lasted for some time.

In treating the condition it is necessary first of all to eliminate anything that causes congestion, and in addition to the factors noted above the use of alcohol should be mentioned. Iron tonics are often useful, especially if magnesium sulphate is added. Douches assist in keeping the parts clean. It may be necessary to have the womb curetted. Injections of pure glycerin into the womb give good results in skilled hands in both the acute and chronic forms of the disease.

See Douche; Genital System; Puerperium; Womb.

ENEMA. An injection of liquid into the rectum, or lower bowel, is called an enema (plural, enemata) and may be used to clear the bowel, to dispel flatus, to introduce nourishment into the body, and for other purposes.

Nutrient enemata are dealt with under the heading Rectal Feeding.

For a purgative enema 16 ounces or more of liquid should be used; for a child of five about 5 ounces, and for an infant about 1 ounce. It may consist of plain or soapy water, or 2 to 4 tablespoonsful of castor oil or 1 or 2 tablespoonsful of oil of turpentine, or both, may be added for an adult. Instead of castor oil, 6 ounces of olive oil may be added, or when there is difficulty in moving the bowels the enema may consist of $\frac{1}{2}$ to 1 pint of olive oil. A soapy enema is made by pouring 1 pint of boiling water over 1 ounce of soft soap, or an equivalent amount of hard soap shavings, and stirring till the soap dissolves. Other ingredients should be thoroughly mixed.

The addition of turpentine to an enema will help to dispel flatus, but this can also be achieved by $\frac{1}{2}$ ounce of tincture of asafoetida made up to 4 ounces with starch mucilage.

An enema should be at a temperature of about 98° F. Sometimes $\frac{1}{2}$ to 1 pint of water at tap temperature is used for constipation, and iced water may be injected for hyperpyrexia or for bleeding from the lower bowel.

In cases of persistent diarrhoea an enema of 4 to 6 ounces of starch mucilage is sometimes used, often with the addition of laudanum, and starch mucilage is also a useful medium for introducing other drugs into the bowel.

Different kinds of apparatus are used for giving an enema; usually it is a Higginson's syringe (q.v.). For the larger enemata an ordinary douche can or bag, of at least 1 pint capacity, will also serve. For children a rubber ball syringe is often used, and this would also serve for an adult

receiving a small nutrient, or a starch enema, though it is more usual to employ for such purposes a funnel with a length of rubber tubing attached.

Whatever the type of apparatus used it is generally provided with a bone or vulcanite nozzle for introduction into the bowel, or it may be that the end of the rubber tube attached to the douche can or funnel is rounded off for direct insertion or a similar piece of tubing is attached to a nozzle. This obviates the risk of injuring the bowel lining, which may happen when a hard nozzle is used. A glycerin enema, consisting of 1 or 2 teaspoonsful of this substance, is given with a small syringe which has a long nozzle.

For receiving an enema the patient is placed on the side, preferably the left, with the thighs bent up on the abdomen. The bed or couch should be protected with a waterproof sheet. All air should be expelled from the tubing before introducing the nozzle, which, having been smeared with soft paraffin, is then pushed into the bowel in an upward and forward direction for a distance of an inch or rather more. Should the liquid not run freely the position of the nozzle should be moved a little. To prevent the immediate return of the liquid the injection should be given slowly.

A douche can or funnel should not be more than $1\frac{1}{2}$ to 2 feet above the level of the patient's body, in order to lessen the force of the flow.

When the enema is to be retained and the patient has difficulty in holding it, it will be helpful if a folded napkin is held against the lower end of the bowel.

See Constipation; Douche; Syringe.

ENTERIC FEVER. See Typhoid Fever.

ENTERITIS. Inflammation of the bowel, or enteritis, may be due to many causes, and commonly pain and diarrhoea are amongst its symptoms. When the stomach is also affected one speaks of gastroenteritis. Inflammation of the large bowel is described as colitis (q.v.).

See Diarrhoea; Intestine.

ENTROPION. The turning inwards of the edges of the eyelids is called entropion, and is usually due to trachoma, a form of conjunctivitis (q.v.). It leads to much irritation of the eye.

See Ectropion; Eye.

ENUCLEATION. Some tumours are contained in a capsule and their removal consists in shelling them out of the capsule. This procedure is called enucleation. The removal of an eyeball is also known by this term.

ENURESIS. The involuntary discharge of urine is called enuresis, and, when the accident occurs at night, nocturnal enuresis.

See Bed-wetting; Bladder; Micturition.

ENZYME. A ferment (*q.v.*) is also called an enzyme.

EPIDEMIC. When a disease assails a number of persons simultaneously or in rapid succession it is said to be epidemic, and when world-wide, as was the outbreak of influenza in 1918, pandemic.

It may be an epidemic of arsenic or lead poisoning, for example, from contaminated food or beverages, of beri-beri or scurvy, from a lack of proper food, but usually the disease is one due to some micro-organism.

The pollution of drinking water with the excreta of some person carrying the infection may cause a widespread epidemic of typhoid fever, cholera or some other water-borne disease throughout the community that uses the water, and each patient may serve as a fresh focus of infection. The provision of a safe water supply prevents such epidemics, however, and, even when the water supply cannot be depended on, inoculation against the diseases goes a long way towards preventing epidemics, as was proved by the slight prevalence of typhoid fever amongst the inoculated troops in the Great War, contrasted with the large number of cases among the non-inoculated troops during the South African War.

Some diseases show a seasonal tendency to epidemicity, and, as in dysentery and infantile summer diarrhoea, this may depend on the earth temperature reaching a certain height or, as in the common cold and influenza, on cold weather causing people to crowd together in a heated atmosphere. Weather conditions may favour an outbreak of certain diseases by increasing the prevalence of flies or other insects which act as carriers.

Some diseases show a periodicity in the recurrence of epidemics not at all, or only partially, dependent on seasons; thus, for influenza it is 33 weeks and for measles 2 years. This can be explained by each epidemic using up the available stock of susceptible persons so that for a period, varying according to the disease, the community is largely immune. The protection of the individual against influenza wears off; children are born and form a sufficient number of susceptible subjects to permit infection from a measles carrier to become effective. Whether this using up of available soil in which the seeds of disease may grow is the whole explanation of periodicity is, however, not established.

Preventive vaccination and inoculation, if thoroughly carried out, would largely control the epidemicity of most infectious diseases. Other safeguards are the notification and isolation of cases which actually occur, segregation of contacts, quarantine of ships, etc., and disinfection.

See Endemic; Infectious Disease; Notification; Vaccination.

EPIDERMIS. *See* Skin.

EPIDIDYMIS. Attached to the back of each testicle is an elongated curved structure, known as the epididymis. It is about 2 inches long and $\frac{1}{2}$ inch broad, and presents three parts, the head, the body and the tail. Into the head pass the afferent ducts of the testicle, carrying away its secretion, while the body and tail consist of a long twisted tube into which all this secretion is gathered, and by which it is conveyed to the vas deferens, or main duct, of the testicle, which begins at the end of the tail.

Inflammation of the organ is called epididymitis and, when acute, is usually due to gonorrhoea. Tuberculous disease of the testicle (*q.v.*) begins in the epididymis.

EPIGASTRIUM. The area on the surface of the abdomen which lies in front of the stomach is called the epigastrium; often it is referred to as the pit of the stomach. Behind the stomach there is the large artery, known as the abdominal aorta, and its pulsations may be visible, particularly in thin and nervous persons, the occurrence being spoken of as epigastric pulsation. As a rule it has no significance.

EPIGLOTTIS. Situated behind and below the root of the tongue, the epiglottis, which is made of fibro-cartilage, looks like a lid for the larynx (*q.v.*), and at one time was supposed to be drawn down over the entrance to the latter during the act of swallowing. Food and drink, however, are prevented from entering the larynx by this being drawn up against the epiglottis and the base of the tongue in swallowing.

EPILEPSY. An old popular name for epilepsy was the falling sickness ; nowadays the disease is usually referred to simply as " fits." There are instances of epilepsy, however, in which the patient neither falls nor has fits. He merely becomes pale, stares in front of him, and for the moment stops whatever he is doing ; if he has anything in his hand, he drops it. Then he resumes talking or whatever he was doing ; for the moment he has been quite unconscious.

This is called petit mal, or minor epilepsy, and it is the seizure of unconsciousness which identifies his condition with the form of epilepsy in which fits occur—grand mal, or major epilepsy.

But the conception of epilepsy must be still further extended to include states akin to that of the sleep-walker, in which a person may commit strange, dangerous and even criminal actions, for, while such states generally follow a seizure of either minor or major epilepsy, they may sometimes occur without them ; in fact they appear to replace them. A patient may be in such a condition for a long while, during which he acts like a different person, an instance of the phenomenon known as dual personality, but when he again finds himself he has no knowledge of what has occurred in the interval, any more than a person who has had a seizure of minor or major epilepsy.

An epileptic fit may be preceded by some alteration in the patient's demeanour, for example, he may be very irritable or irascible or, on the other hand, peculiarly placid ; or by some sign, designated an aura (q.v.), such as flashing lights, ringing in the ears, a feeling of coldness or warmth or tingling somewhere about the body, a smell, a taste, or even an idea. The aura varies for different epileptics, but for any one person it is always the same.

Commonly the fit is ushered in by a loud shout, the so-called epileptic cry, the patient immediately falling to the ground. He is very pale and is in a state of tonic spasm or rigidity, the face being turned t one side with the mouth firmly closed an the eyeballs turned upwards ; the hand are clenched and the legs stretched out This lasts for a few seconds, and then th stage of clonic spasms begins, the fac twitches, the eyes roll, and the head, bod and limbs are jerked about, the hand opening and closing.

The face is dusky. Rapid champin movements are made with the lower jaw and foam gathers at the corners of th mouth ; as the tongue is often caugh between the teeth and bitten deeply the foam may be blood-stained. Fre quently there is an escape of urine an faeces. This stage lasts for one or tw minutes or a little longer, and then th movements gradually cease, the patien becoming limp and breathing stertorously He is now in a state of profound un consciousness, or coma, from which h may awake in a dazed condition, or, i allowed, he may sleep on for some time

In some instances fits only occur a night, nocturnal epilepsy, and the patien and his friends may remain ignoran of his disease, bed-wetting, which is a likely accompaniment of the fits, being ascribed to other causes.

Condition Known as Status Epilepticus

In what is called status epilepticus one fit rapidly succeeds another, perhaps for hours or even days, and this may easily have a fatal ending. Ordinarily there is a considerable interval between the fits, perhaps a fortnight or a month ; but they may occur more or less frequently than this. There is also considerable variation in the length of time, following a fit, during which an epileptic is incapacitated from his ordinary duties. Sometimes serious and constant symptoms of mental derangement manifest themselves, and this may lead to progressive mental decline, or dementia (q.v.).

True epilepsy mostly begins in early life, infantile convulsions sometimes being of this nature ; or, at any rate, the fits lead on from these, and it affects boys and girls equally, though later on males predominate. Many epileptics inherit their disease ; it may be that a parent has been addicted to alcoholic excess, but it is believed that such addiction in the parent of an epileptic is only a manifestation of a neuropathic constitution rather than that alcoholic excess by a person belonging to a sound stock would cause epilepsy in the progeny. Eyestrain, painful scars and other sources of irritation have been blamed for precipitating attacks.

Fits which are indistinguishable from those of epilepsy occur in a large variety of disorders, as, for example, hysteria, anaemia, diabetes, general paralysis of the insane, dementia praecox, and so on.

There is a form of the disease, known as Jacksonian epilepsy, which is caused by local irritation of the brain by depressed bone, inflammatory swelling or a scar, following an injury to the head. Here the spasmodic movements affect a limb or the face, according to the part of the surface of the brain which is irritated. Consciousness is not lost unless the fits are general.

The incidence of epilepsy would be much diminished if epileptics refrained from marrying and having children; every child of an epileptic need not have the taint, but in a family some members are almost sure to have it.

When a child is subject to fits, an examination should be made for possible sources of irritation, and such should be remedied. An operation on the cause of irritation may cure Jacksonian epilepsy, but if the fits are very general it is unlikely that they will be cured even by removal of a possible irritant.

Attacking the Element of Habit

The object in view in the medicinal treatment of epilepsy is to prevent the occurrence of fits for a long period—two years at least—and so attempt to eliminate the element of habit. The drugs most generally used are the bromides, especially the potassium salt; but, as this may be generally depressing when used constantly for a long time, it is often combined with the sodium and ammonium salts, or the sodium salt is given in preference, from 30 to 90 grains of this or of the mixed salts being given daily. This amount is given in three doses, and it may be arranged that the last dose is twice as strong as the others, more especially for nocturnal epilepsy. Each dose is freely diluted with water. This lessens the risk of the drugs irritating the stomach or causing a bromide rash on the skin, particularly if about 10 grains of sodium bicarbonate are given with the dose. If, nevertheless, a rash tends to occur, short courses of arsenic should be taken.

Amongst other drugs given for the disease are borax along with bromides, belladonna and luminal. The instructions of the doctor as regards dosage should be faithfully carried out, though untoward symptoms should be brought to his notice at once. A sudden interruption of the medicine is very undesirable.

Dietetic Principles to Observe

The diet should be simple, condiments and highly seasoned dishes being objectionable, and meat should be taken in strictly moderate amount. No alcohol should be taken, and tea and coffee only sparingly, if at all. No late meals should be indulged in. The bowels should be kept active. Exercise in the open air is desirable.

The general treatment of epileptiform fits occurring in other disorders is discussed under appropriate headings. It may be useful to say here, however, that, as many of the cases of epilepsy which occurred in soldiers during the Great War, and which closely resembled ordinary or idiopathic epilepsy, were shown to be of hysterical origin and susceptible of psycho-therapy, it may be that emotional stress is a factor in some cases occurring in civil life, and that similar treatment might be useful.

When fits are numerous and difficult to control, the best treatment is that received in an epileptic colony, and should symptoms of mental derangement manifest themselves the desirability of early removal to an asylum should be considered forthwith.

The treatment of a fit follows very much the same lines, whatever its cause. The patient is placed on his back, and although the movements should be restrained sufficiently to prevent him from hurting himself, no attempt should be made to suppress them by force. A piece of wood, the handle of a spoon or anything similar, should be wrapped in a fold of a handkerchief and pushed between the back teeth, to act as a gag and prevent the tongue from being bitten. Tight clothing about the neck and chest should be loosened. If the patient vomits, he should be turned on his side. As he is recovering he should be spoken to reassuringly, the possibility of his being in a somnambulic state and capable of sudden, violent action being borne in mind.

See Bromide; Double Consciousness; Ecstasy; Fit; Hysteria; Psycho-therapy.

EPIPHYSIS. A long bone, that is, one possessing a shaft and two articular ends, is at the outset a bar of cartilage or gristle, and becomes bone by centres of ossification appearing and extending until the process is complete. Such occur not only in the shaft, or diaphysis, but at the ends, and a stage arrives when both the shaft and the ends are bone, but the latter are separated from the shaft by a plate of cartilage. Each end is then spoken of as an epiphysis, and the plate of cartilage as the epiphyseal line. The persistence of these plates makes it possible for the bone to grow in length, and by about the twenty-fifth year all have been replaced by bone and no further growth is possible.

Epiphyses are not confined to long bones, however, but occur in any bone which develops from cartilage.

So long as the epiphyseal cartilage exists, it represents a vulnerable part of the bone as, by the exercise of sufficient force, the epiphysis may be dragged or knocked off the shaft (*see* illustration p. 319).

Such an accident may occur from pulling on the limbs of young children, as by lifting up a child by the wrists.

Inflammation of the epiphyseal cartilage, or epiphysitis, may be acute or chronic. The acute disease is due to the invasion of the cartilage by one of the micro-organisms which cause suppuration. The organism is carried in the blood, but its settlement and activity in the cartilage may be favoured by general debility or by an injury to the cartilage, such as might be caused by a wrench. The mischief may spread from the epiphysis to the whole bone, causing the serious condition known as osteomyelitis, and eventuating in acute necrosis, or death of the bone.

Acute epiphysitis has a superficial resemblance to acute rheumatism in the neighbouring joint, but the pain and tenderness are outside the joint, and the patient looks more ill than would be expected in the other disorder. Surgical care is extremely urgent. Chronic epiphysitis is generally due to tuberculosis though sometimes it is syphilitic in origin. Tuberculosis of a joint in children begins usually as an epiphysitis.

See Bone; Cartilage; Joint.

EPISCLERITIS. A patchy inflammation of the superficial part of the sclerotic coat, or white, of the eye is called episcleritis. The disease occurs more often in adults, especially women. Rheumatism appears to be a common cause. The patches have a purple colour and may be elevated above the general surface and hard; often there is no pain. As one patch disappears, another comes out elsewhere, and both eyes may be affected. The site of a patch may show a dark discoloration. A patch may last but a short time and not be followed by others, but generally the complaint is a tedious one.

The disorder commonly referred to as hot eye is rather similar, but there is no hard nodule, as in the other type, nor is there any stain left when a patch disappears. The disease most often attacks middle-aged people, and recurrences usually take place over several years. Both diseases require expert treatment.

EPISPASTIC. A blistering agent is also called an epispastic.

See Blister.

EPISTAXIS. The technical name for bleeding from the nose is epistaxis.

See Bleeding.

EPITHELIOMA. A carcinoma developing in the epithelium (*q.v.*) of the skin or a mucous membrane is called an epithelioma. Chronic irritation, such as that caused by a jagged tooth to the tongue, for instance, may result in an epithelioma.

See Cancer.

EPITHELIUM. The tissue which covers the surface of the body and lines its cavities is called epithelium. The cells of which it is composed are crowded together with very little cement substance to separate them. If they form a single layer, the epithelium is said to be simple, or, if several layers, compound or stratified, except that one generally uses the term transitional when, as in the bladder lining, there are no more than three or four layers.

The cells exhibit various shapes. Those lining the peritoneum and other cavities within the body consist of flat, thin plates joined to each other at the edges so as to produce a tesselated appearance. Such are described as pavement cells, and pavement epithelium is also spoken of as endothelium when found in the blood vessels, lymphatics, serous and other cavities.

Again, the cells may be cubical or columnar in shape. Cubical cells are often found lining the ducts of glands, and columnar cells form the usual covering of a mucous membrane which lines the alimentary, respiratory and other passages. It is so called because it is kept moist by the exudation of a sticky liquid known as mucus. In the air passages, the Fallopian tubes and elsewhere, the free border of the columnar cells is prolonged into a number of hair-like processes, or cilia (*see* page 139). These carry out a lashing movement by which particles are carried along the surface of the membrane. In this way sputum is brought up from the air passages, for example, and with it particles of dust which may have been inhaled.

Sometimes epithelial cells are spheroidal or polyhedral in shape. These are found in the deeper layers of stratified epithelium, such as the epidermis or scarf skin, and in many glands. In glands the cells are sometimes referred to as secreting epithelium.

The hairs, nails and enamel of the teeth consist of modified epithelial cells.

See Cell ; Tissue.

EPSOM SALT. Because it was originally obtained from the mineral waters of Epsom, magnesium sulphate is commonly known as Epsom salt. It occurs as small, colourless crystals, and has a bitter taste. It is freely soluble in water. It acts as a saline cathartic, and is given in doses of 120 to 240 grains, or, if given in repeated

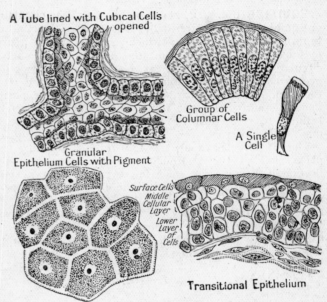

A Tube lined with Cubical Cells opened

Group of Columnar Cells

A Single Cell

Granular Epithelium Cells with Pigment

Surface Cells
Middle Cellular Layer
Lower Layer of Cells

Transitional Epithelium

Epithelium. Various types of cells which make up epithelial tissue

doses, 30 to 90 grains. There is also an effervescent form, and this is given in doses of 240 to 480 grains.

Magnesium sulphate is contained in the compound senna mixture, or black draught, and in the so-called white mixture, and may be taken in these forms.

Magnesium sulphate acts as an antidote in poisoning by lead or carbolic acid. A lotion made by dissolving 1 ounce in 10 ounces of water, if dabbed on the skin and allowed to dry, is a protection against mosquito bites.

See Cathartic ; Magnesium.

EPULIS. The name epulis is given to two tumours found on the gums, though they differ in nature. The simple epulis is composed of fibrous tissue. It only occurs when there is septic mischief, such as pyorrhoea, in a tooth socket, and grows from the periosteum covering the jaw-bone or from the socket. It forms a rounded, red swelling which later may ulcerate.

The malignant epulis is a myeloid sarcoma, that is, one containing a large number of giant cells. Compared with other sarcomata, it has a low degree of malignancy. At first it forms a smooth mass of a purple colour, but soon ulcerates and acquires a fungous appearance.

Removal by operation is the treatment in either case, and it is necessary also to remove tooth-stumps and bone to which the growth is attached; this must be done more freely for the malignant type.

See Gum; Mouth; Pyorrhoea; Tumour.

EQUILIBRIUM. The sense of balance or equilibrium is controlled by the lesser brain, or cerebellum, to which centre messages are carried from the semi-circular canals in the inner ear, from the eye, from muscles and joints, and from the skin. In accordance with such messages, impulses pass out from the cerebellum to the muscles concerned in maintaining posture.

The semicircular canals are tiny tubes placed behind the vestibule or middle portion of the inner ear, one being vertical and from before backwards, another vertical but from side to side, and the third horizontal. Each is filled with fluid, and this is set in motion by movements of the head only or of the whole body in the direction in which the tube is placed.

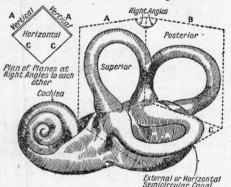

Equilibrium. Rôle of the semicircular canals of the internal ear in the maintenance of balance

At one end of each canal there is an expansion, or ampulla, containing a viscid mass, the cupula, in which are embedded crystals of calcium carbonate or otoliths. Into this mass hairs project, and the movements of the otoliths, occasioned by movements in the canal fluid, excite impulses in the terminals of the vestibular nerve, which pass on into the brain.

When the head or body is rapidly rotated and then brought to a standstill, the continuance of the effect of rotation on the canal fluid may cause so much giddiness that the person is not able to keep erect; also, pressure on the ear-drum, as in syringing, may be communicated to the canals and cause giddiness. Serious giddiness occurs in Ménière's disease, which is caused by bleeding into the canals or some other disturbance of the circulation in the canals.

In the disease known as locomotor ataxia there is a diminution of feeling which affects the soles of the feet, so that an affected person feels as if he were walking on cotton wool, and the sense of the position of joints and muscles is also affected. In this disease, therefore, it may be impossible to stand with the eyes shut or to walk steadily without watching the feet as they are lifted and placed on the ground. With these sensations in good order, however, a blind person is perfectly steady.

Disease of the cerebellum seriously interferes with the sense of balance, the gait of an affected person resembling that of alcoholic intoxication.

See Ataxia; Dizziness; Ear; Gait.

ERECTILE TISSUE. In one or two parts of the body the tissue is very freely supplied with blood vessels, and when stimulated these vessels become engorged with blood, so that the tissue swells and becomes hard; such is called erectile tissue. It occurs, for example, in the turbinate bodies of the nose, which are ordinarily of such dimensions as to leave a free passage for air, but which by the stimulus of cold air are made to expand greatly. By thus lessening the space through which the air can pass, and at the same time increasing the area of warm blood to which it is exposed, the air is properly heated before it passes on into the air-passages.

ERGOT. The spawn of a fungus found growing on rye, ergot causes contraction of the smooth muscle fibres in blood vessels, the uterus, the bladder, and elsewhere in the body. It thus may control bleeding, correct menstrual disorders, or stimulate a sluggish bladder. It is generally given as a routine measure at the end of labour to procure firm contraction of the uterus, the expulsion of clots, and to lessen the risk of undue bleeding. There are several preparations, including the dried extract, which is given in pills or tablets, in doses of 2 to 8 grains ; the liquid extract, dose 10 to 30 minims ; and the ammoniated tincture, dose $\frac{1}{2}$ to 1 drachm.

Poisoning by Ergot. From the continuous use of rye bread containing the fungus, chronic poisoning, known as ergotism, may occur. There may be itching and tingling of the skin, followed by numbness or actual anaesthesia of the hands and feet, and parts of the fingers and toes may become gangrenous, or die. In other instances there may be dimness of vision and some degree of deafness, epileptiform convulsions and perhaps mental weakness. Sickness and diarrhoea may be troublesome symptoms.

An overdose of the drug may cause acute poisoning, characterised by sickness, purging, headache, dizziness, convulsions, loss of consciousness, and perhaps death. An emetic should be given, and thereafter a dose of castor oil and copious draughts of strong tea. The patient should be kept warm.

EROSION. There are many conditions in which body tissues are gradually destroyed or eroded, though the method is not always the same. Continuous pressure or friction will cause erosion even of sound tissues, but much more readily and rapidly if the tissue is softened by disease. Thus, in inflammation of joints the diseased cartilages are often eroded by the pressure of the bones on one another ; they may, in fact, be destroyed altogether. A remarkable instance of erosion is that of the vertebrae by the pressure of an aortic aneurysm ; the constant repetition of pulsations in the dilated vessel gradually wears away the solid bone, and may give rise to excruciating pain. Perforation of the cartilaginous septum of the nose may occur simply from the irritation of dust passing over some projecting spur ; erosion of the septum also frequently followed the use of cocaine snuff.

The so-called erosions of the neck of the womb, so far from representing loss of tissue, are actually due to overgrowth. They look like raw patches on the mucous membrane, but the appearance is generally illusory.

See Bone ; Joint ; Necrosis ; Womb.

ERUPTION. *See* Rash ; Skin.

ERYSIPELAS. An acute infectious disease sometimes referred to as St. Anthony's Fire and " the rose," erysipelas is caused by a streptococcus which invades the lymphatic vessels just beneath the scarf skin and causes inflammation. There results a bright red patch which spreads, the spreading edge not fading into the normal skin like many inflammatory blushes, but being raised and well defined ; usually blisters appear on the patch, the fluid in which is clear at first, but soon becomes turbid. The affected part feels hot and stiff, but rarely actually painful unless it is the scalp, when the pain may be very great. From the absorption of poisons from the erysipelatous skin there is fever, sometimes reaching 104° F. and over, and generally delirium also. The expansion of the patch may cease after about five days, and the temperature fall ; but, on the other hand, the disease may be prolonged up to three weeks.

Protraction of the disease causes great prostration ; the tongue becomes dry, cracked and brown, and low muttering delirium sets in. Sometimes the infection extends to the loose tissue beneath the skin, and there is cellulitis as well as erysipelas. Pus forms freely, and parts of the skin overlying it may die.

Erysipelas begins most commonly on the face, infection being admitted probably through some little crack about the edge of the mouth or nostril, but it may spread to other parts of the body. In other instances infection begins at some wound or ulcer. Cases of wandering erysipelas are described where the disease disappears at one part of the body only to reappear at another. In numbers of cases there is a tendency to recurrence on the face particularly, and in time there is considerable thickening of the skin and more or less deformity.

Erysipelas is a notifiable disease. A person with an open wound or a woman who has just been confined, runs a great risk of contracting the disease if brought into contact with it directly or indirectly. Elderly people and alcoholics are liable to succumb to it.

In the general treatment of the disease anti-streptococcic serum and intramuscular injections of colloidal manganese have been successfully used. The tincture of perchloride of iron, in doses of 20 to 30 minims, is an old remedy. The diet should be easily digested but liberal. Alcoholic and other stimulants, such as strychnine, may be ordered by the doctor.

For the local treatment ichthyol is a favourite remedy. It may be used in watery solution or as an ointment, from 20 per cent. upwards. Sometimes the patch may be prevented from spreading by painting the sound skin, some distance in front of the edge, with a strong solution of silver nitrate or with tincture of iodine. Should cellulitis be present, free incisions will be necessary to drain off the pus.

Complications such as broncho-pneumonia, meningitis, Bright's disease and others will demand appropriate treatment. *See* Dermatitis; Eczema; Erythema; Skin.

ERYTHEMA. Redness of the skin, due to flushing of the blood vessels, may be described as erythema, a Greek word meaning redness or a blush, and indeed blushing is a good example of a transitory erythema. Redness due to an increase in the number or size of the blood vessels, as occurs in birth marks, is distinguished from erythema, and also that due to bleeding into the skin; in the latter pressure on the skin does not cause the redness to disappear as it does in erythema.

The cause of erythema may be something external, such as sunlight, artificial sunlight, X-rays, heat, cold, friction or chemical irritants, the redness occurring on the part exposed to irritation. Thus, blacksmiths or stokers often have the face and arms affected. Erythema due to opposing surfaces of the body rubbing on one another is called intertrigo and may occur in the groin of a fat person, below the breast in women and in other situations. Erythema on the buttocks in infants, the so-called napkin rash, may be due to the napkins not being changed sufficiently often or to their being washed with a strong alkaline soap which is not rinsed out of them. A chilblain is an example of erythema caused by cold.

Erythema from the action of internal poisons may be a symptom of scarlet fever or some other infectious disease. It may be caused also by drugs or poisons which have been swallowed and by poisons generated in the bowel or elsewhere in the patient's body. In this group there are, however, several more or less definitely defined skin affections which deserve more particular mention.

Erythema multiforme is characterised by patches of redness, having different shapes, particularly on the back of the hands and arms, and the extensor surfaces of the feet and legs. Sometimes there are blisters on these patches. The disease most often affects young people, especially females, and may persist for several weeks. Apart from slight burning the patches cause no discomfort and there is no subsequent peeling. At the beginning there may be considerable fever. Sometimes, however, there is sore throat and pains in the joints. A special form of the disease, erythema iris, exhibits lesions consisting of a central vesicle and one or more red rings around it.

The treatment consists of rest in bed on a light diet, sodium salicylate or aspirin and a soothing dusting powder or lotion, such as one containing zinc oxide.

Nodular Form of the Disease

In erythema nodosum, which may occur as part of the multiform variety or independently, there are round or oval nodular patches, most often on the skin below the knees but perhaps also on the arms below the elbows. These have some resemblance to bruises and so the disease is sometimes called erythema contusiforme. The patches are acutely tender. After persisting for some time they show discoloration similar to that which follows a bruise. Sometimes this form of erythema is complicated by endocarditis or pericarditis. The treatment includes salicylates and soothing applications to the patches.

There is another skin condition, erythema induratum, or Bazin's disease, which somewhat resembles erythema nodosum as the same parts are affected, though the most usual site for the patches is on the calves. The patches are, however, very indolent and show a tendency to suppurate. They represent a form of tuberculosis and are treated accordingly.

Erythema scarlatiniforme is a disorder in which the rash bears a strong resemblance to that of scarlatina, or scarlet fever, and the greater part of the surface of the body may be covered. Should the face be affected there is not, however, the zone of pallor round the mouth which one finds in scarlet fever, nor is there the strawberry tongue. The distinction between the disorders can only be drawn properly by a doctor, however.

Lupus erythematosus, despite its name, has no relationship to ordinary lupus, which is a tuberculous disease. It affects youngish people usually, and mostly females. The erythema begins on one or both cheeks as a rounded patch which spreads at its margins, and, as there may come to be a large patch on each cheek connected across the bridge of the nose, the appearance is sometimes designated the butterfly eruption. Often there is a patch on the ear or the scalp.

The patches become scaly, and if a scale be pulled off its lower surface is seen to be shaggy. As the disease spreads healing takes place in the central portions, the healed area consisting of scar tissue.

Though it may occur in an acute form the disease is usually protracted. Salicylates and ichthyol are among the drugs given internally. The external treatment includes plasters of salicylic acid and application of light and electricity.

Erythromelalgia is a disorder characterised by sudden erythema of the hands and feet, the colouration being dusky red ; at the same time there is a sharp burning pain in the affected parts. The disorder is considered to be due to a disturbance of the vaso-motor nerves, similar to what occurs in Raynaud's disease (*q.v.*). Treatment is difficult, but in some cases stretching the nerves of the limb has been successful in curing the disorder.

See Chafing ; Dermatitis ; Eczema ; Intertrigo.

ESMARCH'S BANDAGE. This name is applied to the triangular bandage and also to a rubber elastic bandage used to prevent bleeding in amputation of a limb. The limb is elevated and the bandage is applied from below upwards till well above the intended site of operation ; three or four turns are then made round the limb and the lower part of the bandage is loosened off, leaving that part of the limb bloodless.

See Bandage ; Elastic Bandage.

ETHER. A colourless volatile liquid with a strong odour, ether is used in medicine as an anaesthetic, a stimulant and a carminative. For producing general anaesthesia purified ether is employed, either with a special apparatus, such as a Clover's inhaler, or by dropping the drug on a piece of fabric placed over the mouth and nose. Generally speaking, it is a safer anaesthetic than chloroform, but it tends to cause irritation of the air tubes, and may possibly cause bronchitis or even broncho-pneumonia, though this is not very common. Sprayed on the skin, it chills the surface by its rapid evaporation, and so acts as a local anaesthetic. It may be used to lessen the pain of an incision or over painful points in neuralgia.

Ether is highly inflammable, and no naked light should be brought near it.

Ether may be used as a stimulant in fainting, collapse or cardiac weakness. The dose is 45 to 60 minims, or if repeated, 15 to 30 minims, in water. Sometimes in an emergency it is used hypodermically. It may relieve flatulence and asthmatic symptoms. Spirit of ether and the compound spirit of ether, either of which may be referred to as Hoffmann's anodyne, although the second was originally meant, are given in doses of 60 to 90 minims, or if to be repeated, 20 to 40 minims, and for the same purposes as those just mentioned.

Ether is used as a solvent in collodion and in ethereal tinctures. It is a solvent of fat, and is sometimes used to cleanse a greasy skin, either in a lotion or as ether soap, for which purpose, however, methylated ether may be used.

The spirit of nitrous ether, better known as sweet spirit of nitre, increases perspiration and the action of the kidneys, and is usually included in fever mixtures. The dose is 15 to 60 minims ; for a child of one year, 8 minims. It is often successful in relieving infantile colic, and is given in a little water. It is used as a solvent for silver nitrate when this is to be painted on the skin or a mucous membrane.

Acetic ether, a colourless liquid with an agreeable odour, is sometimes used as a stimulant.

ETHMOID BONE. The ethmoid bone is situated in the fore part of the base of the skull, between the orbits and in the roof of the nose. It consists of a horizontal plate, to which are attached two lateral masses, and a vertical portion projecting upwards and downwards from the middle of the horizontal plate ; the upper part, known as the crista galli, or cock-crest, gives attachment to the forward end of the falx cerebri, the sickle-shaped membranous structure which separates the two hemispheres of the large brain, while the lower takes part in forming the septum which divides the interior of the nose into right and left cavities.

The horizontal plate is perforated by numerous openings, hence it is called the cribriform plate, and hence also the name ethmoid given to the bone, as this means sieve-like. The olfactory lobes lie on the upper surface of this plate on either side of the crista galli, and through the openings come to them the fibres of the olfactory nerves which are distributed over the upper third of each nasal cavity.

The lateral masses help to form the inner wall of each orbit, and, with their other side, the lateral wall of each nasal cavity. From the lateral mass two bony shelves curve over into the nasal cavity. These are the superior and middle turbinate processes. Each mass is a sponge-like structure, the spaces within it being called the ethmoid cells ; these may become infected from the nose and suppuration occur within them. It will then be difficult to get rid of septic mischief from the nose.

See Nose.

ETHYL ALCOHOL. The spirit contained in wines and spirits and used in medicine is known as ethyl alcohol. Wood spirit, or methyl alcohol, is more poisonous, though a purified form has occasionally been used in medicine.

See Alcohol.

ETHYL CHLORIDE. A colourless and very volatile liquid, ethyl chloride is much used as a general anaesthetic for short operations, such as tooth extractions, opening abscesses, the removal of tonsils and adenoids and so on. It is given with a bag inhaler. It is the drug most often used as a spray to produce local anaesthesia.

ETHYLENE. Olefiant, or ethylene, gas is used as a general anaesthetic and appears to be especially useful when the patient is very ill. It is very inflammable and no naked light or cautery is permissible in the room in which the gas is being used.

ETHYL FORMATE. A colourless liquid with an odour of peach kernels, ethyl formate, also known as formic ether, has been used in medicine to relieve pain and as a narcotic. It is sometimes used as a flavouring agent.

ETHYL NITRITE. The solution of ethyl nitrite is a colourless liquid with actions similar to those of amyl nitrite (*q.v.*). It is given in doses of 15 to 20 minims, and the dose should be added to two tablespoonsful of water just before use ; if the drug is mixed with water for any length of time it decomposes. It is used in the preparation of sweet spirits of nitre. It should not be handled near a naked light as it is highly inflammable.

EUCAINE. A synthetic compound, eucaine, or benzamine, is a substance resembling cocaine, and may be used instead of the latter as a local anaesthetic for eye injuries or operations, tooth extraction, etc. It is much less poisonous than cocaine, and has the further advantage that it can be sterilised by boiling without losing its virtues. It can be used in an ointment for the relief of intolerable itching. The preparation which has been most often employed is β-eucaine hydrochloride, but β-eucaine borate appears to have greater anaesthetising power.

EUCALYPTUS. A distillate of the fresh leaves of species of the Australian blue gum, eucalyptus oil acts as an antiseptic, disinfectant and deodorant. It is given inwardly in doses of ½ to 3 minims for fermentative dyspepsia, intestinal parasites and other affections of the alimentary tract, and as it is excreted in the breath it is useful also in infections of the air passages and when the sputum is foul. The dose may be dropped on a piece of lump sugar.

Affections of the air passages, as in a common cold or influenza, may be treated with the oil by using it in a spray or in a steam inhalation, or by dropping it on some such apparatus as Burney Yeo's inhaler, but here it is better rather to use eucalyptol, which is obtained from the oil. Ten drops of the oil shaken up with a half-glass of water provide an efficient mouth wash and gargle. Eucalyptus ointment is a good application for burns and abrasions and equal parts of the oil and of olive oil make a useful embrocation for rheumatism.

The dried garnet-coloured exudate, or red gum, obtained from species of eucalyptus trees has an astringent action. It is also known as kino eucalypti, is given in doses of 5 to 20 grains in powder, tablets or lozenges and is also used as an insufflation, a decoction, a liquid extract and a tincture. The decoction is given in doses of 2 to 4 drachms for diarrhoea; it makes a good gargle for a relaxed throat, for which purpose also the lozenge may be used, being allowed to dissolve slowly in the mouth. The tincture is a good application for arresting bleeding.

See Atomiser; Inhalation; Spray.

EUGENOL. A colourless, oily liquid, eugenol is the main constituent of oil of cloves. It is a powerful antiseptic and also reduces the sensibility of mucous membranes. It is used in dentistry.

EUONYMIN. The root-bark of the spindle-tree contains a bitter glucoside, known as euonymin, which acts as a cathartic, causing copious watery stools. The dry extract of the bark, also called euonymin, is given in doses of 1 to 2 grains and is particularly useful for sluggishness of the liver caused by free living. The drug affects the heart in a similar way to digitalis (*q.v.*).

EUSOL. A solution containing chlorinated lime and boracic acid is known as eusol. It is of great value in cleaning out infected wounds, and the method of slow irrigation with eusol through rubber tubes, known as Carrel's tubes, is sometimes adopted for this purpose. The disinfecting action of eusol is brought about by the chlorine which it liberates. Dakin's solution is a similar preparation.

EUSTACHIAN TUBE. Just behind the posterior opening of each cavity of the nose there is the opening of the

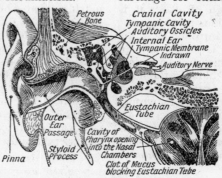

Eustachian tube obstructed by mucus, with consequent retraction of the ear drum

Eustachian, or auditory tube, which connects the cavity behind the nose, the naso-pharynx, with the middle ear. This tube, about 2 inches long, consists of cartilage for rather more than its lower two-thirds, while the remainder is of bone. The tube passes upwards and outwards from the naso-pharynx, and its lowest part is funnel-shaped. If the cheeks are blown out while the mouth is tightly closed there is a sensation of pressure on the ear drums. This is due to air being forced from the naso-pharynx up into the middle ear. The same thing happens when one swallows. The main function of the Eustachian tube, in fact, is to regulate the amount of air in the middle ear. If this is excessive, it presses the drum outwards, and if deficient, on the other hand, the drum is pressed inwards by the air in the external passage of the ear; in either event, hearing is more or less impaired.

Deafness often accompanies a common cold, and this is caused by the extension of the nasal catarrh to the Eustachian tubes, causing their lining to swell and block the passage of air through them. The air present in the middle ear is already diminished by some of it being absorbed, and the lessened pressure in the middle ear leads to the drum being pushed in. With the disappearance of the catarrh in the tubes, when the cold gets better, the hearing is restored.

Chronic catarrhal conditions at the back of the nose, due to adenoids or other disorders, are dangerous because they may be accompanied by chronic catarrh in the tubes, and either by the constant blocking of the tubes, or, more frequently, by the extension of the catarrh to the middle ear itself, permanent impairment of hearing may result.

If there is sepsis at the back of the nose, in connexion with either acute or chronic trouble there, it may spread up the tubes and cause suppuration in the middle ear. Probably the tubes normally serve to allow the escape of mucus from the ear, but it is unlikely that much fluid will escape in this way, so that if there is fluid in the middle ear, it must be given vent by incising the drum, otherwise, unless it breaks through of itself, it is likely to cause more serious trouble.

In view of the risk of introducing septic matter into the ear, it is undesirable to inflate the tubes when this can be avoided. The ordinary method of blowing the nose, that is, by compressing both nostrils and suddenly letting go, is therefore wrong, because it inflates the tubes.

The proper method of blowing the nose is to compress each nostril in turn and blow down into the handkerchief through the other.

When deafness is due to narrowing of the Eustachian tube, an effort is made to relieve it by blowing air into the middle ear. This is done by using a Politzer bag, a rubber ball with a nozzle for putting into the nostril. The patient is asked to swallow, or blow out his cheeks, and at the same time the ball is compressed, and air is forced through the nose and up through the Eustachian tubes. If there is any difficulty in getting the air to enter the tube, an Eustachian catheter is passed through the nose and into the tube, and air is forced up through this. All such procedures can only be carried out by a doctor, however.

See Deafness ; Ear.

EXALGIN. This is the trade name for methyl-acetanilide, a drug which is used as a pain-killer. It must be taken with great care or much depression may result.

See Acetanilide.

EXANTHEMA. *See* Rash.

EXCISION. The cutting out of diseased organs or pieces of tissue is generally referred to as an excision ; for example, the excision of the breast, of a joint, or of a growth.

See Enucleation.

EXCRETA. The faeces, the urine and the sweat are spoken of collectively as the excreta ; they consist of the waste products of the body which, unless completely removed, will clog its mechanism and impair its activities. The process of their removal is called excretion and the organs concerned are excretory organs.

EXERCISE. For the young exercise is essential to a complete and sturdy development of the body and its organs, and most children exhibit a natural disposition for vigorous exercise. So much so that while it could be admitted that a child might have no desire to romp and still be healthy, this should not be assumed until the child has been scrutinised. In adolescents a want of keenness for exercise may be due to sheer indolence, and is often so where older people are concerned, but in either case it may be desirable to have an overhaul of the physical condition before insisting on exercise, certainly of a strenuous character.

The habit of taking regular exercise requires to be cultivated, like every other habit which is at odds with self-indulgence, otherwise, should a sedentary calling be adopted, very little, and probably quite insufficient, exercise will be taken throughout life.

Moreover, if games are not begun in early life, it is not common for one who takes them up later on to acquire sufficient skill to make a game thoroughly enjoyable. The importance of physical training in education for citizenship is better recognized than formerly, but recognition is still far short of what it should be.

Lack of exercise means a relatively poor expansion of the chest, sluggishness of the digestive apparatus, flabbiness of muscles, probably including the heart, and an imperfect removal of waste products from the muscles and related tissues and of excretion by the skin. In course of time health is depreciated by these things and the desire and capacity for exercise lessened ; in fact, a vicious circle is established, to break through which remedial exercises may be necessary, but these will probably only have a limited scope.

The benefits of exercise out of doors is enhanced by the stimulation of the skin, by the movements of fresh air and, in bathing, by contact with water, and by the action of the ultra-violet rays of light, particularly when a considerable part of the body-surface is exposed. To secure these advantages as far as possible, when exercise is taken indoors, the windows should be wide open and a minimum of clothing should be worn.

Hard exercise should not be undertaken except when in training.

It is dangerous, for example, to indulge in strenuous exercise at the week-ends if the employment be sedentary and little or no exercise is taken through the week ; or to go in for hard exercises, such as mountain climbing, at the beginning of the annual holiday without some preliminary training. Indulgence in exercises which call for brisk, rapid movements, tennis and dancing, for example, by those who are out of training for the exercise in question, may readily induce a strain or even rupture of some muscle ; this is especially true for older people.

Walking is a most useful form of outdoor exercise as, by regulating the pace and distance and choosing hilly or level routes, the amount of exercise taken can be graduated. For those whose capacity is small, gentle walking on the level makes a good beginning of an attempt to improve fitness. A sensible choice of clothing will enable more walking to be done ; many people overweight, and so overheat, themselves.

While running is excellent for younger people, long distance running and sprinting require preliminary training, and before engaging in serious athletics, there should be an examination by a doctor. Sprinting becomes dangerous as middle life is approached.

Question of Athletics for Girls

Whatever may have been said at one time about the suitability of athletics for girls, very few will be found in these days to gainsay their value. There is no need for girls to engage in rough-and-tumble games, and it is hardly expedient that they should, but sharp, brisk games, such as hockey, can usually be played with advantage. A girl's frame needs muscular exercise for its development not less than does her brother's, and failure to recognize this has been responsible for much disabling maldevelopment in the past.

Swimming is a good exercise for those whose circulation is good. Contrary to popular opinion, it is not specially useful for chest development ; it helps in this direction mainly by tending to cause deep breathing, as many other kinds of exercise do. This subject is also discussed under the heading Bathing.

Football, hockey, and similar games require training. As a rule, football should not be indulged in before the age of nine or after that of thirty. Such games develop the team spirit, cultivate control of the temper, and are thus invaluable.

Riding develops the sense of balance and calls into play a large number of muscles. It gives a certain sense of exhilaration, and the same applies to motor driving, though this gives hardly so much actual muscular work.

Exercise for the Middle-aged

Golf is the ideal game for the middle-aged, as it can be played as quietly as needs be ; yet there is exercise for many muscles, and need for co-ordinated effort.

Dancing possesses the advantage that it is done to music, rhythm and balance being brought into play. It is the more useful, according to the extent to which a close, hot atmosphere, late hours and loss of sleep are eliminated.

For those who have the opportunity and taste for it, gardening may supply about as much additional exercise as they require.

Drill is useful, especially when practised in the open air, and the exercise is made more agreeable by being done with others and at the word of command ; this applies also to other kinds of physical training. As was demonstrated in the Great War, regular drill may have an extraordinary effect in improving physique. Eurhythmics are the expression of music by rhythmical movements, and are useful for developing the sense of rhythm.

Several exercises may easily be practised in the bedroom when there is no opportunity for anything more. The following are examples (*see* Plate XVI) :

(1) Put the hands on the floor with the arms straight and the body and legs extended so as to rest on the toes. Raise the body and lower it several times by bending the elbows.

(2) Standing erect, lower the body by bending the knees to the full extent, and then rise slowly.

(3) Perform shadow boxing, that is, strike out at any imaginary opponent.

Pieces of apparatus may be used to give variety and interest to exercises. Dumb-bells may be made of wood or metal, and for a young man should generally weigh from 2 to 4 pounds. Some are provided with springs in the handles for strengthening the grip, and dumb-bells may also be provided with elastic straps for resisting the movements made with them. The so-called " strong man " ideal of fitness should be avoided, however, and exercises calling for quickness and elasticity should be mixed with the slower exercises done with dumb-bells. Indian clubs generally weigh from 3 to 4 pounds, but may be lighter or heavier. A skipping rope furnishes a useful means of taking exercise ; the rope should have weight.

Gymnastics formerly meant exercises performed while naked, but now the term means exercises taken on such forms of apparatus as the vaulting-horse, the trapeze, parallel and horizontal bars, and so on. With a skilled instructor fitness can quickly be acquired in a gymnasium by a healthy person. Jiu-jitsu consists of movements for overpowering, disabling or overthrowing an opponent, but, like boxing and ordinary wrestling, its practice requires and fosters a high standard of physical fitness.

Remedial Exercises for the Unfit

When exercises are directed towards the cure or improvement of disorders of any kind they are said to be remedial. Such are the abdominal exercises, breathing exercises, exercises for flat foot, etc., discussed under these headings.

The well-known Swedish, or Ling, exercises are used for general physical training in Sweden, but in other countries mainly as remedial exercises. They are performed with the patient lying, sitting, standing, kneeling or suspended, and may consist of movements by the patient himself, or active movements ; or of movements performed on him by another person, passive movements. Also this other person may resist the movements done by the patient and vice-versa, the former being called concentric, and the latter eccentric movements. Any muscle or set of muscles can thus be exercised.

The Zander method (*see* Plate XVI, 6) consists in fixing the part to be exercised in a moving part of a machine which performs the exercise independently of the patient, and may be of use for stiffness of the joints and other defects, but has the disadvantage that the attention of the patient need not be engaged, and this is a factor which cannot readily be dispensed with in efficient exercise. Except for simple complaints, remedial exercise must not only be prescribed by a doctor, but in many instances be carried out under his immediate supervision.

See Abdominal Exercises ; Bathing ; Breathing Exercises ; Massage ; Sedentary Habits ; Training.

EXHAUSTION. *See* Fatigue.

EXOPHTHALMIC GOITRE. Also known as Graves' disease, and, abroad, as Basedow's disease, exophthalmic goitre is thus named because typical cases present two abnormal conditions, protrusion of the eyeballs, exophthalmos, and enlargement of the thyroid gland, or goitre.

The normal thyroid gland contains an immense number of spaces filled with colloid material which is secreted by cells which line the spaces. This colloid material contains an organic compound of iodine, called thyroxin, which is liberated into the blood circulation for certain purposes, amongst which are the stimulation of general body metabolism and the destruction of poisonous substances. From a variety of causes, including chronic sepsis, and mental stress, an excessive amount of thyroid secretion, or an altered secretion, may be poured into the blood and cause poisoning, which shows itself in the symptoms of Graves' disease.

In most instances the gland is uniformly enlarged, is very freely supplied with blood vessels, and the colloid contents of the spaces are replaced by a thinner liquid ; this is called primary Graves' disease. In other instances, symptoms of poisoning occur in a person who has had a simple goitre for a long time, in whom the gland is irregularly enlarged, or in whom there is no definite enlargement at all ; such are called cases of secondary Graves' disease. Most of the symptoms of the typical disease may be absent except increased rapidity of the pulse.

In connexion with the exophthalmos, certain signs are present which are named after those who first described them :

Von Graefe's sign is the delay of the upper eyelid in following the eyeball when the patient looks down, so that the white of the eye appears or a larger amount is seen ; Stellwag's or Dalrymple's sign is the absence of winking ; and Moebius' sign is the inability to keep the eyes converged, as when looking at a near object. If the eyeballs protrude very much, there is a risk of ulceration of the cornea.

The pulse rate is very rapid, perhaps 120 to 160 per minute, and it is to be noted that Graves' disease may lead to auricular fibrillation and heart failure. There is a fine tremor of the hands and eyelids and increased excitability, and there may be disagreeable sweating. There is loss of weight, the internal combustion which goes on, even when a person is at rest, being increased in this disease. There may be mental disturbance.

Rest is an important part of the treatment of this disease, and in some cases must be absolute. A search must be made for sources of poisoning, infected tooth sockets, diseased tonsils, or nasal sinuses, or some other focus, and anything discovered must be cleaned up. The diet must be liberal, and contain a fair amount of fresh food.

Iodine is a useful drug, although some cases do not tolerate it well. It is desirable to give iodine for a little time prior to operation. This may consist in tying the blood vessels which supply the gland, or in removing a portion of the latter. An operation becomes an urgent matter if the poisoning is severe, if heart disease develops, if the protrusion of the eyes endangers the corneae, or if the patient must keep at work to earn a living. The application of X-rays diminishes the size of the gland and may improve the symptoms, though some doctors are averse to its use.

The disease is one in which relapses are prone to occur and also sudden exacerbations.

See Endocrine ; Goitre ; Heart ; Thyroid Gland.

EXPECTATION OF LIFE. By calculations based on the number of deaths which have occurred in a community, and other data, what is called a life-table can be constructed, showing the number of persons, out of a million born, who can be presumed to be still alive at various ages. Thus there might be 840,000 at the end of the first year, 365,000 at the end of the sixtieth, and 8,000 at the end of the ninetieth.

From such a table it is possible to estimate the number of years which members of an age-group apparently have before them, that is to say, their expectation of life on the average ; at 55, for example, it might be 16 years. It must be observed that this has no application to any individual case, however.

For the population of London the expectation of life at birth was estimated at 34·6 for males, and 38·3 for females on the experiences of the period 1841–50 ; while on those of the period 1920–22 the figures had risen to 53·8 for males and 59·1 for females. Many people seem to think that such figures afford a reliable measure of the health of a community, but as they are based on hypothetical considerations this is not so, though for other purposes they are useful ; in calculating the risks when fixing premiums for life insurance, for example.

See Birth Rate ; Death Rate.

EXPECTORANT. A drug which promotes the expulsion of sputum is called an expectorant. Not every cough mixture is of this nature, however, as the object is sometimes to prevent a cough, and skilled judgement may be required to select the type of remedy required in a particular case or, possibly, at different times in the same case.

See Cough Mixture ; Senega.

EXPECTORATION. The ejection of phlegm from the lower air-passages by coughing or spitting is called expectoration. The process of clearing the back of the throat is described as hawking. Liquid or solid substances are, like air, forced out of the air-cells of the lungs when these contract in expiration ; they pass along the small air tubes, being propelled by the expired air and by muscle fibres in the walls of the tubes. The minute hair-like processes on the lining of the tubes, by lashing upwards, also help to push forward small particles. In the larger tubes the powerful blast of air in coughing comes into operation. In hawking, the movements of the pharyngeal muscles combined with that of the air detach phlegm from the surface of the throat. Overmuch hawking damages the throat. The matter expectorated is called the sputum.

Spitting in public places or on floors is not only a dirty practice, but a very dangerous one.

The sputum of many persons contains disease microbes and when the sputum dries the microbes are blown about in the dust and inhaled by other people. Consumption and other diseases may be contracted in this way. A spittoon, or cuspidor, unless cleansed very frequently does not make spitting any safer, as sputum dries on its margins.

See Bronchitis ; Consumption ; Cough ; Haemoptysis ; Sputum.

EXPRESSION. Various bodily movements are expressive of feeling, but principally those of the face, the muscles of which are usually referred to as the muscles of expression. These muscles are supplied by the seventh cranial, or facial nerve. The state of the facial expression is often of much use in diagnosis.

See Face.

EXTENSION. The straightening out of a limb or part of a limb at a joint is called extension at the joint, at the elbow or knee, for example, but carrying the arm backwards at the shoulder, or the thigh at the hip, represents extension also. When the head is bent back the neck is extended, and the spine when the shoulders are thrown back. A muscle which carries out this movement is called an extensor. The opposite movement is known as flexion (*q.v.*).

Pulling on a fractured limb in order to correct shortening and to bring the ends of the fragments into apposition is also described as extension, and resistance to the pull as counter - extension. Thus, if the thigh bone is broken, one person

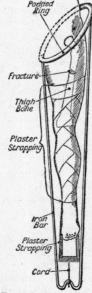

Extension apparatus for fractured thigh

Labels on figure: Padded Ring ; Fracture ; Thigh Bone ; Plaster Strapping ; Iron Bar ; Plaster Strapping ; Cord

grasps the ankle and extends the limb, while another, by grasping the patient at the armpits, fixes his body and so the upper end of the thigh, or, in other words, applies counter-extension.

In order to keep up the extension when the patient is in bed, strips of adhesive plaster are applied to each side of the limb, reaching as high as the site of fracture. The lower ends of the strips are attached to a wooden cross-piece, or stirrup, upon which traction is made by a spring or by a weight attached to the stirrup by a cord passing over a pulley. An extension apparatus might also be used in the treatment of a diseased joint.

See Fracture ; Splint.

EXTRACT. From crude drugs extracts are prepared by soaking them in some solvent, known as the menstruum and consisting usually of water or alcohol ; the active principles of the drug are dissolved and inert substances are got rid of. Various parts of different plants are used for preparing the extract.

An extract may be dry or semi-solid, and is then usually given in pill form. Liquid extracts are solutions of extracts in water and alcohol, or concentrated infusions with alcohol added as a preservative. The liquid extract of male fern is made with ether.

Extracts of animal tissues are also used as drugs, for example, thyroid extract.

See Drug.

EXTRAVASATION. The diffusion of some body fluid amongst the tissues is called extravasation. It is caused by a rupture in the retaining wall of a structure in which a fluid is present, whether this be a blood vessel or something larger. A common instance is the extravasation of blood following a bruise.

See Bleeding ; Bruise ; Hydatid Disease ; Urethra.

EXUDATE. The liquid that flows from the small blood vessels in inflammation is called a serous exudate. It forms the discharge from a wound ; a catarrhal discharge from a mucous membrane, as in a common cold ; the collection of fluid in wet pleurisy, and so on. If, as may happen in pleurisy, for example, a layer of coagulated fibrin forms on an inflamed surface, it is termed a fibrinous exudate ; if lumps of fibrin are floating in serous fluid, it is a sero-fibrinous exudate; and if the fluid contains many pus cells, it is a purulent exudate.

See Inflammation.

EYE. The essential parts of the visual apparatus are the eye, or eyeball, certain nerve cells in the hinder part of the large brain, and nerve fibres connecting the eye with these cells. Vibrations of the ether, which are known as light, produce images of the outside world on the sensitive membrane, or retina, at the back of the eye, thus stimulating the ends of the optic nerve, whence impulses pass back to the brain and cause the sensation of light. Stimulation of no other nerve causes this sensation, but, on the other hand, other stimuli than light, pressure on the eyeball over the retina, for instance, will cause it.

The eye is contained in a bony cavity in the front of the skull, known as the orbit, and is thus largely protected from external violence. Moreover, as the orbit is a roomy space, the eye, which with its attached muscles is embedded in soft, fatty tissue, is afforded a sufficiently free range of movement. In front of the eye are the lids, with their lashes, which can close and protect the eye, while in the outer part of the upper lid is the tear-gland, which helps to keep the surface of the eye moist.

The eye presents to view a circular clear transparent window in front, known as the cornea (*q.v.*), and beyond this, the white of the eye. The latter represents the sclerotic coat, a dense tough membrane, which, except for the corneal surface, covers the eyeball. This is almost spherical, but if the eye is examined from the side, it will be seen that the cornea projects from the sclerotic part, just as a concave watch glass would do were it applied to the surface of a circular orange. The cornea has no blood vessels traversing it, but is plentifully supplied with nerves and is very sensitive. Within the sclerotic coat is another, the choroid, and inside this the retina. The former has a free supply of blood vessels and many pigment cells; it extends forwards to near the

junction of the cornea with the sclerotic coat, where it forms a large number of folds known as the ciliary processes, and beyond these is continuous with the outer circumference of the curtain of the eye, which is called the iris.

The iris may have a brown, a blue or almost a greenish tint in different people, and it is perforated by a central, circular opening, the pupil, which can vary in size. This is because the iris contains two

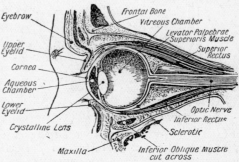

Eye. Section showing principal contents of the orbit

sets of muscle fibres, some circling round it, which contract the pupil, and others radiating outwards, which dilate it. The iris is covered behind by a layer of pigment cells, which prevents light passing otherwise than through the pupil.

Behind the iris is the crystalline lens of the eye which resembles a magnifying glass in miniature. It is enclosed in a capsule, and supported all round its circumference by a membrane, the suspensory ligament of the lens, which, in turn, is attached to the ciliary processes. When the eye is at rest this ligament is tense, and by pulling on the capsule compresses the lens and makes its front surface flatter than the back. All round the front of the ligament, however, are muscle fibres, the ciliary muscles, which, when they contract, draw the ligament forward and relax its tension. This lessens the compression of the lens, which is an elastic body and expands, the anterior surface bulging forwards, and thereby the lens becomes more powerful in focussing. This is necessary when the eye

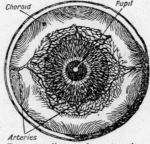

By expanding and contracting, the iris regulates the admission of light to the eye

looks at a near object, and the process is called accommodation (*q.v.*).

If a section were made through an eyeball, it would be noted that the lens and suspensory ligament divide the eye

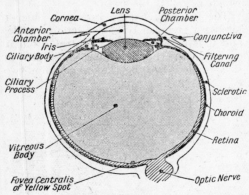

Eye. Horizontal section through the eyeball

into a smaller front and a larger back portion. The former is further divided into what are called the anterior and posterior chambers of the eye : these are filled with aqueous, or watery, humour. The space behind the lens is occupied by a clear, transparent jelly, known as the vitreous humour. The aqueous humour is secreted from the ciliary processes, and is drained into the canal of Schlemm, a minute tube pressing round the eye in the sclerotic coat just behind the junction of the latter with the cornea. If the fluid is prevented from draining into this canal, the eye becomes very hard from the pressure of the pent-up fluid, and this constitutes the dangerous eye disease known as glaucoma (*q.v.*).

When the interior of the eye is examined with an ophthalmoscope, the surface of the retina is spread out to the view. It has a bright red colour, and over it arteries and veins are coursing, which are seen to emerge from a small round or oval area a little to the inner or nasal side of the back of the eye. This area is known as the optic disk, and is the place where the fibres of the optic nerve, having penetrated the sclerotic coat, spread out all over the retina.

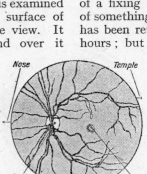

Retina. The optic disk marks the entrance of the optic nerve

This membrane has ten layers, but it will be sufficient to note, in addition to the layer of nerve fibres, that which is known as the layer of rods and cones, and behind these a layer of pigment cells. The other layers are merely concerned with bringing the nerve fibres into relation with the rods and cones, which are the cells upon which light really acts. The names rod and cone are applied to the cells on account of their shape.

These cells are marshalled together in a layer all over the retina, except that there are none of them on the optic disk, and consequently there is no perception of light here. At the centre of the back of the eye there is a little area which, from its colour, is called the macula lutea, or yellow spot. At its centre there is a little pit or depression, the fovea centralis, which represents the part of the retina where visual perception is sharpest in ordinary illumination. It is noteworthy that lining this part, and close around it, there are only cones. On the outlying parts of the retina, however, where vision is best in a subdued light, the rods form a great majority.

The changes induced in the rods and cones must be very subtle and complicated in order to produce vision of the multifarious shades and gradations of colour, but very little is known about them. In the retina of some animals which have been killed in the dark a substance known as visual purple, or rhodopsin, has been seen in the rods which is bleached on exposure to light, and by rapid use of a fixing agent a picture or optogram of something reproduced by this bleaching has been retained on the retina for some hours ; but as there is no visual purple in the cones its existence can only be a partial explanation of what takes place.

Sensation is supplied to the eyeball by branches of the fifth cranial nerve, which also supplies the face. Branches of the third cranial nerve supply the ciliary muscle, which, it has been noted, accommodates the eye to near vision, nd also the circular fibres in the iris, o that when we look at a near object he pupil contracts. The pupil also ontracts when light falls on the eye. ympathetic nerve fibres supply the nuscle fibres which dilate the pupil, and f those in the neck are reflexly stimulated, ay, by pinching the skin of the neck, he pupil dilates.

The exposed surface of the eyeball, vith the exception of the cornea, is covered y a delicate mantle of mucous membrane, he conjunctiva, which also covers the nner aspect of the lids, joining up with the skin at the lid margins. The surface of this nembrane is kept moist by ts secretions, and by that of the lachrymal, or tear, gland. When the eye is open there is a space, known as the conjunctival sac, behind the upper lid, in which foreign bodies may lodge. The ducts of the tear gland open into this space, and when the eye is irritated the copious flow of tears tends to wash out a foreign body from the sac or from elsewhere on the eye into the inner corner.

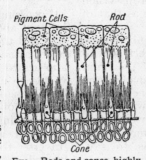

Eye. Rods and cones, highly specialised cells of the retina

Between the skin and conjunctiva covering the outer and inner sides of the eyeballs respectively there are several structures, notably a plate of dense fibres, called the tarsus or tarsal cartilage, which enables the lid to retain its shape, and makes it possible when searching for a foreign body to turn the upper lid outside in. There are also glands, the Meibomian, which lubricate the edges of the lid and the lashes. Circling round the opening of the orbit and on the lids are fibres of the orbicularis muscle which closes the lids ; it is supplied by a branch of the seventh cranial nerve, and one of the signs of facial paralysis is inability to close the eye properly.

The upper lid is raised by the levator palpebrae superioris muscle, which comes forward from the back of the orbit to be inserted into the lid, and is supplied by the third cranial nerve. In the inner part of the edge of each lid is a narrow tube beginning at a tiny opening on the edge, the punctum lachrymale. The secretion

of the tear gland flows into this opening, and along the tube to the lachrymal sac at the corner of the eye, whence it is discharged, through the nasal duct, into the lowest meatus, or passage, of the nose. If the ducts are blocked, tears overflow the lower lid, a condition known as epiphora.

Movements of the eyeball are produced by six muscles. Four of these, the superior, the internal, the inferior, and the external rectus, come from the back of the orbit to be inserted into the upper, the inner, the lower, and outer parts of the globe respectively. Contraction of one of these muscles would rotate the globe towards the position of the muscle ; thus the external rectus would rotate it outwards, the superior upwards, and so on. The other muscles are the superior and inferior oblique, the former directing the gaze downwards and outwards, the latter, upwards and outwards, as in looking over the top of one's spectacles. Paralysis of the superior oblique alone is rare ; it produces double vision when the patient looks downwards.

The external rectus is supplied by the sixth cranial nerve, also called the abducens, because this muscle rotates the eye away from the mid-line of the face ; and the superior oblique by the fourth or trochlear nerve. The word trochlear is derived from a Latin one meaning a pulley, and has reference to the fact that the tendon of the muscle passes through a little ring at the inner and upper angle of the orbit, and then turns outwards to the eyeball, so that the muscle acts as it were through a pulley. All the other muscles are supplied by the third cranial nerve, and this is called the motor oculi, in view of the large share which it takes in producing movements of the eye.

Each optic nerve presses backwards and enters the skull through an opening at the back of the orbit. Just after doing so, the fibres which supply the inner or nasal portion of the retina cross to the other side, the band formed by these and other crossing fibres being known as the optic commissure or chiasma. This lies in a shallow groove on the sphenoid bone just in front of the depression in which the pituitary gland is lodged.

Should the gland become enlarged, as it does in the disease called acromegaly, it may press on the commissure, putting the fibres to the inner parts of the retina out of action, and destroying vision in the parts supplied, so that while the person would see quite well what was in front of him, he would be unable, without turning the head, to see what was going on at the sides. The extent of his vision would be very much the same as that of a horse wearing blinkers.

From the commissure the fibres pass back in the optic tract on either side to flat projections on the base of the brain called the corpora quadrigemina, in the neighbourhood of which are nerve cells forming relay stations on the way to the back part of the brain and which also act as reflex centres for the movements of the pupil. Light, that is to say, falling on the retina, produces a nerve impulse which[1] is carried to these cells, and an impulse comes back causing the pupil to contract.

From the relay stations fibres carry visual impressions to the back parts of the occipital lobes of the brain, to nerve cells in the cortex, or superficial part of the brain substance, where the sensation of light is appreciated; from these cells, what are called association fibres link up with other cells farther forward on the brain concerned with the storage of images and the other intellectual aspects of vision.

When the eye is fixed on an object, the image of the latter is formed about the centre of the retina, and it is upside down ; it is the brain, therefore, which enables us to see things in their correct positions.

If one eye is covered, besides seeing the particular object looked at, one sees more or less of its surroundings, and all that is visible is spoken of as the field of vision of the eye. Although one is not ordinarily aware of it, there is a small area which is not seen. This corresponds to the optic disk, and lies outside the object looked at. If the left eye is closed and the gaze of the right fixed on the square shown here, the page being held about 10 inches away, it will be noticed that as the page is brought near the eye, the round dot disappears, but reappears when the page is brought still nearer. It disappears because rays from it fall on the insensitive optic disk. The area on the field of vision corresponding to the disk is called the blind spot.

Focussing of images on the retina is brought about by the property of refraction. If the end of a stick is pushed into water at an angle, the part in the water appears to be bent forwards. Anything visible to us at all is so because rays of light come from it to the eye, and in this instance of the stick, while the rays of light coming from it are straight while in the water, when they leave the latter and traverse the air they are bent, or refracted, so that to the observing eye they appear to come from another than their actual source of origin.

The same takes place when rays of light pass from the air into another medium, and, as regards the eye, this happens when rays coming from the outer world pass through the substance of the cornea, the aqueous humour, the lens and the vitreous humour. Refraction is further increased, however, by the curvature of the anterior surface of the cornea and the anterior and posterior curved surface of the lens. These surfaces act like glass prisms.

Diagram demonstrating the existence of a blind spot in the retina. See text for method of use

A prism is triangular in cross section, possessing a base from which two sides rise up to one angle or apex, as shown in the diagram. A ray of light which strikes one side of the prism, otherwise than at right angles to it, is bent towards the base, and, having traversed the prism, is bent further in the same direction when it emerges. If two equal prisms are placed base to base, the emerging rays meet at a point on the other side of the prisms from that on which is the source of the light rays.

Now, a structure like the lens, with surfaces bulging away from its centre, corresponds to the two prisms just described, and the surface of the cornea to one side of the two prisms. A bulge like that of the cornea or the surfaces of the lens is said to be convex. Were it in the opposite direction, that is, like two prisms placed with their apices touching

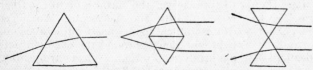

In the eye the curvatures of cornea and lens act like glass prisms, deflecting the light rays in the manner shown in these diagrams

rather than their bases, it would be a concave surface, and a lens with one or both surfaces like this would not bring rays of light to a focus, but would disperse them.

Rays of light coming from a small source about twenty feet away or further are practically parallel, and such rays, when the eye is at rest, are focussed on the retina, the distance between the anterior surface of the cornea and the retina being such that this happens. Such an eye is called an emmetropic eye. If, however, the eye is shorter than the normal, parallel rays will be focussed behind the retina ; if it is longer than the normal, they will be focussed in front of the retina ; in either event there will be a blurring of the image actually formed on the retina. The former condition is called hypermetropia, and the latter myopia, or short sight.

A person with hypermetropia can focus the parallel rays on the retina, however, by accommodating, that is, making the lens stronger by bringing the ciliary muscle into play, but this induces fatigue when constantly in operation as it must be for ordinary vision, and therefore such a person is fitted with a convex lens which will form a clear image on the retina without calling on accommodative effort. A person with myopia, on the other hand, requires concave lenses in order to disperse somewhat the rays of light entering the eye, and thus throw the focus point further back and on to the retina.

After a person has reached the age of forty, changes are apt to occur in the lens which make it less elastic, and therefore less able to become stronger when near objects have to be examined. It becomes impossible to read small print, and again convex lenses are necessary to compensate for lack of strength in the natural lens. This condition is called presbyopia.

All these are known as refractive errors, and there is another which depends usually on the curvature of the cornea not being equal in all planes. Instead of being shaped like a circular watch-glass, it is shaped more like the bowl of a spoon. Rays of light are therefore brought to a focus at different points, and images are blurred. This defect is called astigmatism, and is corrected by putting a prism in front of the eye, so as to compensate for the unequal corneal curvature.

Injuries and Diseases of the Eye. The skin around and below the eye is very lax, and an insect sting in this region is usually followed by considerable swelling. For the same reason a blow on the eye may result in free bleeding beneath the skin and much discoloration, in fact, a black eye. Treatment of a black eye is dealt with under the heading Bruise.

If a foreign body gets into the eye, the worst possible thing to do is to rub it. The eye should be kept closed while the nostril on the same side is blown briskly ; this promotes a rapid flow of tears into the inner corner of the eye, possibly carrying the foreign body with them.

A search should be made for it there and beneath the lower eyelid. If it is not found, the cornea should be inspected both from in front and from the side, and, if still unsuccessful, the upper lid should be turned over. The patient is directed to keep on looking downwards, while with the forefinger and thumb of one hand the person rendering first aid grasps the lashes at their roots and a narrow fold of the adjoining skin about the middle of the lid. A match or something similar is laid along the upper border of the lid, and while it presses downwards and forwards the edge of the lid is turned back over it (*see* Plate XV, 3–5).

Wherever the foreign body is found, it may be possible to lift it off with a clean piece of blotting-paper or the corner of a handkerchief. On no account should an attempt be made to rub a foreign body off the cornea. If it does not come off on blotting-paper, it is probably embedded, and rubbing will only implant it more deeply in the delicate cornea. Medical help should be secured at once.

Metal chippings and cinders may be hot when they reach the eye, and are then commonly referred to as "fires." In addition to any mechanical damage they cause more or less scorching, and the wound is likely to be longer in healing.

After Removal of a Foreign Body

A drop of castor oil is very soothing to the eye after the removal of a foreign body. When there has been a wound of the cornea or conjunctiva the eye should be protected with a loose eye-shade for a few days, and may, with advantage, be bathed with boracic lotion several times a day.

If a foreign body has appeared to strike the eye with some force, but nevertheless cannot be discovered, a doctor should always be consulted, as it may have been driven right into the eye, and, if it is left, will do serious damage by mechanical or chemical irritation or, possibly, by infection which it has conveyed into the eye.

Inflammations of the conjunctiva are described under the heading Conjunctivitis, and inflammation of the edge of the lid under the heading Blepharitis.

The passages conducting the tears into the nose may be stenosed or narrowed, and possibly infected. Dilating probes may have to be passed, and sometimes the tear sac is washed out by using an Anel's syringe. Inflammation of the sac is called dacryocystitis, and pus may be present, the abscess bulging at the inner corner of the eye.

The lashes normally curve away from the eye, but sometimes are turned towards it, and cause much irritation ; this condition is known as trichiasis. It is more likely to happen if there is entropion, the edge of the lid turned inwards. Ectropion means that the edge of the lid is turned outwards, exposing the inner surface. Operative treatment is required to remedy these disfigurements. An enlargement of a Meibomian gland constitutes a chalazion ; it may cause irritation and may become inflamed ; it is to be distinguished from a hordeolum, or stye (q.v.), which is suppuration at the root of a lash.

Inflammation of the cornea, or keratitis, may have several causes. Corneal ulcers are very painful, and tend either to spread over the surface, or to eat their way inwards and perforate. An ulcer causes much pain and intolerance of light, the muscles round the eye contracting firmly, and resisting efforts at opening, a condition styled blepharospasm. When an ulcer heals an opacity is left ; if faint and small it is called a nebula, if more pronounced a macula, and if white and dense, a leucoma. If near the centre of the cornea, it may seriously interfere with vision. If the cornea is weakened by inflammation or ulceration, it may bulge forwards in the centre. A similar bulging due to atrophy of the corneal tissue is called keratoconus. In either case the alteration in the curvature of the cornea spoils the vision more or less, apart from any opacities.

Various Inflammatory Conditions

If the cornea is perforated by a wound or an ulcer, the aqueous humour tends to escape, and the iris may bulge forward and into the wound, where it may be caught if healing takes place. Infection may also get into the eye, and hypopyon, or pus in the anterior chamber, result. Infection may spread along the iris to the ciliary body and, indeed, involve the whole eye, a condition known as panophthalmitis.

Inflammation of the iris, or iritis, besides being caused in this way, may result from blood infections, for example, syphilis, gonorrhoea or rheumatism. Commonly there is inflammation of the ciliary body, or cyclitis also, the condition being known as irido-cyclitis. When irido-cyclitis follows a penetrating injury of the eye, not only is the sight of this eye menaced, but there is great danger of a similar condition in the other eye, sympathetic ophthalmia, and this may not occur till long after the injury.

PLATE XV

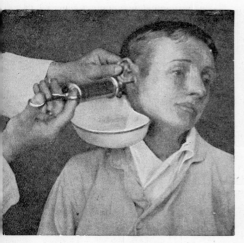

Ear. 1. Syringing to remove wax. The ear is drawn upward and backward and the syringe pointed towards the back of the auditory canal

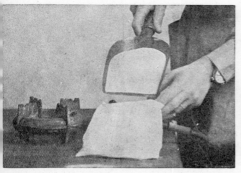

2. A small flannel bag filled with common salt which has been heated in a shovel may be laid over an aching ear to relieve the pain

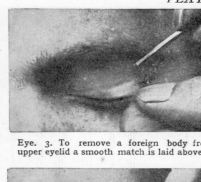

Eye. 3. To remove a foreign body from the upper eyelid a smooth match is laid above the lid

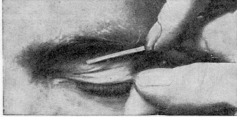

4. The operator gently takes hold of the lashes and draws them forward and up over the match

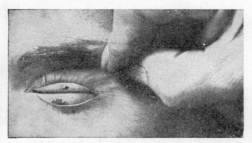

5. By this means the lid is turned inside out and the foreign body adhering to it can be easily removed with a clean silk handkerchief

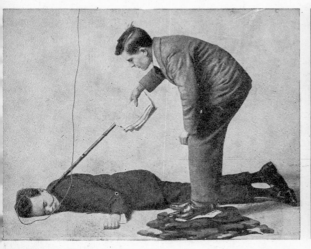

6. Electric Shock. When a live wire is in contact the rescuer must stand on a heap of dry clothing or newspaper and protect his hands with similar non-conducting material

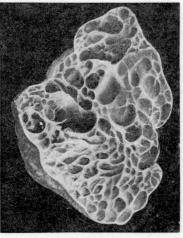

7. Emphysema. Portion of lung showing enlarged air cells due to difficulty in exhaling

PLATE XVI

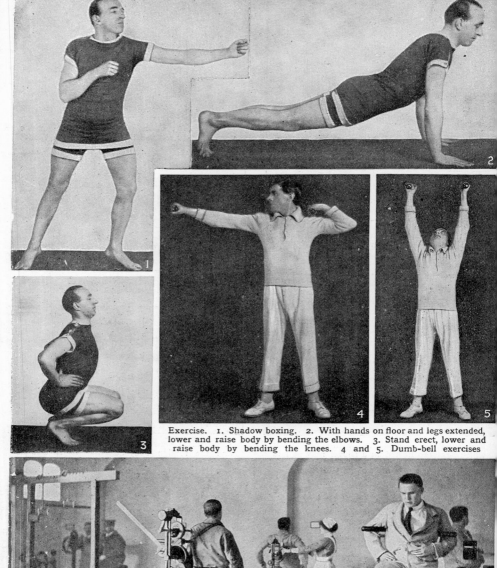

Exercise. 1. Shadow boxing. 2. With hands on floor and legs extended, lower and raise body by bending the elbows. 3. Stand erect, lower and raise body by bending the knees. 4 and 5. Dumb-bell exercises

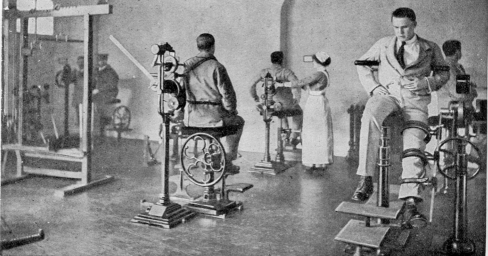

6. Zander system of mechano-therapy which consists in producing passive movements by means of apparatus

Courtesy of Grand Pump Room. Bath

Opacity of the lens constitutes cataract *q.v.*) ; when ripe the lens may be removed from its capsule. Sometimes from an injury the lens is dislocated from its normal position. The absence of the lens, described as aphakia, very much lessens the refractive power of the eye. Floating specks in front of the eye, muscae volitantes, are seen in abnormalities of the vitreous humour, and in old people may be associated with the commencement of cataract ; but they may be due to a disordered liver or other condition apart from the eye.

From wounds perforating the ball of the eye a suppurative and general inflammation of the choroid, or choroiditis, may occur. In another form of choroiditis, from localised exudations into the membrane, white spots form in it ; this condition may be found widely spread over the back of the eye, disseminated choroiditis, or may be localised. Syphilis is a common cause.

Affections of the Retina

A blow on the eye may produce concussion effects in the retina, commotio retinae, or may rupture it. From several causes the retina may be separated off from the choroid, the detached part appearing as a white patch with billowy folds when the eye is examined with an ophthalmoscope. Inflammation of the membrane, retinitis, may occur from kidney disease, leukaemia, haemorrhage and other causes ; it is commonly associated with inflammation of the optic nerve also, when the condition is spoken of as neuro-retinitis. It generally affects both eyes. Retinitis pigmentosa, a degenerative disease of the membrane, is usually associated with night blindness.

A swelling of the optic disk, papilloedema, is associated with increase in the pressure within the skull, say, from a brain tumour. This, or inflammation of the optic nerve, may be followed by atrophy of the nerve, or atrophy may occur independently ; there is progressive loss of vision. Tumours may occur in the eyeball ; one of these, glioma, is a malignant tumour which occurs in young children. Unless the eye is removed at an early stage, there is grave risk of extension to the brain.

Paralysis of one or more of the muscles of the eyeball, or, on the other hand, spasm, causes squint, or strabismus, from which results diplopia, or double vision. Syphilis is a common cause of paralysis of the ocular muscles. When those supplied by the third nerve are involved, there is also drooping of the upper eyelid, or ptosis, though this condition may also be congenital.

Fuller accounts of the commoner disorders of the eye are given under appropriate headings.

See Accommodation ; Asthenopia ; Binocular ; Blepharitis ; Colour Blindness ; Conjunctivitis ; Cornea ; Cyclitis ; Ectropion ; Episcleritis ; Field of Vision ; Glaucoma ; Keratitis ; Nyctalopia ; Nystagmus ; Optic Nerve ; Pupil ; Squint ; Stye ; Vision.

EYE, ARTIFICIAL. The use of an artificial eye is desirable not only to correct the deformity due to the empty socket, but to prevent further deformity from shrinkage of the socket and eyelids. The eye must fit well, however, otherwise it also will tend to induce shrinkage, and the eye and the socket must be well cared for. The eye should be taken out at night, cleaned from discharge and left to soak overnight in boracic lotion ; the socket should be cleansed with a little lotion. An artificial eye is made of glass and in course of time becomes roughened ; when this happens it should be at once discarded.

EYE BATH. The eyes may be washed out by squeezing a lotion from a piece of cotton wool over the eye while the patient holds his head, turned to the side, over a vessel for collecting the liquid. This method should be adopted when there is much discharge in the eye, but otherwise the use of an eye bath is a very convenient method. This apparatus is usually made of glass or aluminium, and its rim is shaped to fit round the socket of the eye. It is filled with warm lotion, say boracic acid, 10 grains to the ounce, and the patient stoops forward and fits it securely over the eye. He then throws the head back, and by alternately opening and closing the eye the lotion reaches all parts of its surface.

See Collyrium ; Conjunctivitis ; Eye.

EYE DROP. An instrument like a fountain-pen filler is used for putting drops into the eye. The patient is told to throw back his head and keep looking

K

up ; the lower eyelid is drawn downwards and one or two drops are squeezed out over the eye, which the patient then closes for a few moments (Plate X, 2).

See Blepharitis; Conjunctivitis; Ectropion; Ptosis.

EYE SALVE. When introducing an eye salve, or ointment, a portion about the size of a pea is taken up, usually on the end of a clean glass rod ; the patient looks up and his lower eyelid is drawn downwards. The ointment is then placed on the lower part of the surface of the eyeball and the eye is closed. By gentle rubbing the ointment is then spread all over the eye. A common salve for inflamed eyes is made up of yellow oxide of mercury ointment and soft paraffin in equal parts.

EYE SHADE. Protection from light and wind is afforded to the eye by some kind of shade. A common type is one made of flesh-coloured celluloid. This is often worn so as to fit over the eye tightly, and in general this is a mistake. Proper ventilation of the eye and a free exit for discharges are desirable. To rest an eye properly it may be necessary to shade both eyes. A suitable shade for this purpose, with a green lining, may be purchased, or one can be cut from a piece of cardboard and lined with some thin green or black fabric.

EYE STRAIN. Inflammation of the eyes, headache, mental irritability and other symptoms may be caused by eye strain. Usually there is some error of refraction present, weak sight or astigmatism, but even sound eyes may be strained by overmuch reading or other kinds of near work, by the lack of sufficient light when doing such work, or by reading much in bed, particularly if the reading is done sidewise. Sometimes the weakness is in the muscles which move the eyeball and strain may cause a tendency to squint.

A lowering of the general health may precipitate symptoms of eye strain, and the use of general tonic treatment must then be combined with that directed specially to the eyes. What direction this should take can only be decided by a doctor after a careful investigation of the visual apparatus.

See Accommodation; Astigmatism; Eye.

FACE. The eyebrows mark the boundary between the forehead and the face, which extends below to the chin and on either side to the ear, the part immediately in front of the ear being called the parotid region. The prominence of the cheek is formed by the malar, or cheek bone, which, with the zygomatic process of the temporal bone (*q.v.*), forms an arch, separating the cheek from the temporal region of the head.

The skin of the face is thin, but is freely supplied with sweat and sebaceous glands, and with blood vessels. Sensation is supplied to it by branches of the fifth or trigeminal nerve. The tissue beneath the skin is loose, except over the chin, where it is especially dense, resembling, in fact, that found in the scalp. Owing to the looseness of this subcutaneous tissue, great swelling may take place from dropsy or from inflammation following a bee-sting, for example.

A large number of muscles are found in the face and, in conjunction with those of the forehead, are concerned in the production of expression ; the buccinator, a muscle in the cheek, aids in keeping food between the teeth when chewing, and in preventing an accumulation of food between the inside of the cheek and the teeth. All these muscles are supplied by the seventh or facial nerve.

The facial artery runs on to the face round the lower margin of the lower jaw bone, about an inch in front of the angle of this bone, and courses obliquely upwards and forwards across the face. It comes from the external carotid, and amongst its branches are one to the tonsil, one along the lower lip and another along the upper lip, which by anastomosing with those from the facial artery on the other side, encircle the mouth. For arresting bleeding from a cut on the lip, it may be necessary therefore to grasp and compress the lip at both sides of the wound.

The facial vein lies near the artery as the latter is passing over the jaw, but elsewhere is at some distance from it. It communicates at one end with the cavernous sinus, which is within the skull, and at the other with the internal jugular vein, which drains off blood from the face. The connexion with the cavernous sinus is an important fact because, should septic mischief occur in the facial vein, say, from carbuncle, the infection may spread to the great venous channels inside the skull. Septic conditions on the face must therefore be treated with especial care.

The appearance of the skin of the face —its colour and texture—is commonly referred to as the complexion, and is dealt with under that heading.

Brown patches, often called liver spots, occur in chloasma, a pigmentation which may occur during pregnancy, disappearing when this is over, but which may occur also in other people ; or such patches may occur apart from chloasma.

Some Causes of Flushing

Flushing of the face is common in fevers, and is a phenomenon often noted in women at the change of life. It occurs also in the disorder known as acne rosacea, affecting chiefly the nose and adjoining parts of the face ; this is usually associated with some digestive disturbance, and the consumption of alcohol may play an important part in its causation, though not so often as is popularly supposed.

Redness of the face may be due to networks of dilated vessels, the dilatation not being merely temporary as in flushing, but a more or less fixed state of the vessels ; and the patches may show a tendency to lividity. Exposure may bring this about, but alcoholic habits are often responsible. Birthmarks (*q.v.*) should also be mentioned as a variety of red patch.

A blue-grey or purple discoloration of the face, known as lividity or cyanosis, may occur in chronic bronchitis, asthma, and other respiratory disorders, in heart disease, and in certain types of poisoning.

Pallor of the face results from anaemia and other diseases. In some persons it is natural, as will be established by observing that the mucous membrane on the inside of the lower eyelid and the gums has a proper red tint.

In addition to those already mentioned, the skin diseases which tend to occur on the face include eczema, especially in children, impetigo, lupus erythematosus, ordinary lupus, rodent ulcer, etc.

There is a considerable layer of fat beneath the skin of the face, and should this be diminished, wrinkles tend to appear, particularly as at the same time the skin may lose some of its elasticity. This happens ordinarily as years go on, but may be due to general ill-health.

Like any other muscle, one that is much exercised in producing some facial expression is likely to become larger, and so, in time, a more or less fixed physiognomy may be acquired. Loss of expression when due to paralysis of the facial nerve (*q.v.*) is usually confined to one side. A wooden expression is characteristic of paralysis agitans, or Parkinson's disease. Typical or, at any rate, suggestive expressions are seen in adenoids, exophthalmic goitre, myasthenia gravis, and a number of other diseases.

What is called the Hippocratic facies, characterised by sharpness of the nose, hollowing of the eyes and the temples, and a brown or livid discoloration of the face, is usually a sign of impending death, but is not necessarily so in acute peritonitis, cholera, or starvation.

Twitching of facial muscles, or tic (*q.v.*) may represent a habit spasm, or have some other significance.

See Acne ; Acne Rosacea ; Barber's Itch ; Blushing ; Cancrum Oris ; Complexion ; Pallor ; Parotid Gland ; Rash ; Skin ; Sycosis.

FACE-ACHE. Pain in the face is generally due to irritation of some branch of the fifth or trigeminal nerve, the source of the irritation being most commonly a decayed tooth. It may be caused, however, by disease of the Gasserian ganglion, which gives rise to the excruciating pains of tic douloureux.

See Neuralgia ; Trigeminal Nerve.

FACIAL NERVE. The seventh cranial or facial nerve comes from a centre in that part of the brain known as the pons. This centre is, however, under the control of other centres in the cortex of the brain. The nerve leaves the brain and travels into the inner ear in close proximity to the eighth cranial or auditory nerve. It now leaves this nerve, however, and passing through a bony canal, the Fallopian canal, beneath the floor of the passage connecting the mastoid antrum and the middle ear, and then downwards through the mastoid process, it emerges through the stylo-mastoid foramen, below and in front of the ear-hole. From here it wends upwards and forwards into the parotid gland, where it divides into superior and inferior divisions, from which branches are supplied to the muscles of the forehead and face

The facial nerve is also known as the nerve of expression, as it activates the muscles by which changes of expression, wrinkling the brows, closing the eyes and so on, are brought about. If, therefore, the nerve is paralysed there will be a loss of expression on the corresponding side of the face. Such paralysis may be due to a lesion in the nervous tract between the cortex of the brain and the nucleus in the pons, or it may be in the nucleus or the trunk of the nerve.

The former is the central type of paralysis and the latter the peripheral type, sometimes referred to as Bell's

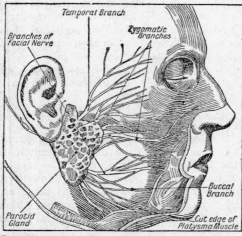

Branches of Facial Nerve
Temporal Branch
Zygomatic Branches
Buccal Branch
Parotid Gland
Cut edge of Platysma Muscle

Paralysis of the facial nerve produces a mask-like appearance on the affected side of the face

palsy or paralysis. In the central type, accompanying a stroke of apoplexy, for example, the muscles on the forehead and those about the eye escape, so that the patient can close the eye, wrinkle his brow and frown. In the peripheral type he cannot do these things nor show his upper teeth ; the whole face is mask-like on the affected side, and the mouth is drawn towards the sound side. Moreover, when eating, food tends to accumulate between the cheek and the teeth, because the facial nerve supplies the buccinator muscle.

This type of paralysis may be caused by cold, say by the play of wind on the cheek when travelling in a railway carriage with the window open. A common cause is suppuration in the middle ear ; or the cause may be syphilis. It may also be caused by a wound of the cheek, penetrating the parotid gland, or an abscess in this gland.

When the paralysis is due to cold, warmth is applied to the side of the face and perhaps blisters are applied. Later recovery is hastened by electrical stimulation of the muscles. In other cases the cause must be treated appropriately. Sometimes after recovery there is a tendency to spasmodic contraction of some of the muscles concerned.

When, from injury or disease, the nerve is divided beyond hope of repair an anastomosis may be made between it and the hypoglossal nerve, the nerve that activates the tongue.

See Tic.

FAECES. The discharges of the bowel are called the faeces, though more commonly referred to as stools or motions. They consist of dead cells from the bowel lining, lime, magnesium, iron and phosphoric acid, bacteria, indigestible and undigested food, and a number of other substances, including stercobilin, a derivative of bile, which gives them a brownish colour. Their odour they owe to the presence of indol and skatol, benzene derivatives formed by the action of bacteria on proteins in the bowel.

The daily amount of faeces discharged by an adult usually is from 4 to 6 ounces, half of which consists of bacteria, most of them dead. The faeces generally have a cylindrical form, and if flattened, or tape-like, obstruction in the lower bowel is suggested. In constipation and some other disorders the faeces may occur as hard balls. To these the term scybala is applied. In diarrhoea, and after taking purgative medicines, the stools are more or less soft. In typhoid fever they are described as a pea-soup stool. In cholera the stools are profuse and watery, with whitish particles floating in the liquid ; such are called rice-water stools.

The colour of the stools may be dark from an excess of meat in the diet, or after taking fruit having a dark red juice, or red wine. Such drugs as bismuth, iron and manganese make the stools black, but where there is no such explanation, black stools are due to the presence of blood. These are sometimes referred to as tarry stools, and to the passing of them the term melaena is applied. The black colour is due to the blood having been altered by the digestive juices, and indicates, therefore, that the blood has come from the stomach or upper part of the bowel. It may, however, have reached the stomach from higher up, when, for example, blood has been swallowed during bleeding from the nose.

Presence of Unchanged Blood

When blood mixed in the stools has its usual colour, it shows either that it has been poured into the lower part of the bowel, or that the blood has been poured out in large quantities in the upper reaches of the bowel and has been hurried through.

Blood may be present in the stools invisible to the naked eye, but discoverable by the use of a microscope. This is called " occult " blood.

The stools are pale when the diet consists mainly of milk, or milk-foods. Clay-coloured stools occur when the entrance of bile into the bowel is prevented, for example, by the obstruction of the main duct by a gall-stone ; in this event the patient is also jaundiced. When the stools of an infant are green when passed the colour is due to the activities of bacteria, not to bile pigment. A soft green stool resembling chopped parsley is sometimes present in typhoid fever.

After eating eggs, the stools may have a disagreeable odour from the decomposition of sulphur, and also when this substance is taken as a drug. The clay-coloured stools of obstructive jaundice are usually offensive from the decomposition of fats. The stools in summer diarrhoea of infants, in dysentery and other disorders may be very offensive.

When a large amount of vegetable food is taken, the stools contain much cellulose, as this is indigestible. The presence of indigestible matter hastens the movement of food through the bowel, and some digestible substances may also be carried through and found in the faeces. If an excess of fat is consumed, there may be fat visible in the faeces, otherwise this circumstance is due to poor digestion of fat, such as occurs in obstructive jaundice and in the absence or insufficiency of the pancreatic juice. If this juice is at fault, microscopical examination also reveals undigested meat fibres.

Normally there is a little mucus or slime coating the faeces, but in some disorders, such as inflammation of the rectum or colon, dysentery, or intussusception (q.v.), there is a large increase of mucus ; in fact, the faeces may largely consist of this substance. Along with the mucus there is more or less blood as a rule. In mucous colitis, casts of the bowel, made of thickened mucus, may be passed. In countries where dysentery is prevalent, the passage of blood and mucus would at once suggest this disease, and in children anywhere the passage of such a stool concurrently with attacks of colicky pains would suggest intussusception, though in either case the opinion would require to be tested by other considerations. In dysentery and other disorders there may be pus or matter in the stools.

Significance of Intestinal Sand

A sandy-looking admixture in the faeces is called intestinal sand. It may be " true " sand, that is, with a large mineral content, or " false " sand, that is, composed of vegetable substances. The former denotes organic disease of the colon, and is most often found in mucous colitis. The latter occurs in those who have consumed large quantities of pears or similar fruit. Other abnormal contents of the faeces include gall-stones and other concretions, undigested pills, foreign bodies in the stools of children or feeble-minded persons, and intestinal parasites. These may be round or flat worms, visible to the naked eye, or their eggs, which can only be discovered by the microscope. Thus only also can be found the eggs of flukes and the protozoal parasites.

The passing of faeces is described as defaecation. The nervous centre for the act is in the lumbar part of the spinal cord, and this is stimulated by the entry of faeces into the rectum ; it may also be stimulated, however, by fear. The expulsion of faeces is brought about by the contraction of the bowel wall, aided by the muscles of the abdominal wall and in the floor of the pelvis. It is a reflex act and can take place during unconsciousness, but ordinarily is under the control of the will, the escape of faeces being prevented by keeping the sphincters at the lower end of the rectum closed. Inability to do this is called incontinence of faeces. This occurs in some nervous diseases, even when the patient is conscious; during fright; when the sphincters have been injured; and in other disorders.

See Constipation; Diarrhoea; Intestine; Rectum; Tenesmus; Worm.

FAINTING. The immediate cause of fainting is a momentary failure of the blood supply to the brain and the usual things that bring this about are pain, fright or other mental shocks, a close, oppressive atmosphere, cold or hunger. These operate by depressing the heart's action. Blurring of vision, ringing in the ears, giddiness or sickness may precede fainting, while bystanders will notice that the patient becomes pale and unsteady looking. He, or she, falls or sinks to the ground sometimes with a prolonged sigh. The patient may appear to be lifeless, as breathing may hardly be noticeable and the pulse may not be felt at the wrist. On the other hand, there may be shallow efforts at breathing and a feeble pulse. Soon, however, as a rule, he begins breathing, some colour flows back to the face and the eyes open.

In view of the cause an obvious essential in treatment is to keep the head low. It may suffice to press down the head between the knees, but it is better that the patient should be lying down. On no account should an attempt be made to hold him up in a sitting position. A free supply of air should be obtained by keeping a crowd back; in a hot meeting-place the coolest air is at the floor. Tight clothing about the neck and chest should be loosened. If smelling salts are available the patient should be given an opportunity of inhaling them. When he is able to swallow, sips of water should be given, or better still, weak spirits or sal volatile.

See Collapse; Dizziness; Unconsciousness.

FALLOPIAN TUBE. The oviduct, or passage by which the ovum, or egg, makes its way from the ovary into the womb, is known as the Fallopian tube.

See Genital System.

FARINACEOUS FOOD. In the group of farinaceous foods are included those derived from grain, roots and tubers which yield a flour or meal and contain a considerable proportion of starch, such as wheat-flour, rice, sago, tapioca, etc. Their chief function as food is the production of energy from their conversion into sugar in the body and utilisation as such. Their consumption in diabetes must, therefore, be strictly controlled, and also in obesity, as starchy foods tend to be stored as fats. In some forms of dyspepsia, too, it is necessary to restrict farinaceous foods on account of their liability to ferment.

See Diet; Food.

FASCIA. The term fascia, which is the Latin word for a bandage, is applied to various structures in the body which invest certain organs and tissues, affording them protection and support. Thus, beneath the skin all over the body there is a layer of loose, open, or areolar tissue which is called the superficial fascia, and beneath this a layer, composed of strong tendinous fibres, which surrounds or covers the muscles, and is called the deep fascia. The fascia lata of the thigh (*q.v.*) is a good example of the latter.

See Aponeurosis.

FASTING. Some individuals have been able to fast for many days. To accomplish this, however, a sufficiency of water had to be taken and throughout the fast the body was at rest and means were taken to minimise the loss of body heat. Even at rest the output of energy in the work of the organs and in producing heat is considerable and during a fast the fuel for this must be provided by the body itself. While it lasts the natural store of fat is drawn on, but other tissues also waste.

Fasting secures rest for the digestive apparatus and a short fast may be undertaken as a treatment for indigestion. It also helps to clear toxins out of the body so long as water is taken freely. When beginning to diet for diabetes a few days' fasting is often enjoined; green vegetables may be allowed, but the supply of actual nutriment in these is small, and their use has the advantage of supplying vitamin, keeping the bowels moving and elping to prevent the sensation of hunger. Even in a strict fast, however, hunger is not troublesome. After the first 24 hours it is not urgent and after 48 hours generally disappears. It is often desirable to begin a strict fast with a sharp purge in order to clear the bowel of possible sources of toxaemia. It is desirable, also, even for a short fast, to keep warm in bed. A fast for longer than a day or two should not be undertaken except under medical supervision. The meal which breaks the fast should be very small. *See* Starvation.

FAT. Adipose, or fatty, tissue is widely distributed throughout the body but is absent from the cavity of the head and from the substance of some glands, such as the liver. With the exception of the eyelids and one or two other places, it forms a layer of varying thickness everywhere beneath the skin. Another layer occurs beneath serous membranes, and is especially abundant over the heart, around the kidney and intestines, and in the fold of peritoneum, the great omentum, which is disposed like an apron in front of the coils of intestine. The bone marrow contains a large quantity of fat.

Adipose tissue forms a storehouse of fuel for the body, which is replenished from fat and a proportion of the carbohydrates and even proteins consumed as food. It also serves to protect the body from external heat and cold and from physical injury. Delicate organs like the eyeball and vessels and nerves, which would otherwise be subjected to pressure, are surrounded by adipose tissue. For other organs, such as the kidneys and bowels, it serves as a support and its rapid disappearance in wasting diseases creates a tendency to visceroptosis, or dropping of the organs.

Adipose tissue consists of tiny globules containing liquid fat, each globule being a distended tissue cell.

A general increase of fatty tissue is called corpulence, adiposity or obesity (*q.v.*). A fatty tumour is called a lipoma ; this is described under the heading Tumour. An accumulation of adipose tissue amongst the essential structures of an organ is called fatty infiltration. This may occur, for example, amongst the heart muscles or amongst the fibres of voluntary muscles and occasions a degree of weakness varying with its amount. Should, however, the protoplasm of the tissue cells undergo an alteration so that tiny droplets of fat appear in them, this is called fatty degeneration. It occurs, for example, in phosphorus poisoning.

Animal fat mainly consists of a mixture of three fats, namely, olein, palmitin and stearin. The first is liquid even at the freezing point of water, while the others remain solid at temperatures above that of the human body, stearin requiring a higher temperature than palmitin for its liquefaction. In the human body, therefore, it is the olein that keeps the other fats liquid.

A fat, if decomposed, splits up into glycerol, or glycerin, and a fatty acid, for example, oleic, palmitic or stearic, acid, or a combination of these acids. If an alkali is present a soap is formed by the combination of this with the fatty acids, the process being described as the saponification of fat. This is an essential part of the process of the digestion of fats and is aided by emulsification, that is, the subdivision of the fat into minute droplets.

In the cells of the body a substance known as lecithin occurs. This is spoken of as a phosphorised fat, and when decomposed produces not only the substances already mentioned but also phosphoric acid and an alkaloid known as choline.

Vegetable fats are similarly constituted, though some contain other fats than olein, palmitin and stearin. An important difference is that vegetable fats do not contain the vitamins present in animal fats and essential to growth. Fat is an important source of body-heat, one ounce producing more heat than two ounces of either carbohydrate or protein. The consumption of fat is, therefore, greater in the colder countries.
See Diet ; Food ; Obesity.

FATIGUE. There are definite limits to the working capacity of the human machine, although there are considerable individual differences in this respect. A certain amount of work can be done at top pressure, but gradually the volume and quality decline, and if the task is continued in spite of these evidences of fatigue, a stage of exhaustion is reached.

The development of fatigue can be studied by using various kinds of apparatus. In one of these, the ergograph, a finger raises a weight which is attached to it by a string passing over a pulley, the height to which the weight is raised being recorded on a blackened paper, fixed on a revolving drum. Intervals of time, seconds usually, can be simultaneously recorded. By alternately flexing and extending the finger, the weight is raised and lowered. A comparison may thus be made between the powers of different persons or of one person at different periods and under varying conditions.

Another apparatus is arranged so that dots pass in front of the person undergoing the test ; he is expected to prick them, and fatigue is shown according to the accuracy with which the pricks are made.

Physiological Explanation of Fatigue

In both of these experiments there are two parts of the body mechanism involved; the muscles which raise the weight or make the pricks ; the nerve cells in the brain and spinal cord, and the nerves through which the movements are brought about. It has been shown, however, that a nerve fibre does not become fatigued, though its ending in the muscle does. A muscle can also become fatigued if stimulated otherwise than through the nerve, but in the living body stimulation is, practically speaking, always through the nerve ; it is, therefore, fatigue of the ending in the muscle which concerns us. In the nervous system fatigue takes place at a synapse, the place where the processes of one nerve cell intertwine with those of another.

There are two factors in the induction of fatigue, the using up of the energy-producing substance, and the accumulation of waste products. This is similar to what takes place in a furnace for raising steam-power. The heat of the furnace may decline either from insufficiency of fuel or from the choking of the fire from an over-accumulation of ash. The ash or waste material which matters most in muscle is lactic acid, and it is an interesting fact that when this acid is washed out of a fatigued muscle in labora-

tory experiments, fatigue disappears. Res does the same for fatigued tissues in th ordinary way ; lactic acid is oxidised an destroyed.

The onset of fatigue is hastened b toxaemic states of the body, presumabl because these lead to an earlier accumu lation of waste products. The toxaemi may be due to chronic constipation or t some septic focus somewhere in th body. Toxaemia is combated partly b the secretions of the ductless glands and, if long continued, these gland may manifest signs of fatigue and ex haustion.

Fatigue is not limited to the part of th organism employed in a particular opera tion, but is experienced more or less by a the parts, so that it is not always correct as used to be said, that the best rest is change of occupation. It is true, however that within limits more work can b achieved with the same expenditure o energy if the element of change is intro duced into work, so long as the fresh worl is quite familiar. In experiments or industrial fatigue it has been found tha the output of work is greater if the worker are put to fresh work in the afternoons work somewhat different from that don in the mornings, but sufficiently familia to the workers.

Value of Good Working Conditions

It has likewise been found that good conditions in workshops, as regards venti lation, lighting, heating and comfort, do much to delay the onset of fatigue in the workers. Moreover, the output when the working hours are unduly long is less than when the hours are reasonable. The mental outlook is an important factor : cheerfulness and interest delay the onset of fatigue; low spirits, discontent and worry hasten it.

The sense of fatigue is removed by caffeine, hence the popularity of tea, coffee and other beverages which contain it. An excessive consumption of such beverages, however, to make possible an undue expenditure of energy, is likely to be followed by exhaustion, probably because there is dissipation of the energy-producing substances in the cells. Consequently it may require a prolonged rest before vigour is re-established.

Excess of work, worry, or drugs may result in neurasthenia or psychasthenia, r in conditions akin to these, though many people are constitutionally in such states ; they are " born tired." In some of these cases, perhaps many, it may well be that there is a dissipation of energy by emotional conflicts.

See Auto-intoxication ; Exercise ; Eye Strain ; Psycho-therapy ; Rest ; Ventilation.

FAUCES. The opening between the cavity of the mouth and the throat is called the fauces. On either side can be noted two folds, projecting inwards, one of which, lying in front, passes from the soft palate to the side of the back of the tongue, while the other, situated further back, passes from the soft palate and loses itself in the side wall of the throat. The former is called the anterior pillar, and the latter the posterior pillar, of the fauces. Between the pillars lies the tonsil, though not extending to the top of the enclosed space, the portion of which above the tonsil is known as the supra-tonsillar recess. It is in this neighbourhood that pus or matter tends specially to accumulate in quinsy. The space between the pillars on the two sides constitutes the isthmus of the fauces. This may be narrowed by tonsillitis, or some other swollen condition of the tonsil, or swelling of the back of the tongue or the soft palate.

See Pharynx ; Tonsil.

FAVUS. A skin disease, uncommon in Great Britain, but prevalent in different parts of Europe, favus is caused by a vegetable parasite, a fungus, known as achorion Schönleinii. It affects children mostly, and is usually found on the scalp, though other parts of the skin and even the nails are occasionally infected.

A crust appears on the skin in the form of a tiny, round cup, or scutulum, from the centre of which a hair projects. The crust is golden-yellow in colour, and when a number are adherent together, an appearance is caused which suggested for the disease the name of honeycomb ringworm at one time applied to it. If the colour is not very definite, it becomes so if the crust is rubbed over with spirit.

When crusts have dropped off, the scalp is hairless and scarred ; this scarring and baldness are permanent. Hairs in the affected areas are lustreless and broken. There is no discomfort beyond some itchiness, perhaps, which may cause scratching, and in this way the nails may become infected. A musty odour, like that of mice, is noticeable from the head.

The disease is spread by contact with infected persons, by wearing their caps, for example, though it may be contracted from animals, for instance, a cat.

The crusts must be removed and, to soften them, a boracic fomentation, or an ointment containing 20 grains of salicylic acid to the ounce, may be used. The hairs must be removed, and the best method is by X-rays in the hands of an expert, or, if this is not available, by pulling out a few at a time with epilating forceps. To kill the parasite, tincture of iodine should be applied freely to the head.

See Ringworm ; Scalp.

FEBRIFUGE. *See* Antipyretic.

FEEBLE-MINDED. In the customary classification of degrees of mental deficiency the epithet feeble-minded is restricted to those who are the least deficient, those whose mental endowments are more scanty being described as imbeciles and idiots. Some notion of what is meant by such terms respectively may be gathered from a comparison with the mental equipment of a normal child. Thus, a person who corresponds mentally to a child of about two years old is called an idiot, to a child of from three to seven years, an imbecile, and to one of from eight to twelve years, a feeble-minded person or moron.

These different degrees of mental deficiency may be encountered in persons who have started out in life with at least an average mental endowment but in consequence of some disorder or another have suffered deterioration ; but the persons who are more particularly included in the above classification are such as have been mentally deficient from birth, though one would probably include also those who, presumably normal at birth, have suffered deterioration in early childhood. Congenital mental deficiency may depend on a constitutional or inherited weakness of the brain, on disease of the brain occurring before birth, or on a brain injury before or during birth.

Addiction to alcohol by one or both parents is cited as one of the possible causes of enfeebling the brain of an unborn child.

In the form of idiocy associated with a defect of the thyroid gland and known as cretinism, the administration of thyroid extract, if begun sufficiently early, may effect a cure, though the drug must be continued throughout life. The only thing to be done for mental deficiency from other causes, however, is to educate the child as skilfully as possible. It cannot be hoped that even the best methods of education can do much for an idiot or imbecile ; the former is incapable of proper speech, and while the latter can be taught to understand and use simple language, he is not capable of much more.

A feeble-minded person, on the other hand, may be trained to do something towards his own support and in the higher grades even to be self-supporting.

No Appreciation of Moral Standards

Amongst feeble-minded persons are included those suffering from so-called moral imbecility, for though such might appear to the ordinary observer to suffer from no mental weakness in the ordinary sense, even, in fact, to be especially well endowed, their inability to understand the ordinary moral standards and their lack of susceptibility to moral claims must indicate some serious defect in the texture of their minds.

The proper control of this type of feeble-mindedness is a most difficult problem. Such people are not fit to be at large, however much some of them may appear to be so ; they bring trouble on themselves, humiliation on their friends and may be guilty of crimes of violence. As, however, in other respects they appear to be quite normal it is extremely difficult to obtain consent to their confinement in an institution. Their friends cling to the hope of moral improvement, a hope which is rendered vain by the absence of machinery in the mind of the unfortunate individual for producing any proper change of feeling to make moral improvement possible.

It is also a disconcerting fact that very many people who are feeble-minded, but of a sufficiently high grade to enable them to earn their living, at any rate in a sort of way, are marrying and producing children who inherit the defects of their parents, so increasing the number of those for whose support society must provide, partly or wholly.

Much has been done by legislation to safeguard the interests of the mentally deficient. The Mental Deficiency Act, 1913, provides for children and young persons, suffering from idiocy, imbecility or, if under twenty-one years of age, otherwise mentally defective, being placed, at the instance of a parent or guardian, in an institution, a course which can also be followed if such a child is neglected or abandoned. The local education authority must give notice to the local authority under the Act of any child over seven years of age who is deemed to be incapable by reason of mental defect of benefiting by special classes or of attending school without detriment to other children. Notice must be given also, when such a person attains the age of sixteen or before this, if he is about to be discharged or withdrawn from a special school or class ; this is done in order that his interests may be supervised. This Act makes it an offence to supply intoxicating liquor to a person who is mentally deficient after warning of the fact has been given.

The Elementary Education (Defective and Epileptic Children) Act, 1914, makes it the duty of the local education authority to make provision for the education of mentally-defective children over the age of seven.

The Mental Deficiency (Amendment) Act, 1925, enables a mentally deficient person to be removed from an institution and placed under guardianship.

See Degeneracy ; Idiocy ; Mental Disease.

FEEDING BOTTLE. The old-fashioned feeding bottle, with glass and rubber tubes through which the milk is sucked, is now rarely seen and is only mentioned to be condemned. It has been responsible for an enormous amount of illness and very many deaths. A feeding bottle should be either of the boat-shaped variety or a plain bottle, rounded at the bottom and at the shoulders, so that it presents no corners. Each of these varieties is furnished with a large teat, and the bottle-shaped one has an opening at the other end, which is closed with a rubber valve. The management of feeding bottles is discussed under the heading Baby.

FEMORAL VESSELS. The main blood vessels of the thigh are called the femoral artery and vein. The artery, which is a direct continuation of the external iliac artery, begins about the middle of the groin. It passes down in front of the hip joint, and then the front and inside of the thigh till it passes behind the lower end of the femur, or thigh bone, and is then called the popliteal artery. Its principal branch is called the deep femoral; this strikes off about $1\frac{1}{2}$ inches below Poupart's ligament, a strong band of fascia stretched along the groin.

The femoral vein is the continuation upwards of the popliteal vein, and for most of its course lies behind the artery, but its highest part lies on the inside of the artery. It drains the blood from the lower limb. On the front of the thigh just below Poupart's ligament, and towards the inner side, it receives the long saphenous vein which passes up the whole length of the limb on the inner side and just beneath the skin. This is the vein chiefly affected in varicose veins.

The fasciae lining the abdominal cavity are continued on to the femoral vessels beneath Poupart's ligament, and form the femoral sheath, as it is called. This has three compartments, one for the artery on the outside, then one for the vein, and on the inside a funnel-shaped space, about $\frac{1}{2}$ inch long, known as the crural canal. Ordinarily the canal is occupied simply by fat, embedded in which are lymphatic vessels and sometimes a lymphatic gland, but some abdominal viscus may be forced down this canal and on to the thigh, constituting a femoral hernia.

Serious bleeding in the thigh must be stopped by compression of the femoral artery at its beginning, the method being described under the heading Bleeding and shown in Plate VI, 10.

Sometimes in long-continued fevers, like enteric, the blood clots in the femoral vein, and so obstructs the exit of blood from the limb, which swells and generally remains swollen, the limb feeling heavy when handled. A somewhat similar condition known as a white leg sometimes follows a difficult labour.

See Groin; Puerperium; Thigh; Varicose Vein.

FEMUR. The thigh bone, or femur, is the longest bone in the body (Plate VII, 4). Its upper end consists of a rounded head and a portion called the neck which unites the head to the shaft of the bone. The head is fitted into a cavity in the pelvic bone, called the acetabulum, to form the hip joint, and from this the neck passes downwards, outwards and slightly backwards to make an angle of about 125 deg. with the shaft. Where it joins the shaft the latter bulges, on the outer side into the great trochanter, and on the inner side into the lesser trochanter. These eminences receive the insertion of important muscles, the lesser trochanter that of the ilio-psoas, a large muscle situated within the abdomen, which flexes the thigh and rotates it outwards.

The shaft of the bone consists of a cylinder of dense bone. The lower extremity is thickened and presents a rounded eminence, or condyle, on its outer and inner aspects which are covered with cartilage and articulate with the upper surface of the head of the tibia to form the knee joint. The space between the condyles in front is also covered with cartilage and articulates with the patella, or knee-cap, while behind the condyles are separated by a notch, the intercondylar fossa, in which lie the popliteal vessels and other structures.

The femur does not occupy a vertical position, being nearer the middle line of the body at the knee than at the hip; this obliquity is even more pronounced in women.

Congenital Dislocation of the Hip

In children and adolescents it may happen that the neck of the bone comes to make a smaller angle with the shaft than 125 deg.; it may become horizontal or even pass upwards to the shaft instead of downwards. This deformity is called coxa vara (*see* illustration, page 221), and is caused by softening of the bone.

It is not uncommon for the neck of the femur to be broken, especially in elderly people, and possibly from mere jarring of the bone. Sometimes the neck is driven into the expanded bone at the top of the shaft, and fixed there. This is called an impacted fracture, and it may permit of the patient walking so that the existence of the fracture might be overlooked. Whenever possible, in an elderly person, the limb is fixed in a Thomas's splint (Plate XXXIII, 4) and a patten provided for the other foot, so that the patient can get about on crutches. If confined to bed, there is a great risk of death, probably from pneumonia. First-aid treatment of a fractured femur is shown in Plate XVIII.

The lower end of the femur is a common site of infective osteomyelitis, a serious disease which may cause large destruction of the bone or even kill the patient, and of a tumour, the so-called myeloid sarcoma.
See Bone; Fracture; Hip; Innominate; Knee; Osteomyelitis; Tumour.

FERMENT. A ferment is defined as a substance which is capable of causing chemical changes in another substance, with which it comes into contact without itself undergoing any change. Yeasts and bacteria are sometimes called living or organised ferments, as distinguished from soluble ferments, such as the pepsin of the gastric juice. The latter are also called enzymes.

Ferments are of enormous importance to animal and vegetable life and very many are produced and exercise activity in the human body. The coagulation of milk in the stomach, for example, is brought about by the ferment rennin, proteins are reduced to an absorbable form by the ferments pepsin and trypsin, fats are split up by the ferment lipase, starch is converted into sugar by the ferments ptyalin and amylopsin, and so on.
See Digestion.

FERMENTATION. The best known instance of fermentation is the production of alcohol. If a little yeast be added to a solution of sugar a froth soon appears, which is found to consist of carbonic acid gas, while alcohol begins to accumulate in the liquid and there is a corresponding diminution in the quantity of sugar. Yeast consists of a minute vegetable growth, or fungus, and from it may be extracted a substance to which the name zymase has been given and which is the active factor in causing the fermentation.

As is well known, beer and wines may become sour and vinegary, and this is due to some of the alcohol being converted into acetic acid by a living ferment known as mycoderma aceti. Milk sugar may be converted into lactic acid by the lactic acid bacillus, as occurs in the souring of milk. Artificial buttermilk is made by the deliberate introduction of such a bacillus. Fermentation may occur in the stomach with the formation of lactic acid, and possibly also of butyric acid, which is formed from fat by the action of another bacillus. Flatulence may be troublesome in such circumstances and is due to the production of carbonic acid gas. Any considerable fermentation in the stomach or bowel is indicative of stagnation of the contents.
See Flatulence; Indigestion.

FEVER. The normal body temperature is usually about 98·4° F., though it may reach 99° F. without anything being wrong, as, for example, during digestion or after hard exercise. When the temperature is higher than this, however, a state of fever, or pyrexia, is said to exist, or if the temperature is over 105·8° F., hyperpyrexia, a dangerous condition because merely to be so hot as this, without other noxious influence, might be sufficient to kill a person.

Fever may arise in different ways; after exposure to great heat, for example, as in heat stroke; in apoplexy, especially when there is bleeding into that part of the brain known as the pons; or when there is inflammation anywhere about the body.

By far the most common cause of fever, however, is the invasion of the body by microbes. The acute infectious fevers constitute a group of diseases marked by a more or less definite course, each fever being characterised by particular symptoms. There is a well-founded belief that when fever occurs in connexion with microbic invasion, it represents part of the effort which the body makes to repel the invasion, and, so long as the temperature keeps within bounds, an attempt to depress it is likely to be mischievous.

The existence of fever may be surmised from the sensations of the patient himself, and when a hand is place on his skin it may feel hot; indeed, in some diseases, such as scarlet fever, it may feel burning hot. On the other hand, a patient may shiver violently and his skin feel cold, and nevertheless a thermometer in his mouth may reveal the fact that he is highly fevered. The only reliable means therefore of discovering fever and its degree is to use a thermometer.

It is usual for the temperature in fevers to be higher in the evening and to fall towards morning, but occasionally this sequence is reversed. When there are intervals of normal or subnormal temperature, lasting from some hours to two or three days, between bouts of fever, the fever is said to be intermittent ; when the temperature does not reach normal, but the difference between the highest and lowest readings exceeds 1·5° F., it is called remittent, or, if the difference is only 1·5° F. or less, continued fever.

In a febrile disease the temperature may rise rapidly, that is, within the course of a few hours, or it may not reach its high level till a few days have elapsed. Similarly, it may decline by a sudden or by a gradual drop, the former being called termination by crisis and the latter, termination by lysis. Sometimes the temperature suddenly falls but again rises ; such a fall is described as a pseudo-crisis. The crisis is usually accompanied by profuse sweating, by a large flow of urine or by diarrhoea. That is what is meant by critical sweating, diuresis or diarrhoea.

What Constitutes the Febrile State

The various acute specific fevers have characteristic symptoms and signs which distinguish each, but there are symptoms common to all, those associated merely with the febrile state. The patient may feel out of sorts and uncomfortable, his condition being aptly expressed in the word malaise. He may feel shivery, and in some cases there are severe shiverings or rigors. In children fevers are not uncommonly ushered in by convulsions, which at this age are the equivalent of a rigor. There may be a general feeling of soreness in the muscles and bones, and sometimes even neuralgia. Bright lights are offensive to the eyes, and loud noises to the ears, and there may be noises in the ears and giddiness.

The pulse rate is almost always more increased, typhoid fever being a notable exception in this respect, and it is generally found that the pulse rate is increased by eight to ten beats for each degree of rise of temperature. The breathing rate is also increased, although, except in lung diseases, the normal ratio of one full respiratory movement to about four pulse beats is preserved.

All the secretions of the body are diminished and so the skin is dry, the mouth is dry, the urine is diminished and high-coloured, and there is a tendency to constipation. The tongue is furred, there is thirst, and, as a rule, loss of appetite. Usually there is some headache, and there may be delirium ; children become delirious in comparatively slight febrile attacks.

Method of Treating Fever

Slight fever does not prevent a person from being up and about, but it disappears earlier if rest be taken, and if there is any decided degree of fever, the patient must go to bed. There should be just a sufficiency of bedclothes, and the room should be well ventilated. For this purpose it is best to have a window always open, and the more widely open it is the less draught. If a draught plays on the bed, a screen should be placed where it will prevent this. Lights should be shaded, and there should be no noise in the sick-room, creaking doors or furniture being very objectionable.

Diet should be light, the main item being milk, which may be diluted with hot water, barley water or soda water. Two pints or more of milk should be taken in the 24 hours, a feed being given every two hours. One or two of the feeds may be replaced by one of beef tea or a meat extract, especially if the bowels are constipated. If the bowels are loose, on the other hand, meat extracts should be withheld, and the milk may be boiled and diluted with lime water. Water should be taken freely, some of it in the form of home-made lemonade, or, if the bowels are constipated, Imperial drink.

A restriction to liquid diet in fevers is not insisted on by many doctors if the patient can digest and relish anything more, when thin bread and butter, cornflour, ground rice, arrowroot and lightly-cooked eggs are given in addition to milk. Sometimes a patient may not appear to digest even milk readily, however, and then he may be put on gelatin, 1½ ounces dissolved in a quart of water, and flavoured with fresh lemon-juice, feeds of this being taken at the same intervals as for milk.

Each day the patient should be washed all over, but piecemeal, so as to avoid unnecessary exposure, first the face, then each arm, then the back, and so on, each part being dried before proceeding to the next. The hair should be brushed through ; in some illnesses it will be desirable to cut it short. The mouth should be cleansed several times during the day. The bed should be shaken up, and, if the patient cannot be transported to another bed or a couch, meanwhile, he can be placed at one side of the bed while the other is being made. In continued fevers it is a good plan to have one bed for day use and another for the night ; here, also, it is especially necessary to guard against bed sores (q.v.).

It is common to give a simple fever mixture such as the following :

Sweet spirit of nitre	½ ounce
Liquor of acetate of ammonium	1 ounce
Syrup of oranges	4 drachms
Camphor water .. .. to 6 ounces	

A tablespoonful for an adult, or a teaspoonful for a child, every 3 hours.

This helps to keep the skin active. At the commencement of the illness 10 grains of aspirin may be given to relieve headache or muscular pains, if necessary ; or if this is unsuccessful, 7 grains of phenacetin with 1 grain of caffeine citrate. As a rule, there should be as little drugging as possible. One or two layers of gauze wrung out of iced water and placed on the forehead will help to relieve headache.

Should the temperature rise above 102·5° F., the patient can be sponged with tepid or cold water, to which has been added a little vinegar or eau-de-Cologne, one part at a time, as in washing. If the temperature continues to rise, he may be placed in a wet pack, made with tepid or cold water. For hyperpyrexia an iced pack or bath may be required, but these should only be used under medical supervision. A patient is always removed from a cold bath or iced pack when his temperature is still two or three degrees above normal, otherwise he might collapse, as the temperature continues to fall after his removal.

If there is much delirium, a tepid or hot pack will be likely to do good, whatever the state of the patient's temperature. Such treatment may also be adopted to procure sleep when necessary. It is important that the patient should have sufficient sleep, and in short illnesses it will rarely be desirable to wake the patient in order to give food ; in prolonged illnesses, however, it may be necessary, but the advice of the medical attendant should be obtained.

Other details of description and treatment are given in connexion with each fever to which they are applicable.

See Bacteria ; Bath ; Beverages ; Cold ; Cold Pack ; Crisis ; Infectious Disease ; Nursing ; Pack ; Pneumonia ; Scarlet Fever ; Temperature ; Thermometer ; Typhoid Fever.

FIBROSIS. The development of fibrous tissue is described as fibrosis. The essential elements of glands and other active tissues are separated, more or less, by connective tissue, which binds them together and supports them. Wounds or gaps in tissues caused by disease are repaired by this connective tissue from which new cells are formed and later developed into fibres.

In the same way a focus of irritation may be surrounded and sealed off, as it were, by new fibrous tissue. This may happen to a foreign body, for instance, and is a common event when tubercle bacilli have invaded the lung.

It may happen, however, that fibrosis is not a limited process, but either is widely diffused through an organ or by gradual extension becomes so. This may take place, for example, in the lung from the irritation of dust and in other circumstances, and also in the liver, kidney, heart wall and other places. This type of fibrosis is also spoken of as cirrhosis.

The new fibrous tissue, if in considerable amount, may cause enlargement of the organ concerned ; but when the tissue contracts, in the manner of scar tissue, the organ becomes smaller and harder than normally is the case. The pressure of the new tissue in the first instance, and later on the compression caused by its contraction, result in the loss of the essential parts of the tissue, the liver cells, for example, so that to the extent to which fibrosis occurs, the functional power of the organ is impaired.

FIBROSITIS. Inflammation of the connective tissue which is widely distributed in the body as fascia, muscle-sheaths and so on, is called fibrositis. Muscular rheumatism, so-called, is of this nature, but, while the rheumatic poison may sometimes be responsible, other poisons produce the disorder and notably that from septic teeth or a septic throat.

The inflamed tissue is first enlarged by an exudation of fluid so that it forms a soft and ill-defined swelling, which may become more defined, however, if it is massaged. New cells are also produced and these accumulate and in time are converted into fibrous tissue forming a strand or knot. When the swelling occurs it presses on nerves and may give rise to intense pain. This abates when the swelling has diminished sufficiently and should the mischief be cleared up there may be no more pain, but should a sufficient amount of new tissue be formed, leaving strands or knots, these are apt to swell up, particularly at a change of weather. This explains the recurrence of pain at the site of an old fibrositis and the apprehension of its victims as regards exposure to cold and damp. The disease in the first instance may possibly be induced by cold and damp as these may favour local congestion and the accumulation of poison at a certain spot. Many people suffer from fibrositis if an electric fan plays directly on any part of their bodies for a short time. Alcoholic indulgence is another thing that may precipitate an attack.

Fibrositis in certain situations receives a special name ; thus when occurring in the lumbar region it is called lumbago, or in intercostal muscles, pleurodynia. It is the commonest cause of stiff neck.

In acute fibrositis the most urgent duty is to relieve the pain, but at the same time a search must be made for some septic focus which should be cleaned up promptly. This will often entail the extraction of teeth.

The most effective agents for relieving pain are heat and massage, or a combina-tion of these. Heat may be applied in a variety of ways such as a hot bath, a hot-air bath, a radiant heat bath, poultices, hot fomentations, or hot-water bags. Massage should be gentle when done over tender spots, but often the pain decreases under gentle massage and permits of firmer movements. An attempt should be made to discover the swellings or nodules above referred to, and these should be rubbed away as it were (*see* illustrations, Plate XVII, 1–2). A useful method of combining heat and massage is ironing the part with a hot iron. The skin is protected by a layer of brown paper or flannel and the pressure of the iron regulated according to the weight able to be borne. This method is often used for lumbago. After the massage the patient should be encouraged to exercise the affected muscles a little.

Drugs may be of some use. The bowels may be cleared by giving 3 grains of calomel at bed-time and 120 grains of Epsom salts in a third of a glass of water in the morning. Aspirin, in 10-grain doses, or 5 grains each of aspirin and phenacetin often give relief. Sodium salicylate is another remedy. Occasionally an opiate will be needed to secure relief. The patient should be kept warm and should avoid draughts ; woollen or flannel under-clothing should be worn.

In slighter cases, or when improvement has occurred in severe cases, rubbing the part with a liniment, such as equal parts of methyl salicylate and olive oil, will generally suffice. After rubbing, the part may be covered with capsicum wool or with flannel. When apparatus is available, electrical treatment or diathermy is sometimes used in treating fibrositis.

When there is a tendency to the disorder the bowels should be kept open and the diet should be simple ; wool, or at least a wool mixture, should be worn next the skin, and there should be no standing about in damp clothes or in draughts.

See Back-ache ; Pleurodynia ; Rheumatism.

FIBULA. The long slender bone on the outer side of the leg is called the fibula. It articulates at its upper and lower ends with the tibia, but, whereas it takes no part in forming the knee joint, its share in forming the ankle joint is an important one. It forms the outer boundary of what might be described as the mortice of the ankle joint, which receives the tenon consisting of the astragalus bone.

Into the head of the bone is inserted the tendon of the biceps muscle, the outer hamstring, and about an inch below the head the external popliteal, or common peroneal, nerve winds round the bone to divide into the anterior tibial and popliteal nerves. A considerable injury at this point might bruise or otherwise injure the external popliteal nerve and perhaps give rise to foot drop.

The lower end of the bone is enlarged to make the external malleolus or prominence of the ankle. When one turns over on the ankle, as in stepping off a kerb for instance, the ankle may simply be sprained, but it may happen that the pressure on the fibula causes a fracture of the bone in its lower third. This is called a Pott's fracture, and it usually takes place about 3 inches above the tip of the lower end of the bone. At the same time the internal lateral ligament of the joint may be torn or even the internal malleolus torn off. The foot is twisted or even displaced outwards. A more severe degree of displacement, upwards as well as outwards, occurs in Dupuytren's fracture, in which the lower end of the fibula is separated from the tibia.

The first-aid treatment of these fractures is to pull steadily but gently on the foot until it is placed at right angles with the leg, with the sole in its natural position, and then fix the foot by inner and outer splints, or, failing splints, by tying the legs and ankles together. If there is any difficulty in correcting the position of the foot it should be left for a doctor to do ; bending the limb at the knee may suffice, but an anaesthetic may be necessary.

See Extension ; Fracture : Leg.

FIDGETS. Jerky and purposeless movements occurring in children may be due to tic (*q.v.*) or habit spasm, to chorea or St. Vitus's dance (*q.v.*) or may simply represent fidgets, movements that are distinguished from those of a true tic by their not being so much confined to one muscle group and by not being so persistent. Fidgets tend to occur in

highly strung children when excited from fear or some other cause and are more likely to occur if the child is over-tired. Fidgets may also be an expression of fatigue in older persons.

FIELD OF VISION. If one eye be closed and the gaze of the other directed to some point in front, there is an area within which things surrounding the point looked at are visible. This area is called the field of vision of the eye in question. Inwards and upwards it is more limited than in other directions on account of the obstruction to inward vision caused by the bridge of the nose, and to upward vision by the eyebrow. Thus, when both eyes are looking at a certain point the central part of the total field of vision will be seen by both eyes, but the portions to the right and left of this will be visible to the respective eye only.

The extent of the field of vision of an eye can be tested in a rough way by directing its gaze on a fixed point, while the vision of the other eye is obstructed, and then bringing a moving finger or a small piece of white paper from all directions towards the line of vision.

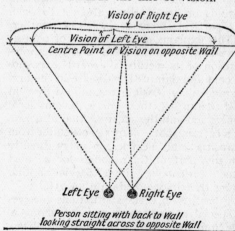

Vision of Right Eye
Vision of Left Eye
Centre Point of Vision on opposite Wall
Left Eye   *Right Eye*
Person sitting with back to Wall looking straight across to opposite Wall

The field of vision of an eye has a greater range on its own side than on that of the other eye

When greater accuracy is necessary an instrument known as a perimeter is used. A small piece of white cardboard is slid round a metal bar in the form of a quadrant which can be rotated round an axis corresponding to the line of vision. The bar is graduated so that the point where the cardboard becomes visible can be noted definitely. This point is marked on a chart prepared for the purpose. Some instruments are fitted up for the automatic marking of these points on a chart.

A chart consists of a number of concentric circles around a central spot and lines radiating at equal intervals from the centre and intersecting the circles. Charts are furnished for the right and left eye respectively, and on the chart a dotted line is usually made to enclose the normal field of vision for the eye. A short distance outside the centre of each chart a small area is marked which is called the blind spot and corresponds to the optic disk, or the part of the retina where the optic nerve enters, which is incapable of vision.

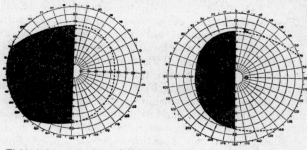

Field of vision of both eyes half obscured (hemianopia), the blackness on the left indicating a defect in the right side of each retina

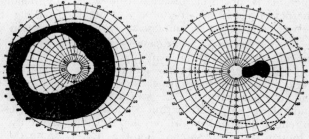

Left, blindness due to glaucoma or to commencing atrophy of the optic nerve.   Right, blind spot or scotoma found in tobacco poisoning

The outer half of each chart is known as the temporal half, but records the vision of the nasal half of the retina, while the inner, or nasal, half of the chart records the vision of the temporal half of the retina. Blindness shown on one half of the chart is called hemianopia, or hemianopsia, temporal or nasal as the case may be. When the nasal half of one chart is invisible and the temporal half of the other, the hemianopia is said to be homonymous. A blind area within the chart is called a scotoma.

A defect in the field of vision may be due to a lesion in the eye itself, in the optic nerve or tract, or in the parts of the brain subserving vision. A general, or concentric, contraction of the field of vision suggests atrophy of the optic nerve. Homonymous hemianopia points to a lesion of the optic tract or the brain on the opposite side from that showing on the chart. A central scotoma is most commonly due to tobacco poisoning.

If coloured objects are used instead of a white one when testing the field of vision, it is found that the field for blue is almost as large as that for white, but is less for other colours, diminishing progressively for yellow, red and green in this order.

See Binocular ; Eye ; Vision.

FIG. Besides being nutritious, in virtue of their content of sugar, figs have a laxative effect and may be eaten to correct constipation. This should not be done, however, if there are piles, as the seeds are liable to collect in the folds at the lower end of the bowel and cause irritation. Figs are contained in confection of senna and a syrup is also made from the fruit, which is especially useful for children. The aromatic and compound syrups of figs contain other laxative drugs and are stronger preparations.

FILARIA. In tropical and sub-tropical countries the human body may be invaded by various species of parasitic roundworm belonging to the genus filaria. One of these is the guinea-worm (*q.v.*). Infestation with species other than the guinea-worm is called filariasis, and, besides occurring in man, may be found in other mammals and in birds.

In man, the embryos of three species are known to occur in the blood, and are collectively known as filaria sanguinis hominis. Of these, filaria diurna, found in West Africa, occurs in the blood during the day, but the usual habitat of the adult worm, known as filaria loa, is beneath the conjunctiva. Filaria perstans is the adult form of a worm, the embryos, or microfilariae, of which appear to invade the blood at any time during the 24 hours. The adults lurk in connective tissue, pericardial fat, the supra-renal bodies and elsewhere. The third species, filaria bancrofti or nocturna, is the most important. Its embryo is known as microfilaria nocturna because it invades the peripheral blood stream only at night between about 7 p.m. and 7 a.m.

A consequence, or a cause, of this periodicity is that there is an opportunity for the digestion of the embryos by mosquitoes when these are sucking blood, and it is necessary that the worm should undergo development within a mosquito to render it capable of full development in a human being. It should be noted, however, that in persons on night duty who sleep during the day the parasites are in the peripheral blood during the day. The time passed in the body of the mosquito is from ten to twenty days, after which, when the mosquito again feeds, the parasites are injected into the skin and, making their way into lymphatic channels, develop into the adult form. The sexes unite and swarms of embryos are produced.

These are about one seventy-fifth of an inch in length, and their presence in the blood does not have any ill effect. The adult worms are from three to four inches long, however, and tend to cause irritation and obstruction of lymphatic channels. Thus there may be lymphangitis, with painful swelling of a limb and irregular fever, described as elephantoid fever. Other results are chyluria or the discharge of milky-looking urine; chylocele, a swelling in the scrotum resembling a hydro-

cele (*q.v.*) but containing a milky fluid; lymph scrotum, or distension of the lymphatics of the scrotum; or enlargements of the glands in the groin. Another possible consequence is the enormous enlargement of a limb, the scrotum or some other part, to which the name elephantiasis is given.

Injections of arsenical preparations and of tartrate of antimony have been followed by a great diminution in the number of microfilariae in the blood and moderation of the swelling and other symptoms caused by obstruction of the lymphatics. Lymphangitis is treated by hot or other soothing applications, and swelling by elevation of the part affected.

See Elephantiasis; Guinea-worm; Lymphatic System.

FILTER. Drinking-water from shallow wells and other unsafe sources should be filtered in order to clear it of suspended impurities and especially of bacteria, and the only filter which can be depended on to do this is one of the candle type. Animal charcoal, flannel, canvas, spongy iron and various iron compounds have been used as filtering agents, but they do not keep back bacteria; in fact, owing to their becoming clogged with organic matter, they may actually cause an increase of bacterial impurity in the water. In army operations in the field, filter-carts are used in which water is pumped through flannel or canvas. This removes sand and clay, or at any rate most of it, but the water must further be either boiled or treated with chemical disinfectants before use.

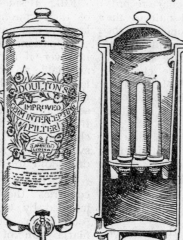

Germ-proof filter of the non-pressure type

In the candle type of filter the candle, which is a hollow cylinder or a conical tube, may be made of biscuit porcelain, as in the Pasteur-Chamberland, of white porcelain, as in the Doulton, or of infusorial clay, as in the Berkefeld. The rate of flow through the last is about twice as fast as that through the Pasteur-Chamberland, the flow through which is also somewhat slower than that through the Doulton.

In all, the direction of the flow is from the outside into the candles, so that any deposit takes place on the surface of the latter. With continuous use this deposit accumulates, and bacteria might grow through into the interior of the candle. It is necessary, therefore, to take out the candles every third day, cleanse them with a brush kept for the purpose, and plunge them for a short time into boiling water.

A disadvantage of this type of filter is its relatively slow delivery of filtered water unless the inflow is at considerable pressure, as when a filter is attached to the delivery pipe of a cistern placed at some height, or the water is pumped through the filter.

If, however, the water is emptied into the large container of the usual household pattern and must make its way through the filter candles simply by the pressure of its own weight, the only safe alternative to waiting on the accumulation of filtered water is to sterilise the water by boiling or by chemicals.

Although ordinary micro-organisms cannot make their way through filter candles there are minute forms which can, such being known as filterable viruses. Rabies, smallpox and possibly influenza are amongst the diseases caused by them.

See Infectious Disease ; Water.

FINGER. There are three bones in each finger, as contrasted with the thumb, which has only two. These bones are spoken of as phalanges (singular, phalanx), and a joint between them as an inter-phalangeal joint. The joint connecting a finger with the rest of the hand is called a metacarpo-phalangeal joint, and resembles a ball-and-socket joint, an inter-phalangeal joint being of the hinge variety.

Of the creases on the palmar surface of the fingers the lower two correspond to the inter-phalangeal joints, but the uppermost are considerably below the metacarpo-phalangeal joints, which correspond with creases passing across the palm of the hand.

The fingers are distinguished as the fore or index, the middle, the ring and the little finger, the first being most highly mobile and most highly developed as regards touch. The fingers may be flexed, extended, abducted and adducted.

Abduction of a finger means movement away from, and adduction movement towards, a line drawn down the middle of the middle finger. These movements are performed by the interossei, small muscles in the body of the hand, activated by the ulnar nerve. This explains why paralysis of this nerve results in a loss of power to spread the fingers.

Flexion is brought about by muscles in the forearm, whose tendons pass down in the palm of the hand to the fingers, and, at the metacarpo-phalangeal joint, by four small muscles known as the lumbricals. Extension is caused by forearm muscles.

Tendons and Their Sheaths

The tendons, or sinews, of the forearm muscles are enclosed in synovial sheaths, but in the index, middle and ring fingers there is a distinct separation between the sheath covering the tendon in the finger itself and that covering the tendon in the palm and wrist. In the little finger, as in the thumb, the sheath is continuous. From this it follows that suppuration, for example, from a whitlow in the little finger, if it reaches the synovial sheath, may spread upwards and cause an abscess in the forearm ; this is unlikely to happen from suppuration in the other fingers.

Various congenital deformities of the fingers occur. There may be an excessive number, or polydactylism ; fingers may be missing, or ectrodactylism ; adjoining fingers may be united, or syndactyly, the connexion being either a thin web or fleshy ; a finger may be of excessive size, or macrodactyly ; or the fingers may be contracted, or bent, a deformity which has to be distinguished from Dupuytren's contraction (*q.v.*). Often such deformities are inherited.

Fingers may also be distorted by the contraction of scars, for instance, following a burn, and sometimes when opposing surfaces of fingers are concerned a thin web unites them. Plastic operations may be successful in restoring function. In what is called a mallet finger the end phalanx is flexed, probably from damage to structures on the back of the finger. A trigger, snap, spring or jerk finger is one in which the straightening of the finger cannot be accomplished at once,

[*Continued in page* 302

BRIEF INSTRUCTIONS FOR EVERYDAY EMERGENCIES

ANIMAL BITE

Animal obviously healthy. Wash wound with warm water or antiseptic lotion : antiseptic dressing.

Animal possibly rabid, or viper bite. Arrest circulation. If limb, apply tourniquet (*see* below) to upper arm or thigh as case may be ; if a finger, grasp at once firmly round the root.

Suck ; encourage bleeding ; wash with warm water or antiseptic lotion. No danger in sucking if no broken surface about mouth.

Warmth and stimulants if necessary.

See a doctor as soon as possible.

Possibly rabid animal should *not* be destroyed at once.

Improvised Tourniquet. Put stone about width of five-shilling piece, or similar hard object, as a pad, in centre of folded handkerchief or triangular bandage. Place pad over main artery ; tie handkerchief loosely round limb ; put stick through loop thus made : twist till bleeding stops.

ARTIFICIAL RESPIRATION

Ascertain that mouth and throat are clear ; loosen tight clothing at neck and chest.

Lay face downwards, head to one side, arms forward as illustrated in Plate IV. Kneel alongside, level of hips, hands on lower ribs, thumbs parallel and near spine. Stoop forward with arms straight ; count slowly, 1, 2, 3, keeping hands on chest, spring back to take off pressure ; count, slowly, 1, 2. Repeat till natural breathing is established.

When breathing established, but not before, give coffee or weak spirits ; chafe limbs ; hot bottles.

BLEEDING

Free external bleeding. Put finger or thumb at once on bleeding spot ; replace finger by firm pad of antiseptic dressing or clean rag as soon as ready ; if necessary, press on main artery of part, first with fingers and then, in case of limb, by improvised tourniquet.

If bleeding from limb, lay patient down and elevate the limb ; remove garters and other constrictions.

Summon doctor at once ; no stimulants meanwhile.

Oozing of blood. Press firmly with pad of antiseptic or clean fabric.

Nose-bleeding. Lay patient down ; cold water on forehead ; do not blow nose ; if necessary, stuff clean white silk handkerchief, gauze or rag into nostril.

Bleeding from socket of extracted tooth. Make firm pad of clean handkerchief and bite on it.

Spitting or vomiting blood. Summon doctor ; lay patient down, shoulders raised ; plenty of fresh air ; warmth to feet ; reassure patient.

BRUISE

Cold application (layer of muslin or other fabric kept moist with water, perhaps with addition of eau-de-Cologne, spirits or vinegar) ; rest injured part by means of sling, etc.

BURN

Skin not broken. Vaseline, carron oil, boracic vaseline, boracic powder, or thick paste of bicarbonate of soda.

Skin broken. Boracic lint moistened or rag dipped in antiseptic lotion.

Severe burn of child. Place in warm bath and then undress ; child seriously burnt is general'y quiet.

To uncover burn. Do not pull away clothing ; first cut round, then soak off. Place severely burnt limb of adult in warm bath.

In case of severe burn. Summon doctor at once, and meanwhile give small doses of stimulants.

Person on fire. Wrap blanket, rug, or coat round and roll on floor.

CHOKING

Pass finger or handle of spoon along inside of cheek to back of throat ; hook foreign body forward.

If teeth clenched, handle of spoon between back teeth and turn on its edge ; slap smartly between shoulders.

When foreign body out, if breathing ceased, employ artificial respiration.

COUGH

Suck pastille ; equal parts hot milk and soda water with pinch bicarbonate of soda ; cold compress to throat (folded handkerchief or lint, wrung out cold water, covered with oiled silk or brown paper) ; inhalation of steam from jug of nearly boiling water to which teaspoonful Friar's balsam added.

CRAMP

In legs, apply cold plate to sole of feet ; massage.

CROUP

If breath.ng difficult and child's face dusky give one drachm of ipecacuanha wine to cause vomiting and repeat this if necessary.

CUT

Arrest bleeding (*see* Bleeding) ; if small, dab with tincture of iodine or Friar's balsam ; any larger cut, cover with antiseptic dressing ; bandage.

EAR

Foreign body (*e.g.* pea or insect) in ; put in a little warm almond or olive oil. Do not syringe, except on doctor's orders. Make *no* attempt to extract by hairpin or any other instrument.

EARACHE

Drop warm almond oil in ear ; roast common salt on shovel, put in small flannel bag and apply.

ELECTRIC SHOCK

Turn off current at main or, to remove patient, stand on pile of dry clothing, hands gloved.

EYE

Foreign body in the eye. Wash freely with warm water ; dip face in basin of warm water, opening and closing eye while under water ; draw down lower lid, remove foreign body with corner of handkerchief. Turn up upper lid over match while patient looks down at his feet, remove as above.

Do not attempt to rub foreign body from clear part of eye.

Irritation after removal of foreign body. Drop of castor oil. If any difficulty, see doctor at once.

FAINTING

Lay flat on floor, loosen tight clothing neck and chest ; snuff smelling salts. When able to swallow, sips of water, weak spirits or sal volatile in water.

FIT

Summon doctor ; meanwhile : *Child*—warm bath, cold cloths to head.

Adult—keep lying down, head slightly raised ; no attempt to prevent movements, but restrain if very violent ; stick or handle of tooth brush between back teeth to prevent biting tongue ; loosen tight clothing, neck and chest ; allow sleep 2 or 3 hours.

FRACTURE

Do not move before broken bone is fixed by splints, etc. Bleeding, arrest (*see* Bleeding). Summon doctor.

Splints : umbrella, walking-sticks, broom handle, cardboard, tightly rolled newspapers, etc. ; if legs, tie together, above and below. Pad splints with coats, etc.

BRIEF INSTRUCTIONS FOR EVERYDAY EMERGENCIES (continued)

FROST-BITE

Or chilling feet, hands, nose, or ears. Do not bring near fire, do not use warmth. Rub with snow or cold water till circulation restored.

GAS POISONING

Don't use naked light. Protect mouth and nose with damp cloth ; turn gas off ; open window or knock out pane with some implement ; remove patient to landing or further if air not fresh. If breathing weak, artificial respiration at once.

GIDDINESS

If stomach upset, induce vomiting by tickling back of throat ; to make vomiting easier give tepid water in large draughts ; dose of castor oil ; and if constipated an enema of soap and water.

If severe, keep lying down, mustard plaster to nape of neck ; darken room.

HEADACHE

Fresh air ; cup of tea ; half teaspoonful sal volatile in water ; mustard plaster nape of neck ; cold applications to forehead (see Bruise) ; aspirin.

HEART-BURN

Half teaspoonful bicarbonate of soda or magnesia in water ; light food ; no greasy food or pastry.

INSECT BITES

Bathe with solution of ammonia, of bicarbonate of soda or of permanganate of potash. Bites sometimes prevented by spraying cuffs and stockings with compound tincture of lavender and dabbing exposed parts with same. Mosquito bites prevented by dabbing exposed parts with solution of Epsom salts. See Sting.

ITCHING

Sponge with water, hot as can be borne ; heaped teaspoonful bicarbonate of soda in pint of water ; weak lead lotion ; apply zinc ointment or zinc dusting powder.

NOSE

If foreign body in nose, cause patient to blow down or sneeze. Do not attempt to extract with any instrument.

POISONING

Doctor at once, saying '' case of poisoning '' : meanwhile, if :

Stains on lips or mouth. Give no emetic.

If from acid, *e.g.* oil of vitriol, give chalk, whiting, magnesia in water, or, except for salts of lemon, bicarbonate of soda.

If from alkali, *e.g.* caustic soda, give weak vinegar or lemon juice.

If from carbolic acid or creosote give dessertspoonful of Epsom salts in water, and repeat ½ hour.

Give water freely in all these cases, also white of egg, gruel, milk, thin arrowroot or cornflour.

Other poisons. Give emetic, tablespoonful mustard or common salt in glass of water ; tickle back of throat ; large draughts tepid water ; strong warm tea freely.

White of egg, gruel, etc., as above.

Patient drowsy—keep awake.

Patient unconscious—pint of warm (*not* hot) coffee by enema in bowel.

Breathing difficult—warm compress or sponge wrung out of hot water to throat ; moisten air with steam from bronchitis kettle or ordinary kettle with long cardboard tube attached to spout ; give ice to suck.

Breathing ceased—artificial respiration.

Abdominal pain—hot fomentations or poultices.

Faintness or collapse—weak spirits.

Preserve all the vomited matter for doctor's inspection.

SCALD

See Burn.

SCRATCH

Dab with tincture of iodine.

SICKNESS

May be due to large number of causes. Obtain medical advice early.

For retching, large draughts of warm water may ease.

Vomiting—sips of hot water ; iced champagne ; mustard plaster on pit of stomach.

SPRAINS

Simple Sprain—cold applications (*see* Bruise) ; put part in position of rest, lower limb elevated on pillow, upper in a sling. Do not prolong cold applications on old or debilitated people. Gentle massage as soon as acute symptoms subside, then gentle moving of joint by the nurse ; elastic bandage.

Severe Sprain—difficult to exclude possibility of fracture or dislocation, consult doctor.

STING

Extract sting, then apply weak solution of household ammonia or sal volatile ; solution of bicarbonate of soda or permanganate of potash.

If necessary give weak spirits or one drachm of sal volatile in water.

Severe inflammation and general illness, see doctor at once.

STOMACH-ACHE

Various remedies : (1) Half-teaspoonful bicarbonate of soda ; (2) bismuth and soda ; (3) peppermint water ; (4) essence cinnamon, or spirit of camphor, 5 drops on sugar ; (5) dilute spirits ; (6) hot-water bag, hot fomentation or poultice.

In Infants. Sips of warm water ; dill water ; warm flannel to abdomen ; warm feet. If not speedily relieved, consult doctor.

TOOTHACHE

Clove oil or spirit of camphor on cotton wool into cavity of tooth.

Dry the gum and paint with tincture of iodine.

Hot-water bag or bread poultice to cheek. Aspirin.

To Destroy a Badly Injured Dog or Cat with a minimum of pain, the best plan is to strangle with a ligature round neck on principle of an improvised tourniquet—a loosely tied pocket-handkerchief or string, tightened by twisting a short stick through it, will serve.

FIRST AID OUTFIT FOR THE HOME

A really adequate outfit should include the items specified below :

Boracic Lint, ½ yard
Oiled Silk, ½ yard
Absorbent Cotton Wool, ¼ lb.
2 Triangular Bandages
Finger Bandage
Clean Scissors
(The above to be kept in their packages in tin box with tight lid)

Tincture of Iodine, 1 oz.
(A teaspoonful in 1 pint water for antiseptic lotion)
Boracic Acid Powder, 1 oz.
(To make eye lotion, etc.)
Sal Volatile, 1 oz.
Boracic Vaseline, 1 oz.
Friar's Balsam, 1 oz.

Permanganate of Potash
(Crystals or Tablets)
Epsom Salts, 1 oz.

Tin of Mustard

Eye Bath

Higginson's Enema Syringe

and when it does take place, does so in a jerky fashion. There are various causes for this state of affairs, but the most common is an excessive size of the sesamoid bone, which may occur in the tendons and ligaments at the front of the root of a finger.

In tuberculosis of the lungs, emphysema and other lung diseases, and in malignant endocarditis, the fingers may be swollen at the ends, or, as it is called, clubbed. In osteo-arthritis little, hard nodules may form on the sides of the end phalanx. Deposits of urate of sodium, or tophi, may occur at the finger joints in gout. The condition known as dead fingers occurs in Raynaud's disease.

See Forearm ; Hand ; Nail ; Poultice ; Sensation ; Thumb ; Whitlow ; Wrist.

FINGER-STALL. Thin rubber finger-stalls are sold for the use of doctors when making certain examinations, and such would be very useful for protecting a finger when the skin is broken by cuts, hacks or abrasions. It might be worn over a thin dressing. It would not be sufficiently strong, however, to withstand the degree of friction involved in hard work, and for this a leather stall should be worn ; if necessary, this might be a finger cut off an old glove.

FIRE-GUARD. Young children should not be left alone in a room with a fire unless there is an efficient fire-guard. If a child under seven years of age dies or suffers severe injury from neglect of this precaution it constitutes a punishable offence as regards anyone over sixteen who has the care or custody of the child.

FIRST AID. Everyone should be acquainted with the principles of first aid, as emergencies are constantly arising in which immediate treatment, pending the arrival of a doctor, may obviate the more serious consequences of injury or sudden illness, and may even be the means of saving the patient's life.

The apparently natural tendency of passers-by to crowd closely round the stricken person must be prevented, and a free supply of air must be procured. Another impulse which must be checked is to make the fallen person sit or stand. As a general rule a man who has fallen does so because he cannot stand, and the effort to make him stand may do him grave injury.

To take the simplest accident, which is fainting—it may easily be shown that the act of falling is part of Nature's mechanism for curing the state of affairs which brought about the faint. Fainting is due to an insufficiency of the blood supplied to the head, and this blood supply is made much more easy when the head is on the same level as the rest of the body than when it is uppermost. Tight clothing about the neck and chest should be loosened.

If there is bleeding the wound should be sought for, and someone should put his thumb on it and keep it there. Many a life has been saved by this simple procedure.

The injured person will certainly be offered water and alcohol. If he has merely fainted the alcohol will do him good, if he is bleeding the alcohol will increase the haemorrhage and so do him harm. This is true whether the bleeding is external and visible or internal and invisible, as in an apoplectic stroke.

Unless the person rendering first aid is quite competent to distinguish between simple fainting and more serious conditions, alcohol should most certainly be withheld.

Except in the case of the slightest injuries, a doctor should be summoned at once, and should there be difficulty or delay in securing the services of one, the patient should not be moved till it is clear that he has no bones broken. If he has sustained such an injury, splints must be improvised and applied before he is moved, otherwise there is a great danger of aggravating his injury.

One result of accidents in general is what is called shock. This is more serious in children, but is observed in some measure in almost every accident, and next to bleeding it is the most important thing to control. To this end efforts must be made to make the patient warmer by extra clothing, chafing his limbs, etc.

In the table in pages 300-301 brief instructions are given for dealing with sudden emergencies. The reader is referred to individual articles for fuller details.

See Artificial Respiration ; Bleeding ; Burn ; Dislocation ; Epilepsy ; Fainting ; Fracture ; Poisoning ; Shock ; Transport of the Sick and Injured, etc.

FISSURE. In anatomy the term fissure is applied to many clefts or gaps separating the lobes or other subdivisions of an organ or separating one structure from another. There are many fissures in the brain, for example, the longitudinal fissure, separating the two cerebral hemispheres, and the Rolandic and Sylvian fissures, separating lobes on the outer surface of each hemisphere. The cleft between the upper and lower eyelid is called the palpebral fissure.

The term fissure is also used for a narrow, elongated sore, and of this there are two common examples—fissure of the nipple and anal fissure. The former nearly always occurs during suckling and is largely due to failure to keep the nipple clean, though a hard, inelastic condition of the skin over the nipple doubtless contributes. To prevent this condition as far as possible, certain precautions should be observed during pregnancy (*q.v.*).

The nipple should always be carefully washed and dried after suckling, and if it appears to lack suppleness a paste consisting of equal parts of the powder of bismuth carbonate and castor oil may be applied. Should a fissure occur the same paste is useful in treating it, the nipple being first washed with boracic acid lotion, however ; and it will usually be desirable to use a nipple-shield for suckling.

An anal fissure occurs at the back part of the lower end of the bowel, and there is generally an external pile, commonly referred to as a sentinel pile, at the lower end of the fissure. There is great pain when the bowels move and considerable straining, while the motion may be streaked with blood or matter. The pain may shoot down the thighs and may last a long time.

The bowels should be kept easy by laxatives, and very soft paper or a soft rag should be used to cleanse the bowel after defaecation. It is a good thing also to wash the anal region thereafter by sitting in a basin of water. After drying, a little ointment of witch hazel may be applied, and should be put as far into the bowel as possible. Often it is necessary to resort to surgery, and the method most in favour is to divide the fissure with a knife and trim its edges ; the incision into the fissure is made sufficiently deep to prevent dragging on the wound, and the rest thus secured allows quick healing to take place.

See Piles.

FISTULA. A Latin word meaning a pipe or tube, the term fistula is applied to an abnormal, narrow passage connecting some body cavity with the external surface of the skin or some such cavity with another one. Any opening into or between body cavities which acts like a fistula, although the passage is not narrow or pipe-like, may be described as a fistulous opening.

A fistula may be congenital, and is then due to a failure in the closure of tubes or gaps which exist in the foetus but which are normally obliterated. Thus there may be an opening at the navel, through which urine discharges, due to the non-closure of the urachus, a foetal tube which in the ordinary individual comes to exist only as a fibrous cord, reaching from the bladder to the navel.

A fistula may be caused by a wound which involves a body cavity ; the wound does not heal because the contents of the cavity pass along the track, and so a fistula becomes established. A more frequent mode of origin, however, is the occurrence of an abscess which opens into a body cavity and also into another cavity or externally on the surface of the skin. Here, again, the passage of the contents of the cavity affected prevents healing. A common instance of this type is the anal fistula.

Three varieties of anal fistula have been described. It may be complete, that is, there may be a passage opening out of the rectum some distance above the anus and burrowing down outside the bowel to open on the surface, generally by the side of the anal opening. An incomplete anal fistula may either be one that has no external opening, a blind internal fistula, or one that communicates with the outer air but does not reach the bowel cavity, a blind external fistula ; but an incomplete fistula would be more properly described as a sinus merely, that is to say, a narrow passage leading to an unhealed abscess cavity.

The abscess is caused by disease germs making their way through some breach in the surface of the bowel lining. If the abscess is opened early the risk of a fistula is greatly lessened. The presence of a fistula leads to a fairly constant discharge of pus, but there is not much pain unless the passage is blocked and the discharge accumulates in it. There may, however, be irritation of the skin around the external opening of the fistula, and possibly itching.

If the fistula has lasted beyond a few weeks cure without an operation is very unlikely. An operation is not readily resorted to if, as sometimes happens, the fistula is due to infection with tuberculosis.

A fistula opening on the abdominal wall may follow an abscess about the appendix which has been evacuated through the wall, but which has been accompanied by sloughing of the appendix. Fistulae between the bladder and vagina or the rectum and vagina sometimes follow difficult childbirth in which the lining of the vagina has been damaged by pressure or otherwise.

Sometimes an abscess forms on the duct of the parotid gland and bursts through the cheek, leaving a salivary fistula.

See Abscess ; Intestine ; Sinus.

FIT. Although it is used for many things that begin more or less suddenly and are more or less intense, such as a fit of coughing, a fit of depression, and so on, a fit is usually meant to imply a seizure in which there are tumultuous spasmodic movements of many muscles, or, in other words, a convulsion.

Of fits of this kind the most common are those that occur in epilepsy (q.v.), in eclampsia (q.v.), and infantile convulsions. The nervous mechanism of a child is relatively unstable, and fits may occur from slight causes and may not have much significance, though sometimes they have. The subject is dealt with under the heading Convulsion.

There is a stage in asphyxia in which convulsions may occur, and although fits are more characteristic of poisoning by strychnine and other poisons of the convulsant group, they may occur in many forms of poisoning.

Tetanus, or lockjaw, causes spasms rather similar to those of strychnine poisoning, and spasms also occur in hydrophobia.

Fits may occur in an apoplectic seizure and in irritation of the brain from other causes, such as meningitis and encephalitis. Anaemia of the brain is responsible for the fits occurring in Stokes-Adams disease, which is associated with an undue slowness of the pulse, and in other instances of slow pulse.

Sometimes, and especially in young women, fits are due to hysteria.

The immediate treatment of an ordinary fit is described under the heading Epilepsy.

See Bright's Disease ; Convulsion ; Eclampsia ; Epilepsy ; Fainting.

FLAT FOOT. The impress of the sole of the normal foot possesses a large depression, or bay, on the inner side, the reason for this being that the inner border of the foot, in consequence of its being arched from behind forwards, does not touch the ground. Dropping of this arch causes the condition known as flat foot, splay foot, or pes planus, and according to its degree the concavity in the normal impress becomes filled up and may entirely disappear.

This might happen suddenly from the arch being smashed down, for example, by the wheel of a vehicle passing over it ; it sometimes comes on very quickly in those who are weakened by disease and have to do much standing, particularly if they are also engaged in weight lifting or carrying. Much more frequently, however, the arch of the foot sags gradually. This sagging, whether occurring quickly or slowly, is due to the structures which maintain the arch, and which are described under the heading Foot, becoming weakened and stretched.

The flattening of the arch is noticeable on looking at the inner border of the foot when the patient is standing, though in the early stages standing on tip-toe causes the arching to reappear, and for long after this it may be possible by ordinary manipulation to put the foot into its normal position. In course of time, however, this cannot be done because adhesions have formed between ligaments, tendons, muscles and bones, and the last have altered in shape, so that any possible rectification can only be accomplished by violent wrenching or even by the removal of bone.

Flat foot causes soreness in the feet, which also are easily tired. The transverse arch also flattens, and from pressure on nerves in the sole of the foot there may be disabling seizures of pain, known as metatarsalgia, or Morton's disease.

Flat foot is often treated by putting a moulded pad or metal plate into the boot, so that the foot is supported in an arched position, but, except perhaps for old people, a better method is to exercise the muscles concerned in maintaining the arch in order to strengthen them, and raising the inside of the sole of the boot, thereby throwing more weight on the outer part of the sole of the foot. In acute cases this treatment must be preceded, however, by sufficient rest, often secured by putting the foot into plaster of Paris, to allow the overstretched structures to recover.

Suitable exercises are as follows: (1) Bend and straighten the toes. (2) In a sitting position, and with the foot off the ground, twist the foot, so that its front part describes a circle in the air (Plate XVII, 3). Each exercise should be repeated a number of times for several days and then the following exercises are introduced: (3) With the feet parallel, rise on tiptoe, with the soles of the feet directed inwards as far as possible. (4) With the feet parallel and on their outer edge, walk forward for half a dozen paces (see Plate XVII, 4).

Even apart from exercises, the feet should always be kept parallel when walking, and the patient should never walk without wearing boots or shoes. Massage, electricity and whirlpool baths may be of service in restoring tone to muscles when the patient is debilitated.

The inner border of the boot should be straight, and the boot should be sufficiently roomy. The heel should be broad and the sole firm. A shoemaker should be directed to put a wedge on the

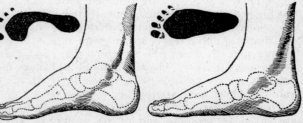

Flat Foot. Left, normal bony arch with the imprint it makes ; right, position of bones and impression of sole in a case of flat foot

inner side of the heel, so as to raise it ⅓-inch and also to prolong the heel forward on this side for ¾-inch. On the sole, just below the ball of the great toe, another wedge should be put, raising this part also ⅓-inch.

There is a variety of flat foot in which the treatment is different, that due to spasm of the peroneal muscles which lie on the outer side of the leg. Here an attempt to manipulate the foot into its correct position causes great pain. The condition is treated by dividing the tendons of the muscles, or sometimes by crushing the nerves supplying them, and so paralysing them for the time being. *See* Ankle ; Foot.

FLATULENCE. A disagreeable amount of air or other gases in the stomach or bowels is described as flatulence. Distension of the digestive tube may give rise to a painful sense of pressure and may even embarrass the action of the heart and of respiration. Excessive distension of the abdomen by gas is called meteorism.

The gas may be brought up from the stomach by eructations or belching, or be passed from the bowel, what is got rid of in these ways being described as flatus.

Although in certain instances flatulence is due to gases evolved by fermentation in the stomach, its usual cause is air, which is swallowed when eating and drinking. This is sometimes called aerophagy.

It is only when there is definite obstruction to the discharge of the contents of the stomach into the duodenum that there is likely to be sufficient fermentation to give rise to enough gas to cause flatulence.

Air may be swallowed incorporated with food or it may be gulped down. Sometimes hysterical people are troubled with belching lasting for hours, but if they are observed it will be noticed that they are simply gulping down air and bringing it up again. To lessen the air which may be mixed with food chewing should be done as far as possible with closed lips and should be done thoroughly.

To relieve flatulent distension remedies are taken to promote and at the same time regulate the movements of the walls of the stomach and bowels and are described as carminatives. Sips of hot water may relieve gastric flatulence, or diluted spirits, but most drugs which act as carminatives owe their virtue to a pungent volatile oil which they contain. To this class belong dill, anise, peppermint, ginger and others.

Intestinal flatulence is apt to follow certain classes of food, beans, for example. It largely depends on bacterial activity, and its occurrence may be prevented, or at any rate made less likely, by intestinal antiseptics, such as salol. It may be relieved by giving carminatives by the mouth or by incorporating something of the kind in an enema (*q.v.*).

Besides promoting the expulsion of gas, carminatives help to relieve the colic which often accompanies flatulence. Hot applications may also serve to this end.

See Asafoetida ; Carminative ; Indigestion.

FLEA. Since the discovery of its connexion with the spread of bubonic plague the flea has assumed great importance in public health administration. The flea specially concerned in carrying the germs of plague is a tropical species, which usually infests the black rat and might readily be brought to seaports, whence an epidemic might spread.

Fleas are blood-suckers and may transmit plague infection either by injecting the bacilli into the wound which they make or by depositing their excrement, which contains bacilli, after a meal taken from a victim of the disease, on the skin ; this may then be rubbed into the skin by the person scratching.

The irritation arising from a bite is caused by the salivary secretion which the creature squirts into the wound. Some people suffer very little from flea bites, while others have extreme irritation of the skin. Many species of flea manifest a distinct preference for certain animals as a host, but may on occasion adopt some other. Thus the human flea may attack dogs, and cats, and, on the other hand, fleas more peculiar to these animals may attack human beings.

Three Stages of Development

A flea passes through the three stages of development of egg, larva and cocoon. The eggs are deposited in cracks, beneath floors, mouse-holes and elsewhere, and are visible to the naked eye as small, waxy, oval bodies. The larvae feed on any organic matter mixed with the dust in the floor cracks, or found wherever the eggs have been deposited. The fully developed fleas may not leave their cocoons for some time, but are ready to do so at once if they are disturbed. This explains instances of persons being attacked by hosts of fleas on entering a building which has been disused for a period. The human flea may pass through all stages of its development, from the egg to the adult, in from four to six weeks, according to whether the weather is warm or cold.

To prevent infestation with fleas it is necessary to destroy rats and mice, to supervise, and when necessary disinfect, the coat of dogs and cats, and to preserve strict cleanliness of the dwelling and of such places as dog kennels. The proximity of stables, fowl houses and other places where fleas may breed freely, makes vigilance all the more necessary.

An emulsion which may be used to destroy fleas on floors, the coats of animals and elsewhere, may be made from soft soap and paraffin oil or kerosene. An ounce of soft soap is dissolved by heat in 5 ounces, by weight, of water, and while the solution is still hot 25 ounces, by weight, of paraffin oil is gradually added, the mixture being constantly and vigorously stirred and shaken throughout. There results an even, milky fluid. The water and oil are weighed by first of all weighing a container, such as a tin, and then putting in the liquid. The emulsion is sprayed or rubbed smoothly over the surface to be treated. It should be worked into the coat of an animal, and the head must be cleansed equally with other parts of the body.

Cats that object to washing should be freely sprinkled with fresh pyrethrum powder. Clothing in store should be treated with naphthalene balls. Flaked naphthalene is a useful thing to sprinkle over the floor of a room which has been shut up and which may be infested with fleas.

The sand-flea, jigger or chigoe is found in the tropics. The female burrows into the skin, particularly of the feet, where she deposits her eggs. This causes intense itching and directs attention to the presence of the insect, which can be ejected with the point of a needle. If allowed to remain, the accumulation of eggs causes a lump, perhaps of the size of a pea. When the eggs mature they are expelled and an ulcer results, which may be considerably enlarged by microbic infection. Care should be taken to dress antiseptically a wound following the extraction of a jigger. Their invasion may be hindered to some extent by refraining from wandering about barefooted over the floor of a bedroom or a verandah.

See Bite ; Infectious Disease ; Plague ; Rats.

FLEXION. Bending a limb or part of a limb is described as flexion. Thus the fingers are flexed in making a fist. A muscle which produces this movement is called a flexor.

See Extension.

FLIES. A great deal of the infection causing human sickness, to say nothing of domestic animals, is conveyed by flies of different kinds. The common house fly, which is distributed all over the world, may carry dysentery, cholera, typhoid fever, bacterial food poisoning, diphtheria, tuberculosis, ophthalmia, anthrax, and possibly leprosy, besides the eggs of different parasitic worms.

Flies are attracted by human excrement, and should this be infected it is likely to be taken up by the insect, either adhering to the hairs on its legs or actually in its stomach. When the fly then alights on food the infection is deposited there ; if it has been swallowed it is deposited by the fly voiding the contents of its bowel on the food, which it habitually does, a disgusting fact which does not appear to be very well known.

In hot countries the domestic fly breeds all the year round, but in colder countries only in the warmer weather. In Great Britain this means between June and October, with the greatest prevalence probably in August and September. In what condition the flies pass the winter is not known. A female fly lays from 120 to 150 eggs at a time, and in her lifetime from 600 to 900, and the interval between the egg stage and that of the adult female capable of breeding may be as short as three weeks.

Conditions Suitable for Breeding

The great bulk of the eggs are deposited in horse manure, but a certain number are deposited in human faeces and in garbage. Moisture and warmth make the substance, whatever it may be, more suitable for fly-breeding, nor will eggs be deposited in horse-manure unless it is fresh, say within 24 hours after it has been voided.

The eggs, which are about $\frac{1}{25}$ inch long, hatch out in from eight hours to three days into maggots or larvae which, in the course of about two to five days more, attain a length of almost $\frac{1}{2}$ inch. These migrate during the dark from the substance in which they have developed and bury themselves in the earth, at depths varying up to several feet. Here they become quiescent and pass through the pupal or chrysalid stage, which lasts from three days to four or more weeks, when the fly hatches out and makes its way to the surface. In about two weeks or rather more it is mature and commences breeding. The variation in the times mentioned for the various stages of development depends on the nature of the season, the longer periods being those occurring when the weather is cold.

In view of the disgusting and possibly dangerous contamination of food the destruction of flies is of the utmost importance.

Horse-manure heaps should not be allowed near dwellings, and should be so dealt with as to discourage breeding. If horse manure is built in stacks about 5 or 6 feet high, each fresh addition being firmly compressed by beating it with the flat of a spade, the fermentation which goes on in the centre of the stack raises the temperature to such a height that larvae are destroyed. The ground on which a stack is to be placed is prepared by spreading cresol or heavy oil on it and this should extend for at least 3 feet beyond the circumference of the stack.

In dry weather the manure should be moistened to encourage fermentation. It should also be noted that if manure is thoroughly spread out, the lumps being broken up with a spade or rake, breeding is prevented if the manure becomes dry.

An earth closet or latrine is only permissible if it is fly-proof, as larvae can burrow up through the soil from a considerable depth. Garbage should be burned in the kitchen fire as far as possible, and if put into a bin this should have a close and firm lid. Sprinkling the contents thoroughly with a solution of borax, $\frac{1}{2}$ pound to 2 or 3 gallons, is an efficient deterrent, but it is necessary to point out that chloride of lime is useless for preventing the breeding of flies.

There are numerous ways of destroying adult flies. Fly-papers may be used or metal rods made sticky with a mixture of 5 parts of castor oil and 8 parts of powdered resin, the resin being dissolved in the oil with the aid of heat. The rods are suspended from a string stretched across a room, but are only useful so long as they are sticky. Periodically they are passed through a flame and then recoated.

It is useful also to have plates standing about in the room, containing a little formalin solution, made up of two teaspoonsful of commercial formalin and lime-water to a pint, two heaped tablespoonsful of sugar being dissolved in this. A piece of bread is placed in the centre of each plate for flies to rest on. Fly traps of various kinds, such as the gauze globe and the Japanese mechanical trap, are also useful, the trapped flies

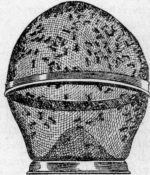

Baited gauze fly-trap, the flies crawling beneath the lower edge and up through the inner cone

being killed with boiling water or petrol vapour. Another method is to kill the flies with a gauze racquet or fly-swot.

In addition to all this, it is still necessary to protect all food-stuffs in cupboards or on the table with gauze or muslin covers.

There are two other flies, the lesser housefly and the latrine fly, which may similarly contaminate food and convey infection.

A certain number of flies, like the blue-bottle and the green-bottle, deposit their eggs in or on meat and are described as blow-flies.

A gauze cover is not sufficient protection against the blue-bottle as the eggs are deposited on the gauze, whence they drop on to the meat. It is therefore necessary to have a piece of closely woven fabric either on the top of the gauze cover or over the meat.

These flies may also deposit their eggs on wounds or sores, which, if neglected, may become infested with maggots. A species of this kind, sarcophaga carnaria, deposits not eggs but living larvae, which proceed to feed upon dead animal matter in the wound.

A blue-bottle may deposit its eggs in the nostrils of man or one of the lower animals, and other flies may also deposit eggs in this or some other of the natural cavities of the body. The larvae of some flies are hatched out in the digestive tract from eggs which have been swallowed, and are passed in the motions. The larvae of other flies are able to penetrate the skin and burrow deeply in the soft tissues or extend for long distances under the skin. One of these larvae, called the screw-worm, is found in most parts of America, though particularly in the more central parts of the continent. Infestation of the living body with fly-larvae or the symptoms caused by their presence is described as myiasis.

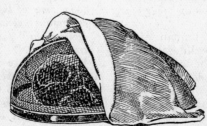

Gauze meat-cover, which must itself be covered by a piece of closely woven muslin

A large number of flies are biting and blood-sucking insects. The ordinary house fly does not bite but only sucks up juices from the surface of the body, and bites sometimes ascribed to this fly are due to some other, probably a stable fly, stomoxys calcitrans. A connexion between the bites of this fly and infantile paralysis has been suggested.

The bites of clegs, or horse-flies, may be very painful ; while that of the tick-fly, hippobosca, a dark, leathery-looking creature with yellow markings, can convey trypanosomiasis to lower animals and, possibly, leishmaniasis to man, in parts of the world where such disorders exist. Tsetse flies communicate trypanosomiasis, more familiarly known as sleeping sickness, to man.

See Food ; Formalin ; Infectious Disease ; Sandfly Fever.

FLOODING. A large discharge of blood from the vagina, or front passage, is commonly described as a flooding. Most frequently it comes from the womb, but its source may be in the vagina itself. It may occur at a menstrual period and such discharges may be both very copious and more frequent than usual, a state of things that is not uncommon at the change of life, or menopause. A flooding may occur in connexion with abortion, miscarriage or childbirth, and the most dangerous is that occurring after childbirth. The measures to be taken to prevent this accident, so far as possible, are described under the heading Childbirth.

The immediate treatment of flooding is to keep the patient lying down with the head low and the legs raised. Douches of water at a temperature of 120° F. may be tried, and ergot is one of the drugs used in this emergency. Other treatment will depend on the special cause of the flooding.

See Abortion ; Change of Life ; Menstruation ; Pregnancy.

FLUORESCEIN. A compound of resorcin (*q.v.*), fluorescein is used in solution to aid in the detection of abrasions of the cornea. A few drops are put into the eye and any abrasion is coloured green.

FLUORINE. A gaseous element, belonging to the same group as chlorine, fluorine occurs in the enamel of teeth and in minute quantities in other tissues of the body. Its compounds are sometimes used in the treatment of goitre, enlarged spleen, tuberculosis, etc. Fluoroform, used for whooping-cough, etc., is analogous to chloroform.

FLUSHING. *See* Blushing.

FOG. Air contains many minute floating particles of solid matter, and a fog or mist is caused by the condensation of the watery vapour of the air round such particles, owing to chilling of the air. In the atmosphere of towns it is a smoke-fog that forms from the presence of multitudes of particles of carbon in the air, including sulphur compounds which make the fog acid.

Much smoke in the atmosphere shuts off a good deal of sunlight, and the presence of the acid compounds of sulphur further damages animal life and vegetation and also damages buildings. Such ill-effects are greatly increased, however, by the existence of fogs which also have a chilling effect on the body, and, if smoke-fogs, cause irritation of the respiratory passages.

The prevention of smoke-fogs can only be achieved by lessening the smoke emitted from domestic and factory chimneys, by using anthracite, coke, and other kinds of smokeless fuel or, where raw coal is used, by improving the efficiency of grates and furnaces, and insisting on proper methods of stoking. Conscientious care on the part of individual householders is an indispensable factor towards securing purity of the air.

See Air ; Climate ; Damp ; Dust.

FOMENTATION. A fomentation is applied to relieve pain and inflammation. The fabric generally used is either flannel or lint, and the piece selected should be large enough, when folded double, to cover the area to be treated. Sometimes more than two layers are used, however ; perhaps as many as eight. The fabric is placed in a basin and boiling water poured over it until it is thoroughly soaked, when it is taken out and wrung almost dry.

The best way to do this is to put the fomentation between the folds of a roller-towel, or an ordinary long towel with its ends fastened together, through each end of which a long wooden stirrer, or something of the kind, is pushed and used to twist the end round, the twisting being performed in different directions at the two ends (*see* Plate XVII, 5-7).

The fomentation is then shaken out and applied, quickly but smoothly, and immediately covered with a piece of thin mackintosh, jaconette or pegamoid, sufficiently large to overlap it by at least an inch all round. It is desirable then to cover with a thick layer of cotton wool and apply a broad roller bandage to keep the fomentation in position.

A fomentation applied in this way will retain its heat for a long time, but if the object is to relieve pain and greater heat is necessary, the fomentation should be renewed every twenty minutes or half an hour. The fomentation should be as hot as can be borne, but great care should be taken not to scald the patient.

The reddening effect on the skin of a fomentation is increased by sprinkling a large teaspoonful of oil of turpentine over it just before it is applied. Sometimes laudanum is sprinkled over a fomentation, or a decoction of poppy heads or of camomile flowers is used instead of plain water, but it is unlikely that any of these additions will be more efficacious than an ordinary fomentation. When renewing a fomentation the skin should always be dried before the fresh one is put on.

Sometimes spongio-piline is used instead of flannel or lint. This consists of a felt, made of an admixture of wool and sponge, with a backing of rubber. The latter would tend to deteriorate if left long in boiling water, or when, as is sometimes done, a hot smoothing iron is passed over a fomentation to augment its effect; also when spirituous solutions of drugs are applied, as in treating lumbago, etc. For these purposes, however, a variety of spongio-piline, having a thinner felt and another kind of backing, is available.

See Dressing; Poultice.

FOMITES. The Latin word fomites, the plural of fomes, meaning tinder, is used as a descriptive term for articles of clothing, food-utensils, toys and other things that come into contact with a person suffering from an infectious disease (*q.v.*) and therefore become capable of conveying contagion.

FOOD. The principles regulating the proper rationing of food are discussed under the heading Diet. The claims of the palate must give way to soundness in dieting, and difficulty, on the score of expense, in providing a proper diet can be overcome quite well by a judicious choice of food-stuffs, as many of the cheap foods are intrinsically as valuable as the more expensive. Skilful cookery can do much to give attractiveness to food-stuffs which are not in themselves very inviting, and this is perhaps the most important factor in solving the dietetic problems of households with very limited resources.

Meat may be (1) home-fed and killed; (2) fed abroad but killed at home; (3) refrigerated, or chilled; or (4) frozen; the last is generally mutton. The second class is that of prime animals but has probably lost fat during the voyage. The third class can be recognized by its pink fat and by the outside of the meat lacking the lustre of fresh meat. The fourth class, if unthawed, will be stiff, and, if thawed, the outside will have a faded or perhaps even a parboiled appearance, while fluid will drip or ooze from the meat, which has not the mottled appearance of fresh meat; the fat has a dull, white colour.

Food Value of Frozen Meat

It should be understood, however, that chilled and frozen meat are quite as nutritious as fresh meat, and that the inferior cuts of any meat are from this point of view quite as good as the better. As regards digestibility, mutton is more digestible than beef and beef than veal. Pork, because of its large content of fat, is difficult to digest. Tripe and sweetbreads are easily digested.

Rabbits are in season from September to February; a young animal is distinguished by its smooth, sharp claws and soft ears. The meat is easily digested. Game derives its flavour by being hung for from five to ten days, until, in fact, decomposition has begun; this, however, has no ill consequences because the meat is dry.

In choosing a fowl an old one will be recognized by its stiff, horny feet, long spurs and dark-coloured thighs. The skin of a fowl should not be discoloured and the flesh should be firm. The meat of duck or grouse contains a considerable amount of fat and is correspondingly harder to digest. The breast of a chicken is the most easily digested kind of meat.

Only fresh fish should be accepted; a fresh fish is stiff, the eyes are prominent and bright and the gills are bright red. Salmon and eel contain a considerable proportion of fat, and so require good digestive powers, and invalids may find that even herring disagree. Owing to their cheapness, herring are, however, one of the most valuable foods. Oysters, if raw, are very easily digested, but they do not contain much nourishment. Crab and lobster are difficult to digest. Many fish are "out of season," or unwholesome, during their breeding times. Among those in season all the year round are included brill, lobster, plaice and sole. Oysters are out of season during the four months of the year whose names do not include an R. Mussels are out of season from May till November inclusive, and herring during the first four months of the year.

Some Farinaceous Food Stuffs

The qualities of bread are discussed under its own heading. Macaroni and vermicelli are preparations of wheat flour and are rich in gluten. Barley has a composition like that of wheat, but it does not form gluten. It is a good food, though barley cakes are less palatable than, and not as easily digested as, bread. To make pearl barley the grains are deprived of the husk, rounded and polished. Barley meal consists of the whole grain ground; in Scotch, mulled or pot barley, the grains are husked and roughly ground; patent barley is merely flour formed from pearl barley. Rye makes a dark, somewhat heavy and acid loaf, which is not so easily digested as wheat bread but otherwise very wholesome.

Oatmeal contains relatively large amounts of protein and fat and, apart from greater difficulty of digestion, is a better food than white bread. It might with advantage form a part of every dietary, and children should be accustomed to its use, as a taste for it seems to be difficult to form and to preserve. Maize resembles oats in composition but is rather harsh in flavour. From it cornflour and hominy are prepared. Rice is deficient in protein,

fat and salts, and therefore is mainly a starchy food. Polishing the rice deprives it of vitamin and a diet of polished rice causes beri-beri.

Arrowroot, tapioca and sago consist of starch simply. There are various kinds of arrowroot on the market, Bermudan arrowroot being the best. Tapioca is got from cassava root, sago from the sago palm. When these are used as milk puddings, protein and fat are supplied by the milk. The pulses, namely peas, beans and lentils, are rich in protein, but peas and beans are rather difficult of digestion and much of the protein is not assimilated. They are deficient in fat, but this lack is remedied in the mixture of pork and beans.

Grammes per ounce Food-stuff.	Protein	Carbo-hydrate	Fat	Calories per ounce
Milk, fresh, average	1·0	1·5	1·0	20
Butter	0	0	25·0	225
Cheese, Cheddar	12·6	0	6·8	115
„ American	9·6	0	9·3	126
„ Stilton	6·9	0·6	10·6	130
„ Cream	5·2	0	7·0	86
„ Camembert	5·3	0·9	6·0	80
„ Skim-milk	9·2	1·9	2·4	69
Margarine	0·2	0	23·2	216
Eggs	3·0	0	3·0	40
Beef, fresh, lean	6·0	0	3·0	51
„ corned	6·6	0	4·0	64
Veal, loin	5·6	0	2·8	49
Mutton, shoulder	4·1	0	5·5	68
Lamb „	5·2	0	4·7	65
Pork, fresh side	2·5	0	14·9	149
Bacon	5·0	0	15·0	160
Chicken	6·0	0	2·2	45
Cod	4·7	0	0	19
Eel	5·3	0	2·6	46
Herring, fresh	5·6	0	2·0	47
„ smoked	10·5	0	4·5	85
Haddock	4·9	0	0	20
Mackerel	5·3	0	2·0	40
Salmon	6·2	0	3·6	59
Whiting	4·8	0	0	20
Flour, family grade	2·3	20·8	0·3	88
Bread, white	2·0	14·5	0·4	76
„ brown	1·4	13·0	0·4	63
Biscuit	4·4	20·8	0·3	106
Oatmeal	4·6	18·0	2·0	111
Rice	2·0	22·5	0·1	101
Peas, fresh	1·5	4·7	0·1	26
„ dried	4·9	17·8	0·2	95
Jam or Marmalade	0	16·6	0	68
Sugar, refined	0	28·3	0	116
Vegetables, fruit, raw A	0·5	1·0	0	6
„ „ „ B	0·4	2·0	0	10
„ „ „ C	0·3	3·0	0	14
„ „ „ D	0·1	4·0	0	17
„ „ „ E	0·3	6·0	0	26

Constituents of some common articles of food

Potatoes contain a large proportion of starch with a little protein. Experimentally, vigorous health has been maintained on a diet of potatoes and vegetable margarine with a flavouring of onion. But the water in which the potatoes were boiled was also taken, the potatoes being very thinly peeled before cooking. The water contains valuable salts and vitamins taken out of the potatoes. The loss of these salts can be prevented, or lessened, by boiling potatoes in their skins.

For convenience vegetables and fruits are grouped in five classes according to their content of carbohydrate, which is their principal constituent as regards caloric value. Their vitamins, salts and acids are of great importance, in many cases of most importance. The carbohydrate content of each group is shown in the table of foods in page 311. The groups are as follows : A. Cabbage, lettuce, cauliflower, sprouts, spinach, tomatoes, watercress and radishes. B. French beans, onions, carrots, turnip and beets. C. Strawberries, gooseberries, oranges, peaches, pineapples and melons. D. Pears, apples, currants, raspberries, cherries, apricots, peas, parsnips and artichokes. E. Bananas, plums, prunes and potatoes.

Construction of Well-balanced Dietaries

By reference to this table and to the particulars given under the heading Diet as to the relative proportions of proteins, carbohydrates and fats in a diet, and the number of calories needed by various people, it should be possible to construct correct dietaries. These can be varied very largely to suit the family purse. It may be said that some of the food-stuffs detailed above as containing none of some constituent, fat, for example, may actually contain some, but so little as to be negligible.

Condiments and beverages are sometimes described as food accessories.

In the storage of food cleanliness and coolness are essential.

On no account should milk, fish, meat or similar food-stuffs be kept on the floor of the larder, and they should always be covered or screened to protect them from dust and from the visits of flies.

A gauze screen is not sufficient protection against the blue-bottle as the female deposits her eggs on the gauze and they drop down on to the meat ; a piece of muslin should be placed over the meat or on the top of the gauze cover. Weighted gauze covers should be put over jugs or other receptacles containing milk, jam, etc. Root and green vegetables should be stored separately.

Coolness may be secured by free ventilation of the larder through a gauze-screened window ; by having a moistened canvas cover over a food container ; by placing ice on fish, meat, etc., or by placing food in an ice-chest ; the last would be of inestimable value in hot weather.

Dangers Lurking in the Tin

Much of the food used nowadays is canned or bottled and a considerable amount of bottling is done in the home. To make such food keep it is subjected to heat in the tin, in the lid of which an opening is left to allow the escape of vapour. This opening is then soldered up, and the contraction which occurs when the tin and its contents cool usually causes the ends of the tin to bulge inwards.

If the end of a tin bulges outwards it should be rejected, as the bulging is due to gases formed by putrefaction. Such a tin is said to be blown.

Unscrupulous traders may perforate the tin, allowing the escape of the gases, then reheat and reseal. The presence of two soldered openings should therefore be viewed with suspicion. Bottled fruit and vegetables are treated similarly. Jam is usually covered after it is cold, and the surface may be sprinkled with some chemical preservative ; indeed, something of this kind may be found in any kind of preserved food.

When a tin has been opened the food should be used at once ; it is dangerous to allow it to stand in the tin or even, having once heated the food emptied from the tin, to allow it to stand.

The use of chemical preservatives for food can hardly be dispensed with, as so much food is imported and both this and home-produced food require to be stored, sometimes for considerable periods. Some chemicals used for preserving are harmful if taken in the amounts which might well be ingested in the course of ordinary

PLATE XVII

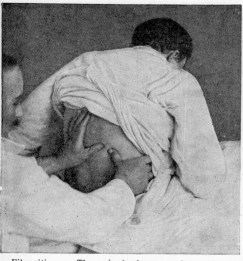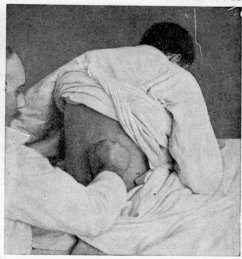

Fibrositis. 1. The pain is due to nodules in the tissues pressing upon nerves. When these have been diminished by light rubbing, deep pressure with the thumbs is used and then (2) massage with the closed fist

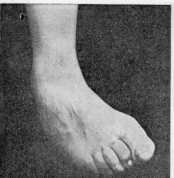

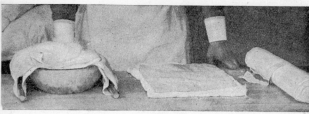

Fomentation. 5. Two or more thicknesses of flannel are spread between the layers of a small roller towel laid over a basin

Flat Foot 3. Rotatory exercise

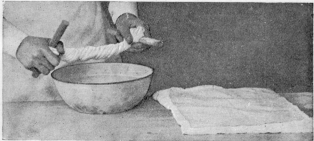

6. Sticks are passed through the ends of the towel, boiling water poured over it, and the sticks then twisted in opposite directions

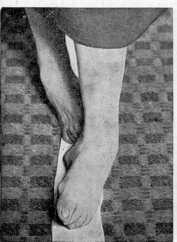

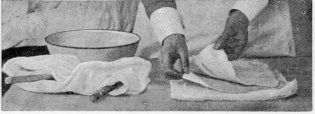

4. Walking along a straight line on the edges of the feet will help to cure flat foot

7. When the fomentation has been wrung nearly dry inside the towel it is shaken out and applied, covered with a slightly larger piece of mackintosh and a still larger layer of cotton wool

PLATE XVIII

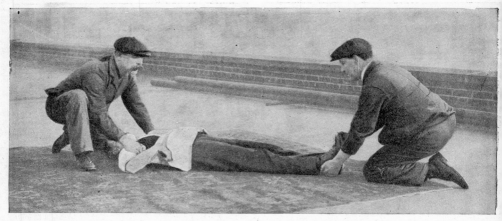

Fracture : first-aid treatment of a broken thigh. 1. The injured limb is first rendered as symmetrical as possible with the sound one. This is done by one man pulling steadily upon it, holding the foot by the heel in the correct upward position. Meanwhile, another man provides counter-extension at the armpit

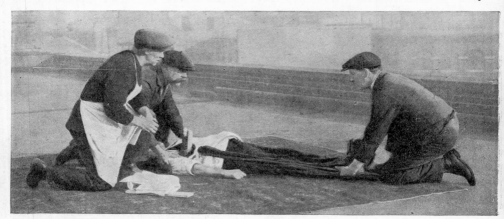

2. A splint can be improvised by taking a stick or a long broom, the head padded, and laying it along the outer side of the limb, with sacking or some other soft material interposed. The broom is fixed to the chest by a broad-fold bandage. A second well-padded splint is placed on the inside of the limb

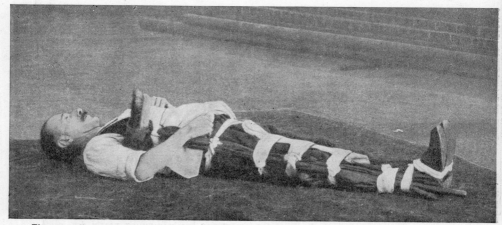

3. The two splints are fixed to the thigh by a bandage above the fracture (applied first) and another below it. Two other bandages are applied, one below the knee, the other just above the ankle. Finally, the feet are tied together as shown. Tightly folded newspapers may be used as splints in an emergency

diets containing a fair proportion of preserved food. Boracic acid is an example.

The Public Health (Preservatives, etc., in Food) Regulations, 1925, in force in part from Jan. 1, 1927, and wholly from July 1, 1928, prescribe the articles which may contain chemical preservatives and the appropriate preservative and amount of it for each. The only preservatives allowed are sulphurous acid and benzoic acid.

Poisoning by Food. Food poisoning may be due to metallic poisons, copper, tin, or lead, from containers or cooking utensils, but is relatively infrequent. Strict care, however, is necessary to keep such utensils clean and not to allow foods containing acids, fatty or otherwise, to remain long in a copper utensil. Defects in the lining of a tin may cause chemical contamination of food.

Most cases of food poisoning are due to the activities of what are called the salmonella group of bacilli, for example, bacillus aertrycke and bacillus enteritidis. The symptoms may be caused by the poisons produced by the bacilli, poisons which remain active even if the food is raised above the boiling point of water ; or by the living bacilli themselves. These bacteria may be present in either canned or fresh food.

Symptoms due to the accumulated poisonous products of the bacilli begin shortly after the food is consumed, and suddenly. There is vomiting, diarrhoea, abdominal pain, cramps in the limbs and some fever. This type of poisoning is most frequent after taking tinned foods. When the living bacilli are swallowed, symptoms do not begin till about twelve hours or longer after the infected food has been taken. Though similar to those of the other type they are less abrupt in their onset, less severe as a rule, but more protracted.

Vomiting and diarrhoea are usually sufficiently severe to clear the bowel, but it will be useful to aid cleansing of the stomach by giving large draughts of tepid water and, if the bowels are not acting freely, a dose of salts or of castor oil. The patient must be kept lying down and be kept warm ; stimulants also may be needed. Pain and cramps should be treated by hot applications.

Another kind of bacterial food poisoning is known as botulism (*q.v.*).

Formerly much importance was attributed to ptomaines, alkaloidal products of putrefactive organisms, but it is now clear that such poisons are destroyed in the stomach and are extremely unlikely to give rise to symptoms.

It must be borne in mind that food capable of causing poisoning is rarely offensive or in fact noticeably altered in any way.

There is another type of food poisoning which occurs in persons who have an idiosyncrasy for some kind of food, the ingestion of which may cause signs of irritation of the stomach and bowels, some skin rash, such as nettle-rash, erythema, eczema, or perhaps, asthmatic symptoms. White of egg is the chief offender, but fish, cheese, tomatoes, pork, shell-fish or some other food-stuff may be responsible. This is known as food allergy.

See Adulteration ; Diet ; Egg ; Farinaceous Food ; Flies ; Fungus ; Milk ; Ptomaine ; Vegetable Foods ; Vitamin.

FOOT. There are three regions in the foot, the tarsus, containing seven bones, the metatarsus containing five, and the toes containing fourteen—that is, three for each toe except the big toe which has only two. The bones of the toes are called phalanges (singular phalanx). The foot is jointed to the leg bones by the astragalus which is perched on the top of the os calcis, calcaneum, or heel bone as it is variously called. These two bones belong to the tarsus, and the others are the scaphoid, which articulates with the astragalus, three cuneiform or wedge-shaped bones, which articulate with the scaphoid, and the cuboid bone which articulates with the forward end of the os calcis.

A glance at the normal foot will show that it has two arches, an antero-posterior, that is from front to back, and a transverse, or from side to side. The posterior pillar of the former is made up of the os calcis and astragalus, and the anterior pillar, of the other tarsal bones and the

L

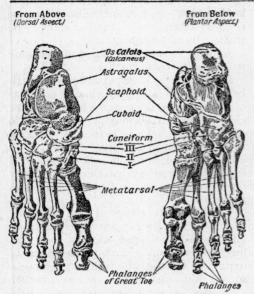

From Above
(Dorsal Aspect)

From Below
(Plantar Aspect)

Os Calcis
(calcaneus)

Astragalus

Scaphoid

Cuboid

Cuneiform
III
II
I

Metatarsal

Phalanges
of Great Toe

Phalanges

Foot. Bones of the upper and lower surfaces

metatarsal bones. This arch, moreover, is more marked on the inner border of the foot which therefore rests, when one is standing, on the heel, the outer border of the foot, and the heads, or forward ends, of the metatarsal bones. Only in walking is much pressure put on the toes, and even then it is only on the inner toes. The toes are more or less retrograde structures in man.

What might be called the keystone of this antero-posterior arch is represented by the head of the astragalus, which rests on a ligament, joining the os calcis and the scaphoid bone, and known as the inferior calcaneo-scaphoid ligament. This structure is very important in maintaining the integrity of the arch. Relaxation of the ligament is followed by collapse of the arch and flat foot. The existence of the arch in the foot of an infant may be obscured by the presence of a pad of fat in the hollow which creates an appearance of flatness, or, as is sometimes called, plainness, of the sole.

An exaggeration of the antero-posterior arch occurs in the deformity known as pes cavus, or claw foot, in which there is also the condition of hammer toes.

The transverse arch of the foot is best seen about the middle, that is, at the cuneiform bones, and contributes to-

wards the elasticity of the forward part of the foot, another factor in this direction being the large number of joints in the anterior pillar of the other arch. If, when jumping, one lands on the fore part of the foot, there is much less shock transmitted up the legs than when one lands on the heels.

The lower surface of the foot is called the sole or plantar aspect, and the upper surface, the dorsum or dorsal aspect; the upper part of this is commonly referred to as the instep.

The skin of the sole is very thick as compared with that of the dorsum, and there is the further difference that in the sole the structures between the skin and the bones are densely packed together, while beneath the skin of the dorsum there is much loose tissue. So, while inflammation in the dorsum of the foot may cause very considerable swelling, there is not, as a rule, very much swelling in the sole, but, on the other hand, this inability to swell results in very severe pain.

Of the muscles which move the foot and toes some are situated in the leg, and prolonged into the foot by tendons, while others are in the foot itself, most of them being in the sole. An important structure in the sole is a band of fascia,

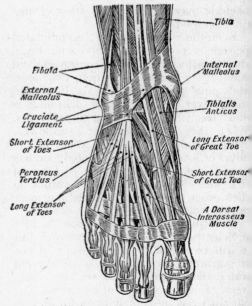

Tibia

Fibula

External
Malleolus

Cruciate
Ligament

Short Extensor
of Toes

Peroneus
Tertius

Long Extensor
of Toes

Internal
Malleolus

Tibialis
Anticus

Long Extensor
of Great Toe

Short Extensor
of Great Toe

A Dorsal
Interosseus
Muscle

Principal muscles and tendons of the foot

the plantar aponeurosis, which is attached behind to the os calcis, and in front about the heads of the metatarsal bones, and assists in maintaining the antero-posterior arch much as a bow string keeps the bend in a bow.

Besides the movements at the ankle joint (*q.v.*), the foot can be turned so that the sole looks inwards (inversion) or outwards (eversion).

Blood is supplied to the foot by the anterior and posterior tibial arteries. The latter runs into the sole beyond the inner prominence, or malleolus, of the ankle, and divides into the internal and external plantar arteries. The former of these runs down the inner border of the foot, while the latter runs to the outer border, and then bends in across the sole, forming the plantar arch. From this digital branches pass forward to the toes. On the dorsum of the foot about midway between the two malleoli of the ankle, the anterior tibial becomes the dorsalis pedis artery. This runs down the foot to the interval between the big toe and the next, where it dips down to join the end of the external plantar. Bleeding from a wound in the sole is best arrested by pressure on the posterior tibial artery (*see* Plate VI, 9). The superficial veins of the foot run into the internal saphenous vein mostly, but some are drained by the external saphenous vein.

Several nerves run into the foot. The posterior tibial which is found on the

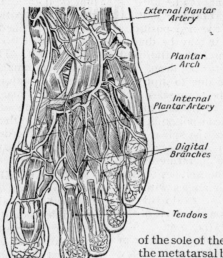

Plantar arterial arch and its branches

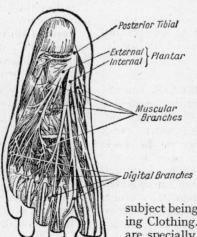

Course of nerves in the sole of the foot

inside of the ankle with the artery of the same name, on passing into the sole divides into the internal and external plantar. The digital branches of these, passing to the toes, are sometimes compressed at the heads of the metatarsal bones, giving rise to severe pain of a neuralgic character. This constitutes Morton's disease, or metatarsalgia, and is liable to affect those who have to stand much. The pain can often be relieved by compressing the foot from side to side, that is, restoring the transverse arch. A bar fixed across the outside of the sole of the foot behind the heads of the metatarsal bones, by taking the pressure off the nerves, may prevent pain.

The tarsus may be the site of tuberculous disease which spreads from bone to bone, this being facilitated by the synovial joint cavities.

Should a foot require to be amputated in the neighbourhood of the ankle, what is called Syme's amputation is usually done ; the lower ends of the tibia and fibula are sawn off and covered by a thick flap from the sole, the stump resting on the skin of the heel.

The care of the feet implies a careful selection and care of boots, this subject being discussed under the heading Clothing. The soles of the feet are specially well provided with sweat glands, and frequent cleansing of the feet is therefore necessary. If sweating is excessive or foul, the feet may be bathed with alum solution, a teaspoonful to a pint, or with a weak solution of permanganate of potassium.

See Ankle ; Blister ; Chilblain ; Claw Foot ; Club Foot ; Corn ; Flat Foot ; Fungus Foot ; Hallux Valgus ; Hammer Toe ; Toe.

FOOT DROP. If the foot cannot be raised to make at least a right angle at the front of the ankle a condition of foot drop exists. This may be due to disease about the ankle or to shortening of the muscles of the back of the leg and the foot be fixed, more or less, in the bad position ; or, on the other hand, it may be due to loss of power in the muscles on the front of the leg, that is, paralytic foot drop.

The paralysis may be due to injury of the nerve supplying these muscles, say by a gun-shot wound, to disease of the nerves, as a result of lead-poisoning, for example, or to disease of the spinal cord, as in infantile palsy.

It may be possible by operating on the ankle joint or dividing the Achilles tendon to put the foot at right angles with the leg, or in a paralytic case to do this by shortening the tendons on the front of the ankle so as to anchor the foot. In a paralytic case, when recovery of power in the muscles is still possible, it is highly important to prevent the foot from dropping and the patient should wear an apparatus to prevent this when he is up and about and should also wear a right-angle splint, sometimes referred to as a bed-shoe, when in bed.

When the deformity cannot be remedied otherwise, a patient with foot drop should wear a spring on the front of the leg to keep the foot up.

See Ankle.

FOOT AND MOUTH DISEASE. Known also as epizootic stomatitis, epidemic stomatitis and aphthous fever, foot and mouth disease chiefly affects cattle, pigs, sheep and goats but it may attack other domestic animals and may even be communicated to human beings. Small vesicles, or aphthae, appear, mainly on the feet and mouth ; in man they occur on the hands also. The disease, which is supposed to be due to a filterable virus, is spread by contact with infected animals, with straw and other things contaminated by such animals or by milk from them. In man, after an incubation period of three to five days, fever and headache occur and, soon after, the vesicles appear.

The treatment is that of fever (*q.v.*), and the application of antiseptics to the vesicles or the shallow ulcers which form

when these rupture. Carbolic acid or silver nitrate may be used for this purpose but in addition a wash containing a hypochlorite (*q.v.*), permanganate of potassium or boracic acid should be used frequently. The patient must be isolated and the disease notified.

See Infectious Disease.

FORAMEN. The Latin word foramen (plural, foramina), meaning a perforation, is used in anatomy for many openings. The foramen magnum, or large foramen, is the opening at the base of the skull through which the spinal cord passes to be attached to the brain ; the foramen ovale is an opening between the right and left auricles in the heart of the unborn child.

FORCIBLE FEEDING. Persons suffering from mental disorders may refuse to take food and make it necessary to resort to forcible feeding. The best method is by a rubber tube passed through the nose or the mouth and on through the gullet to the stomach, though it is not really necessary that it should go all the way ; it suffices if it reaches well below the opening into the air-passages. A gag will be necessary if the oral route be chosen. Liquid foods are then passed in through the tube. If proper skill and care are shown no harm can be done.

Feeding through a tube may be necessary when a patient is unable to swallow, and for children the nasal route would be chosen. It will sometimes be desirable, however, to abandon the attempt to feed through the gullet and adopt rectal feeding (*q.v.*).

FOREARM. If the forearm is stretched out with the palm of the hand forwards, it will be noted that the forearm is not quite in line with the arm, but is drawn outwards, or abducted, at an angle of about 15 deg. The angle so formed is called the carrying angle, and may be increased or diminished after disease or injury of the elbow, interfering more or less with function.

The front of the forearm, also called its anterior, or ventral, surface, is well clothed with muscles, the use of which is to flex the hand, thumb and fingers, and to pronate the forearm. The fleshy mass on the back is not quite so thick, the muscles on this, the posterior, or dorsal, aspect, being concerned with the extension of the thumb and fingers.

The median nerve runs down the middle of the forearm below a superficial layer of muscles and the ulnar nerve along its inner side, at the same depth. About half an inch below the bend of the elbow the brachial artery, which runs down on the inner side of the tendon of the biceps, divides into the radial and ulnar arteries which curve towards the respective bones, and continue on towards the wrist, the radial being easily palpable in front of the radius at the wrist. It is here that the pulse is taken. These arteries anastomose freely in the forearm.

There are three main superficial veins in the forearm. Curving forward, from the outside to the front about the junction of the lower and middle thirds, and continuing on up the middle, is the median vein, while, from the same side about half way up, the cephalic comes forward. About this level also, but from the inner side, the basilic vein comes on to the front of the forearm.

See Arm ; Elbow; Hand ; Ischaemia ; Median Nerve ; Radius ; Ulna ; Wrist.

FOREHEAD. The part of the skull forming the forehead is the frontal bone (*q.v.*). Covering this bone is a broad sheet of muscle, the frontalis, the fibres of which pass backwards to be inserted into an aponeurosis. When this muscle comes into action, the brow is wrinkled transversely. From the upper border of the orbit and passing downwards and inwards are the corrugator supercilii muscles, which wrinkle the brow vertically about the middle line, producing a frown. Both muscles are supplied by the facial nerve.

The supra-orbital nerve winds round the upper margin of the orbit, or passes through a foramen there, about a finger-breadth from the mid-line of the forehead, and passes upwards. A little to the inner side is another nerve, the supra-trochlear. These are branches of the fifth nerve, and supply sensation to the forehead.

This region is the site of a rash (*q.v.*) in different disorders. Apart from infectious diseases, a seborrhoeic rash is common.

See Seborrhoea.

FORMALIN. By passing the vapour of methyl alcohol over red hot copper a colourless gas with an acrid smell is got,

which is known as formaldehyde, or formic aldehyde. Formalin, or formol, is a 40 per cent. solution of this gas in water. Both solution and gas are strong disinfectants and deodorants. From the solution by proper dilution are made lotions for wounds, injections, gargles and sprays. If the solution is very strong, considerable irritation may be caused ; a 1 per cent. solution of formalin is suitable as a general antiseptic.

Formosyl is a liquid potash soap containing formaldehyde, and lysoform is a similar preparation. These are used as lotions, injections, and mouth washes, and may be incorporated in tooth pastes, tooth powders and dusting powders.

Formaldehyde is much used for disinfecting rooms which have been occupied by persons suffering from infectious diseases. A solution may be sprayed over the walls and furniture, as leather and cloth fabrics are not injured, or the vapour may be used. This may be obtained by evaporating formalin by the heat of a lamp or by using formaldehyde tablets, paraformaldehyde, or paraform in a special fumigating lamp. A pint of the solution and about one ounce of paraform should suffice for 1,000 cubic feet of space, and disinfection should be complete in about ten hours.

Formalin has been used for preserving food, but is noxious when so used. As a spray and in other ways it is useful for destroying flies (*q.v.*).

See Antiseptic ; Disinfection.

FORMIC ACID. A colourless liquid with a pungent, irritating smell, formic acid is contained in the liquid injected by ants and bees when biting and stinging. It is the cause of the pain and swelling which follow. Formic acid is also generally stated to be present in the ordinary stinging nettle, though this has been queried. The pure acid blisters the skin. Rheumatic joints are sometimes treated by causing bees to sting the skin over them, and dilute solutions of formic acid have been injected hypodermically for the same purpose. This acid, when taken inwardly, is thought by some to relieve muscular tremors. Sodium formate, calcium formate, and other salts may be used in preference to the acid itself,

There is a compound syrup or elixir of formates, which is used as a tonic, some of the individual salts also being used with this object.

FORMICATION. The abnormal sensation, or paraesthesia, resembling that caused by ants crawling over the skin, is described as formication. This may occur, for example, in peripheral neuritis, an inflammation of nerves, caused by alcohol and other poisons.

See Sensation.

FOSSA. The Latin word fossa, meaning a ditch, is used as a general name for numerous depressions on body structures, as, for example, the antecubital fossa, or depression on the front of the elbow ; the anterior, middle and posterior fossae of the base of the skull, and so on.

FRACTURE. A bone may be broken or fractured by external violence, and this may be direct or indirect, the former as when a wheel passes over the leg and breaks it, the latter as when the wheel passes over the chest and breaks one or more ribs. In the latter instance the break does not occur at the point where violence is applied, but the rib is bent and snaps at its weakest point. A fracture is occasionally due to muscular action simply, as when the humerus snaps during the act of throwing a cricket ball, or a rib is broken by excessive coughing.

Various circumstances predispose a bone to fracture. Thus the bones of an aged person break easily because the earthy constituents have increased very largely, with a corresponding diminution of the tough cartilaginous, or gristly, constituents. Again, some people are born with a weakness in their bones, a condition known as fragilitas ossium, and such during a lifetime may sustain many fractures. Rickets and other diseases weaken the bones ; in nervous diseases like tabes, which may interfere with the nutrition of the bones, these become more fragile. Inflammation, and especially suppuration in a bone, or the presence of a tumour, may so weaken a bone, that what is called spontaneous fracture occurs, merely from the ordinary use of the limb and without any violence.

The damage in a fracture may be limited to the bone, or, at any rate, that occurring to the soft parts may have little significance ; such is called a simple fracture. If the skin is divided, either by the broken bone projecting through it or by a missile, the fracture is said to be compound, and is more serious than a simple one in that there is an opportunity for a free loss of blood, but more so, perhaps, because disease organisms may be admitted to the site of fracture. When a fracture is accompanied by tearing of the main blood vessels, or nerves, or of muscles or internal organs, it is said to be a complicated one.

A comminuted fracture is one in which there is splintering of the bone at the site of fracture, and when a bone is broken in several places, or several bones are broken, the fracture is multiple. In young persons the bones are relatively tough and, as a rule, a fracture is not complete, but the bone is partly bent and partly broken. This is what usually occurs when a fresh twig is broken, so such is known as a greenstick fracture (see illustration page 106). It sometimes happens in fractures near the ends of long bones that the shaft, which is made of dense bone, is driven into the end of the bone, which is made of cancellous, or spongy, bone, and fixed there ; this is an impacted fracture.

In a fracture through the shaft of a long bone, the direction of the break is generally oblique, an important fact because the fragments can readily slip past each other and be displaced by the violence breaking the bone or by the pull of the muscles, and, further, because each frag-

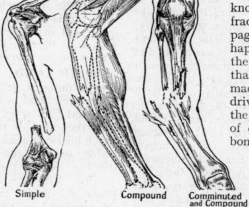

Fracture. Three types of this bone injury : left, simple fracture of the humerus ; centre, skin torn by fractured leg bones ; right, splintered bones in leg fracture.

Simple   Compound   Comminuted and Compound

ment is furnished with a sharp point or edge which may easily damage the soft tissues. If the violence has been partly of a twisting character, the direction may be a spiral one. The direction may be transverse, however or, particularly when the fracture is caused by a missile, say a bullet, or by a stabbing instrument, it may be longitudinal, or vertical ; near a joint it is not uncommon for these to be combined, so that a T-shaped fracture results.

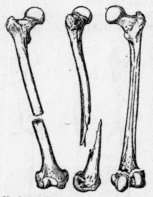

Varied direction of fracture : transverse, oblique and T-shaped

A fracture of a flat bone may consist of a fissure which may be straight or curved, perhaps even semi-circular, and the detached portion may be depressed, or it may consist of several fissures radiating from a centre, such as may be seen when a pane of glass is broken.

In young persons whose bones are still growing an accident resembling a fracture may occur, namely, separation at the epiphyseal cartilage. This is a plate uniting the end of a bone to the shaft, and by which the bone grows in length. Either by hard pulling on the bone, as for example when a heavy child is lifted by the hands, or otherwise, the end of the bone is detached from the shaft. Unless the accident is properly treated, the growth of the bone may be interfered with seriously.

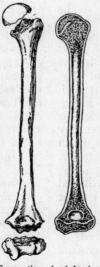

Separation of epiphysis. Right, section showing epiphyseal line

A person who sustains a fracture may be conscious of the snap ; bystanders have even sometimes heard it. At any rate, there is likely to be considerable pain and more or less shock. If it is a limb bone, there is loss of the use of the limb if a main bone is broken, but if, say, the fibula alone is broken, a person may stand fairly well, or if the lower end of the radius, he may use his forearm, especially if the fracture is an impacted one. A person with an impacted fracture of the neck of the femur may also be able to walk. The displacement of the fragments may cause a prominence on the limb, or this may be bent, and very quickly, from effused blood and inflammatory fluid, there is more or less swelling. If the limb be grasped above and below the fracture, it will be observed that there is movement between the fragments, and, if the ends of the latter are brought together, there will be a sense of grating, or crepitus, when they are moved on one another. Such methods of examination, however, should be left to a doctor, as unskilful handling might cause damage to soft parts and possibly convert a simple into a compound fracture.

When only one bone of the arm or leg is broken, there may be little displacement of the fragments, because the other bone acts as a splint. Fractures near a joint may be difficult to distinguish from dislocations, especially an impacted fracture, and indeed in many instances of dislocation, there is fracture as well.

There is likely to be considerable discoloration of the skin over a fracture, and the same succession of colours as is observed after a bruise.

The absorption of effused blood, etc., causes a little feverishness for a day or two, and there may be what is sometimes called traumatic delirium.

A broken bone is mended by a copious formation of new cells, forming a mass known as callus, in which the ends of the fragments become embedded ; the amount of callus is increased by mal-position of the fragments and by movement ; and, on the other hand, when the nutrition of the parts is poor, there may be insufficient callus to effect union. Lime salts are deposited in the callus or in fibrous tissue into which this has been converted, and later there is a development of true bone.

Damage to soft parts is also repaired by new cell formation, and as these cells are in a mass with the callus, muscles and other structures may be fixed to the new bone uniting the fragments. More or less thickening of the bone may persist at the site of fracture. Sometimes there is only fibrous tissue between the ends of the fragments ; this is called fibrous union. Several things might account for this, such as excessive movement, improper setting of the fracture, the presence of ligament or some other soft tissue between the ends of the fragments, and so on. Union of a fracture is usually complete in from four to eight weeks, according to the size of the bone involved.

In the first-aid treatment of fractures the first thing to be attended to may be bleeding, and there is always a certain degree of shock. If the fracture is a compound one, and there is more than slight bleeding, or, if from the rapid and severe swelling of the limb it may be apprehended that serious bleeding is taking place within the limb, a tourniquet (*q.v.*) ought to be applied.

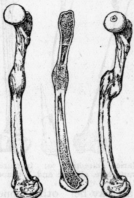

Left and centre, healing of fractured bone in good position. Right, bad position

Shock is treated by warmth ; stimulants may be given, but only in the event of there being little bleeding. If the fracture is compound and a piece of bone is projecting, this may be daubed with tincture of iodine, and if there is soiling by earth or anything else, as much as possible of the dirt should be removed by light rubbing with a clean rag, after which tincture of iodine should be used freely. If a doctor can be on the spot quickly, however, the wound should be covered with a clean rag and the cleaning left for him to do.

Before moving a patient with a broken limb, the fracture must be reduced, or set, that is, the ends of the fragments should be brought into their natural position as far as possible, and the limb should then be splinted to prevent the fragments from moving. Reduction is accomplished by one person pulling on the limb (extension) while another fixes the upper end of the limb or the trunk (**counter extension**). Thus, for a fractured

thigh, someone would pull at the ankle while another fixed the trunk by grasping below the armpits. In extension the pull must be steady and the limb should be held in a correct position, the foot, for example, in fractures of the lower extremity, being at right angles to the leg, and the toes turned slightly outwards. If a doctor is superintending, he may possibly help the reduction by manipulating the fragments.

A splint may consist of anything which is sufficiently rigid and light—a broom handle, umbrellas, walking sticks, battens, even folded cardboard or newspapers. It should be long enough to prevent movement at the joint above and below the fracture, and, before being applied, should be well padded. Extra padding is used over bone prominences, as at the ankle, the haunch, or the elbow. Splints are placed both on the inner and the outer side of the limb and are fixed with bandages, preferably folded triangular bandages or large handkerchiefs. These should be knotted over the splint on the outer side of the limb.

A splint should be broad enough to prevent the bandages from cutting into the flesh, or, if narrow, like a broom handle, additional small splints should be placed round the limb. On the other hand, if splints are too broad, they will not maintain a firm position.

When there is difficulty in obtaining splints, an upper limb may be fixed against the trunk, or the lower limbs can be tied together until splints are available, but a lower limb must be made rigid by splinting before a patient is lifted.

While splinting must be firm enough to control the fracture it must not be tight enough to interfere with the circulation in the limb. To test this, when the splints are applied, the finger or toe nails may be observed ; pressure on the nail should cause it to whiten, but the pink tint should return as soon as pressure is discontinued. Over-tightness of splints is responsible for Volkmann's contracture in the forearm in which there is inability to straighten out the fingers unless the wrist is bent.

A person with a broken lower limb or spine should be carried on a rigid stretcher and be treated on a fracture bed, that is, one which has been made rigid by putting boards over the framework of the bed, beneath the mattress.

If at all possible, the fracture should be examined with X-rays to ascertain its nature and ensure its correct reduction. Varieties of splint are dealt with under that heading. Thomas's splint consists of a round or oval ring of metal padded and covered with leather at its upper end, from which metal bars pass downwards to be joined together at the lower end. This is shaped so that an extension apparatus can be fixed to it (*see* illustration page 274), and the rods themselves may be bent to form a right angle and adapt the splint for the arm (Plate XXXIII).

Extension Apparatus for Fracture

An extension apparatus usually consists of two strips of adhesive plaster, one on either side of the limb and prolonged for 2 or 3 inches below the sole of the foot, or the elbow, as the case may be. To the ends a cross-piece of wood, the stirrup, is attached, in the centre of which is a hole through which is passed a string, retained by a knot. The other end of the string may be fixed to a thick rubber band, forming a spring, and attached to the lower end of the splint, or it may be passed over a wheel at the foot of the bed or the splint and attached to a weight sufficient to keep up a proper tension. The plaster, which should not extend up the limb above the site of the fracture, is fixed by a roller bandage.

Sometimes a plaster of paris bandage is put on a limb, and when quite dry, or in a few days, is divided on each side of the limb so that a moulded splint of two pieces is obtained which can be taken off and reapplied as desired.

Fractures at or near the neck of the femur or the neck of the humerus are put up in an abducted position as a rule, that is, the lower end of the limb is drawn away from the middle line of the body. The lower limb, in a Thomas or other splint, is suspended at its lower end to a wooden frame, known as a Balkan splint, or to something similar. The arm may be placed on a triangular frame, and may be put as high as at a right angle with the body.

After a few days a limb is taken from the splints daily and the joints are gently moved by the doctor ; very soon, too, the patient may be asked to do gentle movements himself. Massage is done regularly, and perhaps electrical treatment is used also, these measures being useful for promoting absorption of swelling and for maintaining the bulk and tone of the muscles. Before much weight is put on a fractured lower limb the patient should get about for some days on a crutch and should use a stick for some time afterwards.

An old person who has fractured the neck of the femur and is treated by confinement to bed runs a considerable risk of dying.

When possible, therefore, the injured limb is fixed in a Thomas's splint, the other foot raised on a patten and the patient provided with crutches and allowed to get about ; the patten is sufficiently high to keep the lower end of the splint off the ground. By the use of special splints other fractures are sometimes treated by this so-called ambulatory method.

How to Give First Aid

The first aid treatment of various fractures may be summarised as follows :

SKULL. Carry and lay in bed with the head raised ; warmth to the feet ; cold, preferably iced, applications to the head. The room should be darkened and kept quiet. Do not give alcoholic stimulants.

NOSE. Put cold applications on the bridge of the nose ; the patient should be in a semi-recumbent position. If there is free bleeding, gently plug the nostril affected.

LOWER JAW. Put the centre of a narrow-fold bandage below the jaw, carry the ends to the top of the head and tie in front of the vertex, or most prominent part. Put the centre of another narrow-fold bandage over the front of the lower jaw, carry the ends to the back of the neck and tie ; now tie each of these ends to the corresponding end of the other bandage.

SPINE. Wait for a doctor, if possible, before lifting. Procure a door or something similar, or place a board beneath the canvas of a stretcher, resting on the traverses so that the stretcher will not sag. For lifting, gently drag a thick sheet or blanket beneath the patient. Four persons stand astride over the patient and, grasping the sheet close to his body, raise him together, someone giving the command, avoiding any bending of the spine ; while another person pushes the stretcher through between the legs of the bearers. The patient is now lowered on to the stretcher, where he lies flat. The same precautions are necessary in removing him from the stretcher on to a bed, which should also be rigid. The patient must be kept warm and should be given stimulants in small doses.

COLLAR BONE. A large pad is put in the armpit. One end of a triangular bandage is put over the sound shoulder, the point of the bandage being also towards the sound side. The injured limb is placed over the cloth, the fingers directed towards the sound shoulder. The other end is then brought over the lower third of the arm, passed below the armpit and knotted to the other end at the back. The point of the bandage is folded in and the loose carried over the hand and pinned off. A narrow-fold bandage is placed with its centre a little above the elbow and the ends are carried round the body and tied. Another method of bandaging is shown in Plate X, 3–6.

SHOULDER BLADE. Support the arm in a greater arm-sling and fix it by a bandage passing round the limb and the body.

HUMERUS. Select two splints, one to reach from the shoulder and the other from the armpit to below the elbow ; pad well, including the upper end of the latter, which goes on the inner side of the arm, the other being on the outer side. Fix the splints by a narrow-fold bandage above the fracture and another below it. Support at the wrist by a lesser arm sling.

If the fracture is near the elbow joint, take a splint reaching from the armpit to the elbow and another from the elbow to the tips of the fingers. Tie or other-wise fix these at one end so as to form an L-shaped splint. This is applied to the inner side of the limb, fixed by a bandage round the arm, and another round the forearm. Support the limb by a greater arm sling (*see* Plate XXXIII, 1).

BONES OF THE FOREARM. Apply the same splint as above, the forearm being placed with the thumb upwards, and put a short splint on the back of the forearm. Fix by bandages above and below the fracture. Use a greater arm sling. It is an advantage, however, to put up the forearm with the palm of the hand looking upwards, and this should be done if an L-shaped splint can be got ready, one limb of which is applied to the back of the arm and the other to the back of the forearm. A short splint is placed on the front of the forearm. Both splints must be well padded.

BONES OF THE HAND. Splint as for the forearm, the first method above described.

RIB. Put a pillow-slip round the chest and fix with pins or apply bandages as described in page 68. The pressure should be sufficient to lessen the breathing movements, but should not cause pain.

PELVIS. Put a pillow-slip or two broad-fold bandages round the pelvis. Carry on a rigid stretcher and lay on a fracture-bed.

THIGH BONE. The splint for the outer side of the limb should reach from the armpit to below the sole of the foot and that for the inner side from the crutch to below the knee ; frequently a short splint is also placed on the front of the thigh. The upper ends of the two former must be well padded. A long broom makes a good outer splint (*see* Plate XVIII). Liston's long splint is a batten with two V-shaped portions cut out of the lower end for the attachment of bandages.

The outer splint is first attached to the body by broad-fold bandages, one round the chest below the armpits, and another round the haunches. The other splints are then applied and fixed with one bandage above the fracture and another below it. The long splint is now fixed to the leg by a bandage just below the knee and another at the ankle ; finally, the two legs are tied together by placing the middle of a narrow-fold bandage at the back of the legs just above the ankles, bringing the ends round, crossing over the insteps and tying opposite the space between the soles of the feet.

When applying a bandage to the limb, it should be folded double and a short splint put into the loop, which is then pushed beneath the limb, when one end of the loop is caught and drawn forward. This obviates any movement of the limb. The lower end of the long splint should be raised off the ground by a block several inches high, and this should be used also on the stretcher and when the patient is put to bed. Later, the limb is slung, as a rule.

KNEE-CAP. A splint reaching from the buttock to below the heel is placed beneath the limb. The centre of a narrow-fold sling is placed above the upper fragment, and the ends carried round beneath the splint, crossed, brought forward and tied below the knee ; this is to drag the upper fragment down. The centre of another narrow-fold is applied below the lower fragment, and the ends of this are tied above the knee ; this is to drag the lower fragment up. The splint is further fixed by a bandage round the thigh and another at the ankle, when the two legs are tied together, the feet being raised.

LEG BONES. An outer and an inner splint are required, each reaching from above the knee to below the sole, and fixed by a bandage above the site of fracture and another below it, or if the fracture is at the ankle, by two above and one below. The legs are tied together and the feet raised. Care in handling is required to prevent perforation of the skin by a fragment of the shin bone.

FOOT BONES. Splints are applied as above.

In fractures of the lower extremity care should be taken to keep the foot at right angles to the leg.

See Bleeding ; Dislocation ; Extension ; First Aid ; Ischaemia ; Joint ; Splint ; Transport of the Sick and Injured.

FRECKLES. The small, light to dark brown areas of discoloration on the skin, which are known as freckles, are caused by the chemical rays of sunlight, and only exposed parts of the skin are affected. Pigment accumulates in the cells forming the deepest layer of the scarf skin, and the purpose of this is to afford protection against further action by the chemical rays. Freckles are more prone to appear in brunettes and in persons with red hair and a delicate skin ; they come out in summer and disappear in winter. Those who are subject to them are not bronzed by exposure to sunlight.

Preventive measures consist in avoiding direct exposure to the sun's rays as far as possible, by using a broad hat, a parasol, a red or brown veil, or a calamine or skin-coloured dusting powder. Ointments containing corrosive sublimate or some other substance to induce peeling are sometimes used to diminish disfigurement caused by freckles, but should not be used on children. Also, while freckles can be removed in this way, they are not prevented from recurring.

See Light ; Pigmentation ; Skin.

FRENUM. A small fold of skin or mucous membrane, which in several situations in the body limits the movement of some structure to which it is attached, is described as a frenum, or fraenum, a word meaning a bridle. The frenum of the tongue (*q.v.*) is an example.

FREUDISM. The contributions of Freud to psychological knowledge can be properly divided into two parts. The first comprises his theories of the nature of mental operations, and the second, his notions of the paramount influence of sex on thought. Indignation against this second aspect of Freud's teaching has prevented many from making a patient examination of the first.

As a warring of the spirit against the flesh, or in some other figure, the notion of the control of behaviour by our ideas of good and evil is a very old one, and our sense of what should be done in any circumstance, involving such conflict, we have been in the habit of calling the conscience. Freud terms this barrier to the untrammelled play of our instincts the censor, and says that it operates even in dreams ; in fact it operates, even while we are awake, against certain kinds of ideas, preventing them from emerging into consciousness, so that it is more than conscience, which is a conscious weighing of two lines of conduct.

According to Freud, the thoughts or desires, thus repressed, go to form the contents of the unconscious mind ; they are charged with dynamic energy which may be transferred to some other idea, as when the unsatisfied maternal instinct creates a passionate fondness for a pet animal. Such a transference may, however, also take place consciously. Dreams, in Freud's view, are a method of satisfying such repressed longings, though, as has been said, the manner of satisfaction must be such as is allowed by the censor and this may involve distortion of the events and feelings of the dream.

The transference of energy from one idea to another may, however, take an abnormal turn and result in disease ; if this is a conscious process, the patient develops an anxiety state, if unconscious, a conversion neurosis, say, palsy of a limb, blindness or some other disability. If a person relates his thoughts as they occur without attempting to guide them in any way, that is to say, allows a free association of ideas, a doctor may be able to trace the connexion between illness and the content of the unconscious mind. This is the method of psycho-analysis, and was devised by Freud.

Another of Freud's opinions is that the mental processes in infancy and childhood are of much importance, so much so that they form the ground work for all later development. He teaches also that sex attraction in a broad sense exists in early childhood, at first for individuals of the same sex (homosexual) and later, but long before puberty, for those of the opposite sex (heterosexual). Further, the attraction is for the parent of the opposite sex, and this so-called " Oedipus complex " he considers to be the cause of subsequent mental conflict and of much neurotic disease. Sexual perversion in the same way may have its origin in early life, say, from a failure to develop beyond the homosexual stage.

See Dreams; Hypnotism; Mind; Psycho-therapy.

FRIAR'S BALSAM. *See* Balsam.

FRIEDREICH'S ATAXIA. An uncommon nervous disease, Friedreich's ataxia tends to affect several members of a family, but, though also called hereditary ataxia, inheritance of the disease is unusual. It begins in early life and in the legs, the gait becoming like that of a drunken man. Soon the feet become deformed, the child walking with the heel raised and on the outer side of the foot, which also takes on the appearance described under the heading Claw Foot. A notable feature is the drawing back of the great toe at the joint connecting it with the foot.

The speech is syllabic or scanning, the eyeballs oscillate to and fro, a condition known as nystagmus, the knee-jerks (*q.v.*) are lost, but the pupil contracts on exposure to light, in contrast to what occurs in locomotor ataxia. The arms also become affected, and the legs become paralysed ; indeed, the patient may never walk. Lateral curvature of the spine is common, and there may also be kyphosis. There is no disturbance of sensation and no wasting of muscles apart from that due to disease. Death occurs from pneumonia or some other intercurrent disease.

The disease is caused by imperfect development of tracts in the spinal cord, and this cannot be remedied. An attempt should be made, however, to prevent contracture, or tightening up, of muscles as far as possible.

See Ataxia ; Nervous System.

FRONTAL BONE. The cavity of the cranium, or brain-pan, is closed in anteriorly by the frontal bone, which also helps to form the floor of the cavity. The bone, therefore, consists of two parts, one more or less upright, and another attached to the former near its lower border and passing horizontally backwards. The upright portion is the bone of the forehead and on either side presents a bulging, the frontal eminence. An illustration is given in Plate VII, 1. In rickets these eminences are much more prominent, due to the thickening of the bone in this region. Sometimes a suture, or joint, persists in the middle line, separating the bone into two parts ; this is called the metopic suture.

Towards the middle line the frontal bone is jointed to the upper jaw bone and the nasal bone, and outside this, on either side, is the superciliary arch, or upper border of the orbit. Towards the nasal side each arch tends to bulge forwards, this being due to the existence of an air space, the frontal sinus, which space communicates with the nasal cavity. The sinus may be infected from the nose, and may become filled with pus—a frontal sinus empyema. To clean out an unhealthy sinus it may be necessary to open up the space from the front.

The horizontal part of the bone roofs in the orbit on either side but presents a gap in the centre which is filled in by the cribriform plate of the ethmoid bone (*q.v.*). The roof of the orbit is very thin.

See Skull.

FROST BITE. A severe degree of cold may arrest the circulation in certain parts of the body, those most often affected being the toes, the fingers, the edge of the ear and the tip of the nose. Tight, ill-fitting gloves and boots increase the risk to the fingers and toes respectively. The part becomes waxy and dead-looking but there is no pain, so that the person may be unaware of what has happened. If the part recovers from the chilling it becomes acutely inflamed and very painful ; blisters may form on the surface, and on rupturing leave ulcers, and the part may die.

The old-established remedy for frost bite in cold countries is to rub the part with snow, as it is considered to be unwise to warm it too quickly. So in treating frost bite it is customary to bathe with cold water and employ moderate friction. In the state of congestion, the plan is to treat the part with hot and cold water alternately and then massage towards the heart, in order to lessen congestion as far as possible. For the same reason the part should be kept in an elevated position, the leg on a pillow or the arm in a sling, with the hand well up towards the opposite shoulder. If ulcers form they are dressed antiseptically, and this is also done if the part actually dies.

Aspirin or opiates may be necessary to relieve pain.

See Chilblain ; Gangrene.

FUCUS VESICULOSUS. Popularly know as bladder or sea wrack, fucus vesiculosus contains considerable quantities of iodine, bromine and chlorine in the form of salts. It is used in the treatment of obesity and other disorders. From the wrack are prepared the extract, B.P.C., the dose of which is 3 to 10 grains, in pill form, given before meals, and the liquid extract, B.P.C., the dose being 1 to 2 drachms before meals.

See Iodine.

FULLER'S EARTH. So called because it is used by fullers to facilitate the washing of cloth, fuller's earth is a native aluminium silicate containing a trace of iron. It has been much used in medicine as an astringent and drying powder in intertrigo, weeping eczema and the like, but its use is not free from danger when the surface of the skin is broken ; it has caused lockjaw in infants when applied to sores on the navel and buttocks.

FUNCTIONAL DISEASE. A disorder is said to be functional when there is no change in the tissues to account for it. Some organic diseases are accompanied by changes which can be readily detected with the naked eye ; to exhibit the changes in others the use of a microscope may be necessary. In conditions labelled as being functional, however, not even the microscope can reveal anything. Hysterical paralysis is an example of this. If a functional disorder persists for some time, on the other hand, it may cause organic changes, as when functional over-action of the heart causes enlargement of the organ.

See Disease.

FUNGUS. The low forms of plant life, known as fungi, are distinguished by the absence of chlorophyll, or green colouring matter. They are either parasitic on living plants or animals or feed on decaying organic matter, when they are called saprophytes. Amongst the plant forms belonging to this class are the moulds, the yeasts and larger types, mushrooms and toadstools.

Fungi consists of tiny threads, or hyphae, which form a network or mycelium, and propagate by spores. What is popularly called a mushroom is really the spore-bearing apparatus which grows up from the mycelium. It consists of a stalk, or stupe, and a cap or pileus. Radiating from the centre of this cap are gills on which the spores are produced. Gill-bearing fungi are called agarics. The upper surface of the pileus exhibits a great variety of colour, and there are differences also in the colour of the gills and of the spores.

From a health point of view, fungi are of importance because some of the smaller types cause ringworm and other skin diseases ; yeasts are used for making bread and fermented liquors ; and some of the larger types of fungus are eaten. In Great Britain it is customary to call an edible agaric a mushroom, and a poisonous one, a toadstool. Bacteria are sometimes classed as fungi, but probably should be excluded from this class.

The common mushroom, agaricus, or psalliota, campestris, and the champignon, agaricus oreades, are the two fungi most often eaten in Great Britain. The common mushroom has a pale brown pileus, and the gills are pink at first but quickly become dark brown. The pileus of the champignon has a light to deep buff colour with brown gills. Poisonous agarics are, however, sometimes eaten by mistake for edible mushrooms, and no one who is inexperienced in the matter should pick fungi for food.

The old test of boiling fungi with a silver spoon and identifying as poisonous those that blacken it, is not at all reliable. Those are probably poisonous which have an acrid, hot taste, a warty speckled cap, or milky juice ; which turn blue or liquefy as they decay, or which grow round the roots of trees.

The fly agaric, amanita muscarius, which has a reddish pileus with white specks, is highly poisonous. It contains an alkaloid muscarine. It owes its popular name to the fact that a fly poison is prepared from it. What is called white or purging agaric, and, from the fact that it grows on old larch trees, boletus larici , is not really an agaric at all. It contains agaricin, or agaric acid, and either this substance, or a tincture or extract from the dried fungus, is used in medicine as a purgative remedy.

The symptoms and treatment of poisoning by fungi are detailed in the table of poisons under the heading Poisoning.

FUNGUS FOOT. In India and other tropical countries a disorder known as tungus, or Madura, foot occurs. The foot becomes chronically enlarged and sinuses form at various parts of it from which matter containing white or black granules is discharged. These granules represent some species of fungus of which several have been found to be responsible for the disease. The fungus is supposed to obtain entrance to the foot through an abrasion ; it then starts to grow, forming a lump which in the course of about eight weeks breaks down and discharges.

The disease very occasionally is found in the hand. Potassium iodide has been tried as a remedy, but the only satisfactory treatment is amputation.

FUNNY BONE. *See* Elbow ; Ulnar Nerve.

FURRED TONGUE. Fur on the tongue consists of bacterial growth, cells cast off from the epithelial covering of the organ and particles of food. A thin, white fur may have no particular significance in some individuals. In others, however, it may imply digestive disorder and it is always present in fevers, though if the fever persists the fur becomes thicker and yellow or brown in colour.

In the typhoid state (*q.v.*) the fur becomes brown and dry. At the beginning of scarlet fever swollen papillae may project as red spots through the white fur, constituting the so-called strawberry tongue. Local patches of furring may be caused by the irritation of a rough tooth or inflammation restricted to some part of the oral cavity. Patches of thrush (*q.v.*) have to be distinguished from furring. The tongue of a sick person should be carefully and regularly cleansed with a solution of bicarbonate of sodium in water, applied with a rag. *See* Tongue.

FURUNCULUS. *See* Boil.

FUSEL OIL. The substance known as fusel oil consists chiefly of amyl alcohol, small quantities of other alcohols also being present, and furfurol. Amyl alcohol is a colourless liquid with the odour of pear-drops ; its action resembles that of ethylic alcohol, but it is much more intoxicating. Furfurol, or furfurane aldehyde, is a liquid with an odour resembling that of bitter almonds ; when fresh it is colourless, but becomes brown on exposure to the air. Fusel oil is present in recently distilled spirits but disappears on keeping. *See* Alcohol.

GAIT. Some diseases produce a more or less characteristic gait. In locomotor ataxia the foot is lifted up suddenly and too far, then jerked forwards and brought down with a stamp, probably on the heel first, the patient meanwhile stooping forward with his eyes fixed on the movements of his feet. These are also widely apart. This is the ataxic gait and is caused by imperfect co-ordination. In disease of the cerebellum co-ordination may also be affected, but the gait is then like that of a drunken person.

In disease affecting the lateral columns of the spinal cord the gait is spastic. The limb moves stiffly, with apparent difficulty in bending the knee, and the foot is dragged forward over the ground. Sometimes each foot is brought in front of the other, this being called cross-legged progression. In hemiplegia, in which one side only is paralysed, the affected limb is swung round and forwards by twisting the body.

When the muscles on the front of the leg are paralysed, causing foot drop, a steppage gait results. The foot is raised well off the ground to clear the toes and the person walks as if among high grass.

In paralysis agitans the patient moves forward with quick, shuffling steps as if he were being pushed, the body being inclined somewhat forwards. This is called festination or propulsion. If he moves backwards the body is inclined backwards as if he were about to fall. This is called retropulsion.

A waddling gait is caused by such disorders as pseudo-hypertrophic muscular paralysis, in which, although the calf and other muscles are much enlarged, they are really degenerated and very weak; and congenital dislocation of the hip. The shoulders are thrown back and the small of the back hollowed out. A similar gait occurs in advanced pregnancy.

Pain, shortening of a limb, or stiffness of joints are suggested by a limping gait.

See Ataxia; Paralysis.

GALBANUM. A gum-resin, galbanum has a greenish-yellow colour and a disagreeable odour and taste. It is given in doses of 5 to 15 grains and is used for chronic bronchitis. The compound pill of galbanum contains myrrh and asafoetida and is known also as the compound asafoetida pill. It is used in hysteria.

GALL. The rounded excrescences or nut-galls, produced on the oak, quercus infectoria, by the deposit of the eggs of a small wasp, contain tannic and gallic acids and are used in medicine as an astringent. Their action is entirely due to the tannic acid, however; gallic acid possesses no astringency, either when used externally or internally. From powdered galls are prepared gall ointment and the ointment of gall and opium, which are often used in treating piles. The ointment of witch hazel may be preferred, however, as it is cleaner looking. Subgallate of bismuth, or dermatol, is used as a dusting powder in eczema, etc.

The term gall is sometimes used as a synonym for bile (*q.v.*).

GALL BLADDER. The pear-shaped bag known as the gall bladder lies on the under surface of the liver, its thicker end, or fundus, when the bag is full, pressing against the anterior abdominal wall just below the cartilage of the ninth rib on the right side. It is about 4 inches long and 1½ inches across at its widest part, and has a capacity of 8 to 10 drachms.

Its wall is composed of plain muscle and fibrous tissue and it is lined with mucous membrane. Its narrower end, or neck, which is directed backwards, opens into the cystic duct and this runs across to join the hepatic duct at an acute angle, the junction of the two forming the common bile duct.

Gall bladder in which bile is both stored and concentrated

Labels: Gall Bladder Laid Open; Cystic Duct; Hepatic Duct; Mucous Lining; Common Bile Duct

Bile passes into the gall bladder from the liver and is stored there till required for digestion. The acid chyme from the stomach passing over the surface of the duodenum causes a reflex stimulation of the muscle fibres in the wall of the gall bladder, and these contract and squeeze bile out of the bladder and into the duodenum.

Bacteria, and more especially the bacillus coli communis, a normal inhabitant of the bowel, and the typhoid fever bacillus, may invade the gall bladder. A chronic catarrhal inflammation may be thus set up and small masses of inflammatory products may form nuclei round which gall-stones grow. Inflammation of the gall bladder is called cholecystitis and, when acute, may result in the bag becoming filled with pus. This would require to be drained.

After typhoid fever the germs of the disease may multiply in the gall bladder, from which at intervals they pass into the bowel to be discharged in the faeces, so that the person becomes a carrier of the disease. To cure this condition it has been suggested that the gall bladder should be removed. This can be done without ill effect as the bag is not indispensable; it may have to be removed also when it is affected with cancer or otherwise constitutes a danger or serious annoyance.

See Bile ; Liver.

GALL-STONE. Brownish concretions, or gall-stones, may occur in the gall bladder or in the bile ducts and may be as large as a hen's egg or no bigger than a grain of sand. They are light, floating in water, and have a soft and almost soapy feel. Their chief constituents are cholesterol and bile pigments, but there is also lime. These are derived from the bile but are deposited around a nucleus, formed by a little mass of bacteria or of inflammatory exudation. Cholesterol is really an alcohol, though it occurs as a white crystalline substance ; it occurs not only in bile, but in blood, nervous tissue, yolk of egg, etc.

If several gall-stones are packed together their mutual pressure causes flattened surfaces, or facets, so that the existence of such on a stone passed by the bowel shows that it has not occurred singly. Stones may long exist in the gall bladder without symptoms, but when a stone of any size moves down a bile duct it causes biliary, or gall-stone, colic. A stone may pass through the ducts and

into the bowel, or may become stuck, or impacted, in a duct, and if this should be the common bile duct, jaundice will ensue.

The pain in biliary colic is in the pit of the stomach and towards the right ; it shoots through to the back on the same level and also up to the back of the right shoulder. It is agonising and may cause the patient to collapse. There is also vomiting and a certain amount of fever. While awaiting a doctor large, hot poultices should be put over the liver, and if vomiting is severe the patient should drink warm water with bicarbonate of sodium dissolved in it ; this will make the vomiting easier. In most instances a dose of morphia is necessary. Sometimes chloroform is used by inhalation.

The attack is brought to an end by the stone becoming impacted or by its slipping back into the gall bladder or through into the bowel. To test the last possibility a close watch should be kept on the stools for a day or two ; these are mixed with water and strained through coarse muslin.

An attempt has been made to dissolve stones in the gall bladder or ducts by giving salicylate of sodium and other drugs, but the only thing likely to be of any use is olive oil. A course of this should be taken, 3 or 4 ounces on an empty stomach, preferably first thing in the morning.

When stones are known to be in the gall bladder or ducts an operation is desirable if the patient is able to stand it, as the presence of the stones involves certain risks, including that of cancer. The gall bladder may be opened and the stones ejected, or the bladder may be taken away altogether.

See Bile ; Gall Bladder ; Jaundice ; Liver.

GALVANIC BELT. Belts containing alternate disks of copper and zinc are sold as galvanic belts and vaunted as sources of vital energy. Any effect they may have is purely by suggestion.

See Electricity in Medicine.

GAMGEE TISSUE. A layer of absorbent cotton wool between layers of gauze constitutes what is called gamgee tissue. Its advantages are that it can be cut and handled more easily and neatly than the ordinary wool and provides a better surface on which to spread ointments. In pneumonia and other chest disorders a gamgee jacket, cut from a sheet of the tissue, is often worn.

See Dressing.

GANGLION. An elastic swelling, connected with a tendon and due to an accumulation of a clear, jelly-like substance in the tendon sheath, is called a ganglion. It occurs in various situations, most commonly on the back of the wrist or hand, and, beyond the disfigurement, is of little account. An old-fashioned treatment was to rupture the sac by striking it with a heavy book, and the same may be accomplished by passing a knife through the skin and transfixing the sac. In either case, however, the swelling tends to reappear, and it may be necessary to dissect the sac out. The strictest antiseptic precautions are necessary in this dissection or when transfixing the sac.

A more serious condition, often referred to as a compound ganglion, sometimes results from tuberculous infection of tendon sheaths, its commonest situation being on the front of the wrist. In the substance contained in such a swelling there is a large number of little granules which are known as melon-seed bodies. The treatment is that of tuberculous infections generally.

The name ganglion is also given to collections of nerve cells occurring in connexion with cranial or spinal nerves or the sympathetic nervous system. These form, as it were, relay stations, whereby nervous impulses can be distributed over a wider area than would be possible for a single nerve, or their cells are concerned with the nutriment of the fibres to which they are attached.

See Gasserian Ganglion ; Sympathetic Nervous System ; Wrist.

GANGRENE. Death of a considerable portion of tissue is called gangrene or mortification, and this may be due to various causes, such as violent crushing, burns, frost bite or wounding of the main blood vessels to a part, cutting off its supply. Some germs are capable of producing a spreading type of gangrene. A piece of strangulated gut becomes gangrenous, the commonest instance of this being a strangulated hernia, and from bacterial action a portion of lung sometimes exhibits gangrene.

Apart from accident, the cause of gangrene is interference with the blood supply. In ergot poisoning, for example, the drug by constricting the arteries may shut off the blood supply to fingers, toes, etc., and these, or portions of them, die. A similar constriction occurs in Raynaud's disease (*q.v.*), possibly with the same result. The constriction may be due to actual changes in the walls of the blood vessels such as occur in arterio-sclerosis, and senile gangrene is of this type. Chronic Bright's disease and diabetes are general diseases which favour the occurrence of gangrene.

If the blood supply through the arteries is cut off, and the venous blood and lymph flow away from the part, what is called dry gangrene results. If, on the other hand, these do not flow away, the condition is one of moist gangrene, more dangerous because of the greater risk of serious putrefactive changes.

Appearance of Mortified Tissue

When a part dies it becomes cold and insensitive, though at the same time there may be severe pain. It may be waxen or livid in appearance, and if dry becomes shrunken, brown and then black ; if moist there may be considerable swelling, the skin may show the colour changes noticed in a bruise (*q.v.*), and blisters may form on it.

Except in rapidly advancing gangrene, at some point above the dead or dying tissue a red line appears which has been called the line of demarcation. It is caused by inflammation, and in the course of some days the tissue here is replaced by granulation tissue, such as is found on an ulcer and a healing wound, and at this line, should the patient survive, a severance would take place between the living and dead tissues. There is always a risk, however, that before this could happen the patient would die from septic poisoning.

As the chief risk is that of bacterial invasion, it is essential that the skin over the dead tissue be kept as aseptic as possible. The skin should therefore be cleansed thoroughly, including the parts about the nails in the case of the hands or feet, and the nails should be clipped short. An antiseptic dressing is then applied and renewed immediately it becomes soiled. This might consist of a thick dusting of boracic acid powder covered with boracic lint or cyanide gauze, cotton wool, and a bandage.

An affected limb should be elevated on a pillow or a sling. As soon as a line of demarcation has formed amputation is done above it, but if gangrene is advancing there may be no time to lose, and amputation may have to be done well above the part which appears unhealthy.

If wounds are invaded by certain bacteria there is a rapidly spreading inflammation of the tissues accompanied by the evolution of gas in their substance, and large portions of tissue die. This condition is known as gas gangrene, and the three organisms most often found are the bacillus of Welch, the bacillus of malignant oedema, also known as vibrion septique, and bacillus oedematiens. These flourish in soil, especially when this is manured, and are anaerobes, or only capable of growing in the absence of oxygen. Affected parts have to be opened up freely and treated with antiseptics, but frequently amputation is necessary.

See Caries ; Frost Bite ; Ischaemia ; Necrosis ; Raynaud's Disease ; Slough ; Wound.

GARGLE. The back of the throat may be cleansed and have drugs applied to it by gargling. A tablespoonful, or more, of the liquid to be used is taken into the mouth, the head is thrown back and the liquid allowed to run backwards, and the patient then breathes out through it. Young children and some adults cannot do this without gulping, so that liquids which may not be swallowed must be avoided. When inflammation is very acute gargling may be too painful, but it will suffice to let the liquid lie for a few moments in contact with the throat.

To cleanse the throat warm water with a pinch of common salt or of bicarbonate of soda, or both, may be used, or, if there is foetor, a weak solution of permanganate of potassium. A pinch of powdered alum in warm water makes a good astringent gargle, or the following may be used :

Potassium chlorate	..		..	90 grains
Tincture of perchloride of				
iron ..	..	..	..	2 drachms
Glycerin	..	..	.. 4	,,
Water ..	..	..	..to 6 ounces	

A tablespoonful to be gargled

Sometimes gargling aggravates irritation in the throat, especially if done too frequently.

See Atomiser ; Inhalation ; Spray.

GARLIC. The garlic bulb contains an essential oil which has the characteristic odour and taste of the plant. Its chief constituent is allyl sulphide, which acts as an antiseptic and expectorant. It is chiefly used for respiratory disorders, such as consumption, foetid bronchitis, bronchiectasis and whooping-cough, but the juice has also been used as an application for infected wounds and sores. Garlic also acts as a sedative, and the juice may relieve nervous vomiting. The dose of the minced bulb is 60 to 120 grains, of the juice, 10 to 30 minims, and of the dried juice, 3 to 10 grains, in pill. Sometimes allyl sulphide is given in preference to the crude drug, in capsules containing $\frac{1}{2}$ to 2 minims, or by inhalation.

GAS POISONING. *See* Carbon Monoxide.

GASSERIAN GANGLION. A large collection of nerve cells, forming a thickening on the sensory root of the fifth cranial nerve, the Gasserian, or semilunar, ganglion lies in a shallow depression on the tip of the petrous portion of the temporal bone in the base of the skull. From it emerge the three divisions of the nerve. In trigeminal neuralgia it is sometimes necessary to remove this ganglion or to paralyse it by injecting alcohol into its substance.

See Neuralgia ; Trigeminal Nerve.

GASTRIC FEVER. This term should be considered as obsolete. It has been applied to quite different disorders, by some to acute gastritis, because this is accompanied by fever, and by others to fever accompanied by notable gastric symptoms, cases of this kind being probably mild enteric or typhoid fever.

GASTRIC ULCER. The lining of the stomach is able, in its normal state, to resist the corrosive, or digestive, action of the gastric juice, but when its vitality is impaired part of the lining is digested off, leaving an acute ulcer. The devitalisation of the lining is almost always due to bacterial poisoning and this may have a definite origin such as septic teeth, a diseased appendix or gall bladder, or chronic stagnation of the contents of the large bowel.

Acute ulcers are usually multiple and may occur on any part of the stomach lining. It may chance that an acute ulcer does not heal, becoming chronic and possibly persisting for months or years ; such an ulcer is usually situated on or near the lesser curvature of the stomach, and there is rarely more than one present. Further, most acute ulcers are under a quarter of an inch in diameter, but a chronic ulcer is commonly an inch across and may be three.

How Tobacco May Delay Healing

The failure of an ulcer in this situation to heal may sometimes be due to coarse, irritating food, but it appears to be definitely associated as a rule with delays in the emptying of the stomach due to spasm of the pylorus. There may be various causes for this, but it is generally believed that excessive smoking may be one of them. The frequency of the occurrence of acute ulcers does not seem to be affected by age, except that they are rather less frequent under twenty, but chronic ulcers are much more frequent in those who are over forty. Gastric ulcers occur with equal frequency in the two sexes, in contrast to duodenal ulcers, which are much more common in males.

An acute ulcer rarely perforates the stomach wall, but there is always a risk of a chronic ulcer doing so. Another risk connected with a chronic ulcer is a fatal haemorrhage, though this is not such a frequent event as perforation ; still another risk is that the ulcer will become cancerous. Acute gastric ulcers may be present without causing symptoms. There may, however, be dyspepsia and vomiting of blood, or haematemesis. On the other hand, even a large amount of blood may be brought up when there is no actual visible ulceration and the stomach lining is merely congested and spongy, a condition described as gastrostaxis and which usually occurs in anaemic young women.

A chronic ulcer causes pain which comes on from a few minutes to one or two hours after eating and is generally relieved by vomiting ; pain may also be felt in the back. There is tenderness over the epigastrium. From time to time there may be vomiting of blood, though this is not invariable. There is always, however, blood in the stools, either in sufficient quantity to blacken them or discoverable by microscopical examination.

The treatment of an acute ulcer consists of rest in bed, a bland diet and a free administration of bismuth and alkalies. What is called the Lenhartz diet is commonly used. In this raw eggs and milk are first given, but in the course of a few days raw minced meat, rice milk, rusks, raw ham and butter are added, and some of the eggs are lightly cooked. This diet may be modified in various ways ; for instance, pounded fish may be substituted for some of the eggs. Chronic ulcers are treated in the same way, but in certain circumstances an operation becomes necessary. This takes various forms, such as making an artificial opening from the stomach into the small bowel or removing a portion of the stomach including the ulcer.

In all cases of gastric ulcer, whether acute or chronic, any focus of infection which is discovered should be cleared up.

See Duodenum ; Indigestion ; Stomach.

GASTRITIS. Inflammation of the lining of the stomach, otherwise gastritis or gastric catarrh, may occur as an acute disorder or may be chronic. Acute gastritis may be caused by overloading the stomach with food ; by taking decomposing food, an accident more likely to occur in hot weather ; by an alcoholic bout ; or by taking some other poison capable of causing irritation. It frequently occurs at the beginning of an infectious fever.

At the beginning the patient feels dull and depressed and usually suffers from headache. There is fullness in the pit of the stomach a sense of weight and perhaps pain. There may be belching of wind. Nausea is felt sooner or later and culminates in vomiting. At first the vomited matter consists of undigested food, but later there is much mucus and bile, and the appearance of the last may lead to the disorder being described as a bilious attack. The bile, however, has nothing to do with causing the symptoms ; it is merely drawn into the stomach from the first part of the small bowel, and this takes place in persistent vomiting, whatever the cause. The tongue is covered with white or yellowish fur, the breath is unpleasant, and there may be a free flow of saliva. In children there is diarrhoea, with colicky pains, as a rule.

Such an attack does not usually last much longer than 24 hours, but severer attacks occur in which there is considerable fever, the temperature rising to 103° F. or more, and with corresponding urgency in the other symptoms; sometimes there is more or less collapse. Such an attack may last for four days or more.

If there is extension of the inflammation to the duodenum it may further extend to the bile ducts and give rise to jaundice.

Rarely inflammation proceeding to suppuration may occur in the walls of the stomach. This is described as phlegmonous gastritis. In diphtheria and in other infections inflammation of the stomach lining may be accompanied by the formation of a membrane in the throat; this is called diphtheritic gastritis.

Treatment of an Acute Attack

In the treatment of acute gastritis it is obviously desirable to clear irritating contents out of the stomach, and this may be done in a natural way by the onset of vomiting, which should be encouraged rather than otherwise. By drinking large draughts of tepid water the patient will make the process of vomiting easier and will help to cleanse the stomach. Should vomiting be delayed it may be brought on by a simple emetic, such as a tablespoonful of mustard or 2 tablespoonsful of common salt in a glass of tepid water. To clear offending substances from the bowel 2 or 3 grains of calomel may be given, to be followed by a dose of salts in the morning. For a child, castor oil is better.

No food should be given if the vomiting tends to recur, but as much plain water or soda water as is desired. Should vomiting persist after the stomach has been cleared, an attempt may be made to stop it by sipping hot water, sucking morsels of ice, or by sips of iced champagne if necessary, and by putting a large mustard plaster or a poultice over the pit of the stomach.

As the symptoms abate, milk in some form should be given, as whey, for example, or with the addition of 1 to 3 grains of sodium citrate to the ounce, or milk and soda water. Thereafter, arrowroot or other milk foods are added, and then sweetbreads or steamed white fish. Ordinary food is not resumed for two or three days. When the gastritis is due to some irritant poison, however, thin arrowroot or some other demulcent drink is given as soon as an emetic has acted, as is described under the heading Poisoning.

Amongst drugs most used for calming the irritation of the stomach preparations of bismuth (q.v.) take the chief place.

If acute gastritis is at all severe, or even when it is mild if the cause is obscure, treatment should always be superintended by a doctor; what looks like acute gastritis may actually be due to brain disease or some other cause unrelated to the stomach.

Chronic gastritis may follow an attack of the acute disorder, but more frequently begins insidiously though subsequently there may be occasional exacerbations. It may be caused by habitual over-indulgence in food or alcohol, in tobacco and, in some parts of the world, in iced drinks. Habitual failure to chew food properly is another cause. Many suffer from the disease from swallowing septic discharges from the teeth, from the sinuses of the nose or from tonsils and adenoids.

Some Causes of Chronic Gastritis

A chronic ulcer or other organic disease of the stomach is likely to be accompanied by chronic gastritis. Constant overfilling of the veins of the stomach, as occurs in cirrhosis of the liver, chronic heart disease and some lung diseases, may cause it, and, finally, it may be a consequence of chronic tuberculosis, chronic nephritis, anaemia and other debilitating diseases.

There is a fullness in the pit of the stomach and perhaps dull pain, worse after food but often almost continuous. The pain may sometimes take the form of a hot burning feeling about the lower end of the breast bone, referred to as heartburn, or of a more acute pain in the heart region, or cardialgia. There is a diffuse tenderness over the pit of the stomach. The appetite is normally poor, but at times may be very keen. Nausea in the morning is common; vomiting sometimes occurs, though this is only common in alcoholics.

The tongue is furred and is usually red at the tip and edges; there is a bad taste in the mouth and the breath tends to be foul ; constipation is the rule.

Headache is common and there may be a liability to giddiness. The spirits are depressed and there may be also irritability of temper. When the disorder has lasted for some time the complexion generally becomes sallow.

There is a form of chronic gastritis, the atrophic or sclerotic, in which the lining of the stomach becomes replaced by fibrous tissue, and in which there is a progressive development of severe symptoms of indigestion and of malnutrition.

The treatment of chronic gastritis cannot be safely prescribed until a careful investigation of the habits and functional condition of other organs besides the stomach permits of a fair estimate of the underlying cause or causes.

Sound dietetic habits must be insisted on ; alcohol should preferably be discontinued, and if tobacco is used at all it should be very moderately. Food should be plain but varied. Spiced food, pastries, pickles and fried food should be avoided. The amount of food should be moderate and meals should be properly spaced, say at four-hourly intervals, the last heavy meal being not later than three hours before bedtime.

If the condition is severe it may be desirable to begin treatment by a few days' rest in bed and restriction to a milk diet ; it may even be necessary to give peptonised milk.

As regards medicinal treatment it will usually be necessary to take a laxative to promote regularity of the bowels. It is often useful to take a pinch of bicarbonate of soda thrice daily, about 20 minutes before the principal meals, or a little Gregory's mixture, say as much as will lie on a sixpence. Digestives (*q.v.*) may be necessary at times and, when the signs of irritation have abated, gentian, quassia or some other bitter may be useful in promoting appetite and digestion.

See Constipation ; Digestion ; Indigestion ; Stomach.

GASTRODYNIA. Severe pain in the pit of the stomach, occurring in paroxysms, is sometimes described as gastrodynia or gastralgia.

See Indigestion.

GASTRO-ENTERITIS. Inflammation involving both stomach and bowels is called gastro-enteritis.

GAULTHERIA. Also known as oil of wintergreen, oil of gaultheria is a fragrant oil containing more than 90 per cent. of methyl salicylate, and with oil of sweet birch is the chief source of natural salicylic acid. In doses of 5 to 15 minims, in capsules, it is sometimes used in the treatment of acute rheumatism ; more usually it is used as an outward application for joint and muscular rheumatism, but, as the natural oil is somewhat expensive, it is generally the artificial, also called methyl salicylate, that is chosen for this purpose. The drug may be rubbed on the skin full strength or mixed with olive oil in equal parts. If the joint is very painful this liniment may be simply applied on lint, covered over with gutta-percha tissue. The spirit of gaultheria B.P.C. is used for flavouring mouth washes.

See Salicylic Acid.

GAUZE. *See* Dressing.

GELATIN. A substance resembling protein and classed as an albuminoid, gelatin is obtained from cartilage or gristle, bone, connective tissue and skin, by boiling. It is readily digested, being converted into a peptone-like substance which is easily absorbed. An animal fed on gelatin loses weight, however, though it thrives on a mixture of gelatin with some protein, so that while it cannot entirely replace protein in the diet, gelatin can do so in part, and is thus what is called a protein-sparer. It can replace half the weight of protein.

Sterile solutions of gelatin are used by injection to increase the coagulability of the blood and arrest internal bleeding in haemoptysis, enteric fever and other instances of the kind. Such injections may also relieve the pain of an aneurysm or even promote its cure.

Gelatin is used in making the glycerin suppositories B.P., also other suppositories and capsules for administering drugs, pessaries and bougies. Treated with formalin, gelatin may be used in place of collodion (*q.v.*). Preparations containing gelatin are sometimes used in place of greasy ointments. Unna's paste (*q.v.*) is of this type.

GENERAL PARALYSIS OF THE INSANE.

The disease described as general paralysis of the insane (popularly termed G.P.I.), general paresis or paralytic dementia, is not, as the first name might suggest, a paralysis liable to affect any person suffering from mental derangement, but a disease in which, from inflammatory and degenerative changes in the grey matter of the brain, both mental disorder and paralysis of muscles occur.

The mental symptoms usually appear first, and at the beginning are slight and indefinite, a slacker attention to the duties of life and loose moral conduct which may go on, however, as far as foolish business transactions, flagrant moral faults or even crime, before the fact of mental disease is appreciated. Indeed, this fact may not be observed even then, the development of the disease being so insidious.

It would be found, however, that the patient's memory was weakening, also his power of concentrating attention on anything, and that mental and physical work soon produced fatigue. Slovenliness and even dirtiness in habits would also probably be noted. The speech might be slow and hesitating, with slight tremor of the lips and tongue, the pupil unresponsive to the action of light, and the knee jerks exaggerated ; the handwriting is unsteady. Sometimes the mental attitude is one of extreme complacency as regards the patient himself, his qualities and powers, his possessions and his family, and in the course of the disease this attitude may reach the degree of grandiose delusions, or megalomania. About this period there may also be great excitement and restlessness. On the other hand, the mental state may simply show a progressive weakening throughout without marked excitement, or the patient may even be melancholic.

As the disease progresses, the speech becomes more slurring and indistinct, the handwriting more shaky and disjointed, words often being left unfinished, until writing is impossible and speech an unintelligible mumble. Standing becomes increasingly difficult until finally the patient is bedridden, helpless, mindless, and the bladder and bowels are uncontrolled. Bed sores are very liable to

form, and some intercurrent disease brings the story to a merciful end.

Generally the duration of the disease is from two to three years, but some patients make a temporary recovery, even from what looks like an advanced stage of the disease, and may be comparatively well even for some years, when the downward course is again resumed. On the other hand, in some instances the disease proves fatal in a few weeks.

The disease usually appears about middle life, and most often in men. Children who are born suffering from syphilis may manifest this disease, however, symptoms appearing when they are between twelve and fourteen years of age. The essential cause of the disease in adult cases is also syphilitic infection, although only a small proportion of those who are infected or who have congenital syphilis suffer in this way. The relatively greater prevalence amongst town dwellers suggests that mental stress and strain may have a predisposing effect. In suspected cases of general paralysis, the blood and cerebro-spinal fluid may give the Wassermann reaction, indicating the existence of syphilitic infection, and other tests applied to the fluid may point to general paralysis, or such tests may be positive even before the Wassermann reaction is detected.

Treatment by Inoculating Malaria Germs

A person suffering from general paralysis should be put into an institution for mental diseases. Drugs that cure ordinary manifestations of syphilis have little effect on general paralysis, though possibly the organic arsenical compounds might arrest the disease at a very early stage. Within the last few years many cases have been treated by inoculation with malaria, and it has been claimed that the disease has been cured when this was done at an early stage, and that in more advanced cases some may improve sufficiently to enable them to be discharged to their homes ; others have improved physically but not mentally, and others still who were maniacal have quieted into dementia.

These effects appear to be due simply to the fever rather than to any other effect of the existence of the malarial parasite in the patient's body, and other infections and vaccines, which consist of dead bacteria, are also used. Some general paralytics are even treated with baths sufficiently hot to raise the body temperature some degrees, that is, to produce a state resembling fever.

See Brain ; Locomotor Ataxia ; Syphilis.

GENITAL SYSTEM. The male elements in generation, spermatozoa, are formed in the testicles, two glands situated in the scrotum, or bag, which is partitioned into two chambers for their reception. Covering each testicle, within the scrotum, is a closed sac of serous membrane, the tunica vaginalis, which is the remains of a tube of the abdominal peritoneum, which accompanies the testicle in its descent from the abdomen into the scrotum, for the testicle is developed in the abdomen and does not make its way out into the scrotum until about two months before birth. Sometimes, in fact, it may fail to emerge, or descend only part of the way.

Behind the body of the testicle there is an elongated mass, the epididymis, representing the tubules that carry the spermatozoa from the gland, and a convoluted main tube into which the tubules pour the secretion. From the lower end of the epididymis the vas deferens, or duct proper of the testicle, passes up out of the scrotum, through the inguinal canal in the front wall of the abdomen, and down into the pelvis as far as the base of the bladder, where it empties into the seminal vesicles, of which there is one on either side.

Accompanying the vas deferens in the inguinal canal and thence into the scrotum are arteries, veins, nerves and lymphatics, some of the veins being collected into what is called the pampiniform plexus. These structures form the so-called spermatic cord, and surrounding the cord are three coverings, superimposed on one another, one of which, the cremasteric, consists of muscle fibres, by the contraction of which the testicle is pulled upwards.

The testicular secretion is stored in the seminal vesicles and is discharged from them through the ejaculatory ducts, which open in the floor of the back part of the urethra, or discharge tube of the bladder, along with a certain amount of secretion from the prostate gland ; the whole constituting the semen.

The introductive organ, or penis, consists of three columns of erectile tissue ; one below, the corpus spongiosum, and two above, lying side by side, the corpora cavernosa ; these terminate in the glans penis. The urethra passes forward through the corpus spongiosum and emerges at the tip of the glans, its opening being called the meatus. Under stimulation by nerves the blood circulation is modified so that the spaces in the erectile tissue become engorged with blood and the organ is made rigid. Apart from the sexual stimulus, this may be brought about by local irritation, such as that from a tight fore-skin or inflammation of the urethra, or from diseases of the nervous system, a persistent erection from this cause being known as priapism.

The skin over the glans is usually prolonged forward to form the fore-skin, but this can generally be retracted to expose the whole glans. Sometimes, however, this is impossible on account of the fore-skin being too tight, a condition described as phimosis, and the consequent difficulty in keeping the glans clean may result in much irritation. The solid, greasy substance which tends to accumulate behind the corona, or most prominent part, of the glans is called smegma. It consists chiefly of effete cells from the mucous membrane covering the parts, but may also contain fatty secretion from glands in the membrane. It is the decomposition of the smegma that causes the irritation.

Condition of Paraphimosis

Sometimes when a tight fore-skin is fully retracted the glans swells and the fore-skin cannot be brought forward again. This is called paraphimosis, and the longer it persists the greater the swelling and pain. It is generally treated by tightly compressing the glans till it is reduced in size, but sometimes a little operation is necessary.

Besides producing spermatozoa the testicles form an internal secretion, or endocrine (q.v.), which has much influence on the development and maintenance of male characteristics, as is shown by the loss of depth in the tone of the voice, the disappearance of hair from the face, and other marks of eunuchism which follow the loss or atrophy of the glands.

The commonest diseases of the male genital organs, apart from phimosis, varicocele and hydrocele, are those of venereal origin, gonorrhoea and syphilis. In view of their possible consequences both are of very great importance. Gonorrhoea causes inflammation of the urethra, or urethritis, and possibly of the seminal vesicles and of the testicle, orchitis. Probably there is inflammation of the glans also, balanitis. The infection may be conveyed to the eyes and may also cause general blood poisoning.

In syphilis a sore, usually on the glans or fore-skin, marks the local infection, but there is a rapid extension by the blood to all parts of the body. In the third stage of the disease there may be an enlargement of the testicle by the development of a gumma.

A varicocele consists of enlargement and varicosity of the veins of the pampiniform plexus ; a hydrocele is a collection of serous fluid in the tunica vaginalis ; sometimes the fluid is milky, a chylous hydrocele ; and sometimes blood, a haematocele, this being caused by an injury. An enlargement of the testicle itself is sometimes called a sarcocele ; it may be caused by inflammation or by a tumour.

Arrangement of the Female System

The external genital organs in the female, known as the vulva or pudendum, are bounded in front by a pad of fat, the skin over which is covered with hair. This is called the mons veneris, and from it proceed backwards, and curving inwards, two folds, also consisting largely of fat, the labia majora. Within these at the front are two shorter folds, the labia minora or nymphae, placed like an inverted V, that is to say, meeting in front, and at the apex is a sensitive, erectile organ, the clitoris. Some distance behind this is the orifice of the urethra, the tube coming from the bladder, immediately behind this orifice again being the entrance to the genital passage, the vagina, sometimes referred to as the front passage. From the close proximity of the two openings it follows that infection readily extends from the vagina to the urethra and bladder.

In a virgin the vaginal orifice is partially closed by a membrane, known as the hymen, the remains of which after its rupture may persist as nodular tags, carunculae myrtiformes, and which sometimes become inflamed and tender. It may chance that the hymen is imperforate, and then there will be retention of the menses, for the release of which division of the membrane by a small operation is necessary. On either side of the vaginal orifice towards the back is the gland of Bartholini. The orifice of the vagina is separated from the anus, or orifice of the rectum, sometimes called the back passage, by the perineum, a mass of tissue which is not uncommonly torn in childbirth.

Formation of a Fistulous Opening

The vagina is about $3\frac{1}{2}$ inches long and leads up to the womb. Its front wall is in close contact with the urethra and, higher up, with the bladder itself, while its back wall is in close contact with the rectum. It follows from this that, from injury or disease, the partition may be perforated and a fistulous opening established between the vagina and the bladder, or the rectum, as the case may be. Also, the bladder may bulge down into the vagina, the protrusion being called a vesicocele, or the rectum may protrude, a rectocele.

The womb, or uterus, is a pear-shaped organ, but is flattened from before backwards. In a woman who has borne children it is generally about 3 inches long, 2 inches broad, and 1 inch thick. The thinner portion, called the cervix, or neck, is directed downwards, projecting in fact into the upper part of the vagina. Through this portion there passes a narrow canal, the outer opening of which is called the os externum and the inner the os internum. The rest of the womb constitutes the body, the cavity of which is roughly triangular in shape, the base of the triangle being uppermost, and at the upper two angles are situated the inner openings of the Fallopian tubes. The part of the womb above these openings is generally referred to as the fundus.

Each Fallopian tube is about $4\frac{1}{2}$ inches long and its outer end opens into the general peritoneal cavity. It is surrounded by a fringe of finger-like processes, or fimbriae. The tube, which is lined with ciliated epithelium, is for the passage of ova, or ovules, from the ovary to the womb, the onward course of an ovum being furthered by the lashing movement of the cilia, or tiny hair-like processes projecting from the epithelial cells.

The womb, which is composed largely of muscular tissue, is covered by peritoneum, folds of which pass out in several directions, attaching the organ to neighbouring structures. Such a fold, stretching out on either side to the wall of the pelvis, is called the broad ligament, and between the layers of peritoneum which compose it several structures are contained, including the Fallopian tube in the upper border of the fold, the round ligament, which passes forward from the womb and through the inguinal canal to be attached to the front of the pubic bone, the ovarian ligament uniting the ovary to the womb, blood vessels, nerves, lymphatics and a mass of loose cellular tissue,

The ovary lies behind the broad ligament and near the pelvic wall. It is 1 to 2 inches long, ¾ inch broad and ½ inch thick. It is covered with epithelium from which are developed the Graafian follicles, within which the ovules develop. When a follicle is ripe, or, in other words, the ovule is ready to be impregnated, the follicle bursts and the ovule is discharged. After this the walls of the follicle thicken and become yellow in colour, the structure being now known as a corpus luteum. This in a short time disappears, however, leaving a scar ; but if the ovum has been inseminated, that is, penetrated by a spermatozoon, a corpus luteum keeps on growing until the third or fourth month of pregnancy, after which it disappears.

Valuable Internal Secretion in Women

Besides producing the ovules, or female cells from which new individuals may be developed, the ovary appears to form an internal secretion, to the existence of which female characteristics are, at any rate in part, due, as the loss of the ovaries may be followed by growth of hair on the face and other male signs. In pregnancy an ovarian secretion also seems to promote development of the womb and breasts, and, by stimulating the posterior part of the pituitary body, to affect the metabolism of sugar, as sugar may appear in the urine during pregnancy. An internal secretion is also produced by the corpus luteum,

and is concerned with the ovarian secretion in the phenomena of menstruation.

Inflammation of the external genitals, or vulvitis, may be caused by friction, by a want of cleanliness, by the irritation of threadworms, which have made their way forward from the bowel, especially in children, or by infection of some kind. In elderly women vulvitis should always suggest an examination of the urine, as the presence of sugar may be the cause of the irritation. Vulvitis may be caused by an irritating vaginal discharge or, on the other hand, infection may spread from the vulva into the vagina. It may happen that one or both Bartholinian glands become infected, causing bartholinitis, and this may go on to abscess, resulting in a painful swelling by the side of the vaginal orifice. This requires opening. An abscess also sometimes occurs in one of the labia majora.

Danger of Vaginal Infections

An active infection in the vagina is a serious matter, as it may extend to the womb and thence to the Fallopian tubes, which open at their outer ends into the peritoneal cavity ; thus general peritonitis may ensue. If the inflammation is limited to the peritoneum on, or in close proximity to, the womb it is described as perimetritis, and if it occurs in the cellular tissue between the layers of the broad ligament it is called parametritis.

Besides infection introduced into the vagina from without, another fruitful source of infection of the genital tract is decomposition of blood-clot or of membranes or other foetal products. Infection may also be brought in the blood-stream, however, as when tuberculosis affects the genital organs ; or it may extend from the bowel, a diseased appendix, for instance. Inflammation of the lining of the womb is called endometritis, and of the wall of the organ, metritis ; of the Fallopian tube, salpingitis, and of the ovary, ovaritis. The womb is one of the commonest sites of cancer.

See Endometritis ; Gonorrhoea ; Haematocele ; Hydrocele ; Ovary ; Perimetritis ; Phimosis ; Prostate ; Syphilis ; Testicle ; Urethra ; Vagina ; Varicocele ; Womb.

GENTIAN. The rhizome and roots of the yellow gentian contain bitter principles which make preparations of the drug useful for stimulating appetite and digestion. The official preparations are the extract, dose 2 to 8 grains; the compound infusion, dose ½ to 1 ounce; and the compound tincture, dose ½ to 1 drachm. The extract is used as an excipient for pills.

See Bitters.

GERM. The minute animal or vegetable structure which is capable of developing into a new individual is called the germ. It constitutes but a small part of the hen's egg, for example, the remainder going to nourish the growing embryo, and the same applies to a grain, say of wheat or rice, or a seed. The word germ is also used as a general name for a bacterium.

See Bacteria.

GERMAN MEASLES. Also known as rubella, German measles is a mild but highly infectious disease, which occurs in epidemics, usually in spring or early summer, amongst both children and adults. The specific cause has not been identified. The period of incubation is from 1 to 3 weeks, and the initial symptoms are slight, perhaps running at the nose and a little soreness of the throat with a slight rise of temperature.

The rash appears after 24 to 48 hours, first on the face, forehead, scalp and behind the ears, and then elsewhere on the body. It consists of rounded, rose-red spots, slightly raised above the ordinary level of the skin, quite separated, as a rule, except that they tend to run together on the trunk, and suggest the rash of scarlet fever. The rash lasts for about three days, and when it disappears there is fine scaling or desquamation.

A notable feature of German measles is that there is enlargement of glands, not only of those at the angle of the lower jaw, which may happen in scarlet fever and other infectious diseases, but behind the ears, in the occipital region of the head, in the armpits and in the groins. The glands never suppurate. The eyes are reddened, but there is not the discomfort caused by exposure to light which is found in measles. The temperature is rarely above 100° F.

The treatment is that of fever (*q.v.*) generally. The patient should be isolated;

he remains infectious for about ten days after the appearance of the rash. While there is fever he should be confined to bed; bronchitis is sometimes a complication, and exposure might induce this, or cause it to become worse. Also, although albuminuria is not common, it may occur.

The patient, on recovery, should have a bath and put on fresh clothing before leaving the sick-room. Bedding and bed-clothing should be soaked in a disinfecting solution. To disinfect the sick-room it usually suffices to air it thoroughly.

Children who have been in contact with a patient suffering from German measles should not return to school until 21 days have elapsed since the last contact.

See Fever; Infectious Disease.

GERMICIDE. Agents such as dry or moist heat, corrosive sublimate, cresylic acid, etc., that are able to kill germs are called germicides.

See Antiseptic; Disinfectant.

GESTATION. *See* Pregnancy.

GIDDINESS. *See* Dizziness.

GINGER. The rhizome of zingiber officinale, or ginger, contains an oily substance called gingerol, a volatile oil, and a resin. The rhizome, scraped and dried, is used to make powdered ginger and other preparations, including the syrup and the tincture, the dose of each of these being ½ to 1 drachm. Ginger acts as a carminative and a flavouring agent. Powdered ginger is contained in Gregory's and other powders. Gingerin, the treacle-like oleo-resin extracted from ginger, is sometimes included in purgative pills, in doses of ¼ to 1 grain, for the purpose of preventing griping.

See Carminative.

GLAND. In its simplest form a gland consists of a short tube, open at one end but blind at the other, or of a little sac or bag, either tube or sac being lined with epithelial cells. Outside the layer of cells are blood vessels, and from materials supplied by these the cells build up a substance, or secretion, which they pour into the cavity of the tube or sac, and which is discharged through the opening.

In more complicated arrangements the tube is long and coiled, the sac is sub-divided into two or more cavities, or acini, the tube is branched, or there is a combination of tubes and sacs, the former acting as discharge conduits for the latter. The last-mentioned type of gland is generally described as being racemose, a term derived from a word meaning a bunch of grapes.

Glands are generally stimulated to activity by nerves, but some are also stimulated by hormones, or chemical messengers, the pancreas affording a notable instance of this.

A large variety of substances are produced by glands, including numerous ferments, such as those of the gastric and pancreatic juices, which initiate chemical changes in the substances on which they act ; the former of these juices is an acid secretion and the latter alkaline. Amongst other secretions are the sweat, the oily secretion on the skin, the urine and so on.

A racemose gland is built up of portions described as lobules, each lobule having a duct by which the discharge of all its acini is drained, and the lobules may be grouped in larger masses, or lobes, each lobe having a duct into which all the lobular ducts drain ; finally, there is a duct carrying off the secretion of the whole gland.

Glands of Internal Secretion

There are some glands, however, which have no such ducts, but which empty their secretions into the blood either by blood capillaries or lymph channels. These are called ductless or endocrine glands, and of this nature are the thyroid, the supra-renal bodies and other all-important glands.

What are popularly called glands, as in the expression " glands of the neck " are really collections of lymphoid tissue, or lymph-nodes, and are described under the heading Lymphatic System.

If the duct of a gland is blocked, say by a calculus, or stone, the secretion goes on, and its accumulation causes a dilatation of the gland behind the obstruction, so that a bag of fluid results ; this is called a retention cyst.

Inflammation of a gland is called adenitis, and a tumour with a glandular structure, an adenoma.

See Endocrine ; Lymphatic System.

GLANDERS. An infectious disease caused by the bacillus mallei, glanders chiefly affects horses and other equine animals. It may be contracted by human beings, and those who handle horses in any way are especially liable. In the horse there is a discharge from the nose, clear at first, but quickly becoming purulent. If the bacilli attack the lymphatics, forming nodules beneath the skin, the disease is spoken of as farcy and the nodules as farcy-buds.

The risk to human beings is increased by having cuts or abrasions on the hands, but infection may take place by air charged with the bacilli depositing these on the eyes or in the nose. The site of infection becomes inflamed, suggesting erysipelas, and the neighbouring lymphatic glands enlarge. There is a nasal discharge resembling that occurring in the horse. Joints may be painful, and may suggest rheumatic fever. Papules form on the face and elsewhere which develop into umbilicated pustules, suggesting smallpox perhaps. The patient is highly fevered, and the general condition comes to resemble the form of blood-poisoning known as pyaemia (*q.v.*). In this acute form of the disease the patient rarely lasts longer than from one to three weeks.

There is a chronic form of the disease, however, which may run on for months, and from which about half of those affected recover. Sometimes the disease resembles a chronic cold in the head, with periodical extensions to the larynx, causing hoarseness and loss of voice ; others suffer from papules on the skin which ulcerate, while others still have multiple abscesses which burst and discharge an oily-looking pus, or matter. Sometimes in the lungs or other internal organs of patients dying from other diseases, nodules are found which are due to glanders. Treatment is almost entirely symptomatic ; the fever is dealt with as described under that heading, while abscesses are opened and treated antiseptically. Mallein, a substance prepared from the bacilli, is an aid to diagnosis, when used like tuberculin (*q.v.*).

GLANDULAR FEVER. A specific infectious disease, occurring in epidemics, glandular fever mostly attacks children. Its onset is sudden, with headache and possibly abdominal pain. Almost at once, and in any case within 24 hours, the glands in the neck become swollen; in many instances glands in the armpits and groins are also enlarged, and possibly the liver and spleen. The throat may be reddened, but the tonsils are not enlarged, and there is no rash. The temperature is commonly fairly high and may reach 104° F., but after three or four days quickly declines; but though the size of the glands lessens they remain palpable for some time. Convalescence is usually rather slow.

Albuminuria occurs in a certain number of cases. At the outset the disease may be mistaken for a common cold or an attack of influenza, and in countries where dengue prevails, this disease may be diagnosed. Diseases like leukaemia, tuberculous adenitis, and other causes of glandular enlargement, may also create difficulty in recognizing the nature of the complaint. The specific cause of glandular fever has not been recognized except when glands have suppurated, and then a streptococcus has been isolated.

The treatment is that of fever (q.v.) generally. The patient should be isolated for a fortnight, and children who have been in contact with cases should remain away from school for the same period.
See Gland; Mumps.

GLAUBER'S SALT. The sulphate of sodium is also known as Glauber's salt. It acts as a saline cathartic.
See Sodium.

GLAUCOMA. An eye disease in which the eyeball acquires a stony hardness, glaucoma is due to interference with the flow of the aqueous humour into the canal of Schlemm, which lies near the margin of the cornea; the humour accumulates therefore, and the tension inside the eyeball is correspondingly raised. This causes deterioration of the delicate structures within the eye, a notable change being cupping or excavation of the optic disk.

Middle-aged people are mostly affected, and especially women. The disease may come on acutely with severe pain shooting through the head from the eye, which looks inflamed, and the vision of which is much dimmed. The pupil is dilated, and the cornea is dulled as if it had been breathed on. Often there is vomiting, and the condition may be diagnosed as acute dyspepsia. The onset of acute glaucoma may be foreshadowed by a sudden increase in the difficulty in reading small type, dimness of vision and the appearance of coloured halos around lights. This acute attack may pass off, leaving more or less impairment of vision, but other attacks follow.

In chronic glaucoma there is no pain, but the patient seeks advice on account of

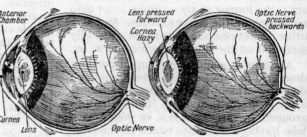

Left, vertical section of normal eye.   Right, changes due to glaucoma

increasing dimness of sight. If the field of vision (q.v.) is investigated, it is found to be contracted. Unless relieved, glaucoma leads to total blindness of the affected eye.

Drugs which contract the pupil lower the intra-ocular tension to some extent, and are indicated in glaucoma. Eserine or physostigmine from the calabar bean (q.v.) is the most powerful of these, but pilocarpine is often used, especially after atropine has been introduced into the eye to dilate the pupil during examination of the eye. There is a risk of atropine precipitating glaucoma, if an eye is predisposed to it, so pilocarpine is used to lessen the risk. Operations are also necessary to cure glaucoma.

There is not the same risk from atropine when used on young people. Glaucoma, however, may occur during the first few years of life, though afterwards and until middle-age it does not occur. Infantile glaucoma leads to the enlargement of the eye known as buphthalmos, or ox-eye.
See Eye.

GLOSSO-PHARYNGEAL NERVE. The 9th cranial, or glosso-pharyngeal, nerve arises partly from nuclei in the medulla, or bulb, of the brain, and partly from cells in ganglia on the nerve trunk itself. Some of the fibres are motor, supplying muscles in the wall of the pharynx, the others being sensory, providing ordinary sensation to the pharynx, tonsil, Eustachian tube, middle ear, and other parts, and taste to the posterior third of the tongue. This nerve leaves the skull along with the vagus or 10th nerve.

GLOTTIS. The upper opening of the larynx, or voice-box, is called the glottis. It is nearly closed when sounds are being produced, but opens up for breathing. The chink, which varies in size, is called the rima glottidis. The space between the ventricular bands, which lie above the vocal cords, is known as the false glottis.

See Larynx.

GLUCOSIDE. In some plants substances known as glucosides occur, some of these being powerful active principles. A glucoside is a body which, when broken up, say by acting on it with an acid, splits into glucose or grape sugar, and another substance. Examples of a glucoside are amygdalin, found in bitter almonds, digitoxin and digitalin, active principles of digitalis, salicin and saponin.

GLUTEUS MUSCLES. There are three large gluteus muscles, the maximus, medius and minimus, which arise from the outer surface of the pelvis, and are inserted into the upper end of the femur, or thigh-bone. The maximus takes a large share in forming the buttock, the fold of the buttock being constituted by the lower border of the muscle. It extends the hip, and conversely raises the body from the stooping position into line with the thigh. The posterior parts of the other two glutei also extend, but their anterior parts flex, the thigh. All the muscles also assist in rotating the thigh.

The superior and inferior gluteal nerves which activate these muscles are branches of the sacral plexus.

The gluteal, or superior gluteal, artery is a large artery which forms the termination of one of the main divisions of the internal iliac or hypogastric, artery. It passes out of the pelvis above and behind the hip-joint, and breaks up into numerous branches. Behind the joint emerges the sciatic artery, which is also called the inferior gluteal artery, and is likewise a branch of the internal iliac. Wounds of the buttock dividing either of these vessels would cause dangerous haemorrhage.

GLYCERIN. A colourless, viscous substance with a sweet taste, glycerin, or glycerol, is produced when fats are broken up; it is a by-product, for example, in soap-making. Chemically it is an alcohol. It is used as a flavouring agent in mixtures and as a substitute for sugar by diabetics. It rapidly absorbs water, and this explains its usefulness for chapping of the hands, the lips, or the nipples, as chapping is caused by excessive dryness of the skin. A useful application for this is glycerin and rose water. If applied to the skin, without dilution, however, glycerin may cause considerable irritation.

Glycerin is added to gargles, as it may keep the drugs contained in these longer in contact with the mucous membrane of the throat. It is a good solvent for iodine and other substances, and so is often used to make a paint for the throat. Pledgets of wool soaked in glycerin are applied to the neck of the womb in order to reduce congestion.

In the British Pharmacopoeia there are a number of preparations consisting of drugs dissolved in this substance and known as the glycerins : glycerin of alum ; of boracic acid, or boro-glyceride ; of borax ; of carbolic acid ; of lead subacetate ; of pepsin ; of starch ; of tannic acid ; and of tragacanth. Glycerin of borax is a better preparation than honey of borax.

GLYCEROPHOSPHATES. Glycerophosphoric acid and its salts were first introduced into medicine because the phosphorus in lecithin, a complex fatty substance found in nervous tissue, blood and elsewhere in the body, is in the form of glycerophosphoric acid, and it was thought that by administering the acid, the nervous and other tissues would be rehabilated after wasting diseases. There is no exact experimental evidence, however, that in this respect glycerophosphoric acid is any better than ordinary phosphoric acid.

Preparations of glycerophosphoric acid are, however, esteemed as tonics, and especially during convalescence from acute diseases. The glycerophosphates of iron and calcium are the most useful salts. The compound glycerol of glycerophosphates B.P.C., the glycerol of glycerophosphates with red bone marrow B.P.C., the yellow syrup of glycerophosphates B.P.C., the compound syrup of glycerophosphates B.P.C., and the syrup of glycerophosphates with formates B.P.C., are used as tonics in doses of 1 to 2 drachms.

A combination of glycerophosphates with casein is found in sanatogen and similar " foods."

GLYCOSURIA. The presence of sugar in the urine is described as glycosuria. As a transient phenomenon this has been found in many different conditions ; when more or less constant it is due to diabetes mellitus. The younger the person in whom glycosuria occurs, the greater the likelihood of its being diabetes.

See Diabetes ; Urine.

GNAT. *See* Mosquito.

GOA POWDER. Araroba, or goa powder, a resinous substance obtained from a Brazilian tree, is the source of chrysarobin, which is extracted from it as a crystalline yellow powder. Purified chrysarobin is usually called chrysophanic acid, though actually the latter substance is chemically somewhat different from chrysarobin. When applied to the skin, chrysarobin has a stimulating action and it is much used in chronic skin diseases, especially psoriasis.

It has to be used with caution, however, as it may cause excessive irritation ; also it has the disadvantage that it causes a deep purple discolouration on the skin and on bed linen. There is an official ointment of chrysarobin.

GOITRE. An enlargement of the thyroid gland is called a goitre or bronchocele. The enlargement may represent what is called a simple goitre, though it

must be understood that in this description are included enlargements in which the microscopical, and even the naked eye, appearances of the gland are different. On the other hand, a goitre may be asso-

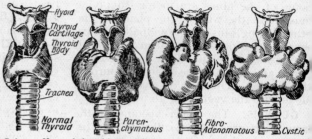

Goitre. Normal thyroid gland (left) and three types of simple goitre

ciated with symptoms of poisoning, as from an overdose of thyroid secretion, a disorder which is described under the heading Exophthalmic Goitre. In a third group the enlargement is caused by a malignant growth.

A simple goitre may be nothing more than hypertrophy of the gland, the normal structure of which is retained (parenchymatous). This type is endemic in many mountainous regions, in parts of the Himalayas and of the Alps, for example ; in Great Britain its prevalence in Derbyshire accounts for its being sometimes called Derbyshire neck. The enlargement as a rule involves the whole gland, that is, both lobes and the intervening isthmus.

Another type of simple goitre, known as the diffuse colloid variety, is especially prevalent in some lowland districts ; this enlargement is also general, but the minute structure differs from the normal. In another type still, the enlargement is localised in a lobe or in the isthmus as a rule ; sometimes swellings occur in more than one of these parts, but the swelling is always irregular, and if not entirely one-sided, is, at any rate, greater at some parts than at others. The swellings may consist of fibrous tissue (fibro-adenomatous) or of cysts containing fluid (cystic).

The enlarged gland in goitre causes a fulness in the neck, more noticeable perhaps when the patient swallows, and in course of time may acquire such dimensions as to cause serious disfigurement. Even when large, however, it may cause no discomfort ; on the other hand, a goitre may press on the windpipe and create a feeling of choking, and this may occur with quite a small goitre. Goitre occurs more frequently in women, and apparently this susceptibility has something to do with other internal secretions, as enlargements of the thyroid may occur at puberty, during pregnancy or lactation, and at the menopause.

The development of a simple goitre has some relation to the supply of iodine to the tissues of the body. The secretion of the thyroid gland contains an organic preparation of iodine, and the most obvious explanation of a simple goitre, certainly of the ordinary hypertrophic type, is that it represents an increased effort to maintain or increase the supply of iodine to the tissues. This might be from a lack of iodine in the diet, or, alternatively, some infection in the body, to combat which an increased flow of thyroid secretion is necessary.

Association with Drinking Water

This infection may be caused by sewage pollution of drinking water, as it has been generally observed that the incidence of goitre seems to be closely connected with drinking water. It has certainly been established that drinking water polluted with the intestinal discharge of persons suffering from goitre has produced swelling of the thyroid gland in man, and definite goitre in lower animals. Another significant fact is that water can be deprived of this unwholesomeness by boiling it.

In districts where goitre is endemic, therefore, all drinking water should be boiled.

Another method of preventing the disease is to give small doses of iodine regularly, say, as iodised common salt or as potassium iodide. The administration of thyroid extract or iodides will also cure the simple goitre in the early stages, but after the condition has lasted for some time, while the further progress of the disorder may be checked, it is very unlikely that the swelling can be entirely removed, or in old-standing cases be materially reduced at all. It is necessary, especially when the goitre occurs away from an endemic centre, that sources of poisoning in the patient's own body, such as septic teeth or tonsils, for example, should be thoroughly cleaned up.

When the goitre is interfering with breathing an operation is needed, and surgical treatment may also be adopted when there is much disfigurement.

A malignant goitre may be either a sarcoma or a carcinoma, but is more frequently the latter ; an early removal by an operation is necessary.

See Cretinism ; Endocrine ; Exophthalmic Goitre ; Thyroid Gland.

GONORRHOEA. A contagious disease, gonorrhoea is caused by a microbe called the gonococcus, and is most commonly contracted from sexual intercourse with an infected person, though a large number of infants have their eyes infected during birth because of infection existing in the mother. In a certain number of cases infection is due to contact with privy seats, clothing, towels, etc., which are polluted with gonorrhoeal discharges.

The period of incubation, that is, the time elapsing between exposure to infection and the first appearance of symptoms, is from three to twenty-one days, the average being five days. In the male there is first of all a burning pain in the urethra when passing water, which is quickly followed by a discharge, thin and clear to begin with, but shortly becoming thick, and whitish or yellow from the presence of pus, or matter.

There is usually feverishness, loss of appetite and constipation. Under proper treatment, and should no complications occur, the discharge gradually diminishes, and generally disappears in the course of four to six weeks, but if complications occur, treatment may have to be continued for many months. Sometimes in the course of the attack a painful erection of the penis, described as chordee, occurs, more particularly when the patient is warm in bed.

If the foreskin is long, and especially if it is at all tight, there may be an accumulation of pus beneath it requiring an incision for its release. Occasionally also infection passes through the lining membrane of the urethra and causes an abscess which bursts outwardly, thereby establishing a fistulous opening from the urethra.

The complications which delay a cure, however, are those due to extension backwards of the infection or its extension into the blood stream. The disease may reach the bladder, causing cystitis, the occurrence of which is signalised by frequent and urgent calls to pass water although there is but little to pass. From the bladder the infection may pass upwards to the pelvis of the kidney and the substance of this organ itself, resulting in pyelonephritis. Inflammation of the prostate gland at the neck of the bladder may also occur.

Another route along which the infection may proceed is to the seminal vesicles and the testicle, inflammation of the epididymis (*q.v.*) taking place, and the testicle becoming swollen and very painful.

Inflammatory Complications that Ensue

Invasion of the blood stream with gonococci constitutes a form of septicaemia, and, as in other forms of this blood poisoning, inflammation of various organs and tissues may result ; for example, of the lining of the heart, of the pleura, of the lungs or of joints. The last-mentioned complication is usually referred to as gonorrhoeal rheumatism, and its cure may be difficult and tedious. One or more of the joints becomes swollen, reddened, hot and very painful and tender. Besides the joints, tendon sheaths and fasciae may be affected, and flat foot may result from the involvement of such structures in the sole of the foot, unless complete rest is taken from the onset of pain there.

If gonorrhoea settles down into a chronic condition there may be little or no discomfort, but the persistence of mischief in the urinary passages is shown by the appearance of a drop of discharge, particularly first thing in the morning, and the urine commonly contains so-called threads, caused by chronic prostatitis. Chronic gonorrhoea is often referred to as gleet. So long as this condition persists the patient is capable of communicating the disease. A possible sequel to an attack of gonorrhoea is a stricture (*q.v.*) of the urethra.

The treatment of gonorrhoea should invariably be supervised by a doctor. There are many free clinics scattered over the country for those whose means are limited. A person affected with the disease should exercise the greatest care against conveying the infection to others or to his own eyes. He should not use a common towel, and should use sufficient cotton wool or clean rags, preferably in a rubber bag, say a sponge-bag, to absorb the discharge, the cotton wool or rags being afterwards burned. It is desirable also to wear a suspensory bandage.

A solution of permanganate of potassium, say 1 grain in 8 ounces of water, should be used as a lotion for cleansing the parts, and would also make a suitable injection for the urethra. This injection is made several times a day after the bladder has been emptied, a small glass syringe with a blunt nozzle being used for the purpose. A common mistake is to have a urethral injection too strong and thereby cause additional irritation. Some drugs for internal use have a reputation for usefulness in this disease, such as oil of sandalwood, cubebs and copaiba, though, as a rule, only the first mentioned is suitable for the very acute stage. Sometimes vaccines are very helpful.

Dietetic Rules to be Observed

A laxative should be taken if there is any constipation, as it is important that the bowels should move every day. The diet should be light and bland during the acute stage ; alcohol and condiments should be avoided. Water, diluted milk or barley water should be taken freely, and it is an advantage to add a pinch of baking soda to the draught. Clothing should be sufficiently plentiful and warm to secure the body from chill. Treatment should be continued conscientiously until, in the opinion of the doctor, the disease is eradicated.

No man who has suffered from gonorrhoea should marry before submitting himself to special tests of his freedom from the disease. These are applied by an expert, if necessary at a clinic.

In the female the disease also invades the urinary passages and may extend to the bladder and kidneys, but it is usually the genital passages that bear the brunt of the disease. There may not be much pain, but there is a thick yellow discharge from the vagina or front passage. The infection may extend to the womb, the Fallopian tubes and the ovaries.

PLATE XIX

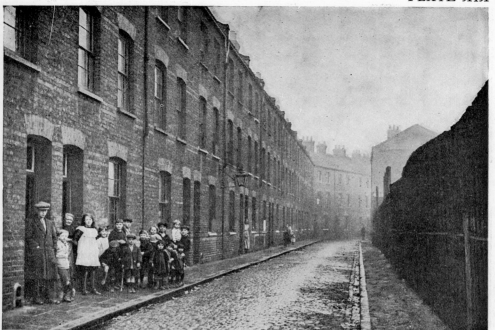

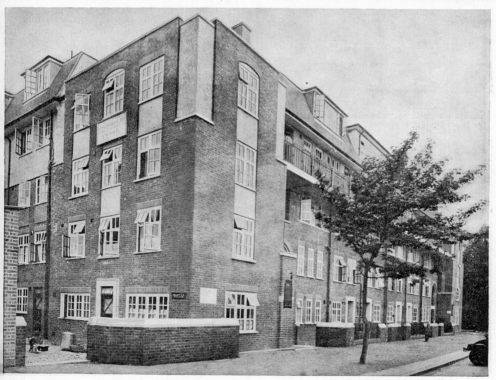

Housing. Above, back-to-back houses in a Bethnal Green slum. Here overcrowding, insanitary conditions, discomfort and ugliness are the source of much ill health. Below, Crosfield House, opened in 1929, the first block of tenements built by the Kensington Housing Trust to relieve working-class overcrowding in that area. It comprises 36 admirably planned flats and maisonnettes, let at rentals of 10s. to 18s. 6d. a week

PLATE XX

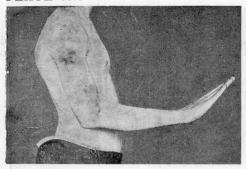

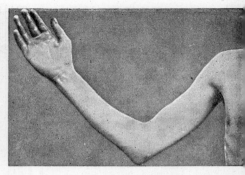

Joint : best positions when ankylosis threatens. 1. Should the wrist joint become ankylosed, the grasp is strongest when the hand is bent slightly backward. 2. When the elbow is ankylosed, the most useful position is with the forearm making an angle of 110° with the upper arm, the thumb pointing upwards

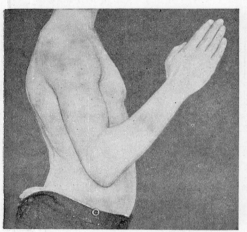

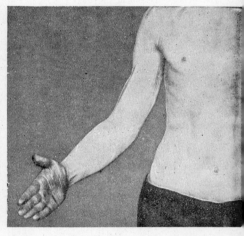

3. If both elbows are ankylosed, one arm can be fixed as shown above in 2, while in the other the forearm makes an angle of 70° with the upper arm. This is the better position for the patient to feed himself. 4. If a shoulder becomes fixed, the arm should be raised so that it forms an angle of 50° with the vertical

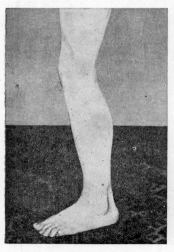

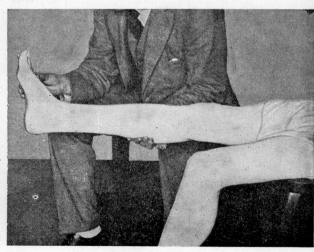

5. The most useful position for an ankylosed knee is with a slight bend, as the patient is able to sit more comfortably than with a straight leg. 6. An ankylosed ankle should be fixed with the foot making a right angle with the leg at the ankle joint. The necessity for a surgical boot will then be avoided

To face page 345

Sometimes the tubes are distended with pus, and always there is likely to be some local peritonitis, which leaves adhesions in its train. Disturbance of menstruation is a frequent result, and also sterility. Medical supervision of treatment is again necessary. Douching with permanganate solution helps towards cleanliness, but more energetic measures are necessary.

Infection of the eyes occurring in infants is discussed under the heading Conjunctivitis. Besides the risk from an infected mother, it should be borne in mind that anyone might have the eyes infected, say, from a towel soiled with discharge.

This disease involves a grave threat to vision, and must be carefully and thoroughly treated.

When one eye only is affected it is customary to try to protect the other by applying what is called Buller's shield ; this is an ordinary watch-glass, kept in position over the eye by strips of adhesive plaster, which are continuous all round the glass.

See Conjunctivitis ; Prostate.

GOULARD'S EXTRACT. The strong solution of lead subacetate is also called Goulard's extract. From it is prepared, by the addition of spirit and dilution with distilled water, the diluted solution, or Goulard's water or lotion, the usual constituent of a lead lotion. The following is very useful for painting on patches of inflammation on the skin, especially when there is intense itching : Goulard's extract, liquor carbonis detergens, and rectified spirit, ½ ounce of each.

See Lead.

GOUT. Also known as podagra, gout is a disorder of metabolism in which uric acid accumulates in the blood and tissues and causes various kinds of manifestations. It may be the short, sharp attacks at long intervals of acute disease, the less sharp but more frequent and prolonged attacks of the chronic disease, critical attacks of disorder of the stomach, heart, brain or lungs in what is called retrocedent or metastatic gout, or the more vague disturbance of many functions and tissues of irregular gout.

The tendency to gout is often inherited and may be transmitted through females who show no signs of the disease themselves. Other causes are an excessive consumption of rich food and of wines, especially champagne, burgundy and port, or of malt liquors. A regular and copious consumption of malt liquor, even when the food supply is spare, results in what is called poor man's gout. Lead poisoning appears also to have a strong influence, though probably only when the other causes mentioned are also at work. Sedentary habits predispose, especially in conjunction with other causes. Women are rarely affected except after the change of life, and not very often even then.

Disease Due to Uric Acid

An acute attack of gout, not so frequent an event as it once was, is due to the deposition of crystals of biurate of sodium in the cartilages of a joint. Normally this is present in the blood and tissue fluids, probably in a colloidal form, and something happens in gout to throw it out of this into a flocculated state. The occurrence is considered to resemble what occurs in anaphylaxis (*q.v.*). A poor circulation in the part, some slight injury or something similar may be the exciting factor, but the excess of uric acid in the blood and tissues, which is the essential feature of gout, alone makes the attack possible.

Prior to an attack there may be irritability of temper, dyspepsia and other premonitory symptoms. Then, suddenly, in the small hours of the morning, a joint, which in a first attack is most often that of the ball of the right great toe, is seized with excruciating pain and becomes swollen, red and hot, while the patient becomes fevered. The pain generally eases off in the course of a few hours, but recurs on the following and several succeeding nights, though with lessening intensity. Another attack may not occur for about a year, or there may be three or four attacks in the year.

The painful joint should be treated by heat in some form ; cold applications are dangerous. The best drug for relieving the pain is colchicum, either the wine or the tincture, in doses of 20 to 30 minims every four hours, until the pain ceases ; but colchicum should only be used on medical advice, as it may cause depression.

Water or gruel containing potassium bicarbonate should be drunk freely. On the night of the attack it is well to take a mercurial purge, say 3 or 4 grains of calomel and follow this up with a dose of Epsom salt in the morning. The diet should be restricted to milk and barley water unless other directions are given.

In retrocedent, or metastatic, gout, the local symptoms may disappear, but the patient is suddenly seized with severe pain in the abdomen, vomiting, diarrhoea and collapse; or with severe pain over the heart, palpitation and shortness of breath; or with alarming asthmatic symptoms; or with symptoms pointing to derangement of the nervous system, such as delirium, coma or an apoplectic attack.

In chronic gout more joints are affected and there is a greater tendency to deposits in the soft parts about the joints and elsewhere, such deposits, or tophi, sometimes ulcerating through the skin, so that a person whose finger joints were affected has been able to write with them on a blackboard. Because of their white, chalky appearance, these deposits are sometimes called chalk-stones; they do not, however, consist of chalk but of sodium urate. The external ear is a common site for a tophus. In a tophus there may also be present the substance known as cholesterol, which in gout is present in excess in the blood.

In chronic gout there is a tendency to arterio-sclerosis (*q.v.*) with enlargement of the left side of the heart and chronic nephritis. The patient often has a sallow complexion and suffers from dyspepsia.

The manifestations of irregular gout are very varied. Biliousness, arterial disease, migraine, hot, itching eyeballs, eczema, urinary gravel, glycosuria, chronic bronchitis, iritis or some other disorder may be found to depend on the gouty habit. Glycosuria, or gouty diabetes, is usually easily controlled by dieting.

A person who is of the gouty habit, or, as it is also put, is subject to the gouty

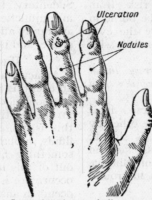

Gouty deposits, or chalk-stones, ulcerating through the skin

diathesis, should be moderate in eating, avoiding fats and rich food, meat extracts, sauces, liver, kidney and sweetbreads, and restricting red meat, starchy foods and sugar.

Fresh fruit and vegetables may be taken, but, as a rule, tomatoes, cucumber, rhubarb, bananas, gooseberries, currants and strawberries are unsuitable. Potatoes may generally be allowed. Asparagus and beans and other pulses should be taken in small quantities only. Alcohol is best avoided altogether, but if any is taken it should be in the form of spirits, claret or hock, in moderate quantities and freely diluted. Sparkling cider may be harmful, though dry, still cider is usually safe. Water should be taken freely.

An active open-air life should be adopted. Clothing should be warm and the skin should be kept active by regular baths and brisk friction with a towel.

When attacks have occurred, or there are manifestations of irregular gout, it may be worth while to have spa treatment, at Bath, Buxton, Harrogate, Aix-les-Bains, Contrexéville, Karlsbad, Homburg or elsewhere.

See Arterio-sclerosis; Colchicum; Diet; Metabolism; Purin.

GRAFT. A piece of living tissue is sometimes taken from some part of the body and transplanted as a graft on another part, to make good a deficiency resulting from injury or disease. When a considerable area of the body is denuded of skin, say, after a burn or other injury, or resulting from ulceration, the prospect of an unduly protracted and troublesome period of healing, or the risk, when certain situations are concerned, of deformity and disablement from undue contraction of ordinary scar tissue, will often raise the question of skin grafting.

Skin grafts may consist of small fragments snipped off with scissors from the superficial layers of the skin, which are planted here and there over the surface to be covered, each forming, as it were, a little islet from which epithelial cells grow out in all directions. Sometimes a large, thin sheet is shaved off the skin. This is known as Thiersch's method and is often used. The line of separation of the graft is calculated to pass through the tops of the papillae of the true skin and no deeper. This leaves sufficient epithelial cells to grow and cover over the surface from which the graft is taken. The third kind of graft consists of the whole thickness of the skin, and is very liable to fail unless the graft is left partly in contact with the part from which it is taken until it has received a supply of new blood vessels.

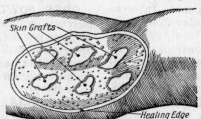

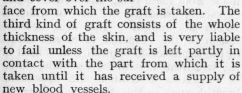

Graft. Rapid repair with small skin grafts

Bone grafts have been of much use in connecting the ends of a broken bone and preserving a correct alignment, particularly when, from extensive destruction of the bone, a considerable gap has been left between the ends. The whole of the graft may be absorbed by phagocytes, however, though replaced by new bone, and almost always a bone graft, even although not absorbed in this way, acts rather as a scaffolding on which new bone can be formed than as a permanent replacement of the missing bone. Cartilage grafts have been used in correcting deformities of the nose.

Muscle grafts are sometimes used to fill up cavities left in bones by injury or disease, but the muscle can only survive if left partly attached to its normal connexions. Tendons are sometimes divided, and the end attached to the muscle is sutured to some other bone when the muscle which normally moves this bone is paralysed ; or the lower end of a divided tendon may be attached to bone above a joint, forming a rigid cord across the joint and thus anchoring it.

Nerve grafts have been used to bridge a gap in a divided nerve. Glands are sometimes grafted, for example, thyroid gland in myxoedema and other instances of thyroid defect. Grafting of the testicle of a higher ape into man has been vaunted as a remedy of senility. Undoubtedly some benefit may accrue from this, but it is not likely to be more than transitory, as the engrafted gland is sufficiently foreign to the human body to be attacked by phagocytes and replaced by fibrous tissue.

Any chance of success in a grafting operation of any kind will be much imperilled if septic organisms obtain any footing in the graft.

GRANULATION TISSUE. Almost invariably a wound is healed by the formation of granulation tissue, which consists of large, round cells derived from the connective tissue in the neighbourhood of the wound. First a mass or layer of these cells is produced, and then vascular loops bud off from adjacent capillaries and thread their way in amongst the cells until the whole mass is freely supplied with blood vessels. The tissue presents a granular surface of a fresh, pink colour and bleeds easily.

Granulation tissue also covers ulcers, lines abscess cavities and sinuses, and forms around foreign bodies embedded in the tissues. Sometimes there is an overgrowth of granulation tissue ; it is then said to be exuberant, or, in popular phraseology, constitutes proud flesh. On

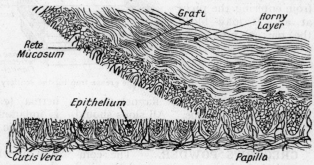

Line of section when removing a piece of skin for grafting elsewhere

the other hand, as in a callous ulcer, the granulations may be pale and watery-looking. If healing proceeds, the round cells become elongated and ultimately form fibrous, or scar, tissue.

A granuloma is a tumour composed of granulation tissue and occurs in tuberculosis, yaws, syphilis and other diseases.

See Caries ; Inflammation ; Proud Flesh ; Scar.

GRAPE CURE. At Montreux, Vevey, Interlaken and other resorts what is called the grape cure is taken for chronic constipation, corpulence, chronic bronchitis and other disorders. The cure consists in taking each day from 1 to 8 pounds of grapes freed from skins and stones. This treatment, when carried out at home, does not achieve the success which it sometimes has at a resort.

GRAVEL. A sandy deposit of uric acid, oxalates, phosphates or other substances in the urine is described as gravel. This may happen for many years without giving rise to symptoms, but, on the other hand, there may be pain and straining after micturition and other signs of irritation of the bladder and passages. The exact nature of the gravel may be determined by microscopic examination and other tests, and dietetic and medicinal treatment be adopted according to the result. The deposits which come down when the urine is allowed to stand and cool must be distinguished from gravel.

See Calculus ; Uric Acid ; Urine.

GREASE TRAP. Drain pipes are provided with traps for grease and other solid and semi-solid substances, but it is important to prevent, as far as possible, grease from entering the pipes at all. It may block the narrow pipe from a sink and also may decompose and become offensive. A simple trap may be made by stretching a piece of flannel over a shallow wooden frame. All slops should be poured through this.

See Drains.

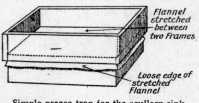

Flannel stretched between two Frames

Loose edge of stretched Flannel

Simple grease trap for the scullery sink

GREGORY'S POWDER. The compound rhubarb powder, commonly called Gregory's powder, contains light or heavy magnesia and ginger, in addition to rhubarb. It is used as a purgative in doses of 10 to 60 grains or 5 grains for a young child. It may be given in milk A tiny pinch three times a day before meals acts as a stomachic.

GREY POWDER. The powder of mercury and chalk is usually referred to as grey powder. A dose of 1 grain is often useful in diarrhoea in young children Grey powder has been extensively used in syphilis, 1 grain three or four times daily

See Mercury.

GRINDELIA. The dried leaves and flowering tops of grindelia camporum are used in medicine, among the preparations made from them being the official liquid extract of grindelia, the dose of which is 10 to 20 minims The drug relieves spasm of the bronchial tubes and assists in the expulsion of sputum, and is used in the treatment of asthma, whooping-cough or bronchitis associated with spasmodic breathlessness. The powdered drug is included in some asthma cigarettes.

GRIPES. *See* Colic ; Flatulence ; Intussusception.

GROIN. The meeting place of the abdominal wall and the front of the thigh is called the groin. In very stout people and in infants the skin of the groin may become inflamed and tender, owing to the decomposition of imprisoned sweat or the rubbing of the folds of skin-covered fat on one another. To prevent this, daily washing of the part is needed, possibly followed by some bland powder.

The femoral vessels pass down into the thigh about the middle of the groin, and wounds here are accordingly very dangerous. The arrest of bleeding from the femoral artery is described under the heading Bleeding.

A lump in the groin may be a rupture or hernia (*q.v.*). Another common cause is inflammation and enlargement of the lymphatic glands, which is described as a bubo. This may be due to a septic sore anywhere on the leg or foot or about the genitals or perineum. The inflammation may go on to abscess formation, but not from a purely syphilitic sore. Amongst other, and less common, causes of a lump in the groin are enlargement of the glands, known as lymphadenoma or Hodgkin's disease, pointing of a psoas abscess, and a hydrocele or tumour of the spermatic cord.

See Femoral Vessels : Iliac Region ; Poupart's Ligament.

GROWING PAINS. The ordinary process of growth causes no pain, and what are called growing pains are really manifestations of acute rheumatism and should be treated as such. If neglected, serious implication of the heart may result.

See Rheumatism.

GROWTH. At birth a child is usually about 20 inches long, and weighs about 7 pounds. This weight, which is doubled in 6 months, is trebled in 12, while the height has increased to about 28 inches. Thereafter growth is not so rapid, but by the end of the fifth year the original height at birth has been doubled, and by the end of the fourteenth it is about eleven-twelfths of the total to which the individual will attain. In the few years preceding puberty girls grow more rapidly than boys, but from about fourteen onwards boys make greater headway.

The height attainable by an individual is more or less fixed for him by his inheritance ; he is not likely to be tall if he belongs to a short family, and vice versa. On the other hand, if the father is unusually tall for his family it has been noted that his progeny tend to be shorter, that is to say, nearer the average for the family, and if unusually short the progeny tend to be rather taller than he is, again also approaching the average.

In the mechanism of growth the thyroid and pituitary glands take a prominent part. Thyroid insufficiency produces a shorter growth, while an increase in the contribution of the anterior lobe of the pituitary during the growing periods leads to giantism. Normal growth is dependent on a sufficient supply of food containing a requisite amount of vitamins, and on free exercise in the open air, though confinement in bed for some time may cause a young person to grow rapidly.

Life in the poverty-stricken areas of towns usually has the effect of stunting growth, though in many instances this may be due to rickets. Congenital syphilis and infantile diseases that interfere with digestion and assimilation tend to cause stunting. In some instances dwarfism is associated with kidney disorder.

In the following table the average height and weight in each sex at different ages are stated.

AGE LAST BIRTHDAY IN YEARS	MALE		FEMALE	
	Height	Weight	Height	Weight
	ft. in.	st. lb.	ft. in.	st. lb.
1	2 5½	1 4½	2 3½	1 4
2	2 8½	2 4½	2 7	1 11
3	2 11	2 6	2 10	2 3
4	3 1	2 9	3 0	2 8
5	3 4	2 12	3 3	2 1
6	3 7	3 2½	3 6	3 0
7	3 10	3 8	3 8	3 5
8	3 11	3 13	3 10	3 10
9	4 2	4 4	4 0	4 0
10	4 4	4 11	4 3	4 6
11	4 5	5 2	4 5	4 12
12	4 7	5 7	4 7½	5 6
13	4 9	5 12	4 10	6 3
14	4 11	6 8	5 0	6 13
15	5 2	7 5	5 1	7 8
16	5 4	8 7	5 2	8 1
17	5 6	9 5	5 2½	8 2½
18	5 7	9 12	5 2½	8 3½
19	5 7½	10 0	5 3	8 9
20	5 7½	10 3	5 3½	8 12
21	5 7½	10 5	5 3½	9 0

The term growth is often applied to a tumour (*q.v.*).

See Baby; Child; Constitution; Diet; Exercise; Heredity; Infantilism; Vitamin.

GUAIACOL. A colourless liquid which forms the active constituent of creosote, guaiacol was introduced as a remedy for consumption, and is often successful in relieving the cough, sweating, loss of appetite and other symptoms of this disease. It does not irritate the stomach so much as creosote. It is best given in capsules, but may be given in cod-liver oil, in a mixture or in pills ; it is sometimes used by inhalation. The dose is 1 to 5 minims.

Guaiacol carbonate is a white, tasteless powder with a dose of 5 to 15 grains. It may be used for consumption instead of guaiacol, and is generally the most useful drug for treating rheumatoid arthritis. For this complaint it is given in 10-grain doses in cachets three times a day for many months. There are several other compounds of guaiacol, some of them having trade names, all of which have similar uses to guaiacol.

See Creosote.

GUAIACUM. The heart-wood of two species of guaiacum trees, sometimes referred to as lignum vitae, or wood of life, and the resin of these trees, are both used in medicine, more particularly the resin. This is powdered, and given in doses of 5 to 15 grains. From it are prepared the official mixture of guaiacum, dose ½ to 1 ounce : ammoniated tincture, ½ to 1 drachm ; lozenges, containing 3 grains each ; and several unofficial preparations.

Guaiacum is an old remedy for chronic rheumatism and similar complaints, and is a constituent of the so-called " Chelsea pensioner " which can be asked for as the compound confection of guaiacum, B.P.C., and contains, in addition to guaiacum, sulphur, rhubarb and other drugs, the dose being a teaspoonful. Guaiacum may be taken for chronic pharyngitis, and the lozenges afford a convenient form of the drug for this purpose. Even in acute sore throat guaiacum may be beneficial, and one way of using it is to take a drachm of the ammoniated tincture in hot milk every two hours until there is slight looseness of the bowels.

Painful menstruation, or dysmenorrhoea (*q.v.*), may be prevented or relieved by the powdered resin, in 10-grain doses in cachets, or a corresponding dose of one of the liquid preparations, three times a day. The course of the drug should be begun seven to ten days before the period is expected.

GUINEA-WORM. On the Guinea coast of Africa and elsewhere in the tropics a parasitic roundworm, known as the guinea-worm, and scientifically as dracunculus or filaria medinensis, may infest human beings, such infestation being described as dracontiasis. The female worm, which is a slender creature from about 20 to 36 inches long, lies beneath the skin or between muscles, usually in the leg or foot, and bores a hole in the skin through which she discharges the embryos in a milky-looking fluid whenever water comes into contact with the skin.

If the embryos are discharged into a pool of water and find some species of minute crustacean—a cyclops—there, they enter its body and grow somewhat. If some of this water containing cyclops is ingested by a human being, the cyclops is killed by the gastric juice, but the embryos emerge in an active condition and mate. The female then bores her way through the tissues to the skin, her course being marked by heat and irritation, perhaps by pain and swelling, and lasting some months. On that part of the skin where the head bores the opening, a blister forms, and when this bursts embryos can be discharged.

When such an opening has been found, cold douches should be applied to the part each day for a fortnight, or until the worm has discharged all her embryos and begins to emerge. The exit of the worm is expedited by rolling up the free part on a match or quill each day. Premature or ungentle manipulation of the worm may tear it, an accident which may readily be followed by inflammation and perhaps an abscess. A doctor can hasten the cure by killing the worm by injecting into it a solution of perchloride of mercury, and then pulling it out.

See Filaria ; Worm.

GULLET. A muscular tube, lined with mucous membrane, and about 10 inches long, the gullet or oesophagus connects the lower end of the pharynx and the cardiac end of the stomach. It begins just behind the larynx and passes down the neck and thorax, piercing the diaphragm to join the stomach. It lies in front of the spine, in the middle line above but inclining towards the left below. In front of it in the neck is the windpipe, and on either side the great vessels and the vagus nerve ; in the thorax it lies behind the heart.

When empty the gullet is flattened from before backwards. Solid food passes down it by peristaltic movements, but liquids may be shot down quickly with little movement of the walls of the tube. Narrowing of the gullet, with resulting difficulty in swallowing, or dysphagia, may be brought about in various ways. It may be by a foreign body, by the contraction of scars following damage to the gullet from corrosive substances, by the presence of a cancerous tumour, by spasm at the lower end of the gullet, a condition called cardio-spasm, or by pressure from the outside, say, of a goitre or an aneurysm of the aorta.

With cardio-spasm, the lower end of the gullet becomes dilated, and food accumulates there. Sometimes there exists a blind canal or diverticulum, opening into the gullet, within which food may gather and decompose.

The investigation of the condition of the gullet, when necessary, is much assisted by the use of the oesophagoscope, a tube which can be lighted up and with which direct vision may be obtained of the state of the walls of the gullet and of any foreign body lying in it. Through this tube, also, it is possible to remove foreign bodies by the use of special forceps. The patency of the gullet and the position of any obstruction can be tested by passing thick round or oval rods, or bougies, down it. X-ray examination is also extremely useful.

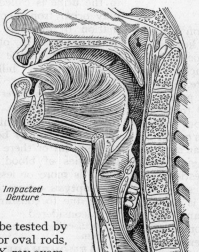

Impacted Denture

Gullet obstructed by a swallowed denture

An instrument for passing down the gullet and drawing out foreign bodies is called a probang (*q.v.*). It is sometimes necessary, however, in order to get the foreign body out, for example, a denture fixed by its hooks, to open into the gullet from the neck, an operation called oesophagotomy. When the obstruction is due to a malignant growth, operation is seldom feasible.

See Digestion ; Larynx ; Swallowing.

GUM. The dense mucous membrane covering the alveolar margin of the jaws and rising up to surround the roots of the teeth, is called the gum, or gingiva. Inflammation of the gum, or gingivitis, may be localised, as in the neighbourhood of a septic tooth, or occur as part of a general inflammation of the mouth, or stomatitis.

The most important disease of the gums from its frequency and its malign influence on the general health, is pyorrhoea ; here pockets filled with pus are found in the gum surrounding the roots of the teeth.

The gums may be caused to bleed by the too vigorous use of a stiff toothbrush, but in scurvy and in mercurial poisoning they become soft and spongy, bleeding at the slightest touch. Sometimes there is an overgrowth of the gum, especially in children, and around carious teeth. This is treated by snipping off redundant tissue.

A fibrous tumour, known as a simple epulis, sometimes grows on the gum, or a myeloid sarcoma, which is called a malignant epulis. A common occurrence is a deep-seated inflammation and suppuration in the gum—an alveolar abscess or gum-boil ; this is discussed under the heading Alveolus.

See Epulis ; Mouth ; Pyorrhoea ; Tooth.

GUM. The juice exuded by certain trees and shrubs and which is chemically related to starch and cellulose, is called a gum. When it dries the juice becomes sticky and then hardens, but may be dissolved in water or form a jelly. The gums mostly used in medicine are gum acacia and gum tragacanth (*q.v.*). Indian gum is often used in the East in place of gum acacia. The latter, also known as gum arabic, occurs as colourless beads or yellowish fragments. Gum tragacanth occurs as whitish flakes. There is an official mucilage of acacia and one of tragacanth, also a glycerin of tragacanth and the compound powder of tragacanth.

These gums are used for suspending heavy powders in mixtures or external applications, except that acacia is not very suitable for suspending bismuth carbonate. Gums are also used for emulsifying fats and oils. Solutions of the gums are sometimes used as demulcents.

A solution of acacia with common salt, when injected into the blood, raises the blood pressure, and may be useful in shock and after a severe bleeding.

Gum benjamin is another name for benzoin (*q.v.*).

See Resin.

GUM RASH. *See* Nettle-rash ; Prickly Heat.

HAEMATEMESIS. The vomiting of blood is technically called haematemesis. The blood may have a natural appearance or, when it has lain in the stomach for some time, be brown—" coffee-ground " vomit. When blood has been brought up it is important to determine whether it comes from the lungs or from the stomach.

See Bleeding ; Haemoptysis.

HAEMATOCELE. A collection of blood in the pouch of Douglas, which lies behind the womb, is called a haematocele. The usual cause is rupture of the sac in extra-uterine pregnancy. There are signs of internal bleeding, pallor, rapid pulse, and so on. If the blood is allowed to remain it may be absorbed in time, but there is considerable risk of suppuration occurring.

In the male a haematocele is an accumulation of blood in the tunica vaginalis, the smooth bag surrounding the testicle, and the usual cause is an injury, such as a kick or a stab. The scrotum is elevated by a bandage or by a cushion and cooling lotions are applied. If tension is great some of the blood may be removed by tapping. As a rule the blood is satisfactorily absorbed.

HAEMATOMA. A swelling caused by a collection of blood is called a haematoma and may occur in different parts, as under the skin, in the cellular tissue of the female pelvis or within the skull. One under the skin may be caused by pressure, as on the face of a new-born child, or by a blow. At first a soft, or at any rate a fluctuant, swelling, it becomes harder when the blood clots. The clot may occupy the margin of the swelling, leaving a soft part in the centre, and on the scalp this condition may feel very like a depressed fracture of the underlying bone.

If suppuration does not take place the blood is generally absorbed, but thickening may persist for a long time, perhaps indefinitely. Bleeding may be lessened and pain relieved by cold applications, but such must be used with caution on old or weakly persons or the skin may be killed.

See Haematocele.

HAEMATURIA. The passing of blood in the urine is called haematuria. This may occur from nephritis, stone, inflammation or growths in the bladder and other causes. In older people a malignant growth in the bladder is suggested. In the tropics bilharziasis (*q.v.*) is a common cause.

See Blackwater Fever ; Urine.

HAEMOPTYSIS. The coughing up of blood is known technically as haemoptysis. There may simply be streaks or spots in the sputum or there may be considerable quantities of blood, in which case the blood is more or less frothy. Whenever haemoptysis occurs the possibility of its being due to consumption must be carefully considered.

See Bleeding ; Consumption ; Haematemesis ; Sputum.

HAEMORRHAGE. *See* Bleeding.

HAEMORRHOID. *See* Piles.

HAIR. At birth the whole body is covered with delicate little lanugo hairs. These soon disappear, however, and are replaced by ordinary hairs in situations mostly determined by the activity of the sex glands.

A hair grows from a little pit, or follicle, in the skin, at the bottom of which is a little rounded elevation, supplied with blood vessels and nerves, on which the hair rears itself. The part of the hair within the follicle is called the root. A hair is a solid structure, contrary to the opinion of the barber, who suggests singeing as a means of closing the

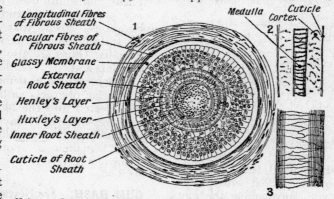

Hair. 1, Cross section of hair follicle, the innermost circle being the hair. 2, Longitudinal section of a hair. 3, Outer surface of a hair

Longitudinal Fibres of Fibrous Sheath 1
Circular Fibres of Fibrous Sheath
Glassy Membrane
External Root Sheath
Henley's Layer
Huxley's Layer
Inner Root Sheath
Cuticle of Root Sheath

Medulla *Cuticle* *Cortex* 2

3

ends of "the tubes" opened by cutting the hair.

Into the follicle is poured the oily secretion of one or more sebaceous glands to keep the hair soft and supple. Colour in hair is due to the presence of pigment cells. Attached to the follicle are tiny muscles, arrectores pilorum, which erect the follicle and with it the hair, a mechanism which also accounts for gooseskin. A hair grows about half an inch in a month, and is estimated to have an average life of 1,600 days.

Alopecia, or baldness (q.v.), may be due to various causes,

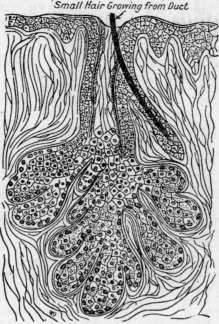

Small Hair Growing from Duct

Hair. Sebaceous gland that opens into the follicle and lubricates the hair

the most common being seborrhoea, which is also the cause of dandruff (q.v.). Hirsuties, or excessive growth of hair, may be disfiguring, and is treated by some form of depilatory (q.v.). Greyness of the hair is a usual result of advancing years, and is then due to atrophy of the pigment cells. This may occur also from general debility occasioned by an acute illness, anaemia, worry, and so on. Sudden blanching of the hair, which may occur from nervous shock, is due to the accumulation of immense numbers of air bubbles in individual hairs.

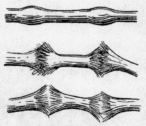

Trichorrhexis nodosa, an atrophic disease of the hair

When greyness of the hair is due to debility, or to local conditions like seborrhoea, benefit may come from treatment which removes or lessens the underlying cause of the greyness. Stimulation of the scalp by light treatment, by electrical methods or by lotions containing pilocarpine, or other drugs which may stimulate the hair follicles, may also be useful. For dyeing the hair, solutions of permanganate of potassium and henna preparations are relatively safe, but those containing paraphenylene-diamene or metallic salts may give rise to severe dermatitis of the scalp, or otherwise cause annoyance. Dyed hair has a diminished lustre.

Beaded hair, or monilithrix, is a rare disorder in which spindle-shape swellings occur on the hairs at regular intervals from the root to the tip, a hair becoming very brittle in the intervals between the swellings. Most cases of the kind are congenital, but some are due to acute illness. Local stimulation of the scalp is the treatment.

In another disorder, trichorrhexis nodosa, at irregular intervals along the hairs whitish bead-like swellings occur, which, when magnified, are seen to be due to the hair breaking up into small fibres, the appearance being described as like that of two brushes put end to end. The hair on the face is usually affected, but the disease may also occur on the scalp in either sex. Various causes have been suggested, such as bacteria, general debility, and roughness in dressing the hair. Treatment depends upon the cause. It will probably be of use to keep the affected part shaved for a time.

See Baldness; Electrolysis; Favus; Ringworm; Scalp; Sebaceous Gland.

HALLUCINATION. A sensory impression for which there is no basis is called a hallucination. This may occur in the field of any sense, sight, hearing, smell, taste, or touch. An illusion differs in having some foundation for the experience. Thus, to mistake a tree-stump for a man is an illusion, but to see a man when there is nothing whatever to suggest one is a hallucination. The vision of rats and snakes is a well-known hallucination in alcoholic delirium, and the hearing of voices in the mental disorder called paranoia.

See Mental Disease.

HALLUX VALGUS. A line prolonged forwards from the inner border of the heel ought to lie along the inner border of the great toe. Commonly, however, the toe is pushed away from this line towards the outer side of the foot, a deformity described as hallux valgus. With a sufficient degree of the deformity the second toe may come to lie either upon or

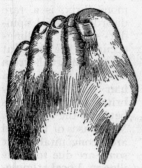

Hallux Valgus. Displacement of the great toe causing a bunion

under the great toe. The main cause of hallux valgus is the boot or shoe with the pointed toe, as such is ordinarily constructed. Once the toe begins to be pushed out by the boot the tendons which move it tend to increase the deformity.

The head of the metatarsal bone on which the great toe is jointed is thus exposed to pressure and to minimise this a bursa, or bag with a smooth lining, develops on the inner side of the joint. Inflammation of this bag constitutes a bunion. The onset of hallux valgus ought to be prevented by fitting children with a shoe which has a straight inner border. Should an outward direction of the toe have been assumed, a suitable pad may be placed between the great toe and the next, so as to force the great toe inwards, or, in worse cases, a post may be fitted into the boot. If, however, the deformity has lasted for years it can hardly be rectified without an operation.

See Bursitis; Foot.

HAMMER TOE. In the deformity called hammer toe the segment or phalanx of the toe which is next the body of the foot is bent sharply upwards, while the other two segments are bent downwards, the toe thus assuming the form of an

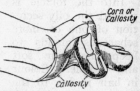

Hammer Toe. Deformity which leads to the formation of corns

inverted V. A corn tends to form over the apex of the V, and also where the point of the toe touches the ground.

Hammer toe is caused chiefly by a badly shaped boot, one that is too short or too pointed. The position of the toe can sometimes be rectified by wearing a splint on the under surface of the toe, but a little operation is the more satisfactory method.

See Claw Foot; Foot.

HAMSTRINGS. The popliteal space, which lies at the back of the knee, is also called the ham, and the tendons bounding the space on its outer and inner sides, the hamstrings. These are the tendons of muscles on the back and inner aspect of the thigh and concerned in bending the knee.

See Knee.

HAND. There are three regions in the hand, the carpus or wrist, the metacarpus or body of the hand, and the fingers. There are eight carpal bones, disposed in

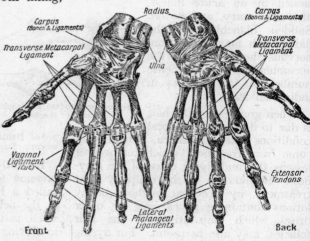

Hand. Bones and ligaments seen from front and back. The metacarpal ligaments prevent the fingers from separating beyond a certain point

two rows, from within outwards, those on the upper row being the cuneiform, on the front of which is the pisiform, the semilunar and the scaphoid, and on the lower row the unciform, the os magnum, the trapezoid and the trapezium. The five metacarpal bones are relatively long and have their shafts bent somewhat backwards. The bones of the fingers, of which there are fourteen, and other relative matters, are described under the heading Finger.

The skin of the palm, like that of the sole of the foot, is relatively thick, freely supplied with sweat glands and always devoid of hairs. Beneath the skin there is a triangular sheet of fascia, the palmar fascia, with extensions to the fingers. It is kept taut by a forearm muscle, the palmaris longus, the long, slender tendon of which is attached to the upper angle of the fascia. Thickening of this fascia is responsible for Dupuytren's contraction (*q.v.*). The skin is attached to the palmar fascia, and the various lines on the palm, to which a prophetic significance is given by the superstitious, are really the product of this attachment working in conjunction with the habitual movements of the hand.

The muscles of the hand are either extrinsic, that is, the tendons of forearm muscles, or intrinsic, that is, placed entirely in the hand itself, and mostly on the palmar aspect of the hand.

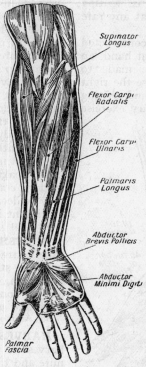

Muscles and tendons used in movements of the hand

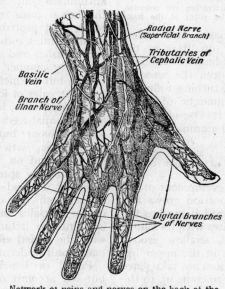

Network of veins and nerves on the back of the hand. The radial is a sensory nerve

Blood is supplied to the hand by the radial and ulnar arteries which form two arches, the deep and superficial palmar arches, from which branches pass downwards; the back, or dorsum of the hand, is mainly supplied by a branch from the radial artery. The superficial arch reaches as low as a line prolonged across the palm from the lower border of the thumb when this is fully abducted and extended, and the deep arch to a point half an inch above the superficial. The principal veins of the forearm (*q.v.*), the cephalic and basilic, have their root in the veins on the dorsum of the hand.

Sensation is supplied to the inner half of the hand, back and front, by the ulnar nerve, and to the outer or thumb half by the median nerve in front and the radial nerve, a branch of the musculo-spiral nerve, behind. The use of the right hand for manipulations requiring dexterity and delicacy is the rule, but a considerable number of children are left-handed. Some of these quickly and easily learn the use of the right hand for such purposes as writing, and become ambidextrous. Others retain the same awkwardness in the right hand as the average person has in the left. It has been noted that weakmindedness not unseldom accompanies this inveterate lefthandedness; the ambidextrous person, on the other hand, is usually more than ordinarily intelligent. A tendency to mirror-writing, that is, writing towards the left, is noted in at any rate some left-handed persons.

As so much machinery is constructed for manipulation with the right hand, an earnest endeavour should be made to teach a left-handed child to use the right for work requiring precision, and writing is probably the best preliminary exercise

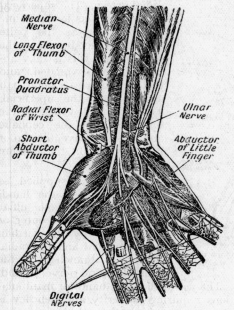

Median Nerve
Long Flexor of Thumb
Pronator Quadratus
Radial Flexor of Wrist
Short Abductor of Thumb
Ulnar Nerve
Abductor of Little Finger
Digital Nerves

Hand. The median nerve, activating the muscles, passes down the arm into the palm of the hand

for this purpose. Patience and understanding are necessary qualities in the teacher ; when a left-handed child is trained with other children the sense of his peculiarity has a disturbing influence on him, and the comments of other children are usually the reverse of helpful, so that nervousness and stammering may readily develop.

See Finger ; Forearm ; Median Nerve ; Musculo-spiral Nerve ; Nail ; Ulnar Nerve ; Wrist.

HARE-LIP. In the development of the face in the embryo a portion grows forward from either side until it reaches the middle line, where it unites with its fellow, but ordinarily a broad, shallow groove marks the line of union in the upper lip. In some children union does not take place through one side failing to come up to the middle line, while in others neither side

succeeds in doing so. In the former case a single hare-lip results, and in the latter a double. The gap may include the whole lip or only part of it, and in some instances besides hare-lip there may be a cleft palate.

Hare-lip is very disfiguring, but besides this it may seriously interfere with suckling. It is therefore necessary to remedy the condition as far as possible by operation, and this may be done on an ordinarily sturdy infant at from six weeks to three months. If the infant is weakly the operation may have to be postponed, but if the weakness is due to inability to take food in consequence of the deformity it may be deemed necessary to operate when the infant is about three weeks old.

See Cleft Palate.

HARTSHORN. Ammonia was at one time extracted from the horns of the hart or stag and was called spirit of hartshorn. The liniment of hartshorn and oil consists of ammonia solution and olive and almond oils.

See Ammonia.

HARVEST MITE. Also known as the harvester, the harvest bug, the mower's mite and the bête rouge, the harvest mite is a minute creature which infests the skin of human beings and domestic and wild animals in late summer and early autumn. It was formerly called leptus autumnalis but has been found to be the larval form of trombidium holosericeum, and probably of other species of trombidium, a mite found on grass, gooseberry bushes and other herbage in spring and early summer.

This mite, which is a vegetable-feeder, has four pairs of legs, but its larval form, the harvest mite, has only three pairs and is an animal-feeder. This has a bright, scarlet colour but is too small to be readily seen with the naked eye. It is chiefly found on the ankles, wrists and neck but may spread out over the body. It is not a blood-sucker but imbibes the juices from the ducts of the skin. It causes papules or wheals on the skin and intense itching and irritation, and with the added effects of scratching this may result in dermatitis.

Petrol or benzine will kill the mite but, on account of their inflammability, these substances must be used with caution. An ointment of white precipitate ointment, one part, and soft paraffin, two parts, or sulphur ointment, will also be effective. Afterwards it may be necessary to use soothing remedies, such as zinc ointment, to clear up dermatitis.

HAY FEVER. Also known as autumnal catarrh, hay fever is a paroxysmal disorder in which the eyes and nose are hot and perhaps itchy and discharge a clear mucous secretion, more or less freely. Sneezing is often troublesome and breathing may be difficult, perhaps to the extent of definite asthmatic seizures. If the catarrh of the eyes and nose is at all severe there is some rise of temperature.

The disorder partakes of the nature of anaphylaxis (*q.v.*) and the usual exciting cause is grass pollen, especially that of Timothy grass. The susceptibility to react to the pollen is largely inherited, and may be accompanied by a tendency to nettle-rash.

Females are more often affected than males, and the first symptoms tend to appear in childhood and recur each summer till middle-age, when the tendency to the disorder often wears off.

The pollen responsible may be determined by noting the reaction of an individual to extracts of various pollens, and when this is done the degree of susceptibility to the particular pollen is tested. This information is got by dropping solutions of pollens into the eye. An attempt is then made to build up the resistance of the patient to the noxious pollen by a series of injections of pollen-extract, the initial dose depending on the patient's susceptibility as decided by the preliminary tests. The injections should begin not later than the end of March.

If a patient has not had the advantage of this treatment residence in town is desirable during the pollen season, and at night wet sheets should be hung in front of the bedroom window to obstruct the entrance of pollen.

Should attacks occur, local sedatives, such as chloretone, may be helpful, and for asthmatic attacks the treatment suggested under the heading Asthma.

HEAD. The shape of the head varies in different races of mankind. In a brachycephalic, or short-headed, person, such as a Malay, the breadth of the cranium nearly approximates to its length, while in a dolicocephalic, or long-headed person, such as a Kafir, the length is considerably greater than the breadth. In a European the head occupies a mean position between these extremes, and he is said to be mesaticephalic. There are other differences, according to how far forward the chin projects, and so on, and there is also a difference in the capacity of the cranium and, therefore, the size of the brain.

The head is balanced on the upper surface of the atlas vertebra on which it can perform nodding movements. Rotation is produced by movement of the atlas vertebra on the axis, the next cervical vertebra in order, and bending of the head towards one or other shoulder by curving of the chain of cervical vertebrae.

See Brain ; Face ; Forehead ; Scalp ; Skull.

HEADACHE. The cause of headache may not be far to seek, as when it occurs as a symptom of fever, acute indigestion, acute nephritis or some other well-marked disorder. Again, when attacks of headache occur, limited to one side, and accompanied by vomiting and certain other symptoms, the existence of sick-headache, or migraine (*q.v.*) is obvious.

Often, however, the cause of the headache must be searched for ; there may be no obvious evidence of general or local disturbance, or concurrent symptoms may be misleading unless skilfully interpreted. Thus, headache accompanied by vomiting may suggest a stomach disorder although actually due, for example, to a brain tumour, to eye trouble, such as glaucoma, or even a refractive error, or to kidney disease.

When headaches are frequent the health requires to be carefully overhauled in at least three directions : (1) any possible source of irritation in the eyes, nose, teeth or ears ; (2) any source of poisoning such as constipation, chronic Bright's disease, pyorrhoea, chronic appendicitis, or, in women, disease of the pelvic organs ; (3) any general weakness, such as anaemia or neurasthenia.

Pain at the root of the nose or in or about the eyes suggests disorder in these organs respectively; a sensation of a tight band round the head, neurasthenia; and a severe, boring pain on the top of the head suggests the clavus of hysteria. Often, however, the situation of the pain is no guide, as headache due to an error of refraction may be felt at the back of the head, or on the top, situations unlikely to suggest the real source of trouble, namely, the eyes. It is often noted, however, that ocular headache tends to be better at the week-ends when the eyes are being rested. Headache which is only present at night, or is worse then, is suggestive of syphilis.

Headache cannot be treated properly unless its cause, or causes, is determined. Immediate relief may be obtained in various ways, as, for example, by putting cold cloths on the forehead or rubbing it over with a menthol cone, or by putting a mustard plaster on the nape of the neck. If there is indigestion or constipation a purge is necessary.

As regards headache powders, pills or potions, it is important to know what one is taking, because secret headache remedies have been found to contain acetanilide, a drug which may cause serious depression.

A useful powder contains 7 grains of phenacetin and 2 grains of caffeine citrate. If a person has had malaria, 5 grains of quinine may be taken alone or with the above. Aspirin, in 10-grain doses, often gives relief, especially in subjects of rheumatism.

See Caffeine; Change of Life; Eye Strain; Fever; Indigestion; Migraine; Neuralgia; Neurasthenia; Teeth.

HEALTH. In general terms health may be defined as the condition in which all the bodily functions, even in the ordinary emergencies of everyday life, are carried out comfortably. The more natural our conditions of life, the more likely is a state of health to be maintained. The countryman has advantages over the urban dweller as regards free exercise in the open air and sunshine, and usually also as to the freshness of his food; on the other hand, he may suffer from exposure to the vicissitudes of weather. Moreover, the urban dweller, by constant exposure to many kinds of air-borne infection, seems to acquire a certain immunity to some disorders as compared with the country dweller. For much disease our excesses are to blame; for example, in the use of alcohol or tobacco, or in excitement.

Many serious disorders begin in an insidious fashion, causing little depreciation of that comfortableness in the process of living which it has been said is indicative of health. A due regard to such slight depreciation is very important, therefore, as appropriate treatment may prevent the development of serious disorders, or at the worst delay their progress. This consideration becomes all the more important when one has passed middle-life.

The wrong way to deal with such slight symptoms, however, is to adopt a fidgety concern with regard to them but do nothing more. If they cannot be removed by simple means which suggest themselves to anyone, a doctor should be consulted.

See Cleanliness; Constitution; Diet; Disease; Exercise; Housing; Mental Hygiene; Ventilation; Sewage.

HEALTH RESORT. A place may be suitable for a health resort on account of its climate, or because it has some natural water which has uses in the treatment of disease. A place selected for some climatic advantage may also possess a natural water, or, on the other hand, the use of the waters at some health resort may be barred by unsuitability of its climate for certain persons or diseases. This, as well as the fact that the waters of different places have different qualities and actions, makes it desirable that anyone contemplating a course of spa treatment should obtain skilled advice before making a choice of a resort.

A marine climate possesses freshness of air, combining purity and movement, an enhanced effect of sunlight from the reflection of ultra-violet rays from the sheet of water, and for inland dwellers there is a freshness of interest which has a stimulating psychological effect. Seaside resorts are, therefore, peculiarly suitable for convalescents as a rule. Tuberculosis often shows an increased tendency to heal, but for acute or debilitated cases warmth, shelter and sanatorium conveniences are necessary adjuncts. Torquay would be most suitable for those with the least reserves of energy, Bournemouth and Ventnor for those with more, but a place like Hastings only for those with a considerable amount of vigour.

On the other hand, the dampness of a marine climate generally makes a seaside resort unsuitable for rheumatism. Many neurasthenics also do not do well at the seaside. The Riviera is a renowned marine resort. Here the cold north wind, or mistral, and the hot south wind, or sirocco, may be disagreeable, more especially from the dust they raise, but the chief drawback to the Riviera is the overcrowding.

Curative Effects of a Mountain Climate

A mountain climate is one at an altitude of over 1,500 feet ; up to 3,500 feet it is ranked as a moderate, and above this, a high, altitude. Purity of air is combined with rarity, this quality increasing the higher one goes. A mountain climate with sanatorium treatment is the most successful form of therapy for consumption, and the stimulating qualities of this climate make it highly useful for other disorders. It is not suitable, however, for old people, for those whose chest wall is inclined to rigidity, for those with valvular disease of the heart or with albuminuria. The Alpine resorts are those usually selected. Leysin has an altitude of 4,760 feet, Montana 5,100 feet, and Davos Platz 5,120 feet. St. Moritz, at 6,100 feet, is rather a place for winter sports than for the residence of invalids. The winter season at these resorts lasts from November to March. In summer, from June to September, St. Moritz and Pontresina, 5,915 feet, are perhaps more frequented.

Of inland climates that of the Egyptian desert has a well-merited reputation as a winter resort for those suffering from chronic nephritis and other maladies. In some circumstances also the high veldt of South Africa has much to recommend it.

Health resorts where the treatment centres round the use of the waters of a mineral spring are described as spas. Patients may be required to drink the waters or use them as baths, douches, etc. ; frequently both the internal and external use of the waters is adopted. The chemical composition of the water of one spa differs more or less from that of another, and even at the same spa there may be springs of different composition. Some of the waters are aerated, and this adds to their palatability. There is a wide range of difference also in the temperature at which the water is delivered from different springs, and to some of the waters superior virtues are ascribed on the ground of their possessing radio-activity.

According to the chemical composition of its water, a spa is considered to be more suitable for some complaints than for others, but differences in this respect may possibly be exaggerated, as much benefit in a large number of disorders may accrue from drinking large draughts of warm water, irrespective of the salts dissolved in it, or even of its having any saline constituents at all ; and the same applies to bathing and douching.

According to their temperature, waters are classified as cold if below 80° F. ; hypothermal, if below 93° ; subthermal, if between 93° and 98° ; and thermal, if between 98° and 105° ; if hotter than this, they are hyperthermal. These differences in temperature are important only as regards the use of the waters for bathing ; and the relative virtues and uses of water at different temperatures, when used in this way, are discussed under the heading Baths.

Turning now to their chemical composition, natural waters are classified in the following groups :

(1) **Simple waters,** that is, not containing a notable amount of any chemical. Amongst spas that have this type of water are Bath, Buxton, Ilkley Wells (Yorkshire), Malvern Wells, and Matlock Bath ; in France, Dax, Evaux-les-Bains and Plombières ; in Italy, Bormio, Fiuggi, and Valdieri ; in Switzerland, Evian-les-Bains, Loèche-les-Bains, and Thonon ; in Austria, Gastein ; in Bohemia, Toeplitz-Schonau ; and in Germany, Wildbad in the Black Forest. At some of the spas there is no drinking of the waters, but bathing simply. Some of the waters are hot and others cold. Bath is the only British spa with hot springs. Simple waters flush the body and remove waste products. They are used to treat catarrhal conditions, chronic rheumatism and gout.

(2) **Alkaline waters,** that is, containing a considerable amount of sodium bicarbonate and free carbonic acid. Some of these contain notable amounts of sodium chloride, and are called muriated alkaline waters; still others contain sulphates. There are thus the following three groups: (a) Alkaline waters, acting as antacids, etc. Amongst the spas with this kind of water are Vichy in France, and Neuenahr in Germany, which have hot springs, and Vals in France, which has a cold spring. Included in this group also are the table waters of Evian, Apollinaris, Johannis, and other sources. (b) Muriated alkaline waters, which to the action of the alkaline water adds the stimulating action of common salt. Amongst spas with this type of water are Châtel-Guyon, in France, and the St. Louis Spring in Michigan, U.S.A. Of this type also are the table waters of Rosbach, Kronthal and other sources. (c) Sulphated alkaline waters, which have a laxative action. Such are found at Karlsbad, Franzensbad and Marienbad in Bohemia, Tarasp in Switzerland, and elsewhere.

(3) **Sulphated or " bitter " waters,** containing magnesium sulphate and sodium sulphate in considerable quantities. These are chiefly used bottled, as purgative medicines. They are found at Cheltenham, Leamington and Scarborough, etc. Of this type also are Aesculap, Apenta, Hunyadi Janos and other waters.

(4) **Muriated waters,** that is, containing common salt. The stronger waters of this type are sometimes called brines. They are much used in the form of baths for chronic joint affections. Such occur at Bridge of Allan in Scotland; Builth and Llandrindod in Wales; Droitwich and Woodhall; Bourbonne and Brides-les-Bains, in France; Homburg, Kissingen and Wiesbaden in Germany; Bex and Rheinhalden in Switzerland; St. Catherine's Wells, Ontario; and the Saratoga Springs, U.S.A. In Harrogate water there is also a considerable amount of common salt, combined with sodium sulphide and sulphuretted hydrogen.

(5) **Sulphur waters,** that is, containing sulphides of sodium, potassium, calcium and magnesium, or sulphuretted hydrogen. These appear to have a special use for chronic joint affections and chronic skin diseases. Such are found at Harrogate, Builth, Llandrindod, Moffat and Strathpeffer; at Lisdoonvarna in Ireland; in France, at Aix-les-Bains, Enghien, etc., and especially at Cauterets, Eaux Bonnes, Eaux Chaudes and many other places in the French Pyrenees; at Acqui, Agnano and Tobiano in Italy; at Baden and Schinznach in Switzerland; at Eilsen and Neuendorf in Germany; at Hercules Bad in Hungary; at Helouan, Egypt; at Banff, a Canadian resort in the Rocky Mountains; and at Rotorua and other resorts in New Zealand.

(6) **Chalybeate or iron-containing waters,** which may be useful in anaemia, but especially in debility, for example, malarial cachexia. Such are the waters at Tunbridge Wells, and Trefriw, in Wales; Bussang and Forges-les-Eaux, in France; Spa, in Belgium; St. Moritz and San Bernardino, in Switzerland; at Schwalbach and Teinach, in Germany; at Val Furva, in Italy; at Caledon, in the Cape Colony, and at numerous spas in the U.S.A.

(7) **Arsenical waters;** these also contain either iron or some saline. The strongest are those of Roncegno and Levico, in Italy. Other springs are at La Bourboule, Mont Dore and Vic-sur-Cere, in France, and Val Sinistra, in Switzerland. These waters are used for debility.

(8) **Earthy or calcareous waters,** which contain the carbonate and sulphate of calcium and carbonate of magnesium. They are antacid and sedative to the gastric mucous membrane. They are also useful in some cases of kidney disorder and of gout and chronic rheumatism. Amongst other sources of such waters are Bath; Bagnères-de-Bigorre, Contrexéville and Pougues-les-Eaux, in France; and Chianciano and San Pellegrino, in Italy.

It should be understood that the waters of many spas might be included in more than one of the groups above mentioned, and that many good spas exist, all over the world, in addition to those which have been named.

Besides the use of the waters, treatment at a spa includes a regulation of the daily life as regards the nature and amount of food, exercise and rest. Moreover, the patient is removed from his ordinary surroundings, duties and worries, while he is enlivened by the new interests in the life at the spa. He is thus placed in the very conditions for cure.

Apart possibly from climate, there is no reason why a patient should not take a cure at a British spa in preference to a Continental one, as at most of the home spas special treatments associated with different foreign spas can be carried out quite as satisfactorily; for example, Nauheim baths, the Aix-Vichy douche, and so on. Volcanic mud packs are also available at home spas, and at one or two peat baths can also be obtained. At all the spas apparatus for giving electrical and light treatment is installed.

See Baths; Convalescence.

HEARING. Waves of air, or some other medium, set in motion by the vibration of some object, are enabled by the mechanism described under the heading Ear to cause impulses to pass along the auditory nerve to the brain, and so give rise to the sensation of hearing. The greater the rapidity of the vibrations the higher the pitch of the sound, but only vibrations between about 30 and 15,000 can be appreciated by the human ear, those used in music ranging from 40 to 4,800.

The power of hearing may be ascertained by observing at what distance a person can hear the ordinary conversational voice, a whisper, the ticking of a watch or the vibrations of a tuning-fork. The sense of relative pitch may be determined by the use of Galton's whistle. It is important to find out the power of hearing by air conduction, by holding the vibrating prongs of a tuning-fork near the ear-hole, and also the bone conduction, by placing the end of the stem of the fork on the mastoid process behind the ear (see Plate XIII, 6). A comparison of the two

is called Rinné's test. Normally the fork should be heard longer by air conduction, but in what is called obstructive deafness, say from outer or middle-ear disease, the bone conduction is better than the air. In applying any test to one ear the other must always be covered over.

If the end of the stem of the fork is placed on the top of the head of a person with obstructive deafness in one ear, the sound is loudest in the bad ear. This is called Weber's test (see Plate XIII 7,).

See Deafness; Ear; Sound.

HEART. The main factor in the circulation of the blood. the heart, is situated between the lungs and rests on the diaphragm, or midriff. It lies behind the breast bone, or sternum, but extends on either side of it, especially towards the left, one-third of the organ being to the right of a line drawn down the middle of the sternum, and two-thirds to the left. The area of the chest wall lying in front of the heart is called the praecordia, but to some extent the heart is separated from the chest wall by the overlapping of the lung on either side.

The heart lies in a fibrous bag lined with a smooth membrane which, however, is reflected on to and covers the heart, these two smooth layers being in contact and gliding over one another during the movements of the heart. The fibrous bag is known as the fibrous pericardium, and the smooth layers are the serous pericardium.

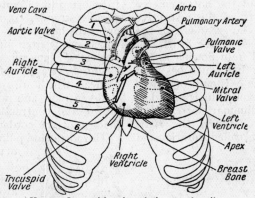

Heart. Its position in relation to the ribs

The heart is roughly pear-shaped and the thicker portion, or base, is directed backwards and to the right, while the narrower, or apex, is forwards and to the left. In an adult the average dimensions of the heart are 5 inches long, $3\frac{1}{2}$ inches broad, and $2\frac{1}{2}$ inches thick, and it weighs 9 ounces; roughly speaking, it is about the size of the closed fist. It is composed of muscle fibres which are peculiar in that although striped, they are also involuntary.

There are four chambers in the heart, two, the auricles, at the base, and below these the ventricles, but while the auricle on each side communicates with the corresponding ventricle, there is no communication within the heart between the auricles or between the ventricles, so that one can speak of the right heart and the left heart, each consisting of an auricle and a ventricle. Before a child is born the two auricles communicate through an opening known as the foramen ovale, but this communication ceases at birth. The heart is somewhat twisted, so that the right chambers are more towards the front than those on the left.

The right auricle receives blood from the veins of the body through two large trunks, the superior and the inferior vena cava, and pumps it into the right ventricle, from which it is sent through the pulmonary artery into the lungs; thence it is returned by four vessels, the pulmonary veins, into the left auricle, and from this into the left ventricle, which pumps it through the aorta and on through the arteries to all parts of the body. The pulmonary artery and the aorta emerge from the upper parts of the respective ventricle, so that all the great vessels are grouped about the base of the heart.

Blood is prevented from flowing in the contrary direction to that which has been just described, by the existence of valves between each auricle and ventricle, and at the orifice of the pulmonary artery and of the aorta. That between the right auricle and ventricle is called the tricuspid

valve because it has three main cusps, or flaps, while the corresponding valve on the left is the mitral, with two main cusps and an outline somewhat resembling a bishop's mitre, whence its name.

A cusp of these valves consists of a thin layer of fibrous tissue covered on both

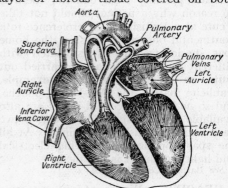

Diagrammatic section of heart showing course of the blood from the auricles into the ventricles

sides by a smooth membrane, the endocardium, which also lines the cavities of the heart. When the valve is closed, the edges of the cusps overlap. A cusp is prevented from being forced into the auricle by little fibrous strands, cordae tendineae, which are attached to its lower surface, and which spring from nipple-shaped muscular processes, musculi papillares, or from elevated strands of muscle, columnae carneae, which are situated on the wall of the ventricle and which, by shortening during the contraction of the ventricle, make taut the cordae tendineae.

The aortic and pulmonary valves consist of three cusps in the form of little pockets, the openings of which face away from the ventricle, so that when blood attempts to pass back into the latter the pockets fill out and close the opening in the vessel which they guard. Each cusp has a half-moon shape, hence the valves are described as the semilunar valves.

The muscular wall of the heart, or myocardium, is relatively thin

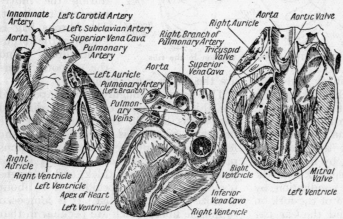

Heart. Left, view from front; centre, from behind; right, internal arrangement

in the auricles as compared with the ventricles, while, of the latter, the thickness of the wall of the left is about three times that of the wall of the right, as might be expected, considering that the left chamber must send blood throughout the whole body while the right only pumps it through the lungs.

Blood is propelled from each chamber by the contraction of its muscle-walls just as water would be expelled from a rubber ball containing it by the hand closing round and compressing the ball. When the muscle again relaxes, blood flows into the chamber which opens out or dilates. The contraction of the heart or any chambers of it is described as its systole, and relaxation as its diastole. In the action of the heart there is a regular cycle ; first there is systole of both auricles together, then systole of the ventricles together, then a period of rest before systole of the auricles begins a fresh cycle. The relative times taken by these events are in the ratios of 1, 3 and 4, so that a chamber is resting for a longer time than it is working. Its strength is thus continuously recuperated, so that it is enabled to go on beating night and day for a lifetime.

The blood in the right side of the heart is dark and venous, that in the left side bright scarlet, purified from carbonic acid gas and charged with oxygen for the use of the body tissues. It is estimated that each ventricle pumps out about three ounces of blood at each beat of the heart. The first branches of the aorta are the coronary arteries, those supplying the tissues of the heart itself, but they receive their blood during the resting period of the heart. Venous blood from these tissues is gathered into a large vein at the back of the heart, known as the coronary sinus, whence it flows into the right auricle.

Owing to the elasticity of the arteries, a wave of expansion, or pulsation, passes

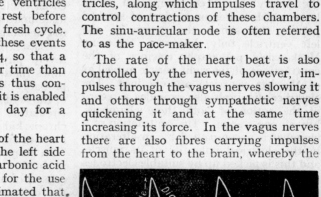

Heart. Section showing the valvular structures

Semi-Lunar Valves — *Pulmonary Artery* — *Aorta* — *Anterior Cusp* — *Inferior Cusp* — *Mitral Valve* — *Medial Cusp* — *Tricuspid Valve*

along them with each beat of the heart. This pulse is usually felt for on the radial artery at the wrist, and takes place here a fraction of a second after the heart beat, the interval representing the time taken by the wave to reach the wrist.

In the wall of the right auricle, between the openings of the superior and inferior vena cava, there is a small particle of altered muscle, about the size of a grain of wheat, which is known as the sinu-auricular node. It originates the rhythmic impulses which control contraction of the auricles. There is a similar node in the lower part of the wall of the right auricle, the auriculo-ventricular node, from which passes the atrio-ventricular bundle, or bundle of His, composed also of pale fibres, to the interventricular septum and other parts of the walls of the ventricles, along which impulses travel to control contractions of these chambers. The sinu-auricular node is often referred to as the pace-maker.

The rate of the heart beat is also controlled by the nerves, however, impulses through the vagus nerves slowing it and others through sympathetic nerves quickening it and at the same time increasing its force. In the vagus nerves there are also fibres carrying impulses from the heart to the brain, whereby the

Curves of heart beats showing the two stages

medium-sized arteries are relaxed and blood pressure lowered, a mechanism which comes into operation when the resistance to the blood flow caused by contraction of these arteries is beginning to embarrass the heart.

When the ventricles contract, the apex of the heart is thrust against the chest wall on the left side, its impact, referred to as the apex beat, being felt most distinctly in the space between the fifth and sixth ribs at a distance of $3\frac{1}{2}$ inches from the mid-line of the sternum.

If one listens over the beating heart two sounds are heard which rather resemble the sound of the words lubb-dup. The first occurs synchronously with the apex beat, and therefore in connexion with the contraction of the ventricles and the closure of their valves ; it is indeed caused by these things and especially by the valves closing. The second sound, which is shorter and sharper, represents the closure of the pulmonary and aortic valves when the blood which has been pumped into the vessels and has distended them presses backwards on the elastic recoil of their walls at the end of ventricular contraction.

In clinical investigations into the condition of the heart, several instruments are used to obtain graphic representations of its action. The sphygmograph furnishes a tracing of the pulse, the movements of the artery being communicated to a lever which writes on a piece of smoked paper ; this shows the action of the left ventricle only, however. By using Mackenzie's polygraph, tracings of the contractions of the right auricle as well as of the left ventricle are obtained. The electrocardiograph also provides a record of the action of both these chambers, but on one tracing. The contraction of a chamber is accompanied by an alteration in the electrical potential of its muscle, and this is picked up by suitable electrodes and carried to a galvanometer, an instrument which measures electrical currents, the changes produced in this being recorded photographically.

Diseases of the Heart. Among the symptoms of heart disease there are some that occur without there being anything organically wrong with the organ ; the symptoms represent a mere functional disturbance, a condition which is sometimes described as disordered action of the heart, or, shortly, D.A.H. Shortness of breath on slight exertion, palpitation, pain over the heart, faintness, giddiness,

and other symptoms may often be so interpreted. Such may follow an acute infectious disease, or arise independently, and particularly in persons of a neurasthenic type. In every case of this kind a search should be made for some source of bacterial toxaemia, at the roots of the teeth, in the nose, in the tonsils, in the appendix, and so on. Any focus of this kind should be thoroughly cleaned up, and beyond this, the treatment mainly consists in following hygienic rules of living. Worry over the heart itself is unnecessary, and does harm.

Heart Disease from Acute Rheumatism

The most frequent cause of organic disease of the heart is acute rheumatism, which is possibly of streptococcal origin. The heart may become affected in the course of an attack of acute rheumatism with joint symptoms, or of chorea, or St. Vitus's Dance. In children the heart may be the sole organ affected in an attack of acute rheumatism, or there may be simply what are called growing pains, and still the heart may suffer. Implication of the heart may occur in tonsillitis, and it is not uncommon in scarlet fever. Other bacterial infections may also cause inflammation of the heart ; syphilis is a not uncommon cause.

Disease of the heart may be induced by severe physical exertion, though sometimes there is also infection of the heart, probably made possible by overstrain of the organ. The effort of carrying on the circulation through arteries narrowed by chronic kidney disease or some other cause, may, in time, induce structural changes.

In some instances heart disease exists at birth. This congenital disease may consist of errors of development whereby the chambers on the two sides are not properly separated, or foetal blood vessels may persist, and in either case there is an admixture of venous blood in that sent from the left heart through the body, so that the skin and mucous membranes are also more or less livid or dusky, a condition sometimes referred to as the blue disease. In other instances from infection, while the child is still within the womb, the valves of the heart are diseased, in which case it is usually those on the right side of the heart that are affected.

Acquired organic disease of the heart may be considered as affecting the walls of the chambers, including the contraction-regulating mechanism, or the valves, or both. Disease of the coronary arteries affects the nutrition of the myocardium ; embolism may cause sudden death, and a more gradual interference is followed by the change of the muscle into fibrous tissue, affecting to a greater or less degree the efficient pumping action of the organ. There is a similar result when the muscle fibres undergo a fatty change (fatty degeneration) or when the fibres are separated by fat (fatty infiltration).

What Constitutes Heart Block

Fibrosis or some other abnormality may interfere with the conduction of impulses to the ventricles along the paths which have been described above. This is known as heart block, and if the ventricle refrains from beating for more than a certain time, say 18 seconds, the patient becomes unconscious and probably has convulsions, this condition being known as the Stokes-Adams syndrome. Sometimes nervous influences are responsible for the heart block. If the block is complete, the ventricle starts beating on its own at a rate of 40 or less, the auricle beating in harmony with impulses from the sinu-auricular node, and this may go on for years. This condition is readily recognized by using one of the instruments mentioned above, which gives a record of auricular contractions.

Sometimes parts of the heart wall may be unduly irritable, and give rise to a rapid action of the organ, perhaps in a long series of beats at the rate of 130 to 200 per minute, constituting attacks of what is called paroxysmal tachycardia, or that kind of irregularity of the pulse distinguished by premature contractions These have no serious significance in sound hearts, though it may be otherwise if the heart is diseased Severe and frequent paroxysmal tachycardia has an exhausting effect, as increase in the rapidity of the heart beat is ordinarily at the expense of the rest period in the cardiac cycle. In some instances the auricles alone are affected, a condition called auricular flutter, contractions taking place at the rate of 200 or more per minute.

Disease of a valve may cause narrowing, or stenosis, so that the blood-flow through it is obstructed ; or incompetence, so that blood flows back, or regurgitates into the chamber from which it has been pumped ; both of these conditions may affect any one valve. In order to drive the blood through a stenosed valve or to deal with the excess of blood caused by regurgitation, the muscle-wall of the chamber affected must thicken, or hypertrophy, in order to acquire greater power. When this happens, compensation is said to have occurred. There is always a little dilatation of the chamber accompanying the hypertrophy, but failing the development of compensation, or consequent on its failure, there is very considerable dilatation of the chamber.

In the course of time compensation does fail, but it may do so at any time from over-stress or from some illness that weakens the muscle. In the early stages of failure, symptoms of back pressure appear, and they become progressively more extensive and severe. For example, in mitral stenosis, that is, narrowing of the mitral valve, the flow of blood into the left auricle through the pulmonary veins is obstructed and the lung becomes congested ; this, in turn, embarrasses the right heart which, on failure of its compensation, transmits the back pressure to the veins, bringing blood from all parts of the body, so that dropsy occurs, and many organs are congested. In aortic regurgitation, the other common form of valvular disease, failure of compensation of the left ventricle leads to regurgitation of blood through the mitral valve, and to the same back-pressure phenomena.

Condition Termed Auricular Fibrillation

In advanced cases of mitral stenosis or in degeneration of the cardiac muscle, a form of heart failure occurs which is called auricular fibrillation. The auricles cease from contracting regularly, but tumultuous, irregular contractions take place in individual muscle fibres in their walls. The stimuli sent to the ventricles are correspondingly uneven, and consequently the pulse, which reflects their contractions, is utterly irregular, that is to say, there is no uniformity at all in the size of successive waves or in their spacing.

Symptoms of cardiac disorders have already been mentioned, and to these may be added those which may indicate congestion of organs, which may occur when compensation fails. Spitting of blood is not uncommon, in mitral stenosis particularly, and anginal attacks may occur, especially in aortic regurgitation. Symptoms pointing to embolism may also occur.

Significance of Heart Murmurs

One of the important signs of valvular disease is a murmur, a new sound heard when listening over the heart, and which may accompany or replace a normal heart sound. The significance of a murmur depends on various facts, including the place where it is best heard, its relation in time to the normal sounds, and so on. It must be added, however, that a murmur may be present although there is no organic, or, in fact, any disease of the heart ; a systolic murmur, that is, one accompanying the first sound, at the apex or at the base, very often has no significance whatever.

The characteristic murmur of mitral disease precedes and leads up to the first sound of the heart, and is called presystolic ; it is often accompanied by a thrill which can be felt by the fingers placed on the chest wall. The murmur of aortic regurgitation accompanies and often replaces the second sound ; as it occurs while the heart is at rest, the ventricles, at any rate, it is said to be diastolic.

Another sign of heart disease is enlargement of the organ. This may mean dilatation merely, or the heart may be hypertrophied, and then the apex beat may be forcible and heaving. Great enlargement may occur, especially in aortic regurgitation, so that the heart resembles that of an ox, cor bovinum. Enlargement caused by great physical exertion is sometimes referred to as athlete's heart.

It may be difficult to say, sometimes, whether the heart is enlarged or displaced, and then X-rays will be very useful.

In aortic regurgitation some of the blood pumped into the arteries flows back into the left ventricle, so that the distension of the vessels is weakly sustained, and they collapse at once, after the heart beat. This produces what is called the waterhammer, or Corrigan's, pulse, best felt at the wrist when the arm is raised above the head.

Valvular disease is caused by endocarditis (q.v.) mainly, and mitral stenosis and aortic regurgitation are the commonest lesions, though mitral regurgitation and aortic stenosis also occur, and, more rarely, similar lesions to all of these on the right side of the heart. More than one valve may be affected, and a lesion of one valve may give rise to others behind it ; thus, aortic regurgitation may lead to mitral regurgitation, then to tricuspid regurgitation.

The treatment of heart disease can only be safely and satisfactorily carried out under medical guidance.

Prevention of heart disease is largely bound up with that of acute rheumatism, but something would be done in this direction were parents fully alive to the possibility of rheumatic inflammation of the heart occurring in connexion with "growing pains," with tonsillitis or with St. Vitus's dance.

Other instances would be prevented were all cases of syphilis subjected to early and thorough treatment. In so far, also, as the incidence of arterio-sclerosis (q.v.) is diminished, will aortic disease, dependent upon this cause, be prevented.

Health Rules for Heart Patients

A person whose heart is damaged must live carefully, punctiliously observing the rules of personal hygiene. Constipation, indigestion or anaemia should be corrected. The mouth should be kept scrupulously clean, and an attempt should be made to clean up sepsis there or elsewhere in the body. Medical advice should be taken on the use of tobacco and alcohol.

Over-exertion should be avoided ; a young person with a damaged heart should choose an occupation which will not subject him to anything of this kind ; persons who are engaged in manual labour should live as near their place of occupation as possible, as a long walk may be too much for them in addition to the exertion involved in the occupation. This becomes a matter for urgent consideration should any signs of difficulty in compensation appear. Rest in bed for a day or two each week may allow work to be done in comfort which would be impossible otherwise. When rest in bed is enjoined by a doctor in heart disease, the patient should on no account get up to go to stool or for any other purpose.

On the other hand, unless he has had orders to the contrary, a person suffering from heart disease should take regular exercise should his employment be a sedentary one, keeping him indoors. Easy walking, or games which do not put one out of breath, should be enjoyed.

The Schott system of exercises for heart disease may be taken along with a course of baths, or independently, but always under medical supervision. These are designed to exercise all the joints and every group of voluntary muscles. Each movement is resisted either by the person superintending the exercises, or by the patient himself bringing into action the muscles which oppose the movement he is performing. Thus, if bending the arm, he brings into action also those that straighten it out. Each movement is done slowly and to the full extent, and there should be a pause of about half a minute between each movement. No movement is done twice in succession.

Exercise flushes the muscles with nourishing blood, and clears out waste products from them. The same results can be achieved by massage, and this is a useful measure, particularly for a patient confined to bed.

The drug most often used in heart disease is digitalis, amongst others being opium, strophanthus, quinidine and general tonics. In expert hands quinidine may be very successful in restoring the heart from the condition of auricular fibrillation.

See Angina Pectoris ; Circulation of the Blood ; Endocarditis ; Murmur ; Myocardium ; Pericardium ; Pulsation ; Pulse.

HEARTBURN. *See* Acidity ; Indigestion.

HEAT. The application of moderate heat to the skin causes redness from dilatation of the capillary blood vessels and an increase of sweating. The introduction of heat into the body in hot drinks has the same effects. Heat may be utilised in either of these ways to stimulate the circulation, for example, in the treatment of faintness and collapse. It should be remembered, however, that while hot baths are stimulating if used for a few minutes only they have a definitely depressing effect when they are more prolonged. The application of moderate heat to the body has also a soothing action on the nervous system, and a warm bath is often used in treating infantile convulsions, to mention one example.

Local applications of heat, by dilating the surface blood vessels and acting on the nerve endings in the skin, may be useful in relieving deeply seated congestion and pain ; spasm may also be relieved. Diathermy, an electrical method of producing heat, has the advantage that it can increase heat actually in the tissues themselves and not merely on the surface.

Excessive degrees of heat cause burning or scalding, and tissues may be killed and destroyed. Thus, by various kinds of cautery or by diathermy, tumours and other forms of unhealthy tissue may be removed. Heat is often used for this purpose when troublesome bleeding is to be apprehended, as considerable degrees of heat arrest bleeding.

See Baths ; Electricity in Medicine ; Fomentation ; Heat Stroke ; Poultice ; Radiant Heat.

HEAT STROKE. Exposure to excessive heat may cause heat stroke, a condition having some resemblance to an apoplectic seizure. When following exposure to the rays of the sun the condition is described as sunstroke, siriasis, or insolation, but exposure to the sun is not the only way in which heat stroke may be caused ; it may occur in stokers and others similarly placed. Its occurrence is favoured by alcoholic habits, inability to sweat freely, by too heavy clothing, and by exposure of the head and neck to the sun.

The patient may suddenly fall unconscious or there may be preliminary symptoms, such as headache, giddiness, vomiting, and sickness. Sometimes there is what appears to be acute asphyxia, with blueness of the face and extremities, and the patient may die in a very short time. Usually, however, the face is flushed, the pupils very small, the pulse bounding, and the breathing stertorous. The skin feels burning, and if the temperature of the body is taken it will be found to be very high, perhaps 107° to 110° F.

The immediate treatment for heat stroke is to take the patient into the shade, or the coolest place available, strip the clothing from the trunk, and souse the trunk and head with cold water. As soon as possible he should be taken home or to a hospital, where an effort will be made to lower the temperature by rubbing him over with ice or giving an iced pack or bath, and possibly an iced enema.

Another effect of excessive heat is what is called heat exhaustion, the patient becoming more or less collapsed. The skin is pale and cool, the pulse small and rapid, and the temperature probably subnormal. There is no loss of consciousness. The patient should be put to bed in a well-ventilated room, and if the temperature is raised the treatment is that of fever (*q.v.*). If, however, the temperature is subnormal, a hot bath or hot-water bottles around him in bed, with stimulants, is the correct treatment. For stimulation a teaspoonful of sal-volatile in a wineglass of water, hot tea or coffee, or diluted spirits may be given.

See Acclimatisation ; Fever.

HECTIC. Fever in which there are daily intermissions and frequent drenching sweats is described as hectic fever. It occurs in advanced consumption and in other conditions in which septic poisons are being absorbed. The flush on the cheeks which may also occur is often called hectic flush.

See Fever.

HEEL. The projection backwards of the os calcis forms the heel (Plate VII, 3). A painful heel may be caused by chafing of the skin by a badly fitting boot, by inflammation at the insertion of the Achilles tendon into the os calcis, by inflammation in the bone itself, or by a spur or outgrowth on the lower surface of the bone. Zinc or boracic ointment will heal chafing, but the boot should be rectified by a shoemaker or changed. For the other conditions rest and sedative applications are indicated, and, sometimes, operation.

See Achilles Tendon; Foot.

HEIGHT. The height of a person is determined by the height of the vertebral bodies and the length of the bones of the lower limbs. Sometimes one or other of these is longer or shorter than the average, so that the individual has a long body and short legs or vice versa. There should be some correspondence between the height and the weight.

See Growth.

HEMIPLEGIA. Paralysis of one side of the body is called hemiplegia. The face may be paralysed on the same side as the rest of the body, or the other side may be affected, a condition described as crossed hemiplegia. With a right hemiplegia speech is commonly affected.

See Paralysis.

HEMP. Indian hemp, which is a narcotic drug, is described under the heading Cannabis Indica. Canadian hemp, or American Indian hemp root, acts as a heart stimulant and diuretic, but is a powerful drug, and should be used with caution. Its active principle is called apocynamarin, or cynotoxin.

HENBANE. The leaves of henbane, or hyoscyamus, contain the alkaloids hyoscyamine, hyoscine and atropine, and are used to make various medicinal preparations, including the following official ones : extract, dose 2 to 8 grains ; tincture, dose $\frac{1}{2}$ to 1 drachm ; and hyoscyamine sulphate, dose $\frac{1}{200}$ to $\frac{1}{100}$ grain. The action of hyoscyamus resembles that of belladonna (*q.v.*). The leaves are sometimes used in making fumigatory powders or cigarettes for the treatment of asthma, the extract is often included in purgative pills in order to prevent griping, and the tincture is used to relieve pain and irritation in inflammation of the bladder.

HEREDITY. Every species of creature has been developed from a preceding type from which it differs in some degree, while differing very profoundly from an ancestor far back in the chain of descent. The characters of a species must, therefore, have been caused by modification, but such would not have availed in the production of new species unless the characters of progenitors were transmitted to the progeny.

That such happens, however, is common knowledge ; a family likeness is stamped on creatures having a common descent and extends to peculiarities which can be ranked as abnormalities. Thus, for example, successive generations of human beings may have an excessive number, or on the other hand a deficiency, of fingers and toes ; or a coarse, scaly condition of the skin known as ichthyosis, or the fish-skin disease. The peculiarity which is inherited may be of a more subtle character, such as the peculiar make-up of the blood in haemophilia, or the bleeder's disease, colour blindness, deaf-mutism, gout, epilepsy or feeble-mindedness.

Although the laws of inheritance are not clear as regards many diseases, it is certain that the method is not haphazard. Mendel, an Austrian monk, showed that some of the characters which are passed on to progeny are what he called dominant, and appear in hybrids, while others are recessive and, although not evident in hybrids, become so in their progeny among which quite definite proportions can be predicted to possess the dominant or the recessive character. This he demonstrated in peas, and it has been found true for other plants and animals, and in human beings with regard to such characters as the colour of the eyes and hair.

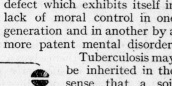

Hybrids resulting from the union of two species show the dominant character (black). But the recessive character (white) appears in their offspring

Sufficient evidence exists for the working of Mendel's laws in some diseases, deaf-mutism, for instance, and it has been suggested that in haemophilia and colour blindness, which may be inherited from a grandfather through a mother who does not manifest the abnormality herself, the abnormality may be a recessive character for a female but dominant for a male.

The inheritance of a character not exhibited by the immediate ancestors, but by one more remote, is described as atavism. It is sometimes asserted that when a female has been mated with more than one male, the progeny by sires subsequent to the first resemble the latter, but this phenomenon, which is described as telegony, is hardly possible.

Another assertion which has been made is that a normal person who has become mentally deranged from alcoholism can transmit his insanity to his progeny. This implies the possibility of the inheritance of

an acquired character. Weismann declared such a thing impossible on the ground that the germ plasm out of which new individuals are developed is itself completely and finally differentiated from the rest of the body at birth, and so could not be given new characters during the lifetime of the individual in whose body it was, but could merely be handed on as a sexual cell to start a new generation. This is the doctrine of the continuity of the germ plasm. It has been found that it does not hold for some lowly creatures, but is thought to be true in the main for such a highly organised creature as man.

The explanation of insanity in the progeny following alcoholism in the parent is that the want of control in the latter is itself due to mental defect which exhibits itself in lack of moral control in one generation and in another by a more patent mental disorder. Tuberculosis may be inherited in the sense that a soil peculiarly susceptible to the growth of the tubercle bacillus is transmitted, but of much greater importance in the genesis of this disease is the opportunity for the infection of young children who are living with consumptive parents, or who drink tuberculous cows' milk. There may be a similar proclivity of tissues to cancer, but here again irritation of some kind is of much more importance in the causation of the disease. Children are born suffering from syphilis— inherited syphilis—which simply means that the sexual cells out of which they develop have been infected, or that infection of the foetus or embryo has taken place ; this is quite a different thing from the inheritance of a constitutional peculiarity like colour blindness or gout.

A distinction must be drawn between inherited disease and a family disease, as, while constitutional tendency may be inherited and manifested by several members of a family, the fact that the same disorder affects several members of a family does not mean that it has been inherited from forbears. Amaurotic familial idiocy, a disease peculiar to Jews, is a case in point, and the same applies to other disorders.

There would appear to be a danger to the race from the inheritance of disease; a multiplication of the numbers suffering from such diseases and an increase in the number of those affected with mental disorder, for example, has been cited as an instance of the effect of the law of inheritance. Hesitation must be shown in accepting statistics which indicate such an increase, however, as it may simply be that by more accurate diagnosis more cases of a particular disease are recognized. Again, even should there actually be an increase in the incidence of a disease, it may be due to environmental effects rather than to inheritance. In any case, the race is protected from severe consequences of the law of inheritance by the working of what is called the law of anticipation. This is that heritable diseases manifest themselves at an increasingly early age in successive generations so that legatees of such diseases come to die before they have an opportunity of transmitting the disease in question.

Whenever it is possible for a child to have inherited a disease, the greatest care should be taken so to adjust its life that things likely to evoke the symptoms of the disorder, or aggravate them, should be eliminated as far as possible. If a child may inherit mental instability, for example, school work should not be excessive either in quantity or quality, and the life-work selected should be such as will impose the minimum of stress and worry. If a gouty tendency may have been inherited, the diet should be such as is suitable for gout (*q.v.*) though it must be observed that even then it may be impossible to prevent the emergence of symptoms of this disease.

See Constitution; Disease.

HERNIA. The protrusion of an organ through the wall of the cavity in which it is contained is called a hernia. Thus, from a wound in the skull a hernia of the brain may occur; from one in the chest wall, a hernia of the lung; or from one in the scrotum, a hernia of the testicle. There are three naturally weak spots in the anterior abdominal wall through which a hernia, or rupture, may occur. These are the umbilicus, or navel; the crural canal, a short passage about an inch long lying on the inner side of the femoral vessels (*q.v.*); and the inguinal canal in the groin, which exists for the passage of the spermatic cord in the male, and the round ligament of the womb in the female.

A weak scar on the abdominal wall, following an operation, for appendicitis for instance, will probably be the site of a ventral hernia. There are other cavities in the abdominal walls into which an organ may push its way, and as some of these are on the posterior wall, the protrusion would not be visible and would constitute an internal hernia.

The organ protruded in an abdominal hernia is usually a loop of bowel (enterocele), but it may be a piece of omentum (epiplocele), the bladder, an ovary, or some other organ. Whatever is protruded derives coverings from the peritoneum lining the abdomen and from the other layers of the wall, all together forming what is called the sac of the hernia.

Hernias Which are Congenital

From imperfection at the navel a hernia here may be congenital, and this may happen also in the inguinal canal from the non-closure of the processus vaginalis, the protrusion of peritoneum, in shape resembling the finger of a glove, which accompanies the testicle in its descent into the scrotum.

Despite its name, a congenital hernia is rarely actually present at birth, but appears very shortly afterwards. Other peculiarities may account for a congenital hernia, or make it easier to acquire one in later life. When the condition occurs on both sides of the body, such as a double inguinal hernia, the existence of a congenital structural weakness is in the highest degree probable. Undue strain is liable to cause rupture, and this may be incidental to many occupations and to the pains of childbirth. A severe cough carries the same danger, as does chronic constipation.

A rupture is usually accompanied by pain, and there may be also a feeling of weakness in the part and perhaps symptoms of indigestion. A lump appears, but this can usually be reduced, or caused to disappear. Frequently an inguinal hernia gets no further than the inguinal canal, when it is called a bubonocele, but if it makes its way through the external ring into the scrotum, it is a scrotal hernia. It is noteworthy that while young males are particularly liable to inguinal hernia, a femoral hernia usually occurs in a woman over twenty-five years of age.

An irreducible hernia is one that cannot be returned into the abdomen by ordinary manipulation, or taxis, as this is called. Sometimes the sac and perhaps also the contents become inflamed, following on some injury, and there is a probability that adhesions will be left by the inflammation and prevent the hernia from being reduced. A more serious risk is that of strangulation from the neck of the hernia being nipped or compressed, so interfering with the blood supply, and in the case of the bowel, the passage of its contents. This causes severe pain, shock and probably vomiting, the symptoms in fact of obstruction (q.v.) of the bowels.

In infancy a hernia can generally be cured by wearing a truss (q.v.) ; the same treatment should be adopted for elderly people, or when, owing to some other disease, an operation is out of the question ; otherwise treatment by operation or what is known as the radical cure, is to be recommended. Should any difficulty in reducing a hernia occur, the matter may be simplified if the patient lies on his back and bends his thighs. The greatest gentleness must be used in handling the hernia.

Hot applications should not be used for pain, which may occur at this time, but iced cloths, or an ice-bag, if left on for some minutes, will not only diminish suffering, but may facilitate the reduction of the hernia.

A doctor should always be called, however, and if there is any sign of strangulation, an immediate operation is necessary.

A ventral hernia may be curable by operation, but if such is not undertaken, a properly fitted belt, with a suitable pad, should be worn.
    See Abdominal Belt ; Femoral Vessels ; Truss.

HEROIN. Diamorphine, diacetyl morphine, or heroin is prepared from morphine, and is generally used in the form of the hydrochloride, a white crystalline powder. It is useful in allaying a troublesome cough, but is a dangerous drug as a habit for it is easily formed, and this produces the same physical, moral and mental degeneration as the morphine habit.
    See Opium.

HERPES. The blisters that sometimes form about the margin of the mouth in those suffering from a common cold, pneumonia, and other disorders, are called febrile herpes, the term herpes being applied to clusters of blisters or vesicles forming on reddened skin or mucous membrane (*see* Plate XXXI, 5). Some children suffer from herpes on the cheeks, which recurs in spring and autumn, or perhaps oftener, and leaves scarring. Herpes may also occur on the genital organs, male and female ; as regards the latter, they appear usually in connexion with menstruation. All of these are examples of simple herpes, and are treated by soothing applications, such as zinc ointment or calamine lotion, and perhaps by giving quinine sulphate, $\frac{1}{4}$ to 1 grain thrice daily.

In a more serious disorder, known as herpes zoster, zona or shingles, the blisters form along the course of a sensory nerve, most frequently an intercostal nerve. There may first be smarting pain along the nerve, suggesting pleurisy or some other deep-seated disorder, and then patches of reddened skin appear on which clusters of vesicles form, the contents of which are at first clear, but become turbid. In about a fortnight they have dried up. There is considerable pain throughout, and this may be of serious moment to elderly persons, and, moreover, such may continue to be troubled with neuralgic pain long after the herpes has disappeared.

A person who suffers from herpes zoster will very often be found to have been in contact with one suffering from chicken-pox, and possibly the causative germ may be the same in the two disorders.

Before the blisters have ruptured the patches may be painted with collodion ; otherwise sedative and antiseptic ointments or lotions are applied. Aspirin is given in 10-grain doses to relieve pain ; opiates are sometimes needed, however. Intramuscular injections of the patient's own blood may be of great service.

A separate mention should be made of herpes zoster affecting the supra-orbital branch of the ophthalmic or first branch of the trigeminal nerve. Here the blisters may form not only on the forehead and eyelids, but on the eyeball itself, and this may leave opacities on the cornea, or even lead to inflammation within the eye and, possibly, to its complete destruction. Besides treatment for the skin as mentioned above, the eye must be frequently bathed with boracic lotion and the pupil kept dilated with atropine, but this serious disorder, and, in fact, all cases of herpes zoster, require expert supervision.

See Chicken-pox ; Dermatitis.

HEXAMINE. Formerly called urotropine, hexamine is an efficient urinary antiseptic when given in doses of 5 to 15 grains, but can only act in an acid urine. If, therefore, the urine is alkaline, 15 to 30 grains of the acid phosphate of sodium is given with each dose of hexamine. The drug acts by liberating formaldehyde in the urine. In retention of urine in locomotor ataxia and other nervous diseases a dose of hexamine may help to empty the bladder.

HICCOUGH. The cause of hiccough, or hiccup, is a spasmodic contraction of the diaphragm, or midriff, producing a deep intake of breath, which is suddenly checked by closure of the glottis. It can usually be cured by such simple expedients as holding the breath as long as possible, drinking from the far side of a glass while stooping forward and holding the breath, holding the arms above the head until tired, putting a pinch of salt on the back of the tongue or by a dose of bicarbonate of soda, bismuth carbonate or rhubarb and magnesia. If such means fail to secure relief a doctor should be consulted.

Persistent hiccough is sometimes a symptom of encephalitis lethargica (*q.v.*).

HIP. The part of the thigh just below the buttock is described as the hip. The hip joint is a ball and socket joint, and is formed by the rounded head of the femur (*q.v.*), or thigh bone, sinking into the cupshaped depression, or acetabulum, on the side of the haunch, or innominate, bone. The greater depth of this cavity, as compared with the corresponding one on the

shoulder-blade, is due to the fact that while the freest movement possible is wanted at the shoulder joint, at the hip joint security is all-important.

The joint is surrounded by a capsular ligament which encloses the neck of the femur wholly in front, but only for about half its length behind, so that, from this point of view, a fracture of the neck of the femur can be either intra-capsular or extra-capsular, according to whether it is divided above or below the attachment of the capsule. The capsule is strengthened by various bands, a very important one being the ilio-femoral ligament, or

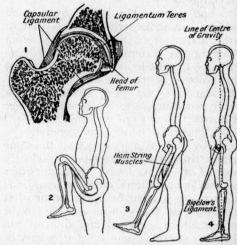

Hip. 1 : Section of joint capsule. 2 and 3 : Flexion at the hip limited by the abdomen and by the hamstrings when leg is extended. 4 : Bigelow's ligament limits backward bending of the trunk

Y-shaped ligament of Bigelow, which is situated in front and owes the second of these names to the fact that as it passes to be attached to the femur it divides into two diverging limbs.

Besides these external ligaments there is another, the ligamentum teres, a round ligament, which is attached to the head of the femur and to the bottom of the acetabular cup. Although its range of movement is less than that of the shoulder joint, the hip joint permits movement in all directions.

In a dislocation of the hip the head of the bone may travel backwards and upwards, backwards and downwards, forwards and upwards, or forwards and downwards. The first is called a dorsal, the second a sciatic, the third a pubic, and the last, an obturator, dislocation. In the backward dislocations the limb is

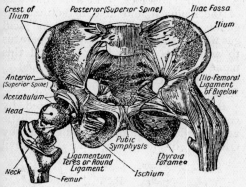

Hip. Ball and socket joint and its ligaments

rotated inwards and in the forward, outwards, the direction of the rotation being indicated by that towards which the toes point. Dislocation occurs usually in young vigorous men, as in elderly people violence tending to dislocate would probably fracture the neck of the femur.

In what is called a congenital dislocation (*see* illustration, page 221), the head of the femur may never have occupied the acetabulum. Up till five or six years of age a cure may be effected by what is called the bloodless method of Lorenz. The limb is abducted, with the head of the bone pressed into the acetabulum and kept in this position by an encasement of plaster of Paris. In older children a cutting operation is usually required.

By hip disease is meant tuberculous arthritis of the joint, although the hip may be the site of synovitis and arthritis from other causes, as described under the heading Joint. Hip disease practically always begins in childhood. A child begins to limp, and on examination it is found that the joint is stiff, the muscles around it being contracted in order to prevent movement and consequent pain. The affected limb looks lengthened, but this is owing to the fact that it is abducted at the hip, and the pelvis is tilted down-

wards, in order to make the sound limb parallel with the diseased one. The thigh is also flexed, but this is concealed by lordosis, or increase of the curve in the small of the back. There is also eversion of the foot, that is, the toes point outwards.

At a later stage the limb appears to be shortened, but only because the thigh is adducted, and the pelvis, therefore, tilted downwards towards the sound side, again in order to make the sound limb parallel with the diseased one. The thigh is still flexed, however, and this tends to increase as the disease progresses, but the toes now point inwards. At a still later stage, from destruction of the head of the bone and displacement from the acetabulum, the limb is actually shortened.

Until pain and other acute signs have moderated, and malposition is rectified, the patient is kept at rest in bed with the limb extended, but afterwards a Thomas's hip splint is applied to fix the joint, and the patient is allowed to get about in the open air with the help of crutches. The general treatment for tuberculosis (*q.v.*) is as necessary as local treatment.

See Dislocation ; Femur ; Fracture ; Joint.

HIVES. The term hives is used for a rash of the nature of urticaria, or nettle-rash (*q.v.*) but is not a good name, as it is also popularly applied to such varying conditions as croup, chicken-pox and catarrh of the bowel.

HOARSENESS. Imperfect apposition or tension of the vocal cords causes hoarseness and may be due to such different things as laryngitis, which is by far the commonest cause, and aneurysm of the aorta, by pressure on the recurrent laryngeal nerve.

See Croup ; Larynx ; Speech.

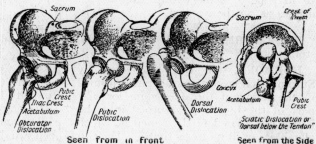

Seen from in front   Seen from the Side
Dislocation of the hip ; the femur can be forced out in four directions

HODGKIN'S DISEASE. The salient features of Hodgkin's disease, also called pseudo-leukaemia and general lymphadenoma, are a progressive enlargement of lymphatic glands all over the body, and a progressive anaemia. The disease, which is not a common one, is oftenest found in young males. The cause is not clearly understood, though many believe that tubercular infection is at the bottom of it. Certainly the course of the disease is suggestive of some infection, though at the same time the enlargements resemble new growths. In fact, the phenomena of Hodgkin's disease are usually cited as evidence for the probability of an infective causation of tumours.

The glands of the neck are usually the first to enlarge, and no others may be affected for several years. At some time, however, those in the armpits and groins are affected, besides other superficial glands and deep glands, including those in the chest and abdomen, the growth of which may press upon important organs and structures. The spleen also enlarges. The red blood cells are diminished to about 50 per cent., and the haemoglobin in the cells to about 40 per cent. There is more or less fever, and sometimes ague-like attacks. Coughing, shortness of breath, and pain may be caused by glandular growths in the chest. As time goes on general dropsy usually supervenes. The disease may run its course in a few weeks or stretch out over several years, and for months at the beginning, although glands are enlarged, the general health is not noticeably impaired. In treating the disease arsenic is the only drug which has any curative effect. In some cases the application of X-rays to the enlargements and to the bone marrow may be beneficial. It may be of some use to excise such masses as can be reached.

See Lymphatic System.

HOOKWORM DISEASE. *See* Ankylostomiasis.

HORMONE. It was discovered by Starling that a certain substance formed in the lining of the duodenum, or first part of the bowel, is absorbed into the blood and carried to the pancreas, which gland it excites to activity. Here a chemical substance has a similar action to an impulse coming through a nerve it is a chemical messenger, as it were and as such, is described as a hormone A similar substance formed in the wall of the stomach and able to activate its glands is called gastrin. Carbonic acid gas which excites the respiratory apparatus to activity is also a hormone, and this name now includes an endocrine (*q.v.*).

HOUSEMAID'S KNEE. *See* Bursitis Knee.

HOUSING. Ill-health is increased by congestion of population, by too little accommodation in the dwellings and by crowding dwellings together. The evi

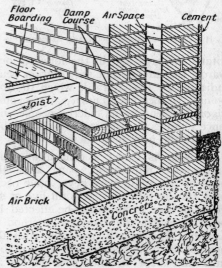

Housing. The foundations should be built on a layer of concrete and efficient ventilation ensured

effects would be mitigated to some extent were the dwellings and common passages constantly and thoroughly ventilated and did the inmates spend a large proportion of their working hours in the open air In the so-called back-to-back houses (Plate XIX) proper ventilation is impossible and the erection of such houses is now prohibited by the Housing Act of 1925.

Not only is a free supply of fresh air necessary but also as much sunshine as possible.

As ultra-violet rays of sunshine, which stimulate health while at the same time destroying micro-organisms, are unable to pass through ordinary window glass, the open window is as necessary for the full benefit of sunlight as of air.

The ground-floor rooms of houses, whether in town or country, are liable to be damp unless the house has been erected on a layer of cement or asphalt or has at least an efficient damp-proof course in its walls. Dampness may come through the walls at any level, however, and especially brick walls, from driving rain or in consequence of an overflow from rain-gutters or defective pipes. A brick, measuring 9 by 3 by 2¾ inches, can soak up and retain a pound of water. A dwelling, moreover, should be dry without the help of constant large fires. Dampness conduces to rheumatism and to chest complaints.

A further advantage of a layer of cement or asphalt beneath a dwelling is that it keeps ground air from rising into it. The interstices of soil are filled either with ground-air or ground-water. At a variable depth below the surface of the ground this water is encountered and it is what is sought to be tapped when a well is sunk. If the depth is less than 10 feet the site is unsuitable for a house and preferably the depth should be from 15 to 20 feet. Heavy rain may cause the level of the water to rise and this will force the ground-air upwards and possibly into dwellings. As the water-level falls air is again drawn into the soil.

It is the movement of ground-air that renders unsuitable what is called a made-up soil, especially one containing faecal or other animal or vegetable refuse, as the products of the decomposition of such substances are mixed with the air. Model by-laws prohibit the use of made-up soil containing such substances for the site of dwellings.

If a site for a house can be selected it should be on an elevation, with the ground falling away on all sides, and preferably on sand or gravel as water quickly drains off from these. Clayey soils are bad unless efficiently drained, and it must be noted that a few feet of sand or gravel on a sub-soil of clay may be as bad as clay itself, unless there is good drainage. Chalk is dry but colder than sand.

If a house can be made to face south east or south-west so much the better for the prospect of a sufficient supply of sunlight for living rooms at the front and of coolness in larders at the back. Rooms should be at least 8½ feet high but need not be more than say 10 feet; if higher there is apt to be a layer of " dead " air on the top. Underground rooms must conform with certain legal requirements to be usable as dwellings.

A chimney is necessary in a room for ventilation unless this is otherwise provided for.

The open fire is objectionable owing to its product of smoke from the raw fuel at present in use; this subject is discussed under the heading Fog. Gas fires have much to recommend them but there should be a free exit for escaping gases. This also applies to anthracite and other stoves; a defect in an anthracite stove may be very dangerous by allowing the escape of carbon monoxide into a room. Charcoal braziers are dangerous unless the ventilation is very free. Electrical heating is admirable but expensive. Electric lighting is better than gas lighting in that the latter pollutes the air; glare should be mitigated, however, by appropriate bulbs or shades.

See Drains; Overcrowding; Ventilation; Water.

HUMERUS. The bone of the arm, or humerus, has an upper extremity, a body or shaft, and a lower extremity. The upper extremity consists of a smooth, rounded articular surface directed inwards, upwards and somewhat backwards, a prominence called the greater tuberosity on the outer side, and another prominence, the lesser tuberosity, in front. Between the tuberosities, which serve for the attachment of muscles,

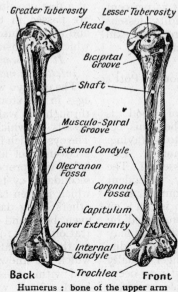

Humerus : bone of the upper arm

is a well marked groove for the long head of the biceps muscle. The junction of the upper extremity and shaft is called the surgical neck of the bone ; a fracture here may simulate a dislocation at the shoulder (*q.v.*).

The shaft is cylindrical in shape above but prismatic below. A shallow groove passing outwards and downwards on the posterior surface is known as the musculo-spiral or radial groove, as it is occupied by the nerve called by either of these names. This nerve may readily be injured in fractures through the shaft.

The lower extremity of the bone is widened out into two prominences, the internal and the external condyle, which, with the ridges above them, give attachment to muscles of the forearm (*q.v.*).

See Arm ; Elbow ; Fracture.

HUMIDITY. The amount of water-vapour present in air, or its humidity, has an important bearing on health. The amount of water-vapour which can be taken up by the air depends on the temperature of the latter ; the higher this is the greater the amount of water-vapour, but at any temperature there is a saturation point, and if the air is then cooled water-vapour is forced out in the form of dew or of rain. Humidity is tested by various kinds of instruments, and the most agreeable amount for healthy persons in temperate climates is about 75 per cent of saturation. Great humidity lessens evaporation of perspiration from the skin and causes depression of vitality.

See Air ; Climate ; Damp.

HUMP-BACK. *See* Backbone ; Pott's Disease.

HUNGER. A desire for food is described as appetite, but when this becomes so keen as to amount to a craving, the sensation is described as hunger. This occurs in fasting (*q.v.*) but passes off. The sensation is not necessarily dependent on the emptiness of the stomach, as it may occur when the stomach is full ; on the other hand it may be prevented by rectal feeding (*q.v.*) when the stomach may be empty for long periods without discomfort. An abnormal hunger usually suggests diabetes mellitus, but may occur in other conditions, for example, excessive secretion of gastric juice, hysteria and epilepsy. In duodenal ulcer (*q.v.*) there is often what is called a hunger-pain which can be relieved by taking food or alkalies.

See Appetite.

HYDATID DISEASE. In the liver and certain other organs of the human body, cysts containing a watery fluid may develop in connexion with the presence of the immature form of a flatworm, known as the taenia echinococcus. These hydatid cysts, as they are called, may attain a great size, specimens having been found to weigh as much as 30 pounds. Unless it presses on some important structure, a cyst, even though large, interferes little or not at all with health.

It may rupture, however, and if this should be into the peritoneal cavity, a fatal peritonitis will supervene. On the other hand, if the rupture should be into a bronchial tube or into the alimentary tract, and if suppuration does not occur, the living contents of the cyst die and are discharged. Suppuration may occur also even without rupture of the cyst ; or the worm may die spontaneously and the cyst shrivel up, possibly becoming calcified by the deposition of lime salts.

The mature worm is a tiny creature, about $\frac{1}{8}$th of an inch long, consisting of four segments including the one which carries the head. It inhabits the intestine of a dog or some allied animal. The eggs are passed in the excreta of the animal and may pollute water or fresh vegetables which are consumed by a human being.

It has been proved, also, that hydatid infestation may occur from kissing a dog.

The embryo worms are set free from the eggs in the stomach, and make their way through the walls of the latter into blood vessels by which they reach some organ. The cyst which forms on the organ acquires a covering of fibrous tissue, inside which is the wall proper of the cyst. Sometimes secondary cysts form within the first, which is then called the mother cyst, the others being daughter cysts ; there may even be grand-daughter cysts (*see* illustration, page 190). On the inner surface of the cyst-walls tiny projections occur, which are known as the brood capsules, and within these a variable number of heads of new worms are produced.

Hydatid cysts also form in sheep and other domestic animals, and by devouring parts of these, dogs ingest the young worms which attach themselves to the lining of the animals' bowel and in a few weeks reach the adult stage.

Hydatid disease is more prevalent in Australia and some other countries than in Great Britain, but as it may occur here, precautions must be taken against the risk of consuming water or vegetables, especially cress, contaminated with the eggs of the parasite. Should the existence of a cyst be recognized it should be removed by operation.

See Worm.

HYDRAGOGUE. Substances that drive water from the body are described as hydragogues. Croton oil, elaterium and jalap are examples of purgatives which are classed as hydragogues. Water may also be removed by giving diuretics to increase the amount of urine and diaphoretics to increase that of the sweat.

HYDRASTIS. The rhizome of golden seal, hydrastis canadensis, contains an alkaloid, hydrastine, which is bitter and constricts blood vessels. On account of its latter action the drug is sometimes used to check bleeding, especially that from the womb. Because it is bitter it is also sometimes used as a stomachic. It has a reputation in the treatment of chronic alcoholic gastritis when liquor has been given up. There is an official tincture, dose $\frac{1}{2}$ to 1 drachm, and a liquid extract, dose 5 to 15 minims.

HYDROCELE. The testicle is covered by a double layer of smooth membrane which forms a closed sac and is known as the tunica vaginalis. An accumulation of clear fluid in this sac is called a hydrocele, and exists as an elastic swelling in front of the testicle. An acute hydrocele accompanies acute inflammation of the testicle, but is usually of small size. A chronic hydrocele is common with a late syphilitic affection of the testicle. Usually, however, a hydrocele occurs from causes not properly understood, except that the testicle appears to be normal. This kind chiefly affects middle-aged men, and the fluid accumulates slowly. Other swellings in the scrotum have to be excluded before diagnosing a hydrocele, and notably hernia ; sometimes, in fact, these conditions may co-exist.

A common method of treating an ordinary hydrocele is to tap it at intervals of a few months. The fluid that runs away is straw coloured. This little operation causes but slight discomfort, as a rule ; a suspensory bandage should be worn in the intervals.

If, however, the patient wishes to avoid this repetition of tapping, he may submit himself to curative treatment. One procedure, which is not very satisfactory, generally speaking, is, after the withdrawal of the fluid, to inject some irritant, such as carbolic acid, into the sac, in order to inflame the inner surfaces and cause them to adhere, thus obliterating the sac. A better method, however, is to cut the sac away.

If the fluid from a hydrocele is milky, the condition is called chylous hydrocele. In tropical countries this is likely to be due to filariasis.

A hydrocele may also occur in the part of the tunica vaginalis in the spermatic cord, and forms a small elastic swelling in the groin ; a similar condition may occur in the female. Behind the upper part of the body of the testicle a cystic swelling known as hydrocele of the epididymis, or spermatocele, may occur from distension of a spermatic duct on one of the developmental vestiges which occur in this neighbourhood. The swelling is not large and can be readily taken away by operation. A cystic swelling, due to distension of lymphatic spaces in the neck or the breast, is sometimes referred to as a hydrocele, but the name is not a good one for such a swelling.

See Filaria ; Haematocele ; Testicle.

HYDROCEPHALUS. An excess of cerebro-spinal fluid in the skull, constituting hydrocephalus, or, as it is popularly called, water on the brain, is usually due to inefficient drainage of the fluid ; otherwise it is caused by excess in production. The fluid, which is derived from cells covering the choroid plexus of veins, normally passes into the ventricles or spaces within the brain, and flows backwards to the 4th ventricle, through openings in the roof of which it reaches the space beneath the arachnoid or middle covering of the brain. From this space it is drained off mainly by the large venous sinuses of the skull.

Hydrocephalus may exist at birth owing to maldevelopment of the parts concerned, or come on later from blocking of the drainage channel by inflammatory products or a tumour. If the onset is before the closure of the fontanelles, or spaces between the skull bones, that is to say, before the end of the second year, the cranium may become very much enlarged by the pressure of the fluid. This, however, also makes room for itself inside the ventricles by compressing the brain substance, and, in later life, when the bony case is firm, an increase of fluid can only exist by compression of the brain. If there is much compression the mental faculties are likely to be impaired.

Slight cases of hydrocephalus are best left alone, but in severe cases an operation should be considered. If there is an interruption in the flow of fluid from the brain into the subarachnoid space a new opening may be made. The choroid plexus is sometimes removed, by which procedure excessive production of fluid would be remedied, but the operation is a very severe one. An operation cannot help if the fluid flows freely into and about the subarachnoid space but is not drained off from there. It may be possible to demonstrate the existence of obstructions by injecting sterilised air into the spinal canal and taking X-ray photographs.

See Brain.

HYDROCHLORIC ACID. Strong hydrochloric acid, which is sometimes referred to as spirit of salt, is a corrosive substance and when swallowed causes serious symptoms, which, with the appropriate treatment, are discussed under the heading Acid.

Hydrochloric acid is a normal constituent of gastric juice, 0·2 to 0·4 per cent. being present. Dilute hydrochloric acid, in doses of 5 to 20 minims, is often useful therefore in dyspepsia, particularly when this depends on a deficiency of the natural acid or on sluggishness of the liver.

HYDROCYANIC ACID. Also known as prussic acid, hydrocyanic acid exists in nature in certain plants, for example, in cherry-laurel leaves and in bitter almonds.

In small doses the dilute acid is used as a gastric and respiratory sedative and is also applied to the skin as a local sedative for itching. In other than small doses hydrocyanic acid is a deadly poison sometimes merely inhaling the strong vapour will give rise to serious symptoms. Emergency treatment, as described under the heading Almond, should be given at once.

HYDROGEN PEROXIDE. Differing from water by containing an extra atom of oxygen in the molecule, hydrogen peroxide gives off this extra oxygen when it comes into contact with organic tissues and other substances, and thus acts as a disinfectant, deodorant and bleaching agent. It is generally used in the form of the official solution in water, which should yield ten times its volume of oxygen.

When this is poured into a wound there is a brisk evolution of gas which may bring to the surface loose particles of clot, etc. As a lotion for wounds and ulcers, a mixture of equal parts of the official solution and water is generally used, but the solution may be used undiluted. This may also be dropped into discharging ears and into an ear blocked by wax, as it may soften and break up hard plugs.

Diluted with three parts of water, the solution of hydrogen peroxide makes a good mouth wash, and is especially useful for cleansing the mouth during fevers. With an equal amount of water which has been boiled and is still warm, it makes a good application for chilblains, used as a lotion for about 15 minutes twice daily.

Hair that is to be bleached with the solution should first be washed thoroughly with soap and water to get rid of grease. The solution is then rubbed in until the hair assumes the required tint, after which it is washed with plain water.

Sodium peroxide gives off hydrogen peroxide when mixed with water, and is used by dentists for cleaning carious teeth. Ozonic ether, a solution of hydrogen peroxide, is used for the same purpose and, in conjunction with tincture of guaiacum, is commonly used to test for blood in urine.

HYDRONEPHROSIS. A sudden, complete obstruction to the flow of urine from a kidney, as when a stone completely blocks the ureter, stops the secretion of urine by the kidney altogether ; but a gradual and incomplete obstruction causes hydronephrosis ; that is, a dilatation of the pelvis and calices of the kidney. If the obstruction is in the urethra the bladder is first dilated, and then by continued back pressure hydronephrosis occurs, affecting both kidneys.

If the obstruction is in a ureter, on the other hand, hydronephrosis only occurs on this side. The obstruction may be due to partial blocking of the ureter by a stone, to kinking of the tube, or to pressure from the outside. The dilated kidney forms a cystic swelling which may be of large size, and the ureter may also be widely dilated, so much so as to resemble a piece of intestine. From time to time there may be the discharge of a large quantity of urine, with a corresponding decrease in the size of the swelling. Sometimes the contents of the swelling become purulent, constituting a pyonephrosis.

Treatment of hydronephrosis is directed to removing the cause, if possible. Frequently, however, the affected kidney must be removed.

See Bladder ; Kidney.

HYDROPHOBIA. Known as rabies when it occurs in dogs or other lower animals, hydrophobia is caused by a micro-organism, not yet identified, which is contained in the saliva of a person or animal suffering from the disease and inoculated into a fresh subject by a bite. The infection passes up the nerves until it reaches the brain, when, sooner or later, symptoms make their appearance. The time elapsing between the bite and the manifestations of the disease is usually from one to three months, but it may be shorter or, it is stated, considerably longer. It varies with the distance of the site of the bite from the brain, so that the disease would be likely to appear much sooner, for example, after a bite on the face than after one on the leg.

Thanks to the quarantine imposed on dogs entering Great Britain, rabies is practically unknown nowadays, and therefore there is no hydrophobia.

Should, however, a dog that has bitten anyone behave queerly, it should not be destroyed at once, but be kept isolated and chained up. If it is suffering from rabies it will be dead within ten days ; if it survives this period, a bitten person need have no fear of hydrophobia.

A dog suffering from rabies becomes morose, irritable and restless, and seeks to bite other dogs, large or small, even although it may have been timid previously. It tends to wander from home. It loses appetite, though it may exhibit a desire to gnaw at mats, woodwork or rubbish of any kind. It does not display any dread of water, as an infected human being does ; on the contrary it drinks greedily so long as it can swallow.

Symptoms of the Infection in Man

The first signs of the disease in a human being are apprehension, restlessness and slight difficulty in swallowing, with a slight rise in temperature. After a time any attempt at swallowing produces very powerful spasms of the muscles of the mouth and larynx, with great difficulty in breathing. The patient therefore develops that terror of water which is implied in the name of the disease, and even the thought of water may bring on a paroxysm, as may noises or even a breath of air on the skin. Saliva cannot be swallowed, so it runs from the mouth, which is kept open. There are attacks of extreme restlessness and sometimes the patient becomes maniacal. This goes on for from about thirty-six hours to three days, after which spasms disappear, unconsciousness supervenes, and in from six to eighteen hours from the onset of this paralytic stage the patient dies.

If there is any possibility that an animal that has bitten someone is rabid, the wound should be cauterised with a red hot wire, or be treated with undiluted carbolic acid or a similar disinfectant.

This cauterisation should be done as soon as possible ; if not done within twenty-four hours after the bite it is probably useless.

It is desirable that treatment should be carried out by a doctor. The matter should be reported at once to the medical officer of health or to the police. Antirabic treatment by vaccines is carried out in Great Britain at St. Thomas's Hospital, London, and should be obtained if the biting animal proves to be rabid.

HYDROTHORAX. The presence of dropsical fluid in the pleural cavity is described as hydrothorax. The fluid, which is clear and watery, is transuded from the blood vessels apart from the inflammatory conditions which cause the accumulation of fluid in a " wet " pleurisy. Hydrothorax may occur when the heart is failing, when a tumour in the chest obstructs the circulation through the veins, in Bright's disease and in other conditions. If the pressure of the fluid is injurious, it may be removed by tapping, but the underlying condition must be attended to in any case.

See Dropsy ; Pleurisy.

HYGIENE. The science of health, hygiene is concerned with the personal habits, such as exercise, rest, feeding and the like, which promote or, on the other hand, diminish health ; and also with questions of housing, sanitation, disinfection, quarantine, water supplies and kindred subjects included in the scope of Public Health. Although the duties in connexion with these larger questions mainly devolve on Public Authorities, much help can often be given by the private citizen.

See Baths ; Cleanliness ; Clothing ; Diet ; Disinfection ; Drains ; Exercise ; Fatigue ; Housing ; Mental Hygiene ; Ventilation ; Water.

HYOID BONE. A small, slender bone, shaped rather like a horseshoe, the hyoid is situated between the lower jaw and the larynx (*q.v.*). The part corresponding to the bend of the shoe, and known as the body, is in front. and from this two processes. the greater horns, project backwards. On the upper surface of the body are two short, pointed projections, the lesser horns, from the tip of each of which the stylo-hyoid ligament passes upwards and backwards to the tip of the styloid process of the temporal bone of the skull.

From the hyoid muscles pass up to the tongue (*q.v.*) to carry out some of its movements, and to enable these to come into action the hyoid bone is fixed by muscles which rise up to it from the breast bone and the thyroid cartilage of the larynx. Owing to its relatively loose connexion to other bones, the hyoid is rarely broken, but this may happen from violent squeezing of the neck.

HYOSCINE. Various species of plant belonging to the natural order solanaceae contain the alkaloid hyoscine, also called scopolamine, or the alkaloid hyoscyamine, or both. These alkaloids are chemically related to atropine (*q.v.*), which they also resemble in their actions, more or less. Hyoscine, generally used as the hydrobromide, is more depressant, however, and is used to reduce cerebral excitement in mania and other disorders. Combined with morphine it is sometimes administered to women in labour in order to bring about the condition commonly referred to as twilight sleep, by which the memory of the suffering undergone in childbirth is abolished or, at any rate, much blunted.

Hyoscyamine, generally used as the sulphate, is also more depressant than atropine, but less so than hyoscine, and less efficacious, therefore, as a sedative. Its chief use is to dilate the pupil for examination of the eye ; it acts more quickly than atropine.

HYOSCYAMUS. *See* Henbane.

HYPERACIDITY. An excessive secretion of gastric juice is called hyperacidity. This is also meant now by the term hyperchlorhydria, the idea of an excessive amount of hydrochloric acid in the juice, implied by this term, having been abandoned, at any rate for all practical purposes. Hyperacidity may occur in a temporary derangement of digestion and is usual in chronic gastritis and when there is a gastric or a duodenal ulcer. It has something to do with the so-called hunger pain of duodenal ulcer, as the pain can be relieved by giving alkalies to neutralise the acidity. Hyperacidity also causes heartburn and acid eructations. Gastroxia is the name given to hyperacidity when it occurs in paroxysms.

A powder consisting of 10 grains of bismuth carbonate, 15 grains of sodium bi-carbonate and 20 grains of magnesium carbonate is useful in hyperacidity, but the actual cause should be determined.

See Acidity ; Digestion ; Indigestion.

HYPERAEMIA. An increased amount of blood in an organ or tissue is called hyperaemia. This is said to be active when there is an increased supply of arterial blood, and passive, when the blood accumulates from slowness in the venous flow. Active hyperaemia occurs in acute inflammation and is often induced artificially by mustard or some other counter-irritant in order to increase the nourishment of the part to which the blood is drawn, or to withdraw it from some congested part. Passive hyperaemia may be induced by an elastic bandage, applied sufficiently firmly to retard the venous flow without obstructing the arterial flow, and known as a Bier's bandage, or by cupping. The objects are the same as those mentioned above.

See Bier's Method ; Congestion.

HYPERAESTHESIA. When merely to touch a part causes a painful sensation, hyperaesthesia is said to exist. This not uncommonly occurs on the scalp, for example, in women at the menopause, and in gouty persons. In hysteria hyperaesthetic areas may occur on different parts of the body, especially below the breast, or the lower part of the abdomen and on the back. Pressure on such a patch may induce a hysterical fit, in which case the patch is said to be hysterogenetic. A general hyperaesthesia all over the body of a young child warrants a suspicion of the onset of rickets.

When a painful sensation is in excess of the cause, a sharp stabbing sensation from a mere prick of a pin, for example, the condition is called hyperalgesia.

See Sensation.

HYPERMETROPIA. Popularly regarded as long sight, hypermetropia is really weak sight, that is, a diminished power of focussing objects on the retina without calling in the aid of the ciliary, or focussing, muscles. This leads to eye strain and requires convex lenses for its correction.

See Eye.

HYPERPIESIS. For the proper circulation of the blood a sufficient degree of blood pressure (*q.v.*) is necessary. Clinically the blood pressure is estimated by an instrument called a sphygmomanometer, which is generally used on a brachial artery. It is estimated in terms of millimetres of mercury which it would support, in the same way as air pressure is measured in a mercurial barometer, though the sphygmomanometer may be of an aneroid type, like some barometers. The blood pressure in the brachial artery is found to vary normally from about 130 millimetres of mercury at twenty years of age to 140 in those above forty years of age.

An increased pressure, judged according to what is usual at the person's age, is described as hyperpiesis. This may be a temporary occurrence, as during excitement or muscular exertion. It may occur, for example, merely from excitement due to the fact that a doctor is applying a sphygmomanometer. Some people are found to have hyperpiesis, on the one hand, or an unusually low blood pressure, on the other, for years without apparent effects on health. Hyperpiesis, however, in conjunction with weakening of the arterial walls, involves a risk of rupture of the vessels, such weakening being caused, as a rule, by micro-organisms or their poisons.

Hyperpiesis leads in time to hypertrophy of the heart and of the muscle coat of the arteries. About middle age hyperpiesis may occur and be associated with indefinite illness, but the increased pressure may not be dependent on kidney disease or narrowing of the blood vessels by arterio-sclerosis (*q.v.*). The condition underlying this rise of blood pressure, or hyperpiesis, is called hyperpiesia. It can be remedied by taking a simple diet, moderate in amount, and sufficient open-air exercise. It is important, also, to get rid of worries, including worry over the increased blood pressure, should this fact be known to the patient. The bowels should be kept open. Bromides are often useful.

See Blood Pressure ; Bright's Disease ; Circulation of the Blood.

HYPERPYREXIA. When fever exceeds 105·8° F. there is said to be hyperpyrexia. This amount of fever is dangerous in itself if it continues for any length of time, and means must be taken to lower it, by cold sponging, a cold pack or iced applications.

See Fever.

HYPERTROPHY. Growth of an organ or tissue beyond what would be proportionate to that of the body generally is called hypertrophy. The arm muscles of the blacksmith and the leg muscles of the racing cyclist are examples of hypertrophy due to the exceptionally vigorous exercise of a tissue. Similarly, if a hollow organ with muscular walls is impeded in discharging its contents, the wall becomes thickened by hypertrophy of the muscle. This happens to the bladder, for example, when the outflow of urine is obstructed by an enlarged prostate or a stricture of the urethra, and to a piece of bowel behind any obstruction.

The heart muscle becomes hypertrophied when the outflow from its chambers is impeded by stenosis of a valve, narrowing of the peripheral arteries or other kinds of obstruction. The increased thickness of the walls of the heart may not be entirely due to new muscle, however, but in part to a new formation of fibrous tissue, and to the extent to which this occurs there is a weakening of the wall, as the fibrous tissue does not contribute to the force of the beat.

Degenerative diseases of muscles occur in which a muscle may become enormously enlarged, but at the same time be much enfeebled, because the enlargement is mainly due to a deposit of fatty tissue. This is described as pseudo-hypertrophy.

In some instances a compensatory hypertrophy occurs. Thus, if one kidney is lost, the other tends to increase in size to enable it to carry on the duty of the kidney that is lost.

Intermittent pressure causes hypertrophy, an ordinary corn being an instance of this. A corn consists of a hypertrophy of the horny layer of the skin due to intermittent pressure by a badly-fitting boot. Constant pressure, on the other hand, causes atrophy (*q.v.*).

HYPNOTIC. A drug that induces sleep is described as a hypnotic or soporific. To this group belong the bromides, chloral, sulphonal, trional, veronal, paraldehyde and allied preparations. Narcotic drugs, such as alcohol and opium, also act as hypnotics, but cause a preliminary excitement ; they can also induce sleep in spite of the presence of pain. The treatment of chronic insomnia by drugs is fraught with grave danger of forming a drug habit.

See Insomnia.

HYPNOTISM. There is no mystery about hypnotism nor is it due to anything of the nature of animal magnetism, as was thought about it when it was known as mesmerism. Its phenomena depend entirely upon suggestion. The operator suggests to the patient that he feels sleepy and he becomes so, that he is asleep and to all appearance he is, though he remains susceptible to the operator's voice and to further suggestions from him.

If the sleep is deep the patient remembers nothing of what takes place during it. Nevertheless, while in this condition he can remember things that have happened, including dreams, the memory of which has been repressed and apparently forgotten. Also, if he receives a suggestion to do something at some particular time after he has awakened from the hypnosis he will do it, although unable to give any reason for doing it.

The ability to expose the unconscious mind makes hypnotism a useful method of discovering repressed ideas or experiences which may be exerting an injurious effect on health, and of dealing with dissociation states, such as dual personality, as by treatment during hypnosis the forgotten or unknown experiences can be remembered by the patient in his waking state, and thus be related to his conscious personality.

The ability to influence conduct during the waking state makes hypnosis sometimes a useful method of dealing with drug-addiction, dipsomania or other injurious habits or impulses. Insomnia may be cured by hypnotic suggestion. Even the action of involuntary muscles may be affected, as, for example, those of the bowel, causing greater activity and thus curing constipation or, conversely, restraining activity and curing diarrhoea, when these disorders are due to nervous influences. Sometimes menstrual irregularities are susceptible of similar treatment. Anaesthesia for small operations, such as tooth-extraction, may be secured by hypnotic suggestion when there is a serious objection to ordinary anaesthetics.

Hypnosis should only be carried out under medical supervision and for purposes of diagnosis or treatment. If the operator is skilful and trustworthy, no harm can result. A person cannot be hypnotised against his will unless he has been hypnotised frequently already, nor, as a rule, will criminal suggestions be carried out if they are grossly repugnant. If a hypnotised person is not awakened by the operator, natural awakening will occur in a few hours.

See Auto-suggestion ; Double Consciousness ; Freudism ; Mind ; Psycho-therapy.

HYPOCHONDRIASIS. The healthy person pays little attention to the ordinary working of his organs. He chews and swallows and breathes without noticing, and so for other functions. A hypochondriacal person is excessively preoccupied with some one or more of his functions, and the conscious performance of a function which is usually done automatically, swallowing, for instance, readily gives rise to the idea that the function is not being done properly ; it is but a step to the further notion that there is some obstruction in the gullet or something of the kind.

The digestive apparatus is the most usual preoccupation of the hypochondriac, but it may be the bladder, the lungs, the heart, the head or some other organ. There is associated depression and perhaps sleeplessness. Sometimes the basis of the trouble may be some little disorder in the parts concerned which would not matter to any ordinary person.

The treatment of hypochondriasis is unsatisfactory. Patient persuasion of the groundlessness of the worry and an attempt to establish an interest in other things than his health may benefit a person suffering in a mild degree. Pyschotherapy of some other kind may sometimes help. There is always the possibility that the condition may progress and become melancholia, a condition in which attempts at suicide are to be seriously apprehended.

See Auto - Suggestion ; Mental Disease ; Psycho-therapy.

HYPOGASTRIUM. The lowest part of the abdomen, towards the middle line, is called the hypogastrium. It is bounded on either side by a line drawn vertically upwards from the mid-point of Poupart's ligament (*q.v.*), and above by a line connecting the most prominent part of each haunch bone. In this part are coils of small intestine and the beginning of the rectum, also the bladder in children, and, when it is full, in adults. When the bladder is distended it can be operated upon through the hypogastric part of the abdominal wall without opening the general peritoneal sac, a matter of some importance.

See Abdomen ; Bladder.

HYPOGLOSSAL NERVE. The twelfth pair of cranial nerves, known as the hypoglossal, which have their origin in the bulb, or medulla, supply the tongue muscles and some other muscles in the neck. If both nerves are paralysed the tongue cannot be protruded from the mouth, but it can be if one nerve only is affected, though then the tip is directed towards the paralysed side, being pushed in this direction by the muscles on the healthy side. The nerves reach the tongue from beneath.

See Brain ; Tongue.

HYPOPHOSPHITE. Salts of hypophosphorous acid, or hypophosphites, are largely used for their tonic properties, especially in nervous debility and wasting diseases. Sodium hypophosphite is official and is given in doses of 3 to 10 grains, but numerous other hypophosphites are in use, including those of ammonium, calcium, iron, magnesium, manganese, potassium, quinine and strychnine.

The compound syrup of hypophosphites, dose $\frac{1}{2}$ to 2 drachms, and the glycerol of hypophosphites, dose 1 drachm, contain a number of the hypophosphites, including those of iron, quinine and strychnine, and Fellow's syrup is said to have a similar composition. The syrup of hypophosphites contains only those of calcium, potassium and sodium with dilute hypophosphorous acid. The average dose is 2 drachms. The benefit derived from such preparations is ascribed, however, rather to the bases, that is, the iron, quinine, etc.; than to the hypophosphorous acid with which they are combined.

HYSTERIA. A young woman who becomes hilariously excited but mixes her laughter with tears is readily identified by anyone as being hysterical, but the manifestations of hysteria are by no means limited to displays of this kind, but may simulate a large number of different disorders. The tumultuous emotional state just mentioned, which is often accompanied by a feeling of a ball rising in the throat — the globus hystericus — and threatening to choke the patient, may be followed by a convulsive seizure, a hysterical fit.

Distinction Between Hysteria and Epilepsy

Sometimes this suggests an attack of epilepsy (*q.v.*) but is usually distinguishable by noting that the patient does not hurt herself in falling, though on some occasions she may do so, that she does not bite her tongue or void urine, and that the eyes are tightly closed, an attempt to open them being resisted, facts that point to the patient not being unconscious as she may appear to be. There is not the coma that follows an epileptic fit, though the patient may not remember the incidents of the fit; sometimes she can. It is sometimes very difficult, however, to determine the true nature of such convulsions.

On rare occasions in hysteria a fixed attitude is taken up, an example being what is called the crucifixion attitude in which the neck, back and lower limbs are rigidly extended while the arms are stretched out on either side. Another attitude is that of ecstasy (*q.v.*). A person suffering from hysteria may also pass into a trance or exhibit somnambulism or catalepsy.

Amongst other manifestations of hysteria the following may be enumerated : muscular paralysis, anaesthesia, loss of voice, deafness, blindness, eructations, persistent absence of appetite, retention of urine, attacks resembling angina pectoris, cough, and so on.

An investigation of these or of any symptoms of hysteria will reveal the fact, however, that there is no organic change to account for such symptoms. Hysterical paralysis may involve a limb or perhaps one half of the body—a hemiplegia. Amongst other signs distinguishing this hemiplegia from that due to an organic cause, say apoplexy, is that the gait (*q.v.*) is different. An hysterical hemiplegic drags the affected lower limb along instead of swinging it round. Again, an hysterical anaesthesia does not involve the area of a definite nerve, or nerves, but when a limb is affected, is of what is called the stocking or glove variety.

Similarly, as hysterical manifestations occur from no apparently adequate reason, a person who has been blind or deaf for years may suddenly recover the lost function, or a person who has been confined to bed for months because he was unable to walk or even stand, might leap from bed and run off, say, on an alarm of fire.

Though things may be so, however, it must not for a moment be imagined that an hysterical patient is a malingerer ; although there is no organic lesion there is a mental lesion, which is none the less definite. This lesion, which is described as dissociation, is seen most completely in the curious condition of dual personality, or double consciousness (*q.v.*). It is similar to what occurs in hypnotism (*q.v.*), in which state, for example, a suggestion that a limb is paralysed, or a part of the skin insensitive, would be acted upon. A hysterical person is extremely open to suggestion, especially such as is favourable to his view of his malady, and this includes auto-suggestion, such as is born of the patient's own thoughts and desires.

Simulation of Physical Disabilities

The genesis of dissociation is well illustrated by the soldier who, exposed to the perils and strain of the trenches, has an intense desire to get away from it all, but who represses the desire because of his sense of duty. He develops, however, hysterical paralysis of the legs, or it may be some other disability, incapacitating him for duty. The sort of person to whom this might happen is thought by many authorities to be already the victim of a mental conflict of which he was unconscious, a conflict dating from childhood, in which repressed desires, according to Freud of a sexual character, were pitted against an acquired standard of conduct.

It is the energy inherent in these childish repressions which directs the solution of the new conflict into such a conversion neurosis as paralysis, or into an anxiety state, marked by such symptoms as introspection, apprehension, tremor, palpitation, shortness of breath, sweating, headache, and so on.

Formerly, hysteria was treated by different kinds of suggestion, including the use of electrical apparatus and the unpleasant drugs asafoetida and valerian, and symptoms were doubtless often relieved, but in view of what is now known of the essential nature of the disorder it is clear that it cannot be satisfactorily treated without some kind of psycho-therapy. In hysteria there is a profound craving for sympathy and an injudicious, though natural, response to this by relatives will but aggravate the complaint. It may, therefore, be necessary to isolate the patient under the care of an intelligent nurse.

See Auto-suggestion ; Double Consciousness ; Epilepsy ; Freudism ; Pyscho-therapy.

ICHTHYOL. A tarry substance obtained by distilling mineral deposits containing fossil fish, ichthyol or ichthosulphol acts as an antiseptic and local sedative. It also causes contraction of the surface blood vessels when applied to the skin or a mucous membrane and, taken inwardly, it often relieves flushing during the menopause and in acne rosacea (q.v.). The dose is 10 to 30 grains a day, and it may be taken in pills, tablets, capsules or a mixture. It is also used internally for rheumatism and for some respiratory disorders. Pessaries or plugs containing it are used for female disorders, and suppositories for treating piles.

For external use, it may be included in a watery lotion, in an oily liniment, in a collodion, in a paste or an ointment. An ointment containing 30 per cent. may arrest the spread of erysipelas, and preparations containing 5 per cent. upwards may prove of benefit in eczema, psoriasis, pruritus, burns, chilblains and other disorders.

ICHTHYOSIS. Fish-skin disease, or ichthyosis, is an abnormality of the skin which is characterised by dryness and scaliness. It is inherited and is one of those diseases which may be transmitted by a mother who does not herself show evidences of it. It makes its appearance in the early months of life. Sometimes the scales are very small, the chief symptom being the dryness of the skin, a condition referred to as xeroderma ; but the scales may be larger and the skin have a dirty-grey colour, and in severer forms there may be thick accumulations of scales giving a blackish colour to the skin. The skin may have a resemblance to that of a reptile or a fish, a fact to which it owes its name. There is no itching.

The skin in front of the elbows and behind the knees is not affected and the face usually escapes. The general health is not affected.

The condition cannot be cured and persists throughout life. Much may be done, however, to mitigate the disorder by frequent warm baths and by keeping the skin greased. If there is thick scaliness soda baths are an advantage. Cold cream may be used as an emollient, or equal parts of salicylic acid ointment and glycerin of starch.

ICTERUS. Jaundice is also called icterus. Jaundice in the new-born, icterus neonatorum, is usually due to breaking down of excessive red blood corpuscles, but may result from septic infection of the umbilical cord or some other serious cause. The severe jaundice of phosphorus poisoning, or acute yellow atrophy of the liver, is sometimes called icterus gravis.

See Jaundice.

IDIOCY. The most deficient degree of mental development, idiocy, may be due to injury to the brain or its membranes in very early childhood. Sometimes it follows a succession of fits. In other instances it may exist from birth without any discoverable cause. It occurs with a very small head, say, one that is less than 17 inches in circumference and in some children who suffer from hydrocephalus (q.v.). Inherited syphilis has appeared to be responsible for other cases.

Idiocy is likely to occur when a child is born blind or deaf, or loses these senses shortly after birth, but such a child has been taught and, in fact, brought to a high degree of mental development. A curious complaint, amaurotic familial idiocy, in which blindness and progressive mental and bodily weakness occur, is usually found in Jews, and, as its name implies, several members of a family may suffer. Mongolian idiocy owes its name to the fact that in those affected the facial expression is of the Mongol type, with slanting eyes and flattened nose. The height is dwarfed, the hands and feet stumpy, and the tongue tends to protrude from the mouth.

In the idiocy of cretinism (*q.v.*) a very striking improvement follows the administration of thyroid extract. In other types very little can be done, and the victims die young.

See Feeble-minded ; Mental Disease.

ILIAC REGION. The portion of the abdomen on either side of the hypogastrium (*q.v.*) is called the iliac region, and it is so called because it lies in front of the ilium, the topmost part of the innominate, or haunch bone. The common iliac arteries, into which the abdominal artery subdivides half an inch below and somewhat to the left of the umbilicus, pass forward to the upper margin of the junction of the ilium with the sacrum, where they themselves divide into the internal and external iliac arteries, the former descending into the pelvis, and the latter continuing round the margin of the pelvis to emerge beneath Poupart's ligament, and become the femoral artery. These vessels are accompanied by veins, the two iliac veins uniting to form the inferior vena cava.

In the right iliac region lie the caecum and appendix, and in the left, a portion of the colon.

See Abdomen ; Groin ; Innominate ; Intestine.

ILLUSION. A misinterpretation of a sensory impression is called an illusion.

See Hallucination.

IMBECILITY. A degree of arrest of mental development intermediate between idiocy and feeble-mindedness is called imbecility.

See Feeble-minded.

IMMUNITY. The usual meaning attached to the word immunity when it is used as a medical term is insusceptibility to some infection. Not every class of animal is vulnerable to an infection which can work havoc in another. The dog and the domestic fowl, for example, are naturally immune to anthrax and lockjaw. Even in one class of animal,

individuals or strains are found to exhibit exceptional immunity to some infections ; amongst human beings, for example, a family may exhibit this freedom for such a disease as scarlet fever.

But, though an individual appears to be naturally immune to an infection, it may be possible to destroy this immunity in some way. Thus, a dog or a fowl may be successfully infected with lockjaw if first given a dose of alcohol, or a fowl with anthrax if it is made to stand for some time in cold water. The liability of a human being to contract a common cold after an overdose of alcohol or a chill is notorious, and so for other infections. Over-fatigue, starvation and other factors which lower the general vitality may also destroy immunity.

Natural and Acquired Immunity

Infection is due to some micro-organism securing a footing in the body, and immunity must depend on some condition, or conditions, in the body inimical to the invasion. If such exist from birth there is a natural immunity, but when this is absent immunity may be acquired in various ways. A person who has had smallpox, for example, is unlikely to take it again ; he has acquired immunity to this disease. Partial immunity may be acquired to other diseases, though the duration of the immunity, instead of being life-long, may last for a very short time, as in influenza, for example. Vaccination against smallpox may also confer immunity ; here the vaccinated person passes through an attack of cow-pox, a modification of the other disease. Again, immunity may be acquired by inoculations with killed disease-germs or their poisons, or with an antitoxin.

The normal resources of the body against bacterial invasion include the activity of the white cells of the blood and a bactericidal action of the serum, which appears to be derived from the white cells. The latter attack bacteria and devour them, on account of which they are often referred to as phagocytes, or cell-eaters. Without attempting to decide whether a special efficiency of these defences could confer natural immunity, it may be noted that in very many instances they are unable to prevent bacterial invasion.

Bacterial poisons, however, whether contained within the organism itself or set free by it, excite the body cells to produce various substances, collectively known as antibodies, which either neutralise the poisons or destroy the bacteria. One of these causes clumping or agglutination of germs ; another, called an opsonin, renders the germs more vulnerable to phagocytes ; and a third, called the immune-body, or amboceptor, in conjunction with complement, a substance normally contained in the blood, breaks up the germs.

It is the formation of such substances that enables a person to recover from the attack of some infection, and it is the persistence of some quantity of such substances that confers immunity against further attacks of the same kind of germ ; not of any other kind, as the antibodies are only effective against the particular germ, or antigen, as it is called, that has led to their production. Vaccines of dead bacteria or their poisons act as antigens, and provoke the formation of antibodies. They therefore create what is called an active immunity to an infection, as opposed to the passive immunity conferred by injections of an antitoxin, which only neutralises the bacterial poison.

With regard to some diseases a relative immunity may exist in various races or peoples. Thus, coloured people, although they suffer from malaria, do not sustain any damage commensurate with that inflicted by the same disease on white people. Similarly, measles and other diseases which have been endemic in a population for many generations have not the virulence that they manifest when they occur in a population which has previously been free from them.

See Antibody ; Antitoxin ; Serum Therapy ; Vaccine.

IMPERIAL DRINK. *See* Beverages.

IMPETIGO. A skin disease caused by infection with a streptococcus, impetigo chiefly affects children, and is usually found on exposed parts of the skin, and especially the face. Blisters form, and at first contain clear fluid, but this quickly becomes cloudy. After a short time the blisters burst, and their contents harden into yellow crusts which rather resemble beeswax. Each crust is surrounded by a narrow line of redness, and from beneath the crust clear fluid may escape, as this continues to ooze from the skin covered by the crust. There may be slight heat and itching, but otherwise there is no local disturbance, nor is the general health affected.

How the Infection is Spread

If the eruption occurs on the scalp, the hair is matted and bound down by the crusts, from beneath which foul-smelling pus, or matter, escapes. It will probably be found that the head is infested with lice. Infection spreads from any impetiginous lesion to sound skin, and the patient may bring this about by fingering a lesion and then touching other parts ; even the eyes or the inside of the nose may be infected. By contact with the patient, or with a towel or anything which has been in contact with him, healthy persons may acquire the disease. The scurfy patches on the face sometimes popularly referred to as tetter are due to the germ of impetigo, and infection may be derived from them. Another source is the fissure which sometimes forms behind an ear.

As washing with ordinary soap and water spreads the infection, it should be discontinued for a few days, and the lesions dusted with some such powder as the following :

Boric acid	60 grains
Zinc oxide	60 ,,
Powdered talc	to 480 ,,

Or a little of the following lotion may be dabbed on each spot :

Powdered calamine	60 grains
Zinc oxide	60 ,,
Precipitated sulphur	5 ,,
Glycerin	½ drachm
Water	to make 1 ounce

When the spots are dry, the separation of the crusts may be hastened by the application of an ointment consisting of one part of white precipitate ointment to three parts of zinc ointment. If there is difficulty in removing crusts, a starch poultice, described under the heading Eczema, should be applied.

A fissure behind the ear or about the lips or nostrils, which constitutes another form of subacute impetigo, should be painted with a one per cent. solution of silver nitrate. When the scalp is affected, the hair should be cut short, and white precipitate ointment applied.

See Eczema ; Louse.

IMPOTENCE. A man may be quite able for sexual intercourse but be impotent to procreate children. The reasons for this state of affairs are discussed under the heading Sterility. On the other hand, a man may be impotent in that he cannot undertake or complete sexual connexion. The penis may be unduly small or be deformed, one kind of deformity being incomplete closure of the floor of the urethra, or hypospadias, with an opening far back through which the contents of the urethra are discharged. Impotence from such causes is uncommon, however. Morbid changes in the corpora cavernosa, usually due to gonorrhoea, may also interfere with erectile power.

Debilitating diseases like diabetes mellitus and chronic Bright's disease are likely to cause impotence and possibly it will occur with obesity. Some diseases of the spinal cord, notably locomotor ataxia, are other causes. The excessive use of alcohol and, it is said, tobacco may have this effect, and addiction to morphine or other powerful narcotics for any length of time certainly has. Excessive sexual indulgence is followed by more or less incapacity for intercourse.

In many instances a functional nervous disorder, such as neurasthenia, is responsible ; here the impediment is psychical. A temporary impotence, also of psychical origin, is quite common just after marriage, but need cause no apprehension as it soon disappears.

Treatment must be guided by the circumstances in each case. Some kinds of deformity can be remedied by operation. Impotence due to excessive intercourse will probably disappear after a sufficient rest of the function, the general health being toned up meanwhile. No alcohol should be taken and tobacco should be used sparingly, if at all.

Quack advertisements should be ignored, as the nostrums they recommend are likely to be useless and may be dangerous.

If progress is not satisfactory a doctor should be consulted ; he will advise as to aphrodisiac drugs and as to the propriety of using them.

See Genital System ; Graft.

INCONTINENCE. Inability to prevent the escape of urine from the bladder or of faeces from the bowel is described as incontinence of the urine or faeces, respectively. The orifices concerned are normally kept closed by a circular ring of muscle fibres, a sphincter, which is innervated from a centre in the lumbar region of the spinal cord. A sufficient filling of the bladder or bowel to create a natural need for emptying sends a nerve impulse to this centre inhibiting its action, and thereby permitting the sphincter to relax.

Ordinarily, however, even when one is asleep, the higher centres in the brain are able to control this reflex mechanism for emptying the bladder or bowel, and prevent such taking place inconveniently. Incontinence may, however, occur during profound unconsciousness, especially when this is accompanied by muscular spasms ; it is therefore a common event in an epileptic seizure.

In what is called the typhoid state (*q.v.*), that is, one of great weakness occurring as a result of long-continued fever, etc., involuntary evacuation of the bladder and bowels is again common. In certain nervous diseases the spinal centre which maintains the activity may be weakened or destroyed, with resulting incontinence. Fright has often the effect of inhibiting this centre, and incontinence from this cause is well known.

Again, through injury or disease, the sphincter may be impeded or prevented from acting, or inflammation of the rectum or bladder may cause sufficient irritation to bring about evacuation in spite of all attempts at control.

See Urinal.

INDIAN HEMP. *See* Cannabis Indica.

INDIGESTION. When discomfort of some kind accompanies or follows a meal it is natural that it should be ascribed to indigestion, or dyspepsia. It may be a sense of weight or fullness in the pit of the stomach or actual pain, either of a dull, steady character or more acute and perhaps spasmodic. This may set in almost immediately or at a variable time after the meal has been taken. There may be a feeling of nausea or perhaps actual vomiting which may, or may not, relieve the pain or discomfort.

Sometimes there is a sharp, burning feeling at the lower end of the breast bone, described as heartburn or pyrosis, and this may be accompanied by the regurgitation of an acid, acrid liquid into the mouth, or water-brash. Sometimes flatulence (*q.v.*) is a troublesome symptom. The tongue may be furred and there may be a nasty taste in the mouth, and, perhaps, an unusually free flow of saliva. There may be headache and possibly giddiness also.

Indigestion a Symptom, not a Disease

It is not enough, however, merely to recognize the existence of indigestion because, in the first place, this may depend on different stomach disorders, demanding widely different kinds of treatment ; in the second place it may depend on disorders of digestive organs other than the stomach, or even on disorders not directly related to digestion at all ; and, in the third place, symptoms such as vomiting and pain in the pit of the stomach, which suggest indigestion, may in fact have nothing to do with this process.

In the first of these groups it will be necessary to distinguish symptoms due to mere functional derangement from those caused by gastritis, dilatation of the stomach, gastric or duodenal ulceration, cancer of the stomach, dropping of the stomach or gastroptosis, and other disorders noted under the heading Stomach or under special headings of their own. It may be pointed out, however, that when indigestion occurs in a middle-aged person who has not had previous trouble of the kind, and which resists ordinary treatment, it suggests cancer of the stomach.

In the second group, in which indigestion is due to disorders outside the stomach, mention may be made of cirrhosis of the liver, cholecystitis or inflammation of the gall bladder (*q.v.*), chronic appendicitis, chronic peritonitis, chronic nephritis, disease of the heart or lungs which causes congestion of the stomach lining, consumption, anaemia and so on. Or some mental condition, such as neurasthenia, hysteria or hypochondriasis, may underlie the symptoms of indigestion.

To the third group, that is, instances in which symptoms may be erroneously ascribed to indigestion, belong such events as vomiting due to brain tumours or other kinds of irritation of the brain, and the so-called gastric crisis of locomotor ataxia (*q.v.*).

In view of such a wide range of possible causes of symptoms of indigestion it is not possible to lay down any simple kind of treatment. It may be said, however, that if a person has too few teeth or has bad teeth, if he chews food insufficiently, if he is in the habit of taking too much food or food that is too rich, if he takes too much condiment, or alcohol, or uses too much tobacco, if he suffers from chronic constipation or takes too little open-air exercise, it is highly possible that by correcting such defects he may cure his indigestion.

See Acidity ; Appetite ; Charcoal ; Constipation ; Diet ; Digestion ; Digestive ; Fasting ; Gastritis ; Hyperacidity ; Liver ; Stomach.

INFANTILE PARALYSIS. The disease known as infantile paralysis is an acute inflammation of the grey matter forming the anterior horn of the spinal cord, what is scientifically described as an acute anterior poliomyelitis. It affects young children mostly, but occasionally occurs even in middle-aged people. It is caused by a filter-passing virus which invades the nose and throat, whence it makes its way along the spinal cord or, sometimes, to the brain. The disease is most prevalent in the hot months, and may occur as an epidemic.

The organism may exist in the secretion of the nose or throat of persons who show no signs of the disease, but who act as carriers. The onset is acute, with fever, perhaps headache and vomiting, and possibly convulsions. There may be pain and tenderness in one or more limbs, and in from one to three days it will be noted that the child has apparently lost the use of one or more limbs and in a short time the affected limbs will begin to waste. Sometimes the initial symptoms are so slight as to be overlooked or attributed merely to a slight chill, and the first thing to cause alarm is the paralysis and wasting of a limb.

The acute stage of the disease lasts from four to six weeks, as a rule, and then more or less recovery occurs, but some muscles are left paralysed, though possibly only a group, probably the extensor muscles of one of the lower limbs, that is to say, the muscles that raise the foot. The affected limb is colder than the other, and is possibly blue ; and, as the growth of the bone is interfered with, the limb is shortened. If the inflammation takes place at a certain level of the cord, the respiratory muscles may be affected, with dangerous results.

Immediately the existence of the disease is noted the patient should be isolated. A notification must also be sent to the Medical Officer of Health. During the acute stage absolute rest in bed is necessary. Aspirin or salicylate of sodium is used to relieve pain, if necessary, and hexamine may be given in the hope that it will have an antiseptic effect against the organisms. Sometimes the withdrawal of cerebro-spinal fluid is necessary for the diagnosis, and this procedure may also be used as part of the treatment.

To prevent affected muscles from being stretched by the action of opposing healthy muscles, some kind of splint may be advised. Thus, to prevent foot drop, what is called a bed-shoe may be worn.

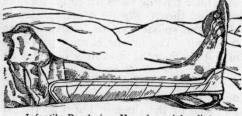

Infantile Paralysis. Use of special splint

This is a splint with a foot-piece which keeps the foot at right angles with the leg. Similarly, a splint on the front of the forearm, and with its lower end bent upwards, in order to throw back the wrist, should be used when the arm is affected.

After about two weeks, as a rule, massage may be commenced, and when the acute stage is over, the patient should be encouraged to move the limb regularly, and electricity may also be used to exercise the muscles. A long, thick stocking should be worn on a lower limb to maintain warmth. When the patient is able to be about, dropping of the foot should be prevented by a spring attached to the leg and the boot. Sometimes the foot is anchored at right angles to the leg by cutting a tendon and fixing the lower end to the shin bone.

See Encephalitis ; Paralysis ; Virus.

INFANTILISM. A person who fails to develop adult characteristics is said to be the subject of infantilism. Usually the general bodily development is of childish dimensions, but it may be greater, and even those who might be described as giants may manifest infantilism in the want of development of the sexual organs and of the secondary sexual characteristics, such as growth of pubic hair, alterations in the voice in a man, and enlargement of the breasts in a woman.

Infantilism may be the result of congenital syphilis or of chronic poisoning with alcohol, morphine, lead or other poisons. In other cases it is due to defects in important organs. Thus, there are types caused by thyroid deficiency. One of these is cretinism (*q.v.*), but in the other, in which the thyroid defect is not so severe, the appearance is more like that of a normal child. The administration of thyroid extract makes a marvellous improvement in either type. A deficiency of pancreatic juice is another cause, and the patient is likely to suffer, also, from severe diarrhoea. Pancreatic extract may be very beneficial but sometimes is useless.

Chronic kidney disease in early childhood gives rise to another type ; such patients do not live long. There is also a thymic type, in which there is obesity and a tendency to syncopal attacks, and a pituitary type, in which also there is obesity and often the patient passes an excessive amount of urine in which sugar may be present. Disease of the heart, of the blood vessels and of the liver are amongst other causes in this group.

Infantilism may occur, however, when neither poisoning nor defects in important organs can be adduced as the cause. One type is known as ateleiosis, and comes on suddenly at any time before development is complete. It usually begins in early childhood, however, and the appearance of the individual remains what it was at the onset of the disorder, except that sexual characters may develop in some cases. In another type, described as progeria, besides the general bodily development of infantilism, there are characteristics of senility, such as loss of flesh, baldness and thickening of the arteries.

See Growth ; Myxoedema ; Thyroid Gland.

INFARCTION. There are two kinds of infarction, the red or haemorrhagic, and the white, but each is caused in the same way, by the sudden arrest of the blood flow in an end artery, that is, one with no anastomotic connexion with other arteries or only a meagre connexion. The stoppage is usually due to an embolus, or plug.

The result is that a wedge-shaped piece of tissue is deprived of blood and may die ; as it contains no blood it is pale and so is called a white infarct, or infarction. This is the common kind in the spleen and kidney, for example. It may happen, however, as in embolism of the lung, that blood from neighbouring veins passes back into the emptied vessels before these have become devitalised, and it does so to the extent of engorging them. This is called a red infarct, and, as the red cells are squeezed out of the vessels into the surrounding tissues, it is also said to be haemorrhagic. This fact also explains the blood-stained sputa from infarction of the lung.

This type of infarction may clear up more or less, but, on the other hand, the tissue may die, or necrose. All necrotic tissue is replaced by granulation tissue and ultimately by a scar.

See Embolism.

INFECTIOUS DISEASE. A disease which is transmissible from one person to another is said to be infectious. If actual contact with the diseased person is necessary to convey it to another, the disease may be called contagious. Some infectious diseases, such as tuberculosis, anthrax, glanders, ringworm, and aphthous fever may be derived from the lower animals. A disease is infectious

because it is due to a living organism which can multiply in or about one person, and be discharged and become parasitic in or on another person.

Some parasites, like those of a common cold or influenza, are discharged in the breath, especially when coughing or sneezing, and in such diseases as tuberculosis and pneumonia the sputum teems with organisms which may be dispersed by coughing, or as a fine dust when the sputum dries. The infection of diphtheria may also be coughed out. The purulent discharge from the nose or ears which may accompany scarlet fever and other diseases is another source of infection. The dried crusts of smallpox and chickenpox are infective, and their dust contaminates the air.

Menace of Contaminated Water

The parasites of other diseases, such as typhoid fever, dysentery and cholera, are chiefly spread by contaminated water, and these are therefore often described as water-borne diseases. Not only may infection come from drinking such water, but from utensils or fresh vegetables or fruit which have been washed with polluted water. Milk may be charged with parasites by being kept in such vessels, or by dilution with the water. Ice-cream may also convey infection. The parasites of these diseases are discharged from the body in the stools and possibly the urine also. Infection often occurs from flies visiting the stools and then coming into contact with food.

Other insects convey infection when they bite ; or infected faeces of an insect may be inoculated into the skin by scratching. By the last method typhus, relapsing fever and trench fever are disseminated by the louse. Mosquitoes, by biting, spread malaria, yellow fever, dengue and filariasis ; the flea transmits bubonic plague ; the bed bug, plague and possibly leprosy and other diseases ; the tsetse fly, sleeping sickness ; the sand-fly, three-day fever ; and the tick, relapsing fever.

Articles of clothing, books and other objects which have been in contact with an infected person may carry the infection, and are referred to as fomites.

Not only may a person actually suffering from a disease be a source of danger to others, but also some who have recovered but still retain a focus of infection in the body. Such a person is called a carrier, and typhoid fever, dysentery, diphtheria, cerebro-spinal fever and other infections may be spread by such. Sometimes a carrier may not have exhibited any signs of the disease at all, though possibly very slight signs may have been overlooked.

Stages in Exanthematous Infections

The infectious diseases which have a characteristic rash, or exanthema, manifest a series of fairly definite stages. There is first a period of incubation, during which the organisms which have entered the body are multiplying and establishing themselves. This period varies for each disease, sometimes within fairly wide bounds. Then follows the prodromal period, in which occur the symptoms of the disease preceding the rash, symptoms referred to as the prodromata. In measles, for example, these resemble those of a common cold, while in scarlet fever there are headache, sore throat and vomiting. Next is the period of rash, or efflorescence, and, following this, the period of decline of the symptoms, or defervescence, which merges into the final stage of convalescence. Infectious diseases which have no characteristic rash exhibit, apart from this fact, a similar sequence of stages.

A person suffering from an infectious disease should be isolated until all danger of communicating the infection has passed.

With respect to a common cold or slight influenza, this will be considered a counsel of perfection, but even in these diseases the patient should try as far as possible to protect others. It may be possible to isolate a patient at home, but if there is any difficulty in doing so, and especially when the disease is one of the more serious infections, the patient should be sent to an isolation hospital.

The room chosen should be at the top of the house, and should have a fireplace. Preferably it should open on to a corridor ventilated by a window, and if the corridor has a sink in it, so much the better. A sheet wrung out of lysol solution, a teaspoonful to the pint of water, or some other antiseptic, and hung over the door, has the advantage of emphasising the fact of the isolation if it does nothing more. Carpets, heavy hangings, and all unnecessary furniture should be removed before the patient goes into the room. Feeding and other utensils used by the patient must be kept for his separate use, and water used for washing the patient or his clothing or utensils, also the stools and urine, should be adequately treated with a disinfectant before being poured into a sink or privy, as the case may be.

Some person must be told off to attend to the patient, and should wear an overall when outside the room, but should mix with other members of the family as little as possible. Books should not be allowed to leave the sick-room. When the period of infectivity is over, the patient must be properly washed all over and dressed in fresh clothing, and the room and all its contents must be dealt with as described under the heading Disinfection.

Not only must the patient be isolated, but also anyone who has been in contact with him, or her, the duration of this quarantine being regulated by the incubation period of the disease, and estimated from the last date of exposure to infection.

Diseases Which Must Be Notified

Some infectious diseases must be notified to the Medical Officer of Health for the district, and this should be done immediately the diagnosis is made. Responsibility for notifying falls both on the doctor in attendance and on the head of the house or any other person in a similar position, but in practice the notification of a doctor usually suffices.

The diseases which must thus be notified are as follows: smallpox, scarlet fever, cholera, diphtheria, membranous croup, erysipelas, typhus fever, enteric fever (including typhoid and paratyphoid), relapsing fever, continued fever, puerperal fever, acute primary pneumonia, acute influenzal pneumonia, tuberculosis, ophthalmia neonatorum, cerebrospinal fever, acute poliomyelitis, acute polio-encephalitis, encephalitis lethargica, plague, dysentery, and, if contracted in England or Wales, malaria. From time to time other diseases, such as measles and chicken-pox, may be made notifiable in a particular district, or throughout the country.

The duration of the incubation, isolation and quarantine periods for each infectious disease is given under the heading of the disease.

See Bacteria ; Disinfection ; Fever ; Flies ; Formalin ; Notification ; Quarantine ; Rash.

INFILTRATION. The spaces between body cells or fibres are occupied by small quantities of lymph or of ground-substance, the amount of these varying with the closeness of the main tissue elements to each other. When there is an excess of fluid, as in dropsy or inflammation, the tissue is said to be infiltrated with the fluid. Infiltration may also occur with other things, such as fat or the cells of a malignant tumour ; in fact, the habit such cells have of insinuating themselves amongst normal cells is one of the distinguishing marks of a malignant tumour.

INFLAMMATION. There are four familiar signs of acute inflammation, namely, redness, heat, swelling and pain. The former two are due to a large influx of blood into the part, which is also in part the cause of the latter two signs, but these are more due to the discharge of a watery fluid or lymph from the vessels which distends the tissues, thus compressing the ends of the sensory nerves and causing pain. This distension may be increased by each beat of the heart, so as to cause a throbbing pain.

The smaller arteries, the capillaries and the veins are all filled with blood, and the circulation through them is more rapid at first, but it slows down, and sometimes to such an extent that the blood, having oscillated several times backwards and forwards, ceases altogether to flow. With the slowing of the rate of flow the white blood corpuscles accumulate along the wall of the blood vessels, and many of them make their way out between the cells forming the vessel walls ; sometimes red blood cells also pass through, but

these are squeezed out, this occurrence being called diapedesis.

The flow of lymph and the migration of the white cells have a salutary purpose, as the former contains substances which are lethal to invading micro-organisms, while the white cells not only devour germs, but also tissue cells, which have been destroyed by the irritant causing the inflammation and clot, or other products of inflammation. From their exercising this function they are called phagocytes. The irritation underlying the inflammation may cease to operate and normal conditions be restored, the processes taking place in the reverse order to what has just been described, that is to say, the blood in the vessels begins to oscillate, then flows more and more rapidly, until all the excess of fluid in the tissues has been removed either by blood or lymph vessels, and the part resumes its usual appearance. Sometimes, however, the fight against invading germs is not so successful, and many white cells are killed, forming an abscess (*q.v.*) ; or a piece of tissue may be killed, as occurs in a boil, for example, the core of which represents killed tissue.

A further possibility is that the irritant may cause phenomena lower in degree

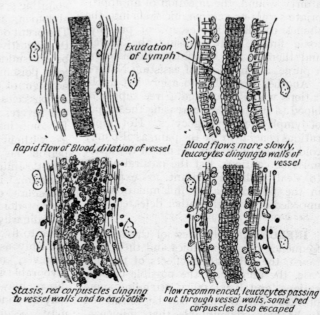

Exudation of Lymph

Rapid flow of Blood, dilation of vessel

Blood flows more slowly, leucocytes clinging to walls of vessel

Stasis, red corpuscles clinging to vessel walls and to each other

Flow recommenced, leucocytes passing out through vessel walls, some red corpuscles also escaped

Inflammation. Stages in the campaign of the blood against injury

than those of acute inflammation, or, having caused acute inflammation, which has lessened in intensity, may continue to operate, so that there is some degree of congestion and filtration of fluid into the tissues. There is then also likely to be new formation of connective tissue cells, which cause the tissue to be denser and firmer. These phenomena constitute chronic inflammation, and may be witnessed, for example, at the edge of many chronic ulcers. The young connective tissue cells may develop into fibres, a process described as fibrosis (q.v.).

Inflammation is most commonly due to micro-organisms, but may also be caused by irritants of other kinds. Thus, severe rubbing of the skin may cause it, an example of a physical irritant ; or a mustard plaster, which is a chemical irritant. Heat might be responsible, as in a burn ; or sunlight, as in solar dermatitis.

In treating inflammation it is important to secure rest for the affected part as far as possible. It may be possible to get rid of the origin at once, as when a foreign body is causing inflammation of the eye. When germs are concerned, the most that can be done in this way is to assist the tissues in their fight. Cleaning up a dirty wound, the injection of an appropriate serum or vaccine, incisions into the tissues to allow the escape of pus and toxic fluids, and cleansing the bowels and thereby the blood by administering a purge, are methods of assisting Nature.

Another method is to apply hot applications which encourage a free supply of blood to the part, so increasing the supply of lymph and of phagocytes. Hot applications generally ease the pain, as also may cold applications, but the use of the latter must be cautious, lest the natural efforts to deal with an irritant, as expressed in the phenomena of inflammation, are impeded or even altogether defeated.

See Exudate ; Lymphatic System.

INFLUENZA. In view of the relative frequency of its epidemics and their wide range, the debilitating effects of the disease, the number of the possible complications, and the fatality attending some of these, few diseases can be considered to be more redoubtable than influenza.

It has been found that epidemics tend to recur every 33 weeks, though if the time when an epidemic is expected happens to fall in the summer, the epidemic will probably not occur. From time to time an epidemic ranges all over the world, the last pandemic being in 1918, and the previous one in the years 1889–90. Such epidemics spread with an impressive and almost incredible rapidity.

Influenza is due to a germ, and there is good evidence for believing that the influenza bacillus of Pfeiffer is the one primarily responsible, though it must be admitted that this question has not been conclusively settled, as other germs, such as pneumococci, streptococci, and a filter-passing virus, have been found in association with the disease, and may be responsible for at least some of the complications.

Variations in Typical Symptoms

The onset of influenza is sudden, and occurs from one to four days after exposure to infection. Running at the eyes and nose may suggest a bad cold, but usually the fever is higher, there is considerable headache and pain in the back and limbs, and more prostration. Often the throat is sore, and there is a dry, irritating cough. The tongue is furred, and there may be nausea and perhaps vomiting ; sometimes there is pain in the abdomen, and there may be diarrhoea. The brunt of the disease may indeed fall on the digestive organs, and the symptoms be so sudden and severe as to suggest food poisoning. Sometimes also there is no sign of irritation of the eyes or the air passages, but the headache and pains are severe, and there may be delirium. In some instances, the onset is unusual as, without feeling noticeably unwell, a person has dropped unconscious in the street. Influenza thus shows considerable variation in type, and in different epidemics one or other of these types may predominate.

Ordinarily, after having persisted from three to five days, the temperature drops, suddenly as a rule. Some complication, however, may interfere with such a favourable issue, and even as the type of disease may vary in different epidemics, so may the kind of complication. Bronchitis may become severe, and from the smallest tubes may spread into the lungs, constituting broncho-pneumonia, with a high temperature, rapid breathing and pulse rates, and lividity or blueness of the skin; in the last pandemic a heliotrope tint was not uncommon. Sometimes the lobar type of pneumonia develops, or, either in association with pneumonia or independently, pleurisy. This may go on to empyema, the accumulation of pus in the pleural cavity.

In connexion with the heart there may be grave weakness of the muscle, or pericarditis may occur, or endocarditis with subsequent valvular disease. Thrombosis may occur in veins anywhere in the body.

Otitis media, inflammation of the middle ear, is not uncommon, and infection may extend into the skull causing meningitis, though this may occur also apart from ear trouble. Inflammation of the brain, the spinal cord or nerves is also possible. Acute nephritis, or Bright's disease, may accompany influenza. Serious eye disorders sometimes occur. Ordinary herpes, or blisters, around the mouth is common, but other skin rashes are sometimes encountered.

Possible Results of an Attack

Apart from legacies left by some of its complications, even an apparently simple attack of influenza may have troublesome sequelae. There may be considerable mental depression, sometimes even melancholia, or serious incapacity for mental and physical exertion. Neuralgia may occur and may be severe. Sometimes there is baldness.

The chance of recovering from an attack of influenza is, generally speaking, good except where young children or aged or debilitated persons are concerned, though in the last pandemic the disease took heavy toll of the young and vigorous.

The general treatment of influenza is that of the state of fever, but special emphasis must be laid on the necessity for rest in bed, abundance of fresh air, and of sufficient time for convalescence.

Aspirin in 10-grain doses is useful for relieving muscular pains and headache. This or salicin, sodium salicylate or quinine may be given at intervals in order to combat the toxaemia of the disease. The treatment of the complications which

have been mentioned is discussed under appropriate headings to which the reader is referred. The patient ceases to be infectious in three or four days after the temperature has become normal. During convalescence a tonic such as Easton's syrup (*q.v.*) may be helpful. A change to the seaside or country should be made if possible when the attack has been more than a slight one.

The infection of influenza is mainly spread by the breath of an infected person, and the danger is increased by his sneezing and coughing.

During an epidemic an infected person should be given as wide a berth as possible. It is a prudent thing to walk to business, for example, or go on the top of a 'bus rather than in a closed vehicle, and rooms and offices should be especially well ventilated.

It may help to lessen the risk to gargle the throat and spray the nose with a weak solution of permaganate of potash twice daily. Should suspicious symptoms make their appearance, 15 drops of essence of cinnamon or of spirit of camphor taken on a lump of sugar may cut them short. Mixed vaccines, containing the influenza bacillus and other germs associated with the disease, are of definite value. If a course of such did not prevent the disease it might mitigate its severity and lessen the risk of complications.

See Cold; Cough; Fever.

INFUSION. Most of the medicinal infusions are made by pouring boiling water over them and infusing for a quarter to half an hour, but for the infusions of calumba and quassia cold water is used. The dose of most infusions is from $\frac{1}{2}$ to 1 ounce; that of infusion of digitalis is 2 to 4 drachms, and of the infusion of buchu, ergot, scoparium and senna (for a single dose) is up to 2 ounces.

See Drug.

INHALATION. Chloroform, ether and other volatile drugs are administered by inhalation as general anaesthetics. For giving ether Clover's inhaler or a modification of it is often used. This consists of a face-piece, a large rubber bag into which the patient breathes and between these a box for containing the drug. The amount of air breathed, and so the amount of the ether inhaled, is regulated by a valve. Ethyl chloride is used with a similar apparatus.

For giving nitrous oxide there is a metal cylinder containing the compressed gas which is allowed to escape from time to time into a bag fitted with a face-piece. Compressed oxygen is also supplied in cylinders and may be given along with volatile anaesthetics, to lessen the risk of asphyxia, or when this condition already exists, as in pneumonia or after gas poisoning.

Method of Giving Chloroform

Chloroform is usually given by what is called the open method, that is, dropping it on a piece of lint, flannel or gauze held over the patient's mouth and nose, and ether may be given in the same way. Sometimes more elaborate apparatus, such as the Junker or the Vernon-Harcourt inhaler, is adopted.

The method of inhalation is used for many other drugs, mostly in the treatment of respiratory disorders. Thus, the more urgent symptoms of asthma (q.v.) may be relieved by inhaling the smoke from fumigatory powders. In whooping-cough the air of the sick-room may be impregnated with the vapour of carbolic acid, lysol, or some similar substance by pouring a teaspoonful of the drug on a large iron spoon or a shovel which has been heated ; or the drug may be placed in a shallow metal saucer or, as in some forms of apparatus, into a porous block, which is heated by a night-light.

Steam may be used to volatilise drugs, as in a Maw's inhaler, which is a porcelain jar with a tube through the cork to admit air, and a mouthpiece at the side by which the patient inspires the drug-impregnated steam. Water which is nearly, but not quite, boiling is put into the jar, care being taken that it does not rise as high as the inner opening of the mouthpiece. Friar's balsam, eucalyptus oil, turpentine and other remedies may be used in this way. An oily substance should be rubbed up with a small quantity of light carbonate of magnesia before being poured on the water as it will then diffuse better.

A useful adaptation of this method is simply to put the hot water and drugs into an ordinary jug and cover the head and jug with a towel while inhaling. Special inhalers are used for inhaling nascent ammonium chloride.

Amyl nitrite is used by inhalation and is contained in a glass capsule which is broken in a handkerchief unless provided with an absorbent cover. Other drugs are used similarly.

Another apparatus used for inhalation is of the type of the Burney-Yeo inhaler. This consists of a perforated zinc mask to cover the mouth and nose. On the top of the mask a strip of flannel or lint is attached, and on this creosote or other drugs may be dropped.

Drugs may be converted into a vaporised form by some kind of spray apparatus. At some spas there is a room, described as an inhalatorium, in which the natural waters may be inhaled as a spray. At some places the emanations of radioactive waters may also be inhaled.

See Atomiser ; Bronchitis Kettle ; Gargle ; Menthol ; Spray.

INJECTION. Some remedies cannot be given by the mouth because they are altered by the digestive juices and become ineffective. They must be injected into the tissues to be of any use. This applies to insulin, for example, and to antitoxic sera and various other substances. Owing to the uncertainty regarding the rate of absorption from the alimentary tract an injection permits of more precise dosage, an advantage when one is dealing with a powerful drug ; also a more rapid effect is secured by injection. Injection is the only method available for most drugs when the patient is unconscious.

An injection may be intradermic, or into the skin. This method is often used when injecting a local anaesthetic as the drug is retained more readily in the injected locality than when given hypodermically, or under the skin. The latter method is, however, the one most used for the general administration of drugs. Some drugs, however, such as quinine and mercury, are liable to cause an abscess when placed beneath the skin and are injected into muscles, an intramuscular injection.

In cases where a drug injected under the skin or into a muscle causes too much pain, the intravenous route is selected.

The solution is injected directly into a vein, generally one at the front of the elbow. The action of a drug is also obtained more rapidly by this route than by any other.

An intraspinal injection, that is, one into the spinal canal, may be given in order to secure anaesthesia below the site of the injection or to secure the action of drugs within the canal, as few reach the cerebro-spinal fluid when given by other routes. An antitoxic serum against cerebro-spinal fever must be given in this way, for example.

For sudden heart failure, say from electric shock or a drug, a solution of adrenalin or of atropine may be injected straight into the heart.

An injection into the bowel is called an enema and into the nose, vagina or other cavities is referred to as a douche.

See Syringe.

INNERVATION. This term simply means a nerve supply. One may speak, for example, of the innervation of a part as consisting of a particular nerve or nerves.

INNOMINATE. The haunch or innominate bone really consists of three bones, namely, the ilium above, the ischium behind, and the pubis in front. In early life these three bones are separated from each other by cartilage, but by the sixteenth year, as a rule, they are all fused into one bone. Each takes part in forming the acetabulum, a deep cup-like depression for the head of the femur, or thigh bone. The reader is referred to the illustrations under the headings Hip and Pelvis.

The ilium forms a broad expanse of bone with a curved upper border, the iliac crest, the front and back terminations of which are the anterior and posterior superior iliac spines respectively. Separated by a notch from each of these, there is an inferior spine. From the outer surface of the ilium arise the three large muscles known as the glutei ; from the anterior superior spine, the sartorius and the tensor fasciae latae ; and from the anterior inferior spine, the rectus femoris which also arises from the upper border of the acetabulum. At the back part of this surface is the surface for articulation with the sacrum (*q.v.*).

The inner surface of the ilium is hollowed somewhat, and constitutes the iliac fossa. Here there is the iliacus muscle and the psoas. The crest of the ilium gives attachment to the muscles of the abdominal wall.

Below and in front of the acetabulum is a large opening, the thyroid foramen, which is covered in by the thyroid membrane. The front boundaries of this are formed by the pubis, and the rear by the ischium. From the outer surface of the arch of bone below the foramen arise the hamstrings and other muscles. The upper border of the front part of the pubis is called the crest of the pubis, and is limited externally by a prominence, the pubic spine, to which the inner end of Poupart's ligament (*q.v.*) is attached.

Projecting backwards from the ischium is the ischial spine, above which is the great sacro-sciatic notch, and below the lesser sacro-sciatic notch. These are converted by ligaments into openings,

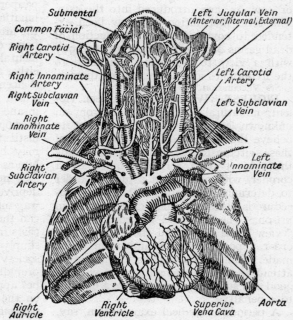

Submental
Common Facial
Right Carotid Artery
Right Innominate Artery
Right Subclavian Vein
Right Innominate Vein
Right Subclavian Artery
Left Jugular Vein (Anterior, Internal, External)
Left Carotid Artery
Left Subclavian Vein
Left Innominate Vein
Right Auricle
Right Ventricle
Superior Vena Cava
Aorta

Innominate. Course of the veins and artery from heart to head or foramina, with corresponding names, and give exit to important structures, the upper foramen, for example, to the great sciatic nerve.

The term innominate is also applied to an artery and to two veins. The artery represents the common origin of the right common carotid and the subclavian arteries from the arch of the aorta ; on the left side of the body these two arteries arise independently from the arch. Corresponding to the innominate artery, there is the right innominate vein, formed by the union of the right internal jugular and subclavian veins, but there is also a left innominate vein formed by the corresponding veins on this side. The innominate veins unite to form the superior vena cava. The artery lies behind the right side of the uppermost part of the breast bone.

See Hip ; Iliac Region ; Pelvis ; Thigh.

INOCULATION. The introduction of disease germs through the skin or mucous membrane is described as inoculation. This may be accidental, as by scratching or pricking with infected nails or instruments, or abrading or piercing an infected skin or mucous surface ; or it may be deliberate, as in inoculation against smallpox, when the living germs of vaccinia, or cowpox, are introduced into the skin. The term inoculation has now been extended to cover also the introduction of dead germs or their poisons into the body with a view to increasing resistance to the living ones and so preventing disease.

See Vaccination.

INQUEST. When death has been violent, unnatural, or sudden and from an unknown cause, or there is reason to believe that it has occurred under any of these circumstances, it must be made the subject of a formal inquiry by a coroner, with or without a jury, in order to determine the cause. The same procedure is necessary when death occurs in prison. The jury and the coroner must " view " the body, and the coroner may order a post-mortem examination to be made. Failure to obey a summons to attend as a witness at an inquest without good and sufficient cause creates a liability to a penalty.

A periodical medical examination, say, at intervals not longer than three months,

of aged or infirm persons, even when there is no particular need for it otherwise, would often enable a medical certificate of the cause of death to be given and thus the necessity for an inquest would be avoided.

INSANITY. Persons who, by reason of mental defect or disorder, are unable to reach what is considered to be a reasonable standard of behaviour, or transgress what are considered to be reasonable limits of conduct, are classed as insane. Mental capacity may be below the average, or there may be mental disorder of some kind, but neither is supposed to constitute insanity unless the conduct of the person affords grounds for such an opinion. This is to say that insanity is not synonymous with mental disease (*q.v.*) ; the term simply connotes some instances of mental disease.

When a person is insane the question of protection must be considered, protection of the individual himself and of others, and of the amount and kind of protection required. As regards congenital mental defects, reference to these subjects is made under the heading Feeblemindedness. As regards those who become insane, apart from special considerations affecting pauper lunatics, wandering and neglected lunatics and criminal lunatics, there are the alternatives of keeping the patient at home or of his entering an institution for mental diseases, which again may be either a private asylum, or licensed house, a licensed hospital, or a public asylum which takes private patients. Again, an insane person may be capable of making a choice and may elect to go into an institution as a voluntary patient, or it may be considered necessary to certify him as insane and send him in.

It need hardly be pointed out that to deprive an individual of his liberty in this way may be a serious matter for him, nor can the fact be ignored that certification casts a stigma upon him, though this simply shows that the understanding of society is not sufficient to overcome a prejudice. The question must, therefore, be approached with earnest solicitude ; on the other hand, neglect or refusal to recognize urgent grounds for certification may be bitterly rued.

A patient is usually admitted to an institution on a reception order made by a magistrate or other competent judicial authority on a petition signed, if possible, by the nearest relative and supported by two medical certificates. When immediate restraint is deemed necessary, as when the patient is very violent or has manifested strong suicidal tendency, he may be admitted on what is called an urgency order. This must be supported by one medical certificate.

See Dementia ; Mental Disease.

INSOMNIA. Sleeplessness, or insomnia, may be incidental to febrile and other disorders and the main line of treatment will be that required for the disease in question. In fever it may suffice to sponge the patient with tepid water. A wet pack will often succeed in producing sleep and this may be a hot pack, particularly if the fever is not high. A pack is especially useful if there is active delirium. In heart disease and other disorders when the patient has difficulty in lying down, sleep may be procured by putting a stool on the bed and over this one or more pillows on which the patient can recline forward.

An occasional fit of insomnia may depend on one or more of a considerable number of disturbing influences, such as a close or overheated bedroom, too many or too few bedclothes, cold feet, an overloaded stomach or, on the other hand, the need for a little food, taking tea or coffee too near bed-time, excitement or worry. The removal or avoidance of any such influence will probably be effective ; in any case a single bad night is not of much consequence.

It is otherwise, however, when insomnia is habitual, as this may lead to serious mental exhaustion, and apprehension of the loss of reason may reduce the patient to a state of desperation. An ever-present worry or anxiety may be responsible for this state of things and prevent a person from going off to sleep. Sometimes, on the other hand, a person goes to sleep but is awakened by terrifying dreams and to prevent the recurrence of these he remains awake. It has been suggested that in other instances, where neither conscious worries nor dreams of this kind can be blamed, dreams which cannot be recalled and of which the person may be unconscious, may be the cause of his premature awakening, or even prevent his going to sleep in the first instance.

In such circumstances it may be of some use to face the cause of worry or anxiety, the magnitude of which may be diminished by looking at it from all points of view. A free discussion of the subject with a friend would be helpful to this end. When the state of health is such that a calm and correct view of business, family or social difficulties is impossible, it will be well to make a change to some place where fresh interests will occupy the mind. When the mental trouble is not apparent help may be got by a resort to psycho-therapy.

A hot bath before retiring for the night often secures sleep, and a course of massage or electricity in an appropriate form are other useful measures.

In many instances it will be necessary to take some drug, but this should only be done under medical supervision. Bromide of potassium, in doses of 30 grains dissolved in half a glass of soda-water, may be used to lessen excitement or the sense of mental strain and thereby allow sleep. Chloral also diminishes cerebral activity. If there is pain, morphine or some other preparation of opium is generally used. In other instances paraldehyde, sulphonal, veronal, or some similar preparation, might be selected.

See Diet ; Neurasthenia ; Psycho-therapy ; Sleep.

INSUFFLATION. The introduction of powdered drugs into body-cavities by blowing is called insufflation, and the apparatus for the purpose, an insufflator. A common type consists of a vulcanite tube attached to a rubber ball. In the tube there is an opening by which the powder is put in and which is then closed by sliding up a movable sleeve. When the bag is compressed the powder is ejected as a fine cloud. Boracic acid powder is often thus blown into the ear when it is discharging. For treating the larynx an insufflator with a bent tube is used.

INSULIN. From the páncreas of the lower animals a substance is obtained which represents the internal secretion of the islets, or insulae, of Langerhans, and it is accordingly known as insulin. It regulates the burning up of sugar in the body, and is deficient in most persons who suffer from diabetes mellitus (*q.v.*). Solutions of insulin are therefore used with benefit in the treatment of this disease. Insulin has been obtained in a crystalline form.

INTERMITTENT CLAUDICATION.

Some persons after walking a short distance are seized with violent, cramp-like pain in the legs, making it necessary to take a short rest. The pain disappears as quickly as it comes on, but tends to reappear after a further short walk. This condition, known as intermittent claudication, is due to spasm occurring in arteries already narrowed by disease in their walls, and either the excessive use of tobacco or syphilis is the probable cause of the arteries being in this state.

The disorder is practically confined to men, and does not often occur before later middle life. A similar spasm may affect arteries elsewhere than in the legs, and may account for a transient numbness in the arm, giddiness, and so on.

The treatment will vary with the apparent cause.

See Arterio-sclerosis.

INTERTRIGO.

Friction between skin surfaces that rub on one another may give rise to redness which is described as intertrigo, or erythema intertrigo. The commonest sites are on the inner surfaces of the thighs, in the groin, in the armpit, or, in fat women, beneath the breasts. In infants, intertrigo may be caused by the rubbing of a napkin. The separation of opposing surfaces by a piece of lint, after dusting them thoroughly with a bland powder, such as one containing zinc oxide and talc (*q.v.*), usually suffices for a cure. From decomposition of imprisoned sweat, there may be maceration of the skin,

and it is important then to make the part thoroughly clean and dry before applying the powder. Infection of the abraded surface by germs may cause dermatitis (*q.v.*).

INTESTINE.

The bowel, or intestine, is a long muscular tube, lined with mucous membrane, extending from the pyloric end of the stomach to the anus. The first part, or small intestine, has an average length of 20 feet, the first 11 inches constituting the duodenum (*q.v.*), and beyond this the jejunum, comprising two-fifths, and ileum, three-fifths, of the length.

The lower end of the ileum joins the large intestine about 2½ inches above the commencement of the latter, the passage between the two portions of gut being guarded by the ileo-caecal valve. The large intestine has an average length of 5 to 5½ feet, and comprises the caecum, ascending colon, transverse colon, descending colon, iliac colon, pelvic colon, rectum and anal canal.

The duodenum is about 2 inches in diameter, but the small gut gradually diminishes in width, until, at the end of the ileum, this is little more than 1 inch. The caecum is about 3 inches across, but the large bowel also diminishes in width, and in the descending and iliac colon, this is only about 1½ inches across.

The jejunum and ileum are completely surrounded by a smooth membrane known as the peritoneum, the two layers of which, reflected off the bowel, pass back to the posterior wall of the abdomen, constituting the mesentery, which anchors this long length of the intestine to the body wall. The line of attachment of the mesentery to the body wall, measuring about 6 inches, extends from the upper part of the abdomen, a little to the left of the middle line, to the lower right-hand corner of the cavity. There is a partial peritoneal covering on the duodenum and the large intestine, but the caecum, the transverse

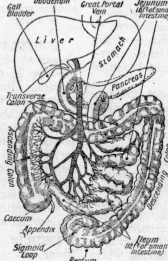

Intestine. **The parts that compose it**

colon, and the pelvic colon have mesenteries. Portions of the gut possessing a mesentery are very freely movable. The ascending and the descending colon have no peritoneal covering behind, and therefore can be operated upon from the back without opening the general peritoneal cavity. There is no peritoneal covering on the lowest third of the rectum.

The muscular wall of the intestine consists of an outer layer of fibres running longitudinally, and an inner layer of circular fibres. The large intestine is constricted at intervals to form a series of dilatations or sacculations. This arrangement, which is preserved by the three longitudinal bands which run along the gut, distinguishes the large from the small intestine. Another feature of the external surface of the large intestine is the existence of small fatty projections, the appendices epiploicae.

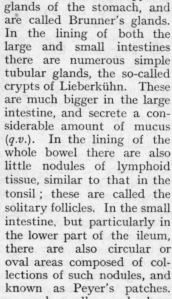

Inner aspect of Gut — *Mesentery*

Valvulae Conniventes

Sectional view of some of the coils of the small intestine

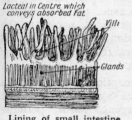

Lacteal in Centre which conveys absorbed Fat — *Villi* — *Glands*

Lining of small intestine studded with villi

Within the muscular coat of the bowel there is a layer of loose connective tissue, the submucous coat, and, within this, the mucous coat. From near the beginning of the duodenum to midway along the ileum, the mucous membrane of the small intestine is disposed in folds at intervals ; these folds, or valvulae conniventes, which do not run entirely round the inner surface of the bowel and have a crescentic shape, are meant to increase the extent of secreting and absorbing surface. The surface of the small gut also has a velvety appearance from the presence of an immense number of tiny, finger-like projections, or villi (singular, villus). In each villus is the beginning of a little lacteal vessel which conveys fatty foods to large vessels and so on to the receptaculum chyli and the thoracic duct (*see* illustration, p. 212).

In the mucous membrane of the duodenum are branched and coiled glands which somewhat resemble the pyloric glands of the stomach, and are called Brunner's glands. In the lining of both the large and small intestines there are numerous simple tubular glands, the so-called crypts of Lieberkühn. These are much bigger in the large intestine, and secrete a considerable amount of mucus (*q.v.*). In the lining of the whole bowel there are also little nodules of lymphoid tissue, similar to that in the tonsil ; these are called the solitary follicles. In the small intestine, but particularly in the lower part of the ileum, there are also circular or oval areas composed of collections of such nodules, and known as Peyer's patches. These become much swollen and ulcerated in typhoid fever.

Intestinal juice, or succus entericus, which is secreted by the lining of the gut, contains a ferment, enterokinase, which is necessary to the activity of the trypsin in the pancreatic juice, and another ferment, erepsin, which aids in the full digestion of carbohydrates. The large intestine

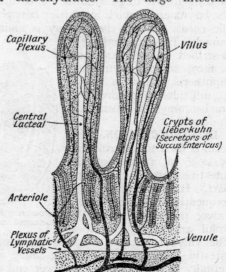

Capillary Plexus — *Villus*

Central Lacteal — *Crypts of Lieberkuhn (Secretors of Succus Entericus)*

Arteriole

Plexus of Lymphatic Vessels — *Venule*

Enlargement of villi showing the central lacteal

hardly contributes to digestion, and very little towards absorption of food. It is an important excretory organ, however, for lime, magnesium, iron and phosphates.

Food is passed along the intestine by wave-like contractions described as peristalsis. What is called segmentation also occurs, that is, contractions take place at short intervals, so that the contents are broken up into a series of portions. Then contractions take place through the middle of the portions, and by a repetition of this process the food masses are broken up and thoroughly mixed with the digestive juices. A meal reaches the caecum about 4½ hours, and the entrance to the rectum about 18 hours, after its consumption.

See Appendicitis ; Colitis ; Constipation ; Diarrhoea ; Digestion ; Duodenum ; Intussusception ; Mesentery ; Obstruction ; Rectum ; Visceroptosis.

INTUBATION. Narrowing of the space between the vocal cords may threaten to cause suffocation, and one way of preventing this is to pass down a tube into the larynx and leave it in position between the cords, so that the air-way is maintained. This operation is described as intubation and is most commonly used in diphtheria, but it is rather a difficult procedure and tracheotomy is generally preferable.

INTUSSUSCEPTION. This term is used to describe the passage of a part of the intestine into an adjoining part. It takes place most frequently at the ileo-caecal valve, the junction of the small and large intestines. The valve is pushed on into the large intestine, and may pass so far along as actually to protrude at the lower end of the bowel. The large bowel is invaginated,

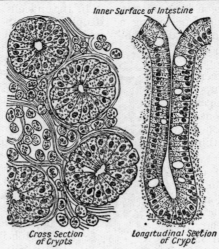

Inner Surface of Intestine

Cross Section of Crypts

Longitudinal Section of Crypt

Intestine. Lieberkühn's crypts in bowel lining

Intussusception. Portion of bowel telescoped into adjacent portion

Entering Layer

Returning Layer

Ensheathing Layer

that is to say, its outer surface becomes its inner one. The process of invagination may be seen if one takes, say, a pencil and presses the tip of an empty glove-finger up into the finger. The outer surface of the finger passes inwards to become the inner surface, until the whole finger is outside in and within the main part of the glove.

Acute intussusception is most common in young children, usually during the first year, and is probably due to straining, caused by irritating food. There is severe pain in the belly, which, at first, occurs in spasms, and there is vomiting. There is straining, as if to pass a stool, but only a little blood-stained mucus comes away. Sometimes, however, nothing is passed, but the severe attacks of pain and also the prostration which ensues point to urgent trouble. An operation is necessary to rectify the condition. Warm enemata sometimes push back the bowel, but cannot be depended on.

Chronic intussusception usually occurs in adults, and the symptoms are not so urgent, until perhaps acute obstruction or acute peritonitis occurs. The treatment of the chronic type is also by operation. *See* Intestine.

INUNCTION. The administration of oils and fats, and drugs incorporated with them, by rubbing them into the skin, is described as inunction. Blue ointment is sometimes used in this way in the treatment of syphilis, a fresh surface of skin being selected each day, so as to avoid undue irritation by the drug. Cod-liver oil can also be given in this way. For infants, a piece of flannel

aturated with the oil may be placed
beneath the binder; the movements of
he child will rub in the oil.

See Ointment.

INVALID COOKERY. Great care must
be exercised in the choice, preparation
and serving of articles of diet for the
invalid and the convalescent. Not only
must food be prepared in such a manner
as to render it easy of digestion, but its
nourishing properties must be retained
and even supplemented, and it must be
taken to the sick-room in so attractive
a form that it will appeal to the eye as
well as to the palate of a patient. The
best materials must always be used for
an invalid's food, and the best methods
of cooking it should be studied.

A patient may be ordered "a little
boiled fish" as a light, digestible dish,
but good sick-room cooks know that to
boil fish is to take away much of its
nutriment and its flavour. It ought
always to be steamed in a little milk,
which can be thickened with flour and
poured over the fish. All fish, poultry
and meat ordered for the sick-room
should be steamed.

Food which is meant to be hot, such
as beef tea, soups or gruel, must be taken
to the sick-room very hot (unless otherwise
ordered by the doctor), and cold food,
such as milk and jellies, must be kept
absolutely cold, on ice during hot weather,
as nothing is more unappetising than
lukewarm food.

The caprices and peculiarities of patients
must be studied. In some cases, when a
liberal milk diet is ordered the patient
rebels, even to the point of active sickness, but will welcome and enjoy and
digest milk if it is merely flavoured with
such simple things as a tablespoonful of
coffee, a teaspoonful of meat extract, or
a pinch of cinnamon, or if it is thickened
with a little arrowroot, or diluted with
soda or potash water. Eggs are disliked
by others, but these can usually be taken
and relished if made into a light custard
or steamed soufflé or omelette. In cases
of debility they should be given raw,
well beaten up in warm milk, sweetened,
and either brandy or a few drops of
flavouring added.

Food must never be allowed to stand
in the sick-room, and after the patient's
meal is over anything left must be removed.

See Arrowroot; Barley Water; Beef Extract;
Beef Juice; Beef Tea; Beverages; Blancmange;
Calf's Foot Jelly; Chicken; Convalescence;
Diet; Egg; Nursing; Sweetbread.

IODINE. An element forming dark,
lustrous scales, iodum or iodine is extensively used in medicine in various preparations. The strong tincture is painted on
the skin as a counter-irritant (*q.v.*). Its
action being sufficient sometimes to
cause blistering, a common practice is
to use equal parts of the strong and of
the weak tinctures. This mixture, or
the weak tincture, may be used as an
antiseptic paint to prepare the skin for
operation. The weak tincture may also
be painted on chilblains, or on the gum,
after it has been dried, for the relief of
toothache. A paint containing iodine
and potassium iodide in glycerin is often
used for unhealthy tonsils.

Iodine ointment, or a stainless iodine
ointment, such as iodex or the unguentum
iodi denigrescens, B.P.C., are used for
various skin diseases requiring stimulating
or antiseptic treatment, and for rubbing
into the skin over chronically inflamed
joints and in muscular rheumatism. The
absorption of inflammatory products in
joints and muscles is thus hastened, and
for this purpose painting with the mixed
tinctures, and rubbing in the ointment
of potassium iodide or the liniment of
potassium iodide with soap, may alternatively be used.

The weak tincture is used inwardly
in doses of 2 to 5 minims. Larger doses
tend to cause irritation of the stomach
and vomiting, though vomiting can sometimes be relieved by giving 1-minim doses
in water, repeated once or twice at half-
hourly intervals. Usually, however, for
internal use, potassium iodide or sodium
iodide, the dose of each of which is 5 to
20 grains, is employed.

Preparations of iodine are given for
the lesions of the tertiary stage of syphilis,
for aneurysm, for chronic bronchitis with
a tough, adhesive sputum, for asthma, for
chronic joint complaints, and as antidotes for poisoning by lead or mercury.
Sometimes, when taking them, catarrhal

symptoms, like those of a common cold, occur, and are more likely to follow small than larger doses. To avoid irritation of the stomach, preparations of iodine should always be taken well diluted and after food. Another effect of taking these preparations may be the appearance of a rash, resembling acne.

The tincture may be swallowed accidentally. An emetic should be given, and then thin starch, arrowroot or bread, freely.

Iodine is normally present in the body in organic combination in the secretion of the thyroid gland (*q.v.*).

IODOFORM. A lemon-yellow crystalline powder, with a characteristic odour, iodoform is used as an antiseptic. A powder consisting of one part of iodoform to three parts of boracic acid is used for dusting wounds or sores, or iodoform may be used alone. Suppositories containing it are used in treating anal fissure and inflamed piles, and bougies for gonorrhoea. There is also an iodoform ointment.

Gauze impregnated with iodoform is a common surgical dressing. A paste consisting of one part of pure bismuth subnitrate, two parts of iodoform, and one part of liquid paraffin, commonly referred to as B.I.P.P., has been used for packing wounds and acute abscesses after they have been opened. The drug has been given inwardly in small doses as an intestinal antiseptic.

Poisoning by Iodoform. Either when swallowed, or from absorption from a large raw surface, iodoform poisoning may occur. There may simply be a persistent taste and smell of the drug, or this may be followed by fever, a rapid pulse, headache, delirium, vomiting and collapse. Sometimes there has been loss of vision. Sometimes the drug brings out a red rash. The use of the drug should be discontinued and any surface to which it has been applied be treated with a solution of bicarbonate of sodium in water. Bromides and other sedatives are given.

IONISATION. When common salt, or sodium chloride, is dissolved in water, a change occurs in it. In the solid state a molecule, the smallest amount capable of independent existence, consists of an atom of the metal sodium and an atom of chlorine gas joined together. But when dissolved in water there is a dissociation of the molecule into the constituent atoms, but the atom of sodium carries a positive charge of electricity, and that of chlorine a negative one. This is called ionisation, and the changed atoms are termed ions. If now a current of electricity is passed through the liquid by dipping electrodes connected with the poles of a battery into it, there will be a flow of the sodium ions to the negative electrode and of the chlorine to the positive, that is, the ions are attracted to the electrode having the opposite kind of electricity, and repelled from that having the same kind.

Acids, salts and bases, when dissolved in such solvents as water or alcohol, all act in this way, and advantage is taken of this in introducing drugs into the body. Metals, alkalies and alkaloids are drawn towards the negative pole, acid radicles to the positive. Thus, if it is desired to drive zinc into the tissues, a solution of the salt is soaked into several thicknesses of lint over the positive electrode, the negative electrode being placed elsewhere on the body. On turning on the current, the zinc (Zn) would pass into the tissues, while the acid radicle (SO_4) would remain in the lint. It is the latter fact which makes it necessary to have several thicknesses of lint, otherwise corrosive substances formed in this way would burn the skin.

Ions are driven into the superficial tissues only, being prevented from going very deeply by the fact that they are caught up by the lymph stream and carried away. Cocaine may, however, be directed into a painful nerve, chlorine and salicylic ions into the structures around joints, and zinc ions into septic tissues, say, in the treatment of middle-ear disease, or infection in deep sinuses or bony cavities. Other drugs are also sometimes used.

IPECACUANHA. Preparations of ipecacuanha root include the powdered root itself, dose 15 to 30 grains; a liquid extract, $\frac{1}{2}$ to 2 minims; ipecacuanha wine, 10 to 30 minims as an expectorant, and 4 to 6 drachms as an emetic; compound ipecacuanha or Dover's powder, 5 to 15 grains; pill of ipecacuanha and squill, 4 to 8 grains; ipecacuanha lozenges, $\frac{1}{4}$ grain in each; lozenges of ipecacuanha and morphine, $\frac{1}{12}$ grain of the former and $\frac{1}{36}$ grain of the latter in each; emetine; and emetine bismuth iodide. Commercial emetine contains not only emetine, the main alkaloid in ipecacuanha, but also another alkaloid, cephaeline.

Ipecacuanha is a depressant to the central nervous system. In small doses it is an expectorant, in larger doses an emetic, and in larger doses still it causes severe vomiting, purging and collapse. Doses of 1 minim of the wine may relieve vomiting, however.

For bronchitis, the wine, the pill, one of the lozenges or Dover's powder may be used. The last is a useful remedy at the beginning of a common cold, as, in combination with the opium in the powder, the ipecacuanha increases sweating.

As an emetic ipecacuanha acts slowly, and is not very suitable for urgent poisoning; it is useful when the bronchial tubes are filled with secretion during bronchitis and breathing is difficult, as vomiting helps to empty the tubes. A teaspoonful may be given to a child and repeated several times if necessary.

Emetine is used in treating amoebic dysentery, from twelve to fourteen daily hypodermic injections of 1 grain being given as a rule. This will not get rid of the dysentery parasite from the bowel of a "carrier," however, but emetine bismuth iodide in daily doses of 3 grains for five or six days will often do so, though the course may have to be repeated.

See Cough; Dysentery.

IRISH MOSS. Carrageen, or Irish moss, which is a seaweed, is used to make a demulcent drink. This is also slightly nutritive. The most convenient preparation is the decoction of Irish moss, B.P.C., the dose of which is 1 to 4 ounces.

See Demulcent.

IRON. The metallic element ferrum, or iron, is a normal constituent of the body. It is found chiefly in haemoglobin, the red colouring matter of the blood corpuscles, which enables these to act as oxygen carriers. A considerable amount of this colouring matter is constantly being broken down and excreted in the urine and faeces, so that it is necessary to replenish the stock of iron by taking foods which contain it. It is found both in animal food and in many vegetable foods; although iron does not occur in chlorophyll, the green colouring matter of plants, its presence in the plant is necessary to the formation of chlorophyll.

In disease, however, when there is a deficiency of iron, some preparation of it must be given to supplement what is contained in food. There are numerous preparations, and a choice is determined largely by the tolerance exhibited by the stomach, as some of the preparations are astringent, and may not be well borne.

Blaud's Pills for Anaemia

Iron pills, commonly called Blaud's pills, which are given in doses of 5 to 15 grains, are good if freshly prepared; otherwise they may pass through the bowel intact. These pills can also be obtained in tablet form. Iron lozenges, containing 1 grain each of reduced iron, are given in doses of 1 to 5 grains.

Ferrous sulphate, which forms pale green crystals, is given in solution in doses of 1 to 5 grains, and is often combined with doses of magnesium sulphate, say, 30 grains to 3 grains of the iron sulphate. It is an astringent preparation. It is contained in the compound iron, or Griffith's mixture, dose $\frac{1}{2}$ to 1 ounce, which is often used for amenorrhoea, but in this mixture is converted into the carbonate by admixture with potassium carbonate. Saccharated carbonate of iron has a dose of 10 to 30 grains, and saccharated phosphate, of 5 to 10 grains.

The scale preparations—so-called because they form crystalline scales: ruby, for citrate of iron and ammonium, yellow-green for citrate of iron and quinine, and deep garnet for tartarated iron—are not astringent, and are usually agreeable. The dose of each is 5 to 10 grains in solution.

Solution of perchloride of iron and tincture of perchloride of iron, or steel drops, are given in doses of 5 to 15 minims. Solution of dialysed iron, which, for ordinary purposes, has a dose of 10 to 30 minims, is given in doses of 1 ounce as an antidote in arsenic poisoning. Syrup of phosphate of iron, dose $\frac{1}{2}$ to 1 drachm, syrup of iron phosphate with quinine and strychnine, or Easton's syrup, dose $\frac{1}{2}$ to 1 drachm, syrup of iodide of iron, dose

½ to 1 drachm, and compound syrup of iron phosphate, B.P.C., or chemical food, dose ½ to 2 drachms, make good general tonics. The last is especially useful for children, and is often given with cod-liver oil. The syrup of iodide of iron is valuable in osteo-arthritis.

Colloidal iron and organic combinations, such as ferratin or haemoglobin, are sometimes used in preference to other preparations, especially when the latter disagree.

The chief use of iron is for anaemia of the chlorotic type, in which the haemoglobin content of the corpuscles is diminished, rather than the number of the latter. After a haemorrhage, however, iron seems to stimulate the production of fresh corpuscles. Perchloride of iron is a useful drug in some kinds of tonsillitis and as a spray in laryngitis. In large doses of the tincture it has long been used as a remedy for erysipelas. The strong solution of perchloride of iron is used to arrest bleeding ; a pledget of wool, soaked in the solution and put into the bleeding socket of an extracted tooth, is usually effective.

Astringent preparations of iron may injure the teeth, and to prevent this the dose may be sucked up through a glass tube or a straw, or the mouth should be rinsed immediately with water.

See Anaemia ; Blaud's Pill.

IRRITABILITY. One of the properties of a living cell, or tissue, is that it responds to stimulation, or, in other words, possesses irritability or excitability. It is this property, for example, that enables muscular contraction to be brought about by nervous stimulation, and which accounts for the phenomena of inflammation.

Used in a popular way, with reference to some organ or the state of the temper, it is over-excitability that is meant by irritability. When the heart is unduly sensitive to exercise and excitement, and beats too rapidly or palpitates, it is said to be an irritable heart ; similarly, of the throat, when there is a troublesome cough ; of the bladder, when calls to micturate are too frequent ; and so on.

A disorder of this kind may be more pronounced when the mind dwells upon it. The cause of the irritability may be in the organ itself, or in the nervous mechanism which regulates its functioning. Thus, irritability of the bladder, for example, occurs from an over-acid urine or gravel, but also in some nervous disorders. Over-fatigue, poisoning of some description, as from septic teeth, or the lack of proper nourishment, are the common conditions underlying irritability whether local or general.

See Nervous System ; Neurasthenia ; Sensation.

ISCHAEMIA. A local anaemia, or lack of blood, may be called ischaemia. It is due to interference, by pressure or otherwise, with the flow of blood through an artery, and if severe may cause the death of the tissue affected. Ischaemia may occur from splints being too tightly applied, though it may also occur where there is no interference by apparatus or otherwise and purely from the nature and extent of the injury, and may interfere with the nutrition of the muscles, causing them to become shortened — ischaemic contracture. In the forearm, for example, the fingers may become bent and incapable of being straightened unless the wrist is flexed, though sometimes this cannot be done on account of the hand being pulled backwards. This condition of the forearm is called Volkmann's contracture. Massage may be tried, or if this fails, a surgical operation.

When splints have been applied, the state of the circulation may be tested by pressing on one of the nails and letting go. The pressure causes the nail to become white, but, if the circulation is good, the pink colour returns at once when pressure is removed. Over-tightness of splints is also suggested by coldness or blueness of the exposed part, and by a sensation of pins and needles. The readjustment of splints should, however, be left to the doctor who should be summoned at once.

See Fracture ; Gangrene.

ITCH. *See* Scabies.

ITCHING. Pruritus, or itching, appears to be due to irritation of the fine terminations of the sensory nerves, and this irritation may be due to a large number of causes. Some people have itching from wearing wool or flannel. The application of some chemical substances to the skin is liable to cause itching, and even an excessive use of soap may have this effect.

Parasites, especially lice and the acarus scabiei or itch-mite, are a common cause, also the bites and stings of insects, There may be some itching in ringworm.

Itching may be a symptom of many skin diseases, such as eczema, lichen planus, nettle-rash and prurigo; it may precede or follow the appearance of the rash, and may be very severe.

Abnormal states of the blood, such as occur in diabetes, gout, digestive disturbances, chronic constipation and jaundice, may also cause it, and in some people the taking of such drugs as morphine, belladonna and arsenic. It may likewise occur in certain diseases of the nervous system, mostly in hysteria and hypochondriasis, but also in organic complaints, such as meningitis, general paralysis, or locomotor ataxia. It may accompany disease of the womb or ovaries.

Sometimes it occurs without any assignable cause, a well-known instance being pruritis senilis which afflicts elderly people, and although in pruritus ani, or itching round the orifice of the bowel, some definite cause, such as piles, fissure or the presence of threadworms, can often be established, it is sometimes impossible to explain the symptom. Similarly, pruritus vulvae may be found to be due to sugar in the urine or to leucorrhoea, or whites, but there may be no such explanation; this type is not uncommon at the change of life.

Itching is usually worse at night when the patient is warm in bed, and may, in fact, be caused by excessive heat; stokers and cooks are prone to it for this reason.

Itching provokes scratching, and scratch marks may exist as red lines, excoriations, or papules. In course of time there may be pigmentation of the skin. In senile pruritus any such disturbances of the surface of the skin are very rare.

The first step in treatment is to determine the cause, if possible, as the substitution of cellular cotton or silk underwear for flannel or wool, or the use of cotton or linen sheets in bed, or the destruction of parasites, may be all that is necessary to do Treatment may be directed to any general or local disorder that is found to be present.

General itching may be relieved, at any rate temporarily, by a warm alkaline bath, made by dissolving 6 ounces of washing soda, or 8 to 12 ounces of bicarbonate of potassium, in a bath of about 30 gallons; or the body may be sponged with a lotion of bicarbonate of sodium, a heaped teaspoonful in a quart of water. Rubbing the skin with a menthol cone which has been dipped in spirit is another good method.

In eczema, and especially the dry variety, relief may be got by painting on the following every few hours:

Starch powder	360	grains
Talc	360	,,
Dilute solution of lead subacetate	1	ounce
One per cent. of boracic acid in water	1	,,
Glycerin	½	,,
Camphor water	2½	ounces
To be well shaken before use		

This lotion may also help in itching from other causes. Carbolic acid lotion, 1 part in 80, and dilute solutions of ichthyol or of tar, are amongst other remedies used. A cream consisting of 30 grains each of prepared calamine and zinc oxide, 3 drachms of lime water, and almond oil to 1 ounce, may have a more prolonged effect than a lotion, and may be improved by the addition of 10 grains of menthol or of camphor to the ounce.

For pruritus ani, when no definite cause can be found, a weak, continuous electric current or diathermy may be of use.

See Basilicon Ointment; Dermatitis; Eczema; Eucaine.

JABORANDI. Preparations of jaborandi leaves increase the flow of saliva, sweat and other secretions. This action is due to pilocarpine, an alkaloid contained in them, and the drug is now mostly administered in the form of a salt of this alkaloid, usually the nitrate. In Bright's disease, when uraemia threatens, a hypodermic injection of a pilocarpine salt may avert the danger by causing profuse sweating. There is always a certain amount of danger from full doses of the drug, however, as the secretion in the bronchial tubes may be made so profuse as to cause suffocation. A solution of a pilocarpine salt, when dropped into the eye, causes the pupil to contract and this action is utilised in glaucoma (*q.v.*) and often after eye examinations, to avert the risk of this disorder when mydriatic drugs have been used. Pilocarpine has also a reputation as a hair restorer. Preferably it should be injected into the bald patch, but external applications are also used, or a lotion containing tincture of jaborandi may be applied.

JACKET. To give support to the spine, what is known as a spinal jacket may be worn. This is often made of plaster of Paris bandages, but poro-plastic, a porous material which is much lighter than plaster of Paris, non-inflammable celluloid, which is also light, and occasionally leather, are also used. While the jacket is being applied or fitted, as the case may be, the spine is kept extended by suspension from a tripod or otherwise. An important requisite in such a jacket is that it should be well applied to the pelvis and give support from there. It is chiefly used for tuberculosis of the spine (Plate XXIX, 4-5) and for lateral curvature-

A pneumonia jacket designed to lessen the risk of chill in respiratory complaints is made of Gamgee tissue (*see* Plate XXIX, 3). Insane patients who are violent may have to be put into a strait-jacket, or waistcoat. This is made of strong canvas, and the sleeves extend well below the hands so that they can be crossed in front of the body and tied behind.

JACONET. A thin waterproof material consisting of linen treated with rubber on one side, jaconet forms a useful covering for a fomentation or poultice. A piece of jaconet may be used to keep dressings dry and clean when they are liable to be soiled by urine, or otherwise, and to keep the patient and the bed dry during such procedure as washing wounds, syringing, etc.

JALAP. A drastic purgative, producing copious watery stools, jalap may be taken in powder, in doses of 5 to 20 grains. It is, however, often taken as the compound powder of jalap, which contains also acid potassium tartrate and ginger, and is used in doses of 20 to 60 grains. Jalap resin may be taken in pills, in doses of 2 to 5 grains. Jalap is especially useful in getting rid of dropsy. It is often given combined with calomel, 2 grains

of the latter with 40 grains of the compound powder. This clears the bowel effectively.

JAUNDICE. The existence of jaundice is shown when both the skin and the white of the eyes are yellow. The tint of the skin may vary from bright lemon-yellow to dark olive-green, and there may be itching, particularly if the condition has lasted for some time, when itching may be severe. The urine is dark in colour, and the stools may be clay-coloured and offensive, more or less natural in appearance or dark-coloured, according to the cause of the jaundice. For jaundice is not a disease in itself, but merely a symptom of a variety of conditions, some of which are not of much, or even any, importance, while others are of grave significance.

Bile, which is formed by the liver-cells, makes its way through ducts into the first part of the small intestine, the duodenum, and, if its passage is prevented, it is absorbed into the blood and gives rise to jaundice, this type being called obstructive jaundice. The obstruction may be due to an inflammatory swelling of the lining of the ducts themselves, constituting catarrhal jaundice ; to blocking of the duct by a gall-stone (*q.v.*), or occasionally by a parasitic worm ; or to pressure on the ducts by a growth in any of the adjoining viscera, most commonly a cancer of the head of the pancreas. In rare instances other organs, as, for example, the pregnant womb, may exert sufficient pressure to cause jaundice.

Catarrhal jaundice usually follows indigestion, and represents extension of catarrh from the duodenum into the bile ducts. Besides the signs of jaundice, the tongue is furred, and there may be pain or heaviness in the pit of the stomach or over the liver ; the appetite is poor, or there may be sickness and vomiting. The pulse-rate may be very slow. There is often also depression of spirits, sometimes to the extent of melancholy. A slow pulse and mental depression may occur, however, in any form of obstructive jaundice.

These symptoms may pass away in a fortnight, and do not often last beyond

PLATE XXI

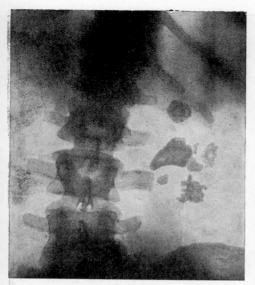

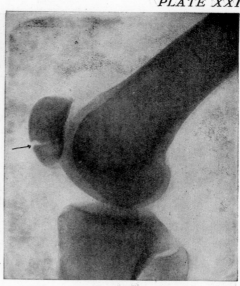

1. Kidney.   Uric acid calculi in the left kidney

2. Knee.   Fracture of the patella or knee-cap

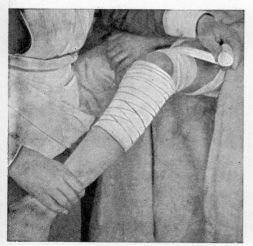

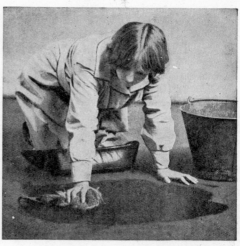

3. Knee.   Figure of 8 bandaging for this joint

4. Use of a mat to prevent housemaid's knee

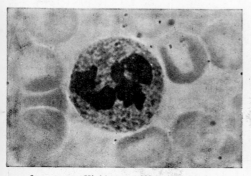

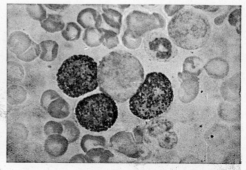

5. Leucocyte.   Highly magnified photograph of a
polynuclear leucocyte or white blood cell

6. Leukaemia. Immature white cells, or myelocytes,
occurring in the blood in this disease

Courtesy of F. Davidson & Co.

PLATE XXII

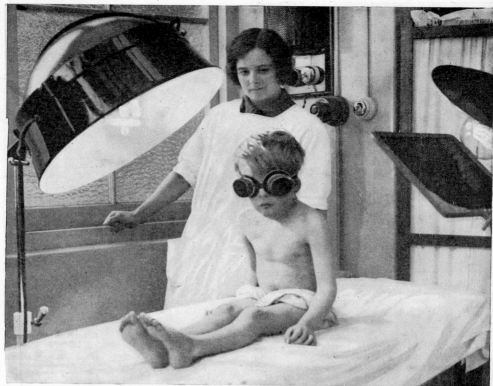

Light Treatment. 1. Application of artificial sunlight, or ultra-violet radiation, as a general tonic

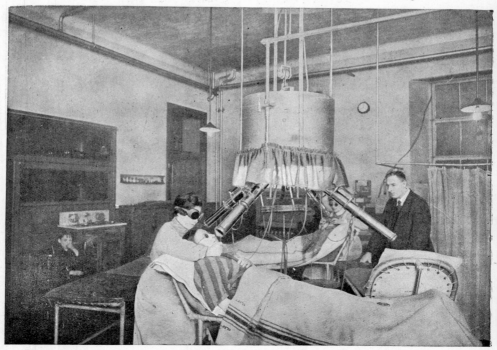

2. Finsen light used in the treatment of lupus and other skin diseases.   The eyes must always be protected

six weeks, though sometimes the catarrh settles down into a chronic state, or such may develop independently of an acute attack. Obstruction due to a gall-stone is likely to be accompanied by other symptoms indicative of a stone, or there may be a history of such ; other facts may point to pressure from a tumour or an enlarged organ.

Acute catarrhal jaundice is treated by putting the patient to bed, where, generally speaking, he should remain till bile is passing freely into the bowel again, as will be shown by the stools. A large linseed poultice or fomentation may be placed over the stomach and liver, especially if there is discomfort. The bowels are usually cleared at the beginning with I grain of calomel at bedtime and a teaspoonful of sodium sulphate in half a glass of water first thing in the morning, the salts being repeated each morning till the motions are normal.

The diet should be limited to milk and hot water at first, and it is an advantage to put a pinch of bicarbonate of sodium in the drinks as it helps to liquefy bile. This purpose may also be served by giving 10 grains of sodium salicylate, thrice daily, dissolved in a little water. After a few days milk puddings and gruel may be added, and, when recovery has begun, white fish and chicken. Fat should be kept out of the diet.

When convalescent, the following may be given :

Dilute nitro-hydrochloric acid 1½ drachms
Glycerin 4   ,,
Compound infusion of gentian to 6 ounces
A tablespoonful in a little water, thrice daily, after food.

The diet should also be light during chronic catarrh, and the bowels must be kept open. Easy open-air exercise is an important consideration.

Treatment may be necessary for itching in jaundice, and for details the reader is referred to that heading. Persons who suffer from jaundice are liable to bleed freely, a fact which must always be kept in mind when there is any question of an operation.

There is another type of jaundice which is due to an excessive breaking down of red blood corpuscles, and is, therefore, called haemolytic jaundice. This is due to

poisoning of some sort. It may occur in malaria, pneumonia, and other infections. It is a feature of Weil's disease (*q.v.*).

Jaundice also occurs in Japanese seven-day fever, which is caused by the leptospira hebdomadalis, infection being caused by the bite of an infected field-mouse. The treatment of these conditions is mainly that of the state of fever (*q.v.*).

A severe acute jaundice occurs in the disease known as acute yellow atrophy of the liver, or it may indicate the action of phosphorus, trinitrotoluene, or other poisons. In haemolytic jaundice, bile pigment is not absent from the stools, which, indeed, may be darker than usual. It sometimes happens that, although there is no staining of the skin or conjunctivae, there is, nevertheless, in the blood an excess of bilirubin, the bile pigment most abundant in man. This is called latent jaundice. On the other hand, people who consume an excess of green vegetable food may manifest a discoloration suggestive of jaundice, although there is nothing of the kind. This is described as pseudo-jaundice.

See Bile ; Liver.

JAW. The upper jaw consists of two separate bones, the right and the left maxilla, which meet at the middle line, while the lower jaw, or mandible, is a single

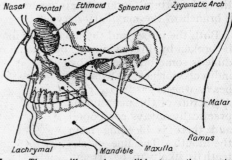

Jaw. The maxillae and mandible form the greater part of the skeleton of the face and carry the teeth

bone, fusion at the middle line taking place in childhood. The part of each jaw which carries the teeth is called the alveolar part.

Each maxilla takes a large share in forming the floor of the orbit and the outer wall of the corresponding nasal cavity, and within it is contained the antrum (*q.v.*), a cavity communicating with the nose and liable to become infected from the nose or from the septic roots of subjacent teeth.

The mandible consists of the body, a horizontal part which is arch-shaped and of two perpendicular portions, or rami (singular, ramus), one at each end of the body. In childhood the ramus is not well marked but in the adult it is so, forming almost a right angle with the body. In old age this angle has become more obtuse, mainly by the wearing away of the alveolar part of the bone. At the top of the ramus are two upward projections with a notch between them. The one in front, triangular in shape, is the coronoid process which gives attachment to the temporal muscle, while the other is the articular process by which the mandible is jointed to the temporal bone in front of the ear, the joint being known as the temporo-mandibular.

The mandible is formed of dense bone, but is pierced by a canal for the inferior dental nerve and by smaller canals for the branches of this nerve to each tooth. The nerve emerges from the bone at the mental foramen which is situated below the second pre-molar tooth. Except for its alveolar part, the maxilla is of more slender construction than the mandible ; on the front of the bone below the orbit is the infra-orbital foramen, giving exit to a branch of the maxillary nerve.

Both the upper and the lower jaws may be broken by direct violence, but the mandible is sometimes broken by indirect violence, as when a heavy wheel passes over it. A fracture of the mandible is practically always compound and there is bleeding from the mouth. The line of the teeth is likely to be irregular. First-aid treatment is given under the heading Fracture. Dislocation of the lower jaw may occur through a blow on the chin, or through opening the mouth too wide in yawning. Emergency treatment is illustrated in Plate XIV, 3 and 4.

The mandible can not only execute a hinge movement but can move from side to side. It should open sufficiently far, as a rule, to separate the edges of the upper and lower incisor teeth by a distance of two inches. Difficulty in opening the mouth may be due to acute inflammation of the tonsil or of neighbouring parts, to inflammation in or about the parotid gland or in the temporo-mandibular joint ; this joint may also be affected by osteo-arthritis, a chronic complaint. Contraction of the skin by scarring may also cause difficulty.

A spasmodic closure of the jaws, or trismus, is found in tetanus, and this fact accounts for the popular name lockjaw given to this disease, but trismus may be due to irritation from teeth and other causes.

See Antrum ; Lockjaw.

JIGGER. The chigoe, or jigger, is a flea, found in tropical countries, which burrows into the skin.

See Flea.

JOINT. The bones and cartilages of the skeleton form with each other a considerable variety of joints, or articulations. They may be grouped into three main classes : immovable, freely movable, and partially movable joints.

The first class includes the suture, the kind of joint uniting the bones of the cranium, or brain-pan. Here, as in the joint between the two parietal bones, the edge of one bone may be fitted into that of the others by tooth-like projections ; or the edges of the bones are bevelled and overlap one another. The latter is called a squamous or scale-like suture because this arrangement is common on scaly surfaces. The joint between the temporal and the parietal bone is an example of a squamous suture.

Another type of immovable joint is exhibited in that between the vomer and the sphenoid. The vomer, which helps to form the middle partition in the nasal cavity, has a groove in one of its edges into which is inserted a ridge of the sphenoid.

A synchondrosis is yet another type, and here two pieces of bone are joined by a

Joint. Suture, an immovable joint, uniting bones of cranium

piece of cartilage. An example of this occurs in growing bones where the epiphysis (*q.v.*) is joined to the diaphysis by a plate of cartilage.

In the course of life any immovable joint may cease to be a joint at all from bone forming across it, but, apart from disease or injury, this cannot happen to a movable joint. This is distinguished by what is called a joint cavity, within which the ends of the bones move on one another. The ends of the bones where they can come into contact with each other are covered with cartilage, known, therefore, as articular cartilage. This softens the play of the bones, prevents friction and lessens jarring. The joint cavity is formed by an outer layer of fibrous tissue, the joint capsule, which is lined by a smooth layer, the synovial membrane.

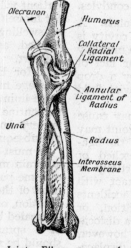

Joint. Elbow, an example of a hinge joint

These together form an airtight enclosure, and the smoothness of the synovial membrane, which is increased by the presence of a clear, thick, lubricating fluid, the synovia, secreted by this membrane, also prevents friction during the movements of the joint. Besides these structures, there are strong fibrous bands, or ligaments, which assist in keeping the ends of the bones in apposition, usually outside, but in some instances actually inside, the joint.

The movements which can be performed at a joint depend upon the shape of the bony parts entering into it, and so a number of varieties of movable joint can be described. The ball-and-socket joint, represented at the shoulder and hip, for example, permits the freest movement of all. This type of joint is well shown in the illustration in page 373.

The possible movements at a joint are abduction and adduction, movement respectively away from and towards the

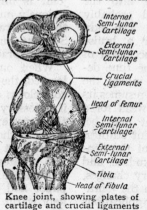

Knee joint, showing plates of cartilage and crucial ligaments

middle line of the body or a limb; flexion, or movement towards the front, or ventral, aspect of the body; and extension, or movement towards the back, or dorsal, aspect of the body. A combination of all these movements is called circumduction, and is performed when the foot or the hand is made to move so as to describe a circle. In addition, at a ball-and-socket joint there is rotation on the longitudinal axis; this happens at the hip, for instance, when the toes are made to point inwards or outwards.

In some joints rotation on this axis is the only movement possible, as in the joint between the uppermost two vertebrae, the atlas and axis, and between the upper and the lower ends of the radius and ulna. On the other hand, in the hinge joint there can only be movement on the transverse axis; this occurs at the elbow, for example. In such joints as those between the small bones of the wrist, surfaces of one bone simply glide on one another; these are called gliding joints.

The description of a movable joint would be incomplete without a reference to the muscles which move it, as by the distribution of muscle fibres or tendons around a joint the latter is more or less strengthened.

The third class of joints, those capable of partial movement, is exemplified by the joints between the bodies of the vertebrae and the symphysis pubis. Here the apposing bones are covered with cartilage, but there is also, separating them, a plate of fibro-cartilage within which is a rudimentary joint cavity. The bones are held together by ligaments. This arrangement must be distinguished from what occurs in some movable joints, such as the knee and that connecting the thumb with the hand, in which there are also plates of cartilage interposed between the ends of bones. These plates, however, have the effect merely of permitting a closer apposition between the bony ends. In the knee the plates are called semilunar cartilages, while those in other joints are referred to as articular disks.

The rounded prominences at the articular ends of some bones are called condyles.

Injuries and Diseases of the Joints. A wound penetrating into a joint cavity is dangerous because septic bacteria multiply very readily in the cavity. The fact of penetration may be disclosed by a drop or two of the thick yellow synovial fluid oozing out.

Violence applied to a joint may cause varying degrees of injury. The joint may be sprained, that is, portions of the ligamentous attachments are stretched or torn, or the bones may be partially or completely displaced from contact with one another, the former of these accidents being called a partial dislocation, or subluxation, while the latter is a dislocation, or luxation. At the knee, however, the injury might otherwise be displacement, bruising or fracture of a semilunar cartilage. Immediately after a sprain full movement will be possible at the joint, though it may be resisted by the patient on account of pain. The joint will swell up rapidly unless the sprain is a slight one, haemorrhage and inflammatory exudation taking place into the tissues around the joint and probably into the joint cavity itself. The skin becomes discoloured as after a bruise (*q.v.*), and shows the same succession of colours. After a few days, the time depending on the severity of the injury, the swelling subsides and the joint resumes its functions, though it remains weak for a longer or shorter period. It may be, however, that there is persistent stiffness due to the binding together of the ligaments by the inflammatory exudate, and sometimes chronic inflammatory changes, or osteo-arthritis, supervene in the joint.

A sprain is treated by cold applications with the object of lessening bleeding into the tissues and relieving pain. After a slight sprain, however, it may be possible simply to strap the joint or apply an elastic bandage. If the injury is at all severe, complete rest is essential, the

injured part being elevated on a pillow; splints may also be required.

After two or three days the joint should be massaged, and passive and active movements begun, that is to say, the nurse will move the joint as far as possible without causing much pain, and also the patient will be encouraged to do the same for himself. To hasten the disappearance of swelling, an elastic bandage may be applied, as firmly as is consistent with comfort. A flannel bandage often does well for this purpose. The benefit of massage may be enhanced by the use of some liniment, say, the acetic liniment of turpentine. Early movement of the joint is very important to lessening the risk of subsequent stiffness.

It must always be borne in mind that a sprain may be associated with fracture of some portion of bone in the neighbourhood of the joint, or there may be a subluxation, occurrences which are sometimes concealed by the swelling. The treatment of a sprain of any gravity, therefore, should be superintended by a doctor, and it will often be advisable to have an X-ray examination made.

When a Joint is Dislocated

A dislocation of a joint causes immediate deformity of a greater or lesser degree, according to the size and position of the joint, and voluntary movement at the joint is impossible, or, at any rate, is seriously impaired. The reader is referred to the X-ray illustrations in Plate XIV. Swelling and discoloration supervene as after a sprain.

When one of the limb joints is dislocated, the first-aid treatment is to apply cold cloths and rest the part, with splints if necessary. A sling should be used for the upper extremity. If the dislocation is of one of the joints of the lower extremity, the patient should be kept lying down, as also, whatever joint is dislocated, if there is evidence of shock, such as faintness, pallor and chilliness, he should also be kept warm. The reduction of the dislocation should be left to a doctor, as unskilled attempts might increase the damage, more particularly if there should be an associated fracture.

A dislocation should be reduced as soon as possible. If it is not reduced, the displaced bone tends to make a fresh socket for itself, what is described as a pseudo-arthrosis, but adhesions form about the ends of the bones. A congenital dislocation, that is, one occurring before birth, is generally due to improper development. Reduction may be difficult, and even when it has been accomplished the dislocation will probably tend to recur, owing to the joint cavity being inadequate to retain the head of the other bone. The methods of dealing with a congenital dislocation are described under the heading Hip.

Inflammation of a joint may be limited to the synovial membrane or practically so, when it is called synovitis, or it may involve all the structures of the joint, when it is called arthritis. Acute synovitis may be due to cold or an injury ; sometimes it is due to the presence of a loose body, such as a piece of cartilage or bone which has been detached in the joint, and which from time to time gets between the surfaces of the joint, causing locking, severe pain and synovitis. A loose semi-lunar cartilage also may cause a recurrent synovitis. Acute synovitis may also be due to some constitutional disorder, such as gout, rheumatism or gonorrhoea, though probably in most of these the condition might rather be called arthritis.

Inflammation of a Joint

Acute synovitis causes pain and swelling of the joint, and, following injury. there will probably be discoloration from effused blood, as described above in the account of sprain. The treatment is also that laid down for sprain. Sometimes on getting up after traumatic synovitis of the knee the joint again swells, and although the fluid disappears after further rest in bed it always tends to recur on getting up. The best thing to do is to wear an elastic bandage on the knee and get about ; although the knee is swollen at night, the amount of fluid gradually diminishes until it disappears altogether. Synovitis due to some constitutional disorder demands primarily treatment for this disorder. The joint should be rested and treated with hot applications or be wrapped up in cotton wool. When the acute stage passes off, movements, mas-sage and a liniment are used to promote absorption of the fluid and flexibility of the joint.

Acute synovitis may be followed by stiffness and limitation of movement from products of inflammation becoming converted into scar-like tissue and forming adhesions inside or outside the joint. These results should be combated by early movements. It is necessary, however, to take care when a joint is inflamed and there is a possibility of ankylosis or fixation that the limb is placed in such a position that, should this occur, its functions will be preserved as far as possible. Such is known as the optimum position in ankylosis. This aspect of treatment will be further dealt with below. Attention to the muscles acting on the joint is very important, as, according to its severity, inflammation in a joint is always followed by wasting of the muscles, to a greater extent also than can be explained by mere disuse.

Chronic Form of Synovitis

Acute synovitis may assume a chronic form or this may exist as such from the beginning, when the cause has not been sufficient to set up severe inflammation. There may not be much pain, but the joint is weak. The synovial membrane is thickened, and its fringes may become enlarged and palpable. There is more or less fluid present as a rule. The movements of the joint are interfered with as regards ease and possibly extent also, and may be accompanied by a sensation of fine or coarse grating.

Blistering and the pressure of an elastic bandage may do good, also hot-air or other baths or diathermy. Operative treatment may be necessary, however.

Acute arthritis is due to bacteria invading the joint, except when such a disease as gout or trauma is the cause. The bacteria may be of the septic type, when suppuration is likely to occur, and if a large joint is involved the patient's life is endangered. Other microbes, such as those of typhoid fever, dysentery, gonorrhoea or pneumonia, may be responsible, however.

As in the more limited condition of synovitis, there is swelling of the joint and pain, which is severe ; merely to touch the limb or shake the bed may occasion intolerable agony, and the patient may be brusquely awakened from sleep by what is called starting pains. There is likely to be a considerable degree of fever, and the patient will probably look very ill ➤ The skin over the joint may be oedematous, and, if suppuration occurs, the pus, or matter, finds its way to the surface by one or more routes, resulting in the presence of discharging sinuses.

Suppurative arthritis, as has been said, may threaten life, but in any arthritis, owing to the destruction of cartilage, etc., there is always an imminent risk of ankylosis of the joint, and if this should take place in an awkward position the utility of a limb may be sacrificed. When effusion occurs into the joint, in synovitis or in arthritis, the joint tends to assume the position of greatest ease, and generally this means that it becomes somewhat flexed, or bent. If left to itself, the flexion or bending is likely to increase. If the inflammation in the joint is severe, the ligaments and other structures binding the ends of the bone together become softened, and partial dislocation may occur, or the limb may be rotated on its long axis. It is necessary, therefore, when there is any risk of ankylosis, to fix the joint in the best position for future service, and for various joints these positions are as follows (*see* Plate XX) :

Best Positions in Ankylosis

SHOULDER, the upper arm making an angle of 50 deg. with the vertical, and the elbow slightly in front.

ELBOW, at an angle of 70 deg., or, if both elbows are affected, one at this angle and the other at an angle of 110 deg. ; the latter is the better position for working and the former for the patient feeding himself. The forearm is placed so that the thumb points upwards or slightly outwards.

WRIST, with the hand drawn backwards, or, at least, in line with the forearm.

HIP, with the thigh in line with the side-to-side plane of the trunk, but drawn a little outwards from the middle line of the body, and the toes pointing somewhat outwards.

KNEE, with the lower limb straight, or very slightly bent.

ANKLE, with the foot at right angles to the leg and the sole directed slightly inwards.

The general condition of the patient requires urgent attention, and treatment will include that for the state of fever (*q.v.*) generally, and probably also the use of vaccines or sera to combat the activities of the microbes concerned. It may be necessary to open and drain the joint, and always will be so if suppuration should take place.

Tuberculosis is a common cause of chronic arthritis, and the disease may begin either in the synovial membrane or the bone ; in children it almost always begins in the epiphyseal cartilage. The synovial membrane swells, and, in course of time, is replaced by granulation tissue, the cartilages are destroyed, bone is softened and disappears, and abscesses form. In the effusion into the joint there are often numerous so-called melon seed bodies floating. The joint swells, and the skin over it is pale, hence the condition is referred to as a white swelling.

Treatment of Hip Disease

The expression hip disease means tuberculous disease of this joint, although other diseases may affect the hip (*q.v.*). It may be necessary for the treatment of a tuberculous joint to evacute an abscess and remove diseased tissue, but more conservative methods of treatment, namely, rest, fresh air, sunlight and feeding, are now thought to be the best routine treatment. Vaccine treatment is sometimes a useful auxiliary.

Chronic arthritis may also be caused by syphilis, and by the organisms mentioned above as causing the acute disease. It may be due to poisons absorbed from septic teeth, from a diseased appendix or from some other focus. It may occur from physical injury, or from metabolic changes. Rheumatoid arthritis and osteo-arthritis are described under their own headings. In cases of chronic arthritis from various causes a joint may be enormously swollen with fluid, though pain and other symptoms are little marked. This condition is called hydrops articuli, or hydrarthrosis.

When in chronic disease the fluid in a joint is at considerable tension, it may cause the capsule to bulge out between the ligaments, giving rise to swellings around the joint ; such are described as Baker's cysts. and are encountered especially in osteo - arthritis and tuberculous disease.

In the treatment of chronic joint disease not due to definite causes, such as gout, tuberculosis or syphilis, it is necessary to search for any focus of infection and clean it up. Rest, or, on the other hand, movement may be needed, and liniments, massage, ionisation, diathermy, hot air baths, light baths and electrical treatment are other useful methods of local treatment. A generous, varied diet with cod-liver oil and other tonics may be required to build up body-energy, and attention to morale must not be neglected ; an attitude of chronic invalidism must be combated. Climatic and spa treatment are often especially helpful.

In locomotor ataxia, signs of disease sometimes appear in a joint, especially the shoulder, hip or knee, and appear suddenly with distension of the joint with fluid. The ends of the bones may become eroded, or, on the other hand, outgrowths of bone, known as osteophytes, may occur. There is no pain. In the wasting, or atrophic form, the joint becomes flail-like, and spontaneous dislocation is common ; in the hypertrophic form, the joint tends to ankylose and probably in a bent position. The disease is known as neuropathic arthritis or Charcot's disease, and also occurs in syringomyelia. A compar-

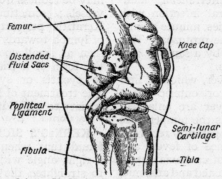

Joint. In Charcot's disease there is rapid swelling and later erosion of the cartilages

Femur
Distended Fluid Sacs
Popliteal Ligament
Fibula
Knee Cap
Semi-lunar Cartilage
Tibia

able condition may also occur in other nervous disorders. It is essential that the joint should be fixed in a correct position.

In neurotic individuals pains may occur in a joint and there may be apparent limitation of movement, suggestive of joint disease. A careful examination may eliminate this possibility, however, and the treatment then adopted is that for hysteria (*q.v.*). Persons affected in this way in the knee have been known to refrain from walking for years, and then have their power restored in an apparently miraculous way, and so for other joints.

See Cartilage ; Dislocation ; Fracture ; Ligament ; Mud Bath ; Osteo-arthritis ; Rheumatoid Arthritis.

JUGULAR VEIN. Most of the venous blood from the interior of the skull drains into the sigmoid sinus on each side, which, through an opening in the skull, becomes continuous with the internal jugular vein. This passes down the neck along with, but on the outer side of, the carotid artery and unites with the subclavian vein to form the innominate vein. On each side of the neck there are also the anterior and the external jugular veins. These lie just below the skin, the former passing down the front of the neck and then passing outwards to join the external jugular : this vein passes obliquely down the side of the neck to enter the subclavian vein. (*See* illustration in page 397.)

Bleeding from the internal jugular vein is very dangerous.

See Innominate ; Neck.

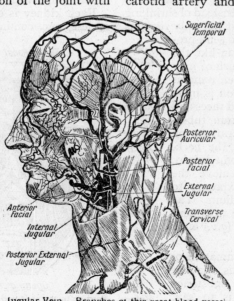

Superficial Temporal
Posterior Auricular
Posterior Facial
External Jugular
Transverse Cervical
Anterior Facial
Internal Jugular
Posterior External Jugular

Jugular Vein. Branches of this great blood vessel

KALA-AZAR. A febrile disease occurring in the East and along the shores of the Mediterranean, kala-azar is due to a general infection with Leishman-Donovan bodies, minute animal parasites belonging to the protozoa. This parasite is transmitted by a sand-fly and possibly by other insects.

There is remittent fever, which at first may suggest malaria or enteric fever, and the spleen and liver are enlarged. After two or three weeks the temperature drops and the patient apparently recovers, but there is a recurrence of fever, and ultimately a condition of cachexia supervenes. The patient is wasted and anaemic, and there is a more or less continuous low fever. The parasites may be discovered in blood drawn from the spleen or liver, or more rarely, in blood from surface vessels.

The disease can be cured by injections of the tartrate or other preparations of antimony.

KAOLIN. China clay, or kaolin, which consists mainly of a natural silicate of aluminium, is purified and reduced to a fine white powder for use in medicine. It is used as an excipient for pills containing phosphorus, permanganate of potassium, silver salts and other substitutes. It is also used as a soothing and absorbent dusting powder for intertrigo, etc.

KELOID. Over-growth of scar-tissue gives rise to a keloid. Instead of shrinking like an ordinary scar, it not only remains prominent but tends to send prolongations along the skin like the claws of a crab. The surface may be white but more often remains pink. Keloid formation is more common in the coloured races and in anyone suffering from tuberculosis ; scars of operations on tuberculous glands of the neck, for example, often become keloid. The best way to remove the disfigurement is by exposure to sunlight, X-rays or radium. The drawback to operative treatment is that the fresh scar (*q.v.*) may also become keloid.

KERATITIS. Inflammation of the cornea, or keratitis, may be superficial, or in the substance of the cornea, that is to say,

interstitial. There is more or less cloudiness of the structure and there may be redness from the presence of blood vessels ; sometimes there is ulceration. Keratitis punctata consists of deposits of lymph towards the back of the cornea, seen as small spots usually arranged in the form of a triangle, and is secondary to cyclitis or sympathetic ophthalmia. The treatment of keratitis depends on the variety to which it belongs.

See Cornea ; Eye.

KERNIG'S SIGN. In meningitis it is found that when the thigh is bent at a right angle with the body an attempt to straighten the limb is resisted by the patient, as this causes much pain. This is called Kernig's sign. It is also present in sciatica.

KIDNEY. Situated on the upper part of the posterior wall of the abdominal cavity, the kidneys, of which there is one on either side of the spine, are partly covered behind by the last ribs, the left being placed rather higher up in the body than the right. A kidney has a characteristic shape, somewhat resembling a flattened bean, the long axis being up and down, but obliquely, as the lower end of the organ is the farther from the mid-line of the body ; the average dimensions are 4 inches long, $2\frac{1}{2}$ inches broad, and 1 inch thick.

Each kidney is embedded in fat, more or less, and coming from the aorta to

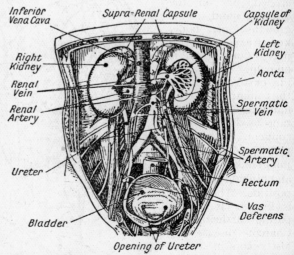

Kidney. Position in the abdomen and relation to other organs

its inner border, almost at right angles, is the renal artery, while from this border the renal vein passes across to the inferior vena cava. Lymphatic vessels also come from it and the ureter, and nerves enter it. All these structures together constitute the pedicle, or root, of the kidney.

The inner portion of the organ is hollowed out into a sinus, within which is attached a membranous bag, roughly triangular in shape, and known as the pelvis of the kidney. Short tube-like prolongations of this bag, known as calyces, surround nipple-shaped projections, or papillae, on the inner border of the kidney. The discharge ducts in the organ itself open on these papillae, of which there are from six to fourteen, and the urine then passes through the calyces into the pelvis and on into the ureter, which begins at the inner angle of the latter.

A section through the kidney reveals the fact that the papillae represent the apices of pyramidal masses of tissue which mainly constitute the inner portion, or medulla, of the kidney substance. Outside the bases of the pyramids, and between them, is the cortex, the substance of which differs from that of the pyramids, even to the naked eye. Under the microscope the pyramids are seen to consist of an immense collection of tiny, straight tubes arranged side by side, between which are small blood vessels, but in the cortex, while there are also some straight tubes, the tubes are mainly convoluted or twisted. Moreover, there is a large number of minute clumps of blood vessels, or glomeruli. Each glomerulus is enclosed in a capsule, the capsule of Bowman, and this is continuous with a length of convoluted tubing which in turn is continuous with a straight tubule in one of the pyramids. The whole kidney substance is enclosed by a fibrous capsule.

The blood vessel entering a glomerulus is larger than that which leaves it, so that

Section of kidney substance, showing the filtering tubes and tufts of blood vessels

the blood in the glomerulus is at high pressure, and, in consequence, water and dissolved substances, like salts and sugar, are squeezed out into the capsule of Bowman. This exudation runs along the tubules, the cells of which reabsorb the sugar and perhaps part of the water and salts also, at the same time passing out into the exudation such substances as urea, uric acid, and probably phosphates. The exudation thus constituted is then delivered into the pelvis of the kidney as urine.

This is the view of the mechanism of urine secretion which has generally been held. The most modern view, however, is that all secretion takes place in the capsules, but that the tubule cells reabsorb certain things.

Sometimes a person is born with both kidneys fused into one, or the organs may be united only at their lower ends, forming what is called a horseshoe kidney. Such an abnormality has no clinical significance except when disease or injury raises the question of operating on the organ.

In some people, and especially women, the kidney may be more or less freely movable. This has no disagreeable effects, as a rule, but occasionally it leads to kinking of the ureter and a sudden

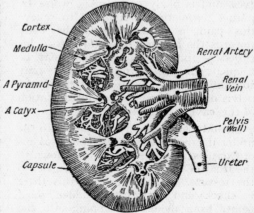

Section of a Kidney. Urine emerges from the tubules into the calyces, whence it reaches the ureter

stoppage of the flow of urine. There is severe pain and probably vomiting, which is relieved by the unkinking through the kidney changing its position ; this is followed by a free flow of urine. This accident is known as Dietl's crisis, and should it tend to recur the kidney may be retained in position by a properly padded belt or may be fixed in position by an operation.

Injuries and Diseases of the Kidney. In visceroptosis (q.v.), or sagging of the abdominal organs, one or both kidneys may share in the displacement. By a severe blow, or by crushing, a kidney may be ruptured. This causes shock and the appearance of blood in the urine.

A renal calculus, or stone in the kidney, may be situated in the pelvis, in a calyx or in the substance of the organ. Lithaemia (q.v.), an increase of uric acid in the blood, or other circumstances which increase the concentration of the acid or of certain other substances in the urine, lead to the precipitation of the crystals out of which calculi are formed. These are usually of uric acid, urate of sodium or ammonium, or of acid phosphate of sodium. Even a large stone may be present in the kidney for a long time without giving rise to symptoms.

A dull pain in the loin is common, however, and is likely to be made worse by jolting ; sometimes, in order to relieve this pain, a patient bends the body towards the affected side and presses his closed fist into the loin. There may be frequency in passing urine and this may contain pus and blood. A stone in the pelvis of the kidney causes inflammation of this cavity, or pyelitis.

Should a stone of any size pass into the ureter it gives rise to renal colic, spasms of excruciating pain which shoot down to the front of the thigh and, in the male, to the testicle. Associated with this there is shock and vomiting. Sudden relief comes from the stone slipping into the bladder or back into the pelvis of the

Kidney displacement due to visceroptosis

Diaphragm
Left Kidney
Supra-renal Capsule
Hip Bone
Ureter
Pelvic Cavity

kidney. Should the stone become stuck, or impacted, in the ureter, it causes arrest of the action, or anuria, of the affected kidney, if the obstruction be complete ; if this is incomplete, there is hydronephrosis, or an accumulation of urine in the passage above the obstruction. If there is a large amount of pus in the retained fluid, the condition is described as pyonephrosis.

The diagnosis is helped greatly by the use of X-rays (see Plate XXI, 1). The treatment is directed to the lithaemia, but it may be necessary to cut down on and explore the organ (nephrotomy), when, if stones are found, the kidney is incised and the stones ejected, or if the organ is much disorganised it may be removed altogether (nephrectomy) ; this can only be done, however, if there is another kidney, which is functioning.

Renal colic is treated by placing the patient in a hot bath or hip-bath and, if necessary, injecting morphine ; the inhalation of chloroform is sometimes necessary.

Inflammation of the kidney substance, or nephritis, is described under the heading Bright's Disease. Septic infection may involve both the pelvis and the kidney substance ; this is called pyelo-nephritis. From such infection an abscess may form in the kidney. Sometimes an abscess forms outside the kidney—a perinephric abscess. Here the infection may pass out from a diseased kidney, but it may come from elsewhere, possibly from a boil somewhere on the body. Abscesses in or around the kidney must be opened and drained

Tuberculous disease may affect one or both kidneys and may be due to the disease spreading upwards from the bladder, or occur independently. The symptoms rather resemble those of stone in the kidney, but a proper examination of the urine is likely to reveal the presence of tubercle bacilli in it. The treatment is that for tuberculosis (q.v.) generally, and tuberculin injections are sometimes useful.

If the disease be limited to one kidney it may be removed.

The limitation of the disease to one kidney may be shown by drawing off urine from each ureter separately. This is done by passing a cystoscope into the bladder and introducing fine tubes, known as ureteral catheters, through this. A cystoscope consists of a metal tube with a little electric bulb at its inner end, by which the interior of the bladder may be illuminated for purposes of examination and treatment.

Various kinds of cysts and tumours may affect the kidney, some of them being congenital. In some cases a cure can be effected by operation.

See Bladder; Bright's Disease; Diuretic; Hydronephrosis; Micturition; Uraemia; Ureter; Urine.

KINO. The evaporated juice of an Eastern tree, and occurring as small, angular, glistening, dark-red fragments, kino contains a large amount of tannic acid, and so acts as an astringent. It is often used in diarrhoea, either as the powdered drug, in doses of 5 to 20 grains, as tincture of kino, dose ½ to 1 drachm, or as compound powder of kino, dose 5 to 20 grains. This powder contains opium and cinnamon bark also.

KLEPTOMANIA. An impulse to steal, evoked by some mental conflict of which the patient is ignorant, and which is irresistible, is described as kleptomania. It occurs more frequently amongst women. It is a different thing from the thieving propensity which may be exhibited by the mentally deficient, and, although in some cases the impulse is to steal particular things, it is a very different thing from the covetousness of the ardent collector. The mental processes underlying the impulse may be brought to light by skilful psycho-analysis.

See Psycho-therapy.

KNEE. To form the knee joint the lower end of the femur rests on the upper surface of the head of the tibia. On this surface there are two areas, an inner, which is oval, and an outer, circular, for the reception of the internal and the external condyle of the femur respectively, these areas being separated by an elevation of the bone known as the spinous process. To this spine is attached one of the two crucial ligaments, so called because they cross one another, which are situated in the middle of the joint and which are important factors in strengthening it and preventing an undue range of movement (*see* illustration in page 411).

The areas above referred to are deepened for additional security by the presence of the internal and external semi-lunar cartilages, which at their extremities are attached to the tibia. In cross section each cartilage is triangular in shape, the thicker part being towards the margin of the joint-surface. A semi-lunar cartilage may be detached by violence, which usually takes the form of a twist of the leg when the knee is slightly bent. This happens most often to the internal cartilage. The cartilage is not only detached but displaced, and so is nipped between the bones.

Injury to a semi-lunar cartilage causes great pain and more or less locking of the joint, which shortly swells up from the accumulation of fluid due to synovitis. As soon as possible after the accident the cartilage should be replaced in position, under a general anaesthetic if necessary. The limb is then rested and hot applications applied in order to remove the inflammation and the fluid. The pressure of an elastic bandage is useful here. Movements of the joint are begun early, but a supporting bandage should be worn when the patient begins to get about

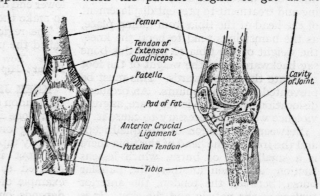

Knee. Left, joint from the front. Right, interior of joint in section

Labels: Femur; Tendon of Extensor Quadriceps; Patella; Pad of Fat; Anterior Crucial Ligament; Patellar Tendon; Tibia; Cavity of Joint

(see Plate XXI, 3). Recurrence of the trouble may take place, however, and it may be deemed advisable to remove the cartilage or, at any rate, the loosened part.

The only movements normally possible at the knees are flexion and extension, or bending and straightening, except that in straightening out there is also slight rotation of the leg outwards and a contrary movement when the limb is again bent. Extension is brought about by the action of the powerful group of muscles on the front of the thigh, described together as the quadriceps extensor. In the ligament by which the quadriceps is attached to the tibia is the small, rounded bone, known as the patella, or knee-cap, the inner surface of which moves on the front of the lower end of the femur. Flexion is mainly due to the hamstring muscles on the back of the thigh.

Some Causes of Instability

Inflammation of the joint, however, may weaken the ligaments and make lateral, that is, side to side, movements possible, and also the end of the tibia may become movable backwards and forwards on the femur when the limb is fully extended. This causes more or less instability of the joint in walking or even standing, and a support of some kind may require to be worn on the knee. Bending backwards of the knee beyond the straight is called genu-recurvatum and implies lengthening of the crucial ligaments. It may be congenital. Unless it is pronounced, or accompanied by general slackness of the joint, it is not of much significance.

A person who is bedridden because of knee-joint disease requires careful watching and treatment to prevent displacement of the head of the tibia from taking place, as the hamstrings tend to bend the knee, the weight of the tibia to make this bone sag backwards, and the weight of the foot to rotate the leg outwards. This must be prevented by proper splints. An ordinary dislocation of the knee is very rare, as great violence would be necessary to cause it.

Between the tendon of the quadriceps and the front of the head of the tibia there is a small bag, or bursa, which lessens friction, and then another, the patellar bursa, between the tendon, the anterior surface of the patella and the skin. It is the accumulation of fluid in the latter, owing to bursitis (q.v.), that constitutes housemaid's knee. This is caused by pressure and so may occur in any person who kneels much. It may be prevented by the use of a cushion (see Plate XXI, 4).

In housemaid's knee the collection of fluid is in front of the knee-cap, while in distention of the joint with fluid the knee-cap is, as it were, floating on the fluid. The synovial cavity extends well above the knee-cap, especially when the limb is extended, so that a stab in the front of the thigh, up to 2 inches above the upper border of the knee-cap, is likely to open the joint.

Knock knee, or genu valgum, is the condition in which the knee is bent inwards towards the middle line of the body, the foot being carried outwards and the toes turned out more than usual. Usually both limbs are affected. It occurs in early childhood from rickets, but may affect a young person with weak ligaments, a condition frequently associated with general debility, or one who does much weight-carrying or habitually adopts a faulty posture in standing. There is usually also flat foot, and the existence of this would predispose to knock knee.

In the earlier stages only the soft parts of the joint are involved, and the condition may be rectified by manipulation and a correct alinement preserved by splints or leg-irons; but when the deformity is of some standing bony changes have occurred, the internal condyle of the femur is enlarged and lengthened and the external condyle atrophied possibly, so that it becomes necessary to break through the lower end of the shaft of the femur in order to make the limb straight.

The region at the back of the knee is called the popliteal space (q.v.).

See Bow Leg; Bursitis; Dislocation; Femur; Hip; Joint; Patella; Rickets; Tibia.

KNEE JERK. In a healthy person, if the tendon connecting the patella with the shin bone is put on the stretch, say, by crossing one leg over the other, and is smartly tapped with the edge of the hand, the foot is kicked forwards. This is referred to as the knee jerk, and is an example of a deep reflex; its existence depends on the integrity of the nervous circle, comprising the nerve from the tendon or extensor muscles to the spinal cord, nerve centres in the cord, and nerves from these to the extensor muscles.

To elicit the reflex, the leg must be hanging loosely, and if the patient's attention is not distracted he may prevent the movement. It is often necessary to ask him to look at the ceiling, and an additional aid is to get him to hook the fingers of one hand in those of the other and pull.

The knee jerk is absent in locomotor ataxia and other diseases in which the sensory path is diseased, and if the motor path is diseased, as when infantile paralysis affects the muscles on the front of the thigh, again it is absent. On the other hand, when the tracts in the spinal cord which bring impulses from the brain to control the activity of motor centres in the cord are diseased, the knee jerk is exaggerated. This happens, for example, in lateral sclerosis. The knee jerk may also be exaggerated, however, in some functional nervous disorders.

See Nervous System ; Reflex Action.

KNOCK KNEE. *See* Knee.

KOLA NUT. The seeds of species of the cola, or kola, tree contain considerable quantities of the alkaloid caffeine (*q.v.*), and are used as a stimulant. In the tropical countries in which the trees grow the seeds are often chewed. There are, however, certain preparations made from the nuts, including the liquid extract of kola, B.P.C., the dose being 10 to 20 minims.

KRAMERIA. Rhatany or krameria root, which is obtained from South America, is rich in tannic acid and its preparations are useful astringents. The official preparations are the extract, dose 5 to 15 grains ; the infusion, dose $\frac{1}{2}$ to 1 ounce ; the tincture, dose $\frac{1}{2}$ to 1 drachm ; the lozenge and the rhatany and cocaine lozenge. Krameria is extensively used for spongy gums and relaxed throat. It may be incorporated in a tooth powder, or a teaspoonful of the tincture in a wineglass of water may be used as a mouth wash and gargle ; some people prefer the lozenges.

KYPHOSIS. An abnormal backward curvature of the spine is described as kyphosis, or, popularly, hump-back. This may be due to a variety of causes.

See Backbone ; Spinal Curvature.

LABYRINTH. The internal ear, comprising parts subserving the function of hearing and others concerned with the maintenance of balance, is described as the labyrinth.

See Ear ; Equilibrium.

LACERATION. A tear through the tissues is described as a laceration or a lacerated wound. There is more damage than when the wound is clean, and consequently a greater risk of infection.

See Wound.

LACHRYMAL APPARATUS. The watery secretion of the eye comes from the lachrymal gland, which is situated behind the outer part of the upper eyelid, and is usually just sufficient to keep the eye moist. When excessive it overflows the lower eyelid in the form of tears. The secretion drains into two tiny tubes situated in the margin of the lids at the inner corner of the eye, by which it is led into the lachrymal sac. This empties by the lachrymal duct into the nasal cavity behind the front part of the inferior turbinate bone.

See Eye ; Nose.

LACTATION. *See* Breast ; Breast-feeding.

LACTEAL VESSELS. The tiny tubes which drain off digested fat from the intestine are called lacteals, because their contents are milky-looking.

See Digestion ; Intestine.

LACTIC ACID. By fermenting lactose, or milk sugar, through the agency of the lactic acid bacillus or certain other bacteria, lactic acid is obtained as a colourless, syrupy liquid. The souring of milk is caused in this way.

Strong lactic acid is used for dissolving the false membrane in diphtheria, tumours and other unhealthy tissue. Dilute lactic acid is sometimes used in catarrh of the bladder, in infantile diarrhoea with green stools and in other disorders. The dose for an adult is $\frac{1}{2}$ to 2 drachms. Various salts of lactic acid are used in medicine, most frequently calcium lactate. Lacto-phosphates are used as tonics.

See Milk.

LACTOMETER. An instrument for determining the specific gravity of milk is called a lactometer. The usual form floats, partially submerged, in the liquid, and has a graduated stem projecting upwards. The graduations are from 1,005 to 1,040, the specific gravity of distilled water being represented by 1,000. During use the instrument must be kept away from the side of the vessel containing the milk, as it might adhere to some extent. The level to which the stem is submerged is read off, the figure representing the specific gravity of the sample.

See Milk.

LACTOPHOSPHATE. A mixture of lactic and phosphoric acids in combination with a base is called a lactophosphate. Calcium lactophosphate occurs as a powder. The official syrup of calcium lactophosphate is given in doses of $\frac{1}{2}$ to 1 drachm in water. There is also a syrup of the lactophosphates of calcium and iron, with the same dose. These preparations are used as tonics.

LACTOSE. Milk sugar, or lactose, belongs to the same group of sugars as cane sugar. It occurs in milk and should be preferred for sweetening milk mixtures used in infant feeding. It is used as a diluent in powders containing strong drugs.

See Milk; Sugar.

LAMELLA. A tiny disk made of gelatin and glycerin, and containing some powerful drug, a lamella is used for introducing drugs into the eye. The lamella is lifted on a glass rod, or camel-hair brush, or with small forceps, and placed on the white of the eyeball while the patient looks up. The eye is then closed, and the disk allowed to dissolve. The official lamellae are those of atropine, cocaine, homatropine and physostigmine.

LAMENESS. Many causes, from painful corns to serious joint or nervous disorders, may account for lameness. In children, infantile paralysis and early hip-joint disease are amongst the possibilities to be considered. The state of the footwear may also require consideration in some instances of lameness.

LANCE. Making a small incision, or cut, is sometimes described as lancing. This is generally done with the ordinary surgical knife, known as a scalpel, though formerly it was customary to use a specially shaped knife, called a lance or lancet, and this may still be employed by some practitioners. The gum is sometimes lanced in teething difficulties, and much relief may be procured if the case is a suitable one ; otherwise, matters may be made worse by lancing.

LANOLIN. Adeps lanae, or wool-fat, obtained from the wool of sheep, is a yellowish, sticky substance. It is sometimes called anhydrous lanolin, the term lanolin being that commonly used for wool-fat with an admixture of about 30 per cent. water—hydrous wool-fat. Lanolin is used as an emollient, and as a basis for ointments. It has the advantage that it does not become rancid. Its stickiness may be lessened by mixing with a little soft paraffin or vaseline.

See Ointment.

LAPAROTOMY. Any operation in which an opening is made into the abdomen by an incision is called a laparotomy.

LARD. From the fat of pigs is prepared lard, or adeps. Adeps praeparatus, or purified lard, is used as a basis for ointments. To guard against its becoming rancid, adeps benzoatus, that is, lard with the addition of three per cent. of benzoin, is generally used.

See Ointment.

LARDACEOUS DISEASE. *See* Amyloid Disease.

LARVA. The young of an insect, when it hatches out of the egg, is called a larva, or, popularly, and especially as regards certain insects, a maggot or grub. A larva is a more or less active creature. The immature form of other animals, when it differs widely from the adult type, is often also described as a larva.

See Fly.

LARYNGISMUS STRIDULUS. *See* Croup.

LARYNX. The organ of voice, which is known as the larynx, is continuous below with the trachea, or windpipe, and opens above into the pharynx, below and behind the base of the tongue. All air entering or leaving the chest passes through the larynx. The pharynx, at the back of the larynx, becomes continuous with the gullet. Food is prevented from entering the larynx by the latter being drawn upwards under the base of the tongue during the act of swallowing (*q.v.*). If a person tries to talk as well as swallow, particles may be drawn into the larynx, but, as they cause much irritation, they are

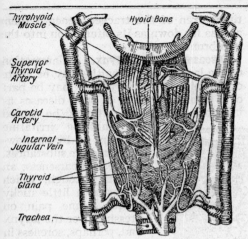

Larynx and related structures from the front

true vocal cord is called the ventricle of the larynx.

On the apex of each arytenoid cartilage is situated a tiny cartilage, known as the cartilage of Santorini, and from this a fold of mucous membrane passes up to be attached to the side of the epiglottis. From its attachments it is called the aryteno-epiglottidean fold. The space between these folds represents the actual entrance into the larynx. In oedema, or dropsy, of the larynx these folds may become sufficiently swollen almost to close the opening and threaten or even cause suffocation.

The vocal cords are formed of elastic tissue and normally appear as two white glistening bands traversing the larynx from front to back. In ordinary breathing they are moderately open, leaving a triangular space, the rima glottidis, the base of the triangle being at the back. This space becomes rather larger during inspiration, diminishing again with expiration.

For the production of voice the cords come together, leaving only a narrow slit for air, which, by throwing the edge of the cords into vibration, produces sound. The pitch of this varies with the closeness of the cords to one another and with their state of tension. The opening and closing of the cords are brought about by rotation of the arytenoid cartilages and by the approximation of these cartilages to one another by little muscles. The

usually expelled by a bout of violent coughing. This accident is familiarly described as a crumb going the wrong way.

The framework of the larynx is formed by a number of cartilaginous structures. The largest is the thyroid cartilage, a plate which is bent sharply on itself so as to make a V-shaped gutter, the point of the V being in front and constituting the prominence in the neck known as the Adam's apple. Below the thyroid is the cricoid cartilage, shaped rather like a signet-ring, the broad part being at the back. There is a space between the thyroid and cricoid cartilages in front, and this is filled in by the thyroid membrane. It is through this membrane that an opening is made in a sudden emergency when an artificial opening for air becomes necessary. This operation is called laryngotomy.

Perched on the upper border of the back part of the cricoid are the two arytenoid cartilages. They are side by side but separated by a narrow interval. Each is a three-sided pyramid and can rotate to some extent on its base. To the anterior angle, or vocal process, one end of the vocal cord is attached, the other being attached at the bottom of the gutter formed in the thyroid cartilage and on about a level with the Adam's apple. A short distance above the vocal cords, but with similar attachments, are two other bands, the false vocal cords. The space between a false and a

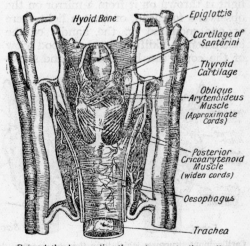

Behind the larynx lies the entrance to the gullet

tension of the cords is varied by rotation of the thyroid on the cricoid, to which it is articulated by means of two prolongations downwards of its posterior border, which are described as the inferior horns. It has been pointed out that there is a gap between the thyroid and the cricoid in front. The existence of this permits the thyroid to rock forward on the cricoid, and this movement will tend to stretch the cords and so increase their tension.

The greater depth of the male voice as compared with the female is due to the larger size of the larynx and consequent greater length of the cords, as everyone knows the pitch of a violin string is raised by shortening it by fingering. The various muscles that operate on the laryngeal cartilages are supplied by branches of the vagus nerve, the inferior and the superior laryngeal nerves, the latter, however, mainly as a sensory nerve.

For examining the larynx an instrument known as a laryngoscope is used. This consists simply of a little mirror mounted at an angle on a metal stem. The mirror is passed to the back of the throat and light is thrown on it from a mirror on the observer's forehead, or from a light there or one mounted on the handle of the instrument. Skilfully used, a good view of the cords can be obtained, and some-

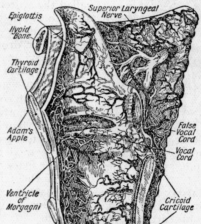

Sectional view of larynx

times even of the trachea beneath then and as far down as its bifurcation into th two bronchi.

Diseases of the Larynx. Inflammatior of the larynx, or laryngitis, may be acut or chronic. Acute laryngitis may be par of a common cold or of such diseases a influenza or measles. It may be caused by inhaling irritating vapours or by swallowing corrosive substances There is hoarseness, ar irritating cough, which brings up a little sticky mucus, some pain or pressing over the larynx and, perhaps, soreness in swallowing. The temperature is raised and the pulse rapid. The voice may be lost altogether and, particularly in children, there may be considerable difficulty in breathing.

The patient should be kept in a warm room, the temperature of which is kept as even as possible. Often it will be desirable to remain in bed. The diet should consist of warm liquids. The patient should refrain from talking. Hot fomentations or poultices over the throat will be useful, and also the use of a bronchitis kettle to keep the air moist ; or steam containing Friar's balsam may be inhaled as described under the heading Inhalation.

Chronic laryngitis may follow one attack or a succession of attacks of acute laryngitis or it may follow over-use or misuse of the voice. It may be associated with chronic inflammation in the nose and throat. Alcoholism predisposes to, and excessive smoking aggravates, the condition. The cords become congested and thickened. The voice is husky or hoarse and easily tired. There is likely also to be a hacking cough with scanty sputum. The voice must be rested as much as possible and those who have to do much public speaking should cultivate

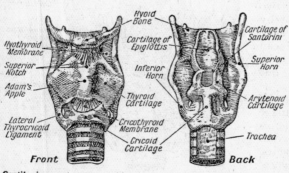

Cartilaginous structures which form the framework of the larynx

an easy style of delivery. Tobacco and alcohol should not be used, nor very hot drinks, condiments or spices. The bowels should be kept regular. Help may be derived by spraying with a solution of perchloride of iron or some other astringent.

The larynx may be subject to some nervous affection either of a sensory or a motor character. In what is called the laryngeal crisis of locomotor ataxia there is a persistent tickling which causes a hard, dry cough. Paralysis of laryngeal muscles may be a manifestation of hysteria or be caused by interference with the nerves, say by the pressure of an aneurysm or tumour in the chest, by the poison of diphtheria or by syphilitic lesions. Laryngeal spasm may be due to local irritation or in children occur as part of a more general nervous disturbance, causing a form of croup (*q.v.*).

Sudden swelling of the mucous membrane of the larynx, or oedema of the larynx, may be due to irritation within the organ or to diffuse inflammation, or cellulitis, in the neck. It may occur in diphtheria (*q.v.*). The risk of suffocation is urgent and medical help should be summoned at once. Meanwhile ice may be sucked and hot applications put round the throat. Laryngotomy or tracheotomy may be necessary.

Laryngeal tuberculosis, also known as laryngeal phthisis, almost always is secondary to the same disease in the lungs, infection of the larynx presumably being caused by the sputa from the lungs. Chronic inflammation goes on to ulceration and destruction of the parts. The treatment follows the lines of that for consumption (*q.v.*), with appropriate local treatment. Swallowing may be difficult on account of great pain, but feeding may be much easier if the vessel containing food, which should be liquid, is placed so far below the patient that he has to stoop down and suck the food up through a glass tube.

Syphilis in an early stage may cause acute laryngitis; in a late stage it may cause ulceration and destruction of the parts of the larynx.

Tumours of the larynx are fairly common and some of them may cause no serious symptoms, at any rate for a long time. A papilloma is the common type of benign tumour and forms a little warty excrescence on the cord. There is not usually much difficulty in removing this or other benign tumours. A malignant tumour is usually a carcinoma and may originate within the larynx or spread in from adjoining parts, the former being considered the less difficult to eradicate. Treatment consists in removing the larynx, in whole or in part.

Larynx. Vocal cords in breathing and phonation

Foreign bodies may be drawn into the larynx and may cause spasm and urgent danger of suffocation. A gulp of water or a slap on the back, if necessary with the patient upside down, may dislodge the object. If this fails and the face is becoming black, the point of a knife may be plunged into the larynx in the middle line of the neck, half an inch, or less in a child, below the most prominent part of the Adam's apple. The edges of the wound are drawn apart by hair-pins. If breathing has stopped artificial respiration (*q.v.*) should be begun. If, however, the foreign body is not causing urgent choking no attempt should be made by any unskilled person to remove it, as this would probably make matters worse.

See Asphyxia; Clergyman's Throat; Croup; Neck; Pharynx; Speech; Trachea.

LASSAR'S PASTE. Various formulae are given for Lassar's paste, which is a preparation used in eczema and other skin diseases. The following is a good example :

Zinc oxide	..	..	120 grains
Powdered venetian talc	..	120	,,
Salicylic acid	..	..	5 ,,
Vaseline	..	..	1 ounce

For seborrhoeic eczema, 20 grains of precipitated sulphur can be added, or for acne, 10 grains each of precipitated sulphur and resorcin. For other affections the formulae can be suitably modified.

LASSITUDE. Occasional attacks of lassitude, or languor, happen to all, be it only from oppressive atmospheric conditions, but habitual lassitude demands a careful investigation of the state of health. In a young person early consumption is always a possibility to be considered, but in many diseases of insidious origin and course, lassitude may be the first notable fact.

See Anaemia ; Consumption ; Fatigue ; Ventilation.

LAUDANUM. The tincture of opium (*q.v.*) is commonly referred to as laudanum. The derivation of the name is obscure.

LAUGHING GAS. *See* Nitrous Oxide.

LAUREL. Cherry-laurel water contains hydrocyanic acid (*q.v.*) and is used, in small doses, as a sedative. It is a dangerous poison.

LAVAGE. Washing out, or lavage, of the stomach may be carried out when its contents are being retained unduly long and are fermenting, when certain poisons have been swallowed, and in other circumstances. A rubber tube is generally used and worked on the principle of siphonage. Lavage of the bowel may be accomplished by passing a long rubber tube, or by the Plombières method. Lavage of the bladder is undertaken in the treatment of chronic cystitis, to facilitate cystoscopic examination, and for other purposes, different kinds of apparatus being used.

See Douche.

LAVENDER. The oil distilled from lavender flowers is used as a carminative in doses of ½ to 3 minims. The dose of spirit of lavender which is prepared from this is 5 to 20 minims. The compound tincture of lavender, which contains other aromatics besides oil of lavender, and is coloured with red sanders wood, has a dose of ½ to 1 drachm. It is often used as a colouring agent in mixtures or lotions, and is contained for this purpose in Fowler's solution and in red lotion.

LAXATIVE. *See* Aperient.

LEAD. Acetate of lead, commonly known as sugar of lead on account of its sweetish taste, is sometimes given in a pill, usually the pill of lead and opium, in order to check severe diarrhoea or haemorrhage from the bowel. The compound suppository of lead, which also contains opium, may be used with the same objects. Lead has been used for treating cancer, but, whatever can be said for its efficacy in any case of the kind, the use of lead internally requires most careful expert supervision, as the drug is a dangerous poison.

As local applications, preparations of lead are astringent and sedative. The strong solution of lead subacetate, or Goulard's extract, is used mainly for making the dilute solution, or Goulard's water. This, often referred to simply as lead lotion, is used to relieve itching and reduce inflammation and discharge in affections of the skin and mucous membranes. It is sometimes used, combined with laudanum, in lotions intended for the immediate treatment of a sprain. Lead lotion is unsuitable for the eye if the cornea is abraded, as an opacity will be caused by deposition of the metal in the abrasion.

As a local sedative the ointment or the glycerin of lead subacetate will sometimes be more suitable than the lotion.

Lead plaster, also called diachylon, or litharge, plaster, is used when not only a sedative but a supporting action is required. It is used as a basis for many other plasters, including resin and soap plaster. A mixture of equal parts of lead plaster and soft paraffin, or vaseline, is known as Hebra's diachylon plaster.

Poisoning by Lead. Lead lotion may be taken accidentally, or liquor or food may contain lead, as the first beer drawn off in the morning at a tap with a lead pipe has been known to do, and symptoms of acute poisoning follow. There is sickness, colic, sometimes diarrhoea, but usually constipation, cramps in the legs, and drowsiness. An emetic should be given, and thereafter milk freely, and $\frac{1}{2}$ ounce of Epsom salts in half a glass of water. The patient should be kept warm.

On account of its extensive use in the arts and for water-pipes, etc., lead is not infrequently a cause of chronic poisoning. Painters, plumbers, pottery-glazers, compositors and others, in addition to those employed in lead-mining and the extraction of the metal from the ore, are always subject to this risk. The poison may be inhaled as dust, but the usual thing is for food to be contaminated by poison adhering to the hands.

Outside such trades the consumption of water containing lead is a common cause of poisoning. A soft water and a peaty water, on account of a certain acid it possesses, are especially dangerous. There is a gradual depreciation of the health ; the appetite fails, and there are signs of anaemia. A stippling of the red corpuscles, as observed under the microscope, is characteristic of lead poisoning. A blue line forms on the margins of the gums; this will be found to be lacking, however, where a tooth has been extracted. The bowels become very constipated and paroxysms of colic, often referred to as painters' colic, occur.

The pain is excruciating, and the abdomen is drawn in and feels hard. Inflammation of nerves, what is called peripheral neuritis, causes cramp-like pains in muscles and paralysis. There may be foot or wrist drop, or the hands may develop a claw-like deformity. The muscles waste, and sensation is impaired. Chronic inflammation of the kidneys, or chronic Bright's disease, and a gouty state of certain joints may also occur. Sometimes there is definite mental disease.

Legislative enactments (1920) against the employment of women and children in certain lead processes, and against the consumption of food, drink or tobacco in places where such are carried on, should do something to diminish the incidence of lead poisoning. The strictest personal cleanliness should be observed by all engaged in occupations involving the risk.

One danger that should be borne in mind is cigarette smoking when the hands may be soiled with lead.

The free use of sulphuric acid, lemonade, or of milk, is an additional way of safeguarding oneself.

Chronic lead poisoning is treated by the free use of magnesium or of sodium sulphate in order to get the bowels acting, and as an antidote against lead in the digestive tract, and then by giving a course of potassium iodide to aid in washing the drug out of the tissues.

LEECH. Once extensively used as a means of extracting blood and relieving congestion, the leech is seldom seen nowadays, though there are some disorders in which the application of one or more of them may be valuable. The skin on which a leech is to be used should be washed clean, and, if the leech will not bite, a little milk may be smeared on the spot. Another expedient is to make the leech crawl over the blanket for a short distance. The creature is left on the skin until it elects to drop off. It should on no account be dragged off, but if it delays unduly, or if a leech has become attached accidentally, a strong solution of common salt may be poured on it.

When the leech comes away, it is put into the fire. Should the bite continue to bleed, firm pressure will usually serve to stop this, but the point may require to be touched with lunar caustic. If there is any repugnance to the use of a natural leech, an instrument known as the artificial leech, or heurteloupe, may be used.

See Bleeding ; Cupping.

LEG. In anatomy the leg is the part of the lower limb between the knee and the ankle, the upper part of the limb being the thigh (*q.v.*) The skeleton of the leg

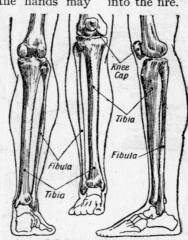

Leg. Relative position of the bones

is formed of the tibia, or shin-bone, on the inner, and the fibula on the outer side, the gap between the bones being filled up by a membrane. The anterior border of the shin-bone and its inner surface are covered by skin only.

The muscles on the front of the leg flex the ankle and extend the toes; those on the outer side, the peronei, assist in extending the ankle, but also twist the foot outwards. The large fleshy bulk of the calf is formed of the gastrocnemius and soleus muscles which are inserted by the Achilles tendon (*q.v.*) into the heel bone; these with other muscles on the back of the leg extend the foot; others flex the toes.

The main arteries of the leg are the anterior and posterior tibial, branches of the popliteal, and the main nerves, the internal and external popliteal, branches of the great sciatic. The superficial veins

Muscles and tendons on the front and inner aspects of the leg

on the front of the leg drain into the long or internal saphenous, which passes up on the inner side, and those on the back into the external or short saphenous vein which passes up the back of the limb and dips in behind the knee to join the popliteal vein.

Varicose veins (*q.v.*) are rather common in the legs and may lead to eczema, ulceration and discoloration. A brownish discoloration may also be due, however, to frequent exposure of the legs to great heat. Apart from such causes, patches of chronic eczema are not uncommon on the shins. In dropsy the legs, being dependent, are early and much affected. Great wasting of the muscles of the leg, especially those in front, may occur from infantile palsy, but may also be found in other nervous diseases. In pseudo-hypertrophic muscular paralysis, on the other hand, the

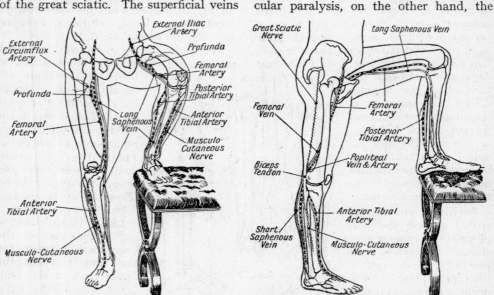

Leg. Anatomical diagrams showing the skeleton and the principal arteries, veins and nerves

calves may be greatly enlarged, though at the same time they are very feeble.

See Achilles Tendon; Artificial Limb; Ankle; Fibula; Foot; Knee; Popliteal; Thigh; Tibia.

LEISHMANIASIS. A genus of animal parasites, belonging to the class of protozoa, causes certain disorders which are described in a general way as leishmaniasis, Two of these disorders, oriental sore and kala-azar, are fairly widespread in the East, while the third, espundia, occurs only in South America. In the latter form, an ulcerative sore forms on a mucous membrane. It may heal, but subsequently there is a destructive ulceration within the nose and mouth which does great damage. Treatment is not satisfactory.

See Kala-azar; Oriental Sore.

LEITER'S TUBES. A flexible metal tube, used for applying continuous cold to some part of the body, is known as Leiter's; it can be twisted into the shape of a cap or otherwise, according to the part for which it is intended. A long rubber tube attaches one end to a water-tap, while a similar tube is led from the other end into a sink to carry off the effluent (*see* Plate IX, 2).

LEMON. Fresh lemon juice contains citric acid, and acts as a refrigerant, or cooling medicine, in fevers, in which it is usually given as home-made lemonade or as imperial drink. The juice is rich in the antiscorbutic vitamin, and is extensively used in the prevention of scurvy; it is also capable of curing the disease. Fresh lemon juice is sometimes used in making an effervescent draught. Syrup of lemons, made from the fresh fruit, is used as a flavouring agent in mixtures.

Oil of lemon, obtained from the fresh peel, is also used as a flavouring agent. In doses of $\frac{1}{2}$ to 3 minims, dropped on sugar, it will relieve colic and flatulence. The tincture of lemon, dose $\frac{1}{2}$ to 1 drachm, is likewise made from the fresh peel, and has the properties of the oil.

See Beverages; Citric Acid; Imperial Drink.

LENS. A piece of glass with one or both of its sides curved is described as a lens. It is a spherical lens if the curved side represents part of a sphere, or a cylindrical if the curve is part of a cylinder, that is, the curve is in one direction only. A lens is convex if it bulges outwards from its centre, and concave if it is excavated towards its centre; or if both sides are curved it is bi-concave or bi-convex. The crystalline lens of the eye is bi-convex.

See Eye; Spectacles.

LEONTIASIS OSSEA. A disease in which there is thickening and enlargement of facial bones is called leontiasis ossea, on account of the leonine expression often assumed. The cause is probably an unidentified microbe. No treatment avails anything.

LEPROSY. An infectious disease caused by the bacillus leprae, leprosy occurs in the tropics and in certain parts of Northern Europe. Infection takes place through the skin or mucous membrane, from actual contact with leprous sores or with clothing and utensils used by lepers, or by the bites of infected insects. Males are more liable than females, and from ten to thirty years is the most susceptible period of life, childhood especially. The incubation period varies from a few weeks to four years or longer, after which there are feverish symptoms and the appearance of reddened patches on the face and other parts of the body. Later these patches are replaced by brown, pigmented areas.

Speaking generally, the disease may now advance in one of two ways, becoming either the nodular or the anaesthetic form. In the former, thickened elevations or nodules, of a purple or earthen colour, appear on the pigmented patches. When this occurs on the face, what is called the leonine facies is produced. Nodules may ulcerate and the ulcers show no tendency to heal. By the advance of this ulceration, fingers, toes, the nose, ears or eyes may be lost and extensive damage done inside the nose, mouth and throat. There is also involvement of internal organs.

In the anaesthetic form there are no nodules but infiltration of nerves. The central part of the stained patches become atrophic and shiny. There is hyperaesthesia in various parts and neuralgic pains; sometimes large blisters, or bullae, make their appearance. Shortly there is loss of sensation in parts supplied by affected nerves, and signs of interference with the nutrition of the parts. Ulceration is readily induced and may lead to the loss of fingers, toes or larger portions of the limbs.

Leprosy runs a prolonged course, tuberculosis or Bright's disease being often the actual cause of death. The duration of the anaesthetic form is usually much longer than the other.

Persons suffering from leprosy should be segregated, though if, as happens particularly in the anaesthetic form, the patient becomes non-infectious, after expert examination he may be allowed his liberty. Children should not be allowed to remain with leprous parents. Thorough treatment with chaulmoogra oil or its preparations usually cures the disease in the early stages and is, at any rate, beneficial later on. But if nerves have been destroyed anaesthesia and trophic changes cannot be removed.

LEUCOCYTE. There are several varieties of white corpuscle, or leucocyte, in the blood, which can be differentiated by staining methods. By the use of an instrument, known as a haemocytometer, the number of cells, both red and white, in a cubic centimetre of blood can be counted and the number of each variety of the white. From variations in the results of such examinations it may be possible to draw important conclusions in diagnosis and prognosis.

More leucocytes are present in childhood and in pregnancy, and in any individual the number varies throughout the day; it may be between 5,000 and 10,000 per cubic millimetre. The average percentages of the varieties are as follows : polymorphonuclear, 60 to 70 ; large mononuclear, including the so-called transitional, 3 to 5 ; lymphocytes, 25 to 30 ; eosinophil, 1 to 4 ; and mast cells, 0·5. All of these are produced in bone-marrow, though a few lymphocytes may come from lymphatic glands and other collections of lymphoid tissue. Cells in the bone-marrow, which are precursors of leucocytes, are called myeloblasts and myelocytes ; in disease these may appear in the blood.

An increase in the white cells is called leucocytosis. This may be physiological,

Lymphocytes   *Hyaline Leucocytes*

Polynuclear Leucocyte   *Eosinophil Leucocyte*

Transitional Leucocytes

Leucocyte. Forms of white blood cells. The polynuclear leucocytes are the most numerous

as after a meal, when lymphocytes abound. Or it may be pathological ; here the increase is usually in the polymorphs and is defensive, to bring the functions of these cells into operation on a large scale. This rôle of the white cells is discussed under the heading Blood. The failure of the leucocytes to increase in a disease when such is to be expected is therefore a bad omen. A highly magnified polynuclear leucocyte is shown in Plate XXI, 5.

Horse-serum and nuclein are sometimes injected into the body to bring about a leucocytosis when this is thought desirable; some drugs, such as quinine, are also useful in this way.

In some diseases, such as tuberculosis, small-pox and whooping-cough, there is an increase of lymphocytes, that is, a lymphocytosis. In infestation with worms, in asthma and some other disorders, there is an increase of eosinophils, a condition described as eosinophilia.

If the number of leucocytes falls below 5,000 per cubic millimetre a state of leucopenia is said to exist. This occurs in typhoid and paratyphoid fever, and also in other diseases.

See Blood ; Leukaemia.

LEUCODERMA. In the skin disorder known as leucoderma, or vitiligo, patches occur which have a convex border and are pale in colour owing to the loss of pigment. The skin surrounding a patch is either apparently or actually more deeply pigmented than the skin generally, and when this darkening is pronounced it is described as melanoderma.

The usual sites for leucodermic patches are the genital organs, the hands, arms, neck and back. If hair grows on an affected patch it also is deprived of pigment. There are no abnormal sensations in the patches, the ordinary sensations are retained and also the activity of the skin-glands.

Leucoderma may occur in connexion with syphilis and may follow other infections, but it occurs apart from any obvious cause to which responsibility might possibly be attached. It is not common in childhood and shows no partiality for either sex.

There is no cure for the disorder, and the most that can be done is to lessen disfigurement by using tinted powders or pastes, or a stain.

LEUCORRHOEA. A discharge from the female genital passage is described as leucorrhoea. This means literally a white discharge and properly designates the discharge which is popularly known as " the whites." It has come, however, to mean any discharge, except, of course, a simple bleeding. Leucorrhoea may occur when there is no local cause or, at most, a slight one, but the general health is below par, notably in anaemia. Even when there is a definite local cause it is desirable to bring the general state of health to as high a level as possible.

A discharge may be due to acute infection of the parts and consist largely of pus. If the inflammation is less acute the discharge will contain pus but also more or less mucus. Congestion of the neck of the womb, which may be associated with laceration following labour, is a common cause of leucorrhoea. The discharge may be clear and glairy, like the white of an egg. Sometimes the inflammation affects the cavity of the womb. In view of the variety of possible causes of a discharge, medical advice should be obtained.

A discharge may be lessened and sometimes cured by a douche (*q.v.*) of water containing sufficient permanganate of potassium to make the solution red,. or common salt or alum, a teaspoonful of either to the pint.

In children a discharge usually comes from the external parts and is due to want of cleanliness or irritation from threadworms.

LEUKAEMIA. A disease characterised by a persistent increase of the white cells of the blood, associated with changes in the blood-forming organs, is described as leukaemia, or leucocythaemia. In one form of this disease the increase is in the lymphocytes and it is called lymphatic leukaemia ; in the other there are large numbers of immature cells in the blood such as in health are only found in the

bone-marrow, and it has been known as spleno-medullary or spleno-myelogenous leukaemia, though these names are being abandoned (*see* Plate XXI, 6).

Either form may be acute or chronic. In the acute cases of so-called spleno-medullary leukaemia, the immature cells are myeloblasts, bone-marrow cells which give rise to other bone-marrow cells, myelocytes, which in their turn give rise to the ordinary leucocytes found in the blood, so that such cases can be correctly described as acute myeloblastic leukaemia. In the chronic cases the cells are myelocytes, and these are described as chronic myeloid leukaemia.

It is not known what is at the bottom of all these changes. The disease is rare, however.

Child Sufferers from Acute Form

Acute lymphatic leukaemia usually affects young children. It begins suddenly and generally with bleeding from the nose or mouth and into the skin. The child is fevered and rapidly becomes waxy-looking from anaemia, the gums become softened and bleed as in scurvy, and bleeding may take place from the bowels or kidneys. Death takes place in from a few days to a few weeks.

Acute myeloblastic leukaemia, which also usually occurs in young children, presents similar symptoms to those of the acute lymphatic form.

Chronic lymphatic leukaemia usually affects middle-aged people. There is swelling of the glands in the neck, the armpits and the groins. The spleen and liver also enlarge, and this may cause a swelling of the abdomen. Lymphatic swellings may also occur in the skin. Anaemia begins and increases, with consequent weakness. Death takes place in the course of a few years.

Chronic myeloid leukaemia is more common at a rather earlier age than the form just described. There is progressive enlargement of the spleen, which may reach a great size, extending right across the abdomen. Bleedings are common. Vision may be affected by bleeding into the retina or by leukaemic plaques there, and deafness and Ménière's symptoms may also occur. The blood has a greyish colour.

There is no useful treatment for the acute forms of leukaemia. In the chronic forms fresh air, wholesome food and rest may help to keep the patient more comfortable. Arsenic and benzol are the most useful drugs. Radium and X-rays are used on the swollen glands and spleen, and, in the chronic myeloid form, on the long bones.

Chloroma, or "green-cancer," is a very rare disease, occurring chiefly in children, but also in young adults. The symptoms resemble those of acute leukaemia, and the spleen and glands are enlarged. There are also peculiar growths in various parts of the body, oftenest about the bones of the face and head, where, by pressure on cranial nerves, blindness, deafness and other consequences may ensue. The growths, when cut open, are of a greenish colour, and on this fact the name of the disorder is based. No treatment can arrest the disease.

See Anaemia ; Leucocyte.

LEUKOPLAKIA. White patches on the tongue and inside of the cheek, occurring usually in middle-aged or elderly men, are described as leukoplakia. They are caused by an overgrowth of the surface epithelium in consequence of inflammation, which can often be related to syphilis, over-smoking, a constant use of raw spirit, or a combination of these. Sometimes, however, there is no evidence of anything of the kind. After a time the patches become painful, especially in swallowing and talking, and later on may become the site of cancer.

Smoking, strong spirits, acid wines, condiments and very hot food must be avoided. A lotion containing sodium bicarbonate may be useful, and also antiseptic applications. The mouth should be kept very clean. Treatment with radium may be beneficial.

LEVATOR. A muscle described as a levator is one that raises something. Thus, the levator anguli oris is a muscle that raises the angle of the mouth, as in smiling.

LICHEN. A considerable number of skin diseases are described as lichens, but this must not be taken to imply any essential connexion between them. At most it means that a disease is characterised by the existence of solid papules, or pimples, throughout its course ; but to this there is an exception, as the papules in the disease known as lichen scrophulosorum often develop a pustule on the top.

In lichen planus the papule is small, polygonal, reddish to purple in colour and with a flat, glancing top (see Plate XXXI, 12). The disease is occasionally acute, with papules scattered over the body ; but usually it is localised and chronic, fresh crops appearing at considerable intervals. The inside of the thighs and the front of the forearms are common sites, but the papules may occur elsewhere, and often on mucous membranes, such as that on the inside of the cheek, where whitish patches are produced.

The papules generally run together to form a patch, but they may occur in circles or have a linear formation. Subjective symptoms may be slight or, on the other hand, itching and burning may be so severe as seriously to interfere with sleep. Old papules tend to become pigmented. Sometimes the papules are so large as to form warty masses ; this is described as lichen planus verrucosus.

Arsenic and mercury are given internally, and tar and other ointments are used on the patches. The high-frequency current is sometimes valuable, and also the expert use of X-rays.

Lichen scrophulosorum occurs in tuberculous people. The papules are brown. Treatment includes that for tuberculosis.

Lichen simplex is a name applied to the papular stage of eczema and other eruptions. Lichen pilaris is a disease in which the back of the arms and the front of the thighs are studded with little brown elevations. These are not proper papules, however, but horny plugs in the hair follicles. Fatty applications with frequent washing, though they may not cure, will improve the appearance of the skin and keep the condition in check. Lichen urticatus, which occurs in children, is related to nettle-rash (q.v.).

LIEBERKÜHN'S GLANDS. Small tubes studding the lining of the intestine, Lieberkühn's glands or crypts produce intestinal juice, a digestive fluid, in the small intestine, and mucus, a glairy lubricant, in the large intestine.

See Digestion ; Intestine.

LIENTERIC DIARRHOEA. The common desire to empty the bowels after breakfast is due to the filling of the stomach stimulating contractions in the lower bowel through a nervous mechanism. This is called the gastro-colic reflex, and takes place to some extent after any meal. If this reflex is too easily excited, the bowels may move several times after breakfast or even after each meal, a state of affairs described as lienteric diarrhoea. Some article of diet may be primarily responsible, and diarrhoea may be prevented by refraining from it. A short rest after a meal will sometimes prevent diarrhoea in those who are subject to it. Belladonna and bromides are amongst the drugs used in treatment.

See Diarrhoea.

LIGAMENT. The bands or cords passing between the ends of the bones forming a joint, and keeping them in position, are described as ligaments. They are formed of interlacing strands of white fibrous tissue and do not stretch, though they are so arranged as to permit of the required movements at a particular joint.

Other ligaments, formed of yellow elastic tissue, are able to stretch, and such are found where, as between the vertebrae, a considerable range of movement is required while the ligament remains taut and keeps the parts steady. These ligaments possess resiliency, like rubber, and, when the movement is discontinued, aid in bringing the parts back into the ordinary position, as when the back is straightened from the stooping position.

Folds of peritoneum (*q.v.*) uniting internal organs to the body wall, or to each other, are also described as ligaments, as, for example, the ligaments of the liver and the broad ligament of the womb.

See Joint.

LIGATURE. To ligature a blood vessel, or any other part, is to constrict it by tying something round it, the cord or thread used for the purpose being described as a ligature. This may be necessary in cutting operations and in accidental bleeding, and is sometimes the method of treatment adopted for piles and warts, or other small tumours which have a slender stalk or pedicle attaching them to the body.

For blood vessels a catgut ligature is usually chosen, as this becomes absorbed after some days and disappears. Linen thread is also used for this purpose. For piles and warts strong linen or silk thread may be used. A ligature should be quite

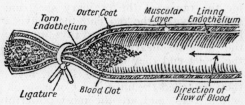
Ligaturing a blood vessel to arrest bleeding

free from germs, and to achieve this thread may be boiled; but catgut would be spoiled by boiling and requires special treatment.

The term ligature is also used to denote a bandage applied to a limb to arrest the circulation, as a tourniquet (*q.v.*) in the case of a dog or snake bite.

LIGHT. Light, which is a form of electrical energy, travels from its source in straight lines. The lines of transmission only maintain their direction, however, so long as the waves are passing through the same medium, say, air. When they strike another medium the direction is changed and the line is then said to be refracted. If a beam of sunlight is made to pass through a glass prism, a bar consisting of a succession of colours is produced, the order of the colours always being the same, namely, red, orange, yellow, green, blue, indigo and violet.

This bar is called the solar spectrum, and represents the disintegration of visible light into its constituent parts, or colours, this disintegration taking place because these different rays of which white light is composed have different wave-lengths, the longer having greater difficulty in passing through the prism, and therefore being more refracted. The longest waves are at the red end of the spectrum, and they become progressively shorter towards the violet end.

Most of the light that falls on a polished surface is reflected; on many surfaces some of the constituent rays may be reflected, while others are absorbed. Thus, if the red rays are reflected, the object will have a red colour; if green, it will be green, and so on. A black surface absorbs most of the light.

Beyond each end of the spectrum rays are passing, although they are not visible, simply because the eye is adjusted for the range of the ordinary spectrum only. Beyond the red end they have a longer wave-length than red rays, and are the invisible heat rays, whilst beyond the violet end they have a shorter wave-length than those of the latter rays; they are called the ultra-violet or invisible actinic rays, and are the most powerful as regards chemical action.

The ultra-violet rays have important functions in the processes of life, and their effect on human health is far-reaching. Those coming to us from the sun, however, are largely prevented from passing through the atmosphere by dust and moisture, and the supply is therefore very restricted in towns. Moreover, they are absorbed by ordinary window glass, so that they are not available in a room so protected. Arc lamps of various kinds, including the Finsen and the Krohmayer, are used to produce ultra-violet rays artificially, so that this method of therapy is readily available. The light from such lamps is sometimes described as artificial sunlight. Different expedients are used to cool the rays.

Exposure to ultra-violet rays will kill micro-organisms, and this explains the long-known disinfecting properties of sunlight. It also largely explains the success of ultra-violet rays in the treatment of skin disorders. An area of skin exposed to the rays becomes reddened, and later there is an increase of pigment in the skin. The rays are absorbed by the blood, increasing its content of calcium, phosphorus and iron, and increasing its germicidal power and the phagocytic capacity of the leucocytes. Tissue activity is also stimulated, and endocrine (*q.v.*) activity. Exposure to ultra-violet rays also increases the vitamin activity of foods.

The value of ultra-violet rays, first demonstrated by Finsen in the treatment of lupus, has now been proved for a large number of other skin diseases, including boils, carbuncles, eczema, baldness, chilblains and psoriasis.

In consequence of their effect on vitamin activity, the rays also afford a powerful means of preventing and curing rickets. They have, in addition, a general tonic effect on the whole body, and can restore vigour and joie-de-vivre when such qualities are deficient or lacking. Often they have a tranquillising effect in states of irritability. Applications of the rays have cured sciatica and lumbago, headaches and neuralgia, and have been beneficial in a large number of other disorders.

Treatment by natural sunlight, or heliotherapy, is carried out at Alton (Plate XXXVIII, 3) and Hayling Island in connexion with the Treloar Homes, and elsewhere in Great Britain, and at Leysin in Switzerland and other places abroad. The value of light in the treatment of surgical tuberculosis was well established at some of those places a long time before its other possibilities were grasped. As ultra-violet rays form such a powerful weapon, however, their indiscriminate use, or, particularly when they are artificially produced, their overdosage, is capable of doing harm. Even moderate doses have been proved to be capable of causing quiescent tuberculosis of the lung to flare up into activity, and of doing other harm, so that this form of therapy is unsafe except under medical supervision. During applications of artificial light patients and nurses should wear goggles to protect the eyes (*see* Plate XXII and XXXVIII, 4).

LIGHTNING. The effects of a lightning stroke on the body are those of a powerful electric discharge. There may be no mark of any kind, or, on the other hand, wounds or signs of scorching. Sometimes an arborescent design is found on the skin. Death is due to shock; if the person is not killed there may be loss of vision, or other paralysis of sensation or of motion, and these results may be temporary or permanent.

LIME. The oxide of calcium is known as lime, or calx, but the term lime is often used as if it were synonymous with calcium, for example, in a reference to salts of calcium as lime salts. Lime, in this sense, is found abundantly in bone, to which it imparts rigidity, but it is present in all body tissues. It is an essential constituent of the blood, as clotting cannot take place without it. The metabolism of lime is regulated, at any rate to some extent, by the parathyroid glands. It is excreted in the urine and by the large bowel.

Lime is a caustic. When treated with water slaked lime is formed, from which several preparations are made, including lime water.

See Calcium.

LINCTUS. A medicinal preparation of a thick, syrupy consistency is described as a linctus. The implication in the name is that the medicine is to be licked off a spoon.

LINIMENT. An external application intended to be rubbed into the skin is described as a liniment, or embrocation. Of the official liniments, those of aconite, belladonna and opium are anodyne; those of ammonia, camphor, ammoniated camphor, croton oil, mustard, soap, turpentine and the acetic liniment of turpentine cause reddening of the skin, or are stimulating; that of chloroform is both stimulating and anodyne; that of lime is sedative to an inflamed surface; and those of mercury and of potassium iodide with soap are stimulating and further the dispersal of inflammatory enlargements.

All of these liniments are liquid except that of potassium iodide with soap, which is a soft solid. Soap liniment is often called opodeldoc, and the liniment of lime is carron oil, except that olive oil replaces the linseed oil of the original formula. This liniment is applied without rubbing, usually on a clean rag or a piece of lint, and the anodyne liniments are usually applied in the same way. Much of the value of the stimulating liniments depends on the vigour used in rubbing in.

LINSEED. The seed of common flax, linseed is chiefly used for making a poultice (*q.v.*). The oil, which is expressed from the seeds without the aid of heat, is sometimes used externally as an emollient. With an equal part of lime water it made the original carron oil. The infusion, or linseed tea, may be taken in irritable states of the bladder.

LINT. By scraping or pulling the surface of a sheet of linen cloth, lint is produced. Usually one side only is treated in this way. Plain white, or surgeon's lint, and pink, or boracic lint, are those most commonly used.

See Dressing.

LIPOID. In the protoplasm of body-cells there are certain substances which are dissolved by alcohol and other solvents of fats and so are called lipoids, that is, fat-like substances. Cholesterol, or cholesterin, which is one of these, is actually an alcohol. This substance is of immense importance to the life and activity of cells. Irradiation with ultra-violet rays confers vitamin-activity on it, and it is to the presence of cholesterol in cells of the skin that much of the benefit of exposure to such rays, whether natural or artificial, is due.

Another lipoid, known as lecithin or phosphorised fat, is abundant in nerve-tissue. Yolk of egg also contains large amounts, and lecithin is extracted from it and used as a tonic in nervous diseases, tuberculosis and diabetes. Interaction with lipoids in the cells of nervous tissue is supposed to explain the effects of chloroform and other drugs.

LIPOMA. A tumour composed of fat is called a lipoma. It may be circumscribed or diffuse. Except when large or in an awkward situation a lipoma is of little account.

See Tumour.

LIPS. Between the skin which covers the outer surface of the lips and the mucous membrane which covers the inner, there is from without inwards a quantity of loose connective tissue, the orbicularis oris muscle and the coronary artery. Both the muscle and the artery form a circle round the mouth. On account of the quantity of connective tissue inflammation of the lip is generally accompanied by considerable swelling.

The artery is more likely to be opened by a wound on the inner side of the lip than an external one. As the artery is a large one bleeding will be very free and for its arrest it is necessary to grasp and compress the lip on both sides of the wound; both ends of the artery will also probably have to be tied to stop bleeding.

The lips are useful in feeding, and a hare-lip (*q.v.*) may seriously interfere with suckling. They are also used in speech, in enunciating the consonants known as labials and in making some of the vowel sounds. Besides, movements of the lips accompany other sounds, and consequently a careful regard to the behaviour of the lips in speech affords a good idea of what is being said. Lip-reading is an extremely useful accomplishment in the deaf and should be taught as soon as practicable.

The inner part of the lips is richly furnished with mucous glands, and dilatation of one of these glands is not uncommon, causing a rounded elastic swelling. Naevi or tumours composed of blood vessels are also found. In a common cold, pneumonia and other fevers, a crop of vesicles or blisters, herpes labialis, frequently forms on the margin of the lips. The upper lip is supplied with sensation by the second division of the trigeminal nerve, and the lower by the third division.

An epithelioma, a type of cancer, sometimes forms on the lip of a man at or past middle age, the usual cause being a rough tooth or the habitual smoking of a short clay pipe. Glands in the neck are implicated very soon. Prompt removal by operation is required. A syphilitic chancre may also occur on the lip.

See Chap ; Herpes.

LIQUOR. A medicinal preparation described as a liquor is a solution of some substance, of vegetable, animal or mineral origin, in distilled water usually, but sometimes in spirit. The strength of the solution is standardised. Thus, the strength of the liquor, or solution, of morphine hydrochloride and of some other liquors is 1 per cent.

LIQUOR AMNII. Popularly known as " the waters," the liquor amnii is the fluid surrounding a child in the womb. It helps to protect the child from undue pressure, and at childbirth forms an elastic wedge for dilating the genital passage.

See Childbirth ; Pregnancy.

LIQUORICE. Glycyrrhiza or liquorice root is a demulcent and in sufficient doses a mild purgative. It is used in the form of the extract as an excipient for pills, and either the dry or the liquid extract, the

dose of which is ½ to 1 drachm, is used to cover the taste of unpleasant drugs, such as senna, aloes, Epsom salts and ammonium chloride. The compound liquorice powder contains also senna, fennel and sulphur. It is used, in doses of 60 to 120 grains, as a laxative, especially for children and for women during pregnancy. Liquorice relieves pharyngeal irritation and is much used in cough mixtures and pastilles. Solazzi juice is a dried extract of liquorice and affords a convenient way of using the drug.

LITHAEMIA. The term lithaemia implies the accumulation in the blood of substances of the uric acid group as a consequence of faulty food or tissue metabolism. This condition is presumed to underlie and precede gouty manifestations and urinary lithiasis. In gout there is an excess of uric acid in the tissues and in the blood, a uric-acidaemia. Lithaemia is caused by excess in eating and drinking, particularly when combined with deficient exercise.

An excess of uric acid and urates in the blood may be caused, however, by excessive exercise, or by extraction of water from the blood in a very hot, dry climate. Treatment consists in a plain, moderate diet, including fresh vegetables and fruit, and a sufficiency of exercise. Lithia salts are beneficial and a liberal consumption of water ; a course of treatment at a spa will often be desirable.

See Kidney ; Uric Acid.

LITHIASIS. The general term used for the formation of stones, or calculi, in the body is lithiasis.

LITHIUM. Salts of lithium, which is a metal in the same class with sodium and potassium, are used for their diuretic and antacid effects. In lithiasis or gout the administration of lithium gets rid of much uric acid from the system. Carbonate of lithium, dose 2 to 5 grains, and citrate of lithium, dose 5 to 10 grains, are the salts most in use. An agreeable way of giving the latter is as the effervescing citrate of lithium, the dose of which is 60 to 120 grains.

LITHOTOMY. The removal of a stone from the bladder by cutting is called lithotomy. The opening may be made in the lower part of the abdomen, the suprapubic route, or in the perineum. A stone may be removed, without cutting, by lithotrity. A crushing instrument, called a lithotrite, is passed into the bladder and the stone is broken up into small fragments, which are then removed by a suction apparatus, called Bigelow's **evacuator**.

LITMUS. The reaction of the urine and other liquids is ascertained by the use of litmus papers. Litmus is a blue pigment obtained from lichens. Contact with acids makes it turn red, but alkalies again turn it blue. Both red and blue papers are supplied. If the solution makes the former blue, it has an alkaline reaction; if the latter red, it has an acid reaction.

See Turmeric.

LITTLE'S DISEASE. *See* Birth Paralysis.

LIVER. The largest gland in the body, having an average weight of 53 ounces in the adult male, the liver is situated in the upper part of the abdomen on the right side. In shape it has some resemblance to a wedge, the thick part being towards the right and the thin part extending towards the left, and reaching a few inches beyond the mid-line of the body. The thick part, or right lobe, as it is called, is tucked up into the right dome of the midriff, or diaphragm, and lies behind the ribs ; but towards the middle line, where it is now the left lobe, the liver passes out from the protection of the ribs. The situation of the organ is shown in the frontispiece and in the illustrations in page 2.

A large vein, the portal, brings blood to the liver from the stomach and bowel, the pancreas and the spleen ; and, contrary to the usual behaviour of veins, this vein breaks up into smaller veins, and these into a large capillary network which traverses the substance of the liver. Blood is also brought to the liver by the hepatic artery. Nerves of various kinds enter the organ. A duct of considerable size, the hepatic duct, drains bile from the liver ; this duct is joined by the cystic duct coming from the gall bladder, and then becomes the common bile duct through which bile is emptied into the duodenum, or first part of the small intestine.

The liver is made up of an immense number of lobules, circular or oval in shape, and consisting of rows of liver cells radiating from a centre which is occupied by the central or intralobular vein. Between the rows of cells are two sets of capillaries for blood and for bile, which communicate with larger vessels at the margins of the lobules. Surrounding and permeating the lobules is a delicate fibrous tissue, known as Glisson's capsule, which is continuous with the fibrous tissue investing the whole organ. It is overgrowth or contraction of this tissue that constitutes cirrhosis of the liver.

Blood flows from the periphery to the centre of a lobule, the hepatic cells meanwhile extracting from it substances for storage or excretion, and by the intralobular vein is conveyed to larger veins, through which it passes to the hepatic veins and is discharged into the inferior vena cava, and so reaches the heart.

Liver cells, which from mutual pressure usually assume a polygonal shape, have many activities. They produce bile, the materials for which they extract from the blood. Bilirubin, the colouring matter occurring most abundantly in human bile, though modified by its passage through a liver cell, is formed by other cells, known as Kupffer's cells, which are found in the lining of the liver-capillaries and elsewhere. It is derived from the haemoglobin of the blood.

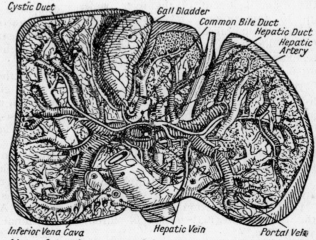

Liver. Internal structure and the course of its great blood vessels

Liver cells also extract harmful substances from the blood, either converting them into harmless ones or excreting them in the bile. If, however, such substances are in excess in the blood, as when the digestion is disordered, they may not be dealt with adequately in the liver, so that a proportion passes on into the blood circulating throughout the body, producing symptoms of " biliousness." Urea is formed in the liver, and is passed into the blood to be excreted by the kidneys. The liver produces fibrinogen, the substance in the blood that forms a clot, and antithrombin, a ferment that prevents clotting in the circulating blood, an accident that might otherwise occur owing to the death and disintegration of white blood corpuscles, as explained under the heading Coagulation.

Another important function of the liver cells is to take up sugar from the blood and store it as glycogen, subsequently reconverting this into sugar to meet the demands of the body. Sugar is the fuel which supplies muscles with their energy. By the use of appropriate tests the modern clinician can measure the capacity of the liver for carrying on some of its functions.

On account of the very considerable amount of oxidation which is part of the chemical activities going on in this large gland, it is quite an important source of body heat. The liver possesses large powers of replacing portions that are thrown out of action by disease by producing fresh cells.

From the umbilicus, a cord known as the round ligament of the liver passes up to this organ ; it represents the obliterated umbilical vein of the foetus. Other ligaments are formed by the reflexions of the peritoneum, covering the organ, on to the body walls.

Diseases of the Liver. Diseases of the liver may or may not be accompanied by jaundice (q.v.). Some diseases cause enlargement of the liver ; others diminish its size. Enlargement may be due to a large number of causes, including the following :

(1) Hypertrophy, or a simple overgrowth of the organ.

(2) Fatty infiltration ; this is usual in the obese, and may occur in chronic alcoholism.

(3) Acute inflammation of the liver, or hepatitis ; here there is acute congestion. The cause may be the poison of a fever, alcohol, etc.

(4) Chronic congestion, which may accompany indigestion ; the so-called tropical liver is of this description.

(5) Passive congestion, or nutmeg liver ; an over-filling of the vesicles and capillaries due to an inefficient flow in the inferior vena cava, such as occurs in advanced heart or lung disease.

Varieties of Liver Abscess

(6) Abscess, which may be due to septic infection or pyaemia, or to the amoebic parasite of dysentery. In the former event the abscesses are likely to be small and multiple, but not causing great enlargement ; a tropical, or amoebic abscess is generally single, and there may be great enlargement. Here there is likely to be a history of previous dysentery, though possibly not, and the symptoms pointing to the liver are preceded and accompanied by a hectic type of fever (q.v.) which may suggest malaria. The contents of such an abscess usually have a resemblance to anchovy paste. Unless evacuated by operation, the abscess may rupture into the abdominal cavity causing general peritonitis, which is likely to be fatal ; or it may rupture through the diaphragm and into the lung, whence it may be evacuated by the bronchial tubes. The existence of the abscess may be revealed by X-rays, but sometimes can only be established by an exploratory operation. Besides evacuating the abscess, emetine is injected subcutaneously.

(7) Obstruction of the bile ducts may cause slight enlargement, accompanied by jaundice.

(8) Cirrhosis. In ordinary cirrhosis, the so-called gin-drinker's or hob-nailed liver, the organ is atrophied, but in some forms of cirrhosis, for example, Hanot's, there is enlargement. This occurs in young people mainly.

(9) Splenic anaemia. In this disease the spleen is enlarged and later the liver, from cirrhotic changes. At this stage the disorder is commonly known as Banti's disease. An accumulation of fluid in the abdominal cavity, or ascites, is a usual accompaniment.

(10) Syphilis. From cirrhotic changes or numerous gummata the liver may be enlarged more or less.

(11) Amyloid disease. Here degenerative changes cause the replacement of the cells by a translucent waxy-looking substance. Syphilis, or long-standing suppuration somewhere, are the common causes.

(12) Hydatid disease (q.v.). Irregular enlargement may occur from the formation of cysts in association with the presence of the hydatid worm.

(13) Cancer. Malignant disease of the liver is generally secondary to the disease elsewhere, say, in the bowel. There may or may not be jaundice, but there is progressive and great wasting with cachexia.

Diminution of the liver in alcoholic cirrhosis is accompanied by the development of knobs on its surface. There may be no symptoms for a long time, but at last the contracted fibrous tissue in the organ obstructs the venous circulation, so that there is congestion of the lining of the stomach and bowel with consequent indigestion, and perhaps vomiting of blood and its passage by the bowel. For the same reason ascites is also common. The treatment is mainly symptomatic, but sometimes fresh channels for the venous blood are procured by operation.

Fatty degeneration of the liver occurs in poisoning by phosphorus and other substances, and in certain diseases, including acute yellow atrophy. This is a rapidly fatal disorder, the cause of which is not clear, though it may follow mental shock. It begins like catarrhal jaundice, but the jaundice becomes intense and there is bleeding from mucous membranes and into the skin. There is fever and nervous symptoms are usual. The liver shrinks in size. Women between twenty and thirty are usually affected, and in association with pregnancy and labour. Treatment is of no avail.

See Bile; Biliousness; Digestion; Gall Bladder; Jaundice.

LIVERISH FEELING. *See* Biliousness.

LIVIDITY. The blue or blackish discoloration of skin or mucous membrane caused by imperfect aeration of the blood, or following a bruise, may be described as lividity.

See Cyanosis.

LOBE. The larger subdivisions of an organ are described as lobes. Any lobe of an organ, as in the lung and the liver, may have the same function as any other but, on the other hand, as in the brain, the functions of the lobes may be quite different. Some lobes, like those of the liver and lung, are made up of much smaller portions, described as lobules. In the lungs are recognized a lobar form of pneumonia and a lobular.

LOCHIA. The discharge from the womb which goes on for two or three weeks after the birth of a child is called the lochia. Consisting at first of almost pure blood, it becomes watery and whitish, and acquires rather a sickly odour.

See Puerperium.

LOCKJAW. Tetanus is popularly known as lockjaw because this symptom occurs early in the disease. The cause of the disease is infection with the tetanus bacillus, an organism which is commonly seen with a rounded knob at one end and so is called the drum-stick bacillus. The knob represents a spore, from which a fresh organism will develop; these spores are very resistant to heat, cold, drying and ordinary antiseptics. The tetanus bacillus is anaerobic, that is, it will not develop in the presence of oxygen. It is a normal inhabitant of the intestine of horses and cattle and is present in manured soil. Contamination of a wound with such soil at once creates a risk of tetanus.

The microbes themselves do not travel far from the site of introduction, but their poisons pass up motor nerves to centres in the spinal cord and brain. Symptoms may begin from a few hours to some weeks after infection. There may be such disturbances as sleeplessness, frequent yawning, stiffness in the throat muscles and difficulty in swallowing. Then the lower jaw becomes spasmodically fixed (trismus) and soon the spasm involves the rest of the face, the neck, the trunk and the limbs.

The patient appears to grin or snarl, the so-called risus sardonicus, the head is drawn back, the neck is fixed and painful and the trunk and limbs are fixed. The back may be bent backwards (opisthotonus), or forwards or to either side. The spasms relax from time to time but rarely completely and are readily brought on by noise, a bright light or a breath of wind ; they are very painful. The mind is quite clear throughout. Death takes place from exhaustion as a rule ; rarely, it is due to spasm of the breathing muscles and consequent asphyxia. The duration of the disease varies from a day or two onwards, and the longer it lasts beyond ten days the better the prospects.

Even more important from the point of view of prognosis is the duration of the incubation period ; the odds in favour of recovery are considerably increased if this lasts beyond ten days and again increased if it lasts beyond three weeks. Symptoms may be quite localised to the neighbourhood of the wound.

Any wound should be cleaned up as a matter of course, but if there is any possibility of contamination with tetanus, as when the wound is got during gardening or on the football field, for example, a prophylactic injection of antitoxic serum should be given as soon as possible. The disease is treated by keeping the patient perfectly quiet in a darkened room. Injections of serum are given, including some into the spinal canal. Sedatives, such as luminal, are given, and chloroform may be needed so that the patient can be fed through a tube.

See Antiseptic ; Serum Therapy.

LOCOMOTOR ATAXIA. Also known as tabes dorsalis, locomotor ataxia is a chronic disease of the spinal cord, the posterior nerve roots and the posterior columns being the parts affected. The morbid changes are brought about by syphilis but do not occur until some years after infection with this disease, not until middle life as a rule. Locomotor ataxia is more common in men than in women and in city, rather than country, dwellers.

Usually the first thing to be noted is loss of the knee jerk (*q.v.*) on one or both sides. It may be noted also that although the pupils contract on looking at a near object, they do not do so on exposure to light, a state of affairs described as the Argyll-Robertson pupil. Severe pains, known as lightning pains, may shoot down the legs and there may be a little difficulty in passing water. Sometimes vision becomes progressively impaired owing to atrophy of the optic nerve.

After some time, possibly many years, the patient finds that he is unsteady in walking if he cannot keep his eyes on his feet, or he manifests Romberg's symptom, that is inability to stand steady with the feet together and the eyes shut. He develops a gait (*q.v.*) which is typical of ataxia. With the eyes shut he may not be able accurately to touch the tip of his nose with his hand. All these are signs of inco-ordination ; the patient does not know the position of his limbs unless he is looking at them, though a normal individual does know this, through sensations coming to the central nervous system from the muscles and joints.

Impairment of Sense of Touch

Ordinary tactile sensation is impaired and also the sense of pain ; a solid object when touched may feel woolly and it may be possible to stick a pin into the skin without its being felt. Sometimes there is a sensation of a tight cord round the waist—the so-called girdle sensation. Another kind of disturbance is what is called a visceral crisis. The most common is the gastric crisis in which pain, sickness and vomiting occur and suggest something seriously wrong in the stomach or bowel. There is also a laryngeal crisis, consisting of a persistent tickling cough ; or it may be dyspnoea ; or a rectal crisis, in which there is persistent and painful although unnecessary straining to empty the bowel ; and so on.

Trophic disturbances are represented by Charcot's joint, a condition described under the heading Joint, and by perforating ulcer of the foot. This usually forms on the ball of the great toe and gets gradually deeper. It is quite painless and, in fact, is due to pressure on and irritation of insensitive tissues. Owing to the difficulty in emptying the bladder inflammation of this viscus, or cystitis, is apt to ensue.

Finally the patient becomes helpless and bedridden. If similar morbid changes have affected the brain the patient will have shown the mental symptoms of general paralysis of the insane (*q.v.*). To this combination of the diseases the name tabo-paresis is given.

If there is any difficulty in recognizing the existence of locomotor ataxia in the

PLATE XXIII

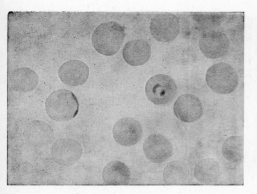
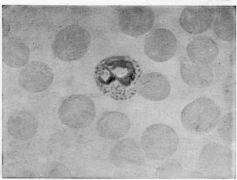

Malaria : life cycle of the benign tertian parasite in man. 1. A parasite which has invaded a red blood cell (left) enlarges and assumes the so-called signet ring shape (right). This stage of invasion by young parasites marks the beginning of fever. 2. Both red cell and parasite have enlarged ; the former is marked by Schüffner's dots ; the latter exhibits amoeboid movements. This stage is reached 18 hours after the first

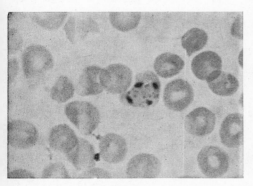
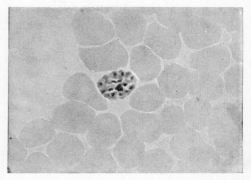

3. At the end of 36 hours from the beginning of the attack the parasite begins to break up, or become segmented. During this and the previous stage the patient is free from fever. 4. At the end of 48 hours segmentation is about complete and a rosette has been formed, after which the red cell ruptures and the young parasites are set free to begin the process over again. At this stage there is renewed fever

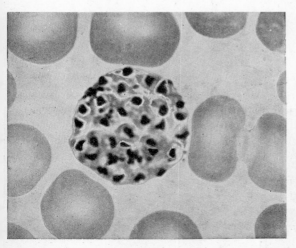
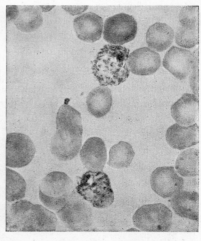

5. Rosette more highly magnified. The dark nuclei and fainter protoplasm of the young parasites are clearly seen. 6. Some of the parasites do not multiply by segmentation but develop into male and female forms known as gametocytes. These are taken up by a biting mosquito and mature and join together in the insect's stomach, the resulting young parasites passing into the salivary glands and thence into man

Microphotographs 1–4 and 6, E. F. Fincham; 5, courtesy of F. Davidson & Co.

PLATE XXIV

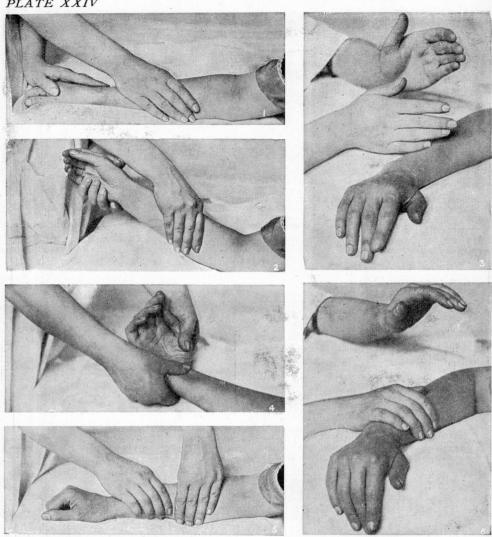

Massage. 1. Effleurage, a light stroking movement for promoting circulation. 2. Pétrissage, for building up muscular tissue. 3. Hacking, to stimulate the muscles. 4. Friction for reducing thickenings. 5. Skin rolling, for treatment of fibrous tissue and fatty deposits. 6. Clapping, for improving cutaneous circulation

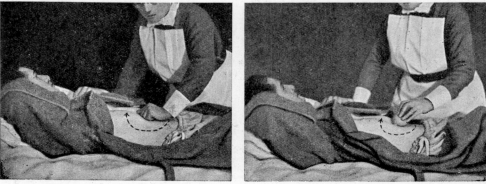

7 and 8. Treatment of constipation by massage of the abdomen with the fist and with a shot ball

earliest stages much help is afforded by a chemical and bacteriological examination of the cerebro-spinal fluid, which is obtained by lumbar puncture—that is, pushing a needle into the spinal canal and allowing a sample of the fluid to drain into a glass tube.

The incidence of this disease would be greatly lessened by thorough treatment of all cases of syphilis, and anti-syphilitic measures form an important part of the treatment. The earlier such treatment is instituted the better. In addition to this, treatment may be required for different symptoms, anodynes for pain, hexamine to assist emptying of the bladder, rest in bed and antiseptic dressings for a perforating ulcer, and so on. Re-education in walking should be undertaken and the system of exercises devised by Frenkel is very useful here.

See Ataxia ; Equilibrium ; General Paralysis of the Insane ; Syphilis.

LOGWOOD. The heart wood of haematoxylon, logwood acts as an astringent, and its red colouring matter, haematoxylin, is used to make a dye for microscopical and general purposes. The infusion of logwood, in doses of $\frac{1}{2}$ to 2 ounces, is a valuable remedy for diarrhoea, and is often included in mixtures for this disorder. There are also a liquid and a dry extract.

LOIN. The part of the back between the last rib and the haunch-bone is called the loin, the two loins together constituting the lumbar region (*q.v.*).

LOOSE CARTILAGE. When reference is made to a loose cartilage one of the semi-lunar cartilages of the knee (*q.v.*) is meant.

LORDOSIS. An increase of the forward curve in the small of the back is called lordosis. This is caused by an effort to improve the balance of the body and is present in the later stages of pregnancy and in hip-joint disease and other disorders.

See Backbone ; Spinal Curvature.

LOTION. A liquid preparation for external application, a lotion may be used to bathe a part, the best thing to use for the purpose being a small piece, usually referred to as a pledget, of cotton-wool or gauze. This is soaked in the lotion and squeezed out over the part ;

sometimes it is used like a sponge to wipe a part clean. For other purposes a piece of lint or gauze is soaked in the lotion, squeezed partly dry and applied. For an evaporating lotion a single layer of gauze is applied and is kept constantly moist by dropping on more lotion from time to time. A lotion may be squeezed on to a part or into a cavity.

Lotions are sometimes classified according to their uses, as antiseptic, astringent or sedative, but a lotion may have more than one action. Lead lotion, for example, is both astringent and sedative.

The official lotions are the yellow and the black lotions of mercury, familiarly known as the yellow and black wash respectively. These are chiefly used for washing venereal sores. Red lotion, or lotio rubra, consists of 1 or 2 grains of zinc sulphate in an ounce of water, coloured red with a few drops of compound tincture of lavender. This has an astringent and stimulating effect on sluggish ulcers.

An evaporating lotion is used for cooling some parts of the body. For headache it may be used on the forehead. It may also be comforting to a sprained joint. A tablespoonful of dilute acetic acid or vinegar in half a pint of water, or one part of eau-de-Cologne to two parts of water, will make a satisfactory lotion for these purposes. An eye lotion is often called a collyrium (*q.v.*).

See Boracic Acid ; Lead.

LOUSE. There are three types of louse, or pediculus, that may infest the human body, namely, the head louse, the

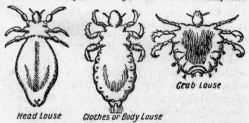

Head Louse   Clothes or Body Louse   Crab Louse

Louse. Three types that affect human beings

body louse, and the pubic louse, usually known as the crab louse. Although the last is most often found on the pubic hairs, it may spread to the thighs, and has been found in the armpit and on the eyebrows and eyelashes.

The presence of lice causes itching, sometimes intense, and the scratching that ensues tends to cause excoriations which may become infected with pus-producing microbes. Thus, there may be pustules on the skin, and scabs, while deeper infection may cause abscesses in or beneath the skin and possibly in neighbouring lymphatic glands. Patches of eczema may also form and in a prolonged infestation with body lice the skin may become pigmented from the scratching. A person who harbours lice or has a skin affection caused by them is said to suffer from pediculosis, or phthiriasis.

Lice are carriers of typhus fever, relapsing fever, trench fever, and possibly other diseases, but although the insects are blood-feeders, infection is not usually caused by the bites but by inoculation, through a person scratching the excreta of the insect into the skin.

The head louse runs freely over the scalp, but the body louse usually haunts the seams of underclothing except when it moves over the skin to feed. The crab louse remains firmly attached to a hair and close to the skin. This creature has a somewhat shield-shaped body and claw-like legs, which distinguish it from the other types. These have oval bodies and resemble one another except that the body louse is rather larger. The eggs of lice, which are known as nits, are tiny, pear-shaped objects and are glued to the hairs. Those of head lice are generally most abundant on the lank hair behind the ears. Little clumps of dandruff may simulate the appearance of nits, but they are easily separated from the hair by brushing, while nits are not.

Sources of the Infestation

Lice may be got from personal contact with an infected person, from a bed in which he has slept or from his clothing; occasionally such agents as wind, flies and domestic animals may be responsible. Crab lice might possibly be got from a privy-seat. A full bath and change of underclothing, at least weekly, will usually protect from the invasion of lice. The head of a child at school should be regularly inspected, however.

To clear off lice from any part of the body it is necessary to deal with the nits as well as the adult insects. The attachment of nits to hair can be loosened by thoroughly damping the hair with a lotion consisting of equal parts of vinegar and water. The nits can then be removed by means of a small-toothed comb. It may be worth while, however, simply to shave off hair in the axilla or on the pubis. When the head is infested the hair should be cut short, and if there is much eczema a close crop is necessary.

Paraffin Oil as a Remedy

Ordinary paraffin oil is an efficient remedy for application to the head, but its inflammability must always be borne in mind. The oil is rubbed into the head, a rag soaked in the oil is then put over the scalp and then a bathing cap. This is left on for ten to twelve hours and the process is twice repeated, after which the head is thoroughly washed with soap and water. If there is much eczema equal parts of olive oil and paraffin should be put on, but the application must be repeated on each of twelve days, after which the head is washed.

Oil of sassafras is an alternative remedy if there is no eczema. It is put on with a stiff brush and the scalp is then covered with a cotton cap. This oil kills both adult insects and nits. If it causes much irritation, olive oil or zinc ointment should be applied. When there is much eczema, stavesacre ointment or an ointment consisting of white precipitate ointment, 60 grains, and zinc ointment to an ounce, may be used.

For body lice the body may be thoroughly rubbed over with a mixture of 5 ounces of petroleum insecticide and 2 drachms of eucalyptus oil, after which a hot bath is taken; or sulphur or stavesacre ointment may be applied for two or three days and then a bath taken.

For the crab louse white precipitate ointment should be used freely on the affected parts.

Clothing should be baked in an oven at a temperature of 160° to 175° F. This may be done by having a good fire, placing the clothing, wrapped in paper, in the oven, and allowing the fire to die down; or the clothing may be soaked in a solution of lysol of a strength of a teaspoonful to the pint of water.

LOZENGE. A pharmaceutical lozenge, also known as a troche or trochiscus, is a small, flat tablet composed of sugar, gum acacia and water with some drug, and usually some flavouring substance, rose, tolu, or black currant paste. This method of administering a drug is useful when a local action on the mouth, fauces or pharynx is required, when a drug is being given to a child, or for convenience in carrying a drug about. The lozenges of potassium chlorate, carbolic acid and krameria are examples of those used for a local effect ; the lozenges of santonin and sulphur are usually well taken by children ; and the compound bismuth lozenge is a convenient method of carrying about bismuth when one is dyspeptic.

LUMBAGO. Pain in the back, due to fibrositis (*q.v.*) in connexion with the muscles of the loins, their tendons or aponeuroses, is called lumbago. It may be very acute and disabling and people who have once suffered from the complaint are liable to a recurrence.

See Backache.

LUMBAR REGION. Corresponding to what is usually described as the small of the back, the lumbar region is built up on the five lumbar vertebrae, this bony column being strengthened behind by the powerful erector spinae muscle, and in front by the psoas muscle. Outside these on either side is a belt of muscle, the quadratus lumborum, between the last ribs and the pelvis. There are besides several sheaths of strong fascia, the lumbar fascia, from the outer border of which the flat abdominal muscles take origin.

The organs lying in front of the lumbar region are the kidneys and the ascending and descending colon. A swelling in this region may sometimes be due to disease of the kidney, a growth or an abscess. When one speaks of a lumbar abscess, however, what is usually meant is one due to caries of the vertebrae, a condition almost always of a tuberculous nature.

Lumbar puncture is the name given to the operation of passing a hollow needle between two vertebrae into the spinal canal and through the arachnoid membrane of the spinal cord. This is done to obtain a sample of the cerebro-spinal fluid. Sera are similarly introduced into the sub-arachnoid space in the treatment of lockjaw and other diseases, and drugs, when inducing spinal anaesthesia.

See Back ; Backbone.

LUMINAL. A synthetic drug, with a sedative action, luminal is used in the treatment of epilepsy, some types of headache and other disorders.

LUMP. The significance of a lump is determined by attention to various facts, such as its situation ; the suddenness, or otherwise, of its appearance ; whether its contents feel solid, liquid, or, in some cases, gaseous ; the presence or absence of inflammation or of pain ; and so on. Often a very difficult problem is presented.

See Abscess ; Aneurysm ; Gland ; Hernia ; Tumour.

LUNAR CAUSTIC. The nitrate of silver is familiarly known as lunar caustic.

See Silver.

LUNATIC. In law a lunatic is defined as being " an idiot, or person of unsound mind." The term is almost restricted to legal usage, though statutes dealing with the insane are called Lunacy Acts and many institutions for mental diseases are described as lunatic asylums.

See Feebleminded ; Idiocy ; Insanity ; Mental Disease.

LUNG. The lungs lie in either side of the chest. The space in the middle of this cavity, known as the mediastinum,

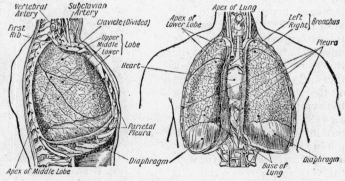

Lung. Sectional views of the chest showing (left) three lobes of the right lung, and (right) both lungs seen from the back, with the heart between them.

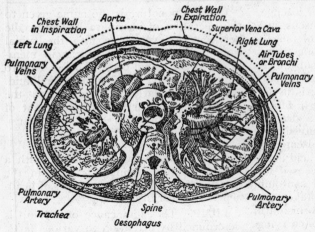

Lung. Cross section of the lungs and chest wall, the expansion of the latter in the act of breathing being indicated by the dotted line

capillaries and the air in the cells, oxygen passing into the blood and carbonic acid in the opposite direction.

Blood is supplied to the capillaries by the pulmonary artery and carried off by the pulmonary veins. Lymphatic vessels also course through the lungs and nerve fibres are supplied by the vagus and the sympathetic nerves. The assemblage of vessels and the bronchus and other structures entering or leaving the organ forms the root of the lung. Here are also lymphatic glands into which are drained the lymphatic vessels coming from the lung. Surrounding the root is a smooth membrane, the pleura (*q.v.*), which also covers the lung, and at the root is reflected on to the inside of the chest wall.

A lung is somewhat conical in shape, the uppermost part forming the apex and the broad lower portion the base. The right lung has two deep clefts in it, dividing it into three lobes, but the left lung has only two lobes. The apex projects $1\frac{1}{2}$ to 2 inches above the collar-bone

is mainly occupied by the heart and great blood vessels, the gullet and other structures, but otherwise the chest is packed with lung. Their relation to other organs is seen in the frontispiece. The general structure of a lung resembles somewhat that of a tree. The stem is represented by a main bronchus (*see* diagram in p. 119) passing to the lung, and this bronchus subdivides into small air-tubes and so on by ramifications, until minute tubes, or bronchioles, are reached. Each of these opens into an expansion, the walls of which are studded with the air-cells or alveoli (*see* Plate XI, 1).

The larger bronchial tubes contain rings of cartilage, but as they become smaller these tubes have fewer rings, then only scattered flakes of cartilage and finally nothing of the kind at all. In the smaller tubes, however, there is more muscle, arranged round the tube; it is the contraction of this and consequent narrowing of the tubes that account for the symptoms of asthma. The air-cells are crowded together, but in the space between adjoining cells is a great network of blood capillaries, and through the very thin walls of the cells an interchange of gases can take place between the blood in the

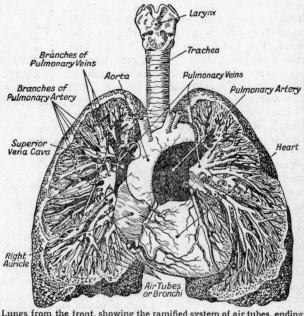

Lungs from the front, showing the ramified system of air tubes, ending in the alveoli, where interchange of oxygen and carbonic acid gas occurs

444

into the root of the neck, and is a usual site of the beginning of pulmonary tuberculosis, or consumption.

The lung of a stillborn child feels solid and sinks when put into water, a condition described as atelectasis, but the first few breaths of a living child fill the lungs with air and, thereafter, there is always so much air in a lung that it floats in water. Consolidation may be brought about by disease, however. Because of its air-content, percussion over a normal lung produces a resonant sound. On listening over a lung a respiratory murmur is heard both in inspiration and expiration, the latter sound, however, being considerably the shorter. When the person speaks also the sound of the voice is conducted through the lung to the ear. Disease produces modifications of these phenomena, and diagnosis is based on the nature of the modifications and on the presence or absence of additional, or adventitious, sounds, known as râles and rhonchi.

Diseases of the Lungs. Acute congestion of the lungs accompanies pneumonia and other inflammatory diseases of the lungs or tubes. Passive congestion is common in disease of the heart when the return of the blood from the lungs is obstructed. In old, bedridden people the bases of the lungs tend to become over-loaded with blood, through feebleness of the circulation there. This is called hypostatic congestion, and to prevent its occurrence as far as possible the position of the patient should be altered frequently. Oedema of the lung accompanies inflammatory and congestive states. Sometimes, as in Bright's disease, it may come on suddenly; the patient is extremely breathless and coughs up large quantities of frothy, watery sputum.

Bleeding from the lung occurs in pulmonary tuberculosis, pneumonia, infarction and other disorders. It may come from a bronchial tube, and is sometimes caused by an aneurysm opening into a tube. The actual cause in some cases is a blood disease. The first-aid treatment is described under the heading Bleeding.

An abscess in the lung may occur in pneumonia, in pulmonary tuberculosis, or from embolism (*q.v.*) with an infective plug. Sometimes an abscess outside, in the liver, for example, bursts into the lung. It may be possible to open and drain the abscess. In severe infections of the lung or of the tubes, as in bronchiectasis, or when the blood supply is interfered with by plugging of the pulmonary artery, death, or gangrene, of a portion of lung may take place. The sputa are extremely offensive, the patient is and looks very ill and the outlook is very bad.

Emphysema (*q.v.*) is the name given to the dilatation of the air cells in the lung. One or both lungs may be affected.

In pulmonary tuberculosis, or after pneumonia, or in collapse of the lung from the pressure of fluid on the pleural cavity, in dust disease and from other causes, a chronic inflammatory process may result in the formation of much fibrous tissue in the lung (*see* Plate XI, 3), with a corresponding amount of consolidation of its tissue. This condition is described as fibrosis and in addition to interfering with lung function it may disturb that of the heart by dragging on and displacing it.

Collapse of the lung, that is, a condition in which the vesicles are deprived of much, or most, of their air content, may affect a whole lung, a large portion or only a small portion. A large collapse may be caused by a chest wound or other conditions, and there is considerable resultant shock and breathlessness.

The lungs may be the site of a malignant growth, either carcinoma or sarcoma. This may be primary, but more often it is secondary to a growth elsewhere.

See Asthma; Breathing Exercises; Bronchi; Bronchiectasis; Bronchitis; Broncho-pneumonia; Consumption; Emphysema; Pleurisy; Pneumonia; Râle; Respiration.

LUPUS. The skin disease known as lupus vulgaris, but often referred to simply as lupus, is caused by the tubercle bacillus. As a rule it begins in childhood. The germs gain entrance through a little abrasion of the skin or a mucous membrane, commonly that lining the nose. The first appearance of the disease on the skin is as a little brown nodule, often referred to as the " apple-jelly " nodule. This is situated in the true skin, but is visible through the epidermis.

Groups of such nodules form a lupus patch, and while nodules may sometimes degenerate and be replaced by scar tissue, others break through the surface of the skin, and the exposed unhealthy tissue is then invaded by ordinary pus-forming microbes, which cause discharge or pustules, and these, by drying up, form crusts and scabs. The surface itself becomes an ulcer, and spreads more or less. Scarring takes place over part of the surface, but the scar is always liable to break down.

When the face is affected there may be hideous disfigurement, and in the nose the disease may cause much destruction of the parts and may even pass through and invade the palate. On the limbs it may cause mutilation. Sometimes the surface of a lupus patch may become covered with warty growths or even a horn-like structure. Neighbouring, or even distant, lymphatic glands may be infected and may suppurate and rupture, causing infection of adjoining skin.

It is all-important that lupus should be recognized and treated in its earliest stages.

The general health is usually fairly good, but the point must be considered and, when necessary, improved hygienic conditions, a generous diet, cod-liver oil and tonics should be resorted to.

As regards local treatment, the diseased patch should be cut out and the wound repaired by stitching, or skin grafting when such treatment is feasible. Other operative treatment includes scraping, scarification, cauterisation and the use of carbonic acid snow. Very good results are achieved by Finsen light treatment, but this is very expensive. Other lamps, which produce ultra-violet rays, are being used and also diathermy. Encouraging results have been got by ionisation. Some doctors use radium. The treatment of lupus needs expert supervision. There is a tendency for carcinoma to form on surfaces that have been ravaged by lupus, and excessive irritation by caustics or otherwise might provoke this occurrence.

Lupus erythematosus, which has no connexion with ordinary lupus, is considered under the heading Erythema.

See Light ; Tuberculosis.

LYMPHATIC SYSTEM. Besides the circulation of the blood, there is another circulation going on throughout the body, namely, the circulation of lymph. This fluid, which in composition resembles a diluted blood plasma, transudes from the blood capillaries and fills the spaces between body cells. From these spaces part returns to the veins, but part is taken up by tiny lymphatic capillaries which open on the spaces and is conveyed to larger lymphatic vessels. These, like veins, possess valves, so that lymph can only flow in one direction. The large serous spaces, the pleural, the pericardial, the peritoneal, and others, are also drained by these vessels.

Interposed in the course of the lymphatic vessels are structures, varying in size from that of a pinhead to a bean, known as lymphatic nodes or glands. These contain spaces through which the lymph percolates, but also masses of

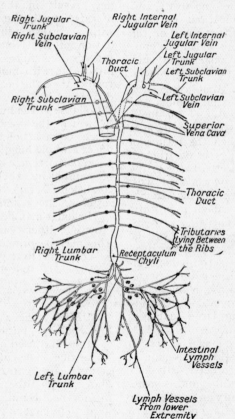

Right Jugular Trunk
Right Subclavian Vein
Right Internal Jugular Vein
Left Internal Jugular Vein
Left Jugular Trunk
Thoracic Duct
Left Subclavian Trunk
Right Subclavian Trunk
Left Subclavian Vein
Superior Vena Cava
Thoracic Duct
Tributaries lying Between the Ribs
Right Lumbar Trunk
Receptaculum Chyli
Intestinal Lymph Vessels
Left Lumbar Trunk
Lymph Vessels from lower Extremity

Lymphatic System. Diagram of main branches

cells resembling the lymphocytes in the blood ; in fact, such cells in the blood may be produced to some extent in lymphatic glands. The glands to a large extent clear the lymph of bacteria and other noxious substances which have made their way into it, and so prevent their reaching the blood stream.

Glands occur in groups of two to fifteen, and are embedded in connective tissue. There is a superficial set and a deep set. There are no superficial glands below the elbow or the knee. All the lymphatic vessels of the body drain into two main vessels, known as the thoracic duct and the right lymphatic duct. The former begins near the right kidney as the receptaculum, or cisterna, chyli, and passes up through the diaphragm and chest cavity to the root of the neck, where it opens into the angle of junction of the left subclavian and internal jugular veins.

The right lymphatic duct opens into the junction of the right subclavian and internal jugular veins. It drains the right side of the chest, the right upper limb, and the right side of the head, all the rest of the body draining into the thoracic duct. After a meal the lymph in the thoracic duct is very milky from the presence of emulsified fat, absorbed from the meal.

Besides that contained in the lymphatic glands, it should be said that numerous collections of lymphoid tissue occur along the course of the digestive tract and some in other situations.

The circulation of the lymph is not helped by the pumping of the heart, but only by the movements of

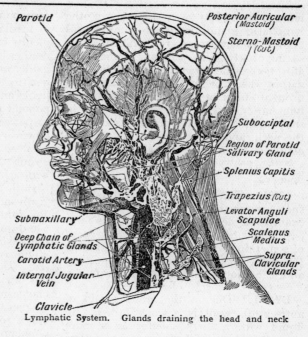

Lymphatic System. Glands draining the head and neck

Labels: Parotid; Posterior Auricular (Mastoid); Sterno-Mastoid (Cut); Subocciptal; Region of Parotid Salivary Gland; Splenius Capitis; Trapezius (Cut); Levator Anguli Scapulae; Scalenus Medius; Supra-Clavicular Glands; Submaxillary; Deep Chain of Lymphatic Glands; Carotid Artery; Internal Jugular Vein; Clavicle

Labels (arm): Axillary Glands; Gland; Superficial Lymphatic Vessels

Inflammation of lymph glands, termed adenitis, can occur in the armpit though due to a septic finger

muscles, the existence of valves in the vessels and the suction action of breathing, in the same way as the inflow from the veins is helped.

Diseases of the Lymphatic System. Inflammation of a lymphatic vessel, or lymphangitis, may be acute or chronic. The acute form may be seen often when a finger is septic, it being possible to trace the course of the inflamed vessels by the thin red lines passing up the forearm. Inflammation of the glands is called lymphadenitis, and may also be acute or chronic. When it occurs, it is necessary to scrutinise the area which drains into the inflamed glands. Thus, inflammation of glands in the groin may be due to a septic sore on a toe or anywhere on the limb above this. Chronic lymphadenitis is often due to tuberculosis.

A tumour consisting of an overgrowth of lymphatic vessels sometimes forms, and is called a lymphangioma. Cysts also may be formed by the dilatation of lymphatic vessels. A tumour of the lymphatic glands may be simple and known as lymphoma, or maligant, consisting of a lympho-sarcoma. Glands may also become enlarged from the growth within them of malignant tumour-cells brought from a distance through the lymphatic vessels. Thus, carcinoma in the mouth leads to enlarged glands in the neck, and, in the breast, to enlarged glands in the armpit.

See Elephantiasis; Hodgkin's Disease; Inflammation; Leukaemia; Thoracic Duct; Tumour; White Leg.

LYSIS. The gradual decline of a fever, such as occurs in typhoid fever, for example, is described as lysis. This term is also used, however, for the breaking down of something. Thus, haematolysis means the disintegration of red blood corpuscles, and bacteriolysis, that of bacteria.

See Fever.

LYSOL. One of the cresol group of antiseptics, lysol is a dark brown oily liquid with a tarry smell. It is more powerful than carbolic acid, and less poisonous. It is generally used in the strength of a teaspoonful to a pint.

See Cresol.

MᶜBURNEY'S POINT. A spot on the anterior abdominal wall, in a line between the umbilicus and the anterior superior spine of the iliac bone and about two inches from this spine, is designated McBurney's point. In appendicitis tenderness is commonly present when pressure is made over this spot.

MACULA. A Latin word meaning a spot, macula or its English form, macule, is a name applied to a place on the skin where the colour is altered, without other change. A port-wine stain, a patch of erythema or reddening, a freckle and a patch of leucoderma are examples of a macule. The term macula is also used in anatomical descriptions, as, for example, the macula lutea or yellow spot of the eye.

MADURA FOOT. Fungus foot (*q.v.*) is also called Madura foot. Another name is mycetoma.

MAGNESIUM. A whitish, silvery-looking metal belonging to the group of alkaline earths, magnesium burns with a brilliant flame and is used as an illuminant in indoor photography. Several of the compounds of the metal are of importance in medicine. Magnesium sulphate, commonly called Epsom salt (*q.v.*), is much used as a purgative, and magnesium oxide, or magnesia, and magnesium carbonate, each of which is prepared in a light and a heavy form, are likewise popular remedies of this class, though not so powerful as the sulphate. They have, however, an antacid quality which is not possessed by the latter. They are very useful, therefore, in dyspepsia associated with acidity.

Both the oxides and the carbonates are given in doses of 30 to 60 grains, or 15 to 30 grains if the dose is to be repeated. Fluid magnesia, which is a solution of the bicarbonate, is given in doses of 1 to 2 ounces, or ½ drachm for a child a year old. The so-called white mixture, or mistura alba, consists of 30 grains of magnesium carbonate and 15 grains of magnesium sulphate dissolved in an ounce of peppermint water. It is a popular laxative. Milk of magnesia and magnesia cream are pleasant preparations of magnesia.

The solution of magnesium citrate, a sort of magnesium lemonade, can be taken freely, and the effervescent citrate of magnesia is a similar preparation. The oxide, the carbonate and the citrate are useful remedies for lithaemia (*q.v.*). Magnesium hydroxide, in repeated doses of 60 grains, is a useful antidote for arsenic. Magnesium lactate is sometimes given instead of calcium lactate to increase the coagulability of the blood. Magnesium carbonate in water causes hardness, though there is much less of this salt than of calcium carbonate in fresh water. The magnesium salt is largely responsible for the hardness of sea water.

MALAISE. An indefinite sense of illness is referred to as malaise. It often ushers in an acute disease, especially the eruptive fevers.

MALAR. The malar, or cheek bone, forms the outer part of the margin of the orbit, and a backward projection of this bone, by joining with the zygomatic process of the temporal bone, forms a bony arch on the side of the skull, to which is attached the masseter muscle below and the temporal fascia above. The muscle is important for chewing, and the fascia is so strong and taut that a tear in it has been mistaken for a fracture of the skull.

See Jaw; Skull.

MALARIA. The fevers described as malaria, ague, marsh fever, jungle fever and by other names, are caused by the invasion of the blood by species of a minute animal parasite belonging to the class of protozoa. These fevers ravage the populations of tropical and sub-tropical countries and also exist in some countries within the temperate zone. On their conquest or control depend the restoration and maintenance of vigour to many large communities, the spread of civilisation, the success of schemes of colonisation and the full exploitation of the natural resources of the tropics.

The parasites are picked up from the blood of an infected individual by a mosquito (*q.v.*) of the genus anopheles (*q.v.*), and after a process of development in the body of the insect are injected into the body of another individual.

Young malarial parasites thus introduced into the blood make their way into red cells and grow at the expense of the cells. After a time the parasite subdivides into a number of young parasites, the mass assuming what is called a rosette form (*see* Plate XXIII, 4 and 5), and then the red cell ruptures, setting free the young parasites, each of which makes its way into a fresh red cell to begin the process over again. The discharge of the parasites into the blood stream coincides with the onset of fever.

Some of the parasites do not follow this course, but develop into sexual forms, male and female (Plate XXIII, 6). If these are taken up by a mosquito they join together in the insect's stomach, producing an active cell with two pointed ends, which makes its way into the stomach wall of the insect, where it grows for a time and then subdivides into a number of young parasites. By the rupture of the containing capsule these are liberated, and they then make their way into the salivary glands of the insect, ready to be discharged wherever the insect bites. This development in

the mosquito occupies about ten to twelve days, so that after taking up infected blood a mosquito may take several meals of blood without infecting its host.

Three species of the malarial parasite are found in human beings, namely, plasmodium vivax (Plate XXIII), plasmodium malariae and plasmodium falciparum. The cycle of development in the blood of the first takes 48 hours and of the second 72 hours, so that bouts of fever occur every third and every fourth day respectively; these fevers are therefore described as benign tertian, and quartan, fever. The development of plasmodium falciparum is more irregular, and the fever produced is called malignant tertian or sub-tertian fever. The temperature may not reach normal in the intervals of the bouts, the fever assuming a remittent form. A daily rise of temperature may occur from two separate infections with the tertian parasite. In sub-tertian fever the sexual forms of the parasite are not developed in the blood, as in the other two, but in the tissues and especially the spleen and bone-marrow, this fact accounting for some of the difficulty encountered in treating this fever.

Three Stages of an Attack

In a typical attack of ague there are three more or less clearly defined stages, namely, the cold, the hot and the sweating stage. At the outset the patient feels chilly and may shiver violently with his teeth chattering. This may last from ten to thirty minutes, and then he feels hot and inclined to throw off bedding that he was grateful for in the first stage. There is headache commonly and perhaps sickness and vomiting. This stage, in which the temperature reaches its maximum, perhaps to 104° or 105° F., may last for four or five hours, after which free perspiration breaks out and the temperature falls rapidly, with a great access of comfort to the patient.

The spleen is enlarged in malaria and there may be tenderness over it. During the apyrexial stage the patient may be well enough to go about his ordinary duties, but after a succession of attacks there is more or less weakness.

In the remittent type symptoms may be severe. The patient may be delirious or stuporose, and coma may supervene. Sometimes there is deep jaundice and there may be blood in the stools and urine. Albuminuria is not uncommon. Sometimes the condition may suggest dysentery or cholera, and cases have been mistaken for appendicitis. In other instances symptoms have pointed to respiratory disease, bronchitis, pleurisy or pneumonia.

In chronic malaria the spleen is enlarged, probably considerably, and hard, a condition sometimes referred to as ague-cake. There is a progressive anaemia and the skin may have a clayey tint. The appetite is poor and there is wasting and weakness. Sleeplessness is sometimes a troublesome symptom, or palpitation and shortness of breath, or neuralgia. There may be lesions in the eyes or ears and impairment of sight or hearing. Mental depression may reach the degree of melancholia, though sometimes maniacal attacks occur.

Quinine as a Preventive

Preventive treatment, in so far as it is concerned with protection from mosquitoes by nets and otherwise, is considered under the heading Mosquito. As some time elapses between infection and the onset of symptoms, eleven days, on the average, for benign tertian, fourteen for quartan and six for malignant tertian, additional protection is afforded by taking quinine regularly, 5 to 10 grains daily or 20 grains twice a week, 10 grains in the morning and 10 at night. A pregnant woman should take smaller doses, but more frequently.

The diagnosis of the existence and variety of malaria is most exactly made by a microscopic examination of the blood, but as this means may not be available, and possibly even on examination no parasites might be found in a specimen of blood, it should be presumed that fever occurring in a malarious country is of this nature and quinine should be given in order to test this presumption. Quinine sulphate is the salt generally used, and preferably it should be dissolved, though a good brand of tablet may be satisfactory. The dosage should be 30 grains daily while there is fever and for three days afterwards, and then 10 grains daily before breakfast for three months.

If the patient is vomiting and does not retain his medicine, 20 grains of quinine hydrochloride dissolved in a little water should be given in a starch enema. When there is a difficulty of this kind, or when symptoms are very urgent, a doctor would give quinine by an intramuscular injection or, in some cases, by an intravenous injection.

It is important that the bowels should act well, and it is desirable to give calomel, 1 to 3 grains, at the outset, and a saline each morning. A tabloid, popularly known as the Livingstone rouser, affords an excellent method of using calomel.

As regards dietetic and general treatment, it should be that laid down for the state of fever (*q.v.*). During the cold stage, hot-water bottles, hot drinks, and additional blankets will be required, and when the sweating stage has ceased the patient should be sponged with warm water, put on dry pyjamas and have fresh bedding. It will generally be desirable during convalescence to give a mixture or tablet containing iron and arsenic as a tonic.

See Anopheles; Blackwater Fever; Diaphoretic; Fever; Mosquito; Quinine; Tropical Hygiene; Warburg's Tincture.

MALE FERN. An oily extract of the root of male fern is given to destroy tapeworms.

See Worm.

MALIGNANT. As applied to a tumour, malignant means that it partakes of the nature of cancer; as applied to an infection, that its virulence is overwhelming; this may sometimes be due, however, to the poor quality of the resistance of the body. Malignant types of scarlet fever and other infections occur, and may kill the patient in a few hours. Malignant endocarditis is a variety of this disease which is progressive, and associated with septicaemia. Malignant pustule is a synonym for anthrax. Malignant tertian fever is a severe type of malaria.

See Benign.

MALINGERING. A deliberate attempt to simulate disease or disability is described as malingering. Its object is to escape some duty or obtain a pecuniary or other advantage, and when such motives can be easily suspected it is natural to imagine that ill-defined or unusual symptoms are nothing more than malingering. The possibility of hysteria or hypochondriasis or even of some obscure organic disease must be carefully excluded, however, before forming such an opinion. Also an element of malingering may have some actual disability associated with it.

MALLEIN. A substance prepared from the bacillus of glanders (*q.v.*), mallein is used in diagnostic tests for this disease.

MALNUTRITION. A person may be ill-nourished because the diet (*q.v.*) is insufficient or improper. If the diet is satisfactory the digestion may be defective. Otherwise malnutrition may be due to metabolic disturbances.

See Atrophy ; Emaciation.

MALT. Barley which has been allowed to germinate and sprout, and is then heated over a kiln, so stopping the germination, is known as malt, or byne. It contains a ferment, diastase, which converts starch into maltose, or malt-sugar, and malt itself has a sweet taste from the conversion of some of the starch in the grain. By adding yeast to malt alcohol is formed, and this is the main process in making beer. Ground malt is added to flour in making malt-bread, and to flour, other cereals or milk in making foods for children and invalids.

Extract of malt is produced by making an infusion of ground malt, filtering and evaporating down to a syrupy consistency. This also contains diastase, but the amount varies, so that it is necessary to procure a good brand. Apart from its diastatic power, however, malt extract has a considerable food value on account of its maltose. It is given, in doses of a teaspoonful to a tablespoonful, to those suffering from debilitating and wasting diseases, but to get the full effect on the starch in the food it should be taken before a meal. Malt extract is often mixed with cod-liver oil and sometimes hypophosphites also are added.

MALTA FEVER. Around the Mediterranean and in other warm countries occurs a febrile disease which is best known as Malta fever, but is also called Mediterranean fever, Italian fever, Neapolitan fever and, at Gibraltar, Rock fever. As the temperature chart commonly shows a succession of curves, the fever is sometimes called undulant fever, though such undulations may occur in other fevers, paratyphoid, for example.

The disease is caused by a germ known as the micrococcus melitensis, and it was established at Malta that this is introduced into the body in goat's milk. Boiling the milk destroys the infection. The presence of the disease can be demonstrated by an agglutination (*q.v.*) test with a sample of the patient's blood.

The incubation period is usually about a fortnight, and fever, when it begins, does not, as a rule, reach its maximum until about the seventh day, the temperature being a little higher each night until then. It often reaches to 104° F. and remains high, with remissions in the mornings, for a few days, when it begins to fall gradually, probably reaching the normal in a few days. During the fever headache is severe, and there may be neuralgic pains, especially sciatica. Constipation is the rule, though in severe cases there may be diarrhoea, with blood and mucus in the stools. Sickness may be troublesome. At night there is commonly copious sweating. Swelling of joints with great pain sometimes occurs and, occasionally, orchitis.

In mild cases the temperature may not go up again, but usually, after some days, there is a relapse, the characters of which resemble those of the first attack, though they are less severe. A succession of such attacks may occur and the patient may be ill for months. Death seldom occurs, but the patient may become much debilitated.

Treatment is that for fever (*q.v.*) generally, with measures to relieve troublesome symptoms. A vaccine may be serviceable. Hot fomentations will often give relief for painful conditions, but drugs may be needed for this purpose. A change to a cooler climate is useful during convalescence.

MANDIBLE. *See* Jaw.

MANGANESE. A metallic element with properties resembling those of iron, manganese, in the form of the prepared oxide of manganese, is used in the treatment of anaemia and amenorrhoea, the dose being 3 to 10 grains. The metal is used much more extensively, however, as a permanganate, especially that of potassium. This occurs as purple crystals, which dissolve readily in water, giving a pink to a dark purple solution, according to the amount used. The drug is a powerful oxidising agent, and so acts as a disinfectant, antiseptic and deodorant. As ordinarily used it is perfectly safe.

The dose of the crystals is 1 to 3 grains in a kaolin pill or a capsule, being given as an intestinal antiseptic in cholera, infective diarrhoea and dysentery. A solution of the same dose in water may also be used, especially when an action in the stomach is wanted, for example, in opium poisoning ; a doctor would probably wash out the stomach with a solution of the drug, and this procedure may also be beneficial in fermentative dyspepsia and in the summer diarrhoea of infants.

Solutions of permanganate of potassium are used for douching, especially when there is foetor, as in ozoena or septic sore throat, and as injections in gonorrhoea. Wounds may be washed with a solution, but this is not suitable for moistening dressings. Light hair when washed with a solution of potassium permanganate becomes a chestnut brown. Staining of skin or fabrics by permanganate of potassium can be removed by washing with sulphurous acid.

The official solution of potassium permanganate has a strength of 1 per cent., and dilutions for various purposes can be made by mixing with warm water ; thus, a tablespoonful of the solution in half a pint would give a strength of 1 in 2,000. For inward use the official solution is given in doses of 2 to 4 drachms in water. Other permanganates have similar properties, but that of zinc has an additional astringent effect. The permanganates of calcium and sodium are also used. Sodium manganate forms a green solution and is used as a disinfectant.

See Antiseptic ; Douche.

MANGE. Occasionally mange is contracted from one of the domestic animals. The treatment is that of scabies (*q.v.*).

MANIA. Insanity characterised by excitement is called mania.

See Mental Disease.

MARGARINE. Some brands of margarine, or butterine, as it is sometimes called, are prepared from vegetable oils, others from animal fats, chiefly beef and mutton, and still others contain fat from both sources. For adults who have a mixed diet, including meat, fish or eggs and green vegetables, margarine is an excellent substitute for butter, but this does not apply to children. These should receive butter, as margarine should not be depended on to supply the vitamin so necessary to their growth.

See Food ; Vitamin.

MARMITE. The proprietary preparation known as marmite, which is made chiefly from yeast, affords an excellent means of supplying what is called the anti-neuritic vitamin, when the diet is otherwise deficient in this way.

See Diet.

MARROW. Preparations of the red bone-marrow of oxen, calves and sheep are used in the treatment of pernicious anaemia and other blood diseases, of rickets and, especially in children, of wasting and general debility. Red marrow consists mainly of marrow cells, which are the precursors of blood corpuscles, with a few fat cells, while yellow marrow is mostly composed of fat cells.

MARTIN'S BANDAGE. *See* Elastic Bandage.

MASSAGE. Skilfully used, massage may be very beneficial in a large variety of disorders and injuries, the different manipulations being employed according to the purpose in view (*see* Plate XXIV, 1-6). Effleurage is stroking with the palmar surface of the hand, fingers and palm, in the direction of the venous blood flow ; if sufficiently firm, it aids the circulation of blood and lymph, improving the nutrition of the tissues. A similar movement in the opposite direction is referred to as stroking ; it should be very light, and is said to have a sedative effect, and to relieve insomnia, when done over the body and limbs.

Tapotement is a tapping movement with the pads of the inner three fingers in turn, each hand being used alternately, and striking with the inner edge of the hand is called hacking. These movements, the former of which are done from the wrist and the latter from the elbow, are stimulating to the tissues. Pétrissage is the name applied to rolling and kneading movements, which are done mainly on muscles and without an emollient unless the skin is very hairy. Pétrissage stimulates the nutrition of a muscle, and may prevent wasting or improve its development, having the same effects, in fact, as light exercise, for which it may be substituted when a patient is confined to bed.

Clapping means striking the surface of the body with the hands hollowed or cupped. It has a stimulating effect on the skin, reddening it and increasing the activity of its glands. Beating and pounding are strong movements designed to reach the deeper tissues. Vibration is performed by placing the hand flat on the surface of the body and inducing a trembling movement in the hand, which is communicated to the tissues beneath as a vibration. Mechanically and electrically worked machines, known as vibrators, are sometimes used for the purpose of tapotement ; the tapping may be rendered very rapid and more powerful than that done by the fingers.

To apply massage successfully a man or woman specially trained in massage is generally necessary, and often medical direction also. But for certain conditions massage by an untrained person may be serviceable, if a skilled person is not available. Effleurage might be used, for example, to improve the circulation of a limb affected with varicose veins, and to promote the absorption of swelling after a sprain. In fibrositis, pain may be relieved by effleurage, begun very gently, and then carried out more firmly, and finally combined with pétrissage.

In infantile paralysis a combination of these movements is also useful ; likewise in heart disease, when a patient can take no exercise. Convalescence from acute diseases can often be shortened if the limbs are massaged as soon as the patient is able to bear it. Massage should not last for longer than twenty minutes, as a rule, and its application once a day will probably be sufficient.

See Exercise.

MASTICATION. The act of chewing, or mastication, includes a biting movement and also a side-to-side movement, the effect of which is to grind food between the teeth. The masseter, the temporal and other muscles on each side of the face bring about these movements.

See Digestion ; Eating ; Jaw.

MASTITIS. Inflammation of the breast (*q.v.*) is called mastitis.

MASTOID. The blunt, bony projection behind and below the ear, known as the mastoid process, is part of the temporal bone (*q.v.*). It gives attachment to the upper end of the sterno-mastoid muscle and the occipital artery runs backward beneath it. It is undeveloped at birth.

Disease of the Mastoid. One of the risks of suppuration in the middle ear is the extension of infection to the cavities —the antrum and cells—that exist within the mastoid process of bone, setting up what is usually referred to as mastoid disease. An acute condition may be caused by the discharge from the ear becoming blocked, by an injury or by reason of some other cause.

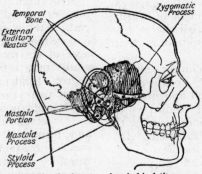

Mastoid : the bony region behind the ear

There is generally then severe pain at the back of the ear, shooting over the head and down the neck, and generally also a very profuse discharge from the ear. There may not be much swelling behind the ear, but should the matter make its way through the bone there is likely to be considerable swelling and redness in this situation, and the skin will be dropsical. The pus may burrow down the neck. The escape of matter through the bone causes inflammation of the periosteum covering the bone, but this mastoid periostitis can also, though rarely, occur apart from suppuration in the mastoid or the ear, when the cause is usually an injury.

The periostitis may disappear with rest and the application of heat, but often it becomes necessary to make an opening and give vent to pus. This will always be required where there is pus in the mastoid, and it will be necessary then to perforate the bone also and allow free drainage of the pus.

Disease in the mastoid may lead to necrosis of pieces of bone, or to the slower destruction of bone known as caries, and

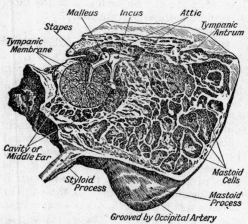

Mastoid. Section showing connexion with the middle ear, thus allowing extension of disease from the latter

there may also be destruction of the small bones in the middle ear and of portions of the bony capsule of the inner ear, with more or less impairment of hearing. In these circumstances a discharge from the ear will continue, in spite of all treatment.

In both acute and chronic mastoid disease there is also a danger of the disease extending within the skull and involving the large venous channel, known as the lateral sinus, the membranes covering the brain and even the brain substance. It is necessary, therefore, that the mastoid process should be opened up and all diseased bone taken away as far as possible. *See* Ear.

MASTURBATION. Though the practice of self-abuse, or masturbation, is generally suggested to younger by older children, it may begin in early childhood through irritation of the external genital organs. In boys the usual cause of such irritation is a tight foreskin, or phimosis (*q.v.*) ; in girls, the presence of threadworms or the decomposition of discharges owing to lack of cleanliness. These are things that should be attended to, apart from any question of self-abuse. Children should be warned against the practice as part of their instruction in sexual hygiene by parents or teachers. Vigorous open-air exercise and an ambition to excel in games should be encouraged.

The practice is generally discontinued as a person grows older, and, contrary to the pernicious teaching of quacks, no evil effects are to be apprehended. Some adults are addicted to it, however, and suffer from evidences of mental exhaustion in consequence, but where actual mental derangement occurs it is not from the practice itself, but rather from brooding on moral guilt and possible mental and physical penalties ; often it is the dread of impotence. Illicit connexion is no remedy for self-abuse, while it is accompanied by an imminent risk of contracting venereal disease. The advice of a doctor should be sought by anyone unable to extricate himself from the toils of the habit.

MATERIA MEDICA. The science dealing with the sources of drugs, the methods of obtaining them, and their physical and chemical properties, is known as Materia Medica.

MAXILLA. *See* Jaw.

MEASLES. A highly infectious fever, measles, morbilli or rubeola, is caused by a germ that has not yet been identified. The disease mostly affects children between the ages of six months and two years, but adults may suffer from it, and in severe degree. Epidemics appear to occur about every two years, and in England these reach a maximum in June and December.

The secretion of the eyes, nose, mouth and throat of a person suffering from measles contains the germs, which are therefore disseminated by breathing, and especially by coughing and sneezing, not to speak of more intimate contact. Should they reach the eyes, mouth or air-passages of a healthy person who is vulnerable to the disease, there is a period of incubation of from seven to fourteen days, usually about ten, and then symptoms resembling those of a common cold occur. The temperature may be 101° or 102° F. ; sometimes it is higher.

About two days later, small spots, with a white centre and a pink margin, and known as Koplik's spots, may be seen on the inside of the lips and cheeks, and reddish patches on the palate. On the second day also it is common for the temperature to drop. From three to four days after the onset the rash appears. This consists of tiny flat, dusky red or perhaps pink papules, which are grouped together to form patches, often of a crescentic shape (Plate XXXI, 2). These appear first on the face and then on the neck and trunk, and may be very itchy. With their appearance the temperature again rises.

Meanwhile, the running of the eyes and nose and the cough have been going on unabated. Sometimes there is diarrhoea. The rash usually begins to disappear in two days, and there may be a fine scaling, or desquamation. The temperature now falls rapidly. Often enough, however, some complication occurs. Severe bronchitis is a common one, and it may go on to the lung disorder called bronchopneumonia ; or the patient may suffer from the other type of pneumonia, lobar pneumonia, or from pleurisy, and perhaps empyema. Increased rapidity in breathing, duskiness of the face, and a sharp pain in the side are some of the symptoms suggestive of chest complications.

The cough may become croupy and the breathing stridulous, showing that there is laryngitis. It must be borne in mind when such symptoms occur that they may be actually due to diphtheria, as this disease sometimes exists along with measles. Earache may indicate an extension of catarrh to the middle ear, and not infrequently this is followed by suppuration and a discharge of the ear. Occasionally there is extension of infection within the skull, amd meningitis.

Complications from Intercurrent Disease

The catarrh of the eyes may be severe, with a copious discharge containing matter. In severe cases of measles there may be bleeding into the skin, the spots not disappearing when they are pressed by the finger, as they ordinarily do. Another disease which may coexist with measles is scarlet fever, and it is not uncommon for whooping-cough to follow an attack of measles, and conversely.

As regards the outlook in measles, it may be said that the younger the patient the greater the risk. Also, when measles has invaded a community which has previously been free from it, the mortality has been high.

A person suffering from measles should be isolated at once. The steps to be taken in this connexion, and as regards disinfection during the course of the disease and after recovery, are described under the heading Infectious Disease. The treatment is that of fever (*q.v.*) generally, while complications should be dealt with according to the instructions given under appropriate headings. It may be said, however, that the room should be kept at a temperature of about 65° F. and the air should be kept moist by means of a bronchitis kettle. At the same time a plentiful supply of fresh air by the window is also necessary.

Treatment of Eyes and Mouth

A screen should be placed so as to prevent light falling directly on the eyes, as the patient often displays marked intolerance to light, a condition described as photophobia. If there is much discharge from the eyes, they should be bathed frequently with warm boracic acid solution.

It is very important that the mouth should be kept clean, and to ensure this it should be washed out several times daily with water containing a little glycerin of borax.

A patient should not be allowed out of bed until the temperature has been normal for a week, and the greatest pains must be taken to ensure a good convalescence by means of fresh air, good food and, when required, tonics. It is necessary to protect against sudden changes of temperature. There is always a risk that tuberculosis of the lungs may be a legacy from an attack of measles. The patient should not be allowed to mix with others until at least two weeks after the disappearance of the rash, and only then if quite better.

Children who have been in contact with a person who has developed the symptoms of measles should not be allowed to return to school for sixteen days after the last exposure to infection.

Meanwhile a close watch should be kept on them. Even before the catarrhal symptoms of measles actually appear, it may be found that a child taking measles displays a reddening of the lining of the eyelids, and has a slight rise of temperature at night. Should such evidences be found the child should be isolated at once.

Blood serum from a person convalescing from measles, if injected into another person, will generally prevent the occurrence of the disease, and this procedure is sometimes practised on young children for whom, as has been said above, the disease carries special risks. One attack of measles generally confers immunity for life, but second, third or more attacks do occur. These are, however, milder, as a rule, than the first attack.

See Cancrum Oris ; German Measles ; Infectious Disease ; Rash.

MEASLY MEAT. Meat containing immature parasitic worms in the form of cysts is said to be measly. Such meat has a mottled appearance. If eaten without being sufficiently cooked the parasites develop in the body into their mature form. Chilling the meat, or soaking in brine for a sufficient time, say, three weeks, will probably kill the parasites.

See Food ; Worm.

MEAT. The qualities of the various kinds of meat are discussed under the heading Food.

MEATUS. Derived from a Latin word meaning to flow, the term meatus is used for various openings and passages in the body.

MECKEL'S DIVERTICULUM. In some people there is a blind tube opening off the small intestine about two or three feet above the junction of the latter with the large intestine. This is called Meckel's diverticulum. Usually it is a few inches long, and the end is free, but it may be attached to the umbilicus by a fibrous cord, and in a few instances the diverticulum has formed a tube opening at the umbilicus and causing a faecal fistula.

It represents, in fact, a tube which, in the embryo, connects the intestine with

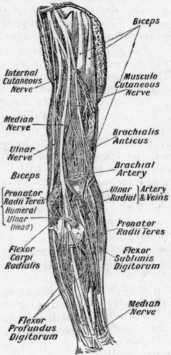

Median Nerve. Its course from the brachial plexus to the hand

the yolk-sac which lies outside the embryonic body, but this tube entirely disappears in most people. The importance of Meckel's diverticulum is that it may cause obstruction of the bowel in various ways, or may become inflamed, when the condition resembles appendicitis.

MECONIUM. The earliest stools of a new-born child consist of a dark-green, sticky substance, which is known as meconium.

MEDIAN NERVE. A branch of the brachial plexus, which is a network formed by certain spinal nerves in the neck, the median nerve runs down the arm on the inner side of the biceps muscle in company with the brachial artery, but it gives no branches to the arm. From the elbow it runs down the middle of the front of the forearm, supplying branches to most of the muscles that flex the wrist and fingers. It breaks up into branches in the hand, some of these supplying muscles in the hand, and others sensation.

Most of the small thumb muscles are supplied by the median, but one or two by the ulnar nerve. Thus, if the median nerve be paralysed, it is impossible to oppose the thumb to the fingers, but the thumb can be drawn along the palm of the hand, as this movement is promoted by the ulnar nerve. Sensation is given by the median to the outer part of the palm, to the palmar surface of the thumb, the index, the middle, and half of the ring finger, also to part of the dorsal surface of these fingers towards the ends. The median nerve is near the surface at the wrist, and can easily be injured by a cut on the front of the wrist.

A vein passing up the front of the forearm (*q.v.*) is called the median vein.

See Musculo-spiral Nerve ; Ulnar Nerve.

MEDIASTINUM. The region of the chest between the breast-bone and the backbone is called the mediastinum. It is bounded at the sides by the pleural sacs containing the lungs, and contains the heart and great blood vessels, the large air-tubes, the gullet, and other important structures, including groups of lymphatic glands, which are referred to as the mediastinal glands.

These are frequently the site of tuberculosis, and a chronic abscess may arise in this way, though it might also be due to tuberculous disease of the spine. Such an abscess might pass through the diaphragm and form a psoas abscess (*q.v.*), or it might burrow on to the front wall of the chest or in other directions. An acute abscess might occur from septic infection from a cancer of the gullet or in other ways.

Inflammation of the structures in this region is called mediastinitis, and a growth a mediastinal tumour. The latter gives rise to pressure symptoms, such as cough, dyspnoea, loss of voice, difficulty in swallowing and so on, but pressure in this region and similar symptoms may also be due to an aneurysm of the aorta or of one of the large vessels springing from it.

MEDICATED WINES. In the British Pharmacopoeia are included preparations called wines, or vina (singular, vinum). Some of these, like ipecacuanha wine, contain considerable quantities of powerful drugs, and resemble tinctures rather than wines in the ordinary sense ; the alcohol in the ordinary doses is relatively small, and large doses could not be taken without causing disagreeable or even dangerous symptoms.

Other wines mentioned in the pharmacopoeia, such as those of iron and of quinine, are taken in larger doses, and the dose of alcohol becomes material. The same applies to proprietary medicated wines. There is a definite risk in the use of medicated wines, as they may develop or foster an alcoholic habit.

Drugs should be given in a safer way, and this need not be unpleasant, and if it is desirable and expedient that a patient should have wine also, then let this be given undisguised. This course affords a better guarantee of the quality of the wine and will be more economical.

See Alcohol.

MEDICINES. The household stock of drugs and dressings should be kept clean and dry in a cupboard, drawer or box placed at some distance from a fireplace or other heating apparatus.

Liquid poisons and liquids intended for external use should be in bottles readily distinguishable by shape and preferably coloured.

All poisons should be kept locked up, but other drugs, and dressings, should be easily got at when required in an emergency.

The medicine being given to a sick person should be kept where it cannot be tampered with and should be out of the patient's reach. Before pouring out a dose of medicine the label on the bottle should be scrutinised. This ensures that the right bottle is being used and that the correct dose is borne in mind.

The dose should be measured with a proper graduated measuring glass, and not by means of a spoon, as spoons of the same category vary in capacity.

The bottle should be thoroughly shaken before pouring out the dose. The cork of the bottle is removed by grasping it between the little finger and the palm of the left hand, the measuring glass being held by the thumb and the other three fingers. When pouring out the medicine the bottle should be held so that the label is uppermost, otherwise some of the medicine might run down on to the label and not only soil it but possibly obscure the instructions. The bottle is corked as soon as the medicine is poured out.

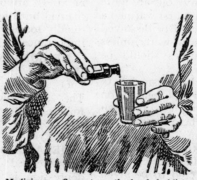

Medicines. Correct method of holding bottle and cork when measuring a dose

Usually it is stated on the label that the medicine is to be taken in a little water, but, if not, water should be added nevertheless, and definite instructions obtained from the doctor at the earliest opportunity. If medicine is given in a feeding-cup, it should, if possible, be in one kept for the purpose, as the use of the cup employed for feeding the patient might create a distaste for his food. When the dose has been given the measure and the cup or glass used in the administration should be washed out at once.

Some powders can be administered by placing them on the tongue and washing over with a draught of water, but others, such as light magnesia or Gregory's mixture, have to be thoroughly mixed in water before giving them. Light powders tend to fly back into the throat when the patient inhales, and this is very unpleasant. Nauseous powders should not be mixed with milk when a patient is on milk diet. There is no objection to milk being used at other times. Powders may be given to children mixed well in jam or marmalade, unless for any reason these substances are objectionable. Powders may also be given between thin pieces of bread and butter, or in rice papers or wafers.

How to Administer Pills

A pill, capsule or tablet is more easily swallowed if placed well at the back of the tongue. If there is still difficulty it may be given in jam or butter, and, if necessary, cut or broken up, bearing in mind, however, that some pills and capsules must be taken whole, as they are intended to pass through the stomach and dissolve only in the bowel.

Castor oil and other heavy oils are more easily poured out if they are first warmed a little. Purgative salts should be dissolved in about a third of a glass of water unless otherwise directed. Gargles should be diluted with a little water.

When a child cannot be persuaded to take its medicine it may be placed on someone's lap, its legs being fixed between the knees and the arms held fixed by an arm thrown round them. The child's nose is held till the mouth is opened and the draught has been swallowed.

When medicine is directed to be given three times a day it should be given after the three principal meals; when four times, it will be convenient to give it at 8 a.m., noon, 4 p.m. and 8 p.m. The times of giving drugs to a patient requiring systematic nursing should be noted down. If the nurse should forget to give a dose at the proper time on no account should she increase the next dose when it falls due.

See Apothecaries' Weights and Measures; Domestic Measures; Dose; Drug; Enema; Inhalation; Injection; Suppository.

MEDULLA. A Latin word meaning marrow, the term medulla is used for bone-marrow. It is also used for the internal portion of some glands, the kidneys, for example, the outer part of such glands being described as the cortex. The spinal cord is sometimes referred to as the medulla spinalis, or spinal marrow, and the part of the brain which is continuous with the cord is called the medulla oblongata or bulb. In fact, when the term medulla is used without qualification it is usually this part of the brain that is meant.

In shape the medulla oblongata resembles an inverted and truncated cone, its exterior presenting, however, certain groovings and bosses. The posterior surface is excavated to some extent by the lower half of the space known as the fourth ventricle of the brain. From the surface of the medulla emerge the 9th to the 12th cranial nerves, and from the groove between this and the next part of the brain, the pons, appear the 6th, 7th and 8th nerves. Within the medulla are centres for breathing, swallowing, heart-control and other functions.

See Brain; Nervous System.

MEGALOMANIA. Insane delusions of greatness are often referred to as megalomania, but the term is also used colloquially for any unwarranted ideas of self-importance.

MEIBOMIAN GLAND. In each eyelid there are tiny, elongated glands with ducts opening along the edge of the lid. They are known as Meibomian glands or follicles. A cyst formed by distension of one of these glands is called a chalazion.

See Eye.

MELANCHOLIA. Insanity which is characterised by persistent mental depression is described as melancholia.

See Mental Disease.

MEMORY. The faculty by which past experiences, what we have seen, heard, thought and so on, are reproduced in the mind is called memory. Any experience is linked up more or less with others, and recollection of one idea is likely to recall other ideas that are linked or associated with it. When the mind is allowed to wander, the idea with which one begins is often, usually, in fact, far separated from that in the mind when one again becomes attentive to what one is thinking, but it is possible to trace back along the line of thought and discover the links.

These links, or associations, are of various kinds. It may be that the two ideas have been considered closely together, or perhaps relate to things closely connected in time or space, or they may even be cause and effect ; or they may exhibit a striking similarity or contrast. In systems of memory-training much emphasis is laid on the recognition of such links, and, when no obvious link exists, on their artificial creation.

The effort to remember, then, means to rummage in a deliberate way along lines of association, although the process is often accomplished unconsciously and with incredible swiftness. An experience is more easily remembered if it has made a deep impression in the first instance, or has been often repeated. Accurate observation is therefore a powerful aid to memory, and in saying this one is reminded that memory or any other so-called faculty of the mind cannot be clearly separated from other faculties ; the mind works as a whole.

Experiences strongly coloured with emotion are easily remembered, but, if the emotional crisis appears to demand it, all memory of the experience may be entirely repressed This happened frequently enough to soldiers in the Great War and happens to other people. It has to be recognized that barriers to remembrance come to exist in the mind, and though experiences may appear to be forgotten they may often be brought to light by hypnotism.

Another evidence of the existence of active barriers to remembrance is furnished by the phenomena of double consciousness, in which the experiences in one phase are not remembered in another, and vice versa, although it is, of course, the one brain that does the thinking for both.

As regards remembrance generally, the usual state of affairs is that a person is able to recall recent events, while others become more elusive the more distant they are in point of time ; but in old people the memory for recent events may be very poor, while the experiences of early life remain quite vivid.

The loss of memory is called amnesia. *See* Double Consciousness ; Mind.

MÉNIÈRE'S SYNDROME. A group of symptoms which are habitually associated is called a syndrome or complex. In Ménière's syndrome the symptoms are giddiness, deafness and noises in one or both ears, and sickness and vomiting. Such symptoms come on suddenly and with great severity when bleeding occurs into the internal ear, or labyrinth, in which case the condition is described as Ménière's disease. This is not at all common, but the occurrence of similar symptoms, though probably not so sudden in their onset, from causes other than bleeding into the labyrinth, is fairly frequent. Between the attacks the patient may be free from giddiness, but sometimes more or less unsteadiness persists.

The treatment during an attack is to keep the patient at rest in a darkened and quiet room and restrict him to a light diet. People who are liable to such symptoms should avoid alcohol, tea, coffee and tobacco.

See Dizziness ; Ear.

MENINGES. The coverings of the brain and spinal cord, known as the meninges, are three in number. In order from without inwards, there is the dura mater, the arachnoid and the pia mater, the meninges of the brain being continuous with those of the cord through the foramen magnum of the skull. The dura mater, which is a thick, strong membrane, lines the skull and the spinal canal, but in the former consists of two layers which are separated in various directions to form the large venous sinuses, conduits taking the blood away from the brain.

The arachnoid and the pia mater are more delicate membranes, the latter being

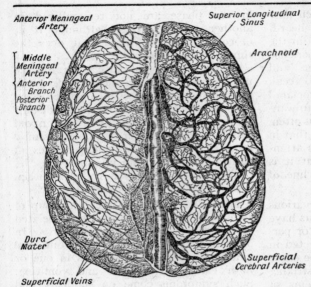

Anterior Meningeal Artery

Superior Longitudinal Sinus

Middle Meningeal Artery
Anterior Branch
Posterior Branch

Arachnoid

Dura Mater

Superficial Cerebral Arteries

Superficial Veins

Meninges. Here the left side of the brain is covered with the dura mater, but this has been cut away on the right side, revealing the arachnoid membrane, beneath which lies the pia mater

closely applied to the surface of the brain and cord and dipping into the fissures and sulci. Between these two meninges is the sub-arachnoid space, filled with cerebro-spinal fluid which can circulate freely in this space, while through an opening in the membranes, known as the foramen of Magendie, and situated at the back of the bulb, the fluid in this space communicates with that in the cavities within the brain and cord.

See Brain ; Skull.

MENINGITIS. Inflammation of the coverings of the brain is known as meningitis, but, for practical purposes, when one speaks of meningitis it is inflammation of the innermost membrane, the pia mater, that is meant. Meningitis may be caused by extension of sepsis from a diseased middle ear, from the orbit, the nose or the face or scalp ; or the infection may be brought by the blood, in pyaemia. This is called the suppurative type. Resembling it is the meningitis occurring in pneumonia, typhoid fever, influenza, measles and other infectious fevers. The meningococcus is the cause of epidemic cerebro-spinal meningitis, and of posterior basal meningitis, which occurs, almost exclusively, in young infants. Tuberculosis is another cause, and chronic

meningitis may occur from alcoholism and from syphilis.

Suppurative meningitis is often fatal in two or three days, and lasts at most one or two weeks. Tuberculous meningitis, which occurs usually in children under ten, though it may occur in adults, rarely lasts beyond two or three weeks. Posterior basal meningitis may run on for two or three months, and the patient may recover. Recovery is rare in the suppurative and tuberculous forms.

In the suppurative type of meningitis there is headache, giddiness, fever, which is often high, intolerance of light, sound and touch, delirium and vomiting. There may be twitching and spasm of muscles, and convulsions, especially in children. The head is usually drawn back and Kernig's sign (*q.v.*) is generally present. There may be squinting of the eyes, drooping of the upper eyelid, inequality of the pupils, and possibly facial paralysis. Sometimes there is paralysis of a limb or of one side of the body. Unconsciousness deepens into coma, and the pulse, which has been slow in comparison with what might have been expected from the amount of fever, becomes very rapid towards the end.

Tuberculous meningitis forms part of a general infection with the tubercle bacillus, and the mischief is mainly situated

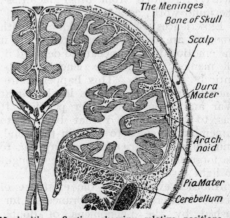

The Meninges
Bone of Skull
Scalp
Dura Mater
Arachnoid
Pia Mater
Cerebellum

Meningitis. Section showing relative positions of brain membranes in which inflammation may arise towards the base of the brain, thus involving the cranial nerves. For a short time before the onset of symptoms definitely pointing to meningitis a child shows signs of ailing, goes off its food, loses flesh and is peevish. Symptoms resembling those above described then supervene. Often the child utters a wailing cry, commonly referred to as the hydro-cephalic cry. The temperature as a rule is not very high. There is flattening or even hollowing of the belly. After some days the child sinks into profound un-consciousness.

Epidemic cerebro-spinal meningitis is discussed under the heading cerebro-spinal fever. Posterior basal meningitis resembles the epidemic form. Opisthotonus, or curving of the back, may be extreme, the heels approaching the back of the head.

What is called serous meningitis is rather inflammation of the lining of the ventricles of the brain, an ependymitis. It mainly affects adults, the symptoms of the acute form resembling those of the suppurative type of meningitis and those of the chronic type a brain tumour.

Recognition of the existence and nature of meningitis is greatly assisted by a chemical and bacteriological examination of the cerebro-spinal fluid.

The treatment of meningitis consists in keeping the patient quiet in a darkened room and keeping the head cool. The head is shaved, and cooling lotions applied or an ice-bag or Leiter's tube (*q.v.*). By lumbar puncture cerebro-spinal fluid is allowed to drain away sufficiently to relieve tension, and in the meningococcal types serum may be injected. In posterior basal meningitis this is not useful, however, except during the first week. Feeding may have to be done through a nasal tube. If the temperature is high it must be lowered by sponging. Drugs may be required for symptoms, and sometimes hexamine is given in the hope that it may exert an antiseptic effect in the cerebro-spinal fluid, as it is one of the few drugs that finds its way into this fluid.

See Brain ; Cerebro-spinal Fever ; Meninges.

MENINGOCELE. A swelling in a new-born child consisting of a protrusion of the dura mater containing cerebro-spinal fluid is called a meningocele. It may affect the skull or the spine, but is uncommon. In the head the swelling usually appears at the root of the nose or in the occipital region. It becomes larger when the child coughs or cries. A similar swelling occurs from protrusion of brain substance. It is called an encephalocele and pulsates synchronously with the heart. A swelling containing both brain substance and fluid is called a hydrencephalocele. These occurrences are of serious significance. Often the child is still-born or dies shortly after birth. If it lives it is mentally deficient. The swelling may increase in size and burst, or it may remain stationary. Operation may be useful in favourable circumstances.

MENOPAUSE. *See* Change of Life.

MENORRHAGIA. An excessive loss during menstruation (*q.v.*) is described as menorrhagia.

MENSTRUATION. The periodical discharges in women referred to as " the monthlies," the menstrua, the menses, the periods, and by other names, are associated with the function of child-bearing. The lining of the womb undergoes changes to fit it for the reception of a fertilised ovum, but when pregnancy does not occur part of the lining is shed and this occasions more or less bleeding. As contrasted with an ordinary bleeding, however, the blood shed at this time usually shows no tendency to clot.

Menstruation goes on from puberty to the change of life, lasting probably about thirty years. In temperate climates it begins about the age of fourteen as a rule, but may be earlier or later in some girls ; in hot countries it usually begins at an earlier age. Generally the time elapsing between the beginning of one period and that of the next is twenty-eight days, but some women normally menstruate every three weeks, and others at intervals just short of five weeks. If, however, the intervals are longer or shorter than these limits there is something wrong.

The ordinary duration of a period is four or five days, and the amount of discharge usually lost may vary from two to eight ounces. Sometimes it is more, but if very profuse or if it causes exhaustion the possibility of some abnormality must be considered. A period may be preceded and accompanied by a feeling of fulness in the lower part of the abdomen and by a feeling of lassitude. Sometimes there is definite pain, or dysmenorrhoea.

Although a woman who is menstruating commonly refers to herself as " unwell," this is not to be taken literally, as formerly it very often was. Menstruation is a physiological process and calls for no great change in the ordinary habits. A moderate amount of open-air exercise is more beneficial than otherwise, but chilling of the feet and legs should be avoided as far as possible. Baths, provided they are not cold, may be taken throughout the period.

Vicarious menstruation is the name applied to a discharge of blood from the nose, the stomach or elsewhere which sometimes replaces a discharge from the womb when there is some gross maldevelopment of the genital organs.

Cessation of menstruation, or amenorrhoea, is a normal incident in pregnancy and lactation. Otherwise it may be due to a local or a general disorder.

See Amenorrhoea ; Change of Life ; Dysmenorrhoea ; Flooding ; Pregnancy ; Womb.

MENTAL DEFICIENCY. The various degrees of mental deficiency are discussed under the headings Feeble-minded and Idiocy.

MENTAL DISEASE. The majority of people can be described as sane, but that is not to say that they enjoy perfect mental health. Probably this could only be said of a few, the rest presenting some degree of depreciation, slight in most cases, but in others quite considerable. Insanity thus forms but a portion, and a relatively small one, of the province of mental disease.

In the study of mental diseases it is necessary to bear in mind that there is an organic continuity between body and mind, and this connexion means more than merely the part taken by the brain, as mental processes are largely influenced by the general activities and states of the body, and notably by the action of the internal secretions or endocrines (*q.v.*). Mental disorder may be merely symptomatic of some bodily disorder, of inflammation, tumour, or other disease of the brain, for example, of the action of poisons, such as alcohol or Indian hemp, on the brain, or of general diseases, as in the delirium of fevers. Consumption, hear disease and other disorders may also b attended by mental disturbance of on kind or another.

There is, however, a large amount o mental disease which cannot be connecte with any gross or even minute changes i the organs of the body, nor with any kin of poisoning. Another fact to be born in mind in the study of mental diseases i that the mental life of an individual is con tinuous ; for example, much help in inter preting the delusions of an insane perso might be at hand did one know what ha been the current of his normal thought.

Causative Rôle of Heredity

Heredity plays an important part in th causation of mental disease, and especiall in the first half of life ; in the second hal its importance rapidly declines before tha of other causes. As regards mental diseas which can be classed as insanity, importan factors besides heredity are the in fection of syphilis, which causes genera paralysis of the insane and other menta disorders, and alcohol, which leads to variety of disorders.

The state of the bodily health and eas or otherwise in obtaining a living are als significant, and especially in the latte half of life ; there is evidence that th incidence of mental disease at this perio in a community is relative to the incidenc of other diseases, or, in other words, tha circumstances such as poverty and ba sanitary conditions, which increase th latter, increase the former also.

Sex is another important factor. T mate with a member of the opposite se is the natural destiny of a sexuall mature individual, and the frustration o this design may occasion mental disorder The incidence of insanity, it has bee pointed out, is considerably greate amongst the unmarried than it is amongs the married. In some of these cases menta unfitness will have prevented marriage but this is only a partial explanation of th difference. Insanity is also more commo amongst those who have been widowe so that, besides satisfying the biologica claims of sex, the married state ma conduce to sanity by helping towards better general adjustment of the persor ality to the difficulties of existence.

Insanity is more apt to occur at the great epochs of life, namely, puberty, the menopause or change of life, and the onset of old age. At puberty the body comes under the strong influence of the secretions of the sex glands, while at the menopause this influence is diminished and withdrawn; in either instance there may be some interference with the balance normally maintained between the actions of other internal secretions. The danger at the onset of old age may possibly be due to similar chemical changes, but arterial degeneration, by impairing the nutrition of the brain, is of greater importance.

The main point noted in the classification of mental diseases is a particular causation, special prominence of a certain state of feeling, or of some other symptom, or a usual assemblage of symptoms. Broadly speaking, there are three classes, namely, neuroses, psychoneuroses and psychoses. In the first are comprised neurasthenia, the chief characteristic of which is that mind and body are easily fatigued; anxiety neurosis, which is a constant state of nervous apprehension; and hypochondriasis. In a mild degree neuroses do not differ much from occasional experiences of a normal individual, and the bodily state has much to do with their causation.

Forms of Psycho-neurosis

The psycho-neuroses include hysteria, which may either take the form of conversion hysteria or of anxiety hysteria, and the obsessional or compulsion neurosis. In these disorders the state of the body is of little account as regards causation. The diseases included in these two classes are described under their own headings.

The third class, the psychoses, which are usually described as the mental diseases proper, are those which may lead to such conduct as will label the sufferer with insanity (*q.v.*). Here are included the following types:

(1) ORGANIC CHANGES IN THE BRAIN. Mental diseases resulting from general paralysis of the insane (*q.v.*) and other disorders dependent on syphilis or on arterial disease, tumours or encephalitis, or which follow an apoplectic seizure or an injury to the brain. Such are mainly of the nature of dementia.

(2) IDIOCY (*q.v.*) and FEEBLE-MINDEDNESS (*q.v.*).

(3) TOXIC PSYCHOSES, that is, disorders due to poisoning, usually chronic poisoning, and especially with alcohol, lead, morphine or cocaine; occasionally insanity is due to mercury poisoning. Ordinary alcoholic drunkenness may present definite signs of mental disorder, but in some persons, especially those with a neuropathic inheritance, even small quantities of alcohol may produce a state of wild excitement with delusions and hallucinations, perhaps a suicidal or homicidal tendency, and sometimes gross moral perversion. This state is described as mania à potu, and is usually recovered from in a few days; sometimes, however, it proves fatal.

Some Results of Chronic Alcoholism

Various kinds of mental disorder may arise from chronic alcoholism, the best known being delirium tremens (*q.v.*). In another form hallucinations, commonly of touch and hearing, are the prominent features, and may give rise to delusions. A third form, known as Korsakow's psychosis or syndrome, is characterised by weak-mindedness, irritability, mental confusion, forgetfulness, especially as regards times and places, along with inflammation of various nerves, causing muscular weakness and wasting, loss of sensation and so on. In still another form there is mental dullness and general inefficiency, then delusions and hallucinations, the patient finally passing into dementia.

(4) EPILEPSY. Insanity may be associated with epilepsy (*q.v.*).

(5) DEMENTIA PRAECOX. This form of insanity may be manifested from the age of fifteen onwards, but the tendency is much lessened after the age of forty. This and manic-depressive insanity are the forms of mental disease in which inheritance is paramount in causation. The patient begins to show a lack of interest in his surroundings, and becomes more and more apathetic. The habits are dirty. Memory deteriorates, and there are hallucinations and delusions. In some cases there is great depression, and a strong suicidal tendency, in others well-marked delusions, while in a third type there is a curious muscular rigidity. The

patient may stand for hours at a time in a fixed position, and if someone places the head or limbs in a particular position, this position will be maintained. Only about 15 per cent. of cases recover.

(6) MANIC - DEPRESSIVE INSANITY. When insanity is marked by violent excitement it is described as mania ; marked by painful mental depression it is melancholia. A patient may suffer from one or other of these or from each alternately. Mania may be acute and may come on without warning, or there may be premonitory symptoms, such as sleeplessness, depression and so on. There is intense restlessness of body and mind, hallucinations, delusions, incoherency of speech and sleeplessness. In chronic mania there is restlessness, but also weak-mindedness ; there may be outbursts of violence or, on the other hand, fits of melancholia.

In melancholia the patient generally sits in a huddled-up position, showing little tendency to move. There is great depression, which differs from ordinary depression in the intensity of the mental suffering, anxiety or fear, which accompanies it. There are delusions, and these generally refer to faults of which the patient deems himself to have been guilty ; sometimes, however, the patient imagines that he is suffering from some severe bodily affection. Food may be refused. In some instances the patient is stuporose, or only partially conscious, but, on the other hand, there may be restlessness and agitation. There is a special tendency to suicide in melancholia.

There is a greater prospect of recovery from manic-depressive than from most other forms of insanity, but there is also a considerable risk of relapse.

(7) PARANOIA. In this type the chief characteristic is a delusion of persecution, though it may be of grandeur. Delusions occur in other forms of mental disorder, of course, but they are fleeting and change in character. In paranoia the patient clings to his delusion, whatever it may be ; he finds reasons for it and regulates his conduct by it. Such a delusion is said to be systematised. To escape or remove the persecution an attempt at suicide or homicide may be made. Before his condition is recognized, a paranoiac may do much harm by false accusations, or even engaging in litigation.

(8) CONFUSIONAL INSANITY. After influenza or some other debilitating disease, childbirth, or a surgical operation, or excessive fatigue, a person may suffer from great confusion of thought, especially as regards dates and persons, waking up from sleep in a dazed state. In conversation there is a failure to complete sentences. There may be delusions, but generally there is neither excitement nor depression. There is no fever. Proper and liberal feeding is of great importance in treatment, and rest in bed if the case is severe ; mild cases, on the other hand, may benefit from going out. Recovery within a year is the rule.

(9) ACUTE DELIRIOUS MANIA, OR BELL'S DISEASE. In some circumstances, such as those mentioned above as causing confusional insanity, or from auto-intoxication (*q.v.*), a person may suddenly become intensely restless and excited, with hallucinations which are of a terrifying character. There is usually fever, commonly up to 103° F., but sometimes as high as 106°. Control of the bladder and bowels is lost. There is confusion of thought as to surroundings, and delusions which change in character quickly. The patient is sleepless. Again feeding is of first importance, and sleep must be secured. The bowels should be freely opened. Early treatment may save life, but the complaint is very dangerous.

(10) DEMENTIA. A damping-down or loss of all the mental faculties, or dementia, is the outcome of many of the disorders described above, but it may occur as a primary condition, as in senile dementia, though in the earlier stages of this there may be confusion of ideas and delusions. In the latter stages, the patient leads a vegetable existence ; there is no volition, and no control of the bladder or bowels.

A large amount of mental disease is preventable. That due to heredity, however, could only be prevented by suitable marriage. The marriage of a person from a tainted stock with one belonging to a sound stock is said to be one of the ways in which a taint is destroyed for subsequent generations, but, whatever are the chances of this happening in a marriage of this kind, it is thoroughly established that if both parties come of neuropathic stock the outlook is very bad for their progeny.

Persons who suffer from alcoholic insanity have also an inherited tendency to mental disease, so that, without discussing the public benefits which might be derived from a general prohibition of the use of alcohol, it can safely be said that any person with a neuropathic inheritance should be a total abstainer.

The modern treatment of syphilis, if effectively carried out, will diminish enormously the incidence of general paralysis of the insane, and of the other mental disorders due to the infection.

Public health measures, by diminishing disease generally, and educational and economic measures which raise the standard of comfort of the poorer classes and lessen the stress of their struggle for existence, will also be beneficial. The stress of living for many persons, whatever their social position, would often be lessened by a more judicious choice of vocation; this applies with special force to those in whom the mental staying power and elasticity have been weakened by inheritance. Young people often need help in establishing easy social relations with their neighbours and in regulating the conditions of the sexual life.

Advantages of Institutional Treatment

Some insane persons can safely be kept at home, but when restraint and skilled nursing are needed the expense and worry involved usually makes institutional treatment necessary. This has the further advantage, however, that the routine of an institution generally has a tranquillising effect on a disordered mind. There has been widespread concern regarding the way in which inmates of such institutions are treated, but this should be removed by the report of a Royal Commission in 1926 that patients, on the whole, are well treated, and that deliberate or systematic ill-usage could only happen in isolated instances. Doubtless increased vigilance will reduce such abuses to a minimum.

In some forms of insanity, dementia praecox for example, psycho-therapy may prove useful.

See Delusions; Dementia; Depression; Feeble-minded; Hysteria; Idiocy; Insanity; Neurasthenia; Neurosis; Psycho-therapy.

MENTAL HYGIENE. It is generally recognized that a proper development of the body and sound bodily health depend upon the maintenance of good hygienic conditions, but the fact that there is a need for a careful mental hygiene is not so well appreciated. The influence of bodily on mental health is recognized, of course, and, so far as a healthy mind can be secured by making and keeping the body healthy, much public and personal effort is being directed towards mental hygiene.

It is clearly established, however, that much mental disease is purely, or mainly, psychical in origin, that is to say, it comes from wrong thinking and is more or less uninfluenced by the state of the bodily health, though, on the other hand, it may cause derangement of the functions of the body. It may be said that secular and religious education are directed towards building up a healthy mind, and certainly when the methods and aims of such instruction are properly directed good hygienic habits are inculcated.

This result is attained more or less when the main object in view is not so much what a child will know as what it will become. The lamentable failure that too often attends years of effort in education does not so much consist in the fact that most of what has been taught is speedily forgotten as that the young person emerges on life without mental or moral interests and with a very inadequate capacity of taking his, or her, place as a social unit. It has been said of some great public schools that, while their products might be ignorant of a good many things when they left school, they were, however, men of the world. Using this phrase according to its best significance, one finds in this statement a correct appreciation of what the mental hygienist looks for from education.

It is in the nature of things that an individual should be profoundly interested in his own personality, but a good education and training will keep him from being wrapped up in himself. Also it is in the nature of things that an adolescent will be subjected to a strong sexual urge, but a sound training will help to control his importunate impulses and turn them into channels that are expedient.

Mental energy is not inexhaustible, and much harm is due to forgetting this. Overwork may leave wounds in the mental constitution that are not easily healed. Also many people are born with less than the average reserve of mental energy, and it is necessary that this point be kept in view when they choose a vocation. This should not be one that will call for a very large expenditure of mental energy nor one to which much worry is incidental.

See Brain Fag ; Mind.

MENTHOL. A colourless, crystalline substance with a pungent taste and smell, menthol is obtained by cooling the oil distilled from several varieties of mint herb, including peppermint. It is sometimes called peppermint camphor. Menthol is a powerful antiseptic, though not much used for this purpose. It is also an anaesthetic, and may remove neuralgia or itching. For these purposes it may be rubbed on the skin in a solid form, applied in an alcoholic solution, or used in the B.P. menthol plaster. A menthol cone forms a convenient means of rubbing the drug on the skin. The application of menthol in any form causes a sensation of coldness.

Equal parts of menthol and of carbolic acid or of thymol, or three parts of menthol and two of camphor, if rubbed up together assume a liquid state and can be painted on the skin or a mucous membrane. One of these, rubbed on the gum, may relieve toothache, or a little menthol may be put into a cavity, if such exists, in the offending tooth.

Solutions of menthol are sprayed into the nose and throat by means of an atomiser (*q.v.*). This relieves the stuffiness of the nose and irritation in the throat. Other methods of using it are with hot water as an inhalation (*q.v.*), or menthol snuff or menthol lozenges. An ointment containing 5 or 10 grains of menthol to an ounce of vaseline is sometimes put into the nose with a camel-hair brush in order to clear the air passage, but this should not be done to infants as it may upset them seriously. Menthol is not often given internally.

MERCURY. A metallic element, which is in a liquid state at ordinary temperatures, mercury, quicksilver or hydrargyrum is extensively used in medicine. It is a valuable remedy for syphilis, and in the treatment of this disease preparations of the drug may be given by the mouth, by intra-muscular injections and by inunction. The powder of mercury and chalk, commonly known as grey powder, dose 1 to 5 grains, is often selected for the oral administration, in doses of 1 grain three or four times daily.

Grey powder is a favourite remedy for diarrhoea in children, with offensive stools, 1 grain for a child one year old, the drug clearing the bowel of its contents and putting a stop to the putrefactive process. Other preparations of mercury used as purgatives are the mercury pill, or blue pill, and subchloride of mercury, or calomel, dose $\frac{1}{2}$ to 5 grains. It is customary to combine other purgatives with these, often a saline, the mercurial preparation being taken at bedtime and the saline in the morning. The compound pill of calomel, or Plummer's pill, is a feeble purgative and is usually given to procure an alterative effect. The official solution of perchloride of mercury, or corrosive sublimate, is also given internally, in small doses. The solution of the iodides of arsenic and mercury, or Donovan's solution, is sometimes used in syphilis.

Antiseptic Solutions of Mercury

Corrosive sublimate and the biniodide are used for preparing antiseptic (*q.v.*) solutions and are powerful agents of this kind. They are, however, extremely poisonous. The yellow and the black mercurial lotions are chiefly used for washing syphilitic sores. The acid solution of mercuric nitrate has a caustic action.

Lotions of the perchloride or of the biniodide of mercury may be used to destroy skin parasites, or, if an ointment is preferable, that of mercury, often referred to as blue ointment, or that of ammoniated mercury, or white precipitate ointment. The latter is a cleaner-looking preparation than blue ointment, but when mercury is to be introduced into the body by inunction, blue ointment is generally used. The repeated application of this or of other strong mercurial preparations to the skin is liable to cause dermatitis.

White precipitate ointment is used in treating chronic skin diseases, such as eczema or psoriasis ; also useful here is the weak nitrate of mercury, or citrine, ointment. The yellow oxide of mercury, or Pagenstecher's ointment, is much used in treating chronic inflammation of the lids or conjunctiva.

The compound mercury or Scott's ointment is sometimes used as a resolvent, that is, to remove chronic inflammatory swellings. Other mercurial ointments are used for this purpose, as are the liniment and the plaster of mercury.

Poisoning by Mercury. A person taking mercury in medicinal doses may suffer from symptoms of over-dosage, either because of an idiosyncrasy to the drug or because too much has been taken. The signs of this condition, which is called mercurialism, are an excessive flow of saliva, a coppery taste in the mouth, a foul breath, soreness and perhaps ulceration of the gums, loosening of teeth and possibly necrosis of the jaw. This condition is less likely to occur if the teeth and mouth are thoroughly cleansed after each meal, and if the patient does not smoke. Treatment consists in discontinuing the drug and the use of a mouth wash containing potassium chlorate.

Acute mercury poisoning from swallowing one of the preparations, most commonly corrosive sublimate, is characterised by a burning pain in the mouth, throat and stomach, vomiting, abdominal pain, diarrhoea and collapse. An emetic should be given and the white of one or two eggs. Milk, flour and water and lime water may also be given. The patient must be kept lying down and warm. Stimulants are likely to be needed.

Chronic poisoning from inhalation of mercury vapour sometimes occurs in thermometer makers and others following certain occupations. The symptoms are mainly those of nervous disorder. There is a tremor of the facial muscles extending to those of the arms and of the legs, paralysis supervening in the muscles. In other cases of chronic poisoning the patient becomes anaemic and loses flesh, and the joints become swollen and extremely painful. Mercury poisoning has occasionally caused insanity. The remedy for chronic poisoning is potassium iodide, which aids its excretion from the body.

See Antiseptic; Corrosive Sublimate; Poisoning.

MESENTERY. The peritoneal fold attaching the small intestine to the posterior abdominal wall, is called the mesentery. It consists of two layers, and between these are the blood vessels, nerves and lymphatics, including lymphatic glands which supply the bowel. The fact that a loop of intestine escaping from the abdominal cavity in a rupture can descend into the scrotum may be due to lengthening of the mesentery, or to the root, or attachment to the posterior abdominal wall, of the mesentery slipping downwards; otherwise it keeps the coils well in place.

There are two arteries, the superior and the inferior mesenteric arteries. The former supplies all the small intestine except the upper part of the duodenum and also the large bowel as far as the middle of the transverse colon, while the inferior supplies all the rest of the large bowel except the lower part of the rectum. Embolism (*q.v.*) of a mesenteric artery is therefore a serious accident.

See Intestine; Peritoneum.

MESMERISM. The notion of animal magnetism underlying the phenomena of mesmerism has now been given up. The phenomena are simply those of hypnotism (*q.v.*).

METABOLISM. Living tissues assimilate foodstuffs and build them into their own substance, a process described as anabolism, or building up. For the exercise of their functions, on the other hand, a certain disintegration of their substance is necessary. This is described as katabolism, or breaking down. The sum of these activities is called metabolism. Carbonic acid gas is a product of katabolism, and the amount breathed out is a measure of metabolic activity, as building up must keep pace with breaking down, at any rate in health. In some diseases, such as fevers and exophthalmic goitre, katabolism is excessively active and the patient loses flesh.

Basal metabolism means the amount of tissue change necessary simply to carry on life, or what goes on when a person is at complete rest mentally and physically. This can be estimated in various ways. The estimation of the basal metabolic rate may be useful in studying disturbances of the thyroid and pituitary glands and for other purposes.

See Diet; Growth; Vitamin.

METACARPUS. *See* Hand.

METASTASIS. The transfer of disease from one organ to another by means of blood vessels or lymphatics is called metastasis. Thus, a sarcoma in the lung may be due to tumour cells being conveyed by the veins from a sarcoma in the leg or elsewhere.

See Tumour.

METATARSUS. *See* Foot.

METCHNIKOFF'S THEORIES. To Professor Elie Metchnikoff we owe the theory of phagocytosis, that certain blood and body cells seize upon bacteria and devour them, thus contributing to the resistance of the body to disease. Another of his theories is the basis of the sour-milk treatment. He supposes that lactic acid bacilli in the bowel war against the putrefactive bacteria, and by thus diminishing the poisons manufactured in the bowel conduce to health.

See Blood; Inflammation; Milk.

METEORISM. Distension of the abdomen with gas is called meteorism. This condition may seriously impede the breathing.

See Flatulence.

METHYL. A hypothetical chemical, containing carbon and hydrogen, methyl forms the basis of a large number of organic compounds, including methyl alcohol, or wood spirit, methyl chloride, etc.

METHYLATED SPIRIT. What is now sold as methylated spirit consists of a mixture of ethyl alcohol with small quantities of methyl alcohol, or wood spirit, crude pyridine and mineral naphtha or petroleum, coloured with methyl violet. This is more properly referred to as mineralised or denatured spirit. This is suitable for burning in spirit lamps, but whereas the old form of methylated spirit could be used freely on the skin with perfect safety, denatured spirit, if so used, may cause dermatitis. Therefore, when spirit is required for the prevention of bed sores or for skin applications generally, what is called surgical spirit should be used. This also is a mixture of the two alcohols, but contains castor oil, or some other substance which renders it unfit for internal use. For the manufac-

ture of liniments another mixture of the alcohols is permitted. This contains quassia, and must not, under a penalty be dispensed in preparations intended for internal use.

When mineralised spirit is taken it effects are like those of ordinary alcohol but more slowly produced and more lasting. Moreover, very dangerous effect may be manifested, such as convulsion or blindness. The stomach should be emptied, by an emetic if the patient i conscious, and hot tea and coffee give freely, warmth being maintained by blankets and hot-water bottles.

METHYLENE BLUE. Methylthionin chloride, which is better known as methylene blue, is extensively used as a dye in histological and bacteriological investigations, and also, both internally and externally, as a remedy. It is a feeble antiseptic, and is used as a lotion for washing infected surfaces or, when injected, for washing out the bladder or other cavities. Inwardly it has analgesic and antipyretic effects, the dose being 2 to 5 grains, preferably in a capsule When the drug is being taken the urine is coloured green or, perhaps, blue.

METHYL SALICYLATE. A synthetic product, methyl salicylate is identical with the active constituent of oil of wintergreen or gaultheria (*q.v.*). It is a remedy for rheumatism.

METRITIS. Inflammation of the wall of the womb (*q.v.*) is called metritis.

METRORRHAGIA. Bleeding from the womb, except that associated with menstruation, is called metrorrhagia. It is important to distinguish such bleeding from menstruation, especially about the time of the change of life. An early investigation into the cause of the bleeding would prevent many deaths from cancer.

See Womb.

MICE. As mice share with rats responsibility for the destruction of millions of pounds' worth of foodstuffs, and may act as carriers of disease to human beings and domestic animals, their destruction is an urgent duty. The domestic cat is of great assistance in clearing out mice, or traps may be used. If necessary, poison may be laid down.

See Rats.

MICROBE. Although literally applicable to any micro-organism, animal or vegetable, the term microbe is generally used as being synonymous with bacterium, that is, a micro-organism belonging to the vegetable kingdom.

MICROCOCCUS. A spherical type of bacterium is called a coccus, or micrococcus.

See Bacteria.

MICROSPORON. Certain diseases of the skin and hair, both in man and the lower animals, are caused by a fungus known as a microsporon. The microsporon audouini is the parasite found in most of the ringworm affecting children attending school.

MICTURITION. The act of passing urine is called micturition, or urination, and is accomplished by the simultaneous contraction of the muscular wall of the bladder and accelerator urinae and the relaxation of the circular muscle, or sphincter, which surrounds the neck of the bladder and retains its contents. The accelerator hastens the stream and expels the last drops of urine. This mechanism is controlled by a centre in the lumbar region of the spinal cord, so that micturition can occur during unconsciousness, but ordinarily, even during sleep, the centre is controlled by the brain. Voluntary micturition is aided by the abdominal muscles, the diaphragm being retained in a fixed position in order to increase their force.

The bladder is normally emptied three or four times a day, and it is not necessary to get up at night. The frequency of micturition is usually greater in cold weather, as more liquid is excreted by the kidneys and less by the skin ; excitement may also increase the frequency. Undue frequency of micturition may be due to inflammation in the urinary tract, in the kidney, the bladder or the urethra, or the irritation of the tract may be due to a stone or a growth. In elderly men an enlarged prostate may necessitate getting out of bed during the night several times to micturate. The undue frequency may be caused by an excessive amount of urine passing through the kidneys, as in diabetes, mellitus or insipidus, and in chronic Bright's disease, or to excess of acid or the presence of other irritants in the urine. Irritation outside the urinary tract, as in the lower bowel and, in females, the womb, is sometimes responsible.

When the act of micturition is painful and spasmodic, with a feeling of urgent necessity to pass water although there may be little or none in the bladder, it is described as dysuria, strangury or bladder tenesmus. This may be caused by the irritative conditions above mentioned, whether within or outside the urinary tract. It has a purely nervous origin, however, in what is called the vesical crisis of locomotor ataxia.

Inability to hold the water, or incontinence of urine, may actually be due to overfilling of the bladder, what comes away representing merely the overflow. Incontinence in children, which may be caused by threadworms, a tight foreskin, and so on, is discussed under the heading Bed-wetting. Circumstances which cause undue frequency in micturition may also cause some incontinence. The bladder is often emptied involuntarily in states of deep unconsciousness, an apoplectic or an epileptic seizure, for instance, but this may occur in other nervous disorders in which, while consciousness is retained, there is loss of the control of the brain on the centre for micturition in the spinal cord.

The stream of urine is diminished in enlargements of the prostate and in stricture (*q.v.*) of the urethra ; in the latter disorder it may be also forked or twisted.

Inability to pass urine may be due to its retention in the bladder because of weakness in the latter or obstruction to the flow, or it may be due to anuria, a cessation of urine formation by the kidney (*q.v.*). The treatment of disorders of micturition depends on the cause, and this can usually only be determined by expert examination. Pain may be eased, at any rate temporari y, by putting hot poultices or fomentations over the bladder, or by the use of a hot hip, or even full, bath.

See Bladder ; Strangury ; Urine.

MIGRAINE. A paroxysmal type of headache, migraine or megrim is usually accompanied by sickness and vomiting, and so is called sick-headache also. Another name for it is hemicrania, as the headache is generally limited to one side. Heredity often plays a part in its causation, and there may be a gouty habit. Eye strain, carious teeth and nasal or aural disease sometimes are responsible, at any rate in part.

Attacks may occur every few days, or at intervals of months, and may last from a few hours to two or three weeks. Warning of an attack may be given by tingling sensations in the limbs, impairment of vision, flashing lights, a vision of battlements, noises in the ears, mental depression or other phenomena. A patient wakes in the morning with a feeling that an attack is impending.

Site and Nature of the Pain

The pain is described as being of a sharp, boring character, and may begin in the temple, in the eyeball or in the forehead, and it tends to spread. Vomiting may relieve it, but in any case the patient is prostrated. In some persons, while the visual phenomena above described are present, there is no headache ; in others there may be only periodical attacks of vomiting, which may be ascribed to biliousness, though actually migrainous in nature.

If there is warning of an attack, a sharp saline purge may avert it. During an attack the patient should lie down in a quiet room with hot-water bottles at his feet. Sometimes hot or cold applications to the head, or a mustard plaster at the nape of the neck, may be beneficial. Phenacetin, antipyrin and similar drugs are given, but repeated doses should not be given without medical advice, as in migraine the drug may not be absorbed during the attack and dangerous symptoms of over-dosage by these powerful drugs may manifest themselves when the patient begins to recover.

In the intervals of attacks the state of the eyes, nose, mouth and ears should be examined to determine whether or not there is any local cause for the headache. The diet should be like that given for gout in many instances, and in every case the quantity of meat should be restricted. A strict vegetarian diet is often most suitable. The bowels should be kept freely open. The course of life should be as free from worry and strain as possible, and a fair amount of open-air exercise should be taken.

Such drugs as solution of trinitrin and bromides are often taken with advantage, and in some inveterate cases more relief has been got by the use of a seton (*q.v.*) than from anything else.

See Headache.

MILIARIA. Two skin affections, characterised by tiny vesicles or blisters, are described as miliaria. In acute fevers, and possibly at other times when there is free sweating, tiny clear vesicles resembling droplets of water may appear, especially on the chest, abdomen and neck. The skin around the blister has a normal appearance, and there is no itching or other disagreeable sensation. Such blisters are called sudamina, and the eruption is sometimes referred to as miliaria crystallina. The blisters may become milky in appearance, but in any case they rupture spontaneously and disappear, leaving no trace of their presence. No treatment is necessary. Miliaria rubra or papulosa is another name for prickly heat (*q.v.*).

MILIARY. The term miliary means having a resemblance to a millet seed. A miliary aneurysm is a minute aneurysmal dilatation of a small artery, or arteriole. Miliary tuberculosis is a name given to generalised tuberculosis because of the minute lesions, or tubercles, scattered throughout the body. Miliary fever is the name given to a fever which has occurred in epidemics from time to time. A rash rather resembling that of prickly heat (*q.v.*) appears on the skin and mucous membranes. There is high fever, and the disease is often fatal. The cause is unknown, and treatment is simply that of fever generally.

MILIUM. A milium is a small, round, white, opaque swelling in the skin, especially frequent in that of the face or in scars. It is supposed to be due to an accumulation of cells round the roots of the small, downy hairs. Only a few milia may be present, but, on the other hand, they may be extremely numerous. The only treatment is to incise and clean out each swelling.

MILK. The young of all mammals depend on the mother's milk for their entire subsistence during the earliest period of life, and milk must therefore contain all the ingredients of a diet, namely, proteins, fat, carbohydrate, salts and vitamins, in addition to water. The milk of different animals varies, however, in the relative proportions of these substances which enter into its composition, and the milk of lower animals, which is used as human food, is, generally speaking, not suitable for infants until it has been modified in some way.

In the following table the average percentage composition of human milk and of others in use is set out.

	Human	Cow's	Goat's	Mare's	Ass's
Proteins	1·70	3·55	4·30	1·31	2·25
Carbohydrate	6·45	4·88	4·46	5.67	6·00
Fat ..	3·78	3·69	4·78	1·21	1·65
Salts ..	0·20	0·71	0·75	0·36	0·50
Water ..	87·87	87·17	85·71	91·45	89·60

The protein content of cow's milk is at least twice that of human milk, but the relative indigestibility of the former as a food for infants depends rather on the quality than on the quantity of protein. There are two proteins in milk, one that forms the curd when milk is acted on by rennet, this being known as caseinogen, and another which coagulates when milk is boiled and is known as lactalbumin. The latter is the more easily digested and the more suitable form, therefore, for young infants. In human milk the two proteins are about equal in quantity, but in cow's milk the proportion of caseinogen to lactalbumin is about 5 or 6 to 1. Dilution of cow's milk does not always get over the difficulty, therefore, and it may be necessary to peptonise milk in order to get it partially digested before giving it to an infant.

The milk of the ass has a large proportion of lactalbumin, 2·3 to 1 of caseinogen, and may be useful for an infant with a weak digestion, but it cannot be continued for long as it has too little fat.

In milk the fat is in tiny droplets diffused through the liquid, which is in fact an emulsion. On standing, the larger drops of fat adhere and rise to the surface as cream, the residuum, or skim milk, retaining most of the other contents of the milk and therefore having a considerable food value. It may be used when fats are not easily digested. The carbohydrate of milk consists of milk-sugar, or lactose. The souring of milk is due to the conversion of this sugar into lactic acid (*q.v.*).

The salts in milk include the chlorides of sodium and potassium, calcium phosphate and salts of iron. Lime salts are necessary to the curdling of milk by rennet. Milk is rather deficient in iron, and a lengthy restriction to a milk diet may cause anaemia. Milk contains all the vitamins necessary for healthy growth. For an adult, milk is not a sufficiently concentrated food, as it would take about 8 pints per diem to afford the energy necessary for light work.

The quality of a sample of milk is sometimes tested by ascertaining the specific gravity by means of an instrument known as a lactometer (*q.v.*) ; ordinarily the specific gravity is 1028 to 1034. There is a fallacy in this test, however, as the removal of cream, which is a light substance, as may be gathered from its rising to the top, makes the specific gravity of milk higher, and water might then be added to bring down the specific gravity to the average figure. It is necessary, therefore, besides taking the specific gravity, to let the milk stand and observe the thickness of the layer of cream that forms on the top.

Grave Dangers of Contamination

The cows from which our milk supply is obtained are often unhealthy, and slovenliness in the management of byres, in milking, and in the handling of milk and milk utensils at the farm and on its way to the consumer, may lead to contamination with dirt and possibly disease germs. Tubercle bacilli of the bovine type are often found in milk, and other germs which may be readily carried in milk are those of diphtheria, scarlet fever, typhoid fever and the summer diarrhoea of infants.

Abroad, cholera may be carried, and the danger of goat's milk conveying Malta fever is discussed under the heading of this disease.

Two views of a model dairy farm are given in Plate XXV.

To further the purity of the public milk supply in Great Britain, the Ministry of

Health has arranged for the licensing of dairy-farms and dairies to sell various categories of milk which fulfil the requirements laid down in the Milk Special Designations Order, 1923. These categories are Certified ; Grade A (tuberculin tested) ; Grade A ; Grade A (pasteurised) ; and Pasteurised. Tuberculin tested means that the cows must be examined by a veterinary surgeon at intervals and be pronounced free from tuberculosis. This applies to Certified milk as well as to the first category of Grade A milk. Certified milk must be bottled at the farm, and the word " certified " must be stamped on the stopper of the bottles. Pasteurisation must be carried out in an approved apparatus, and milk must be kept at a temperature between 145° to 150° F. for at least half an hour and then be cooled to a temperature not exceeding 55° F.

It must be pointed out, however, that contamination of milk may easily occur in the home unless it is kept in clean

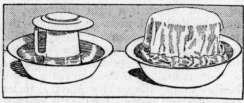

Milk. Two methods of keeping it cool and clean

utensils in a clean, cool larder and efficiently covered to protect it from dust and flies. When brought to table it must also be covered if flies are about. If the milk is not of the tuberculosis-free categories, it should be boiled before being given to young children. In hot weather milk should be kept on ice.

Nothing short of boiling will kill tubercle bacilli, but other forms of infection may be destroyed by pasteurisation. This can be done in an apparatus sold for the purpose or in a double saucepan, according to the instructions laid down above. The cooling must be rapid, and the milk must be stored in a cool place.

To peptonise milk, two-thirds of a pint is diluted with one-third pint of water and heated in a saucepan to a temperature of 140° F. If a thermometer is not available, the correct temperature can be obtained by

bringing one half of the diluted milk to the boil and then adding the other half. The heated milk is put into a jug and two drachms of Benger's liquor pancreaticus and 20 grains of sodium bicarbonate are added and stirred in. The jug is then covered with a cosy and left for from ten to twenty minutes, according to the amount of action required, when the milk is brought to the boil to stop the action. Another method is to use Fairchild's peptogenic milk powder, following the instructions given with the bottles in which the preparation is sold.

Value of Curds and Whey

If rennet be added to milk the caseinogen is converted into casein, and this forms a curd in which most of the fat is entangled. The liquid which remains, the whey, has a slight food value and is sometimes used in feeding infants and the sick. To obtain whey, a pint of milk is warmed to 100° F. and a teaspoonful of rennet added. The milk is kept warm until a proper curd has formed, when the curd is broken up with a fork and the whey is then strained off. The curd, sometimes called junket, forms a nutritious food. Cheese is prepared from casein.

When milk is churned, some of the fat remains in the buttermilk, but there is little or no fat in separated milk. Buttermilk can often be taken by those who dislike ordinary milk, and sometimes a mixture of equal quantities of sweet milk and buttermilk is better taken than sweet milk alone. Tablets or powders containing the Bulgarian or the Caucasian bacillus are used for the artificial souring of milk, these being added to milk which is kept at a temperature of about 110° F. for eight to ten hours. Owing to the trouble in making it, however, artificially soured milk should preferably be obtained from a reliable dairy.

The sour-milk cure is based on the probability that the growth of the lactic acid bacilli in the bowel will lessen the activity of the bacilli which give rise to harmful products from the decomposition of proteins in food. Either soured whole milk or skimmed milk may be used, the latter preferably. A pint of milk, or more or less according to the patient's toler-

PLATE XXV

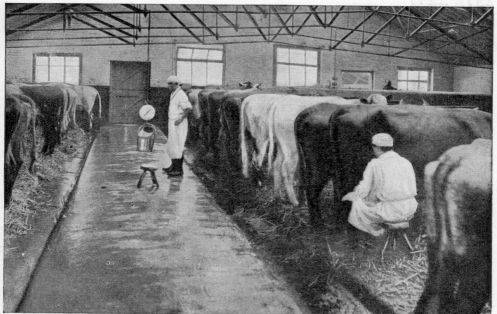

Milk.   1. Hygienic conditions in the cowshed of a Rayleigh model farm.   The walls are of glazed brick and the stalls are slightly sloping to facilitate sluicing.   The cows are inspected at frequent intervals and their flanks, udders and teats are cleansed before milking.   The milkers wear clean overalls and caps

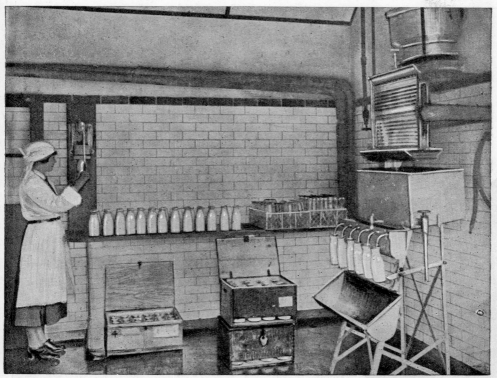

2. When the milk, in its covered bucket, has been weighed, it is passed through the wall into the dairy, where it is first pasteurised.   It then flows through a cooler into a tank-like receptacle, from which the bottles are filled.   Sealing (left) is done mechanically, the hands never touching the mouth of the bottle

PLATE XXVI

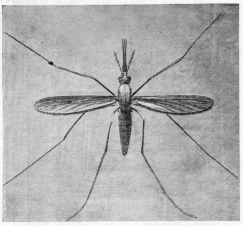

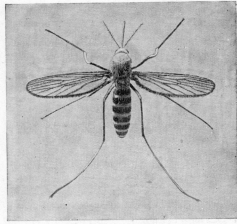

Mosquito. 1. Anopheles maculipennis, a carrier of malaria. It is characterised by spots on its wings and, like other anopheles, rests with the hind part of the body humped up. 2. Culex pipiens, the common gnat

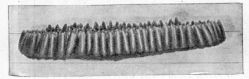

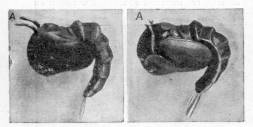

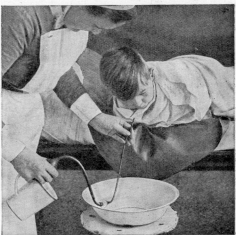

Mosquito. 3. Above, eggs of culex pipiens grouped in characteristic raft-like formation. Below, pupa of culex (left) and anopheles (right). A, air tubes. The pupa succeeds the larval stage

4. Nose. Douching with a Higginson's syringe

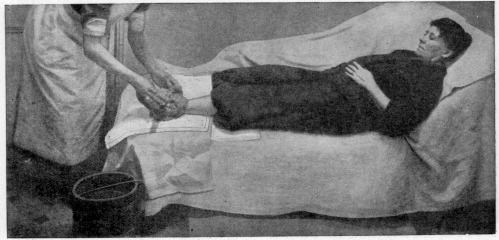

5. Mud Bath. Hot packs of a special mineral content are used for treating rheumatic and stiff joints
Courtesy of Grand Pump Room, Bath

ance, is taken each day, in two or three portions, and this should go on for about three weeks.

Constipation sometimes occurs in the second week, but this will soon disappear as the treatment goes on. The cure is often useful in the summer diarrhoea of children, in diarrhoea or constipation in adults, in migraine, in eczema and other disorders. The course may have to be repeated. During the cure such foods as white of egg, fat meat, meat extracts and high game should be avoided.

Koumiss in its original form is mare's milk which has undergone alcoholic fermentation, besides being soured. It is now made by putting yeast into cow's milk to which glucose has been added. Kephir is a similar preparation made with cow's, goat's or sheep's milk. These foods are easily digested, and may be useful when the digestive powers are enfeebled.

Condensed milk is milk deprived of water until it is of a syrupy consistency. Dried milk is milk deprived of most of its water, so that it is in powder form. Public Health Regulations fix a required amount of fat in condensed and dried milk. Citrated milk is milk to which citrate of sodium has been added, usually in the proportion of 1½ grains to the ounce. The curd is thus rendered more digestible.

See Casein; Condensed Milk; Food; Invalid Cookery; Lactic Acid; Lactometer; Tuberculosis; Whey.

MILK FEVER. The rise of temperature which may occur in a woman about the third day after childbirth, and which is commonly referred to as milk fever, is usually due to absorption of septic matter from the genital passage rather than to disturbances in the breast or other associations with lactation.

See Breast; Puerperal Fever.

MILK SICKNESS. In some parts of the United States of America an acute form of poisoning, known as milk sickness, occasionally occurs. It is due to consumption of the flesh, the milk, or of butter or cheese made from the milk of cattle suffering from a disease popularly described as " the trembles." The bacillus lactimorbi is thought to be the cause of the disorder. There is pain in the stomach, vomiting and intense thirst. Usually there is obstinate constipation, and the breath has a foul odour. Muscular tremors appear and perhaps convulsions and coma.

The bowels should be opened freely with castor oil or salts. During convalescence any exertion must be avoided, as it is likely to bring on tremor.

See Poisoning.

MILK SUGAR. The sweetness of milk is due to the presence of a sugar of the same group as cane sugar and known as lactose (*q.v.*), or milk sugar.

See Sugar.

MIND. The brain is the organ of mind. Mental activity is associated with the discharge of energy by brain cells, and its conduction along the nerves, formed by the processes of these cells, in numerous directions. Some of the impulses go to other cells in the brain, which in turn themselves discharge energy or manifest some other metabolic change, while others pass to or from organs and tissues throughout the body.

The existence of this relationship between mind and the brain is established by definite evidence, but the precise nature of the relationship is not known. It could not be asserted, for instance, that thought is related to cerebral activity merely as the secretion of a gland is to the activity of the cells of the gland ; nor, on the other hand, that the brain cells are like the passive keys of an instrument through which an extrinsic force produces sound.

The groundwork of our minds is knowledge, derived through the senses, of what goes on outside our bodies and, to some extent, within them. This knowledge is registered in the brain in some way and is utilisable in the processes of thinking. In fact, some states of feeling and actions to which these give origin are registered in the ovum, or egg, from which a human being springs, and are distinguished as instincts. There is the ego instinct, the sexual instinct, the parental instinct, the herd instinct and so on.

The urge towards the satisfaction of instinctive and acquired desires exercises a profound influence on the processes of thought. There is, however, a kind of mechanism in the nervous system known as inhibition, that is, a power to control or regulate bodily activities of some kind, and something of this sort grows up in the mind as notions of what is right and expedient, conjoined more or less with a sense of disagreeable consequences attaching to the disregard of such notions. Thus, there is in the mind a conflict of ideas, desires for the satisfaction of animal cravings, for example, or a desire to turn one's back on dangers and difficulties conflicting with the desire for self-respect or for the respect of one's neighbours.

Now, although a person may imagine that he successfully tramples on what would diminish his respect for himself, and that he regulates his life conformably to his ideals, it can by no means be implied that he obliterates all traces of inconvenient desires.

Dissipation of Mental Conflicts

If a desire be sufficiently urgent, it and the network, or complex, of ideas associated with it are simply repressed and the desire continues to press for satisfaction. It obtains this in various ways. One way is through dreams, but, as the barrier to untrammelled thinking extends even below the surface of conscious thought, the dream experience through which satisfaction is achieved may be purely symbolical; in fact, it usually is so.

A second method in which satisfaction may be had is by what is known as sublimation, that is, the transfer of the energy inherent in repressed ideas to such as can be entertained, for example, to mysticism, to philanthropy and so on, though this does not mean that such activities are always, or even very often, mere solutions of mental conflicts.

A third method is the process of rationalisation; the wish is allowed satisfaction but the fact is concealed from the individual by the tissue of argument which he weaves around it. Thus he justifies the expediency of his thought or action to himself, though he may not be so successful in convincing his neighbours. An immense amount of our thinking could be described as mere rationalisation.

A fourth method by which a truce is called to mental conflict is by the development of some kind of psycho-neurosis. The performance of a dangerous or very disagreeable duty may be avoided by paralysis of an arm or of a leg, for example,

the mental and nervous processes through which this is brought about taking place unconsciously and thus differing altogether from pure malingering.

Not only are many of our beliefs, which appear to us to be soundly reasoned, mere rationalisations, but some of them have no reasoned basis at all. They are simply suggestions accepted from others, the general opinion of the community in which one lives or the opinions of persons whose minds happen to dominate our own. Suggestibility is a quality of every mind, more or less, and often enough auto-suggestion (*q.v.*), or a suggestion to oneself, occurs.

For successful thinking there must be adequate concentration, or attention, and this implies a considerable mobilisation of nerve energy which expresses itself not only in the mental effort but affects the whole body. This is shown in the musculature, as the attitude of an attentive person is very different from that of one who is inattentive or allowing his mind to wander. This explains why concentration causes fatigue, sooner or later.

The old-fashioned way of describing the structure of the mind as consisting of various faculties, intellectual, volitional and emotional, has some uses, so long as one realises that these so-called faculties are all closely inter-related. The mind works as a whole and the faculties are simply aspects of this working, not separate machines, as it were, the working capacity of any one of which could be increased or diminished without affecting that of the others.

See Auto-suggestion; Double Consciousness: Dreams; Freudism; Memory; Neurosis; Psycho-therapy.

MINDERERUS SPIRIT. The liquor, or solution, of ammonium acetate is sometimes called spirit of Mindererus. It promotes perspiration and is generally included in a fever mixture. The dose is 2 to 6 drachms.

See Fever.

MINERAL WATER. The varieties and uses of mineral waters are discussed under the heading Health Resort. The beverages often referred to as "minerals" have nothing in common with mineral waters, which are water containing some medicinal substances in solution.

MINER'S ANAEMIA. *See* Ankylostomiasis.

MINER'S ELBOW. Prolonged pressure on the elbow, which may be entailed in a miner's occupation, may cause chronic inflammation and swelling of the bursa at the back of the olecranon process, a condition sometimes described as miner's elbow. *See* Bursitis.

MINER'S NYSTAGMUS. Oscillatory movements of the eyeballs, or nystagmus, are rather common in miners. Usually there are other nervous manifestations associated with the eye trouble, and sometimes there is serious impairment of vision. Inefficient lighting and awkward positions in which a miner may have to carry on his work are two of the suggested causes. *See* Nystagmus.

MISCARRIAGE. What is usually meant by the term miscarriage is termination of pregnancy before the end of the 27th week, though strictly it means an accident of this kind between the end of the 12th week and the end of the 27th, the loss of the foetus before the end of the 12th week being called an abortion. *See* Abortion ; Childbirth ; Pregnancy.

MITRAL VALVE. The valve between the two left chambers of the heart is called the mitral valve from a fancied resemblance to a bishop's mitre. Mitral disease generally consists in narrowing of this valve, though the valve may also become incompetent. *See* Heart.

MIXTURE. In pharmacy a mixture, or mistura, is a preparation intended to be swallowed, and consisting of a solid substance rubbed up with water and, if necessary, kept in suspension by mucilage or something of the sort ; or it consists of two or more liquids added together. If, however, the suspended substance is an oil or a resin the preparation is usually called an emulsion. A mixture intended to be taken all at once is called a draught.

The official mixtures are : almond mixture, ammoniacum mixture, chalk mixture, guaiacum mixture and compound iron mixture, which are given in doses of $\frac{1}{2}$ to 1 ounce, and castor oil and compound senna mixtures, which are given in doses of 1 to 2 ounces.

MOLE. A variety of birth mark is called a mole, or pigmented mole. Sometimes it is covered with hair, when it is usually referred to as a hairy mole. A mole is a tumour formation in the skin, consisting of cells containing pigment and covered by normal epidermis. It may be of minute size or may cover extensive areas, and may occur anywhere on the body. Persons exhibited in shows as ape-women or something of the kind really owe their peculiarity to the fact that large portions of the skin are covered by hairy moles.

A mole may take on malignant characters in later life, especially if it has been irritated much by rubbing or otherwise, and the cells may be disseminated throughout the body. As they are pigmented this dissemination is sometimes called melanosis. When feasible it may be desirable, therefore, to get rid of moles, but this should be done by a doctor, as unskilful treatment might precipitate malignancy.

The term mole is also applied to a mass which may be formed in the womb in the earlier months of pregnancy, replacing the normal contents. One formation of this kind is called a fleshy, or blood, mole and consists mostly of old blood clot. Another is called a hydatid mole, though it has nothing in common with hydatid disease. Signs of abortion (*q.v.*) usually appear before the fifth month of pregnancy. *See* Birth Mark ; Electrolysis ; Skin.

MOLLUSCUM. Two types of soft growth are described as molluscum. One occurs in the disease known as molluscum contagiosum, in which tiny, hemispherical swellings appear on the skin, usually on the face or external genitals, but perhaps on the hands or elsewhere on the body. They grow to about the size of a pea and the colour may be like mother-of-pearl or yellowish brown.

The top of the little tumour is rather flattened, and there is a depression through which a plug of a whitish substance is extruded when the tumour is squeezed in the proper way. This substance consists of degenerated epithelial cells, and the morbid changes are caused by a germ, apparently a filter-passing virus. The disorder is communicable from one person to another. The tumours are not troublesome unless they suppurate, and only in this event do they leave a scar when they disappear. The disease, which is more common amongst the poor, is successfully treated by squeezing out the plugs and disinfecting the cavity that remains.

Molluscum fibrosum, or fibroma molluscum, is quite a different disorder. Here a growth formed of soft tissue occurs in the connective tissue surrounding nerve trunks, and from this may result rounded swellings, which may remain below the skin level or protrude from prominent folds of skin. Tumours that protrude commonly become pedunculated, that is to say, develop a narrow neck attaching them to the skin. The skin over them may be wrinkled, but it preserves its normal tint unless, as often happens, there is an overgrowth of blood vessels, forming a naevus, within the tumour, when a bluish tint is acquired.

Sometimes there is an extensive growth of hairy moles over the body with small whitened areas of skin between them and portions with a light brown or café-au-lait staining.

In conjunction with these changes in the skin there may be thickenings on the nerves beneath it, and some of these may be very tender and give rise to considerable pain.

Molluscum fibrosum is also known as neuro-fibromatosis and as Von Recklinghausen's disease. It is probably always congenital in origin. Small growths may be removed, but nothing can be done to prevent the occurrence of the growths. Sometimes a growth takes on the characters of a sarcoma, a form of cancer.

See Mole ; Skin.

MONOMANIA. Insanity supposed to be limited to a single subject or a group of subjects used to be called monomania. An insuperable objection to this term, however, is that the kind of insanity it connotes cannot well exist, since it is now known that the mind works as a whole, and any unsoundness must permeate the whole, more or less. The possession of delusions of the sort once described as monomania is now called paranoia.

See Mental Disease ; Obsession.

MONSTER. An imperfect development of the embryo (*q.v.*) may result in the production of an individual differing so

widely from the normal type as to constitute a monster or monstrosity. An ovum can divide into two and produce well-formed twins resembling each other in all particulars. If, however, this division takes place only at one end, an individual may be produced with two heads or four legs, as the case may be.

In other instances a monstrosity results from certain parts, the brain, for instance, failing to develop ; in others there is a transposition of viscera, but in this event the appearance and health of the individual may be in no wise affected. The differences from the normal in most monsters, however, are incompatible with life, or at any rate with long survival. Where separation of two individuals is nearly complete, however, as happened to the Siamese twins, life may be prolonged for a number of years.

Sometimes a second individual formed by partial division of an ovum fails to develop any human shape at all, but simply exists as a tumour mass in the body of the individual developed from the remainder of the ovum. Such a tumour is called a teratoma.

Some monsters may occasion serious difficulties in the process of childbirth.

MONTHLY SICKNESS. *See* Menstruation.

MORBUS. A Latin word meaning disease, the term morbus is sometimes used in the name of a disease, cholera morbus, for example. Morbid is the corresponding adjective.

MORPHIA. The chief active principle of opium is the alkaloid morphine, or, as it is popularly called, morphia. Very often this alkaloid is selected as a medicine in preference to opium itself. Chronic poisoning from the morphia habit is called morphinism.

See Drug Habits ; Opium.

MORNING SICKNESS. In the early months of pregnancy (*q.v.*) there is a tendency to sickness on first rising in the morning, and this is usually referred to as morning sickness. There are, however, some diseases in which sickness in the morning is not infrequent, consumption, for example, and chronic alcoholism.

MORTIFICATION. *See* Gangrene.

MORTON'S DISEASE. Severe pain in the front part of the foot from pressure on nerves is called Morton's disease, or metatarsalgia. The treatment is discussed under the heading Foot.

MORVAN'S DISEASE. A person suffering from the disease of the spinal cord known as syringomyelia (*q.v.*) may develop painless whitlows on the fingers, a condition described as Morvan's disease. There is first neuralgic pain in the hands and then a loss of the sensations of heat and pain in the fingers, brought about by the disease in the cord, and, consequently, injuries to the fingers may be overlooked. Infection may thus occur, and this is facilitated by the poor nutrition of the tissues. The whitlow may be superficial or deep, when it may be accompanied by necrosis of the bone.

See Whitlow.

MOSQUITO. An important part is taken by different species of mosquito in disseminating certain diseases. The species concerned belong to two great groups of mosquito, the anopheline and the culicine. The female mosquito sucks blood, because this contributes to the maturation of her eggs, and in the process may inject disease organisms she may happen to be carrying.

The anopheles maculipennis and other anophelines are malaria-carriers. Of the culicinae, culex fatigans carries the filaria worm and possibly dengue; stegomyia or aëdes fasciata carries yellow fever, and other species of stegomyia carry the filaria worm. Septic germs are also sometimes inoculated by mosquitoes.

Anopheles as a rule bite at night, but stegomyia are most active in the early afternoon.. Other characteristics which distinguish the two great groups of mosquitoes are detailed under the heading Anopheles (*see* Plate XXVI, 1-3).

The first protective measure against mosquitoes is to prevent their breeding by getting rid of stagnant water, by drainage and by filling in pools (Plate XXXVII, 4 and 5). If this is not possible, paraffin may be poured on the surface of the water so as to cover the pool. Wells or open cisterns should have a cover of close gauze or netting. When it is necessary to have the legs of a table standing in tins of water to protect them against white ants the water should contain some antiseptic.

A dwelling-house should be as far as possible from marshes or other collections of stagnant water, and the ground around it should be cleared of brushwood. The doors and windows should be efficiently screened by netting or gauze. Should a house have been infected already it may be cleared by fumigation as described under the heading Disinfection. Unless the house is sufficiently protected the inmates should always sleep under a mosquito net.

Should it be necessary to go out at night the face may be protected by a net attached to a helmet or suitable framework, and the hands by gloves. Bites are often received on the legs through thin stockings, so that thick stockings or puttees are advisable. Treatment is discussed under the heading Bite. A solution of an ounce of magnesium sulphate in 10 ounces of water daubed over exposed skin and allowed to dry on is said to prevent bites; or the skin may be smeared with vaseline, with which has

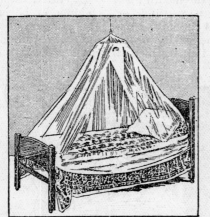

Mosquito net for use in the tropics. It should be well tucked in at the sides

been mixed a little oil of citronella, of cloves or some other fragrant oil.

See Anopheles; Bite; Filaria; Malaria; Tropical Hygiene; Yellow Fever.

MOTOR AREA. The part of the cortex of the brain in front of the fissure of Rolando is called the motor area. Voluntary movements are caused by discharges of energy from cells in this region, but the area on the right side of the brain is responsible for movements on the left side of the body, and vice versa.

See Brain.

MOUNTAIN SICKNESS. Persons who climb mountains to a certain height are liable to be seized with a group of symptoms described as mountain sickness. There is intense headache, air is breathed in by gasps and there is a sense of great muscular feebleness. Sometimes there is nausea and vomiting, but such symptoms are much more likely to be found when there is a pre-existing dyspepsia; in other instances it may be due to fatigue.

Mountain sickness is caused apparently by a diminished supply of oxygen owing to the rarefaction of the air at high altitudes, and occurs also in persons who attain such altitudes in aircraft. The height at which mountaineers have generally begun to be affected is about 16,500 feet and upwards, but in the Mount Everest expedition it made its appearance at 7,000 feet. The inhalation of oxygen, carried in an apparatus, was of much service during this expedition.

MOUTH. Two parts of the mouth may be distinguished, namely, the vestibule, or space between the lips and cheeks and the teeth and gums, and the cavity of the mouth proper, behind the teeth and reaching to the fauces (*q.v.*), where the mouth becomes continuous with the pharynx. The roof of the mouth proper is formed by the hard palate and on the floor lies the tongue. The whole cavity of the mouth is lined with mucous membrane.

From the mucous membrane comes a secretion which helps to keep the mouth moist, but this is chiefly the work of the saliva (*q.v.*). This juice, the product of several glands, also assists in mastication and has important uses in digestion. Dryness of the mouth is common in mouth-breathers. It may occur from fear and in fevers and other disorders. A disorder characterised by constant and excessive dryness of the mouth is called xerostomia.

Inflammation of the mouth is called stomatitis and may assume various forms,

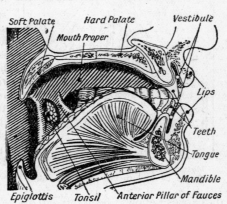

Mouth. Diagram showing the principal parts

Soft Palate · Hard Palate · Vestibule · Mouth Proper · Lips · Teeth · Tongue · Mandible · Epiglottis · Tonsil · Anterior Pillar of Fauces

according to the cause. Generally there is some soreness when chewing. Simple stomatitis may be caused by excessive smoking, by condiments or other irritants, or by indigestion; or it may have a bacterial cause, as in an ordinary cold or an eruptive fever. The lining becomes red and is dry at first, but afterwards there is excessive secretion. The tongue is furred, enlarged and indented by the teeth. The mouth should be kept clean, and a solution of bicarbonate of sodium will help towards this.

In aphthous, follicular or vesicular stomatitis, which affects children mostly, little vesicles or blisters form on the inside of the lips and teeth and on the edges of the tongue, and may even occur on the fauces or in the pharynx. The vesicles, which are surrounded by a red margin, soon rupture, leaving little ulcers. Errors of digestion should be corrected and the mouth should be kept clean.

Ulcerative stomatitis tends to affect children in poverty-stricken households. The gums swell and become ulcerated, sores also forming on the lining of the cheeks. There is a free flow of saliva and the breath is foul. The glands below the jaw may be enlarged. A mouth wash (*q.v.*) containing potassium chlorate should be used, small doses of the drug also being swallowed. The general health must be improved by better hygienic conditions and good food.

Gangrenous stomatitis is also called cancrum oris (*q.v.*); mercurial stomatitis is discussed under the heading Mercury. Thrush is a form of stomatitis caused by the growth of a fungus, the oidium albicans. It usually affects infants, poor health and want of cleanliness in feeding being contributory; but it is not uncommon in debilitated people of any age. Pearly-white spots form on the tongue and spread to the cheeks and fauces; sometimes they spread down the gullet into the stomach and bowel. The mouth is dry, contrary to what occurs in other forms of stomatitis. Strict cleanliness should be observed as regards bottles and other apparatus for feeding, and the mouth should be cleansed at intervals with glycerin of borax diluted with a little water. The general health should be improved as far as possible.

Ulcers on the cheeks may also be caused by a jagged or septic tooth, and on the hard palate may be due to the breaking down of a syphilitic gumma. White patches on the cheeks occur in leukoplakia (*q.v.*). The rashes of various specific fevers, such as measles and chicken-pox, are found in the mouth.

See Cancrum Oris ; Gum ; Lips ; Palate ; Ranula ; Salivary Gland ; Teeth ; Tongue.

MOUTH WASH. The cleanliness of the mouth ordinarily depends mainly on that of the teeth, and this in turn on the use of food requiring thorough mastication, crisp fruit, such as apples, being especially useful for this purpose. The use of a tooth brush is usually necessary also. It will sometimes, however, be desirable to use some kind of wash for the mouth.

When it is merely to relieve a dry, sticky feeling, a pinch of common salt, sodium bicarbonate or borax, or of a combination of each, in half a glass of water will suffice. When the breath is foul a solution of permanganate of potassium, enough of the latter to make the solution red, is useful, though it may be desirable to gargle with this also.

In ulcerative stomatitis the following should be used :

Potassium chlorate	..	..160 grains
Glycerin	.. ..	.. 6 drachms
Water ..	..	..to make 8 ounces

A teaspoonful to a tablespoonful, according to the age of the patient, should be swallowed thrice daily.

Hydrogen peroxide, diluted with 3 parts of water, makes a good wash, and also the compound solution of thymol B.P.C. in the same dilution.

MUCILAGE. In pharmacy a mucilage is a solution of a gum in water. The official mucilages are those of acacia, of tragacanth, and of Indian or ghatti gum. These are used to suspend heavy powders in mixtures and as excipients of pills. A solution of starch is usually called starch mucilage. Mucilages have a demulcent action on mucous membranes, and are sometimes used as demulcents.

MUCO-PURULENT. A mucous discharge mixed with pus, or matter, is said to be muco-purulent. A common instance is the discharge in the later stages of a cold.

MUCOUS MEMBRANE. The digestive, the respiratory, the genito-urinary, and other passages and hollow organs have a delicate lining, known as mucous membrane, which is kept moist by a sticky secretion called mucus. A mucous membrane has a covering of epithelial cells, which vary in shape in the various organs and passages. These cells generally rest on a basement membrane, and beneath this is connective tissue.

Mucus may be derived from some of the superficial epithelial cells, or from mucous glands, sunk in the connective tissue but opening on the surface of the mucous membrane. Amongst the epithelial cells are found some which, from their shape, are called goblet-cells, and whose function is the secretion of mucus. The superficial cells of some mucous membranes, that of the respiratory tract, for example, are ciliated, or have a fringe of tiny, hair-like processes, on their free margin. By a wave-like motion the cilia propel particles resting on the mucous membrane in a particular direction.

Beneath some mucous membranes there are glands of various kinds which open and discharge their secretions on the surface of the membrane. This occurs, for example, all along the stomach and bowels, the secretions of the gland constituting digestive juices.

Inflammation of a mucous membrane tends to increase the secretions of mucus, a condition described as catarrh.

MUCUS. The secretion of a mucous membrane, mucus owes its stickiness to a mucin which it contains. Mucins are viscid substances, compounded of a protein and a carbohydrate. Mucus is rendered less adhesive by solutions of weak alkalies, hence the value of sodium bicarbonate in lotions or sprays for cleansing a mucous membrane.

See Mucous Membrane.

MUD BATH. Chronic skin diseases and chronic joint affections are sometimes treated by means of mud baths, the mud used at some places being of volcanic origin, and some being radio-active. At Bath, hot mud, made by mixing a fuller's earth found locally with the mineral water, is used in the form of packs (Plate XXVI, 5). Local mud is also used at Woodhall. Mud baths are employed at Dax, near Biarritz, in France, at Acqui in Italy, at Rotorua and other places in New Zealand, and at other spas throughout the world. Volcanic mud is imported into this country and used for mud baths at Llandrindod Wells and elsewhere.

See Baths ; Peat Bath.

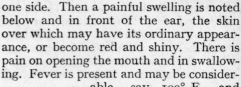

Mumps. Situation of the glands affected in this inflammatory disease

MULTIPARA. A pregnant woman who has already borne one or more children is described as a multipara.

MULTIPLE NEURITIS. Inflammation of several nerves is described as multiple or, sometimes, peripheral neuritis. All four limbs may be involved and possibly nerves in the trunk and face, though these usually escape. The inflammation is usually caused by poisons circulating in the blood, and may occur in diphtheria or, less frequently, some other infectious fever. Alcoholism is a common cause and lead or arsenic poisoning is also a fairly frequent cause. Multiple neuritis also occurs in diabetes and other metabolic diseases.

See Beri-beri ; Neuritis.

MUMPS. An acute infectious disease, mumps mainly attacks children, boys more often than girls, but adults are not immune, and may suffer severely. Inflammation of the parotid salivary glands is a characteristic feature of the disease, which, therefore, is also known as epidemic parotitis. The causative organism appears to be a spirochaete which lurks in the mouth of infected persons. The period of incubation is from ten to twenty-two days.

Malaise and soreness about the ear and throat may then occur, and tenderness may be found on drawing the finger along the under surface of the lower jaw on one side. Then a painful swelling is noted below and in front of the ear, the skin over which may have its ordinary appearance, or become red and shiny. There is pain on opening the mouth and in swallowing. Fever is present and may be considerable, say 100° F., and the patient may become delirious.

Usually, and within a few days, the parotid gland on the other side also becomes swollen, and sometimes the salivary glands below the lower jaw and beneath the front part of the tongue are also affected. Amongst other glands which may also become inflamed are the lachrymal gland, the testicle, the breast and the pancreas. The acute symptoms generally last for four or five days.

The possibility of the inflammation of the parotid gland being septic in origin must be excluded before the condition is accepted as being mumps, this possibility being stronger in adults than in children, however.

A person suffering from mumps should be isolated at once, the measures to be taken in this connexion being outlined under the heading Infectious Disease, and should be kept in bed for at least eight days. Treatment includes that for fever (*q.v.*) generally, but hot, or sometimes cold, applications are used over the swollen glands. It may be necessary to use anodyne remedies also. Several times a day the mouth must be cleansed with a solution of permanganate of potassium, or some other antiseptic mouth wash ; this is most important.

Should inflammation of the testicle (*q.v.*), or orchitis, supervene, it must be carefully treated, as there is a risk of the organ subsequently becoming atrophied. Inflammation of the pancreas, or pancreatitis, may cause abdominal pain, vomiting and diarrhoea, for which warm applications will be necessary ; sometimes, however, there is no discomfort. In a few instances diabetes has followed involvement of the pancreas in the course of mumps. Ear, eye and brain complications may occur, but are rare ; nephritis is not uncommon, especially in adults.

Injection of blood serum, taken from a convalescent from mumps, has been used successfully as a prophylactic measure.

A person who suffers from mumps should not be considered to be free from infection until three weeks have elapsed since the appearance of swelling, and only then if the swelling has been gone for at least one week.

As infection does not last very long on fomites, that is, articles which the patient has handled, disinfection (*q.v.*) is hardly necessary, though it may be worth while to disinfect handkerchiefs, night raiment and bedding which has last been in use.

The quarantine period for persons who have been in contact with anyone suffering from mumps, and who are not considered to be immune, is twenty-five days.

See Gland ; Glandular Fever ; Parotid Gland.

MURIATED WATERS. Mineral waters containing chlorides are commonly referred to as muriated waters. Those with a large amount of sodium chloride, or common salt, are called brines.

See Health Resort.

MURMUR. A sound, other than the ordinary heart sounds, which is heard when listening over the heart, and which appears to be connected with the heart's action, is described as a murmur, or bruit. A rubbing or creaking sound may be heard over the heart, but have no relationship to the normal sounds caused by the heart's action, though it has to the movements of the chest in breathing. This is not a murmur, but a pleuritic friction sound.

Murmurs may be described according to their place in the cardiac cycle as systolic, diastolic or presystolic; according to the valve which appears to be affected, as mitral, aortic, and so on ; according to their characters, as

soft, blowing, harsh, etc.; and, according to whether they appear to be produced inside or outside the heart, as endocardial or exocardial respectively. A systolic murmur may occur without there being organic or indeed any disease of the heart. An exocardial murmur may occur in pericarditis, but often has no pathological significance.

See Auscultation ; Heart.

MUSCAE VOLITANTES. The literal meaning of the term muscae volitantes is flies in flight, and it is applied to the floating specks that sometimes appear before the eyes. These may occur when the liver is disordered, or when there are opacities in the lens or vitreous humour of the eye, but usually they are produced by the movements of the corpuscles in the capillaries of the retina, and have no sinister significance.

MUSCLE. There are three kinds of muscle in the body, namely, striped, voluntary or skeletal muscle, plain or unstriped involuntary muscle, and the heart muscle, which is a striped but involuntary muscle. A striped muscle is one whose fibres show cross-striping on microscopical examination, and a voluntary muscle is one which is under the control of the will.

A skeletal muscle is described as having an origin and an insertion. Thus, the biceps muscle has its origin on the shoulder blade and is inserted into the radius, a bone of the forearm. The origin of the muscle may be direct, that is, the fleshy fibres may be attached to the periosteum, or fibrous covering, of the bone, but, on the other hand, the attachment may be through a tendon or an aponeurosis. The same applies to the insertion ; this may be into another bone, or something else, the eyeball, for example.

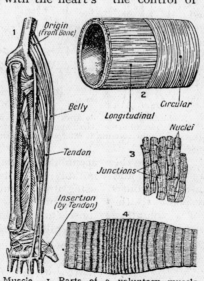

Muscle. 1. Parts of a voluntary muscle. 2. Smooth involuntary muscle. 3. Fibres of heart muscle much enlarged 4. Change in a muscle fibre during contraction

The fleshy part of a muscle is generally referred to as the belly of the muscle. In some, as in the muscles of the forearm, this is prolonged into a long, slender tendon of insertion. Muscles are of various shapes. Some, like the biceps, are rather spindle-shaped, others, like the sartorius, form long, narrow ribbons, and others still, like those in the anterior abdominal wall, form broad, thin sheets.

A muscle is enclosed in a sheath and is found to be made up of bundles separated by connective tissue. The bundles are composed of fibres about one inch long and $\frac{1}{500}$ inch across, each fibre being enclosed in an elastic sheath, known as the sarcolemma. Plain muscle, which is composed of long, spindle-shaped cells, forming fibres which are arranged in bundles, is found in the walls of the hollow organs, that is, the alimentary tract, the ureters and bladder, the Fallopian tubes and womb, and so on. It also occurs in the walls of the trachea and bronchial tubes and in blood vessels, besides many other situations. The fibres commonly surround a tube or hollow organ, but some organs have longitudinal fibres as well, and in the stomach there are also oblique fibres.

Heart muscle is composed of striped cells, forming fibres which are carried round the chambers.

Muscle possesses irritability, that is, it responds to some kind of irritation. Normally, the excitation is nervous energy, but an electric current, the striking of a muscle, and other causes will also evoke a response. This takes the form of contraction; a muscle fibre, and therefore the whole muscle, becomes shorter and thicker in response to the excitation. In the case of a voluntary muscle the shortening causes movement of the bone or anything else to which the muscle is attached. Thus, the contraction of the biceps causes the forearm to move towards the arm.

In a hollow organ or tube the shortening of circular fibres narrows the lumen, or cavity, and by a rhythmical series of such contractions in the bowel the contents are pushed forward; contraction causes the emptying of such organs as the bladder or the gall bladder. Contraction of the heart fibres causes the emptying of the chamber round which the contracting fibres are spread.

It will be appreciated, therefore, that muscles perform a large volume of work. They are enabled to do this by the oxidation, or combustion, of sugar supplied to them by the blood, of which they receive a generous supply. But just as the combustion of fuel may not only supply energy for an engine, but also heat, so the combustion of sugar in a muscle liberates heat, so that blood coming from a muscle is hotter than that which goes into it. This, in fact, is the chief source of the heat of the body, and explains why a person who is cold desires to move about.

Fatigue supervenes sooner or later when a muscle is being continuously exercised, and is due rather to the

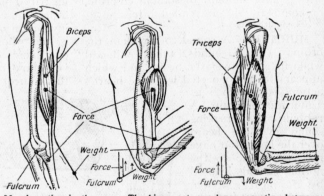

Muscle action in the arm. The biceps acts as a lever operating between the fulcrum (the elbow) and the weight. When the triceps is in action the fulcrum is interposed between the force and the weight

accumulation of waste products, and, notably, sarco-lactic acid, than to the using up of available fuel. Massage, by improving the circulation through a muscle and washing out this acid, helps to remove the sense of fatigue.

The nerve fibres coming to skeletal muscles are derived from cells in the grey matter of the spinal cord, and leave by the anterior root of a spinal nerve, while other fibres pass from the muscle into the spinal cord. The arrangement of these fibres is described under the heading Spinal Cord. The nerve supply of plain muscle is connected with the sympathetic nervous sytem (q.v.), while that of the heart is described under that heading.

Although an effort of will and a consequent impulse along a motor nerve is required to make a skeletal muscle come into action, there is some steady nervous influence constantly on the muscle, as this is always ready to contract, a state of preparedness described as tone. A nervous impulse to a muscle may have an inhibiting effect instead of an activating one. Thus, when one desires to bend the arm at the elbow, impulses must go along the nerves to the muscles on the front of the limb calling them into action, but other impulses must pass along nerves to muscles on the back of the limb, preventing contraction, and allowing them to stretch.

Besides controlling the movements of a muscle, the nerve cells in the spinal cord which send it the motor fibres also control its nutrition, and if the cells become diseased, or the fibres are cut, or cease to carry impulses, the muscle wastes or atrophies. In infantile paralysis, inflammation causes the destruction of such cells, and the wasting of the affected muscles may be very marked.

Injuries and Diseases of the Muscles. Overstretching of a muscle is described as a strain. There is pain and stiffness. The muscle should be rested, and, if necessary, hot or cold applications will relieve pain. Early massage and gentle movements are necessary. A muscle may be ruptured by violent stretching when it is contracted, or by a blow when it is in this condition. The severed fibres contract and leave a gap which is more evident if an effort is made to move the muscle, the severed ends gathering into knots. The limb should be placed in such a position as to put the muscle at rest and shorten it as much as possible. .

Thus, if the large muscle on the front of the thigh is ruptured, the limb should be straightened out and the foot elevated on a high pillow. It may be necessary for a doctor to cut down on the muscle, however, and fasten the ends together by stitching. If the sheath of a muscle be torn, the muscle tends to project through the rent, particularly when in action ; this is called a muscle hernia. The tendon of some muscles works along a definite groove, and it may chance that it becomes displaced from this groove through violence. This accident, which is popularly described as a " rick," causes pain and stiffness, and it may be possible to feel that the tendon is in an abnormal position. The malposition must be rectified by a doctor, and the limb kept at rest, probably from six to eight weeks. It may be necessary to operate, however.

Inflammatory Conditions of Muscles

Inflammation of a muscle, or myositis, may be due to one of the causes of inflammation (q.v.) in any situation, and if this cause be a microbe an abscess may result. The general symptoms and treatment of these conditions are described under their respective headings. A chronic myositis of a tuberculous nature is exemplified in a psoas abscess, and syphilis is another infective cause of chronic myositis. A long-continued and frequently repeated mechanical irritation of muscle or tendon may result in fibrosis and ossification of muscle ; rider's muscle is an instance of this. A rare disease in which there is a progressive ossification of muscles all over the body is called myositis ossificans ; its cause is unknown. The invasion of muscles by the trichina worm or by a hydatid also causes chronic inflammation. Muscular rheumatism is inflammation in the connective tissue mingled throughout a muscle—a fibrositis (q.v.).

It is not common for a tumour to originate in muscle, but a simple tumour, such as a lipoma or angioma, or a sarcoma, which is a malignant tumour, may do so. A tumour composed of muscle is called a myoma.

A painful spasm of a muscle is usually referred to as cramp (q.v.). Pain in a muscle without obvious signs of inflammation is spoken of as myalgia ; it is generally due to rheumatism. An intensive use of muscles leads to an increase in their size, or hypertrophy (q.v.). Disease, on the other hand, causes a diminution in size, or atrophy. As explained above, in connexion with the innervation of muscle, disease in the nerve cells controlling a muscle or interruption of the impulses through the nerve by cutting it or by disease, which is usually neuritis, also results in atrophy. There may be a progressive muscular atrophy involving all parts of the body. The disease known as pseudo-hypertrophic muscular paralysis is a primary disease of muscle, and is of a degenerative character. The hypertrophy is mainly due to a large accumulation of fat, the muscles themselves being very weak.

See Back-ache ; Cramp ; Fibrositis ; Hypertrophy ; Myasthenia ; Myopathy ; Progressive Muscular Atrophy ; Rheumatism ; Sprain ; Thomsen's Disease.

MUSCULO-SPIRAL NERVE. Derived from the brachial plexus of nerves in the neck, the musculo-spiral, or radial, nerve passes across the armpit into the arm, where it winds round the back and outer side of the humerus, dividing into two terminal branches in front of the external prominence of the lower end of the humerus.

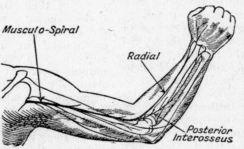

Musculo-spiral Nerve. Its course in the arm and wrist

The musculo-spiral nerve supplies the triceps and anconeus muscles, which straighten the forearm at the elbow, and, by one of its terminal branches, the muscles which extend the wrist and the fingers. The other terminal branch supplies sensation to the back of the thumb and of the index and middle, and the outer half of the ring, fingers.

Paralysis of the nerve may occur from pressure on the axilla, as in crutch paralysis, or by pressure on the back or outer side of the arm, as in the so-called Saturday-night paralysis. It may also be paralysis as a result of inflammation in the nerve from lead or other poisoning. One consequence of paralysis of this nerve is wrist drop.

See Crutch ; Median Nerve ; Ulnar Nerve.

MUSHROOM. See Fungus ; Poisoning.

MUSK. A dried secretion of the musk-deer, musk or moschus acts as a stimulant to the medulla, or bulb, of the brain and is sometimes used in prostration due to acute diseases. It is also an anti-spasmodic and has been used for obstinate

hiccough and other spasmodic affections. The dose is 5 to 10 grains. Synthetic substances are sold as artificial musk.

MUSSEL. Typhoid fever germs may be conveyed by mussels, though it has been found that if the shell-fish are put into pure sea-water they clear themselves of this infection within a fortnight. Poisoning of other kinds may be caused by mussels, however. Sometimes there is severe abdominal pain, with vomiting and diarrhoea, but in other people the symptoms are those of nervine poisoning ; there may be a sensation of heat, itching or prickling, difficulty in breathing, jerky movements of the limbs, especially the arms, muscular feebleness or paralysis and, perhaps, coma and death. Symptoms may come on early or be delayed for several hours, and a fatal result has sometimes occurred within two hours.

Mussels may be poisonous although they appear to be fresh enough, and, if so, cooking at home cannot be depended upon to make them safe. The first-aid treatment of poisoning is to put the patient to bed and keep him warm with hot-water bottles. If he has not vomited freely, and less than four hours has elapsed since taking the mussels, an emetic of mustard and water should be given, and when the patient has vomited he may be given 2 tablespoonsful of castor oil. Brandy and water, or, failing this, strong hot tea, should be given if there is collapse. Medical assistance should be summoned immediately poisoning is suspected.

MUSTARD. The familiar yellow mustard powder consists of mixed white and black mustard seeds which have been ground. The addition of water to this mustard leads to the formation of volatile oil of mustard, to the pungency of which the stimulating properties of mustard are due.

As a condiment it stimulates the flow of the salivary and gastric juices and so aids digestion. It will also dispel flatulence. But in large doses irritation of the stomach is such that mustard is an effective emetic, the dose for this purpose being a tablespoonful in a glass of water.

Mustard is much used as a counter-irritant, but the effect sought from it should be restricted to reddening of the skin, as the blisters and subsequent ulcers caused by mustard are difficult to heal.

The usual way to apply it is as the charta sinapis, or mustard paper, or by making a plaster. This is done by taking a tablespoonful of mustard, or more, according to the surface to be covered, and making it into a thin paste with cold water.

This is spread out thin on a piece of brown paper and covered with a layer of muslin or other thin fabric. It is left on for ten to twenty minutes, or until it has reddened the skin properly. For children the mustard should be mixed with an equal part or more of flour. When the plaster is removed the skin should be washed and dried gently. If this is not done the severer effects of the application may ensue.

When making a mustard poultice a paste should be made as above, and then mixed with the poultice formed by adding the boiling water to linseed. The liniment of mustard, which is made of oil of mustard, castor oil, camphor and alcohol, may be rubbed in for sprains, muscular rheumatism and similar purposes. A hot bath containing an ounce of mustard to the gallon is a common remedy for aborting a cold, relieving painful menstruation and other purposes.

From the essential oil of mustard is obtained a substance called thiosinamin, which has the property of removing an excess of cicatricial tissue. As fibrolysin, and in various combinations, it is injected hypodermically for strictures, lupus, keloid and other disorders. It must be used cautiously, however, as it may cause poisoning.

See Counter-irritant ; Poultice.

MUSTARD GAS. Dichlorethyl sulphide is an oily liquid which vaporises, the vapour being deadly if breathed for some time and also causing blistering of the skin. Hence, during the Great War this substance was referred to as mustard gas. It has been found that to have been gassed with this vapour does not create any special proclivity to consumption. Blisters should be dressed at once.

MUTISM. Dumbness, or mutism, occurs in those who are born deaf or become so in the early years of childhood, when the condition is referred to as deaf-mutism (*q.v.*). Brain disease of different kinds may also cause mutism. In some forms of insanity, such as dementia praecox, the patient remains mute, although there is the power of speech, and in hysteria, though the mechanism for speech is quite in order, there may be inability to use it at all, though more often the patient can speak in whispers. Psycho-therapy, if practised early, may cure the condition, otherwise it might last for years, speech sometimes being restored, however, by some emotional shock.

MYALGIA. Muscular rheumatism is sometimes called myalgia.
See Back-ache ; Fibrositis ; Rheumatism.

MYASTHENIA. As myasthenia is simply another name for muscle-weakness it might be applied to such weakness, whatever its cause, but the term is usually meant to imply a disease characterised by progressive weakness in muscles all over the body, the full name of which is myasthenia gravis.

This disease usually begins in the earlier years of adult life and the muscles of the face and eyes are generally the first affected ; then there is an extension to the trunk and limbs. There may be difficulty in keeping the eyes open and a tendency to squint, the lower jaw may tend to drop, and when the patient smiles the expression may appear to be sneering.

Chewing may be difficult and also swallowing.

Weakness in the arms may make it difficult for a woman to dress her hair without resting the elbows on something. It may be impossible to walk very far without taking a rest. The patient is always fresher in the morning, the expression being more alert, and muscular efforts may be performed apparently quite well. Also there are sometimes intermissions in the disease. For these reasons the nature of the condition is sometimes overlooked and the patient is supposed to be suffering from hysteria.

The cause of myasthenia gravis is not known and treatment is unsatisfactory, though life may be prolonged for years. There is a risk of laryngeal trouble and of death from asphyxia ; such an attack may occur quite early in the disease. The patient should receive the principal meal of the day in the morning, as chewing is easier then.

MYCETOMA. *See* Madura Foot.

MYCOSIS. The literal meaning of the term mycosis is infection of the body with some form of fungus (*q.v.*), which is a higher type of plant growth than bacteria. The disease which is most frequently referred to as mycosis, however, namely mycosis fungoides, is not caused by a fungus. This is indeed about all that can be said about its causation. It is a skin disease in which, after a first stage in which lesions resembling eczema occur, there is a second stage characterised by the appearance of tumours in the skin ; sometimes the tumours appear without a preceding eruption. The disease progresses to a fatal conclusion.

In the first stage there are usually red or livid circular or oval patches, which become scaly and are generally associated with great itching. They resist all efforts at treatment. The tumours are sometimes said to be tomato-like. They may break down and infection with bacteria then occurs, with consequent toxaemia.

The first stage usually lasts for several years but the disease may run its course in some months. Males are more frequently attacked, and usually when between forty and fifty years of age. The application of X-rays may mitigate the disease to some extent.

In the sense of being an infection with a fungus there are various mycoses which may occur on the skin or mucous surfaces of the body, or even in its deeper tissues and its organs, including ringworm and other skin diseases, thrush, actinomycosis and other disorders which are dealt with under separate headings. The leptothrix buccalis, a fungus found in the mouth, in some instances has caused the appearance of white patches in the throat, usually on the soft palate and uvula. These patches are easily detachable in contrast with white patches found on the tonsils and elsewhere in the throat in the disorder which was formerly known as pharyngomycosis leptothricia, though it is now known that such patches are due to an overgrowth of horny cells in the lining of the parts concerned and not to the invasion of a leptothrix or any other fungus.

Infection with the aspergillus fungus, or aspergillosis, is rare in man. The lungs are affected and the course of the disease resembles that of consumption.

MYDRIATIC. Excessive dilatation of the pupil is called mydriasis, and a drug which brings this about, a mydriatic. Atropine and homatropine are the drugs mostly used for this purpose.

See Eye ; Pupil.

MYELITIS. Certain inflammations and softening of the spinal cord are described as myelitis. Such changes may occur in connexion with an infectious fever, in syphilis, from the action of other poisons, probably bacterial, and from pressure on the cord through disease of the vertebrae or by tumours or thickenings within the spinal canal. Syphilis is the commonest cause.

When the whole thickness of the cord is involved the condition is called transverse myelitis. The symptoms will depend on the level at which the disease occurs, but when it is in the dorsal region, as most often happens, there is paralysis and wasting of the legs with loss of sensation, paralysis of the bladder and rectum, causing retention of urine or perhaps incontinence of urine and faeces, and, frequently, the appearance of bed sores. Higher up, the disease would involve the arms also and possibly cause vomiting, shortness of breath, hiccough and difficulty in swallowing.

If the disorder is diffused along the length of the cord the symptoms will appear with great rapidity, perhaps ushered in by convulsions, and death may occur in from five to ten days.

The possibility of pressure may be suggested by deformity of the spine, but in any case an X-ray examination would reveal anything of the kind. Extension of the spine when caries exists, or operation when a tumour or other mass can be removed, may be very beneficial, and also antisyphilitic treatment, should the existence of this disease be established. Otherwise, the most that can be done is to keep the patient at rest and take precautions against the formation of a bed sore (*q.v.*) and infection of the bladder.

See Paraplegia ; Poliomyelitis ; Spinal Cord.

MYELOMA. A tumour growing from the spongy tissue of a bone, a myeloma is found in young people, the commonest sites being the upper end of the tibia and the lower end of the femur. The growth of the tumour causes a thinning of the outer bony covering, and so there may be a sensation, called egg-shell crackling, imparted to the hand when examining the swelling. A myeloma is usually benign. It should be removed by operation.

See Tumour.

MYOCARDIUM. The heart wall is called the myocardium. Inflammation of the myocardium, or myocarditis, is likely to be associated with that of the inner lining, endocarditis, or of the outer lining, pericarditis, and consequent on such inflammation there may be myocardial degeneration. This, however, may occur from other causes, especially in elderly people. Interference with the blood supply from changes in the coronary arteries may lead to fibrosis (*q.v.*) in the myocardium. Fatty degeneration, or infiltration, are other possibilities, and, when there is chronic sepsis, amyloid degeneration. In any of these circumstances there is feebleness of the heart's action according to the extent of the degeneration.

See Heart.

MYOMA. A tumour composed of muscle is called a myoma. In the womb such a tumour may grow to a large size.

MYOPATHY. A progressive wasting in muscles due to some cause operating in the tissue itself is described as a myopathy or a primary dystrophy. The disease is usually hereditary, and, though boys are more affected, the inheritance is generally through the mother.

The disease may begin in the face, causing a constant smoothness of the brow and, from weakness of the muscles of the mouth, protrusion of the lips, the so-called tapir-mouth. In other instances the muscles of the shoulder girdle are first attacked. In still other instances there is an apparent overgrowth of certain muscles, those of the calves, of the

buttocks and others, while other muscles are notably atrophied. The enlargement of the muscles concerned is due to infiltration with fat, the muscle fibres themselves being atrophied and showing signs of degeneration.

This form of myopathy is called pseudo-hypertrophic muscular paralysis. When the disease begins it may be noted that the child has an uncertain gait, and stumbles easily. Then a waddling gait is developed, and when the disease is established the child has to adopt a particular method of getting up off the ground. It gets on its hands and feet, then brings its hands back and raises itself, so to speak, by climbing up its legs.

In this form life is rarely prolonged beyond the age of twenty ; the others have a rather more favourable prognosis. The general health should be maintained at as high a level as possible and massage and electrical treatment applied to the muscles. As time goes on the joints of the limbs tend to be flexed by contracture of the muscles. This should be prevented from occurring in awkward positions.

See Electricity in Medicine ; Massage : Muscle ; Progressive Muscular Atrophy.

MYOPIA. Short-sightedness is also called myopia. It is caused by undue lengthening of the eye from behind forwards and begins in childhood. Excessive use of the eyes on very fine work and wrong postures when engaged on such work are detrimental. Special classes for myopic children at school are desirable when at all practicable. Myopia is generally arrested by the age of twenty, but sometimes it increases, and there are degenerative changes in the retina and great impairment of vision.

See Eye ; Vision.

MYOSITIS. Inflammation of muscle (*q.v.*) is described as myositis.

MYOTIC. Excessive contraction of the pupil is called myosis, and a drug which causes contraction of the pupil, a myotic. The drugs of this class most often used are pilocarpine, the alkaloid in jaborandi leaves, and eserine or physostigmine, the alkaloid in Calabar beans.

See Eye ; Pupil.

MYRRH. A gum-resin, occurring in brownish-yellow or red drops or masses, myrrh is used as a carminative, an expectorant and in menstrual disorders. It is often used also in a mouth wash or a gargle. The dose of the tincture of myrrh is ½ to 1 drachm. The following is a useful formula for a mouth wash:

Tincture of myrrh	..	..	2 drachms
Borax..	..	..	.. 120 grains
Eau-de-Cologne	..	..	5 ounces

A teaspoonful in two tablespoonsful of water.

MYXOEDEMA. When the disease known as myxoedema has had time to develop, the appearances are quite characteristic. The skin is thickened and roughened, the features are coarsened, there is fullness of the eyelids, the complexion is sallow or muddy, except for a pink flush over the cheek-bones, the hair on the scalp and eyebrows is coarse and scanty and the hands are spade-like. Probably there are accumulations of fat above the collar-bones, in the breasts and in the abdominal wall. Speech and movements are slow and there is mental deterioration.

The swelling in myxoedema is not due to fluid in the tissues, as in ordinary oedema, but to the presence of a gelatinous-looking substance. This accumulation and the other symptoms of the disease are due to faulty metabolism occasioned by failure of the activity of the thyroid gland. The disease may begin in childhood, following an acute illness, but is usually found in elderly persons, and more frequently in women. Here, also, it may follow an acute illness, but more often comes on insidiously, apparently from a gradual exhaustion of the thyroid gland.

Many persons who do not manifest typical signs of myxoedema nevertheless show signs of an inefficient action of the gland.

The treatment for myxoedema, or for the less definite shades of thyroid inefficiency, is to administer the extract of the thyroid glands of lower animals, usually that of the sheep, beginning with small doses. The results appear to be miraculous, so great is the improvement in the appearance and mentality ; but the patient must continue to take the drug

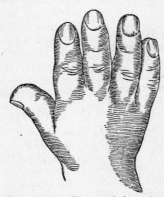

Myxoedema. Characteristic spade-like appearance of the hand

throughout life. Over-dosage must be avoided or unpleasant symptoms, such as palpitation, breathlessness, flushing or diarrhoea, may ensue.

See Endocrine ; Infantilism ; Thyroid Gland.

MYXOMA. A myxoma is a tumour composed of soft, mucous tissue, resembling that known as Wharton's jelly, which occurs in the umbilical cord. It may be found in the subcutaneous tissue, the brain, glands and elsewhere. The mucous tissue is often mixed with other tissues, such as cartilage, fibrous tissue and fat.

NAEVUS. Literally a birth mark (*q.v.*), the term naevus is generally reserved, however, for such marks when caused by an overgrowth or dilatation of blood vessels.

NAIL. A horny structure consisting of a thickening of the middle layer of the epidermis, a nail grows on true skin, somewhat modified from that found in the skin generally, and known as the bed of the nail. The root of the nail grows from a groove in the bed, the part from which it grows being called the matrix. Just in front of the root is a whitish semilunar area, known as the lunula, and covered by a thin membrane prolonged from the adjoining skin. Sometimes this membrane is dragged forward by the growing nail, and then becomes ruffled and detached in the form of tags, a condition described as hang-nail. The division between the tags may be carried back into the skin behind the nail, causing painful fissures, through which infection may occur.

When the membrane extends too far on to the nail, it should be pushed back, and redundant, loosened portions should be snipped off, but if there is no liability to hang-nail the membrane may well be left alone. Care should be taken to guard against infection of fissures on the skin about the root of the nail.

A septic infection at the root of the nail is called onychia. The matrix becomes converted into granulation tissue, from which comes a purulent discharge, and the overlying nail becomes separated. The loosened nail must be removed, and the unhealthy nail bed cleaned up. Poulticing may be necessary for the relief of pain.

When a nail has been struck or squeezed violently, it becomes dark purple or black. This is due to the effusion of blood beneath the nail, and it is likely that the nail will be detached from the bed. If there is severe pain, a doctor may be able to give relief by allowing the blood to escape. Splinters of wood, thorns, or other sharp objects are sometimes pushed up beneath the nail, and cause severe suffering. In order to extract the foreign body, it may be necessary to split the nail. When the foreign body has been taken out, the finger should be dressed antiseptically.

An ingrowing nail may occur in the foot, the nail of a great toe being most often affected. An over-tight boot is the main cause, by forcing the edge of the nail into the adjoining skin. This causes inflammation and ulceration, the unhealthy part sometimes being covered with proud flesh. A square-toed boot should be worn to give more room to the toes. The corner of the ingrowing nail should not be snipped off, as this leaves a sharp corner behind, but a little piece of cotton wool, covered with boracic acid powder, may be pressed up under the nail along the offending edge. It will be possible to push this further up each day, and thus the edge of the nail will be raised up. It may be necessary, however, to cut away a half, or the whole, of the nail and, possibly, diseased skin also.

A curious overgrowth, forming what is called a claw or ram's horn nail, sometimes occurs, almost always on the great-toe nail. The nail may be softened by

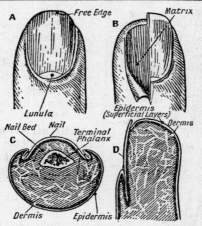

Nail. A, outer view. B, showing the folds of the matrix beneath the nail. C, cross section. D, longitudinal section

prolonged soaking, and the projections trimmed off, but to effect a cure the nail must be removed and the nail bed and matrix cauterised.

Acute fevers and other constitutional diseases may interfere with the growth of the nails and cause a transverse groove, which, however, moves downwards as the nail grows. The movement is a slow one, as the nail may take six months to grow its full length. White spots or "gifts" on the nails may also be caused by constitutional disturbances. Various skin diseases, such as ringworm, favus, psoriasis and eczema, may affect the nails, interfering with their growth and deforming them.

See Finger ; Toe.

NAPHTHOL. From naphthalene, a by-product of coal-tar and the substance contained in moth-balls, are prepared alpha and beta naphthol. The latter is used in medicine and is a white crystalline substance with an odour resembling that of carbolic acid. It is given inwardly as an antiseptic, in doses of 3 to 10 grains, in gastric fermentation and in typhoid and other infections of the bowel. Excessive doses cause symptoms like those of poisoning by carbolic acid (*q.v.*).

Externally it is used as an antiseptic and stimulant in scabies, eczema and other skin diseases, usually in an ointment containing 10 to 15 per cent. of the drug.

NARCOLEPSY. Sudden and irresistible attacks of deep sleep, described as narcolepsy, may occur in people suffering from certain brain diseases, disorders of the internal secretions or endocrines (*q.v.*), and other organic diseases. They may occur apart from anything of this kind, however, as hysterical or epileptic phenomena. The sleep may last from a few minutes to some hours. The general health may be otherwise good.

NARCOTIC. A drug that produces profound unconsciousness, following a stage of excitement, is described as a

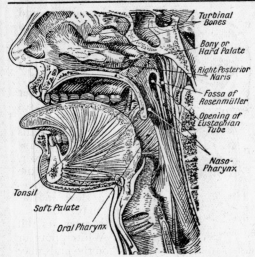

Naso-pharynx.   Its relation to the mouth and nose

narcotic. Amongst the narcotics are included opium, Indian hemp, alcohol, and the general anaesthetics, chloroform and ether.

See Hypnotic.

NASAL FEEDING. *See* Forcible Feeding.

NASO-PHARYNX. The portion of the pharynx behind the nose is called the naso-pharynx. When one breathes through the nose this space communicates freely with the space below it and behind the mouth, but during swallowing or vigorous breathing through the mouth the communication is blocked by the ascent of the soft palate, which then becomes the floor of the naso-pharynx.

The roof is formed by the base of the skull, the posterior wall by the uppermost two cervical vertebrae, and in the anterior wall are the two posterior nares, through which there is communication with the nose (*q.v.*). In each lateral wall is the inner opening of the Eustachian tube.

There is a considerable amount of lymphoid tissue in the mucous

membrane lining this cavity, particularly in the roof, posterior wall, and around the openings of the Eustachian tubes. Inflammatory overgrowths of this tissue constitute adenoids (*q.v.*). A fibroma is sometimes found growing from the roof of the naso-pharynx; when large, it interferes with swallowing.

See Nose ; Palate ; Pharynx.

NAUHEIM TREATMENT. The method of treating heart diseases by a combination of special exercises and baths, originated at Nauheim in Germany, is practised at Bath, Buxton, Harrogate, Strathpeffer and other British spas. The baths contain certain mineral salts and are aerated with carbonic acid gas.

See Heart.

NAUSEA. A feeling of sickness or an inclination to vomit, with a loathing for food, is described as nausea. It may arise from various disorders of the digestive tract or of other organs. It may be provoked by unpleasant sights and smells, or even by the remembrance of these.

See Sea-sickness ; Vomiting.

NAVEL. The separation of the umbilical cord (*q.v.*) leaves a puckered scar, known as the navel or umbilicus.

See Hernia.

NEBULISER. *See* Atomiser.

NECK. In the skeleton the neck is represented by a column composed of the seven cervical vertebrae, but in the clothed skeleton this column is strengthened by strong muscles, which also carry out the movements of the head. Two of these muscles, the sterno-mastoid, stand out prominently on either side of the neck, especially in muscular men ; in women the neck is rounded off, as a rule, by subcutaneous fat. This may be overdeveloped in stout people of either sex, and is the cause of a double chin.

Just beneath and attached to the skin on either side of the neck is

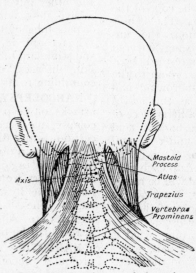

Neck.   Position of the cervical vertebrae

a thin sheet of muscle, the platysma myoides, which represents the muscle beneath the skin all over the body in lower animals, whereby the skin may be twitched and flies driven off. Beneath the skin there are also veins; these are described under the heading Jugular Vein.

In the front of the neck from above downwards are the hyoid bone, the larynx and the trachea. In front, and on either side, of the upper part of the trachea is the thyroid gland. Behind these structures are the lower part of the pharynx, and part of the gullet, or oesophagus, and on either side of the digestive tract there is a fibrous sheath containing the carotid artery and internal jugular vein, and behind and between these the vagus nerve.

From the spinal nerves emerging in the neck are formed two plexuses, the cervical and the brachial. One of the nerves from the former, the phrenic, passes down on either side to supply the corresponding side of the diaphragm. Branches from the brachial plexus supply the upper extremity. In some people an additional rib may extend out from the seventh cervical vertebra, and sometimes also from the sixth one. The branches of the brachial plexus may be stretched

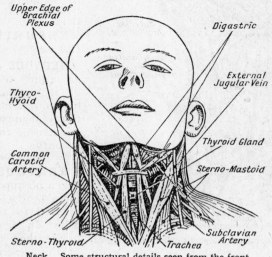

Neck. Some structural details seen from the front

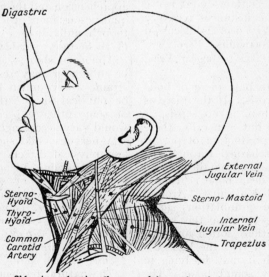

Side view, showing the powerful muscles of the neck

over such cervical ribs, and pain, wasting and weakness of the limb may be caused in this way. The subclavian artery may also be pushed up and suggest an aneurysm at the root of the neck.

In the neck are several groups of lymphatic glands, and a swelling in the neck in young people is generally due to inflammation of these glands. A swelling may also be due to a branchial cyst which is formed from a space persisting from one of the branchial, or gill, clefts found in the embryo; the space may even open on the surface of the neck, constituting a branchial fistula. An extensive swelling of the neck may be caused by inflammation in the loose tissue between the different layers of structures, that is to say, a cellulitis, which is likely to be associated with abscess formation.

In this circumstance the pus does not escape readily, as the neck is enclosed by a sheet of fascia, and is, moreover, divided into compartments by sheets of fascia passing across the neck; an abscess may therefore be diverted down into the mediastinum (*q.v.*). One of these sheets lies in front of the vertebral column, and an abscess behind this, which is usually tuberculous and connected with

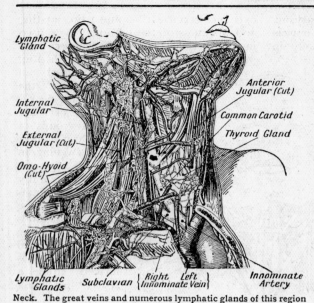

Neck. The great veins and numerous lymphatic glands of this region

Labels on image: Lymphatic Gland; Internal Jugular; External Jugular (Cut); Omo-Hyoid (Cut); Lymphatic Glands; Subclavian; Right Left {Innominate Vein}; Innominate Artery; Anterior Jugular (Cut); Common Carotid; Thyroid Gland

the bodies of the vertebrae, may not burst forward into the pharynx, but be guided by the fascia out to the side of the neck.

A broken neck is almost sure to be fatal, owing to the proximity of the bulb of the brain, which contains vital nerve centres, but in some instances recovery has taken place. Wry neck is discussed under the heading Torticollis.

See Goitre ; Hyoid Bone ; Jugular Vein ; Spine ; Thyroid Gland.

NECROSIS. Death of a piece of bone is described as necrosis. If the piece is quite small, and there is no sepsis, it may be absorbed, but generally there is sepsis, with the production of pus or matter which is discharged through the skin. The passage leading from the opening on the skin to the dead bone is usually narrow, and is called a sinus. Around the piece of bone granulations (*q.v.*) form, and separate it from the sound bone. The granulations soften and disappear in the pus, so that the bone becomes loose, though it may be lying in a cavity formed by sound bone. The loose piece of dead bone is called a sequestrum. So long as it persists, there is likely to be a discharge from the wound ; even should the discharge dry up for some months it will reappear. The seques-

trum must therefore be removed, though to accomplish this it may be necessary to cut in through the sound bone.

See Bone ; Caries ; Erosion ; Gangrene.

NEPHRITIS. *See* Bright's Disease.

NERVOUS BREAKDOWN. According to the popular use of the expression, a nervous breakdown may mean anything from neurasthenia or some other neurotic state to actual insanity.

See Mental Disease ; Neurosis.

NERVOUS HEADACHE. When no apparent reason exists for a headache it is sometimes referred to as a nervous headache. In neurasthenia, for example, there may be a headache of this description. A search for some definite cause should always be made, however, before labelling a headache as nervous.

NERVOUSNESS. Different characteristics are popularly described as nervousness : shyness and timidity, excitability, apprehension and the anxiety state. These qualities are more or less related, however, though individuals exhibit one or other of them more particularly.

Abnormal shyness or excitability may be inborn or may result from excessive strain, worry, much excitement, mental or physical shock, the abuse of drugs or some other experience ; the remedy would vary accordingly.

A nervous child should be overhauled and physical defects put right ; it may be eye strain, adenoids, worms, commencing chorea or something else.

When the disposition is nervous the fact that there is no discoverable cause of this kind is no reason for regarding the child as capable of living the life of ordinary children or of attempting to bully it into doing so.

The natural tendency of ordinary children to tease a sensitive, diffident child and make its life a misery should be borne in mind, and any risk of the sort should be avoided in the choice of a school and otherwise. At the same time a hot-house existence is undesirable, and the child should be encouraged to exercise freely in the open air and to mix with children who are congenial to it. A child should not be forced to sleep in the dark or do anything else that terrifies it. A sense of confidence may be fostered, but it cannot be forced.

See Anxiety; Freudism; Hypochondriasis; Neurosis.

NERVOUS SYSTEM. Under their own headings accounts are given of the brain and the spinal cord, which together with their nerves form the central nervous system, and of the sympathetic nervous system; also of disorders that affect them. Here it is proposed to take a general survey of the nervous system, the principles of its construction and of the working of its various parts, the morbid changes that occur in nervous tissue and the alterations of function resulting from these.

Nerve cells, with their fibres, are the units of the nervous system. These are of various shapes and sizes, but each consists of a mass of protoplasm, the body of the cell, containing a nucleus and a long, slender prolongation outwards of its substance, known as the axon, which forms the conducting part of a nerve fibre. Most of the cells have also other processes connected with their body, relatively short and with numerous branches. These are called dendrons, or dendrites, and do not conduct impulses away from the cell, as the axon in general does, but into the cell. They may also have to do with the nutrition of the cell.

The axon is known as the axis cylinder in a nerve fibre, and is covered with a thin sheath, the primitive sheath, or neurilemma, but many of the nerves have, in addition, within this sheath, a coating of a complex fatty substance,

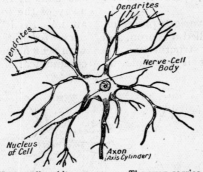

Nerve cell and its processes. The axon carries impulses from the cell; the dendrites to it

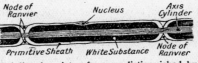

Medullated variety of nerve, distinguished by the white sheath (here darkly stained)

which is known as the white or medullary sheath. This sheath is interrupted, however, at intervals, such points being described as the nodes of Ranvier. Nerves with a white sheath are called medullated nerves, the others, non-medullated. When many medullated nerves are massed together in the brain or spinal cord they form what is called white matter.

Grey matter, on the other hand, consists mainly of nerve cells and non-medullated fibres. In the brain and spinal cord the cells and fibres are supported by a peculiar tissue known as neuroglia, in which are numerous cells with small bodies and a large number of radiating processes, and known as spider cells.

Metabolic changes in the body of a nerve cell can produce a current of energy along the nerve that springs from it, and this may excite movement in a muscle, activity of a gland and so on. The nature of this energy, which is termed nerve impulse, is not known, but, although it possesses certain analogies to electrical energy, it is not an electric current. For one thing, it travels more slowly than the latter. The rate of travel, it may be noted in passing, is faster in a medullated than in a non-medullated nerve.

An electric shock will, however, provoke a current of nerve impulse in a nerve, as will thermal, chemical or mechanical stimulation, and the impulse may go in either direction, up or down a nerve. Normally, however, the impulse will only flow in one direction. In one nerve it flows towards the nerve centres and is called an afferent nerve, in another it flows away from the cell and is called an efferent nerve. A motor nerve, that is, one activating muscle, is efferent, a sensory nerve is afferent. A peculiar effect of an

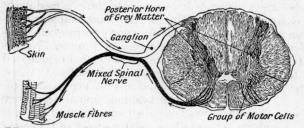

Efferent nerve. The fibres shown here in black carry impulses from the spinal cord to a muscle fibre, and are termed efferent

impulse along an efferent nerve is not activation of anything but the reverse, inhibition or restraint of activity; this power may be called into operation as and when required.

A nerve cell with its various processes, axon and dendron, is called a neuron, and a characteristic of the structure of the nervous system is that it is made up of relays of neurons. The large cells in the cortex of the brain which originate voluntary movements, for example, are not directly in contact with the muscles, but the terminations of their axons come into relationship with other nerve cells in what is called the anterior horn of the grey matter in the spinal cord, and it is the axons of the latter cells that actually come into contact with the muscles, through structures, known as end-plates, on the fibres of a muscle.

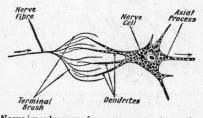

Nerve impulses pass from one neuron to another through the intertwined terminal tendrils

The brain cell with its processes is called the upper motor neuron, and the spinal cord with its processes the lower motor neuron. An impulse in the upper is communicated to the lower neuron, and thus a muscle is called into action. But, when necessary, an impulse in the upper may inhibit the activity of the lower neuron, either altogether or partially.

One neuron is not actually joined to another but effects a communica-

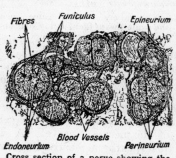

Cross section of a nerve showing the coverings of the fibres

tion through its axon, at its termination, breaking up into fine tendrils, forming a sort of brush; these tendrils surround the cell body of the second neuron or, at any rate, intertwine with its dendrons. Such an arrangement is described as a synapse.

The simplest form of nervous activity occurs in what is called reflex action. If the sole of the foot of a sleeping person is pricked the foot is drawn away, although the person may be unconscious either of the pain of the prick or of the drawing away of the foot. What happens is that an impulse is carried along an afferent nerve to motor cells in the spinal cord with which the fibres of the nerve are in communication by synapses. The cells are provoked to activity and in their turn cause a movement of the muscles to draw away the foot.

This movement is co-ordinated and purposive. It is meant to withdraw the foot from what is hurting it, but it is not voluntary. If the person were awake he would be aware of what is taking place and would probably also withdraw his foot, the withdrawal taking place unless the person willed strongly that it should not do so.

Reflex actions of many kinds, such, for example, as the blinking of an eye, the movements of the intestines, the secretion of saliva and changes in the size of the pupil, are always going on more or less. In numerous instances there are chains of reflex actions, one setting another in motion. Some of the instances of such action are very complicated, and when one moves into the psychical sphere it will be observed that impulsive acts partake largely of this character. Even inhibition may be reflex, as when, for example, the muscles which bend an arm are at work it is necessary that those which straighten it should be relaxed, this being brought about by reflex action.

Reflex action was at one time spoken of as sympathetic action, and therefore the name sympathetic system was applied to those ganglia, or masses of nerve cells, which, with their fibres, appeared to control the activities of the internal organs, the dilatation and contraction of blood vessels, and so on. Whether the cells in the sympathetic ganglia can act as true reflex centres is doubtful, however, though it is possible.

A nerve consists of bundles, or funiculi, of nerve fibres. The whole nerve is surrounded by a sheath of connective tissue, the epineurium, and there is also connective tissue, the perineurium, between the funiculi and even, the endoneurium, between the fibres. A nerve is supplied with blood vessels, with lymphatics and with nerves of its own. A nerve may be purely afferent, purely efferent or be mixed. The optic nerve, for example, is purely afferent, the 3rd cranial nerve purely efferent ; but the 5th cranial nerve is mixed, having both afferent and efferent fibres.

Injuries and Diseases of the Nerves. If a nerve be divided, the part which is separated from the nerve cells undergoes changes, referred to as Wallerian degeneration. The axis cylinder and the white sheath break up and are absorbed, but the primitive sheaths of the fibres remain alive. The regeneration of the nerve is made possible by two circumstances. In the first place, new nerve fibres grow out from the divided end which is still connected with the nerve cells, and, in the second place, the survival of the primitive

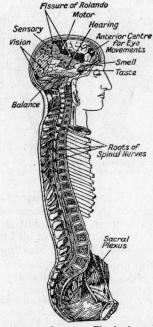

Nervous System. The brain and spinal cord, with their nerves, form the central nervous system

sheaths in the other portion of the nerve provides a scaffolding along which the new fibres may grow. Regeneration may not take place, however, if the space between the divided ends is too wide, or if they are separated by scar tissue. When it does take place it is many months before it is complete, though the time varies for different nerves. Division of fibres within the brain and spinal cord is not followed by regeneration.

The activity of nerve cells may be diminished by certain drugs, bromides, for example, and can be increased by others, such as strychnine. Similar effects are produced by the toxins of various bacteria. If a poison is sufficiently virulent the nerve cells may actually be killed. Nervous tissue may also be damaged by physical or other kinds of violence.

Inflammation in grey nervous matter is associated with dilatation of blood vessels, exudation of lymph and possibly overgrowth of the connecting substance, so that the nerve cells are damaged by compression, apart from any damage caused by the toxins which may be responsible for the inflammation. If these damaging causes are removed sufficiently early the nerve cell may recover, and its function, which was weakened for the time being, may be regained. If the nerve cell is destroyed, however, it cannot be replaced, a fact exemplified in infantile paralysis (q.v.).

An overgrowth of the supporting tissue in the brain or spinal cord, whether due to chronic inflammation or to degeneration of the nervous tissue proper from other causes, is called sclerosis.

In a nerve also inflammation may similarly cause pressure or the nerve fibres may be affected by poisoning, with impairment or actual loss of function. Sometimes the whole nerve is converted into a mere fibrous cord. Nervous tissue may be damaged also by pressure from tumours within it or from tumours or other swellings of adjoining structures.

A poverty of the general nutrition may weaken nervous tissue, though in prolonged starvation it is the tissue which suffers last of all. Deprivation of the blood supply, however, from blocking of the arteries causes a degenerative softening of nervous tissue. The metabolism of nerve cells may also be affected by disorders of the endocrine (*q.v.*) glands.

The symptoms of nervous disorder depend upon the situation of the mischief and upon whether the irritability of the nerve cell is increased, lessened or destroyed, or upon whether or not the conductivity of nerve fibres is maintained.

Disease of the upper motor neuron, if irritative, leads to spasms of the muscles supplied by the affected cells, and possibly general convulsions ; if depressive it leads to weakness or loss of voluntary movements, reflex actions being preserved and, in fact, exaggerated ; the muscles are in a stiff or spastic condition and their nutrition is maintained, apart from the consequences of disuse. An irritative lesion of the lower motor neuron also causes spasm, but a destruction of the nerve cells leads to loss not only of voluntary but of reflex movements, and the muscles waste because good nutrition of the muscles depends on the integrity of these nerve cells.

The effects of irritation of sensory centres in the brain has not been so definitely marked out as those of the motor centres. Destruction of the centres causes paralysis of sensation, and this follows also if the sensory tracts in the brain and cord are affected. As, however, the various kinds of sensation, tactile, heat, pain and so on, run in different tracts in the cord, there may be a loss of

Muscular Branches

Branches to Skin

Nervous System. Here is shown the abundant nerve supply to muscles and skin

some kinds of sensation but not of others. In some instances of disorder of the sensory nerves or tracts there are alterations of sensation, or paraesthesia (*q.v.*).

The cortex of the brain exercises a controlling influence over cells in the optic thalamus, as regards sensation, for if certain fibres passing from the cortex to the thalamus are blocked by disease there is a great increase in the intensity of sensations, whether pleasurable or not.

Diseases affecting the bulb of the brain are very dangerous, as here are the affecting centres for the heart, respiration and blood pressure, in addition to others for various important functions.

Disease of a mixed nerve may cause pain, but if the nerve is blocked there is loss of all kinds of sensation and paralysis and wasting of muscles. There is also atrophy of other tissues, such as the skin and its appendages, the hairs and nails.

See Ataxia ; Brain ; Disseminated Sclerosis ; Friedreich's Ataxia ; Infantile Paralysis ; Neuralgia ; Neuritis ; Paralysis ; Parkinson's Disease ; Sciatica ; Sensation ; Spinal Cord ; Sympathetic Nervous System.

NETTLE-RASH. In the skin disorder known as urticaria, or nettle-rash, there is a sudden appearance of white or pink elevations on the skin. Such elevations are termed wheals and may also be caused by insect stings or by nettles. Probably there is preliminary itching, but, in any case, the presence of wheals is accompanied by a sensation of violent itching, tingling or burning.

Only one or two wheals may appear, or they may affect a considerable area of skin, the commonest sites being the buttocks and the front or back of the chest. Wheals may also form on mucous membranes. As a rule, the wheals disappear in an hour or two, but they may last much longer and then leave some pigmentation of the skin. In a type of the disorder called urticaria pigmentosa, the wheals are more or less persistent and are pigmented.

During the course of nettle-rash, scratching or rubbing the skin tends to bring out wheals.

Sometimes nettle-rash is preceded by digestive disturbances, and in some cases there is a definite connexion between the skin manifestations and the ingestion of fish, strawberries, or less frequently eggs, meat of some particular kind or some cereal food. That is to say, the disorder may be of the nature of anaphylaxis (*q.v.*). If, therefore, nettle-rash is chronic, a search should be made for some food to which the patient is sensitised. Test outfits for this purpose are used by doctors.

When nettle-rash occurs, if the patient knows that he has taken something which has been responsible for a previous attack, it will be worth while to empty the stomach by giving an emetic. In any case, the bowels should be cleansed by giving a dose of castor oil or salts, and it may be well to take a course of alkalies. A heaped teaspoonful of the following powder might be taken three times daily in a little milk :

Sodium bicarbonate..	6 drachms
Bismuth carbonate	4 ,,
Magnesium carbonate	8 ,,

A dusting powder containing zinc oxide, or a weak lotion of vinegar, warmed, or some other sedative lotion may be used.

There is a form of the disease called giant urticaria, or angio-neurotic oedema, in which large swellings form, usually on the face, the only sensory disturbance being perhaps a little warmth. If the swelling should occur in the larynx there would be grave danger of choking. The causes and treatment are the same as those of the ordinary type of urticaria.

One of the varieties of the so-called gum-rash which affects young children is known as lichen urticatus, strophulus, and by other names. It is a disease similar to urticaria. The trunk and limbs, especially the legs, are the chief sites of the eruption, but it may also occur on the face and scalp.

Little pimples about the size of a pin's head make their appearance, each being surrounded by a zone of reddened skin. In the centre of the pimples there may be a little blister, which ultimately forms a crust. The blisters have sometimes a resemblance to those of chicken-pox. There is intense itching, worse when the child is warm in bed, and the rash may be complicated by the presence of scratch marks and blood crusts. Crops of the pimples come out every two or three days, and this may go on for three to five weeks, or longer.

The diet must be scrutinised and anything obviously unsuitable eliminated. The regularity of the bowels should be maintained, say with liquid magnesia ; one grain of grey powder every two to three days is often useful. The affected parts may be sponged with a lotion consisting of two parts of warm water and one part of vinegar, or this lotion may be improved by adding a little spirit of camphor. A paste consisting of equal parts of zinc oxide, talc, soft paraffin and lanolin may be applied if necessary. If the vesicles become filled with matter an ointment of equal parts of white precipitate ointment and soft paraffin is useful.

It is sometimes possible to make wheal-like marks on a person's skin with a blunt pencil or something of the kind. Broad red lines appear along the track of the pencil, and in a moment or two a white, elevated line. This is spoken of as dermography. Though it resembles urticaria it is quite different, though it also depends on a vasomotor disturbance. This in turn may depend on a neurosis, alcoholism, epilepsy, or some disturbance of the endocrine glands or some other cause. The marks last from fifteen to twenty minutes and leave no trace on disappearing. Treatment should be directed to the cause in each case.

See Lichen ; Prickly Heat.

NEURALGIA. Paroxysmal pains of a stabbing, darting or burning character, occurring along the course of a nerve in which no structural changes could be recognized, even with a microscope, are described as neuralgia. The paroxysms may occur every few minutes or at longer intervals, even many weeks. The pain gradually becomes worse during a paroxysm until it reaches its acme, when as a rule it fades away, but sometimes intolerable pain may last for a long time.

A sensation of tingling or numbness may precede the pain, and sometimes redness or other changes in the skin over the affected nerve accompanies it. There are tender spots, usually where the nerve becomes superficial.

Anaemia or the presence of poisons in the blood, as in the infectious fevers, malaria, gout, rheumatism or diabetes, creates a liability to neuralgia, but often there is a local source of irritation which might cause neuralgia even without any constitutional disturbance. Carious teeth, eye trouble or disease in the throat, nose or ears, for example, may provoke neuralgia in some branch of the fifth cranial nerve, and the pressure of a cervical rib might cause neuralgia in the arm. In some instances an hereditary predisposition is an important factor in causing neuralgia.

It should be borne also in mind that pain of a neuralgic character may occur in inflammation of the nerves or nerve roots.

Neuralgia may be classified according to the nerve affected. Thus, for example, there is supraorbital neuralgia, trigeminal neuralgia, intercostal neuralgia or pleurodynia, occipital neuralgia, coccydinia, metatarsalgia, sciatica and visceral neuralgia, including stomach-neuralgia or gastralgia, kidney-neuralgia or nephralgia, and so on.

The immediate treatment of neuralgia consists in applying hot or cold applications and if necessary giving aspirin, phenacetin or some similar drug. Counter-irritation by a mustard plaster, a blister or some other means may be tried, but the application should not be made over the painful part but at some little distance

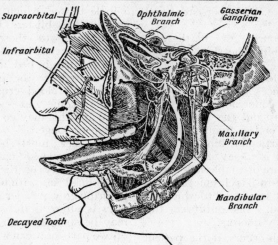

Neuralgia. Pain from a tooth in the lower jaw may be felt in the forehead or above the cheek-bone, being transferred by branches of the trigeminal nerve and the Gasserian ganglion

from it. A search must be made, however, for any constitutional or local cause. The extraction of a bad tooth, for example, or the provision of spectacles may work a cure, or, on the other hand, a course of iron in anaemia or a vegetarian diet for the gouty.

Electrical methods, ultra-violet rays and hot-air baths are used in treatment, and sometimes ionisation is successful when other methods have failed. Sometimes the method of nerve-stretching is adopted, the nerve being cut down upon for the purpose.

See Gasserian Ganglion; Neuritis; Tic Douloureux; Toothache; Veratrine.

NEURASTHENIA. The significant thing in neurasthenia is the poverty of mental and physical vigour, an incapacity for effort. The sense of incapacity may be constant, but some neurasthenics look fit enough, and may get to work quite briskly, only to find, however, that their energy is soon exhausted. Concentration on work cannot be sustained for any length of time, if at all, and efforts in this direction cause much discomfort. The sense of tiredness induced by attempts at thinking is often referred to as brain fag.

Headache is a usual accompaniment, and takes the form of a dull pressure, which has been likened to the sensation of wearing a leaden cap. Sleeplessness is common. The patient has difficulty in rousing in the morning and rises unrefreshed. Digestion is sometimes poor, and there may be a tendency to palpitation and giddiness. There may be a difficulty in holding the urine, and some neurasthenics may complain of a sexual disability. A pain in the back is not uncommon, and there may be a feeling of weakness in the legs.

Symptoms such as these may occur after an acute illness, notably influenza, but they also occur independently of any other disease, and it is then that the appellation neurasthenia is properly applicable. The cause here is sometimes said to be overwork, worry, or sexual excesses. Some persons, however, inherit but a scanty reserve of nervous energy, and in them neurasthenia may be readily induced. More men than women suffer from neurasthenia, but the number of women is considerable. The disorder may sometimes be found even in children.

Obsessions and phobias, or morbid fears, sometimes occur in neurasthenia, especially when it has lasted for some time.

It may require a careful examination to eliminate the possibility of symptoms suggestive of neurasthenia being actually due to some latent disease, such as consumption, malignant disease, or diabetes, but a sound opinion can be given as to the existence of these or other organic diseases, and the patient be relieved of groundless fears.

In treatment it is necessary to build up the general health. If the disorder is severe, rest is necessary, and the best way of obtaining this may be a course of Weir-Mitchell treatment (*q.v.*). In mild cases, however, an agreeable occupation in some kind of creative work is preferable. Relapses are prone to occur, and the outlook is worse if the disease has been of slow and gradual development.

Traumatic neurasthenia is rather of the nature of hysteria (*q.v.*) than of neurasthenia as properly understood. Psychotherapy is essential to its adequate treatment.

See Anxiety ; Auto-intoxication ; Hysteria ; Neurosis.

NEURITIS. Inflammation of a nerve, or neuritis, may be limited to one nerve, or affect several, when it is referred to as multiple neuritis. If it is a purely motor nerve there may be cramps to begin with and then weakness ; actual paralysis is not common when a single nerve is damaged, but does occur, as in facial, or Bell's, paralysis. There may be also marked wasting of muscles concerned. If the nerve is purely sensory there may be pain,

sometimes referred to the nerve-endings, tenderness along the source of the nerve, tingling, numbness, and loss of the sense of touch and of temperature and pain.

When a mixed nerve is affected there is a combination of such effects, and there may be interference with the skin glands, causing dryness, glossiness of the skin, and other trophic changes. Neuritis in a single nerve may be due to injury, cold, inflammation in adjoining parts, or some constitutional disorder, such as influenza, syphilis, rheumatism or gout.

Poisoning a Source of Neuritis

Multiple neuritis, which usually affects the limbs and occurs on both sides, is due to some kind of general poisoning. This may be lead, alcohol, arsenic, or, more rarely, a similar poison ; or it may be the poison of some infectious disorder, such as diphtheria, influenza, malaria, typhoid fever, leprosy, and so on. In other instances the cause is a poison due to some disturbance of metabolism, as in diabetes, anaemia and beri-beri, which is a disease caused by a vitamin defect.

These various poisons show a certain selective tendency. Thus diphtheria commonly affects the nerves of the soft palate, and lead involves motor fibres but spares sensory. Alcoholic neuritis is more common in women and in those who drink spirits regularly than in those who have bouts of spirit-drinking or are regular users of beer or wines. Foot drop is common, and occasions a high-steppage gait to clear the toes from the ground. Painful cramps are also common. Mental symptoms may also appear, as explained under the heading Mental Disease. Arsenical neuritis may follow a large dose of the drug, but is usually due to a prolonged ingestion of minute doses.

Recovery from neuritis may take from one or two months to many, and is sometimes incomplete. In some forms, such as diphtheria and beri-beri, there is a danger to life.

The treatment of neuritis must include that of the cause, but, apart from this, is much the same in any instance. Rest is very important, and unless in slight cases is best taken in bed. Hot fomentations assist resolution of the inflammation and relieve pain, though aspirin, phenacetin, or similar drugs, or sometimes opiates, may be required. When the acute stage has passed, massage should be begun. In some cases special methods, such as diathermy, light-therapy, and electrical stimulation are of great service.

See Nervous System ; Sciatica.

NEUROMA. A tumour connected with a nerve is called a neuroma. Most neuromata contain a considerable amount of ordinary connective tissue.

NEURON. A nerve cell together with its various processes constitutes a neuron ; this is the unit of nervous structure.

See Nervous System.

NEUROSIS. A nervous disorder which is unaccompanied by structural changes in the nerve tissue to account for it is termed a neurosis. It is also said to be a functional nervous disease as distinguished from an organic disease, that is, one in which there is inflammation, degeneration or some other morbid alteration of tissue.

The neuroses comprise the neuroses proper, the causes of which are fatigue, under-nutrition, toxaemia or something else of a physical nature, and the psycho-neuroses, in which the cause is entirely mental. Though such a distinction can be recognized in the causation of the two groups of disorders, there is no such difference in the character of the morbid processes resulting from these causes. Whether it is a neurosis or a psycho-neurosis it is a mental disorder.

The neuroses proper are neurasthenia, or fatigue neurosis, anxiety neurosis and hypochondria ; and the psycho-neuroses are hysteria, including the conversion and the anxiety forms of this disease, and obsessional, or compulsive, neurosis. An occupational neurosis, such as writer's cramp, is akin to a psycho-neurosis, and so also what is called a traumatic neurosis, or traumatic neurasthenia, as a disorder of this kind is hysterical in nature.

A neurosis may be curable by physical methods, rest, tonics, massage and so on, but a psycho-neurosis can only be satisfactorily dealt with by some kind of psycho-therapy.

A fuller account of these disorders is given under individual headings. A person who suffers from a functional nervous disease, or who seems to possess a tendency in this direction, may be said to be neurotic.

See Freudism ; Mental Disease ; Obsession ; Psycho-therapy.

NEW SKIN. A proprietary preparation known as New Skin has similar uses to collodion (*q.v.*) in sealing up clean cuts and abrasions.

NICTITATION. Involuntary winking, or nictitation, may occur in chorea, hysteria and other nervous disorders. It may be set up reflexly by teething, worms, etc. A foreign body in the eye or conjunctivitis may initiate what is called the blinking tic, which goes on long after the cause has disappeared.

See Tic.

NIDUS. Literally meaning a nest, the term nidus is used for a focus of infection or for any substance, such as blood-clot or dead tissue, which is prone to harbour bacteria and promote their multiplication, and thus become an infective focus.

NIGHTMARE. In adults the kind of dream described as a nightmare is usually due to a heavy meal taken late at night, especially if indigestible foods, such as lobster, cucumber or something of the sort, have been included. Those who have suffered from any terrifying experiences may have such dreams, however, apart from any exciting cause ; the so-called war dreams are not uncommon experiences, for example.

Similar causes may operate in the case of children, but in them adenoids, intestinal worms or febrile disorders are frequently found to be responsible. Children who have a neurotic ancestry are especially liable to such dreams, which may sometimes be such as to deserve the description night terrors. In such children also over-pressure at school may be sufficient to cause these alarming experiences.

See Dreams.

NITRATE. A salt formed by nitric acid and a base is called a nitrate. In medicine the nitrates in common use are potassium nitrate, or nitre, and silver nitrate, or lunar caustic.

See Potassium ; Silver.

NITRIC ACID. By the interaction of sodium nitrate and sulphuric acid one obtains nitric acid, which is a colourless liquid. It fumes when its vapour passes into moist air. What is called "fuming" nitric acid is a brown liquid and contains nitrogen tetroxide in solution. Both forms of the acid have a corrosive action and are employed for destroying warts and other unhealthy tissue. If taken internally they act as a corrosive poison.

Dilute nitric acid is sometimes used for some kinds of dyspepsia and dilute nitro-hydrochloric acid also, a combination of nitric and hydrochloric acids which has been kept sufficiently long to allow of the liberation of a considerable amount of free chlorine gas. The dilute nitro-hydrochloric acid is credited with a stimulating action on the liver. Its dose is 5 to 20 minims and that of dilute nitric acid the same.

NITRITE. A salt formed with nitrous acid is called a nitrite, and differs from a nitrate in containing an atom less of oxygen. Nitrites cause relaxation of plain muscle fibres. Their use is followed by dilatation of blood vessels, therefore, and this causes flushing of the skin, increase of sweating and an increased flow of urine. They may be useful in bronchitis associated with asthmatic effects, in colic and other instances of spasm. Nitrites may change the oxyhaemoglobin of the blood corpuscles into a substance called methaemoglobin, the blood assuming a chocolate colour. Examples of nitrites are amyl nitrite and sweet spirit of nitre, otherwise spirit of nitrous ether.

See Amyl Nitrite ; Ethyl Nitrite.

NITROBENZENE. The substance know as nitrobenzene has a variety of other names, nitrobenzol, oil or essence of mirbane and, on account of its odour, artificial oil of bitter almonds. It is a pale yellow oily liquid used for scenting cheap soaps, but more particularly for making other important chemical products.

Poisoning by Nitrobenzene. It is very poisonous, and injurious effects may arise from drinking or inhaling it or even from its application to the skin. It causes headache, drowsiness, difficulty in breathing, extreme blueness of the face and hands, and possibly coma. There is an odour of bitter almonds from the breath and urine. If the patient is conscious an emetic of mustard and water should be given if the poison has been swallowed, and then salvolatile diluted. If the patient is unconscious artificial respiration should be used and smelling salts may be held below the nose.

See Poisoning.

NITROGEN. About four-fifths of the bulk of the atmosphere consist of nitrogen, which is a colourless gas and quite inert, its whole use, as regards the respiratory needs of animals and plants and combustion, being to dilute the oxygen. Nitrifying bacteria are able, however, to extract nitrogen from the air for the building up of nitrogenous substances in plants, though these also obtain a supply of nitrogen from compounds in the soil.

Thus from plants, or from the flesh of animals fed on plants, human beings obtain their necessary supplies of nitrogenous, or protein, foods.

NITROGLYCERIN. The action of trinitrin, or nitroglycerin, resembles that of amyl nitrite (*q.v.*), but is slower. Trinitrin is a nitrate of glycerin, but in the body is converted into a nitrite. It is administered by the mouth and is used to prevent angina pectoris, being more suitable for this purpose than amyl nitrite, though the latter should be chosen as the remedy during an attack.

Nitroglycerin is also useful when there is a tendency to migraine, and in some cases of high blood pressure. There are two official preparations, the tablet and the liquor or solution of trinitrin, the dose of the former being 1 or 2 tablets, and of the latter $\frac{1}{2}$ to 2 minims.

NITROUS OXIDE. Also known as laughing gas, or simply gas, nitrous oxide is a colourless gas with a sweetish taste. It is used as a general anaesthetic for short operations, such as tooth extraction, or, mixed with oxygen, in longer operations. It is a very safe anaesthetic (*q.v.*).

NOCTURNAL EMISSIONS. Seminal emissions may occur periodically during sleep. They are generally accompanied by dreams. Unless they happen very frequently or are followed by depression in the morning they are quite harmless and natural. Their frequency varies in individual cases, but intervals of ten days to a fortnight may usually be regarded without apprehension. A lack of open-air exercise, constipation and sexual excitement provoke their occurrence. Plain food and a cold tub in the morning are helpful in reducing their frequency.

NOISES IN THE EAR. Tinnitus, or noises in the ear, may be due to many causes. Some of these are serious general diseases, or diseases of the brain in which tinnitus is unimportant as compared with the other symptoms. Some drugs, such as quinine, ergot, and sodium salicylate, cause tinnitus, but it ceases as the effects of the drugs wear off. It is also transitory when it occurs as an aura in epilepsy or in indigestion.

When associated with deafness, tinnitus may be due to wax, eczema or a polypus in the external passage of the ear, or to mischief in the middle or internal ear. In these conditions it may occur without noticeable deafness, and, moreover, may continue even when the patient is quite deaf. The noise may be hissing, ringing, blowing, or some other. The combination of giddiness, deafness and tinnitus is known as Ménière's syndrome.

The treatment of tinnitus, when any is called for, depends on the cause.

See Deafness ; Ear ; Hearing.

NORMAL. From a consideration of a large number of individuals an idea may be formed of the behaviour of some function in the ordinary healthy individual. Thus we speak of a normal pulse rate, a normal number of evacuations of urine or faeces per diem, and so on. Individuals may vary from what is the rule, however, without being unhealthy, and it is often more useful to ascertain what is the normal for the individual then whether he conforms to an accepted standard.

See Constitution.

NORMAL SALINE SOLUTION. Normal saline solution is a solution of common salt in distilled water, of a strength of 0·9 per cent. It is called normal saline because the percentage of salt resembles that of the crystalloids in the blood plasma. Another way of stating this is to say that normal saline is isotonic. If the proportion of salt were less it would be a hypotonic solution, if more, hypertonic.

Applied to a wound an isotonic solution causes no increase in the flow of lymph from the capillary blood vessels, but a hypertonic solution may cause a large increase so that the wound is flooded with lymph. As this contains natural antitoxic substances, such an application may be a useful one in preventing and clearing up infection. An isotonic solution is desirable when liquid is being injected into the blood stream.

An isotonic solution is less irritating to the body cells, and this is the reason, for example, of normal saline being a more comfortable solution for the eyes than plain water. A sufficient approximation to normal saline is got by dissolving 80 grains of common salt in a pint of boiled water.

See Transfusion.

NOSE. The external protuberance of the nose forms but a small part of the organ. The nose consists of a cavity, opening in front and behind, for the inspiration of air, the upper part of the cavity also being adapted to subserve the sense of smell. From front to back the cavity is divided into two by the nasal septum, two openings, therefore, being situated in front and behind, the anterior and the posterior nares respectively.

The protuberance of the nose has a framework of cartilage, except at the bridge,

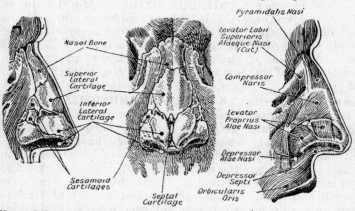

Nose. Left and centre, showing plates of cartilage loosely connected to each other and to the two nasal bones which form the bridge. Right, the muscles

which is formed by the two little nasal bones. The cavity in each side of the septum in this part of the nose is called the vestibule, and from its lining hairs project. The side wall of the vestibule is called the ala.

Beyond the vestibule is the nasal fossa, the cavity proper of the nose. Its inner wall is formed by the septum, which is made up of the plough-share, or vomer, bone behind, the central plate of the ethmoid bone (*q.v.*) above, and elsewhere by plates of cartilage. The floor of the cavity is formed by the hard palate, and the topmost part of its roof by the cribriform plate of the ethmoid, a thin sheet of bone containing many perforations. The outer wall has three shelves, running from before backwards and curling downwards into the fossa.

These shelves, known as the turbinated bodies, are covered with mucous membrane, beneath which is erectile tissue, that is, tissue which can become engorged with blood. Thus, the surface area of the lining of the cavity can be increased, though, of course, the space is lessened. When the external air is cold, this engorgement takes place, so that the air is rendered warmer before it passes on into the air-tubes. Besides being warmed in its passage through the nose, air is moistened, and, to some extent, dust is filtered out from it.

The bones forming the basis of the upper two of these bodies, though called the superior and middle turbinated bones, are part of the lateral mass of the ethmoid bone, but that in the lowest body, the inferior turbinated bone, is a separate bone. The turbinated bodies project inwards almost as far as the septum, and

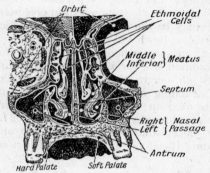

Nose. Cross section of the cavities showing the relative positions of antra and orbits

thus make a sort of division of the cavity into four passages, the three of these lying beneath the bodies being described as the superior, the middle and the inferior meatus of the nose.

In the middle meatus, that is, the one between the middle and the inferior turbinated bodies, are found the openings of certain important cavities, namely, the antrum (*q.v.*) of Highmore, the frontal sinus and some of the ethmoidal cells. Into the space above the superior body opens the sphenoidal sinus, into the superior meatus some ethmoidal cells open, while in the inferior meatus is the opening of the nasal duct through which tears are drained from the lachrymal sac into the nose.

The antrum may be infected through tooth sockets, or any of the spaces above mentioned may be infected from the nose, and when such infection occurs there may be a persistent purulent discharge into the nose, causing chronic inflammation, or rhinitis, and possibly the formation of polypi.

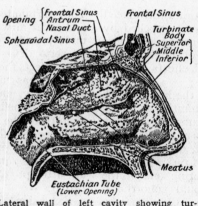

Lateral wall of left cavity showing turbinated processes and sinus openings

The lining of the lower part of the nasal fossa is covered with ciliated epithelium, like the lining of the air-tubes; that of the upper part, however, is different, and contains a large number of special cells, known as the olfactory cells. At the end projecting into the cavity, such a cell is stimulated by odoriferous substances in the air inhaled into the nose, while the inner end is prolonged into a nerve which passes through one of the perforations in the cribriform plate of the ethmoid, and on into the olfactory bulb, which lies on the top of the plate. Thence fibres pass back to the parts of the brain concerned with the sense of smell.

Injuries and Diseases of the Nose. A blow on the nose may cause a fracture (*q.v.*) of the nasal bones or septum, and perhaps subsequent deformity and nasal obstruction.

The skin over the nose may be the site of common acne, acne rosacea, lupus vulgaris, lupus erythematosus, or some other eruption. It is also a common site for a chilblain. Rosacea may go on to the development of great thickening of the skin, which may be disposed in folds, a condition described as rhinophyma. Bleeding from the nose, or epistaxis, is discussed under the heading Bleeding.

Chronic rhinitis may be either of the hypertrophic or the atrophic variety. Hypertrophic rhinitis may follow a repetition of acute attacks. It may also occur in persons much exposed to irritating vapours or sudden changes of temperature, or who have some chronic source of irritation within the nose, such as discharges from an infected sinus, or a spur or prominence on the septum. Changes occur in the turbinated body so that it ceases to contract properly to normal dimensions. The effect of this kind of rhinitis is to obstruct the passage of air through the nose. There is also a muco-purulent discharge from the nose. In some cases of hypertrophic rhinitis, however, there is a disagreeable dryness of the lining.

Atrophic rhinitis is also known as ozoena, a name derived from a Greek word meaning a stench, because crusts form in the nose, and, decomposing, emit an extremely foul odour.

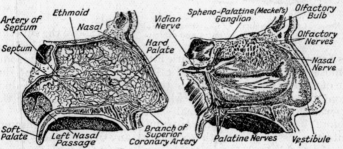

Nose. Left, free blood supply to the lining of the nose. Right, fibres of the olfactory nerve which run from the upper part of the nasal cavity to the olfactory bulb in the skull. The other nerves supply ordinary sensation

A foreign body is sometimes introduced into the nose. If it can be expelled by blowing the nose or by sneezing, good and well, but if not its removal should be left to a doctor, as unskilled efforts may be dangerous.

Acute inflammation of the lining of the nose, otherwise acute rhinitis, or acute nasal catarrh, is what occurs in a common cold (*q.v.*). In some cases of acute rhinitis the discharge is purulent, or at any rate contains a large amount of pus. This may happen, for example, during one of the infectious fevers, or should gonorrhoeal infection reach the nose. Children who have adenoids may also have such a discharge. A foreign body in the nose is another cause, but then the discharge is likely to be from one side of the nose only. In disease of the antrum a purulent discharge may flow into the nostril, particularly when the patient turns the side of the head with the diseased antrum uppermost. Discharges from diseased nasal sinuses may be constantly swallowed, however, and cause chronic poisoning.

The turbinated bodies are shrunken, and the airway through the nose is unduly wide. The interior of the nose is very dry, and dryness and crusts may affect the naso-pharynx also. The patient has usually lost the sense of smell early, and is therefore unconscious of the smell, but this makes the vicinity of the patient so objectionable to other people that his society is shunned. The patient is troubled with a hacking cough and constant hawking in an attempt to clear crusts out of the throat.

Extension of infection from the nose to the throat takes place, more or less, whenever the former is affected, and as the lower opening of the Eustachian tube lies just behind the posterior opening of the nose, extension to the ear also may readily occur.

The treatment of acute catarrhal rhinitis is discussed under the heading of Cold, Common. Before suppurative rhinitis can be treated it is necessary to determine the precise cause. When chronic

PLATE XXVII

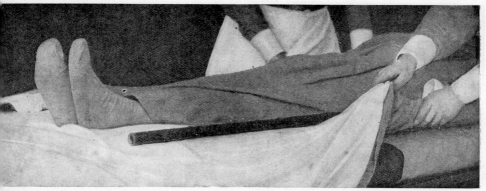

Nursing. 1. To move a helpless patient, two poles are rolled up in the sheet and blanket on which he lies

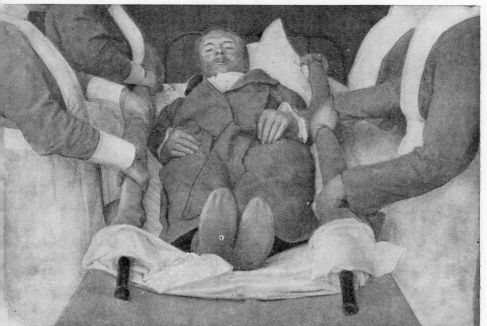

2. Four bearers lift the patient clear of the bottom rail and carry him feet first over the end of the bed

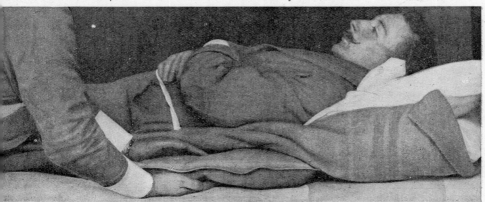

3. A water bed should be filled just enough to prevent the sides of the bed from meeting when indented

PLATE XXVIII

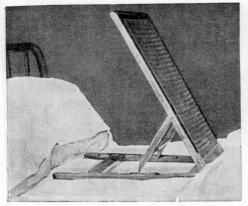

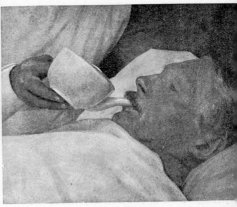

Nursing. 1. Light but strong bed rest having a wooden framework and adjustable cane back

2. China feeding cup. The patient's head should be gently raised by a hand beneath the pillow

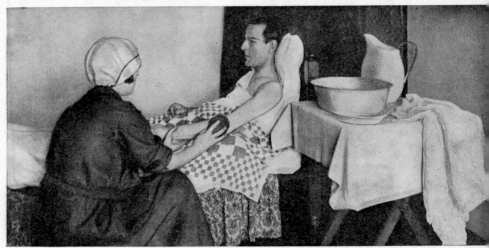

3. Washing the patient. The whole body should be cleaned piecemeal, exposing only one part at a time

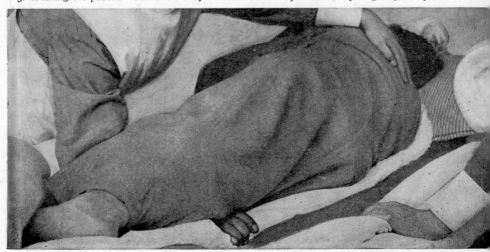

4. Changing a sheet beneath a patient. The fresh sheet is rolled along its length and the patient turned on his side. The soiled sheet is then rolled and passed beneath him, followed by the clean one

rhinitis occurs, it will generally be necessary to improve the general health of the patient by a sufficiency of open-air exercise, proper ventilation of the bedroom, a sufficiency of good, mixed food, avoiding an excess of carbohydrate substances, and, possibly, by giving tonics.

The nose should be cleansed once or twice a day, and lotions for this purpose can be used as a spray or a douche. A simple and effective one can be made by dissolving in a glass of warm water a teaspoonful of a powder consisting of equal parts of common salt, borax, sodium bicarbonate and white sugar, or a teaspoonful each of common salt and sodium bicarbonate. The compound solution of thymol B.P.C. diluted with 3 or 4 parts of warm water also does well. When there is foetor, a solution of potassium permanganate, sufficient of the latter to colour the solution deep red, is desirable. In ozoena, a pint of this should be injected through the nose by means of a Higginson's syringe three times a day (Plate XXVI, 4).

Douching of the nose may be carried out in other ways than by using a syringe. One of these is by using a rubber tube through which the fluid runs by siphonage, and another is by using a small glass vessel with a nozzle at one end, and an opening in the side through which the vessel is filled. By keeping this opening closed with the thumb, the liquid is prevented from running out until the patient is ready. Whichever method is used, the patient breathes in and out through the mouth, thus closing the naso-pharynx by the soft palate, and the liquid runs in through one nostril and flows out at the other, this process being assisted if the patient stoops a little over the basin for receiving the outflow.

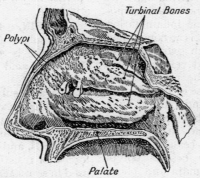

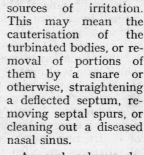

Nose. Polypi are liable to form between the middle and lower turbinated processes

In hypertrophic rhinitis, however, it may be necessary to have an operation in order to relieve obstruction or remove sources of irritation. This may mean the cauterisation of the turbinated bodies, or removal of portions of them by a snare or otherwise, straightening a deflected septum, removing septal spurs, or cleaning out a diseased nasal sinus.

A nasal polypus denotes disease of the bone underlying its site. These growths are usually multiple in the nose, and come from the outer wall. They cause more or less obstruction and discharge, with loss of smell, and often impairment of hearing. The voice loses its resonant quality. Polypi should be removed, this being accomplished usually by means of a wire snare, and the part from which they spring should be cleaned up.

Tuberculosis may occur in the nose, usually in people who have the disease in the lungs, but in rare instances as an independent infection. More frequently lupus (*q.v.*) is found, and this may cause much destruction. Syphilis of the nose may occur, both in the inherited and the acquired disease. It is responsible for the catarrhal condition in the nose referred to as snuffles, which is found in infants born suffering from syphilis, and for the sinking of the bridge of the nose which appears later on. Acquired syphilis may be found in the nose in any of its three stages. It may cause much destruction within the nose, and also of the

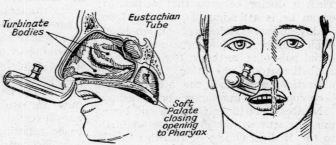

Nasal douching of one nostril at a time by means of a special container

external protuberance; it is the commonest cause of the perforation of the hard palate.

Progressive nasal obstruction may be caused by a rare disease called rhinoscleroma, in which chronic inflammation of the walls of the nose is accompanied by the formation of much scar-tissue, in which bone is ultimately developed. This condition may involve the pharynx and the larynx also. The cause of the disorder is not known. X-rays and radium have produced some benefit, but the removal of obstructing masses and the divisions of strictures are often necessary.

Other simple tumours besides polypi occur in the nose, osteomata and chondromata, for example; malignant tumours are very rare, however. Rough spherical concretions, usually of phosphate and carbonate of lime, may be found in the nose. They are known as rhinoliths, and are formed round a nucleus of blood-clot or dried mucus. They act as foreign bodies, and should be extracted by suitable means. In the tropics maggots may be found in the nose, and should be dislodged by douching with a solution of common salt.

See Acne; Adenoids; Cold, Common; Ethmoid Bone; Eustachian Tube; Lupus; Naso-pharynx; Respiration; Smell.

NOSTALGIA. Homesickness, especially a sufficient degree of it to cause mental and bodily depression, is called nostalgia. It may amount to a serious disability.

NOTIFICATION. Under the heading Infectious Disease there is a list of diseases, notification of the occurrence of which must be sent to the Medical Officer of Health of the area.

Similar notification on a prescribed form must be sent to the Chief Inspector of Factories, at the Home Office, London, when a doctor believes that a patient, whom he is attending, is suffering from lead, phosphorus, arsenical, carbon bisulphide, aniline, chronic benzene, or mercurial poisoning, anthrax, toxic jaundice, epitheliomatous ulceration, or chrome ulceration, and that the affection has been contracted in a factory or workshop.

Notices of birth, including a still-birth, must be sent within 36 hours after birth to the Medical Officer of Health; this is in addition to the ordinary registration.

NOVOCAINE. Introduced as a substitute for cocaine, novocaine is a safer drug and is a good anaesthetic for short operations when used in combination with adrenalin.

NUCLEIN. Derived from yeast, yolk of egg, spleen and other sources, nuclein, or nucleol, is a compound of nucleic or nucleinic acid with albuminates and carbohydrates. It always contains phosphorus and sulphur, and sometimes iron also. That used in medicine is usually obtained from yeast. If injected into the body it increases the number of white blood cells, and thus augments the natural forces for resisting infections. It has been used in septicaemia, tuberculosis and other diseases.

Nucleinic acid is sometimes referred to as nuclein, and a purin (q.v.), although quite another substance, is sometimes called a nuclein body.

NUCLEUS. A mass of differentiated protoplasm in an animal or vegetable cell is described as the nucleus. This term is also used for collections of nerve cells in the lower parts of the brain, processes from which constitute the cranial nerves.

See Cell.

NUISANCE. The proximity of foul cess-pools, pig-styes, collections of rubbish and other nuisances are prejudicial to health. A householder who cannot otherwise have the nuisance satisfactorily dealt with should report the matter to the Medical Officer of Health for his area.

NUMBNESS. The term numbness, as used by doctors, refers to an altered state of sensation resembling the feeling in a limb which is " sleeping " from pressure on a nerve. There is not a total loss of sensation, or anaesthesia, but a dulling of sensation. Numbness occurs in various circumstances in which nerve fibres are injured or irritated, and in certain brain and spinal cord diseases. It occurs in poisoning by aconite and may be general. There may be a premonitory numbness before a paroxysm of neuralgia. Numbness in the hands and feet is not uncommon in osteo-arthritis. Frequently a person complaining of numbness is found to be suffering from hysteria.

See Nervous System; Paraesthesia; Sensation.

NURSING. Many a person owes his or her life to good nursing, and at any time good nursing may hasten recovery, prevent complications, or at any rate shorten the period of convalescence. Good nursing consists in securing as much physical comfort as possible for the patient, in rendering prompt and efficient first aid in any emergencies that may arise, and in soothing and cheering the patient's mind.

A good nurse co-operates loyally with the doctor in attendance, and can help him much in two ways. In the first place, a nurse should faithfully carry out all the instructions for treatment ; in the second place, by close and accurate observation, a nurse may furnish valuable information of what happens to the patient in the intervals of the doctor's visits.

When there is a choice of a room for the accommodation of the patient, a large one should be selected, and preferably one with an exposure to the south or south-west. Other matters may have to be considered, however, such as freedom from noise and the necessity for isolation, the requirements for which are detailed under the heading Infectious Disease. The room should be cleaned, dried and aired before the patient goes into it, and unnecessary furniture should be removed. Large pieces of furniture take up valuable air-space. The best preparation of the floor is to have it waxed or covered with linoleum, and provided with one or two light rugs.

The Bed and Its Furnishing

The bed should be a single one, placed with its head against the wall, so that the nurse has free access to it from either side. It should not be too near the fire, nor in such a position as to be exposed to draught. An iron bedstead, 6½ feet long, 3½ feet wide, and 2½ feet high, furnished with a good spring mattress, is the best kind of bed. In any case there should be a spring mattress and, if possible, over this a hair mattress. A straw mattress might serve if it were well packed, but a flock mattress is objectionable, because the cleanliness of the flock cannot be depended upon, and a feather mattress is undesirable because it is too hot and liable to become lumpy.

Over the mattress is placed a blanket and a sheet, cotton for preference, and to cover the patient a sheet, one or two blankets and a cover, cotton or linen being better for this purpose than silk. An eider-down quilt is often useful. The bolster and pillow should not be too soft.

The bed should be made daily, the mattress being aired and turned. The under-sheet should not be placed over the bolster, but beneath it, and the slack brought over the bolster. The blanket and sheet should be perfectly smooth, and should be tucked under the mattress at the sides. This should be done also with the upper sheet and the blankets when the patient is in bed, but the cover should be allowed to hang at the sides.

Often a draw-sheet will be necessary. This consists of a piece of an old cotton sheet long enough, when doubled, to reach from the back of the shoulders to the knees of the patient, and broad enough to be tucked beneath the mattress. An india-rubber sheet may have to be placed beneath the draw-sheet, or, in an emergency, clean brown paper or newspapers.

How to Change a Sheet

When a patient cannot be taken out of bed, the under-sheet may be changed in this way. The clean sheet is rolled up for half its width. The patient is turned on one side and supported by an assistant. The nurse then rolls up the soiled sheet till the roll is at the patient's back. Against this roll she places the roll of the clean sheet. The patient is then turned on his back, and the assistant removes the soiled sheet and unrolls the clean one (Plate XXVIII, 4).

Should it be necessary to change or turn over the mattress, or remove the patient to another bed, a light pole may be rolled up in either side of the under-sheet until about touching the patient's body. One or two people on each side then grasp the poles, preventing the sheet from slipping, and raise the patient up. He is then carried over the bottom of the bed and over the top of another bed or couch placed in position (Plate XXVII, 1-2).

A sick-room should have a fire-place, and, even if no heating is required, it may be desirable to place a lighted lamp in the fire-place to cause an upward draught and help the ventilation of the room. The temperature of the room should not be less than 55°, and for bronchitis and other disorders may have to be about 70°. It should be kept as even as possible. To achieve accuracy in this respect a thermometer should be placed on the wall near the patient's head, though the part of the wall selected should not be specially heated by the fire nor cooled by draughts. When a coal fire is used, each piece of coal in the scuttle should be wrapped up in a piece of paper, so that it can be noiselessly placed on the fire.

Importance of Free Ventilation

The proper inlet for fresh air is the window, and the top sash should be well pulled down to admit the air. A narrow chink causes the air to rush in with greater force and is more likely to cause a draught. Screens may be placed, when necessary, to prevent the air blowing directly on the patient, and special precautions should be taken when the patient is exposed for washing or when changing sheets.

If practicable, the patient should be washed all over every day with warm water and soap. Only one part of the body is exposed at a time, washed and dried with a warm towel before proceeding to the next. Bedding should be protected with another towel (Plate XXVIII, 3). If the patient is very weak the face and arms should always be washed, and, in any case, parts liable to form bed sores (*q.v.*) must be washed. The teeth and mouth should be washed several times each day. The hair should be brushed. The best time for carrying out this full toilet is about an hour after breakfast.

A feeding cup with a spout is used in feeding a helpless patient. The nurse places one arm beneath the patient's pillow and raises his head and neck on this when he is taking his meal (Plate XXVIII, 2). The method of administering medicines is descibed under that heading.

When a patient is suffering from fever, a chart should be kept for noting the temperature at such times as it is taken. On this chart are also noted the pulse rate, sometimes also the respiration rate and the number of times the bowels move. In any case of illness it may be desirable to keep a record of the food and medicine given to the patient, the amount and character of sleep and other relevant facts. The keeping of a chart ensures precision as to feeding and giving of medicine, and prevents the nurse from forgetting facts which it might be important for the doctor to know.

It will often be necessary for various kinds of apparatus to be provided, an account of which is given under such headings as Bed Cradle, Bed Pan, Bed Rest, Thermometer, and so on. A water-bed may have to be used. This consists of a large rubber bag, 3 feet across and 2, 4, or 6 feet long. The larger sizes require a bed with a specially strong framework to support them, and also planks should be placed on the framework beneath the hair mattress.

A water-bed has a nozzle at one corner, or perhaps at each of two opposite corners. The patient should not be lying on a water-bed when it is being filled. For filling, the upper end of the bed should be raised by blocks placed beneath the legs. Water at a temperature of 90° F. is then poured in through the upper nozzle, from a large jug. Sometimes the rubber is brought up round the nozzle to form a filler, but, if not, a filler will be needed. Enough water should be run in to prevent the sides of the bag meeting when firm pressure is made (Plate XXVII, 3). An over-filled water-bed is very uncomfortable. If safety-pins are being used to fix a draw-sheet, or for other purposes, care must be taken not to perforate the water-bed when the pins are stuck into the bedding lying upon it.

Sometimes cushions inflated with air are used to take the pressure off tender parts. These cushions are of various shapes, a favourite one consisting of a ring, so that pressure is taken around the part to be protected and not on it.

See Bed Sore ; Beverages ; Convalescence ; Diet ; Eau-de-Cologne ; Fomentation ; Infectious Disease ; Invalid Cookery ; Medicines ; Operation ; Poultice, etc.

NUTMEG. The dried nut of an Eastern tree, nutmeg, or myristica, contains a fragrant volatile oil, which acts as a carminative, and a principle, known as myristicin, which has a narcotic effect, and is capable of causing poisoning. The dose of oil of nutmeg is $\frac{1}{2}$ to 3 minims. There is an official spirit of nutmeg, the dose of which is 5 to 20 minims.

NUX VOMICA. The button-shaped, dried seed of an Eastern plant, nux vomica contains, and owes its properties to, the alkaloids strychnine and brucine, more especially the former. Both alkaloids are bitter, and nux vomica is a most useful digestive tonic both on this account and because it increases at the same time the tone of the muscles of the digestive tract.

Strychnine increases the tone and vigour of striped muscle by its action on the spinal cord, though it appears to influence the motor cells of the cord indirectly, through its action on the sensory parts of the cord. The drug is therefore used in treating paralysis of muscles, but its use here is only in selected cases. It stimulates the contraction of plain muscle also, and is of service in constipation and bladder weakness.

Strychnine increases the rapidity and extent of the respiratory movements, and may be of service sometimes in bronchitis and other respiratory troubles. To some extent it also improves the action of the heart.

Another effect of this drug is to sharpen the special senses. The action of brucine is somewhat similar to that of strychnine, but it is less poisonous.

There are official dry and liquid extracts, and a tincture of nux vomica. Strychnine is generally used as the hydrochloride, and of this there is a liquor, or solution.

Poisoning by Nux Vomica. Nux vomica is a very powerful drug, and excessive doses may have dangerous and often fatal consequences. Effects of over-dosage may occur when the drug has been taken in ordinary doses, but for some length of time, say, in Easton's syrup. There is a jumpy feeling and general excitability, sudden noises like the banging of a door making the person start violently.

Poisonous doses cause convulsions rather like those of tetanus, except that they do not begin as lockjaw, nor are they constantly maintained, as in this disease. The whole body is thrown into a rigid spasm in the same way, however, and there may be arching of the back. Symptoms may appear very quickly after taking the dose, and death supervene in a short time, but in some cases either event may be delayed.

If there is time, the stomach should be emptied by an emetic of mustard and water, and then strong tea given freely. A doctor should be summoned at once, being informed of the nature, or suspected nature, of the poisoning, so that he may bring narcotic drugs, such as chloroform, etc., the prompt use of which may be successful.

NYCTALOPIA. A lessened ability to see in a dim light is called night-blindness, or nyctalopia, though some writers use this term for the opposite condition, namely, lessened ability to see in a bright light, which is more properly described as day-blindness, or hemeralopia. Night-blindness occurs most frequently in those suffering from the eye disorder known as retinitis pigmentosa, but may also occur from quinine poisoning, a thickened and dry state of the conjunctiva, known as xerosis, and other disorders. It may follow much exposure to a bright light. Where improvement is possible, it may be obtained by keeping the eyes covered for a length of time and giving general tonics.

Day-blindness occurs in albinism (*q.v.*) in which case nothing can be done for it, nor when it is due to opacities in the clear media of the eye, unless when the opacity is caused by a removable cataract. Tobacco-poisoning, the commonest cause of day-blindness, is treated by breaking off the use of tobacco and giving tonics. The patient may be made more comfortable by remaining in a darkened room, or otherwise shading bright lights.

See Eye ; Vision.

NYSTAGMUS. Involuntary oscillations of the eyes are described as nystagmus. The movements, which are rapid and jerky, may be from side to side (lateral), up and down (vertical) or rotatory, the eye turning on its front-to-back axis. The condition usually affects both eyes and may date from infancy. It arises from difficulty in fixing the eyes on an object ; this difficulty may be created by congenital cataract, inflammatory diseases, which leave obscurity of vision, or the condition of albinism.

In later life nystagmus may arise from ear disease ; merely syringing the ears may cause temporary oscillations. It also occurs in disseminated sclerosis, Friedreich's ataxia, and other diseases of the central nervous system. It may be an occupational complaint, the commonest example being miner's nystagmus. Sometimes the patient is unconscious of the movement of the eyes, but in miner's nystagmus and that due to ear disease, external objects may appear to move, and there may be giddiness. The existence of nystagmus should be brought to the notice of a doctor.

See Eye.

OBESITY. An excessive development of adipose or fatty tissue throughout the body is called obesity. Besides accumulating in the anterior abdominal wall, the buttocks, the back and other superficial situations, there is an accumulation of fat over the internal organs, the heart, for example, the muscular fibres of which may be interspersed with fat.

Certain races, such as Jews, Hindus and Negroes, are especially prone to obesity, but possibly the diet is often responsible. A similar tendency may be noted in some families, and in a considerable proportion of all individuals who have passed middle life. A gouty habit may explain its occurrence in some families. In certain cases obesity is due to lack of activity of glands of internal secretion, notably the thyroid, the pituitary, the testicle, and the ovary.

Fat in the body is derived mainly from carbohydrate foods, but may be formed from fats or proteins. Obesity may result, therefore, from consumption of an excessive amount of food, particularly of carbohydrates, especially when an insufficient amount of open-air exercise is taken, as exercise helps to burn up carbohydrates. Over-indulgence in malt liquors is a notorious cause of obesity. In some persons, usually women, the existence of anaemia accounts for obesity, as the tissues are not properly oxygenated.

An obese person tends to be short of breath on slight exertion. The interference with the contractile power of the heart is mainly responsible, and this organ may become dilated and very feeble. Many of the obese also develop emphysema (*q.v.*), and this is another cause of shortness of breath. Active exercise thus becomes difficult and the enforced sedentariness of the habits increases the obesity. The bowels are sluggish, the liver is much enlarged and is also sluggish, and therefore the digestion may be poor and there is a special tendency to the formation of gall-stones. Some persons develop glycosuria, but this is generally controllable without much difficulty ; others suffer from nephritis.

The treatment of obesity due to definite defects of internal secretions may be most successful when it consists in giving extracts of the gland at fault, but this will only happen in properly selected cases. Thyroid extract is sometimes used indiscriminately, and undoubtedly by speeding up metabolism it has a powerful influence in removing fat, but it is a dangerous remedy without medical control. Fucus vesiculosus (*q.v.*) is also used and may be beneficial, probably on account of the iodine it contains. Citric acid is another remedy, but is likely to be unsuccessful unless taken in sufficient quantities to upset the digestion. Both this acid and fucus are contained in quack remedies for obesity. When there is anaemia iron will be of use.

Ordinarily the treatment of obesity consists of a controlled diet and more exercise. The changes required in the diet are to cut down the carbohydrates, that is, sugars and starches, to a minimum, to eschew very fat flesh foods and to restrict the total amount of food. An example of a strict diet for obesity is given under the heading Banting. Ebstein's and Van Noorden's diets are somewhat similar, but both include fresh fruit, and the former a considerable amount of fresh butter. Strict diets can only be employed temporarily, however, and it will be found that more food can be taken than is allowed in such a diet, but it should be restricted to what provides sufficient energy for one's duties. Under the headings Diet and Food guidance is provided for framing suitable diets. Sufficient liquid may be taken to relieve thirst, but no malt liquor or sweetened drinks.

If a person can take exercise with any comfort, he should get into the open air daily and take progressive amounts of exercise, walking for a beginning. The Schott exercises described under the heading Heart are suitable for those whose hearts are considerably enfeebled. When exercise cannot well be taken, it may be replaced at first by massage or by the use of the Bergonié chair, in which muscles all over the body are made to contract against a weight. After such preliminary treatment ordinary gentle exercise will probably become possible.

See Abdominal Exercises ; Banting ; Change of Life ; Constipation ; Diet ; Exercise ; Food ; Oertel's Treatment ; Thyroid Gland.

OBSESSION. Some people have ideas which keep springing up in their minds, a vision of some particular object, for example ; others have fears of one thing or another or doubts of this or that duty having been performed ; and still others feel impelled, from time to time, to do something which may be trivial or, on the other hand, unpleasant or disgusting. The persons concerned quite realize the want of substance in the ideas and fears and in the motives for their actions, but nevertheless they are unable to suppress or avoid them. Such ideas, fears, doubts and impulses to do certain things are described as obsessions.

Probably everybody has had experiences of this kind at some time or another, but mostly of a slight and very transitory character. When, however, an obsession is very definite and is persistent it constitutes what is called a compulsion, or obsessional, neurosis.

Now, although an obsession is always irrelevant to the ordinary trains of thought and character of the person whom it afflicts, it must be linked up in some way in his unconscious mind, as the mind is a continuous texture, and the proper way to reach an explanation of what lies behind an obsession, if this be possible at all, is by a skilful psycho-analysis.

See Neurosis ; Psycho-therapy.

OBSTETRICS. The branch of medicine dealing with pregnancy and the lying-in is called midwifery or obstetrics.

OBSTRUCTION. Any tubular structure in the body may become the seat of obstruction, but when this term is used without qualification what is meant is obstruction of the bowel. This may occur suddenly, sometimes when a person is making a strong exertion. Severe pain of a colicky nature is felt about the navel and is accompanied by more or less collapse—pallor, faintness, and so on. The collapse is usually recovered from, however, but pain persists and vomiting begins and keeps recurring at intervals. The vomited matter sooner or later acquires a faeculent character. Unless the condition is relieved, the patient dies from exhaustion or peritonitis.

This acute obstruction may be due to strangulation of a hernia, the pressure of bands or adhesions on the bowel, volvulus or twisting of a loop of gut, intussusception (*q.v.*), impaction of faeces or of some foreign body in the gut, or acute kinking. Sometimes the person has been suffering from chronic obstruction.

Acute obstruction demands immediate operation. Severe abdominal pain, especially when it continues and makes the patient feel and look ill, should be brought to the notice of a doctor without delay. On no account should purgatives be given without his advice.

Chronic obstruction is characterised by increasing constipation with bouts of diarrhoea, caused by irritation due to stagnant bowel contents. The belly tends to be distended constantly, more or less, and peristalsis, or movements of the intestine, may be observable. From time to time there are attacks of colic, the pain probably occurring always about the same spot. Vomiting may occur at the same time.

Chronic obstruction may be caused by impaction of faeces, scarring of the bowel, the growth of a tumour in the bowel and other disorders. Here also medical advice should be got without delay.

See Colic ; Constipation ; Hernia ; Intestine ; Intussusception ; Meckel's Diverticulum.

OCCIPITAL BONE. The back of the head, or occiput, as it is called, is mainly closed in by the occipital bone, which consists of a curved, plate-like portion, articulating with the parietal bones above and the temporal bones at the sides, and a narrow, thickened portion, which projects forward below to join the sphenoid bone and form the central part of the base of the skull.

Between these portions there is a large opening, the foramen magnum, through which the junction of the brain and spinal cord is effected. On either side of this opening is a curved elevation, or condyle, for articulation with the atlas, or uppermost cervical vertebra. By means of this joint nodding movements of the head are made possible. The most prominent part of the bone at the back of the head is called the occipital protuberance.

See Skull.

OCCLUSION. As applied to tubular or other hollow organs of the body, the term occlusion means that the cavity is closed or shut off. Occlusion, as applied to the teeth, means that in the position of rest the chewing parts of the upper and lower teeth are fully in contact.

OCCUPATIONAL DISEASE. Various diseases are incidental to certain occupations. Miners, steel-grinders, porters and others who work in an atmosphere charged with dust are liable to dust disease (*q.v.*), a fibrosis of the lungs due to irritation from the dust. Miners, cement workers, alkali workers, those employed in the manufacture of high explosives and in aniline industries, copper and zinc smelters and others are subject to poisoning from gases or volatilised metals.

Poisoning may also occur from handling lead preparations and other poisonous substances and conveying them to the mouth. Aniline and other poisons may even be absorbed through the skin.

In some occupations there is an especial tendency to irritation of the skin from substances which are dealt with. Thus, paraffin workers often have dermatitis, and others who may have it include grocers from handling sugar, polishers from varnish, cabinet-makers from certain kinds of wood, potters from the fine clay, gardeners from primula obconica and other plants, cotton-spinners from oil, and chimney-sweeps and others from handling soot. Paraffin workers may develop cancer, and cancer of the scrotum is particularly common in chimney-sweeps and also in cotton-spinners, when it is called mule-spinner's cancer.

Infection with ankylostomiasis (*q.v.*) is an especial risk for miners, tunnel miners and brickmakers, more especially in some parts of the world. Ostlers may contract glanders from horses; cattlemen, actinomycosis; and those who handle hides, anthrax.

Persons who have to make violent exertions frequently, and thus have to hold the breath, are prone to develop emphysema. Bridge-makers who have to work under water may suffer from caisson disease (*q.v.*). Miners often develop the spasmodic eye affection known as nystagmus (*q.v.*). Clerks, telegraphists and others are liable to neurosis, affecting their capacity for work.

By legislative enactments, concerning ventilation and other matters in mines, workshops and factories, much occupational disease is prevented. More can be prevented by precautions, such as wearing masks when necessary, and by strict personal cleanliness on the part of the workers themselves. Instances of certain industrial diseases must be notified, and a list of such is given under the heading Notification. Under separate headings an account will also be found of the symptoms and treatment of poisoning by the various substances encountered in different employments and of the other occupational diseases.

See Dermatitis ; Writer's Cramp.

OCULO-MOTOR NERVE. The 3rd cranial or oculo-motor nerve supplies most of the muscles that move the eyeball, the fibres in the iris that contract the pupil, the ciliary muscle which produces accommodation (*q.v.*) for near vision, and the muscle that raises the upper eyelid. It is a purely motor nerve.

See Eye.

OEDEMA. Dropsy in a tissue may be called oedema. Its existence may be shown by the phenomenon known as pitting.

See Dropsy.

OERTEL'S TREATMENT. Obesity and certain kinds of heart disease may be dealt with by the régime known as Oertel's treatment. This consists of dieting and exercise, and sometimes effervescent baths. Small meals are given, with a restricted allowance of carbohydrates and fat, and liquids are also limited. As for exercise, a beginning is made with passive movements, that is, the limbs are moved by a nurse without help from the patient. Then gentle movements are made by the patient against resistance made by the nurse. When a sufficient capacity for it has been developed, walking exercise up a slope is undertaken. The duration and vigour of the exercises must be strictly controlled.

See Heart; Obesity.

OESOPHAGUS. *See* Gullet.

OIL. The oils are divided into two main groups. The first consists of the fixed oils, that is, oils which do not volatilise. They are sometimes called expressed oils, because they are obtained by squeezing the substance containing them. Amongst the fixed oils used in medicine are almond oil, castor oil, cod-liver oil and olive oil. A fixed oil has a greasy feeling. Most fixed oils are emollient and nutritive, but castor oil and croton oil are purgative, and the latter is very irritating to body tissues.

The second group is that of the essential or volatile oils. These are aromatic substances and are not greasy. Many oils of this kind are used in medicine, including oil of peppermint, oil of lemon, oil of citronella, oil of cloves and so on. The essential oils are obtained by distillation, except oil of lemon, which is expressed from the rind.

Essential oils act as carminatives and antispasmodics. In large doses they stimulate at first, but later cause depression. They are powerfully antiseptic, and have a stimulating effect on skin and mucous membranes, causing redness. The usual dose is $\frac{1}{2}$ to 2 or 3 minims, and this may be taken by dropping it on a lump of sugar.

OIL OF VITRIOL. *See* Sulphuric Acid.

OINTMENT. The basis of an ointment usually consists of benzoated lard or soft paraffin, but may contain lanolin, beeswax, spermaceti or oil; whatever it is, the consistency is about that of butter. With the basis are incorporated liquid or solid drugs. An ointment is intended for external application and, unless it contains some stimulating drug, it exerts an emollient action on inflamed surfaces.

The drug incorporated may increase this soothing action, as, for example, in the case of the zinc and the lead ointments. Drugs mixed with fats may be absorbed through the skin, however, and an ointment may have a sedative effect beneath the skin. This happens for example, with the aconitine and the cocaine ointment. Mercury ointments are sometimes rubbed into the skin in order to get the drug into the system. Other ointments are antiseptic, astringent, stimulating and alterative.

An ointment should be spread thinly on a clean piece of linen or cotton or on lint. Care should be taken to keep ointments stored at home quite clean, and an admirable way to do this is to have an ointment in a collapsible tube with a screw nozzle through which the contents are squeezed. For the treatment of piles and other anal disorders, say, with hamamelis or gall and opium ointment, it is convenient to have such a tube with a vulcanite tube, or applicator, for screwing on to its nozzle. This enables the ointment to be introduced for a short distance into the bowel. As a rule an ointment is unsuitable for a surface from which there is much discharge as it tends to prevent the escape of the latter.

See Inunction.

OLD AGE. The changes brought about by advancing years are discussed under the heading Age Changes.

OLEATE. A compound of a base with oleic acid is called an oleate. Such a preparation, mixed with soft paraffin or benzoated lard, etc., is used as an ointment. There are oleates of atropine, lead, mercury, veratrine, zinc and other bases.

OLECRANON. The bony projection forming the point of the elbow is called the olecranon process. In the groove between it and the internal prominence of the lower end of the arm bone runs the ulnar nerve.

See Elbow; Fracture; Ulna.

OLFACTORY NERVE. The 1st pair of cranial nerves are called the olfactory nerves. They are concerned with the sense of smell. The olfactory nerves begin as specialised olfactory cells in the lining of the upper part of the nose (*q.v.*).

Fibrils from these cells pass up into the olfactory bulbs, lying on the base of the skull. From the bulbs the olfactory tracts, thick bands of white brain matter, pass backwards to enter the brain, and the fibres contained in the tracts are brought into relationship with nerve-cells in certain parts of the cortex of the brain.

See Smell.

OLIVE OIL. The pale greenish-yellow oil expressed from ripe olives has a considerable place in the dietary, especially in some countries. It has also medicinal uses. In doses of 2 drachms to 1 ounce it has a laxative action. It is also soothing to the lining of the digestive tract, and may be given freely by the mouth in irritant poisoning, except when oils are barred.

Large quantities may be injected into the bowel for colitis or to relieve stubborn constipation. Large doses of olive oil are sometimes given to people suffering from gall-stones in the hope that it will dissolve these out. Olive oil is included in some plasters, ointments and liniments, and has an emollient action on the skin. Mixed with lime-water it forms Carron oil.

OMENTUM. An apron-like structure in the abdomen, consisting of layers of peritoneum and hanging down over the coils of intestine, is described as the great omentum. It is suspended from the lower border of the stomach, and is usually loaded with fat. Sometimes it passes through the inguinal ring and forms a hernia. The lesser omentum is another fold connecting the stomach and liver.

See Peritoneum.

OPEN-AIR TREATMENT. The value of keeping a patient as much as possible in the open air was first emphasised in the treatment of consumption (*q.v.*). Open-air treatment is now used, when practicable, in treating other kinds of tuberculosis and certain other disorders, febrile and otherwise. Sunlight and the free circulation of air about the body are all-important agents in maintaining and restoring health.

See Light ; Ventilation.

OPERATION. It is highly desirable that any but a slight surgical operation should be performed in a hospital or nursing home, as the cleanliness and conveniences of a proper operating theatre might make all the difference in determining the success of the operation. It may be necessary, however, for a sufficient reason to carry out an operation in the patient's home.

The room chosen for the purpose should be large and well lighted. The furniture, pictures and knick-knacks should be removed. If the floor is covered with linoleum, so much the better ; but if there is a heavy carpet its removal might load the air with dust, and it is probably safer to cover over the carpet with clean dust sheets which have been wrung out of lysol solution, a teaspoonful to a pint of water.

To avoid a cloud of dust it may be better also to leave heavy curtains in position and to refrain from touching the walls. Any attempt to remove dust should be done with a moistened cloth.

Improvising an Operation Table

Two kitchen tables, placed end to end, or a long, narrow dining-room table, will make a suitable operating table. They should be thoroughly scrubbed with soap and water, and dried with a clean towel. A blanket, folded double, is placed on top, and over it a waterproof sheet and then an ordinary sheet fresh from the laundry. A side-table and two or three small tables, also scrubbed clean, on which to place lotion bowls, dressings, etc., should also be in the room.

A number of large bowls or pudding dishes should be available for holding lotions and instruments, and are best sterilised by boiling. A large stew-pan or fish-pan should be at hand for sterilising instruments, if necessary. Two or three towels may be boiled in a stew-pan with a tight lid and left in the pan till required by the surgeon ; they can be wrung out, and will serve for surrounding the site of the operation. Sterilised towels, aprons, etc., can be hired in suitable containers, and should be obtained whenever possible.

The room should be well ventilated, and should be kept at a temperature of about 70° F., a thermometer being placed on a wall and not near the fire, to ensure accuracy in this respect. If, as is preferable, the fireplace is an open one, the pieces of coal for replenishing it should be wrapped separately in paper in order to facilitate handling. If the patient is to remain in the room after the operation the temperature should be allowed to fall to about 65° F.

A single bedstead should be placed by the wall, and prepared for his reception by putting in one or two hot-water bottles. The same applies to the operating table, but the bottles must be carefully protected by clean flannel coverings, and should be placed at some little distance from the patient. Serious burning has resulted from using unprotected hot bottles, or from placing them too near a patient who was under the influence of an anaesthetic.

To prepare a patient for operation the skin over the site proposed is shaved, washed thoroughly with soap and water, then with ether, and finally is smeared with tincture of iodine and covered with a sterile dressing. This is done the day before, but if there is greater urgency the skin should be washed well and smeared thoroughly with the iodine. The patient should receive no food for three or four hours before taking an anaesthetic. Directions will be given by the doctor as to whether or not a dose of opening medicine is to be given the night before the operation.

Any person who assists in any way should wear a large sterile or, at any rate, clean apron, and the hands should be washed thoroughly and soaked in lysol solution before touching any bowl or other utensil to be used.

A large pail, well washed and rubbed over with lysol solution, should be available for the reception of soiled swabs, etc.

When the patient has been put back to bed someone must remain by him lest he become sick when recovering from the anaesthetic.

See Antiseptic ; Dressing ; Nursing ; Shock.

OPHTHALMIA. *See* Conjunctivitis.

OPHTHALMOSCOPE. An instrument for examining the interior of the eye is called an ophthalmoscope. Light is thrown into the eye from a little mirror on the instrument, and observation is made through an opening in the centre of the mirror. Some of these instruments are furnished with a tiny electric bulb, which is lit up by a dry cell placed in the handle of the instrument.

See Eye.

OPIUM. The juice of a poppy, which has been rendered solid by evaporation of most of the water, opium contains a large number of alkaloids, including morphine and codeine. Though the main action of the drug is sedative and depressant to muscular activity, some of the alkaloids are capable of causing convulsions when given alone.

Opium is at once one of the most useful and one of the most harmful of drugs, as it readily creates a craving for itself. Accordingly it has been found necessary, by the Dangerous Drugs Act, to hedge round with certain restrictions the sale to the public of opium and morphine, and, with certain exceptions, of preparations containing these.

Opium procures sleep, but the onset of somnolence may be preceded by a certain amount of excitement, and in some persons moderate doses may cause prolonged excitement and actually prevent sleep. Opium is also one of the most powerful remedies for relieving pain, and when used as a hypodermic injection of morphine the effect is very rapid. Caution is required in using opium to relieve abdominal pain, as it may mask the presence of appendicitis or some other condition requiring operation.

Opium is a common ingredient of cough mixtures, as it prevents an irritating cough, but its use is dangerous when coughing is required to clear phlegm from the bronchial tubes.

All the secretions of the body, except the sweat, are diminished or dried up by opium. The drug is often, therefore, of use in checking diarrhoea ; but a drawback to its continued use is that it may dry up the digestive juices, causing indigestion and constipation. Opium is also of use in checking internal haemorrhage.

A dose of Dover's powder, in which opium is mixed with ipecacuanha, is often useful in checking a common cold. Its action here may be threefold, as it increases perspiration and thus diminishes fever, it dries up the catarrh, and it limits inflammation, this last being another of the effects of the drug.

Codeine, one of the alkaloids of opium, diminishes the amount of sugar in the urine and has been used in treating diabetes.

There are many preparations of opium and others containing it or its alkaloids. Tincture of opium is better known as laudanum, and the compound tincture of camphor as paregoric. Ammoniated tincture of opium is sometimes called Scotch paregoric. Opium is the most important ingredient in Dover's powder or compound powder of ipecacuanha, and the drug is also contained in other powders. Opium is present also in the pill of ipecacuanha and squill and other pills. There are three salts of morphine, the acetate, the hydrochloride and the tartrate. Of each of the latter two there is an official liquor, or solution, and the hydrochloride enters into the compound tincture of chloroform and morphine.

Of preparations for external use there are the liniment and the ointment of gall and opium, which is a common remedy for piles.

Some proprietary preparations, such as Battley's solution, chlorodyne and nepenthe, also contain opium or morphine. Some soothing syrups have been found to contain opium, and deaths have occurred from their use, as opium in any shape is very badly borne by young children. It should never be given to them except under medical supervision.

Poisoning by Opium. Poisonous doses of opium cause no noticeable preliminary excitement but a drowsiness which deepens into profound sleep, from which, however, the patient may be roused, and then into coma, when it becomes impossible to rouse him. The skin is pale, cold and perhaps covered with perspiration. The breathing becomes slow, then irregular and shallow. The pupils contract until hardly visible, becoming what is called the pin-point pupil.

The patient must be aroused, if possible, and given an emetic of mustard and water. The best antidote is permanganate of potassium, and sufficient of this should be dissolved in half a glass of water to make

a deep red solution, which the patient should drink. Then hot strong coffee should be given freely, and, if the patient is unconscious, half a pint of coffee should be injected into the bowel ; this may be repeated once or twice. The patient must be kept awake, if necessary by walking up and down, though not to the stage of absolute exhaustion. If breathing is weak, artificial respiration should be carried out.

The victim of the opium habit or morphinism loses his appetite and powers of digestion, and as a rule his moral sense is progressively sapped until he becomes a liar and probably a thief. Sometimes he loses his reason. The condition is best treated by isolation in an institution, though when the patient retains sufficient will-power it is sometimes possible to allow him to go about his work and to treat him by giving progressively diminishing doses of the drug, what De Quincey called " unwinding the accursed chain."

See Apomorphine ; Drug Habits ; Poisoning.

OPTIC NERVE. The second pair of cranial nerves are called the optic nerve and subserve the function of vision. The fibres of an optic nerve are spread out all over the retina of the eye and are gathered up into a rounded bundle which passes back through an opening in the back of the eye. It then passes back through the orbit till within the skull, when the fibres are split up, those from the outer, or temporal, side of the retina passing backwards to the same side of the brain, while those from the nasal side pass to the opposite side of the brain.

The crossing of the fibre from the two sides makes a connecting bar, as it were, between the two nerves, which bar is called the optic commissure or chiasma. This lies immediately in front of the pituitary body and may be compressed when the latter becomes enlarged.

Behind the commissure the band of fibres on each side is called the optic tract. This passes back to masses of cells in the corpora quadrigemina and elsewhere in the same neighbourhood, which act as relay stations, some of the cells also acting as reflex centres for the contraction of the pupil under the influence of light. From these stations, fibres, the optic radiations, pass back to the posterior pole of the cerebrum and the adjoining surface of the inner side of the hemisphere. Disease or injury of this part of the brain will therefore cause blindness in each retina on the same side to that of the lesion.

Inflammation of the optic nerve is called optic neuritis.

See Eye ; Field of Vision.

OPTIC THALAMUS. In the base of the brain are certain masses of grey matter known as the basal ganglia. One pair of these, lying on either side of the 3rd ventricle of the brain, is called the optic thalami. Each thalamus acts as a sort of relay station for sensory fibres coming from the opposite side of the cord, fibres from cells in the thalamus sending on sensory impressions to the cortex of the brain.

Fibres also pass from the brain cortex to the thalamus, apparently controlling activity in the latter, for it has been noted that when such fibres are interrupted the intensity of sensations is greatly increased.

See Brain ; Sensation.

ORANGE. Both the fresh and the dried rind of the bitter orange are used for making medicinal preparations. There is an official infusion, a compound infusion, syrup, tincture and wine of orange. An essential oil distilled from orange-flowers is called oil of neroli and is contained in the official orange-flower water and syrup of orange-flowers. These preparations are chiefly used for flavouring, but the infusions, dose ½ to 1 ounce, the tincture, dose ½ to 1 drachm, and sometimes the wine, may be of use as aromatic bitters. In the materia medica orange is described as aurantium.

ORBIT. The bony cavity which forms the socket of the eye is known as the orbit. It is made up of several bones and is pyramidal in shape, the apex being directed backwards and perforated for the admission of the optic nerve.

See Eye.

ORCHITIS. Inflammation of the testicle is called orchitis. Should the back portion of the organ be first affected, however, the condition is called epididymitis.

See Epididymis ; Testicle.

ORGANIC DISEASE. When disorder of function depends on structural changes in tissue which can be seen by the naked eye or by microscopical examination, the disease is said to be organic. A disease in which no such changes can be found is said to be functional.

ORGANO-THERAPY. *See* Endocrine.

ORIENTAL SORE. In certain localities on the Mediterranean shores and further east there occurs a chronic ulcerative disease which is known as Oriental sore and by other names, according to places in which it is found. Thus it is also called Aleppo button, Baghdad sore, Biskra boil, Delhi boil, Sahara chancre and so on.

It is caused by infection with a minute protozoal parasite, leishmania tropica. This can be conveyed by contact, but insects would appear to play some part in dissemination. There is strong presumptive evidence implicating sand-flies, for example.

The disease begins as a papule. This breaks down, leaving an ulcer which runs a very chronic course, during which it spreads out from its original situation. As a rule there are two or more of such sores. When the ulcer heals it leaves a depressed and probably pigmented scar, so that if the disease has occurred on the face there may be much disfigurement. After the ulcer has healed there is immunity from subsequent attacks.

The disease is usually successfully treated by intravenous injections of antimony. The sores are dressed with antiseptics or with strong salt solution ; healing has been hastened in some cases by injecting emetine into the hard base of the sores.

See Leishmaniasis.

ORTHOPAEDICS. The branch of surgery devoted to the rectification of deformities of the limbs or spine, whether congenital or acquired, in children or adults, is described as orthopaedics.

See Flat Foot ; Spinal Curvature, etc.

OS. In Latin the word os, according to pronunciation, means either a bone or a mouth, the corresponding English adjectives being osseous and oral, respectively. The Latin name for some bones is frequently used when referring to them, for example, os calcis, or the heel-bone, and os innominatum, or the haunch-bone. A tiny bone, like those in the middle ear, is called an ossicle. Similarly, the opening, or mouth, leading into the womb is commonly referred to as the os.

OSMOSIS. The passage of crystaloids, such as common salt for example, through parchment or other permeable membranes is called osmosis. A colloid, of which white of egg may be taken as an example, will not pass through such membranes.

OSSIFICATION. The formation of bone is called ossification. In the skeleton, as it first exists, the bones are represented by cartilage, or gristle, with the exception of a few in the skull, which are represented by membrane. When the embryo is a few weeks old, however, bony tissue begins to be laid down at various points in the bones, such points being called centres of ossification. At birth considerable progress in ossification has been accomplished, but it is not till after the age of twenty that all the cartilage has been converted into bone.

See Bone ; Epiphysis.

OSTEITIS. Inflammation of bone may be called osteitis, or ostitis, though in practice these terms are restricted to inflammation affecting the dense shaft of long bones, the cancellous tissue in their ends, or the tissue of short or flat bones. The commonest cause of osteitis in this sense is tuberculosis, but it may be caused by trauma, syphilis, the organisms of some of the infective fevers or septic organisms of low virulence. There is always some degree of osteitis accompanying osteomyelitis or periostitis. The treatment depends on the cause.

Osteitis deformans, also known as Paget's disease, is a chronic inflammatory bone disease affecting the long bones and those of the brain pan. The bones become thickened and the long bones lengthen. At the same time they become softer, so that those that carry weight become bowed. The spine is kyphotic. The increase in size of the head makes it necessary to get a larger and larger size in hats. There may be neuralgic pains, but otherwise the health is unaffected, though the disease goes on progressively. Aspirin and similar drugs may be used to relieve the pain, but otherwise nothing can be done as the cause of the disease is not known.

See Bone ; Osteomyelitis ; Periosteum.

OSTEO-ARTHRITIS. Middle-aged and elderly people may suffer from progressive changes, described as osteo-arthritis, in the bones and cartilages of joints. The cartilage softens and is rubbed off, the exposed end of the bone becomes smooth and polished, or eburnated, but at the margin of the joint surface, on the other hand, the bone shows overgrowth, either in the form of general accentuation of its edge, that is to say, lipping or in the forming of localised projections, or osteophytes.

The joints most frequently affected are the hip, the knee and the shoulder. Fairly frequent also are enlargements on the back of the last joint of the fingers, known as Heberden's nodes, which are caused by overgrowth at the proximal end, that is, the one nearest the wrist, of the terminal phalanx. It will be noted that the joints mentioned are those exposed to most strain on the whole, so that strain may be a factor in causation. It is thought, however, that toxaemia from foci in the bowel, teeth or elsewhere may also play a part.

At the outset pain may be slight and intermittent, but later may become more severe and be continuous. There is also a limitation of movement which tends to be progressive. From time to time the joint may fill up with fluid.

Other conditions which may have to be distinguished are rheumatoid arthritis, gout, tuberculosis, Charcot's disease and chronic arthritis from gonorrhoea and other specific germs. An X-ray examination may be helpful in determining the nature of the affection.

In treatment the general state of health must be considered. The bowels must be kept freely open. Any possible source of toxaemia should be cleared up as far as possible. As regards the affected joint it may be said that moderate exercise is desirable, though rest may be necessary if the symptoms are acute. The general and local treatment for rheumatism (*q.v.*) may be useful in relieving pain. Sometimes prolonged treatment at a spa will appear to be the wisest course to take. The results of the disease cannot be removed by such general treatment, but further progress may be stayed. It is sometimes desirable to operate and remove osteophytes or other causes of limitation of movement.

See Joint ; Rheumatoid Arthritis.

OSTEOMALACIA. A disease of bone, characterised by softening of its structure, osteomalacia is almost always limited to women and generally begins during pregnancy or the nursing period. The bones bend and may undergo spontaneous fracture. Those of the pelvis are amongst the first to be affected, and the deformity caused by the bones being pressed inwards may occasion serious difficulties during labour, perhaps making Caesarian section necessary. A large proportion of those affected manifest the spasmodic nervous disorder known as tetany (*q.v.*).

Little is known about the causation of the disease, but unhygienic surroundings, including a lack of sunshine, appear to be factors. Cod-liver oil and calcium phosphate have proved capable of doing some good, as has treatment by glandular extracts, including parathyroid.

OSTEOMYELITIS. The literal meaning of the word osteomyelitis is inflammation of the bone marrow, but the name is more commonly used with reference to acute inflammation of the bone marrow in the shaft of long bones, and here the bony case is also involved and, probably, the periosteum or fibrous covering of the bone.

Acute osteomyelitis generally occurs in children, the lower end of the femur or the upper end of the tibia being very common sites, though the other extremities of these bones, the bones of the upper limb or other bones may sometimes be the site of the disease. The immediate cause is the activity of a microbe, usually a staphylococcus, but often there has been some injury, though this may have been so slight as to be overlooked.

The child complains of pain above or below a joint and soon looks very ill, with a high temperature and probably delirium. There is swelling and tenderness over the affected part. The condition is often mistaken for acute rheumatism, though it ought to be distinguished easily from this disease by the fact that the mischief is not in the joint. Unless immediate surgical treatment is undertaken the child may die in a day or two from septicaemia (*q.v.*) or blood-poisoning, or, if it should escape from the immediate risk, a large portion of the body may die and life may be threatened by chronic suppuration unless the limb is amputated.

Treatment consists in boring into the bone and giving free exit to the poisonous discharges.

See Femur ; Osteitis.

OTITIS. Inflammation of the ear is called otitis.

See Ear.

OTORRHOEA. A discharge from the ear is called otorrhoea. The discharge is usually purulent.

See Ear ; Mastoid Disease.

OTOSCLEROSIS. A disease consisting of changes in the bony walls of the labyrinth, or internal ear, otosclerosis causes a progressive loss of hearing and noises in the ear.

See Ear.

OVARY. Under the heading Genital System an account is given of the position, relations and functions of the ovary and of the causes and symptoms of inflammation of this organ, that is, ovaritis or oöphoritis. This is generally associated with inflammation of the Fallopian tube also, and the same applies to tuberculous disease of the ovary.

Displacement of the ovary may occur, and, from congestion of the organ, there is great tenderness and pain during intercourse, and in some cases when the bowels move or when

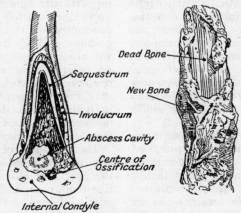

Dead Bone

Sequestrum

New Bone

Involucrum

Abscess Cavity

Centre of Ossification

Internal Condyle

Osteomyelitis. Left, child's thigh bone attacked by acute necrosis. Right, example in shaft of a bone

walking. The cause of the displacement may have to be dealt with by operation.

Tumours of the ovary are generally cystic, and if allowed to do so they may grow to huge dimensions. The contents of some cysts are watery, of others a thick glairy fluid. Both organs may be affected by cystic growth. A dermoid cyst of the ovary contains such structures as hair, bone, brain, teeth and so on, and actually represents the abortive development of a second individual in the body of the first. Ovarian growths should be removed as early as possible.

The removal of one ovary makes no difference, as the other functions for both, but if both ovaries are taken away there results an artificial menopause.

OVERCROWDING. The incidence and spread of infectious diseases is much increased by overcrowding. A certain number of apparently healthy folk are carriers of one infectious disease or another, and the closer they are herded with others the greater the risk of their communicating the infection ; when this has happened the disease spreads rapidly. The physique of an overcrowded population deteriorates ; but, on the other hand, it is difficult to estimate how much of the impaired health is actually due to overcrowding itself, because the feeble in mind and body and the vicious are more likely to drift into overcrowded areas. There are legislative enactments against overcrowding.

See Death Rate ; Housing.

OVERFEEDING. An habitual excess of food not only disturbs the digestion but interferes with metabolism and throws an undue strain on the excretory organs. Obesity, glycosuria and disease of the liver, kidneys and blood-vessels are some of the immediate consequences, and out of these others may flow.

Most people who have passed middle age eat too much.

In some diseases overfeeding, or forced feeding, has been deliberately practised, and by overfeeding in this connexion what is meant is inducing the patient to take more food than his appetite warrants. This has been done in consumption, for example, but here the aim should rather be to improve the appetite.

OVERLYING. A large number of infants are suffocated by being lain upon or covered with bedclothes when sharing the parents' bed. An infant should always sleep in its own cot, which can easily be constructed from a suitable box when the cost of a proper cot cannot be considered.

OVUM. The reproductive cell produced in the ovary is called an ovum, and if fertilised by a spermatozoon it is capable of developing into an animal of the same type as the parents. A mature human ovum is a spherical body about $\frac{1}{125}$ inch in diameter, surrounded by a membrane, the zona pellucida, a narrow space separating the two. In the protoplasm there is a large round nucleus. At the menstrual period an ovum escapes from the ovary and passes along the Fallopian tube.

See Embryo.

OXALIC ACID. In the form of calcium oxalate, oxalic acid is a normal constituent of urine. Its source is mainly food, as tea, rhubarb, tomatoes, gooseberries and other things contain a certain amount, but some of what is excreted is formed within the body. In certain circumstances the calcium oxalate is deposited as crystals in the urine, an occurrence described as oxaluria. The crystals are tiny, colourless and octahedral in shape ; they rather resemble tiny envelopes in their surface appearance.

The deposit of the crystals may have no particular significance, but it has some importance when symptoms point to the possibility of the presence of a renal calculus, and when there is irritability in the urinary passages, as a calculus may be composed of calcium oxalate, and oxaluria, even when no stone is deposited, may irritate the passages. Bed-wetting in children may be due to this, and possibly nocturnal emissions in children. Sufferers from dyspepsia may exhibit oxaluria.

The treatment of oxaluria is to correct any dyspepsia and avoid foods containing the acid, and also to limit milk because it is rich in calcium. Meat, bread, butter, milk puddings and coffee should be the main items of diet. A small amount of apple may be taken. Magnesia and citrate of potash are used to keep the oxalic acid in solution.

Poisoning by Oxalic Acid. Oxalic acid is used in the household as a cleansing agent, and as such is commonly known as salt of sorrel. Its crystals rather resemble those of Epsom salt, and accidental poisoning may occur. Oxalic acid is a corrosive poison, destroying tissues with which it comes into contact. It causes burning pain in the mouth, throat and stomach, vomiting and collapse.

An emetic must on no account be given. The best antidote is lime, such as powdered wall plaster, chalk or whiting, mixed with a little water.

Neither sodium nor potassium carbonate should be used, as they form soluble oxalates with the acid, and these pass into the circulation and poison the heart. For the same reason as little water as possible should be given.

See Poisoning.

OXYGEN. A colourless, odourless and tasteless elemental gas, oxygen constitutes about one-fifth of the bulk of the atmosphere, in which it is mixed with other gases, but mainly nitrogen. Water consists of a chemical combination of oxygen and hydrogen. Animal and vegetable life would be impossible but for the presence of oxygen in the air, or, as regards aquatic animals and plants, dissolved in water. Ordinary combustion also is made possible by oxygen. A lighted splinter of wood burns fiercely in pure oxygen and is quickly consumed, and a similar precipitate chemical activity would take place in animal bodies were the oxygen in the inspired air not diluted with nitrogen.

Pure oxygen, compressed in steel cylinders, is supplied for inhalation in appropriate circumstances, more particularly to prevent or remove asphyxia. Thus, inhalation may be beneficial in pneumonia and in heart disease with lung complications. Oxygen is often useful in carbon monoxide poisoning, and in acute uraemic poisoning. When general anaesthesia is being induced by chloroform and similar drugs, oxygen is always at hand for use when necessary, and a combination of laughing gas and oxygen is often used.

A chemical union between an element and oxygen is called oxidation, the product being an oxide. Thus, in the rusting of iron an oxide of this metal is produced. Freshly liberated or nascent oxygen is a very powerful disinfecting, deodorising and bleaching agent.

OXYMEL. A thick, syrupy liquid, composed of clarified honey, acetic acid and water, oxymel is sometimes taken for bronchial complaints, the dose being $\frac{1}{2}$ to 2 drachms. There is an official oxymel of squill and one of urginea, each of these being also an expectorant and used in doses of $\frac{1}{2}$ to 1 drachm.

OXYURIS VERMICULARIS. The scientific name of the tiny threadworm often found to be infesting the lower bowel is oxyuris vermicularis.

See Worm.

OZOENA. *See* Nose.

OZONE. In the neighbourhood of an electrical machine when it is working the air has a penetrating odour due to the presence of ozone, which is a gas consisting of oxygen but containing three atoms in the molecule instead of two as in ordinary oxygen gas. Ozone is produced in a thunderstorm also.

The benefits of a seaside holiday are not due to ozone, as was once thought, but to the fresh air and sunlight. If there is much ozone in the air breathed in, it causes great irritation, possibly resulting in serious bronchitis. Ozone is a powerful bleaching agent.

PACK. As a means of reducing temperature in fever or promoting sweating, a pack may be used. The method of applying a cold pack is described under that heading; a hot pack is applied in the same way, haste being required, however. The water out of which the sheet is wrung for a cold pack is usually at a temperature of from 60° to 80° F., and for a hot pack 110° F.

PAGET'S DISEASE. Two separate disorders are described as Paget's disease. The first is osteitis deformans, a disease of bones, which is discussed under the heading Osteitis, and the other is Paget's disease of the nipple, discussed under the heading Breast.

PAIN. Irritation of certain nerve endings or of the trunk or root of a sensory nerve causes a sensation of pain, which, in the main, is to be regarded as a salutary occurrence, directing attention to something that threatens the well-being of the body or some part of it.

Pain has not always the same quality, but in various instances may be described as boring, gnawing, cutting, stabbing, crushing, burning, throbbing, and so on. The special quality may give some hint of the cause of the pain, a throbbing pain being often associated with suppuration, for example, or a burning pain with herpes zoster.

The situation, even more than the nature of the pain itself, is usually of greater significance as a clue to the cause. There are instances, nevertheless, when the situation of the pain may give a misleading idea of the cause, unless the distribution of nerves is borne in mind. A pain in the temple, for example, may be caused by a carious tooth, as shown in the illustration in page 498. This is known as referred pain, and visceral pain is of this nature. The organs are for the most part capable of being handled without pain, but, although irritation in an organ may not cause pain actually in it, pain may be experienced at some part of the surface of the body. Irritation in the liver, for instance, may cause a pain at the back of the shoulder.

The explanation of this is that sympathetic nerve fibres from the liver pass into the spinal cord in the posterior root of the nerve supplying the skin over the back of the shoulder, and in the root the impulse travelling up the former is transferred in some way to the fibres of the latter and carried to the brain, where it is interpreted as coming from the endings of the sensory nerve at the back of the shoulder.

Of course, should the irritation reach the surface of an organ and be communicated to the body-wall with which it is in contact, then pain is felt exactly over the organ and it is tender on pressure.

Different people manifest varying degrees of susceptibility to pain and of ability to bear it. Distraction of mind may cause insensibility to pain. People suffering from hysteria sometimes complain bitterly of pain, and this may be accompanied by extreme hypersensitiveness of the skin over the site of pain, the slightest touch being intolerable. This hypersensibility is suggestive of hysteria, but not by any means conclusive evidence of it.

Pain has a wearing effect on the sufferer, and if sudden and very severe may occasion collapse.

A remedy that relieves pain is described as an anodyne or analgesic. The causes and treatment of pain are discussed under such headings as Inflammation ; Neuralgia ; and Neuritis. The expression labour pain is used for the periodical attacks of pain caused by contractions of the womb in the process of childbirth (*q.v.*).

See Sensation ; Spinal Cord ; Sympathetic Nervous System.

PALATE. The rigid arch which forms the roof of the mouth and the floor of the nose is called the hard palate. The front, and larger, part of it consists of portions of the upper jaw bones ; that at the back, of the horizontal plate of the palate bones. The palatal arch may be higher than usual in certain people. It is one of the so-called stigmata of mental degeneracy, but it may be caused by the existence of adenoids or other sources of nasal obstruction in early childhood, without any impairment of mental faculties.

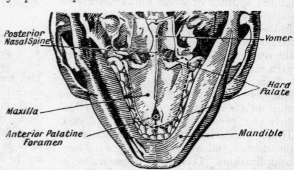

Palate. The hard palate is mainly formed by the two maxillae. Behind it is formed by the two palate bones

From failure of the bones to come together during development a cleft palate (*q.v.*) may exist at birth. Subsequent perforation is usually due to syphilis.

The fleshy curtain hanging downwards from the posterior border of the hard palate is called the soft palate. In the middle line it is prolonged into a narrow projection, the uvula. During swallowing or deep mouth-breathing the soft palate is drawn up so as to shut off the naso-pharynx (*q.v.*). In disease of the base of the brain or of the medulla oblongata one side of the soft palate may be noticed to lag behind the other when the palate is raised. This does not usually affect speech or swallowing much, but in bilateral paralysis, which is generally due to diphtheria, speech has a nasal quality, and fluids that are being swallowed may be partly returned through the nose.

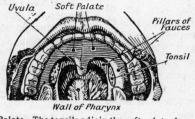

Palate. The tonsils adjoin the soft palate, from which there is a medial projection, the uvula

Sometimes the uvula is unduly long, when it tends to tickle the back of the throat and cause cough and, perhaps, nausea. The application of astringents may improve matters, but it is often necessary to have a part of the structure snipped off.

See Cleft Palate; Mouth; Naso-pharynx.

PALLIATIVE. Any treatment that relieves symptoms merely, without affecting their prime cause, is said to be palliative.

PALLOR. In some healthy people there is pallor or paleness of the face, while the mucous membranes, for example, the lining of the lower eyelid and the gum, retain a good colour. Should these parts, however, also be pallid some departure from the ordinary is indicated. A sudden pallor may occur from faintness or fright, and is then due to contraction of blood vessels, but when it is constant pallor is indicative of anaemia (*q.v.*).

PALPITATION. A sensation of fluttering or throbbing of the heart is called palpitation. It may indicate organic disease, but much more frequently is purely functional.

PALSY. *See* Paralysis.

PANCREAS. One of the most important organs in the body, the pancreas is an elongated gland which is described as having a head, a neck, a body and a tail. The head is tucked into the loop formed by the duodenum, while the body stretches across the abdomen in front of the aorta and behind the stomach, so that the tail comes into contact with the spleen.

The larger part of the glandular tissue is concerned in manufacturing the pancreatic juice, the uses of which are described under the heading Digestion. The main duct, which pours the juice into the bowel, is called the duct of Wirsung. Scattered throughout the pancreatic substance, however, are little collections of cells, known as the islets of Langerhans, the function of which is to produce the internal secretion known as insulin, which accelerates the burning up of sugar in the body.

Diseases of the Pancreas. Inflammation of the pancreas, similar to that occurring in the parotid and other glands, may occur in mumps (*q.v.*). In acute haemorrhagic pancreatitis, which usually occurs in adult males, there is free bleeding into the pancreas. There is severe colicky pain in the upper abdomen, vomiting and collapse. The abdomen is swollen and tense, and there is constipation. This disorder may

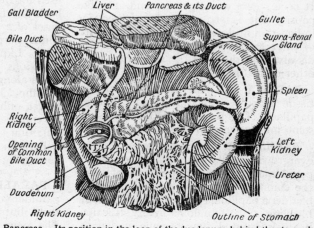

Pancreas. Its position in the loop of the duodenum, behind the stomach

cause sudden death, or the end may be delayed for a few days ; in a few instances, however, the patient has recovered.

In chronic pancreatitis the glandular tissue is replaced by fibrous tissue, and consequently there is impairment in the digestive functions, though the appearance of such may be delayed for a time by the work being done by the gastric and other juices. There tend to be lumps of fat in the faeces, however, showing the lack of digestion of the food. Another consequence is the loss of the insulin supply, and the supervention of diabetes. Alcoholism, syphilis and arterial disease appear to be the main causes of chronic pancreatitis.

Cancer, which is much the most usual new growth found in the pancreas, usually occurs in the head portion. It causes indigestion, pain in the pit of the stomach and rapid wasting. An early operation has sometimes been successful in eradicating the disease.

A cyst sometimes forms in the pancreas and may become sufficiently large to cause a bulging in the upper part of the abdomen. There may be attacks of indigestion and pain, suggestive of the presence of gallstones. Calculi may form in the pancreas itself and may give no trouble, though they may cause inflammation or lead to the development of a cyst.

The pancreas of animals used for food is called the sweetbread ; it is easily digested.
See Abdomen ; Diabetes ; Digestion ; Insulin ; Trypsin.

PAPAIN. A ferment obtained from the juice of the papaw fruit is known as papain. It occurs as a white powder and acts like pepsin, but is stronger. It is used for indigestion in doses of 5 to 10 grains, with or after food, and is also used locally to dissolve off diphtheritic membrane and other unhealthy tissue.

PAPILLA. A small conical elevation of tissue may be called a papilla (plural, papillae). This formation is found in skin, some mucous membranes and elsewhere.

PAPILLOMA. A tumour resembling an overgrown papilla, or papillae, is called a papilloma. It is a benign growth, of which the common wart is an example. In the bladder a papilloma may cause troublesome bleeding, and a papilloma in any situation, if much irritated, may become malignant.

PAPULE. A small, solid elevation on the skin or a mucous membrane is called a papule. Commonly it is referred to as a pimple. Sometimes it develops into a blister, or vesicle, or perhaps into a pustule, a vesicle containing matter.

PARACENTESIS. Puncturing the wall of some body-cavity. in order to evacuate fluid, is known as paracentesis.

PARAESTHESIA. An alteration of sensation, such as tingling, burning, chilliness, numbness or formication, without any obvious cause, is described as a paraesthesia. Formication means the sensation of ants crawling over the skin. A paraesthesia may occur in various nervous diseases.
See Numbness ; Sensation.

PARAFFIN. Various paraffin substances are obtained from shale by distillation and some of them are used in medicine. Hard paraffin, or paraffin wax, is a colourless, semi-transparent, waxy-looking substance without smell or taste. Soft paraffin, also called petroleum and petroleum jelly, is white or yellow and is semisolid. Vaseline is a proprietary brand of soft paraffin.

These paraffins are used for making ointments, the official paraffin ointment being an admixture of the hard and soft varieties. Paraffin wax candles are used in treating burns ; they are lit and the liquefied wax is dropped on the burn

Liquid paraffin is a clear colourless and odourless oily liquid. It must be distinguished from the paraffin oil, or kerosene, used for burning in lamps. It is used as a basis for fluids used in atomisers and in doses of 2 to 4 drachms as a laxative, for which purpose soft paraffin may also be used. Liquid and soft paraffin are used as emulsions for debilitated states sometimes along with hypophosphites. All the paraffin, however, passes through the bowel, unlike what happens with cod-liver oil emulsion, but nevertheless the general nutrition is often improved.

Paraffin oil, or kerosene, is used for destroying lice.
See Ambrine ; Ointment.

PARALDEHYDE. A liquid hypnotic, paraldehyde has a disagreeable odour and taste, but is relatively safe and efficient. The average dose is 2 drachms.

PARALYSIS. Loss of power in a muscle is called paralysis. If the loss is only partial, however, the condition may be referred to as paresis. Paralysis may be due to disease or injury of the nerve cells or nerves controlling a muscle, or, less frequently, to degenerative changes in the muscle itself. Under the heading Nervous System an account is given of the connexions of the nerve cells in the brain and in the cord with each other and with muscles, and of the differences in the character of the paralysis caused by damage to each of these kinds of nerve cell.

Paralysis due to damaged brain cells is likely to be a stiff or spastic paralysis, and that due to damaged cord cells or nerves a limp or flaccid paralysis. When the lower limbs are affected, each of these types produces a characteristic gait (*q.v.*).

Disease of the cortex of the brain on one side may cause hemiplegia, that is, paralysis of one side of the body. Hemiplegia on both sides is called diplegia. Hemiplegia may also be due to damage at lower levels in the brain, but, if sufficiently far down, there may be what is called crossed hemiplegia, that is, paralysis of the face on one side of the body and of the arm and leg on the other. A limited damage to the cortex of the brain may only cause a monoplegia, that is, paralysis of an arm, a leg, or of one side of the face. Paralysis of both legs is called paraplegia, and is usually due to damage to the spinal cord by injury or disease.

In many instances the possibility of a paralysis being functional or hysterical in character will have to be considered. The discrimination is assisted by regard to various circumstances in the case, but it can be said that if what is called the reaction of degeneration is present the paralysis is certainly organic in nature, that is, due to actual damage to nerves or nerve cells. The reaction consists in particular kinds of response to faradic and galvanic electric stimulation.

Treatment of paralysis has two aspects, namely, that of the cause and that of the muscles themselves. As regards the first, it may be necessary in some cases to remove by an operation a source of pressure on nervous tissue or to repair a nerve. Generally rest in bed will be required to promote a return to health of the damaged nervous tissue. When syphilis or some other infection or poison is the cause, special treatment, directed to this, will be required.

A paralysed muscle is liable to be stretched either from the effects of gravity or by contraction of the opposing muscles. Thus, when the muscles on the front of the leg are paralysed, the foot tends to be bent downwards at the ankle merely from its weight, and in bed the bed-clothes cause or increase bending by pressure on the toes. In addition, the muscles of the calf are not resisted as they normally are, so they tend to contract and pull down the toes.

One effect of this is to prevent recovery of power, as a stretched muscle has great difficulty in recovering. Another is that

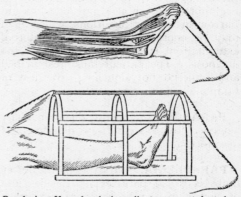

Paralysis. Use of a bed cradle to prevent foot drop in a case where the leg muscles are paralysed

the contracted muscles tend in time to shorten and to assume a position of contracture, so that, in order to put the foot in a natural position, it might be necessary to divide the tendons of the calf muscles close to their insertion into the foot. A similar thing might happen at other joints of the limb, at those of the upper limb, or elsewhere.

To prevent these consequences a paralysed limb is splinted, so that stretching of the paralysed muscle cannot take place. It is necessary to take care that the splinting is never removed during treatment, as merely to let a paralysed muscle be stretched for a moment may undo the benefit of many weeks of treatment. To prevent the pressure of bedclothes on a foot an apparatus called a bed-cradle (*q.v.*), or bed-cage, is employed.

A paralysed limb must be kept warm by means of a thick stocking or a flannel bandage. When any acute mischief responsible for the paralysis has settled down, gentle massage is used, and as time goes on this may become more vigorous, and other means of restoring tone, such as electrical stimulation and whirlpool baths, may be added (Plate XXIX, 1).

See Birth Paralysis ; General Paralysis of the Insane ; Infantile Paralysis ; Nervous System.

PARAMETRITIS. Inflammation of the loose, or cellular, tissue lying on either side of the womb is called parametritis or pelvic cellulitis. Infection takes place in connexion with childbirth, as a rule, and usually from a tear in the neck of the womb. The patient becomes fevered, but there may be little pain, at any rate at the beginning. An abscess may develop and burrow in various directions, when there may be considerable pain. An internal examination is required to make the diagnosis. The patient must rest in bed and undergo hot douching, the use of tampons and other treatment.

See Perimetritis ; Womb.

PARANOIA. A mental disorder, characterised by systematised delusions, is described as paranoia.

See Mental Disease.

PARAPLEGIA. Paralysis of the lower limbs is called paraplegia. Besides loss of power in the limbs there are other symptoms, which vary according to the cause or type of the paralysis.

See Nervous System ; Paralysis.

PARASITE. Animal parasites within the body are called entozoa and include amoebae and various kinds of worms. Those on the surface are called epizoa ; lice and mites, for example. Some of the mites, however, burrow in the skin, and the larvae of flies may penetrate much more deeply.

Similarly, vegetable parasites within the body are called entophyta and include bacteria and various fungi, and those like ringworm, and other fungous parasites which infest the surface, are called epiphyta.

See Amoeba ; Bacteria ; Protozoa.

PARATHYROID. Two pairs of glands, lying behind and in close relationship to the lateral lobes of the thyroid gland, are known as the parathyroid glands. They appear in some way to influence calcium metabolism in the body, and when they are removed or diseased a nervous disorder, known as tetany, supervenes.

PARIETAL. The roof of the skull is formed mainly by the right and left parietal bones, thin plates of bone hollowed out like a saucer. The most prominent part of the bone is called the parietal eminence.

The term parietal is also used for something related to the wall of a body cavity. Thus the layer of pleura covering the wall of the chest is called the parietal layer as distinguished from the visceral layer, which covers the lung.

PARKINSON'S DISEASE. Paralysis agitans, or Parkinson's disease, is a chronic nervous disorder, which usually occurs after middle life and is more frequent in men than in women. Its onset is insidious, and its course is characterised by the development of muscular weakness, rigidity and tremors. The face has a wooden expression, described as Parkinson's mask, and the body is held stiffly. There is a peculiar gait (*q.v.*), which goes by the name of festination. The hands exhibit a coarse tremulous movement, as if rolling pills, and there may also be tremor of the rest of the upper limb, the head, the tongue and the legs.

The part of the brain affected is that known as the corpus striatum, and the disease in some instances dates from a severe nervous shock. Symptoms resembling those described sometimes occur as a sequel to an attack of encephalitis lethargica, or sleepy sickness.

There is no cure for Parkinson's disease, but some relief may be obtained from doses of hyoscine hydrobromide.

PAROTID GLAND. The largest of the salivary glands, the parotid lies in front of, and beneath, the ear. Its main discharge tube, known as Stensen's duct, passes forwards and opens on the inner surface of the cheek, opposite the second upper molar tooth. Through this duct a thin salivary juice is poured into the mouth. The branches into which the facial nerve divides traverse the gland and may be damaged when it is diseased or injured.

Inflammation of this gland is called parotitis. Epidemic parotitis is better known as mumps (*q.v.*). In this disease the gland does not suppurate, but it may do so in ordinary parotitis. Sometimes an abscess forms in Stensen's duct and, bursting through the outer surface of the cheek, causes a salivary fistula. Infection in these cases comes from the mouth.

A simple parotid tumour contains masses of cartilage and of mucous tissue in addition to glandular tissue. It grows slowly and does not affect the health except in so far as it interferes with chewing, but it may become malignant and therefore should be removed.

See Digestion.

PAROVARIUM. Certain tubes in the broad ligament of the womb constitute what is called the parovarium. From these tubes a cystic growth may develop and reach great dimensions. It is filled with a watery fluid.

See Womb.

PAROXYSM. A symptom which is of a clamant character and appears suddenly, such as pain, coughing, convulsions, etc., may be described as a paroxysm. The term is also used for the periodical intensification of a symptom. Another application of the term is to the febrile periods of malaria or some other intermittent fever.

PARRISH'S SYRUP. The compound syrup of iron phosphate, B.P.C., is also called Parrish's syrup and chemical food. It is a useful tonic, especially for children, and is given in doses of ½ to 2 drachms, frequently in conjunction with cod-liver oil.

PASTEURISATION. A method of diminishing the number of microbes in milk (*q.v.*) by the use of heat is called pasteurisation.

PASTILLE. A lozenge with a basis of glycerin and gelatin is called a pastille, though this name is also used for other things.

See Lozenge.

PATELLA. The small rounded disk of bone known as the patella, or knee-cap, is interposed in the tendon attaching the quadriceps extensor muscle of the front of the thigh to the upper end of the tibia, the extension of the tendon from the patella to the tibia being called the patellar ligament.

The skin over the patella is stretched when the knee is bent, and in this position a blow or fall on the bone usually causes a long wound, resembling a cut. The bone may be broken (*see* Plate XXI, 2) by a blow or by a violent attempt to straighten the leg. The first-aid treatment is discussed under the heading Fracture.

See Bursa ; Knee.

PATENT MEDICINE. A secret remedy is a patent medicine only when it has been actually patented, in which case it carries a special label. This label, however, does not imply any recommendation of the preparation by the Patent Office. A proprietary medicine is one protected by a trade mark or trade name, whether or not it has been patented. Secret remedies are in this category, but some proprietary preparations are not secret. They may be either new drugs produced in a laboratory or skilful or elegant combinations of old and known drugs.

The statement that a secret nostrum contains some superlatively valuable medicinal agent, unknown to medical science, can be discounted, as the therapeutical resources of the world in the way of drugs have been thoroughly examined and a judicious selection made by the compilers of the various pharmacopoeias. Moreover, it is a fairly simple matter to discover the contents of any preparation by analysis, and this has been done for most at least of the secret remedies ; if anything new and really valuable had existed it would have been discovered and added to our stock of known remedies.

The composition of some of the secret remedies for which large claims have been made has been altered without changing the name, and the composition of some of them varies in different parts of the world, presumably to conform to the law, but the name remains the same.

Proprietary remedies that are extensively advertised encourage the habit of self-drugging, a vicious habit when carried to excess and possibly dangerous at any time, unless the nature of the complaint is quite simple and the remedy likewise.

See Drug.

PEAT BATH. At Strathpeffer, Harrogate and other spas, baths resembling in appearance and consistency those made from mud are prepared with peat. This bath retains a very even temperature for a considerable time, and is of use in general irritability, rheumatism and similar disorders, and in certain skin diseases. *See* Baths ; Mud Bath.

PEDICULOSIS. Lousiness may be described as pediculosis, a louse (*q.v.*) being called a pediculus.

PELLAGRA. In Italy, the Southern States of America and other countries, mainly those with a warm climate, a disease known as pellagra occurs. It is found amongst poor people whose diet largely consists of maize, and the most probable cause is a lack of protein and especially of particular kinds of protein in the food ; maize is very deficient in this respect.

The disease, which has a gradual onset, is characterised by inflammation and ulceration of the mouth, diarrhoea, vomiting and loss of appetite, redness and subsequent thickening of the skin on the backs of the hands and forearms, and possibly on the face, neck and chest, headache, giddiness, muscular weakness and mental depression, perhaps leading to melancholia and dementia. Sexual perversion is sometimes noted.

The condition tends to improve during the colder part of the year, but gets worse, especially the nervous symptoms, when the weather gets warmer.

Treatment consists in a generous diet and, if possible, removal to a colder climate. Arsenic and bone marrow will probably be helpful.

PELVIS. The skeleton of the lowest part of the trunk is formed by a basin-like structure, the pelvis, which is made up of the innominate bones at the sides and in front, and a triangular mass of bone known as the sacrum behind. The sacrum consists of five vertebrae fused together and has at its tip the coccyx. The gaps which exist in the skeleton are filled in by muscles and membranes, so that a closed basin is actually formed.

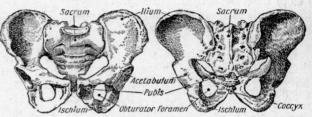

Bones composing the pelvis seen from the front (left) and back

The floor of the basin is pierced by the urethra and anus, however, and in the female by the vagina as well. The pelvis is described as consisting of two parts, the true pelvis and the false pelvis. The latter is the part on a level with the expanded portions of the iliac bones which is bounded below by a definite ridge or margin, beneath which is the true pelvis. In the true pelvis are the bladder and rectum, and in the female the womb and its appendages. Coils of intestine also are disposed over the top of these organs.

Round the brim of the true pelvis run the iliac blood vessels, and on either side the ureter dips in over the brim to join the bladder. On the left side the large bowel also dips down to become the rectum. At the back of the pelvis, lying on the front of the sacrum, is the network of nerves known as the sacral plexus. The pressure of the child's head on these nerves during labour may cause severe pain and cramp.

Deformity of the bones of the pelvis, caused by rickets and

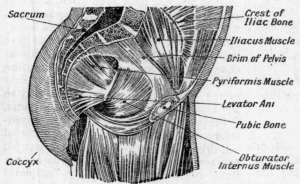

Pelvis, Sectional view showing the muscles that line its cavity and contribute to forming its floor

other disorders, may interpose a serious and sometimes complete obstruction to the birth of a child. Fracture of the pelvis may happen when a person is run over by a heavy vehicle. The bladder or other internal organs may be crushed or torn in this event.

See Fracture ; Hip ; Innominate ; Sacrum.

PEMPHIGUS. A burn or some other kind of irritation, including microbic, may cause large blisters, or bullae, on a skin or mucous surface, but when bullae occur from some obscure reason the condition is described as pemphigus (Plate XXXI, 6).

Butchers and others who handle dead animals are liable to be infected through cuts or abrasions on the hands and suffer from what is called acute febrile pemphigus. Fever occurs with headache and great thirst, and 24 to 48 hours afterwards bullae appear, usually on the neck and limbs. The disease may be subacute without much fever, but bullae form on mucous membranes and then on the skin, and there is an early development of profound general depression, described as the typhoid state. In either form recovery is very exceptional, and the possibility of the disease occurring makes it very necessary to disinfect cuts, etc., most carefully.

A chronic form of pemphigus occurs, bullae first appearing on mucous membranes, especially on that of the mouth, and later on the skin. There is no pain and the general health does not suffer at the beginning, but later it does in a serious way. The bullae rupture and crusts form on the raw surface. Skin lesions of other kinds may form, as in Duhring's disease, or dermatitis herpetiformis. When lesions heal a reddened surface is left. Quinine, in large doses, or organic arsenical preparations, are used internally, and sedative and antiseptic lotions and drying powders are applied externally.

Some persons inherit a tendency to develop bullae from slight irritation of the skin as by the pressure of clothing. Another hereditary skin affection, epidermolysis bullosa, manifests itself from birth. Bullae form chiefly on the face and limbs, and portions of skin may show atrophic changes, the nails possibly being lost in the process. Treatment by organo-therapy has been of use in these disorders.

Two very rare forms of pemphigus may occur. In one of these, pemphigus foliaceus, after bullae have formed the skin becomes reddened all over and large flakes peel off. In the other, pemphigus vegetans, cauliflower-like tumours form on the raw surfaces exposed by the rupture of bullae. Treatment in either form is unsuccessful.

Pemphigus of the new-born is simply a form of impetigo (*q.v.*).

See Dermatitis ; Skin.

PENNYROYAL. Oil of pennyroyal is used as a domestic remedy for flatulence and colic, but should not be given to women except on medical advice, as in certain circumstances it may be dangerous. A half to one teaspoonful in an ounce of olive oil or vaseline, if smeared on exposed parts, may ward off midges and other troublesome insects.

PEPPER. In addition to its use as a condiment, pepper has some medicinal value. It contains a neutral principle, piperine, an acrid resin and a volatile oil. Piperine has the same actions as pepper itself, namely, carminative and stimulant. The confection of pepper, B.P., contains black pepper, and in doses of 60 to 120 grains may be of benefit to people suffering from piles and other rectal disorders.

Piperidine, a drug prepared from piperine, is given to diminish a tendency to the excessive formation of uric acid. Cayenne pepper is powdered capsicum (*q.v.*), and Jamaica pepper, allspice.

PEPPERMINT. From the peppermint plant there is distilled the essential oil of peppermint, which is used as a carminative and anti-spasmodic, the dose being $\frac{1}{2}$ to 3 minims. From this oil are prepared peppermint water, dose 1 to 2 ounces, and spirit of peppermint, dose 5 to 20 minims. From oil of spearmint, which has the same dose and uses as the other, is prepared the water of green mint. Its dose is the same as that of the other water, and either may be given to a child of one year in a dose of 1 drachm.

See Menthol.

PEPSIN. The main digestive ferment in gastric juice is pepsin, which acts on protein foodstuffs. This ferment is extracted from the gastric mucous membrane of the pig, sheep or calf, and is used to assist digestion. It is a light, yellowish-brown granular or scaly substance, and is given in doses of 5 to 10 grains. It may also be used as the glycerin of pepsin, the dose of which is 1 to 2 drachms. The drug can be obtained in tablets, but a good brand should be selected.

PEPTONE. The ferments pepsin and trypsin in the digestive juices convert protein foodstuffs into a simpler protein known as peptone. This is obtained artificially from meat and occurs as a whitish powder. It is sometimes injected into the body in the treatment of asthma.

Food is peptonised by admixture with trypsin, the ferment of the pancreatic juice, the process as regards milk being described under that heading. Meat is peptonised by taking 4 ounces of minced meat, adding ½ pint of water and gradually bringing to the boil. Another ½ pint of cold water is then added and a peptonising powder. The mixture is kept warm for about three hours. The product is not very pleasant to take, however, and peptonised milk is preferable. There are some proprietary peptonised meat preparations on the market.

PERCUSSION. The investigation of the state of the body cavities by tapping their surface with the point of the finger or a special instrument is called percussion. Another finger, or a special plate for the purpose, is generally laid on the surface to be examined and the percussion is done on the finger or the plate. Consolidation of lung, emphysema, the presence of tumours in cavities, the size and position of the heart are amongst some of the subjects about which information can be obtained by percussion.

PERFORATION. The wall of a hollow viscus may be perforated by injury or disease, and when this occurs suddenly there is usually acute pain and collapse. Perforation of the stomach or bowel, occurring in connexion with chronic ulceration, may give rise to no more than slight symptoms owing to the site of the perforation being walled off by peritoneal adhesions resulting from the precedent inflammation.

PERICARDIUM. The heart is enclosed in a bag known as the fibrous pericardium, but inside this is another bag formed of a tough, smooth membrane, which lines the fibrous bag and is reflected on to the heart. This second bag is the serous pericardium and it permits of the heart working without friction.

Inflammation of the serous pericardium is called pericarditis. The surface of the membrane becomes roughened so that a scraping or shuffling sound, caused by the movement of the two roughened surfaces over each other and synchronous with the movements of the heart, is audible on listening over the organ. There may also be pain and a rise of temperature.

The process may not stop short here, but go on to the effusion of fluid into the serous bag, and this may seriously interfere with the heart's action, causing dyspnoea.

The most frequent cause of pericarditis is acute rheumatism, but it may occur in other infectious fevers, from tuberculous infection or from other causes. The causative disease must be treated and counter-irritation applied over the heart. A large fly-blister is often effective. Sometimes fluid should be drawn off by tapping.

Parts of the two surfaces of the membrane may remain stuck together, such being called pericardial adhesions, and may hamper the heart's action, leading to hypertrophy.

See Heart ; Serous Membrane.

PERIMETRITIS. Inflammation of the peritoneum covering the organs in the pelvis is called perimetritis or pelvic peritonitis. Infection usually comes from the genital tract, but it may come from a diseased appendix or from some other part of the bowel. When acute there is severe pain and tenderness, high fever and probably vomiting, while the abdomen is swollen and tympanitic. The condition may gradually lessen in severity and in about a fortnight settle down into a chronic condition ; or at any time there may be an extension of the infection and general peritonitis.

In chronic perimetritis there is an extensive formation of adhesions, matting the organs together and probably displacing them. From dragging on these adhesions there may be irritability of the bladder and menstrual pain, some obstruction of the bowel and other troubles.

The treatment of the acute disorder resembles that of parametritis (*q.v.*), but if a diseased appendix is suspected an operation will be necessary, and also if there is much pus. Later, an operation may be desirable to remove a diseased Fallopian tube or to divide adhesions. Spa treatment is sometimes successful in lessening chronic inflammatory trouble and improving the general health.

PERINEUM. The area on the lower part of the trunk, corresponding to the outlet of the pelvis, is called the perineum. It extends from the arch of the pubis in front to the top of the coccyx behind, and to the tuberosity of the ischium on either side. In this region is the opening of the bowel, or anus, and the external genital organs.

In females there is a wedge-shaped mass of tissues, consisting of skin, muscles and fascia between the lower portions of the vagina and rectum. This is called the perineal body, the skin covering it usually being referred to simply as the perineum. These tissues stretch during childbirth to allow the passage of the child and sometimes tear. The laceration may extend right into the rectum. All such lacerations, however slight, should be stitched, as they afford an entrance to bacteria, and if at all considerable they favour prolapse of the womb.

PERIOSTEUM. The fibrous membrane covering the surface of bone, except where this is clothed with cartilage, is called the periosteum. It contains a free supply of blood vessels which contribute to the nourishment of the bone, and a piece of bone, denuded of its periosteum, necroses or dies if the uncovering is at all extensive.

Inflammation of this membrane, or periostitis, may be acute or chronic. Simple acute periostitis may be caused

Periosteal Vessels

Artery Entering Bone

Part of femur with turned-up flap of its periosteum

by an injury, say a kick on the shin. There is a hot, painful swelling, largely caused by effused blood. Rest is required, and if the part affected is in the lower limb the limb should be put in an elevated position. If the skin is not broken cold applications may be applied, otherwise hot boracic fomentations are indicated.

Acute inflammation from septic infection occurs as a rule in connexion with the inflammation of the bone itself. Chronic inflammation results in thickening of the periosteum and of the underlying bone, the elevation being described as a node. Syphilis, or a chronic ulcer adjacent to the periosteum, is the usual cause ; but a chronic periostitis may also occur from tuberculosis.

See Bone ; Osteitis ; Osteo-myelitis.

PERIPHERAL NEURITIS. Multiple neuritis is also called peripheral neuritis.
See Neuritis.

PERISTALSIS. The movements of the stomach and bowels, which mix their contents and drive them along, are described as peristalsis.
See Digestion ; Intestine.

PERITONEUM. The smooth, thin membrane that lines the abdomen is called the peritoneum. It forms a closed bag, except for the opening of the Fallopian tube in the female, but from the posterior wall of the abdomen and the floor of the pelvis the organs push forward into this bag and fill it up, notably the bowel, of which the peritoneum forms the mesentery (*q.v.*). Ordinarily, therefore, there is no actual space in the bag, but when the abdomen is opened at an operation the cavity becomes apparent.

The outer surface of the peritoneal bag is very resistant to infection, and an operation on an abdominal or pelvic organ which avoided opening the bag would generally be adopted in preference to one that involved opening it, as the inside of the bag is readily infected and the consequences may be very serious. At the same time, it must be added, the risk of opening the bag has been reduced to a minimum by aseptic methods of surgery.

Inflammation of the peritoneum is called peritonitis, and may be acute or chronic and localised or general. A localised peritonitis may occur when a chronic inflammatory process, such as a gastric ulcer, or infection of low virulence, as in some cases of appendicitis, affects the peritoneum. On the adjoining surfaces of the peritoneal bag lymph is poured out and glues the surfaces together, thus shutting off the cavity of the peritoneum. Should, however, the stomach rupture into the cavity, or an appendix abscess burst into it before this shutting off could take place, there would be general peritonitis, the whole of the inside of the bag, more or less, being implicated.

General peritonitis may also be caused by wounds of the abdomen, by obstruction or rupture of the gut, by extension of infection from the Fallopian tube, by rupture of the womb and so on.

Chronic peritonitis, whether localised or general, is characterised by gluing of the surfaces of the membrane, resulting in the formation of adhesions and the matting together of adjoining viscera. Abscesses may form at any time. The more usual sites for localised chronic peritonitis are the appendix and the pelvis. The first is discussed under the heading Appendicitis. Besides depressing the general health the pelvic disorder causes pain, especially in connexion with menstruation, probably sterility and possibly other troubles.

A more extensive chronic peritonitis may result from cancer affecting one of the abdominal organs, leading to adhesions and the accumulation of fluid in the abdomen. Otherwise the usual cause is tuberculosis, children being the usual victims. In some instances thickening of the peritoneum, adhesions and matting of the intestines are the prominent features, but in others it is the accumulation of fluid or ascites. The abdomen is more or

Peritoneum. Principal folds of this lining membrane in the female abdominal cavity

less swollen in all cases, however. The general treatment for tuberculosis, including fresh air and sunlight, is required. In some cases the mere opening of the abdomen has caused a wonderful improvement.

Acute general peritonitis is a very serious disorder. There is great pain in the abdomen, which becomes distended and tender. The bowels are paralysed, and there is stagnation of their contents. The patient looks poisoned and very ill and tends to develop what is called the Hippocratic facies, described under the heading Face. Vomiting is troublesome. The risk of a fatal termination is very great. Generally an operation is required to deal with the source of infection and provide for the drainage of the abdomen. The patient is usually put up in a half-reclining posture, referred to as Fowler's position. Hot applications or ice, and probably drugs, are used to relieve pain. Food must be very light and possibly nutrient enemata may be necessary.

See Abscess ; Appendicitis ; Lymphatic System ; Serous Membrane.

PERITYPHLITIS. Inflammation of the caecum is called typhlitis, and of its peritoneal covering, perityphlitis. An independent inflammation of the caecum may occur from the irritation of worms and other causes, but, generally speaking, inflammation in this region is associated with appendicitis (*q.v.*), and should be treated as such.

PERNICIOUS ANAEMIA. *See* Anaemia.

PERSPIRATION. *See* Sweat.

PERVERSION. An unnatural inclination or habit is called a perversion. A perverted appetite, a desire to eat cinders or other unsuitable things, often occurs in pregnancy, and is encountered in certain nervous disorders. Sexual perversion is believed by many to proceed usually from a suppressed mental complex, and perhaps remediable by psycho-analysis.

See Freudism.

PESSARY. An apparatus for supporting the womb and preventing its displacement is called a pessary. Different types are used according to the circumstances of each case. One consists of a round ring with a core of watch-spring and a soft rubber covering, and is much used. Others commonly used are vulcanite rings moulded into various shapes. All pessaries of the types which have been mentioned should be inserted and removed by a doctor. They should not be worn for longer than three months without renewal, as they tend to become corrugated and corroded and may irritate. Also, while a pessary is being worn the patient should douche every day with lysol solution, a teaspoonful in two pints of warm water.

When one of those types fails to prevent prolapse, or falling, of the womb, the cup and stem variety will probably do so. This is supported by elastic bands attached to the waist. It is taken out at night and cleansed, and reinserted in the morning.

The term pessary is also used for large suppositories intended for introducing drugs into the vagina. Some contraceptive pessaries are of this kind, but another, the check pessary, is an apparatus intended to cover the neck of the womb. Neither of these types is quite satisfactory for the purpose, however.

Pessaries containing ichthyol and other drugs are often of great use in the treatment of internal inflammatory disorders.

PETECHIA. A small round spot caused by bleeding into the skin is called a petechia.

See Purpura.

PEYER'S PATCH. In the mucous lining of the small bowel, opposite the line of attachment of the mesentery, there are collections of lymphoid tissue, known as Peyer's patches. They are oval or elongated in shape, from ½ inch to 4 inches long and about ½ inch across. They become inflamed and ulcerated in typhoid fever. Nodules of the same tissue dot the bowel and are called solitary follicles.

PHAGEDAENA. A rapidly spreading ulceration associated with sloughing, or gangrene (*q.v.*), is described as phagedaena. It sometimes occurs in connexion with a venereal sore, or chancre, but might complicate any wound. This, however, is rare nowadays except in the tropics, where an ulcer of this description is variously termed a tropical ulcer, tropical phagedaenic ulcer, or, according to places where it more commonly occurs, Aden ulcer, Cochin sore, Guiana ulcer, Mozambique sore and so on.

The condition may be due to the combined activities of Vincent's fusiform bacillus and a spironema. Diabetes, alcoholism and other debilitating factors favour the activity of these organisms. The condition is treated by cutting away sloughs and disinfecting the area with pure carbolic acid or cauterising it. Continuous irrigation of the wound or prolonged warm antiseptic baths are also used. Organic arsenical compounds and other drugs are administered, and the general state of health is improved by fresh air, a generous diet and tonics.

PHAGOCYTE. Certain blood corpuscles and body cells attack and destroy bacteria and other harmful bodies by ingesting them. Such a cell is called a phagocyte, and the process, phagocytosis. Antibodies in the blood plasma, known as opsonins, facilitate the ingestion of germs. Phagocytosis is an important factor in causing immunity (*q.v.*).

PHALANGES. The bones in the fingers and toes are called the phalanges (singular, phalanx). There are three of these, the proximal, the middle and the distal, in each finger and toe, but the thumb and the great toe have each only two.

See Finger ; Toe.

PHARYNX. The cavity behind the nose, mouth and larynx is known as the pharynx. When one breathes through the nose, as is proper, the pharynx forms a continuous tube, but, in swallowing, the portion behind the nose, called the nasopharynx (*q v*), is shut off from the rest by the ascent of the soft palate. The portion behind the mouth and larynx, to which this account will be limited, has behind it the cervical vertebrae, from which it is separated by ligaments and muscles.

In front it has the fauces (*q.v.*) and the base of the tongue, and below this the epiglottis and the entrance into the larynx. At the level of the cricoid cartilage of the larynx it becomes continuous with the oesophagus, or gullet. The wall of the pharynx consists of a membranous bag, outside which are three flat muscles, the constrictors of the pharynx, and inside, a lining of mucous membrane.

Inflammation of this lining, or pharyngitis, may be acute or chronic.

Acute pharyngitis, a form of acute sore throat, may be due to a common cold, to a rheumatic poison, to other infections, to irritation by vapours or hot or otherwise irritating food or liquor, and so on. The mucous membrane is red and angry-looking, and white or yellowish mucus adheres here and there in patches. Swallowing and speaking are painful and there is usually a dry, irritating cough.

The general treatment will depend on the cause. If this is judged to be rheumatism it should be on the lines of that for acute rheumatism, and the fact that heart complications are possible should be borne in mind. In all cases talking should be avoided and the food should be at most semi-solid, and should be bland and not too hot. Hot applications to the neck may be useful. The inhalation of steam from a jug of hot water to which a teaspoonful of Friar's balsam has been added is often very soothing. The throat may be gargled with a warm, weak solution of permanganate of potash or some other gargle (*q.v.*), or it may be sprayed with menthol. Lozenges of menthol or krameria may also be sucked.

Chronic pharyngitis may be caused by the excessive use of alcohol, tobacco or condiments. It is common also in those who have to talk much, especially when the voice is misused, and in those who work in an atmosphere charged with dust or with irritating vapours. Anaemia, gout, constipation and other general disorders predispose to the occurrence of pharyngitis.

The mucous membrane may be reddened, with dilated veins showing here and there, and there may be patches of dry mucus which the patient tries to get rid of by frequent hawking. Sometimes there are little red elevations dotted over the surface, and in clergyman's throat (*q.v.*) these may occur without other signs. The voice is easily tired, and commonly there is an irritating cough which may excite nausea.

Treatment must be directed to any general disorder, or to dyspepsia or constipation if such exist. Tobacco, alcohol and condiments should be stopped. The voice must be rested when necessary, and, when daily work involves much talking, lessons in voice production from a reliable teacher may be invaluable. The inhalation, gargle and lozenges above mentioned may be useful for relieving irritation. Sometimes the back of the throat is painted with silver nitrate or some other astringent, and it may be necessary to burn

Pharyngeal Tonsil

Naso-Pharynx

Soft Palate

Buccal Pharynx

Uvula

Tonsil

Laryngo Pharynx

Tongue

Epiglottis

Oesophagus

Pharynx. Its three parts seen from behind

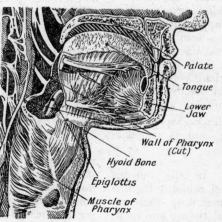

Palate

Tongue

Lower Jaw

Wall of Pharynx (Cut)

Hyoid Bone

Epiglottis

Muscle of Pharynx

Side section showing position of epiglottis

off the little red granules with an electro-cautery.

An abscess behind the pharynx, which is referred to as a retro-pharyngeal abscess, may be acute or chronic. An acute abscess is commonest in children, and, though the prick of a fish-bone or some similar accident may sometimes account for the infection, the cause may be obscure. A child suffering from such an abscess adopts rather a characteristic attitude, with the head thrown back and towards one side and the mouth open. A cold abscess is generally due to tuberculosis. In either case the posterior wall of the pharynx is seen to be bulging forward. Surgical treatment is necessary.

See Clergyman's Throat ; Fauces ; Mouth ; Naso-pharynx ; Neck.

PHENACETIN. A coal-tar derivative, phenacetin occurs as colourless, scaly crystals, without smell or taste. It is but slightly soluble in water, and is usually given in cachets, tablets or a little gruel. The dose is 5 to 15 grains. Phenacetin is mainly used to relieve headache and other pains, and as it may cause some depression a little caffeine (*q.v.*) is often combined with it.

If an overdose has been taken the patient should lie down and have warm bottles at the feet and by his side. Dilute spirits or sal volatile should be given, or some strong coffee.

PHENOL. *See* Carbolic Acid.

PHIMOSIS. Undue length and tightness of the foreskin, so that it cannot be pulled back clear of the glans penis, constitutes phimosis. The passage may be so narrow as to obstruct the flow of urine, but in any case there is an accumulation of smegma, the thick white, or yellow, secretion from the membrane behind the corona, or prominent edge, of the glans, and this secretion causes much irritation and possibly inflammation of the glans, or balanitis. Phimosis is usually congenital. It may cause a habit of bed-wetting and perhaps of self-abuse. It is frequently a cause of rupture. Its existence throughout life predisposes to cancer of the penis after a certain age. Phimosis should be treated by circumcision (*q.v.*).

It sometimes happens that when the foreskin is retracted behind the glans it cannot be brought forward again. This is called paraphimosis, and leads to much swelling of the glans and other parts in front of the constriction. Firm and steady pressure on the swollen parts by grasping them through a towel may so reduce the swelling as to permit of the foreskin being brought forward, but a little operation is sometimes needed. In any case circumcision should be done as soon as possible.

PHLEBITIS. Inflammation of a vein is called phlebitis.
See Vein.

PHLEGM. Sticky mucus, brought up by coughing or vomiting, is commonly referred to as phlegm.
See Sputum.

PHLEGMASIA. The most common use of the term phlegmasia, which means inflammation, is in the name phlegmasia alba dolens, applied to a disorder of the leg, or legs, which may occur in the lying-in period. It is better known as milk-leg, or white-leg (*q.v.*).

PHOBIA. Certain individuals have a dread of some situation, action or thing ; for example, of being in a closed space or, on the contrary, an open space, of sitting or of running, or of a black cat. These fears do not depend on a lowered state of health, nor can the individual find any explanation for his fear in any of his experiences.

Such a fear is described as a phobia. It may depend on some childish experience which has been repressed or forgotten. In other instances it may depend on some mental conflict, the real character of which is unknown to the patient and which is merely symbolised in his phobia.

The only treatment likely to be quite satisfactory is psycho-therapy, and especially psycho-analysis.

PHOSGENE. Carbonyl chloride, or phosgene, is an irritating gas which causes a choking sensation, coughing and oedema of the lungs, with the discharge of a copious, thin, frothy sputum. The victim becomes blue, or cyanosed. Death usually occurs within 48 hours, or, if the early effects are not fatal, death may occur later from broncho-pneumonia. If the patient escapes those risks he may, however, be subject to emphysema and bronchitis.

Phosgene may be present in small quantities in an operating theatre from the decomposition of chloroform. It was one of the poison gases used in the Great War. Full protection is afforded by an efficient gas-mask containing charcoal and soda-lime. A victim of gassing should be placed in a position in which he can get rid of the sputum most easily and should have oxygen to inhale. Bleeding may be of assistance.

PHOSPHORIC ACID. Concentrated phosphoric acid forms a clear, syrupy liquid which acts as a caustic. Dilute phosphoric acid is used internally in doses of 5 to 20 minims, sometimes in an acid mixture for dyspepsia, at other times as a general tonic. Salts formed with this acid are called phosphates; many are used in medicine, including those of iron, calcium, sodium, etc.

See Easton's Syrup; Glycero-phosphates; Hypophosphite; Parrish's Syrup.

PHOSPHORUS. A non-metallic element, phosphorus occurs in two forms, the white and the red. The former rather resembles wax in appearance and consistency. It gives off fumes in the air and is luminous in the dark; it readily ignites. The fumes have an odour of garlic. Red phosphorus is hard and brittle; it does not fume nor is it luminous.

Phosphorus is a constituent of protoplasm, and also occurs in the body as phosphates, in bone and other tissues. Its usefulness as a drug in nervous disorders is doubtful, to say the least, but it is capable of hastening and consolidating the repair of a fracture and may be of service in rickets and osteomalacia. It is given as phosphorated oil or in a pill.

Poisoning by Phosphorus. Acute phosphorus poisoning has generally occurred from consuming match-heads made with white phosphorus or rat-paste. There is a feeling of heat in the mouth, throat and stomach, vomiting and occasionally diarrhoea. The vomited matter and faeces are luminous in the dark and smell of garlic. The patient may apparently recover, but in from three to five days jaundice occurs, with renewed vomiting. There may be convulsions and coma or severe bleeding from the stomach and bowels. The heart is greatly weakened.

The first-aid treatment consists in giving an emetic of mustard and water and washing out the stomach by giving large draughts of a weak solution of permanganate of potassium at a tepid temperature. No oils or fats should be given. The best emetic for phosphorus poisoning is copper sulphate, 3 to 10 grains in solution, and a doctor would probably use this or wash out the stomach with permanganate solution through a stomach tube. Permanganate of potassium is the best antidote, but old oil of turpentine is also used, in doses of 10 minims.

Chronic phosphorus poisoning generally occurs in the form of phossy jaw, but there may be signs of irritation of the alimentary tract and cachexia. Phossy jaw means necrosis of the lower jaw. This can occur when teeth are carious or a tooth has been extracted, the direct cause being the fumes given off from white phosphorus. The action of the fumes lays the affected bone open to the attack of microbes and especially the tubercle bacillus, so that the resulting disorder is almost always tuberculosis of the jaw.

Phossy jaw has become very rare since the manufacture of matches from white phosphorus was forbidden by law. Red phosphorus or sesquisulphide of phosphorus are now employed. When, however, anyone is much exposed to phosphorus fumes a respirator should be worn, and careful attention paid to the cleanliness and integrity of the teeth.

See Phosphoric Acid.

PHOTOPHOBIA. Intolerance of light, or photophobia, may be caused by conjunctivitis, foreign bodies in the eye, corneal ulcers or inflammation within the eye. Sometimes it is accompanied by a spasmodic closure of the lids, or blepharospasm. The treatment depends on the cause, to determine which a skilled medical examination is often necessary.

PHOTO-THERAPY. *See* Light.

PHRENIC NERVE. Each half of the diaphragm, or midriff, is supplied by a phrenic nerve, which arises from the cervical plexus of nerves in the neck.

PLATE XXIX

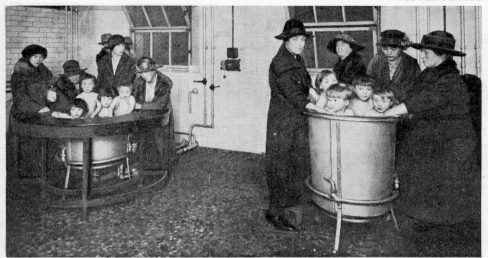

1. Paralysis.   A whirlpool bath, taken by immersion or locally, helps in the restoration of wasted muscles

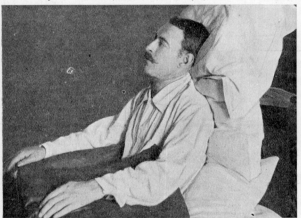

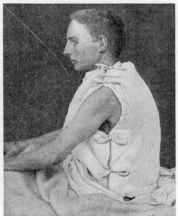

Pneumonia.   2. The patient should be well propped up, the hands resting on cushions to lessen the strain on the heart.   3. Pneumonia jacket of flannel lined with cotton wool, for wearing over a poultice

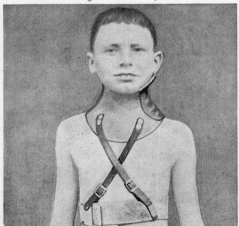

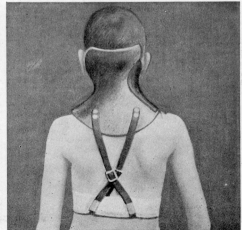

Pott's Disease of the Spine.   4 and 5. Collar which supports the head and prevents movement of the neck

Courtesy of Princess Mary's Hospital for Children, Margate

PLATE XXX

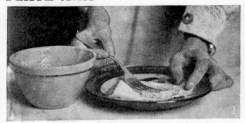
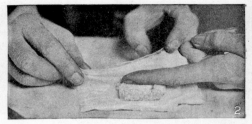

Poultice. 1 and 2. Festered finger treated with a poultice made of bread and a little boracic acid powder

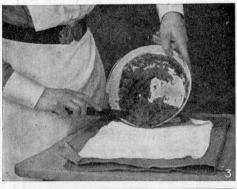
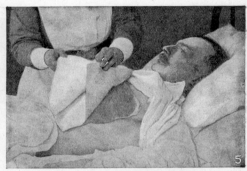
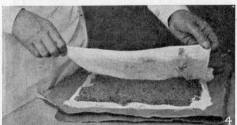
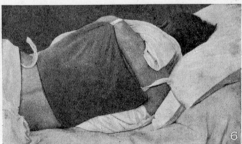

3. To make a linseed poultice, boiling water is poured into a bowl and linseed added gradually while stirring. When the mixture is such that it leaves the bowl clean, it is spread on a piece of linen. 4. A second piece of linen is placed over it and the margins pressed together. 5. When applied to the chest it is covered with a piece of jaconet and a layer of cotton wool. 6. Poultice bag for the back

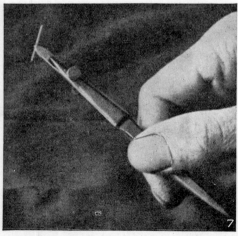
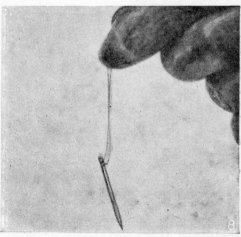

Radium Needle. 7. Three-quarter inch length of capillary tube containing radium emanation. 8. The glass needle is now placed inside a sterilised steel needle which may be inserted into cancerous growths

PHRENOLOGY. The doctrine that the configuration of the skull, or, as the saying goes, the arrangement of the bumps, is indicative of the moral and intellectual qualities of the individual is described as phrenology. There is no basis in fact, however, for any such hypothesis.

PHTHISIS. Meaning wasting or consumption, the term phthisis was once commonly used to denote tuberculosis of the lungs. Fibroid phthisis is a name given to this disease when there is a large development of fibrous, or scar-like, tissue in the lung. Such tissue represents an effort of Nature to wall off and restrict the activities of the disease-germs, and occurs in other instances of chronic irritation of the lung. Thus, miner's phthisis, stonecutter's phthisis and grinder's phthisis may exist apart from tuberculosis, though in the two latter conditions tuberculous infection is highly probable.

The term phthisis is also applied to general wasting, whatever its cause, and to wasting of organs other than the lung, for example, wasting of the eye, or phthisis bulbi, and of the stomach, or phthisis ventriculi.

See Consumption.

PIA MATER. The innermost of the coverings of the brain and spinal cord is called the pia mater, literally, tender mother, in view of its delicacy.

See Brain.

PICRIC ACID. A yellow, crystalline substance obtained from carbolic acid by inter-action with fuming nitric acid, picric acid is sometimes used, in watery solution or ointments, for burns, chilblains, erysipelas, eczema, etc. It must be used with caution, however, as poisoning may result.

PIGEON BREAST. A deformity of the chest, consisting of a pushing forward of the sternum and flattening of the sides of the chest, is described as pigeon breast. It is caused by rickets (*q.v.*).

See Chest.

PIGMENTATION. Certain cells of the skin and of other parts of the body contain granules of a pigment known as melanin. An increase in this pigment occurs in negroes and other coloured people, and is a result of sunburn in white races. Whether natural or acquired, the effect of the browning of the skin is protective. A congenital absence of this pigment is called albinism (*q.v.*).

In various disorders, such as Addison's disease, chloasma, exophthalmic goitre and others, there is an increase of pigmentation. In leucoderma, on the other hand, there is a lessening of the normal pigmentation, and this may happen in some other disorders.

The pigmentation in jaundice is caused by bile pigment in the blood, and that which follows a bruise is due to disintegration of blood effused beneath the skin. Pigmentation from taking silver salts internally was once not uncommon but is now rare.

PILES. Haemorrhoids, or piles, consist of dilated and varicose veins at the anus or in the lower inch or two of the rectum. An external pile forms a little brownish fold of skin, radiating from the anus, and is often referred to as a perianal tag. It may cause no trouble or only a little itching, and perhaps a sense of tightness when the bowels are moved.

Internal piles may consist of thickened folds or of rounded masses with more or less of a stalk, covered with mucous membrane which is reddish-blue in colour. Both varieties cause a sense of fullness and weight in the bowel. The first variety is apt to cause prolapse, or falling down, of the lining of the bowel, so that it protrudes through the anus ; the second are liable themselves to prolapse, and also cause bleeding, perhaps to a serious extent.

Internal piles sometimes become inflamed and the blood in the veins may clot, or thrombose. These occurrences give rise to considerable pain and distress. Sometimes the neck of a prolapsed pile is compressed by the circular muscle, or sphincter, of the anus and the pile is strangulated. It swells up and is very painful and tender, and if not replaced may slough off. An external pile may also become inflamed, when it forms a tense, bluish swelling, which is painful and tender.

Piles may be caused by chronic constipation, sedentary habits, congestion or cirrhosis of the liver, the pressure of the pregnant womb or of a tumour, and in other ways.

Bleeding from the bowel may have other causes than piles, and, especially after middle age, it should not be assumed that the bleeding is necessarily due to this cause.

When piles exist, whether internal or external, constipation (*q.v.*), if present, should be corrected. No preparation of aloes should be used as a purgative, however. The anal region must be kept very clean ; it should be washed once a day at least. Only a soft, smooth toilet paper should be used and sometimes a soft rag is the best thing. A little witch-hazel or hamamelis ointment should be smeared round the anus if there is irritation, and, when there are bleeding internal piles, this ointment or gall and opium ointment should be introduced into the bowel by the method described under the heading Ointment.

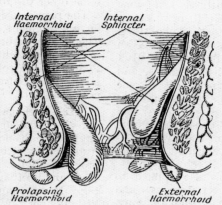

Piles. Diagram of both internal and external forms. Internal piles may prolapse

Care should be taken against getting the feet wet and cold, and cold seats should be avoided.

Should an external pile become inflamed rest in bed for a day or two, opening the bowels thoroughly by means of a large enema, and the use of hot fomentations will probably cause the inflammation to subside, though sometimes the pile should be incised.

Inflamed internal piles require similar treatment but it will be more prolonged. When internal piles are troublesome, however, it is desirable to get rid of them. This generally means cutting them away, but sometimes the method of injecting a few drops of carbolic acid in glycerin is adopted.

See Fissure.

PILL. A small, globular mass containing one or more active drugs, a pill is intended for internal use. Some substance, called the excipient, is used to give cohesion to its contents and, often, size also. This may be hard soap, breadcrumb, tragacanth, syrup of glucose, kaolin or something else. Most of the official pills have a dose of 4 to 8 grains, but this generally means that one or two pills, as the case may be, should be taken, as, except when it contains a very heavy ingredient, a pill should not weigh more than 4 or 5 grains. The methods of giving a pill are described under the heading Medicines.

PIMPLE. Small inflammatory elevations of the skin, pimples may be solid structures, or papules, or, on the other hand, may have a pustule at the top.

See Acne.

PINE. The oil obtained from pinus pumilio, commonly referred to as oil of pine, is a colourless liquid, with a pungent taste and aromatic odour. It is chiefly used as an inhalation in catarrh of the respiratory passages. It acts as an antiseptic.

See Turpentine.

PINEAL. A small structure situated in the middle of the brain, the pineal body is glandular in early life but later does not appear to have any function. A tumour of this gland may cause sexual precocity and perhaps other symptoms.

PINGUECULA. In an old person a triangular yellow swelling, known as a pinguecula, may form on either side of the cornea of the eye. It is of little importance.

See Eye ; Pterygium.

PINK EYE. The redness of the eye caused by conjunctivitis (*q.v.*) is sometimes referred to by the popular name of pink eye.

PINS AND NEEDLES. The sensation of pins and needles is a form of paraesthesia (*q.v.*).

PITUITARY BODY. The small structure called the pituitary body is situated in the base of the skull, in a cavity in the sphenoid bone, known from its shape as the sella turcica, or Turkish saddle. It consists of an anterior lobe, a posterior lobe and an intermediate part connecting the two.

The anterior lobe is glandular in structure and its secretion stimulates growth, as over-activity of this lobe during the growing period causes giantism and later in life the disease called acromegaly (*q.v.*). Deficient activity, on the other hand, results in failure of bodily and sexual development, a condition described as infantilism.

The posterior lobe produces an internal secretion which causes contraction of all arteries except those of the kidney, and of plain muscle in the bowels, the bladder, the womb and other organs. It also has something to do with the metabolism of carbohydrates, as over-activity leads to excessive secretion of urine, or polyuria, and possibly to the presence of sugar in the urine, or glycosuria. Deficiency of the secretion, on the other hand, leads to obesity. The intermediate portion appears to act in conjunction with this lobe.

An extract of the posterior lobe, known as pituitrin, is used, by injection into the body, in a variety of disorders, including shock, in which it raises blood pressure, in paralysis of the bowel following an operation, and in weakness of the uterine muscle during or after labour.

See Endocrine.

PITYRIASIS. Various skin disorders, in which fine branny scales appear, are described as pityriasis.

In pityriasis rosea, which occurs usually in late spring or early summer, a patch, known as the herald patch, appears on the front or side of the chest. It is oval in shape and has a slightly raised rose-coloured border with fine scales, the centre being of a yellowish colour. After a week or two similar patches, but smaller, and also little red, scaly spots, appear in crops on the trunk and upper parts of the lower limbs. There is no general and little, if any, local discomfort. The rash disappears in about six weeks. All the treatment necessary is to dust with talc or some other bland powder.

Pityriasis simplex is discussed under the heading Dandruff. Pityriasis versicolor is the name given to a rash which is most often seen on the front or back of the chest. It is light to dark brown in colour and slightly scaly, and is caused by a fungus, microsporon furfur. The parasite may be killed by painting with tincture of iodine or by sulphur ointments or baths. The rash is illustrated in Plate XXXI, 9.

Pityriasis rubra of Hebra, also known as dermatitis exfoliativa, is characterised by universal redness of the skin and peeling of the skin in large, thin flakes. It is sometimes secondary to other skin diseases, but may occur independently. It is very debilitating and death may occur. Confinement to bed is necessary during the acute stage, and the diet should be generous but easily digested ; alcohol and coffee are best omitted. Sulphur baths, a free use of lead lotion, and, later, sedative ointments usually constitute the local treatment.

Pityriasis rubra pilaris is quite a different disease. There are also redness and scaling, but in addition there are papules. The course of the disease may last for weeks only or for years. Rest in bed may be necessary at the start. Various internal remedies such as arsenic and thyroid are used, and externally ointments containing ichthyol or tar with salicylic acid.

See Dandruff ; Lichen ; Psoriasis ; Seborrhoea.

PLACENTA PRAEVIA. The after-birth (*q.v.*) is technically known as the placenta. When this organ is situated in the lower part of the womb, an occurrence described as placenta praevia, contractions of the womb tend to loosen the attachment of portions of the placenta and so cause bleeding. This may occur from the end of the second month onwards, and dangerous amounts of blood may be lost. The difficulties and dangers of labour are also increased.

See Accidental Haemorrhage.

PLAGUE. Endemic in the East, plague, or the pest, breaks out in epidemics from time to time. It was this disease that ravaged Europe in former centuries and was known as the Black Death. It is caused by a microbe, the bacillus pestis, which may infect rats and the fleas which feed on them. The disease may therefore be carried on ships to European ports and be disseminated by fleas. This is the usual mode of infection in what is called bubonic plague, but in pneumonic plague infection takes place from breathing in particles carrying the microbe.

The period of incubation is about three days as a rule, after which the victim is suddenly smitten with high fever and prostration. Very soon a gland, usually one in the groin, becomes enlarged and tender, and then other glands. A mass of such glands constitutes a bubo, whence the name of this form of plague. The glands often suppurate and may slough, or die. The general condition may begin to improve on the fourth or fifth day, or may go on worsening to a fatal issue. Even when the temperature has come down, sudden heart failure may occur.

In pneumonic plague the symptoms and signs resemble those of a virulent attack of pneumonia (*q.v.*). There is another type of plague in which neither buboes nor lung involvement occurs, but there is simply profound toxaemia. This is called the septicaemic type, and probably occurs when the infectious material is swallowed.

The treatment of plague is mainly symptomatic. The state of fever (*q.v.*) must be dealt with, precautions detailed under the heading Infectious Disease being observed. Sera, such as Yersin's, are used, but opinions vary widely as to their usefulness. This is true also of Haffkine's prophylactic serum, and much stress must be laid on the destruction of rats as a preventive measure. Rubber gloves and the adjustment of clothing so as to diminish the risk of flea bites is important for those who are in attendance on plague patients. A respirator made of cotton wool and gauze is also important, especially when dealing with pneumonic plague ; it must be burnt immediately on being taken off.

PLASTER. An emplastrum, or plaster, is a solid, adhesive preparation for external application. The plaster is spread on cotton, linen, or some other kind of backing. Most plasters contain a proportion of lead plaster. Resin or adhesive plaster and soap plaster are used mainly for giving support, but other plasters, like those of belladonna, cantharidin, menthol, etc., contain powerful drugs which are intended to act on the skin. To lessen the risk of imprisoned sweat irritating the skin, plasters with many perforations are made and are sold as porous plasters.

The removal of a plaster is facilitated by warming it, or moistening thoroughly with surgical spirit.

See Adhesive Plaster ; Court Plaster.

PLASTER OF PARIS. Powdered gypsum when mixed with water and allowed to stand sets into a hard mass. Bandages impregnated with the powder are called plaster of Paris bandages and are used as immovable bandages for fractures and other injuries and for making plaster jackets, which are put on as spinal supports. The method of applying an immovable bandage is described under the heading Bandage.

PLETHORA. An excess of blood in the vessels is described as plethora. A plethoric person has a red face, and is liable to bleeding at the nose and, if a woman, to a very free monthly flow. There is usually a sense of fullness in the head, and after middle life plethora much increases the risk of apoplexy. The condition should be combated by a restricted, though adequate, diet, the avoidance of alcohol and by taking open-air exercise.

Some people suffer from an excessive number of red cells in the blood, polycythaemia or erythrocythaemia. Here, again, the face is very red, or perhaps purple, and there may be blueness of the fingers and toes. Headache, giddiness, noises in the ears and shortness of breath are often complained of, and there is a liability to a severe internal haemorrhage. The spleen is often enlarged. Most benefit has been derived from the old operation of bleeding.

Persons who live in high altitudes or who suffer from congenital heart disease, asthma and other disorders may also exhibit polycythaemia.

See Blood ; Congestion.

PLEURA. The inner surface of the wall of the chest is lined by a smooth membrane known as the pleura, which, at the root of the lung, is reflected on to this organ and completely covers it, even dipping into the fissures which divide the lung into lobes. The pleura on either side thus forms a closed bag, although normally its walls are always in contact. These rub over one another during the expansion and deflation of the lung in the process of breathing, and by their smoothness friction in this operation is reduced to a minimum. The existence of the bag is shown in some diseases or injuries by the accumulation of fluids or air in its cavity.

From a chest wound, from rupture of an aneurysm and other causes, blood may accumulate in a pleural cavity; this is called haemothorax. Unless there are reasons against it, the blood is aspirated from the chest in order to relieve the lung. An accumulation of more or less clear fluid occurs in pleurisy with effusion, commonly referred to as wet pleurisy, or it may be dropsical, as in some cases of nephritis or heart disease, when it is called hydrothorax.

Air in the pleural cavity is called pneumothorax. It is generally due to the rupture of a tuberculous cavity in the lung into the pleura. Usually there is sudden, severe pain and great breathlessness. The air is reabsorbed, but generally there ensues a wet pleurisy which develops into empyema. A pleural empyema (*q.v.*) consists of a collection of purulent fluid.

See Serous Membrane.

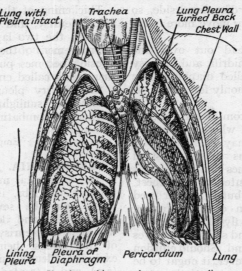

Pleura. Showing this membrane surrounding a contracted left lung

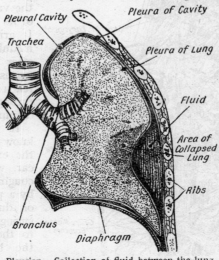

Pleurisy. Collection of fluid between the lung and chest wall, constituting wet pleurisy

PLEURISY. Inflammation of the pleura is called pleurisy. It may be due to extension of inflammation from some part covered by the pleura, notably from the lung in pneumonia or tuberculosis. It may also occur in acute rheumatism and in some of the specific fevers, in Bright's disease and so on. A primary inflammation of the pleura, however, is presumably tuberculous.

The opposing inflamed surfaces of the pleura become covered with a fibrinous exudation which causes friction when the surfaces move over each other. This gives rise to the sharp, stabbing pain felt in pleurisy and increased by coughing and deep breathing, and to the friction sound heard by the doctor when listening over the chest. It is called dry pleurisy.

Often, however, following on this there is the effusion of fluid into the pleural cavity, what is called wet pleurisy. The fluid separates the two layers of the pleura and pain and coughing probably cease. The effusion may be very large, perhaps sufficient to displace the heart, but breathing may not be interfered with as much as might be expected from its size.

The temperature usually rises in pleurisy, though not often above 101 deg. F. When pain is troublesome the patient may prefer to lie on the sound side, as pressure may increase the pain, but when there is effusion he prefers to lie on the disordered side, so that the other side may move more freely in breathing.

The pleura is spread out over the upper surface of the midriff, and pleurisy in this situation is called diaphragmatic pleurisy. Pain is commonly felt in the pit of the stomach.

A person suffering from pleurisy should be confined to bed, whether there is fever or not. Pain may be relieved by poultices, fomentations or a mustard plaster, but sometimes an opiate is required. Iodine, painted on the chest, may also be of value, but is oftener used to promote absorption of the effusion, for which purpose also fly-blisters may be employed. Diuretics and saline purgatives may be helpful to this end. Should effusion persist for a week, however, it ought to be drawn off, preferably not entirely at a sitting, but sufficient to allow the lung to expand to some extent.

By subsequent tappings, if necessary, the chest may be cleared. Expansion of the lung may be furthered by making the patient blow up balloons or blow water from one bottle into another to which it is connected by tubing.

Thickening of the pleura may remain after pleurisy, and sometimes adhesions between the two layers, interfering with the movement of the lung. Sometimes the effusion becomes purulent, the condition then being called empyema.

As primary pleurisy is likely to be tuberculous, sunlight, fresh air and other methods of combating this disease should be employed.

See Aspiration; Empyema; Lung; Pleura; Pneumonia.

PLEURODYNIA. Muscular rheumatism in the intercostal muscles, that is, those between the ribs, is called pleurodynia. There may be severe pain, increased by coughing and deep breathing. This will suggest pleurisy and the possibility of this disease being present must be excluded. Pleurodynia is a form of fibrositis (q.v.), and is treated accordingly.

PLEXUS. A network of vessels or of nerves is called a plexus. Some plexuses, the solar plexus, for example, include masses of nerve cells, or ganglia.

See Nervous System.

PNEUMOCONIOSIS. The constant inhalation of dust is liable to produce a fibrotic disease of the lungs, the general name for which is pneumoconiosis.

See Dust Disease.

PNEUMOGASTRIC NERVE. The 10th cranial, or pneumogastric, nerve is also called the vagus nerve, on account of its long, wandering course. It arises from the bulb, or medulla, of the brain, and after leaving the skull traverses the neck and chest to reach the abdomen by passing through an opening in the diaphragm.

It sends a little branch, know as Arnold's nerve, to the external passage of the ear, which accounts for the coughing sometimes caused by a plug of wax in the ear or during the operation of syringing. It sends branches to the pharynx, the larynx, the heart, the lungs, the stomach, the liver and the

Glosso-Pharyngeal
Spinal Accessory
Pharyngeal Branches
Hypoglossal
Superior Laryngeal
Left Vagus
Cervical Loop
Right Vagus
Brachial Plexus
Recurrent | Right
Laryngeal | Left
Inferior Cervical Ganglion
Arch of Aorta
Pulmonary Branches
Oesophagus
Gastro-Hepatic Branches
Diaphragm

Pneumogastric or Vagus Nerve. Its course from brain to abdomen

spleen. Impulses down this nerve to the heart slow its rate of beating, and if the nerve is sufficiently irritated the heart may be stopped altogether.

In view of its connexion with the heart and the other organs which have been enumerated, the pneumogastric must be regarded as a very important nerve.

PNEUMONIA. Two morbid conditions in the lungs are described as pneumonia. In one there is an involvement of the smaller subdivisions of lung tissue, the lobules, and this is called broncho-pneumonia (q.v.). In the other, one or more entire lobes of one or both lungs is concerned, and this is called lobar pneumonia ; when the word pneumonia is used without qualification it is generally this type that is meant.

Lobar pneumonia is properly regarded as a general disease, a specific fever, with a special involvement of the lungs. It is caused by germs circulating in the blood, the most usual one being the pneumococcus, though the typhoid bacillus, the plague bacillus, the influenza bacillus, and other organisms, when they cause a general infection of the body, may also cause changes in the lung similar to those occurring in pneumonia.

In this disorder the infection is generally acquired from the breath of a person suffering from the disease or from that of a carrier (q.v.). The incubation period is from one to seven days and the onset is sudden, generally with a chill, perhaps in the severe form called a rigor, especially in children, in whom also convulsions might occur. The temperature rises quickly, and soon there is a short cough, which, however, the patient may try to suppress because it causes a sharp, cutting pain in the side ; for the same reason the breathing may be shallow.

The pulse is rapid, but the respiratory rate is more so in proportion. The normal ratio of the pulse and respiratory rates is 72 to 18, or 4 to 1, but in pneumonia it may only be 3 or even 2 to 1. The patient looks ill. The sputum brought up by coughing is very sticky and brownish in colour. It is referred to as a rusty sputum. Sometimes, however, it is blood-red. The cheeks are flushed, perhaps one more than the other, and frequently there are crops of blisters, or herpes, round the mouth. The tongue is furred, and as the disease goes on may become dry and brown. Sleeplessness is apt to be troublesome, and delirium is common and may be violent ; unless he is watched, the patient may get out of bed and hurt himself by falling.

After some days the fever begins to abate, and usually terminates by crisis, that is to say, the temperature falls within a few hours to normal, or subnormal. The patient commonly falls into a deep sleep while this is taking place, from which he awakes feeling very much better. The crisis often occurs on the odd-numbered days, say, the fifth, seventh, or ninth.

In adults the disease usually affects the base of the lung, but it may be at the apex, when it is called apical pneumonia. This is the commonest site in children. It may extend to other lobes and possibly to the other lung, when one speaks of double pneumonia.

Changes in the Lung Tissue

The changes in the lungs consist of acute congestion, followed by filling up of the air cells with fibrin and red cells, a state of affairs described as consolidation (see illustrations of lung tissue in Plate XI). Later this red substance is invaded by a host of white blood cells, and becomes greyish in colour. The contents of the air cells are also softer, and soon become liquefied and are discharged through the air tubes, or absorbed ; this is the stage of resolution.

There is usually an extension of the inflammation to the adjoining pleura, and it is the accompanying pleurisy that accounts for the sharp pain. The pleurisy usually clears up when resolution takes place, but it may not do so, and a collection of purulent fluid, or empyema (q.v.), may occur in the pleural cavity. Again, resolution may be delayed, and sometimes it is incomplete, so that a chronic inflammatory process goes on which leads to fibrosis (q.v.) of the lung. Sometimes, instead of resolution, an abscess of the lung occurs, or even gangrene. Complications affecting other organs may occur, as, for example, meningitis, nephritis, and so on.

The general treatment of pneumonia is that of fever (q.v.), but as it is infectious the provisions for isolation described under the heading Infectious Disease should be carried out. The existence of the disease must be notified to the Medical Officer of Health for the area, but this duty can be left to the doctor.

In no disease is good nursing of more importance, and as the patient must be constantly under observation both a day and a night nurse will be necessary.

Pain is usually relieved by a poultice (*q.v.*), but an injection of morphia may be necessary. Often the patient is put into a pneumonia jacket (Plate XXIX, 3). He should be propped up in a sitting position to aid circulation through the lung (Plate XXIX, 2). Stimulation of the heart by alcohol, digitalis, etc., may become necessary. Sometimes a sleeping draught must be given, and paraldehyde is commonly selected. If the patient tends to become livid, the inhalation of oxygen is of value. If the type of organism responsible has been discovered by bacteriological examination, a serum prepared for this type may be injected with advantage. To aid in the expulsion of the sputum, a cough mixture containing ammonium carbonate and other drugs is often given.

Those in attendance on the patient should bear in mind the possibility of infection, and should gargle the throat several times with some antiseptic, say, a weak solution of permanganate of potassium. A gauze respirator may usefully be worn, especially when it is necessary to come close to the patient. The sputum should be received in a jar containing lysol solution, a teaspoonful to the pint, and should not be allowed to adhere to the sides of the jar. The mouth should be wiped with paper handkerchiefs, which should be burnt at once.

See Broncho-pneumonia ; Lung ; Nursing.

PODOPHYLLUM. The root of podophyllum acts as a purgative, causing profuse watery motions. Like calomel, it clears out the duodenum, and consequently is sometimes called vegetable calomel, but it possesses none of the alterative qualities of the latter drug. Podophyllum is generally used as the resin, dose ¼ to 1 grain in pill, or the tincture, dose 5 to 15 minims. It is rather uncertain in its effects on different individuals.

POISON. Certain substances are statutory poisons. They are enumerated in the Schedule to the Poison Act. Any preparation which contains a statutory poison must be labelled as " poison." A medicine prescribed for internal use may be thus labelled, but this fact need not alarm the patient ; care must be taken, however, to adhere to the instructions.

Poisonous substances must be dispensed in containers which are easily distinguishable by colour and shape, and on no account should they be transferred to plain containers in the home. All poisons should be kept under lock and key. It is illegal to send poisonous substances by post, except such as are contained in medicines prescribed by a registered doctor and dispensed by a registered chemist and druggist. Opium, its alkaloids and cocaine are classed as Dangerous Drugs, and dealings in them, by prescription or otherwise, are subject to strict regulations.

POISONING. In few emergencies can sagacious first aid be of such service as in that of poisoning. The need may arise in a variety of circumstances. It may be definitely known that poison has been swallowed or otherwise may have got into the body, and the nature of the poison may even be known. Without this knowledge, however, the probability of poisoning would be recognized when a person becomes ill shortly after taking food, drink or a dose of medicine. If several persons who have taken the same food are affected, the presumption is very strong.

Some poisons destroy tissues with which they come into contact, and are known as corrosives. There is evidence of destruction of the lining of the mouth, and possibly marks on the face and clothing. Such poisons cause an immediate burning pain in the mouth, throat and stomach, also vomiting, and perhaps purging. The vomited matter may contain shreds of stomach lining. From irritation of the entrance to the larynx there may be difficulty in breathing. The patient is more or less collapsed.

Amongst the corrosive poisons are the strong mineral acids, such as oil of vitriol ; the caustic alkalies, such as strong ammonia, corrosive sublimate, formalin, oxalic acid, certain metallic salts, etc.

Carbolic acid and creosote also cause a burning pain, but vomiting is uncommon, and there is a sense of giddiness and intoxication, followed by unconsciousness.

Irritant poisons may or may not occasion a hot feeling during swallowing, but they cause nausea, vomiting, abdominal pain, purging, and more or less collapse. Some cause difficulty in breathing, and some cramps in the legs. They include antimony, arsenic, copper, lead, mercury, zinc, croton oil and other strong purgatives, arum, cantharides, etc.

Narcotic poisons may, like opium, cause immediate somnolence, deepening into sleep and coma ; or, like belladonna, there may be pronounced delirium for a time and then coma ; or, like alcohol and nitro-benzene, they may cause signs of intoxication, followed by coma.

Some poisons, including aconite, diluted oxalic acid, prussic acid, etc., cause great depression of the heart, while others, such as hemlock, calabar bean and curare, cause muscular paralysis. Nux vomica and its alkaloids, strychnine and brucine, cause convulsions, without impairing consciousness or producing signs of irritation of the alimentary tract, but poisons of other descriptions and giving rise to such signs may also cause convulsions.

Cantharides, or Spanish fly, turpentine and potassium chlorate cause bloody urine, amongst other symptoms.

How to Render First Aid

In the event of poisoning a doctor should be sent for at once, and should be told what poison has been taken if this fact be known. In the meantime, first aid should be rendered promptly. If the nature of the poison is known, instructions as to its treatment will be found under the appropriate heading in this book, but, if not, treatment should be along the lines to be now laid down.

If the poison is a corrosive, on no account should an emetic be given, as vomiting might cause perforation of the stomach, but in all other cases, if the patient can swallow, an effort should be made to empty the stomach.

To this end, a tablespoonful of mustard, or two tablespoonsful of common salt, may be given in a tumbler of warm water. Vomiting may be hastened by tickling the back of the throat with a feather or a paper spill, and when it begins the patient should drink large draughts of tepid water in order to wash out the stomach.

In the next place, or in the first, when dealing with a corrosive poison, something should be given to neutralise the activities of any drug remaining in the stomach ; a list of the appropriate things to use for each poison is given under the heading Antidote. A strong infusion, or decoction, of tea is usually a good thing to give, as not only does it stimulate, but the tannic acid which it contains is an antidote for alkaloids, the active principle of most vegetable poisons, and for some metals.

Dealing with Corrosive Poisoning

The irritation caused by a corrosive or irritant poison may be lessened by giving demulcent drinks, such as milk, thin gruel, thin cornflour or arrowroot, olive oil, or white of egg in water. Oil should not be given, however, in poisoning by cantharides or phosphorus, and as little water as possible in poisoning by oxalic acid or lysol. When poison has been in the stomach for some time some of it may have passed into the bowel, in which case one or two tablespoonsful of castor oil, or a tablespoonful of Epsom salts in a tumbler of warm water, should be given.

For difficulty of breathing caused by corrosive poisons, hot cloths should be put on the neck, and the air may be moistened with steam by means of a bronchitis kettle (*q.v.*), which can be improvised if necessary. Pieces of ice should be given to the patient to suck.

Faintness and collapse are treated by keeping the patient lying down in bed and promoting warmth by blankets and by putting hot-water bottles, covered with flannel, at the feet and by the sides. Stimulants should be given in the shape of sal volatile, a teaspoonful in a wineglass of water, whisky or brandy, a teaspoonful or more, according to age, etc., well diluted, or strong tea or coffee. If the patient is unconscious, one or two tablespoonsful of diluted spirits, or, when a narcotic poison has been taken, a pint of coffee, may be injected into the bowel. No alcohol should be given in poisoning by aniline, nitro-benzene, or related poisons.

Pain or cramps are treated by placing large hot fomentations or poultices over the affected parts.

If breathing ceases, artificial respiration should be started at once.

Any bottles found near the patient, or any vomited matter, should always be kept for the doctor's inspection.

See Antidote; Artificial Respiration; Asphyxia; Collapse; Emetic; Fainting; Shock.

POLIOENCEPHALITIS. Inflammation of the brain in which the grey matter is particularly affected is called polioencephalitis.
See Encephalitis.

POLIOMYELITIS. Inflammation of the grey matter in the spinal cord is called poliomyelitis. Acute anterior poliomyelitis is better known as infantile paralysis (q.v.). Chronic anterior poliomyelitis resembles progressive muscular atrophy.

POLYPUS. The term polypus is used for a tumour which hangs by a stalk from the surface of a body cavity. As regards its structure and nature, a polypus in one situation may differ widely from one in another situation. An aural polypus, for example, consists of granulation tissue, the overgrowth of this tissue being caused by chronic irritation in the ear. A nasal polypus consists of a soft overgrowth of the mucous lining, also due to chronic irritation. A rectal polypus, on the other hand, is usually a growth of the nature of an adenoma, or gland tumour.

Polypi should be removed, a simple matter when they are readily accessible, but in some cases the base to which the stalk is attached must also be cleaned up.
See Nose.

POMEGRANATE. The bark of the roots and stem of the pomegranate contains pelletierine and other alkaloids which are extracted and used for destroying tapeworms. Pelletierine tannate, which is generally given, has a dose of 2 to 8 grains. The rind of the pomegranate is rich in tannic acid, and is given in powder or made into a decoction, in chronic diarrhœa and dysentery.

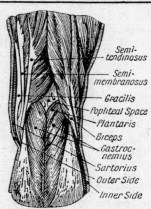

Semi-tendinosus
Semi-membranosus
Gracilis
Popliteal Space
Plantaris
Biceps
Gastrocnemius
Sartorius
Outer Side
Inner Side

Muscles surrounding the popliteal space at the back of the knee

POPLITEAL. When the knee is bent a hollow appears at the back between the outer and inner hamstrings above and the heads of the gastrocnemius below. This is called the popliteal space. The femoral artery as it traverses the space is called the popliteal artery, and it is accompanied by the popliteal vein. The great sciatic nerve within this space divides into the internal and external popliteal nerves.

The popliteal artery is sometimes the site of an aneurysm, which forms a pulsating swelling. Other swellings may be due to enlargement of a bursa, of which there are several at the back of the knee, an abscess and other causes.
See Bursa; Knee.

POST-MORTEM. In many instances the correct cause of death can only be established by a post-mortem examination of the body, and in certain events such an examination will be ordered by a coroner or, in Scotland, by a Procurator-Fiscal.

POTASSIUM. An elemental metal, belonging, like sodium, to the alkaline group, potassium is a normal constituent of the body, being especially abundant in the solid tissues. Some of its compounds are used in medicine and act similarly to those of sodium, except that potassium, if given in large doses or over a long period, is depressing to the heart and nervous system.

Potassium carbonate, also known as salt of tartar, the dose of which is 5 to 70 grains, and potassium bicarbonate, dose 5 to 30 grains, are used as alkalies in dyspepsia. Crude potassium carbonate is sold for cleansing purposes as potash, potashes or pearl-ash. It acts as a corrosive alkaline poison.

Potassium hydroxide, or caustic potash, is sometimes used in the form of a pencil as a caustic. A solution of this, liquor potassae, is given internally as an antacid, and may be used locally to soften off a thickened or deformed toe-nail.

Potassium sulphate, 15 to 45 grains, potassium tartrate, 30 to 240 grains, and acid tartrate of potassium, or purified cream of tartar, 15 to 60 grains, are used in solution as mild purgatives ; potassium acetate and potassium citrate, the dose of each being 15 to 60 grains, have also a slight action of this kind, but are usually given for a diuretic action.

Potassium nitrate, also called nitre and saltpetre, dose 5 to 20 grains, is sometimes included in mixtures given to encourage the flow of urine, or sweating. It is much used in fumigating powders for asthma (*q.v.*).

Potassium chlorate, 5 to 15 grains, has a remarkable effect in restoring health to disordered mucous membranes, and is a common constituent of a mouth wash, though it may be useful also to other mucous membranes than that of the mouth. It acts as a diuretic, but in excessive doses may cause inflammation of the kidney and bloody urine. There are lozenges of potassium chlorate, containing 3 grains each, which are sucked for relief to a sore throat.

Potassium permanganate is discussed under the heading Manganese ; potassium bromide under Bromide ; and potassium iodide under Iodine.

Potash water is simple aerated water containing a small quantity of potassium bicarbonate.

See Sodium.

POTT'S DISEASE. Tuberculous disease of the spine is called Pott's disease. The bodies of the vertebrae are the parts most often affected, and, as bone is destroyed, the spine gives way at the site of the disease, the vertebrae above and below coming closer together and so causing a sharp backward projection of the spine, usually referred to as hunchback. The bending of the spine may be sufficient to cause compression of the spinal cord and paralysis. There may also be a lateral curvature of the spine.

The softening of tissues leads to the formation of a cold abscess, the nature and course of which are described under the heading Abscess.

Pott's disease is more common in children, but is not uncommon in adults. Pain occurs in the back, and may date from a fall or a blow. Tenderness may also be detected over the affected vertebrae, and the back is held rigid. The general health may be good in the early stages, but as time goes on it fails rapidly, fever and perhaps discharge from an abscess being material factors in causing this decline.

Pott's disease should be recognized early, an X-ray examination being an excellent means of determining whether the disease is or is not present, when pain is felt in the back. Early treatment may be successful in preventing deformity. Absolute rest in bed is necessary, and for a space of two years at least, so that treatment should properly be carried out in an institution. It may be possible to correct deformity or to fix the spine and so hasten recovery by apparatus (Plate XXIX, 4-5), and, possibly, operation. The general treatment of tuberculosis by sunlight, fresh air, etc., is indispensable.

Pott's disease is also known as spondylitis and spinal caries.

See Backbone : Spina Curvature; Tuberculosis.

POULTICE. A prolonged application of moist heat is most easily secured by the use of a poultice, and this is generally made with linseed. The materials required are one or two pounds of linseed, a large bowl, a spatula or blunt-edged knife, boiling water, a piece of calico of the proposed area of the poultice with an inch to spare all round, and a piece of jaconet, or thin macintosh, sufficiently large to overlap the poultice all round by an inch at least (Plate XXX, 3-6).

The bowl is warmed and a sufficient amount of boiling water for the size of poultice required is poured in ; for an adult it will be about three-quarters of a pint. Linseed is then slowly added, being constantly stirred with the knife, previously dipped in boiling water, until the mass has the consistency of thick porridge. The poultice is then emptied out on the calico and quickly spread, leaving a margin of an inch, which is then turned over the poultice (Plate XXX, 5). This is now tested against the cheek or the skin of the forearm of the nurse, to prevent scalding, then applied and covered with the jaconet or macintosh. Sometimes a layer of cotton wool is put over this. Such a poultice should retain its heat for many hours.

An alternative method is to have a flannel bag with a broad flap, and, when for use on the back, with tapes attached to the four corners. The poultice is emptied into the bag and spread out in a layer. The tapes serve to keep the bag in the required position (Plate XXX, 6).

Bread, cut up into little cubes, may also be used to make a poultice (Plate XXX, 1-2). Instead of an ordinary poultice one might use the kaolin poultice B.P.C. The method of making a starch poultice is described in the account of the treatment of eczema (q.v.), and a mustard poultice under the heading Mustard.

POUPART'S LIGAMENT. A strong, fibrous cord stretching from the anterior tip of the haunch bone to the pubic bone, and therefore lying in the groin, Poupart's ligament forms the junction between the aponeurosis of the external oblique muscle of the abdomen and that encasing the muscles of the thigh. At its inner end it supports the spermatic cord, while beneath it here is the femoral sheath containing the femoral vessels and the femoral canal. An inguinal hernia thus passes out above the ligament and a femoral hernia beneath it.
See Groin.

POWDER. A drug prepared in a finely powdered form is called a powder, or pulvis (plural, pulveres). There are many such powders, official and otherwise, some of them containing more than one drug and called compound powders. Some of these have special names. Thus, the compound powder of ipecacuanha is also called Dover's powder, the compound rhubarb powder Gregory's powder, and so on. Instructions for giving powders appear under the heading Medicines.
See Insufflation.

PRECIPITATE. The solid substance thrown down out of solution in a liquid by the addition of a reagent, or by the action of heat or cold, is termed a precipitate. This happens, for example, when common salt is added to a solution of silver nitrate. Ammoniated mercury is commonly called white precipitate.

PREGNANCY. Conception, or impregnation of the ovum by a spermatozoon, which initiates the series of developmental changes resulting in the formation of a child, creates a condition, also marked by many changes, in the mother described as pregnancy, or gravidity.

Fertilisation of an ovum may take place in the womb, the Fallopian tube or the ovary, but wherever it occurs, unless in exceptional instances, the ovum makes its way into the womb, on some part of the lining membrane of which it comes to rest. It acquires coverings, some from the lining of the womb and others through its own development. The progress subsequent to fertilisation is discussed under the heading Embryo.

For a first conception the most likely period of a woman's life is between twenty and thirty years of age, and intercourse is most often fruitful just after a menstrual period or during the week preceding it. From the seventeenth to the twenty-fourth day after the beginning of a period it is very unlikely to be fruitful.

In certain circumstances a woman ought not to become pregnant, on account of danger to her own life or the likelihood of bearing a diseased child, possibilities which would exist much less frequently were people with bad personal health or bad family histories to refrain from marrying. When necessary, advice should be got from a doctor about the methods of contraception, as the prevention of pregnancy is usually called.

Signs of the Condition

A woman who conceives almost always misses her next period and does not menstruate again until after the child is born. Some women continue to menstruate, however, although they are pregnant. On the other hand, amenorrhoea (q.v.), or cessation of menstruation, may be due to anaemia or other causes, but a sudden cessation in a healthy woman, after intercourse, is very significant. In the sixth week morning sickness may begin ; there may be actual vomiting on getting up, or only nausea. This symptom usually persists till the fourth month, but may continue longer. About the time that sickness begins it will probably be found that the breasts are beginning to enlarge, that the veins on them are more prominent and that the areola round the nipple is enlarging and becoming darker in colour, while little nodules, Montgomery's tubercles, appear over its surface.

From the end of the sixteenth week fluttering or thumping movements, referred to as quickening, may be felt in the lower abdomen, and a doctor, by listening, might be able to hear the sounds of the foetal heart from the fourteenth week. During all this time the womb has been enlarging and undergoing certain changes which a doctor could detect by examination, and after the first few months there is a quite definite enlargement of the abdomen.

Impoverishment of Teeth and Bones

Pregnancy is quite a normal process, of course, and usually proceeds throughout without upsetting the health, but in certain circumstances disagreeable and sometimes dangerous incidents attend it. The claims of the growing child, for example, on lime salts may starve the teeth and bones of the mother. Thus, dental caries is common in pregnancy, and, though the occurrence is not at all common, a softening of the bones, known as osteomalacia (q.v.) may result from the same cause.

Sickness also may be so frequent and severe as to menace health or even life, a condition described as pernicious vomiting. Some pregnant women have a desire for raw oatmeal, unripe green apples and other unsuitable things. Constipation is common in pregnancy and piles may be troublesome. Frequently also there are varicose veins in the legs. Pressure on the veins in the pelvis is responsible for piles and for varicose veins.

The state of the veins may cause dropsical swelling of the legs, but dropsy may also be due to kidney disease, to which pregnant women are especially liable. Frequent headache or dimness of sight are symptoms very suggestive of kidney disease. Such symptoms may precede convulsive seizures, referred to as eclampsia (q.v.).

Bleeding from the womb may occur. This points to the necessity for rest, quiet and care, as it may mean a threatened abortion and sometimes is due to the dangerous condition known as placenta praevia (q.v.).

Mental disturbances of some kind may occur in pregnancy and may take the form of actual insanity.

A complication which is annoying but of no particular consequence is the pigmentation of the face known as chloasma.

Most of the dangers that threaten a pregnant woman and her child can be avoided or greatly mitigated by timely advice and treatment.

As, however, the early stages of these disorders may only be detectable by a doctor, it is necessary that a pregnant woman should keep in touch with her doctor or with an ante-natal clinic until her child is born. If she does this, some serious difficulties that sometimes present themselves during labour may also be avoided.

It is very important, for one thing, that the urine should be examined by a doctor from time to time.

A pregnant woman should keep to a plain, good diet, with meat once a day only, and strict moderation in starchy and sugary foods. Milk should be taken freely, as it is rich in the lime that she requires. Plenty of green vegetables and of fruit should be included in the diet. Alcohol should be avoided. While there is a tendency to sickness it is advisable to have a light breakfast in bed and to rest in bed for half an hour afterwards. Open-air exercise is necessary if at all possible, and the best form is walking. Any kind of violent exercise is undesirable. If the veins of the legs are swollen, bandages should be put on from the feet upwards before getting up, and it will be well to lie down, with the legs elevated on a cushion, several times during the day.

Aperients that are Safe

The bowels must be kept regular, and for this purpose many women prefer to take a teaspoonful of castor oil each evening, but cascara sagrada, confection of sulphur and the compound liquorice powder are also good. Strong purgatives should not be taken. Sexual intercourse is best avoided ; in the earlier months of pregnancy it may easily provoke abortion.

The elasticity of the skin of the abdominal wall can be increased by massaging daily with olive oil. During the last few weeks of pregnancy an attempt should be made to bring the nipples into the best condition possible by drawing them out gently each day, and the skin over them will be made tougher by smearing with a preparation consisting of 2 ounces of compound tincture of lavender with ½ drachm of glycerin.

The usual duration of pregnancy is about 280 days. One way of calculating the probable date of childbirth is to count three months back from the beginning of the last menstrual period and add ten days. The actual date may be a few days on either side of the date thus ascertained. The calculation may be checked by noting the date on which quickening occurs, and other methods are available for a doctor.

See Abortion ; Bacilluria ; Childbirth ; Eclampsia ; Ectopic Gestation ; Embryo ; Presentation.

PRESBYOPIA. The inability to focus small objects clearly at a distance less than about a foot from the eye is called presbyopia, when the defect is due to age. It becomes apparent usually about forty-five years of age. It is corrected by glasses or spectacles with spherical lenses, stronger ones being required at intervals, often of about five years, as the age increases.

See Eye.

PRESCRIPTION. A medical prescription consists of several parts. First there is the sign ℞, which, originally an invocation of the planet Jupiter, is now taken to represent the Latin word recipe, meaning " take." Then follows the inscription, or body of the prescription, in which the names of the drugs are generally written in contracted Latin words and the quantities represented by signs or contractions, as follows : grain, gr. ; minim, ℨ ; drachm, ℨ ; and ounce, ℥.

The third part is the subscription, consisting of instructions to the chemist, which are generally in Latin, and the fourth part the signature, or instructions to the patient, which are generally in English, or, if written in Latin, are translated by the chemist for the label of the preparation.

See Apothecaries' Weights and Measures ; B.P.

PRESENTATION. The part of an unborn child which is opposite the mouth of the womb is called the presentation. The most common is the vertex presentation, that is, the back of the top of the head. There are four so-called positions of this presentation, according as the back of the head is toward the front or back of the mother's body and towards the right or left side. Usually it is towards the front, the more favourable position. Other presentations are described as brow, breech, shoulder, frontal, transverse and so on. A transverse position means that the child's body lies across the mouth of the womb.

See Childbirth.

PRICKLY HEAT. In the tropics, and especially during the hot season, a rash known as miliaria rubra papulosa, lichen tropicus, or, popularly, prickly heat, is a common event. It is caused by excessive warmth, over-heavy clothing perhaps contributing to this, and is commonly preceded and accompanied by profuse sweating. A similar eruption from the same circumstances may occur in temperate climates, an instance being the rash which sometimes forms on the cheek of an infant from one side of its face being kept pressed against the nurse's body.

The rash, which comes out suddenly, consists of little papules and vesicles, due to distension of sweat glands, around which there is at the same time some degree of inflammation. The trunk, back and front, is mainly affected. The part is reddened, and there is heat, tingling and itching. The blisters are clear at first, but become milky in a few days. Unless infected by scratching they soon disappear, leaving minute scabs which scale off.

Heavy food, especially in large meals, alcohol and iced drinks are prone to provoke an outbreak of prickly heat, and should be avoided. Flannel underwear is also provocative, and, if a rash appears, should be replaced by cellular cotton. Alkaline baths and soothing lotions, details of which are given under the heading Itching, will be of service. Rubbing the body over with soft paraffin after the morning bath is a useful preventive precaution for those who are subject to this disorder.

See Miliaria.

PRIMIPARA. A woman who is pregnant for the first time is called a primipara.

PROBANG. An instrument used for removing foreign bodies from the gullet is called a probang. That generally used is the umbrella-probang, which has an arrangement of bristles at one end which remain elongated while this end of the instrument is passed beyond the foreign body. Then, by pulling out a stout wire passed through the stem of the probang, the bristles are made to double on themselves and spread out to form a disk, which carries the foreign body in front of it when the probang is withdrawn from the gullet.

See Choking ; Gullet.

PROBE. A slender rod of flexible metal for sounding wounds, sinuses and other cavities or passages, natural or pathological, is called a probe. Except in expert hands it may prove a dangerous instrument.

PROCESS. Many projections or prominences about the body are referred to as processes.

PROGNOSIS. An opinion regarding the progress and result of an illness is called a prognosis. In arriving at a prognosis many facts have to be considered, such as the general reputation of the disease, the previous health and the habits of the patient, his response to treatment, etc.

See Diagnosis.

PROGRESSIVE MUSCULAR ATROPHY. There are many circumstances under which one or more muscles may atrophy progressively, but an uncommon disease in adults in which wasting begins in the hands, and then involves the forearms, the arms, the legs and the remainder of the body, is specially named as progressive muscular atrophy. The wasting is due to degeneration of the nerve cells in the spinal cord which control the muscles, but the cause of this change is not known.

The disease begins in the ball of the thumb, the corresponding eminence on the inner side of the palm, and the little muscles between the bones, so that the latter become very prominent, while the whole hand becomes claw-like. Then other parts are affected in succession, but the disease progresses slowly. There is no pain or other disturbance of sensation throughout the disease.

There is a similar disorder in which the motor cells in the bulb, or medulla, degenerate. It is called bulbar paralysis, and here the muscles of the tongue, lips, pharynx and larynx are affected. First of all there are defects of speech and then difficulty in swallowing. In an affection known as amyotrophic lateral sclerosis, the atrophic changes in the upper limbs, which are described above, are accompanied by rigidity, tremors in the legs and exaggerated knee-jerks.

In children, often in several members of one family, a progressive muscular atrophy occurs which is known as the peroneal type, because it affects first the peroneal muscles and those on the front of the leg. Consequently a club foot (*q.v.*) develops, either talipes varus, or equino-varus. There is no curative treatment for any of these conditions, although gentle massage may produce some temporary benefit.

See Muscle ; Myopathy.

PROLAPSE. The protrusion of the lining of a body cavity through a natural opening, or of an organ through a wound, is described as prolapse of the part in question. To the first variety belong prolapse of the lining of the bowel or of the vagina. In connexion with the latter of these it may be said that a falling of the womb is also called a prolapse.

Instances of prolapse through wounds might be furnished by the bowel or the lung, when the abdominal wall or the chest wall, respectively, is penetrated. When a corneal ulcer perforates there is a danger of prolapse of the iris, or curtain of the eye.

PROPHYLAXIS. The preventive treatment of disease is described as prophylaxis. Thus, quinine is a prophylactic remedy against malaria, and vaccination against smallpox.

PROSTATE. In the male the first part of the urethra, or discharge tube of the bladder, passes through a structure shaped rather like a chestnut, and known as the prostate. This is made up of three lobes, right, left and middle, the last lying beneath the urethra. The structure is made up of glandular tissue mainly, but there is also plain muscle tissue. The glands secrete a clear, glairy substance.

Inflammation of the prostate, or prostatitis, may be acute or chronic, and the commonest cause of both is gonorrhoea. Acute prostatitis is a very painful affection. There are frequent calls to pass water, and this causes pain and straining ; considerable pain may also be caused by defecation. Frequently an abscess forms in the prostate, and may aggravate the symptoms, so that bodily movements, or even sitting, cause intolerable pain.

Strict rest, restriction of diet to bland drinks, and the application of heat, preferably as a hot hip bath, will probably bring relief in acute prostatitis, but if pus forms it must have vent. If it bursts through into the bowel, or externally, it is likely to leave a fistula, so it should be evacuated by operation.

Chronic prostatitis is the usual cause of gleet, the chronic type of gonorrhoea (*q.v.*). Amongst other details of treatment for gleet, massage of the prostate through the rectum takes an important place.

Enlargement of the Prostate

An elderly man may suffer from an enlarged prostate; this may happen under the age of fifty, but only rarely. Generally the enlargement makes the flow of urine slower by causing some obstruction. In the earliest stages it may simply be a little delay in the starting of the flow, but it will be noticed that any effort to press the urine out rather hinders than helps. The patient will next find that he has to pass water more frequently and get up once or twice in the night for the purpose.

After a time, when the urine is passed some will be left in the bottom of the bladder. This is known as residual urine, and, sooner or later, it begins to decompose and become irritating, thus giving rise to inflammation of the bladder lining, or cystitis. At any time, a chill or overmuch alcohol may cause retention of urine altogether. There is always a likelihood also of the inflammation passing up the urethra to the kidneys.

One way of dealing with the situation is for the patient to use a catheter (*q.v.*) regularly; another, and a better way, is to have the prostate removed by the operation described as prostatectomy. This is entirely satisfactory, as the bladder begins to function as in a normal individual.

Sometimes, however, an enlargement may be due to a sarcoma or a carcinoma, but these tumours are not very common in this situation. The only kind of treatment which, as a rule, is available when the enlargement is discovered is that by radium or by X-rays. Sometimes, as a result of chronic inflammation in the prostate, stones, referred to as prostatic calculi, form in the organ. These are revealed by the use of X-rays.

See Bladder; Gonorrhoea; Urethra.

PROSTRATION. Severe weakness of the vital functions, or prostration, if it occurs suddenly from an accident or an operation, is called shock; if suddenly from other causes, collapse. Prostration may have a gradual onset, however, as a result of severe and prolonged febrile disorders or other debilitating diseases, and may assume the form of the typhoid state. Exhaustion from an excessive expenditure of nerve energy is commonly referred to as nervous prostration.

The treatment of prostration depends to some extent on its type; that for shock, for collapse and for the typhoid state is described under those separate headings. In nervous prostration, rest, physical and mental, is very necessary, and mental rest may have to be prolonged far beyond the time when the patient is fit for fairly active bodily exercise. Diet at the beginning should be light, but may be increased liberally as the digestive powers improve.

See Neurasthenia; Weir-Mitchell Treatment.

PROTARGOL. A combination of protein and silver, protargol has been used in the treatment of conjunctivitis and, more particularly, gonorrhoea. It is used in watery solution, ointments, bougies, and as a jelly.

See Silver.

PROTEIN. In the chemical composition of living structures a most important position is occupied by complex substances, containing nitrogen, and described as proteins. Plants build up such substances from nitrates contained in the soil, and animals obtain their necessary supplies of proteins from plants or from the flesh of other animals.

In the process of digestion the complex proteins are split up into simpler forms and ultimately into substances known as amino-acids. These are absorbed from the digestive tract and carried in the blood to the body cells, which use them for building up again the complex protein substances. Again, these are broken down in the course of the activities of living cells and are discharged as urea and other substances which in the soil are converted into nitrates and again utilised by plants. Besides nitrogen, the other constant elements in proteins are carbon, hydrogen, oxygen and sulphur.

In view of the fact that they are used to build up protoplasm, proteins are commonly referred to as flesh-forming foods, but it must be observed that all the proteins used as food do not split up into the same amino-acids. Now, as regards human beings, some of the amino-acids are more important than the others. In fact, if one or two of them are not forthcoming, health is impossible. Proteins which, on being split up, furnish these necessary amino-acids may be called " good " proteins, and those which do not, " bad " proteins. Animal foods, meat, eggs, milk and fish furnish the former, and vegetable foodstuffs the latter, but it should be added that a relatively small amount of good protein would appear to be all that is needed.

There are numerous classes of protein. Two very important ones are the albumins and the globulins. White of egg consists largely of albumin, but it also contains a globulin, and both are also contained in the blood plasma. Fibrinogen, out of which blood clot is formed, is also a globulin. The protein of wheat known as gluten consists really of two proteins, one of which enables dough to be formed. This one is absent from rice, for example, so that bread cannot be made with rice. Legumin, the protein of the pulses, consists of globulins. Myosin, of meat, consists of globulins also.

A very important group of proteins are called nucleo-proteins. These, in addition to protein, contain an organic acid of which phosphorus is a constituent. Some nucleo-proteins also contain iron. The proteins in protoplasm (*q.v.*), the substance of living cells, are chiefly in the form of nucleo-protein.

See Diet ; Food ; Peptone.

PROTOPLASM. The substance of which animal and vegetable cells are composed is described as protoplasm. It differs from all other substances in possessing the properties which are distinguished as manifestations of life. There are numerous variations of protoplasm according to certain differences in the chemical constitution.

About three-fourths of its substance consists of water, and the bulk of the remainder of the complex nitrogenous compounds known as proteins. Small quantities of lipoids and of mineral salts, the chlorides and phosphates of calcium, sodium and potassium, also occur.

Complex chemical interchanges go on within a mass of protoplasm ; from so-called foodstuffs it can select materials for building up its own substance and a host of other substances, including the numerous alkaloids which are found in plants. Its own chemical activities can be modified in different ways by many substances, and this accounts for the activities of many drugs and their beneficent or poisonous effects on health.

See Cell ; Lipoid ; Protein.

PROTOZOA. The simplest forms of animal life consist of a single cell, and are known as protozoa. These are divided into four classes according to their means of locomotion. The first includes the amoeba, which moves by protruding a portion of its substance into a finger-like process, or pseudopodium. Several amoebae, including the dysentery parasite, are found in man. The second class move by means of a slender process, like a whip lash ; they are called flagellata, and in this class some authorities include the trypanosome, the kind of parasite that causes sleeping sickness. The third class, the ciliata, move by means of little hair-like processes, called cilia. Of this class the balantidium and other species are sometimes found in man. The fourth class, sporozoa, multiply by forming spores, and in this class is included the malaria parasite.

See Amoeba ; Parasite.

PROUD FLESH. Excessive or exuberant granulation tissue (*q.v.*) is commonly called proud flesh. The cause of the exuberance is the existence of sepsis, and measures must be taken to clean up the wound when proud flesh forms. Astringent lotions are also used, and sometimes the granulations are rubbed over with a crystal of copper sulphate, or blue stone.

PRURIGO. Several types of itchy eruption are described as prurigo, the two most important being what is called Hebra's prurigo and common prurigo. Hebra's prurigo usually begins during the first year of life, either as lichen urticatus, an affection described under the heading Nettle-rash, or simply with itching. It leads to much scratching, so that the skin is broken, and infection with pus-forming microbes occurs. The back of the arms and front of the legs are principally involved, but later the trunk and face may share. After about a year the surface of the skin is covered with straight scratch marks, crusts, pustules and papules, many of which have their tops torn. Portions of the skin are also thickened. The lymphatic glands in the groins, the armpits, and possibly elsewhere, are enlarged, and there is general debility.

Sometimes the disease gradually lessens in severity at puberty or in adult life, but often it persists. Local remedies include such as are described under the heading Itching. The diet must be strictly regulated ; sometimes a purely vegetarian one is the best, though milk may also be taken if it appears to agree. Cod-liver oil is often a valuable addition to the diet.

Common prurigo usually begins about the age of thirty. It may be generalised over the body, or it may be localised at the back of the neck, between the buttocks, or in other situations.

The latter form is usually found in women. Either form may last for months or years. Treatment is similar to that described above, but in the localised form X-rays or radium give the best results.

See Itching ; Nettle-rash.

PRURITIS. *See* Itching.

PRUSSIC ACID. *See* Hydrocyanic Acid.

PSOAS MUSCLE. A large muscle, arising from the front and side of the lower part of the spine on either side of the body, the psoas is inserted, along with the iliacus muscle, which clothes the inner surface of the iliac bone, into the lesser trochanter of the femur (*q.v.*). These muscles bend the thigh on the abdomen and rotate it outwards, or, alternatively, bend the trunk on the thigh.

A psoas abscess, which is a type of the so-called " cold " abscess, is described under the heading Abscess.

PSORIASIS. A rather common skin disease, psoriasis occurs as papules, covered with scales, the papules sometimes being separate, but more often crowded together to form patches of varying size. The disease, of which the cause is unknown, begins in early life as a rule, probably with a general distribution of the eruption over the body. It then clears away except for one or two places, where it is likely to persist, namely, the back of the elbow, the front of the knee, and possibly the scalp. From time to time outbreaks involving more or less of the body surface are apt to occur. Only exceptionally is there any itching or any other discomfort, and the general health is not affected. The scales on the top of a psoriasis papule are white, and can be removed from a patch in layers ; scraping them produces a silvery sheen. Sometimes inflammation of the small joints occurs in a person subject to psoriasis.

In some cases of psoriasis a change in the diet is beneficial. Thus, an improvement may follow a reduction of protein foods, such as meat and eggs, to a minimum, especially in acute cases. Arsenic is the drug most often used inwardly, but potassium iodide, thyroid extract, and others are also tried in certain cases.

Alkaline or sulphur baths, and a subsequent application of salicylic acid in vaseline, will help to clear off the scales, after which preparations of such things as ordinary tar, chrysarobin from goa powder (*q.v.*) and mercurials are applied. Treatment, however, should be under medical supervision, as drugs, when applied over a large surface, may be absorbed in unpleasant amounts ; also over-energetic treatment might provoke an acute outbreak.

PSYCHOLOGY. Often defined as the science of the mind, psychology, in the present state of our knowledge, is better defined, following McDougall, as the science of the behaviour of living things. *See* Mind.

PSYCHONEUROSIS. A neurosis (*q.v.*), which has, like hysteria, a purely mental origin is called a psychoneurosis.

PSYCHOSIS. A mental disease is sometimes called a psychosis. A psycho-neurosis is sometimes referred to as a minor psychosis.

PSYCHO-THERAPY. The influence of conscious thinking on the functions of the body has long been recognized; also that faith in a physician, or a particular remedy, may be an important factor in bringing about a cure. Every doctor may thus be said to practise psycho-therapy, and certainly the success of many a vaunted patent or secret remedy is an example of it.

As described under the heading Freudism, however, it is now known that unconscious thought processes have also an influence on health, and that some disorders are entirely due to such influences. Some of these disorders were at one time treated by ordinary physical methods, but, as the root of the trouble is purely mental, it is but common sense that the treatment should be directed to the mental trouble, and it is to the special methods of doing this that the term psycho-therapy is more properly applied.

The simplest method is sometimes referred to as a therapeutic conversation. The patient discusses the state of his health with his doctor, who explains the nature of his symptoms to him, and may be able to show that fears entertained by the patient are perfectly groundless. Merely to talk over things in this way may effect a cure. Possibly the doctor may have to appeal to the patient's reason, or, in other words, use the method of persuasion.

Sometimes a doctor authoritatively lays down a proposition which is not directed to the patient's reason, but which is expected to be accepted in the unquestioning fashion of a little child receiving statements from its elders. This is called the method of suggestion, and it may be used with the patient in his ordinary or in a hypnotic state. The method is ten enough used, for good or ill, by a person on himself, this being known as auto-suggestion (*q.v*).

When it is apparent that a disability due to some repressed thought, the only way to cure the patient may be to reveal the thought to the patient by the method of psycho-analysis. The patient is requested to relate his thoughts as they occur to him, not directing them or holding anything back, a process described as free association. The doctor watches narrowly for clues to the nature of the repressed ideas. The process may take a long time from the existence of conscious or unconscious bars, or resistances, to free association.

Sometimes, by uttering a list of key-words to a patient and noting the readiness or otherwise of the patient's responses as to what a word suggests to him, a clue may be obtained to a repression. Information may also be got from the interpretation of dreams, and repressed memories may sometimes be recovered by hypnotism.

By putting a repressed idea or memory into its proper relationship to the patient's thinking and his disability, the latter may be successfully removed. Also, the realization of the circumstances of a repressed memory of some mental shock may be accompanied by an outburst of emotion, associated with the incident, this relief of pent-up emotion being described as abreaction, or catharsis; it may be of much service to the patient.

Psycho-analysis has the serious disadvantage that it is apt to be a lengthy and therefore costly method of treatment.
See Auto-Suggestion; Dreams; Freudism; Hypnotism; Mental Disease; Mind; Neurosis.

PTERYGIUM. A triangular, fleshy looking fold of conjunctiva which extends on to the cornea from the outer or inner side of the eyeball is called a pterygium. It develops from a pinguecula (*q.v.*) and usually occurs in elderly people, especially those exposed to much irritation of the eyes by cold winds, dust, etc. If it passes to the centre of the cornea it interferes seriously with sight, and otherwise may keep up slight irritation in the eye. If necessary, it can be removed by operation.

PTOMAINE. An alkaloidal substance produce by the action of putrefactive bacteria on protein food, a ptomaine was at one time considered to be the main cause in all cases of food poisoning. It is now recognized that in most cases of poisoning from this source a disease-producing microbe is responsible, and that the poisonous toxins are produced actually within the body, and are not often ptomaines.

Ptomaines, if absorbed into the blood, cause symptoms of poisoning, which is referred to as sapraemia, but few ptomaines are poisonous when taken by the mouth. A poisonous ptomaine may, however, occur in cheese, ice-cream and some other foodstuffs, the usual symptoms being those of irritant poisoning, though there are often nervous symptoms also.

The symptoms and treatment of food poisoning are discussed under the heading Food.

See Botulism ; Food ; Poisoning ; Sapraemia.

PTOSIS. Drooping of the upper eyelid is called ptosis. A double ptosis may exist from birth and is due to imperfect development of the muscle that raises the eyelid. Later, ptosis is usually due to paralysis of the oculo-motor nerve (*q.v.*). In some cases drugs may avail, but often an operation is necessary.

See Eye.

PTYALIN. The ferment in saliva is called ptyalin ; it converts starch into sugar. An excessive flow of saliva, or salivation, is sometimes called ptyalism.

PUBERTY. The period when childhood first begins to merge into adult life is described as puberty.

See Adolescence.

PUBIS. The front portion of the innominate body is called the pubis, or pubic bone. An expanded part of the bone, known as the body of the pubis, helps to form the acetabulum, the joint cavity for the head of the thigh bone. From the body a bar, the superior ramus, passes downwards and inwards towards the middle line, meeting the ramus from the opposite side in a joint, called the symphysis pubis. From the lower part of the superior ramus at the symphysis, the inferior ramus diverges in a downward and outward direction. The angle made by the diverging inferior rami is filled in by the triangular ligament, which is pierced by the urethra.

The hairy region over the pubic bones is commonly referred to as the pubes.

See Pelvis ; Urethra.

PUBLIC HEALTH. The department of medicine concerned with the activities of the State in the promotion of health is described as Public Health or State Medicine. Legislative enactments dealing with the subject of health are put into force by central and local authorities. The Ministry of Health is the central authority for England and Wales. Public Health comprises such subjects as housing, sanitation, the prevention of infectious diseases, pre-natal and maternity care, infant welfare, the health of school children, the purity of food and water, the health in mines, factories and workshops, the treatment of venereal diseases and so on. A large amount of research is also carried out.

See Birth Rate ; Death Rate ; Drains ; Food ; Housing ; Infectious Disease ; Notification ; Occupational Disease ; Quarantine ; Sewage.

PUERPERIUM. After childbirth the womb, which has been much enlarged for the reception of the child, must return to ordinary dimensions. The period during which this is taking place is called the puerperium, and lasts for six weeks at least. In the earlier stages blood-clot, and possibly shreds of membrane, are discharged, sometimes giving rise to after-pains ; the raw surface on the lining of the womb caused by the removal of the after-birth heals ; and the genital passages recover from bruising and perhaps lacerations to which they have been subject.

Till the lining of the womb has resumed its ordinary condition more or less, a discharge, known as the lochia, continues. In the first three days following labour this is reddish in colour, and then for three or four days longer it is watery. If the redness continues it suggests the retention of a piece of after-birth, clot or membrane in the womb. The odour of the lochia becomes rather sickly, but should not be stinking. If the discharge suddenly ceases, puerperal infection should be suspected.

After childbirth a woman should be dried and put into a dry, warmed nightdress as quickly as possible, and, when made comfortable, should be allowed rest for some hours. When she has rest sufficiently, the child should be put the breast, as, although for three da the breast secretes only a watery flu known as colostrum, the act of nursi is beneficial, to the mother at least.

The greatest care must be taken to keep the private parts thoroughly clean, lysol solution, a teaspoonful to the pint, being used for sponging. No soiled diapers or clothing should be allowed to remain in the room. *Particular care should be shown in cleaning the teeth and mouth, as a septic mouth may cause puerperal infection.*

Diet for the first day or two should be light. On the third day a dose of opening medicine, castor oil or liquorice powder, is given, and afterwards the diet should be more liberal. If the breast milk is scanty, the patient should take milk freely, but not stout nor alcohol in any form, unless ordered by a doctor.

Sometimes after labour there is a retention of urine. This may be relieved simply by making the patient listen to running water or by hot applications to the private parts, but the use of a catheter may be necessary.

Over-exertion and its Penalty

The patient should remain in bed for ten days at least ; a fortnight is desirable, and it may require to be longer. During the next fortnight she should lie down from time to time, and avoid any exertion. Bleeding in the 24 hours after labour is called post-partum haemorrhage, and after this time puerperal haemorrhage. Its first-aid treatment is given under the heading Flooding, but a doctor should be summoned at once.

There is a considerable risk of infection during the puerperium, especially the earlier part, and for the first two or three weeks the temperature should be taken at least night and morning. Fever due to septic infection at this time is called puerperal, or child-bed, fever, but it may take several forms. The placenta, etc., retained in the womb may putrefy, and the products of bacterial action may be absorbed into the blood, causing a condition described as sapraemia. The cleansing of the womb from these offensive substances is usually followed by a very rapid improvement in the general state of the patient. The fever in this condition is likely to begin early, perhaps from the third to the fifth day, but might occur earlier or later, and the same applies to the next form of infection, namely, puerperal septicaemia.

Here there are bacteria actually circulating in the blood. The onset of fever may be gradual, but often is sudden and accompanied by rigor. The fever is high, possibly with delirium, and there may be sickness and vomiting. The lochia may cease or become offensive. There may or may not be pain, tenderness and swelling of the abdomen. This is a very dangerous condition. Amongst other possibilities is that of the development of septic endocarditis. Similar symptoms occur in puerperal pyaemia. Another form of infection is inflammation of the bladder (*q.v.*), or cystitis. Others are parametritis (*q.v.*) and perimetritis (*q.v.*), which usually occur in the second week, as does also the last form of infection to be mentioned, namely, white leg (*q.v.*).

Puerperal fever is a notifiable disease, and immediate medical supervision of treatment is required. Sometimes douching is depended on to remove infection from the passages, but at other times more energetic and thorough measures are necessary. Otherwise the treatment is mainly that of fever (*q.v.*). Antistreptococcic serum is useful in some cases, especially if used early.

See After-birth ; Breast-feeding ; Childbirth ; Womb.

PULEX IRRITANS. The scientific name of the common flea (*q.v.*) is pulex irritans.

PULMONARY. The adjective pulmonary means that any word which it qualifies has reference to something related to the lung, as, for example, pulmonary disease, pulmonary circulation, pulmonary artery and pulmonary valve.

PULSATION. A throbbing caused by the beating of the heart is called a pulsation. Sometimes it can be seen ; at other times it can only be felt. Visible pulsation in arteries may mean an aneurysm, but more often it does not. What is called epigastric pulsation, that is, a throbbing in the pit of the stomach, is common in thin individuals, and in persons who have been doing hard and prolonged mental labour, and in neurotic persons. Pulsation in the neck is common in anaemia.

Pulsation in a swelling may be due to the beating of a large artery which underlies the swelling. This is called communicated pulsation. Pulsation may occur in veins, as when the liver is passively congested in disease of the right side of the heart. Pulsation in the capillaries, which may be visible in the lips and nails, occurs in aortic regurgitation.

See Heart ; Pulse.

PULSE. Each beat of the heart sends a wave of expansion along the arteries. This wave, referred to as the pulse, can be felt at numerous places on the surface of the body, but the artery usually selected for the examination of the pulse is the radial, where it lies just beneath the skin and over the radius bone a little distance above the wrist.

When examining the pulse, a doctor notes its rate, its regularity, its force, the blood pressure and the state of the vessel-wall. The rate is usually that of the heart-beat, but sometimes some of the heart-beats fail to cause an appreciable wave along the vessel, so that the pulse-beats are fewer than those of the heart and not a true indication of the rate at which the heart is working. Beats that fail to appear at the wrist are referred to as missed beats.

The average rate of the pulse in an adult is 72 beats per minute, but in some healthy people the rate is constantly slower or faster than this. In the early weeks of life the rate is 120 to 140, and it gets progressively slower as the child grows older.

The pulse rate is increased by exertion ; even to get up from a sitting, and especially a recumbent, posture puts it up for a short time. After brisk exercise, such as running upstairs, the rate should return to the ordinary one within about two minutes at most. The rate is also increased by excitement and by a full meal. It is increased in many diseases. In fever the increase is usually about 8 to 10 beats for every degree of fever.

Undue rapidity of the pulse is called tachycardia, undue slowness, bradycardia.

The normal pulse is regular, the beats being of the same size and occurring at the same intervals of time. When there are missed beats, the pulse is more or less irregular, but this occurrence often has no particular significance. As a rule, and especially in children, the pulse is faster when air is being inhaled and slows down while it is being exhaled. The serious disorder called auricular fibrillation produces a pulse which is altogether irregular.

A graphic record of the pulse can be obtained by an instrument called a sphygmograph, the record itself being called a sphygmogram. This exhibits not a simple up-and-down stroke, but a plain up stroke, and several little secondary curves on the down stroke, one of these being caused by the closure of the aortic valve.

The force of the pulse-beat may vary. In conditions associated with great physical depression, the pulse may have what is called a thready character. To estimate the blood pressure, it is necessary to note not only the force of the beat, but the extent to which the blood vessel is filled in the intervals between the beats. The state of the vessel walls is determined by rolling the vessel between the fingers and the bone. If thickened, the vessel feels cord-like. Thickening of the vessels may be sufficient to make their walls more or less rigid, a state of affairs described as arterio-sclerosis (*q.v.*).

See Blood Pressure ; Heart.

P.U.O. The letters P.U.O. stand for pyrexia of unknown origin, and are sometimes used as a label for fever when the precise cause has not been diagnosed.

PUPIL. The round, black opening in the centre of the iris, or coloured curtain of the eye, is called the pupil. If the iris is drawn outwards, the pupil enlarges or dilates ; if the iris, on the other hand, moves inwards, the pupil becomes smaller, or contracts. The pupil is often said to be active or sluggish, as the case may be, but what is really meant is that the iris moves briskly or otherwise.

The pupil contracts when the eye is exposed to light—the light-reflex, and also when a near object is looked at—the accommodation-reflex. When the latter reflex exists, but there is no response to light, what is called the Argyll-Robertson pupil is said to be present. It occurs most frequently in locomotor ataxia, but is found also in one or two other diseases.

Usually, in health, the pupils are equal in size, but they may be unequal in healthy persons, though, on the other hand, inequality may be indicative of some disease. The same applies to a condition known as hippus, which consists of alternate rapid contraction and dilatation of the pupil on exposure to light.

After inflammation of the iris the outline of the pupil may be irregular. This is due to the posterior surface of the iris being adherent to the front of the lens ; such adhesions are called posterior synechiae.

Excessive dilatation of the pupil is called mydriasis, and excessive contraction, miosis.

See Eye.

PURGATIVE. *See* Cathartic.

PURIN. Certain substances found in animals and plants are related chemically in that they each contain a substance composed of carbon, hydrogen and nitrogen, and known as purin. Substances into the composition of which purin enters are described as purin bodies. Such are hypoxanthine, xanthine, adenine, guanine, and, lastly, uric acid, into which the others are converted by the action of ferments in the various tissues of the body. Caffeine, found in tea and coffee, and theobromine, found in cocoa, are also purin bodies but are not converted into uric acid.

The purin bodies occurring in animals result from the destruction of nuclein, a substance found in the nuclei of cells. The cells may be consumed as food, glandular substances such as liver and sweetbread being especially rich in nuclein, and the purin bodies thus formed are said to be exogenous in origin ; or the bodies may be derived from the destruction of nuclei of cells in the body tissues, when they are said to be endogenous in origin.

Some foods, such as meat, contain a considerable quantity of purin bodies, especially hypoxanthine.

As purin bodies are converted into uric acid, it follows that in certain diseases in which many body cells are being destroyed, leukaemia, for example, there will be an increase in the uric acid formed in the body, and there will also be an increase if liver or sweetbread or much meat is taken. Such foods should therefore be avoided by the gouty, in whom there is an increase of uric acid in the tissues and blood. As regards meat, it will suffice to restrict red meat in favour of the white kinds of flesh. Meat extracts and soup are rich in purin bodies.

See Gout ; Uric Acid.

PURPURA. Bleeding into the skin is described as purpura. The marks on the skin are red at first, then become purple, and finally brown or yellow. At no time can they be removed by pressure, and this fact distinguishes the condition from that of erythema (*q.v.*). The marks vary in shape and size. They may be small, round spots, like flea-bites, when they are called petechiae, large patches, or ecchymoses (*see* Plate XXXI, 10), or lines, as if caused by a whip lash, these being known as vibices.

Such patches may be due to insect bites, to sprains or other injuries, to poisoning by snake-bite, or by mercury or other substances, or they may occur in connexion with measles, smallpox, or some other specific fever, or with jaundice, however it may be caused. They are also seen in debilitating diseases, such as chronic nephritis, in pernicious anaemia and other blood disorders, sometimes in hysteria, and in other diseases.

In all the conditions enumerated purpura is simply a symptom which may or may not occur, but there are several diseases in which it is the most prominent fact, and such a disease is called a purpura.

Simple purpura is a disease which mainly affects children. Petechiae form mainly on the legs, and may run together to form large patches. The petechiae come out in crops each day. There is at most a trifling constitutional disturbance, possibly slight fever and pains in the joints. In one or two weeks the spots cease to form, and the condition then clears up.

In rheumatic purpura, also called peliosis rheumatica, and Schönlein's disease, the joints are also affected, and crops of petechiae or of ecchymoses appear on the legs and other parts of the body, commonly on mucous membranes as well as skin. Occasionally there is bleeding from the nose, bowels or other cavity.

Henoch's purpura resembles that just described, but is characterised in addition by attacks of severe pain in the abdomen with vomiting and diarrhoea, blood often occurring in the stool and sometimes in the urine. This disorder mainly affects children, and tends to recur, though not beyond about the age of puberty.

Haemorrhagic purpura, or Werlhof's disease, usually occurs in young and delicate girls. There is bleeding into the skin and almost always into mucous membranes as well. There may be bleeding from the nose, throat, kidneys and other parts. Sometimes death occurs in the 24 hours, but in the larger number of cases the patient survives, the disease abating in from six to eight weeks.

The treatment of purpura is to keep the patient in bed on a light nutritious diet, the bowels being kept open. A search should be made for any source of poisoning. Calcium, in the form of the chloride or the lactate, iron and quinine are the drugs mostly used.

PUS. The liquid contained in an abscess is called pus. The way in which it is formed and its characteristics are described under the heading Abscess. A discharge containing pus is said to be purulent.
See Pyogenic Bacteria.

PUSTULE. A small blister containing pus is called a pustule. Acne, impetigo and smallpox are some of the diseases in which pustules may occur. When a pustule dries it forms a scab.

PUTREFACTION. The decomposition of dead animal and vegetable matter, with the formation of foul-smelling substances, is called putrefaction. This is caused by bacteria, mainly by those of the anaerobic type, or such as thrive in the absence of oxygen, and the source of the disagreeable substances is the protein in the putrefying mass. Ptomaines are also formed in the process. A certain amount of putrefaction constantly goes on in the contents of the bowel.

PYAEMIA. A form of blood-poisoning, pyaemia is characterised by the fact that infected particles of thrombus, or clot, are circulating in the blood and giving rise to numerous small abscesses in various organs, notably the lungs. This may occur when there is a suppurative lesion anywhere in the body; thrombosis takes place in a vein at the site of the lesion, and, by softening of the thrombus, portions are detached and pass into the circulating blood. Symptoms of pyaemia usually occur suddenly with a chill or rigor.

The fever is high and there may be vomiting, and possibly diarrhoea. After some hours the temperature falls, and there is free sweating. This occurs each day, or there may be several rigors in a day, the temperature going up and down. The patient is soon prostrated. If the lungs are affected by abscesses, there are signs of bronchitis, or of consolidation, the condition found in pneumonia. Joints may become inflamed and swollen, and there may be evidence of involvement of the heart or of some other organ.

It is often impossible to locate the lesion which is the source of the poisoning, but if it can be found it is cleaned up as well as possible. Vaccines and sera are sometimes of value in fighting the infection. Otherwise, the treatment is that of fever (*q.v.*). Free stimulation with alcohol may be necessary, and as much light food as the patient can take should be given.
See Embolism ; Septicaemia ; Thrombosis.

PYELITIS. Inflammation of the pelvis of the kidney (*q.v.*) is called pyelitis.

PYLORUS. The portion of the stomach which joins the duodenum, or first part of the bowel, is called the pylorus.
See Stomach.

PYOGENIC BACTERIA. Microbes that produce pus, or matter, are said to be pyogenic. In this group are included staphylococci, streptococci, the bacillus coli communis, gonococci and others.
See Abscess ; Bacteria.

PYONEPHROSIS. An accumulation of pus in the pelvis of the kidney is called pyonephrosis.
See Hydronephrosis ; Kidney.

PYORRHOEA. A chronic discharge of pus from the gums is described as pyorrhoea alveolaris, or Rigg's disease. The pus forms between the neck of a tooth and the collar of gum which surrounds it, loosening the contact of the gum with the tooth. Pockets form in the gum and exude pus, and septic inflammation spreads down the socket, softening the bone that forms it, and gradually loosening the tooth. In later stages the gum becomes very spongy and bleeds easily ; the gum may even be destroyed and the root of the tooth exposed.

A considerable quantity of pus is constantly being swallowed, and this causes indigestion and may infect the lining of the alimentary tract somewhere. The absorption of the poisons produced by the pus-forming bacteria causes anaemia, nerv-

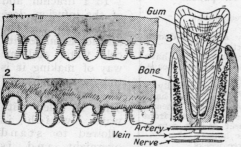

Pyorrhoea. 1. Normal gum and teeth. 2. Thickening of gum between teeth through pyorrhoea. 3. Section of tooth in socket showing pouch behind the gum

ous irritability, nervous exhaustion, inflammation of joints and possibly other troubles. The bacteria themselves may enter the blood, and cause the kind of blood-poisoning known as pyaemia (q.v.).

It should be understood that pyorrhoea may exist and damage the system while the appearance of the gums and teeth may give no hint of the condition, though an X-ray photograph will reveal it.

The formation of tartar at the neck of a tooth favours the occurrence of pyorrhoea. One of the best natural methods of keeping the teeth clean is the regular consumption of crisp salads and fruits. This should be supplemented, however, by the regular use of a tooth brush.

The existence of pyorrhoea makes it necessary to wash out the mouth frequently each day, an antiseptic mouth wash (q.v.) being used for two or three of the washings. More energetic treatment is also required, however. Ionisation, vaccine injections, and ultra-violet rays are amongst methods of treatment that are tried, but often it is necessary to have the teeth extracted.

See Epulis ; Gum ; Teeth.

PYRETHRUM. A dusting powder made from the dry flowers of species of pyrethrum is used to keep away insects. The tincture of pyrethrum, B.P.C., prepared from the flowers, is used as an insecticide lotion. The root of another species of pyrethrum is usually called pellitory root. When chewed it excites a free flow of saliva. The official tincture, made from the root, is sometimes used in a mouth wash ; it should not be swallowed.

PYREXIA. An abnormal elevation of the body temperature is described as pyrexia, or fever (q.v.).

PYRETIC TREATMENT. The treatment of rheumatic complaints by artificially raising the body temperature by means of hot baths is sometimes called pyretic treatment. Part of the value of this kind of treatment is due to the free sweating which it induces.

PYROGALLIC ACID. A crystalline substance obtained from gallic acid by heating, pyrogallic acid, or pyrogallol, is an antiseptic and is slightly stimulating to the skin. It is used in an ointment in psoriasis, chronic eczema, ringworm and other skin affections. If spread over a large surface of skin, however, it may cause poisoning. It also stains the skin. In conjunction with silver nitrate it is used as a hair-dye, various tints up to jet black being obtainable.

PYROSIS. Popularly known as heartburn, pyrosis is a symptom of indigestion (q.v.).

PYURIA. The presence of pus, or matter, in the urine is called pyuria ; its existence is established by easy tests. *See* Urine.

QUARANTINE. The period during which a ship on which an infectious disease has occurred is kept out of port, or, at any rate, from free personal communication with the shore, is called the quarantine period. The word quarantine has, however, also come to mean the period of isolation of persons suffering or convalescing from an infectious disease, and of others who have been in contact with such persons, wherever they may be.

The question of quarantine, in the general experience, mostly arises in connexion with the attendance of children at school. In the table in page 562 the dates

Disease	Quarantine Period (Period of Exclusion from School)	
	Patient	Contacts
Cerebro - spinal meningitis	Three months at least from onset of disease	Three weeks
Chicken-pox ..	Until all scabs have gone; usually three weeks	For those who have not had the disease, three weeks
Diphtheria	Depends on bacteriological tests	As for patient
Encephalitis lethargica	Until recovery (at least six weeks)	Three weeks
Erysipelas	Until rash and peeling gone	May attend if doctor certifies
German measles	Not less than a week from appearance of rash	For those who have not had the disease, three weeks
Influenza	Until recovery	May attend usually
Measles	Until morbid discharges have ceased (three weeks at least)	For those who have not had the disease, three weeks from onset of last case in the house
Mumps	A week after the subsidence of swelling (at least three weeks)	Three weeks
Poliomyelitis ..	Until pronounced free by a doctor	Three weeks
Scarlet Fever ..	Two weeks after release from isolation or from hospital	Ten days; seven days after patient is removed to hospital or released from isolation allowed by some authorities
Smallpox	Until free from scabs (at least six weeks)	If not recently vaccinated, sixteen days
Typhoid Fever ..	Depends on bacteriological tests	May attend
Whooping - cough	Until six weeks from commencement of whoop	For infants only, three weeks from last exposure
Impetigo .. .. Ringworm .. .. Scabies	} Until cured	{ If free on inspection, may attend

at which a convalescent or contact may return to school are duly set out, but children who have actually been ill will probably require a little holiday before going back to school.

The date from which the quarantine of contacts is to be calculated is that of the last exposure to infection. A certificate of fitness to attend school should be got from a doctor, both for patients and contacts. Most of the above particulars do not apply to adults except in special circumstances. Further information is given under the heading of the separate diseases.

See Infectious Disease.

QUARTAN FEVER. *See* Malaria.

QUASSIA. Shavings or chips of quassia are used in medicine for the sake of a bitter principle which they contain. The drug is used in the form of the tincture, dose $\frac{1}{2}$ to 1 drachm, and of the infusion, dose $\frac{1}{2}$ to 1 ounce. The infusion is made with cold water, and one way of making it is to have a cup formed of quassia wood. This is filled with water, which is allowed to stand overnight and is taken in the morning.

Quassia is used as an appetiser and in dyspepsia. It forms a clear solution with iron preparations. A strong infusion is often used to kill threadworms, by injection into the bowel. After washing out the bowel with a plain soap-and-water injection, half a pint of the infusion of quassia is injected three or four times as high up as possible.

See Bitters.

QUICKENING. The sensations caused by the movements of a child in the womb are described as quickening.

See Pregnancy.

QUICKLIME. The oxide of calcium is commonly known as quicklime. It is used to make lime water. When quicklime gets into the eye it should be washed out with a strong solution of cane sugar or with olive oil ; plain water slakes the lime and increases its caustic action.

See Calcium.

QUILLAIA. Also known as soap bark and Panama bark, quillaia bark is sometimes used as an expectorant, its properties in this respect resembling those of senega. It has other medicinal uses, but, as it may cause gastro-intestinal irritation and other poisonous effects, its use is mainly restricted to that of an emulsifying agent.

QUININE. An alkaloid obtained from cinchona bark, quinine is an indispensable drug in the treatment of malaria. It is sometimes used as an antipyretic in other fevers. It may also relieve neuralgia, and, in small doses, is a bitter tonic.

Many salts of the alkaloid have been produced, though most are not much used. That most often employed is quinine sulphate, but the hydrochloride and the bihydrochloride of quinine are also much used, the last being the preparation chosen when quinine is to be injected into the body. The dose of each of these three salts is 1 to 2 grains as a tonic, and up to 10 grains or more for fever.

When the temperature is raised, it is preferable to give quinine in solution, as follows :

Quinine sulphate	10 grains
Dilute sulphuric acid	10 minims
Syrup of lemons	1 drachm
Water..	..to 1 ounce

This makes one dose.

There is a tincture of quinine and an ammoniated tincture, the dose of each being ½ to 1 drachm. The latter, commonly referred to as ammoniated quinine, is often used at the beginning of a common cold or of influenza. There is also a wine of quinine, dose ½ to 1 ounce, and a pill of quinine sulphate, dose 4 to 8 grains.

Considerable doses of quinine, or even small doses, when there is an idiosyncrasy to the drug, cause symptoms of poisoning, referred to as quininism. These include ringing in the ears, headache, deafness and dimness of vision, or actual blindness. Permanent damage may be done either to hearing or sight. To lessen the tendency to headache and noises in the ears, quinine is often combined with dilute hydrobromic acid, as follows :

Quinine hydrochloride	10 grains
Dilute hydrobromic acid.. ..	15 minims
Simple syrup	1 drachm
Water..	..to 1 ounce

This forms one dose.

There is a hydrobromide of quinine, but it is a very expensive preparation.

The sulphate and the hydrochloride of quinine are used in watery solutions of a strength of 1 in 400 to 1 in 1,000 as antiseptic lotions for cleansing wounds, washing out an infected bladder and for other purposes. A combination of quinine hydrochloride and urea, commonly referred to as urea-quinine, is sometimes used as a local anaesthetic.

See Cinchona Bark ; Malaria.

QUINSY. Suppurative tonsillitis is commonly called quinsy.

See Tonsil.

QUOTIDIAN FEVER. *See* Malaria.

Q.V. After many words in technical books, as in this volume, the initial letters of the Latin words quod vide, meaning " which see," are inserted within brackets thus, (*q.v.*). This means that further information on the subject under discussion is given under the heading of the word in question. Much repetition is thus avoided.

RABIES. The disease which is called hydrophobia when it affects human beings is known as rabies when it occurs in the lower animals. Dogs, cats, horses, cattle and other animals may suffer from rabies.

See Hydrophobia.

RADIANT HEAT. One method of applying dry heat to the body is to use the heat radiated from electric lamps, either one large lamp or a number of small ones, arranged in rows in a special cabinet, in which the patient lies or is seated. In this way pain in rheumatism and other affections is relieved. In addition to this, when a cabinet is used sweating is prompted and injurious substances expelled from the body and, in fever, the temperature lowered.

See Heat.

RADIO-ACTIVITY. Certain substances, including the elements radium, uranium, thorium, polonium and actinium, emit rays which are chemically and electrically active, ionising air, forming ozone in the atmosphere, affecting a photographic plate and so on. Such substances are said to be radio-active. Mud baths and natural waters may possess radio-activity from the presence in them of a gas, known as radium emanation, or radon, and some of their good effects are attributed to radio-activity. While, however, it has been shown that a definite dosage of radon certainly has a beneficial effect on a variety of disorders, whether there is any appreciable effect from the quantities present in mud and natural waters is still largely a matter of opinion.

See Radium.

RADIOGRAPHY. The taking of photographs by means of X-rays is called radiography. The print obtained from the negative is variously known as a radiograph, radiogram, skiagraph, skiagram, sciagraph and sciagram. A radiogram is not a photograph of actual things but only of the shadows cast by them, and the pictures may be distorted more or less according to the direction from which the rays fall on an object.

See X-rays.

RADIO-THERAPY. The treatment of disease by X-rays, radium and similar means is called radio-therapy.

RADIUM. A white metallic element belonging to the group of alkaline earths, which also includes barium, calcium, magnesium and strontium, radium is found in pitch-blende and other mineral deposits. It occurs in conjunction with uranium and a heavy gas, known as radium emanation, radon or niton. This conjunction is due to the fact that radium is formed from uranium by the irradiation of atoms of helium gas from the latter, and by a similar process the emanation is formed from radium. The emanation decays similarly, and, by a series of changes occurring within definite periods of time, lead is finally reached as the last product.

From radium three different kinds of rays, distinguished as the alpha, beta and gamma rays, are emitted. The first are the atoms of helium gas referred to above, and are charged with positive electricity ; the second are electrons, or disembodied particles of negative electricity ; while the third are similar to the X-rays.

When the skin is exposed to a sufficient dosage of radium, redness, or erythema, appears in from seven to fifteen days. This may be followed by peeling. Larger doses may cause blistering also, and, larger still, ulceration, which is slow to heal.

These severer effects, when caused inadvertently, are referred to as a radium burn. When a deep effect is required from a surface exposure the radium is screened by a layer of gutta-percha or lead in order to cut off the alpha and beta rays and allow only the more penetrating gamma rays to pass through. Silver is used as a screen in some cases.

Radium is an important instrument in the treatment of malignant tumours when an operation is out of the question. It is sometimes used in the area of operation after the removal of such a tumour so that isolated small portions of tumour tissue which might chance to be present would be killed. It is also used in treating some kinds of birth mark, keloid, lupus and other chronic skin diseases. Some cases of chronic joint disease have benefited considerably from drinking water containing a measured dose of radon.

Radium is generally used in the form of one of its salts, as such are more stable than the element itself. Different kinds of tubes are used for inserting radium into body cavities and tumour tissue, including platinum needles (Plate XXX, 7–8) and tiny glass tubes, known as " seeds," which are filled with radon. These seeds are permanently buried in tumour tissues.

In addition to radium burns alluded to above, other occasional consequences to the skin are telangiectasis, or dilatation of the superficial blood vessels, and pigmentation, both conditions being, however, susceptible of improvement at least by appropriate treatment. After exposure of the skin to large doses there may be symptoms of depression, but these usually pass off in a few days at most.

RADIUS. The bone on the outer or thumb side of the forearm is called the radius. At the elbow it articulates with the humerus, and its lower end, which is more massive than the upper, takes a much larger share than the ulna, the other bone of the forearm, in forming the wrist joint. The radius articulates with the ulna at both its extremities and consequently can rotate on the latter in the movements of pronation and supination.

The upper end of the radius is diskshaped and below this is a rounded portion called the neck of the radius. Just below the neck on the inner and front aspect of the bone is a prominence called the radial tuberosity, into which the tendon of the biceps muscle is inserted. The pull of the biceps on the radius causes supination and flexion of the forearm. The outer aspect of the lower end of the radius is prolonged into a narrow pointed portion called the styloid process, which gives attachment to the upper end of the external lateral ligament of the wrist joint.

A fracture through the lower end of the radius is known as Colles' fracture. It most often occurs in elderly women and from falling on the palm of the hand with the arm stretched out. The deformity caused by the fracture is often referred to as the dinner-fork deformity; the hand is drawn towards the thumb side, and there is a swelling on the back of the wrist and another on the front, below which there is a notable depression. In a young person a separation of the lower epiphysis of the radius may resemble a Colles' fracture. The first-aid treatment of fractures of the radius is described under the heading Fracture.

The word radial may be used as an adjective qualifying anything related to the radius. Thus, the corresponding side of the forearm is called its radial side. The radial artery is the outer of the two branches into which the brachial artery divides. It crosses the forearm obliquely, beneath the muscles, until at the wrist it lies in front of and on the lower end of the radius. It passes into the hand, where

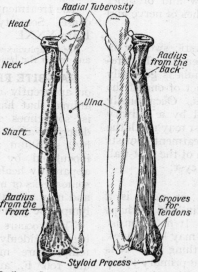

Radius. Its parts and position relative to the ulna, the inner bone of the forearm

it joins the ulnar artery to form the palmar arch.

The name radial nerve is used in two senses. It may apply to a branch of the musculo-spiral nerve which is distributed to the skin on the radial side of the back of the hand, but is more often used for the whole musculo-spiral nerve (*q.v.*), in place of the latter name.

See Elbow ; Forearm ; Ulna ; Wrist.

RAILWAY SPINE.
The nervous disorders that may follow a railway collision or any similar accident are usually of a hysterical nature. The fact that the patient often recovers very quickly after his claim for compensation has been finally dealt with does not necessarily imply malingering.
See Hysteria.

RÂLE. When listening over a healthy lung, sounds caused by the inflow and outflow of air—and known as the breath sounds—are heard. If, from disease, the air tubes or the air cells of the lungs should be occupied by liquid substances, or if abnormal cavities containing fluid exist in the lung, additional or adventitious sounds occur, caused by the flow of the air through the liquid, and described as râles. They may have a clicking, crackling or bubbling character. Crackling râles are also called crepitations.

When the air tubes are narrowed by swelling of their lining or by a sticky discharge, a sound known as a rhonchus may be produced ; if caused by the passage of air through one of the larger tubes it is sonorous in character, if through one of the smaller tubes it is sibilant. A rhonchus is sometimes

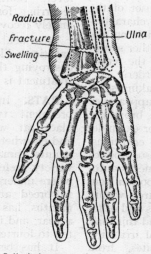

Colles' fracture of the radius, causing displacement of the hand

called a dry rále, the other type being a moist rále.

See Lung.

RAMUS. A Latin word meaning a branch, the term ramus is applied to portions of the lower jaw and of other bones, and to some branches of nerve and blood vessels.

RANULA. A small cystic swelling in the floor of the mouth, beneath the fore-part of the tongue, a ranula is generally due to blocking of the duct of one of the sublingual salivary glands. Occasionally the obstruction is caused by a salivary calculus, or stone. The cyst may reach the size of a pigeon's egg. Treatment consists in dissecting out a portion of the cyst-wall or, if necessary, the entire cyst.

See Tongue.

RASH. An eruption, or rash, is a breaking-out on the skin and perhaps mucous membranes also. It may consist merely of redness or there may be papules, vesicles, pustules or something else. It is important to recognize the primary lesion or essential feature of a rash, whether it be redness, a papule or some other, as later on there may be obscuring of the real nature of the condition by the effects of scratching, infection, etc. Thus, a widely spread eczematous condition may actually be due to scabies, or itch.

A rash may be due to one of the specific fevers, in which case it usually occurs at a definite time after the onset of the illness. It has a more or less character-istic appearance and distribution on the body, and is accompanied by other symp-toms which may help towards the recog-nition of the nature of the disorder.

A rash may also be due to taking some drug, and here again the appearance may be suggestive. Antipyrine, bromides, iodides, copaiba and arsenic, for example, produce fairly typical skin eruptions. The injection of serum may also produce a rash. Sometimes a rash is due to auto-intoxication, the absorption of poison from the bowel or some other source within the body. Syphilis, tuberculosis and other infections may cause a rash, and this may be acute or chronic. External irritation from lice and other parasites, from chemical or mechanical irritants or from the sun, is another possible cause of a rash. Sometimes a rash is produced arti-ficially by the sufferer, as may happen in hysteria or in malingering. Finally, a rash may represent some particular skin disease.

The treatment of a rash depends on the cause. Some types of rash are shown in Plate XXXI.

See Anaphylaxis ; Infectious Disease ; Skin ; and under the headings of individual diseases.

RAT-BITE FEVER. The bite of a rat, or apparently of a cat or some other animal that has recently worried a rat, is sometimes followed by a disorder described as rat-bite fever. This is caused by a spirillum, a micro-organism, which is inoculated by the bite. The wound apparently heals, but after an interval of some weeks or months it becomes inflamed and may ulcerate, while the neighbouring lymphatic glands become enlarged.

Then occurs a bout of fever which begins suddenly, often with a rigor. The temperature may range between 102° and 106° F., and the patient is more or less prostrated. With the onset of fever a rash appears, usually measly in character but sometimes resembling nettle-rash, and there is pain in muscles and probably in joints also.

The fever lasts for a few days and then disappears. The patient feels well for some days, when there is a recurrence of the fever. Bouts of this kind may keep on recurring for many months, but ulti-mately recovery takes place.

Treatment with organic arsenical pre-parations, like salvarsan, is successful in destroying the infection. Otherwise the treatment is that of fever (*q.v.*).

RATS. In Europe the brown rat is the prevalent type, having displaced the black rat, which still abounds in India and elsewhere in the East. The black rat haunts human dwellings, but the brown variety prefers to live in sewers and else-where underground. A female rat begins to breed at the age of three to four months, has five or six or more litters in a year, and in each of these there may be ten to fourteen or more young.

It has been estimated that in Great Britain the annual bill for foodstuffs consumed or destroyed by rats amounts to about £52,000,000, and beyond this there is damage to other kinds of merchandise, to buildings and to fowls. In addition, however, to all this, rats play a considerable part in disseminating disease, the disorders which may be attributable to their agency including rat-bite fever, haemorrhagic jaundice, plague, a tapeworm, ringworm, foot-and-mouth disease, and a virulent form of equine influenza.

Rats become a very serious menace in the presence of plague. Although the different kinds of rat may suffer from plague, the black rat is the chief danger on account of its presence in dwellings and ships. Fleas that feed on the rats pick up the plague germs and transfer them to human beings.

The destruction of rats about one's premises is a legal duty, enforceable by a penalty. Concerted efforts to this end take place each year, during what is called " rat-week." There is a variety of methods of destroying rats. That of pumping prussic acid vapour into ricks and rat-holes is dangerous except when employed by experts. Fatality has occurred from using it in an enclosed space. Other methods are ferreting, the use of dogs, poisons and traps. Preparations containing arsenic or barium are satisfactory for poisoning, but should be placed in boxes, the lids of which are raised a few inches on bricks, so that dogs or cats cannot get at the poison.

For trapping, it is recommended that a five-inch rabbit trap should be used. This is placed on a run known to be used by rats, and should be sufficiently covered to prevent danger to other animals. It should never be handled with the naked hands, otherwise rats will not go near it, and if it has been so handled should be boiled to remove the traces.

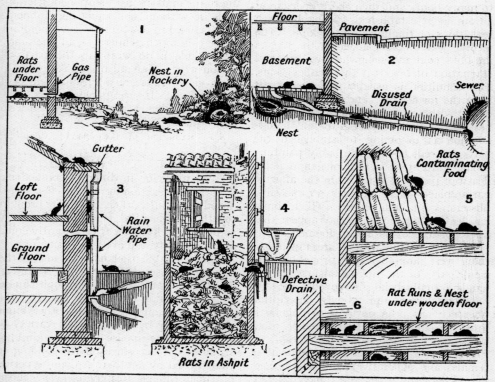

Rats : how they may effect entrance into a house. 1. Nesting in the garden, they may come through the aperture around a gaspipe. 2. Disused drain used as a nest. 3. Use of a roof gutter or rainwater pipe. 4. Defective drains and the old-fashioned type of insanitary ashpit encourage their inroads. 5. How rats contaminate grain. 6. Wooden floors in a warehouse where only concrete should be used

Courtesy of Liverpool Public Health Department

It is important to prevent the entrance of rats into premises by keeping doors shut, blocking up disused drains and holes of any kind, putting netting over the lower ends of water pipes, and so on. It is advisable also to trap a likely run, even though rats appear to have been destroyed, and to continue to do so all the year round.

See Flea ; Plague ; Rat-bite Fever.

RAYNAUD'S DISEASE. The disorder which passes by the name of Raynaud's disease is characterised by a disturbance of the circulation in various parts, especially the fingers and toes, the primary disturbance apparently being a spasmodic contraction of the small arteries. The effects of this disturbance may vary, and three degrees are recognized.

The first is that popularly known as dead fingers, in which the fingers become white and waxy-looking and feel numb. This state may persist from a few minutes to many hours and then the proper circulation is re-established, probably with sensations of tingling and pricking. The second degree is one in which the fingers are blue, cold and somewhat swollen from stagnation of blood in the smaller veins. This condition is usually more persistent than the former one, and it may be associated with severe pain and much tenderness in the affected parts. When the circulation is becoming re-established the parts are red, hot and probably painful.

The third stage is that of gangrene, or death of pieces of tissue. On the affected parts black areas appear or possibly blisters, containing blood, which burst and leave ulceration. It may appear that large portions of tissue are doomed to die, but generally the results are much less than were apprehended, probably only small parts of the tips of fingers on both hands actually being destroyed.

Although in the above description reference has been entirely to fingers, it must be understood that toes or other parts may undergo similar changes.

Raynaud's disease is more frequent in females and generally begins in the age-period between fifteen and thirty. Heredity is a fairly common factor in causing it, but the liability to the disease may be acquired, numbers of cases occurring, for example, after some acute illness. Others follow mental shock and worry. Cold is the immediate cause, and affected persons suffer most in the winter.

In some instances the tendency may disappear altogether, and in others, in whom gangrene has occurred, there may be subsequently only the slighter manifestations of the disease. The severer forms of the disease are not common.

A tendency to exhibit Raynaud's symtoms should be countered, if possible, by warm clothing during the colder weather, warm and roomy gloves and boots being worn. The use of calcium lactate, nitroglycerin or sodium nitrite may be serviceable in some cases, and in most it is desirable to take cod-liver oil throughout the winter. If there is any general debility, iron and arsenic are useful drugs. Neither cold nor hot water should be used for washing.

If manifestations occur, besides attending to the matters just mentioned, friction, with or without a stimulating liniment, may be used to restore the circulation, but if there is much tenderness all that may be possible is to wrap up the parts in cotton wool. Galvanism and exposure to ultra-violet rays are additional kinds of treatment. If gangrene occurs, the parts affected must be kept covered with antiseptic dressings.

See Circulation of the Blood ; Cyanosis ; Gangrene.

REACTION. The term reaction is used in medicine in different connexions. A chemical reaction means the effects produced when different chemicals are brought together. Chemical reactions of a very complicated character are constantly going on in the body and are very numerous.

Again, by reaction may be meant the response of some tissue to a stimulus. Thus, the contraction of the pupil caused by light shining on the eye is called the reaction to light. Similarly, other kinds of tissue may be tested with a variety of stimuli, the response to one kind of stimulus not necessarily corresponding to that caused by another. A definite period of time, though it may be very short, elapses between the application of the stimulus and the response ; this is called the reaction time.

PLATE XXXI

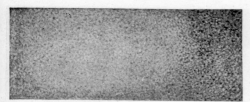

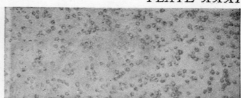

Rash. 1. Scarlet Fever : innumerable dark red dots on a flushed background of skin

2. Measles : small dusky red papules occurring in patches which are often crescentic

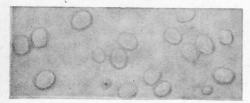

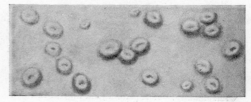

3. Chicken-pox : round or oval blisters, like tiny pearls, filled with a clear fluid

4. Smallpox : oval yellow blisters depressed or umbilicated in the centre

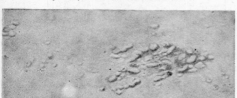

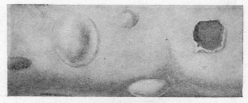

5. Herpes : crops of clear or yellow blisters, which may coalesce, on a dusky red skin

6. Pemphigus : large blisters or bullae, the contents of which may be clear or turbid

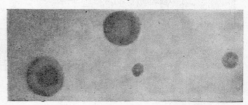

7. Nettle-rash : evanescent wheals and raised patches which may be white or pink

8. Antipyrine rash due to overdosage : reddened circular areas with raised margins

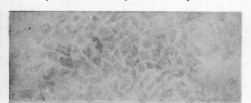

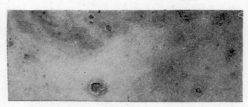

9. Pityriasis versicolor : brownish-yellow scaly lesions in patches tending to coalesce

10. Purpura : large patches of livid discoloration due to bleeding into the skin

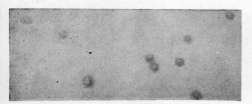

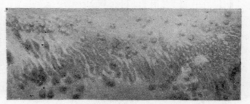

11. Typhoid Fever : raised pink spots, the size of lentils, occurring in crops

12. Lichen ruber planus : tiny, flat-topped papules, forming purplish-red patches

PLATE XXXII

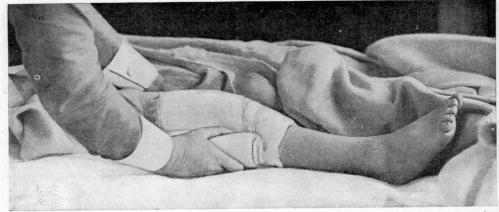

Rheumatism.   1. A painful joint may be smeared with methyl salicylate and covered with hot cotton wool

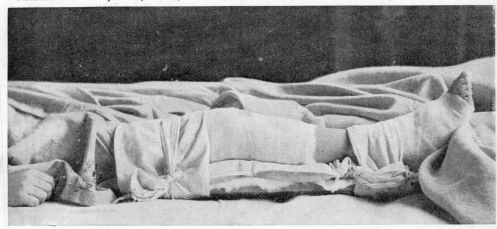

2. When a patient is restless the joint may be immobilised by placing the limb on a well-padded splint

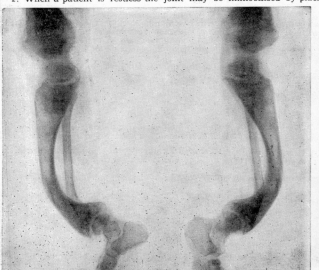

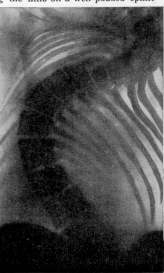

3. Rickets. Radiogram showing the deformity of bow legs resulting from softening and twisting of the long bones in infancy

4. Spinal Curvature.   Severe lateral curvature or scoliosis

The quality of the mental powers of attention and decision may be tested by directing a person to do something on being given a certain signal, his powers being judged according to the length of the reaction time. Similarly, when probing for hidden mental complexes by getting a patient to utter the mental associations of a list of test-words spoken to him, the desired information may be furnished by noting a lengthened reaction time in the response to certain words.

Reaction is sometimes used to indicate an opposite and contrary state ; a person who is first unduly excited and elated and then becomes depressed is said to suffer from reaction. Also, in concussion, after a time the temperature, which has been subnormal, becomes unduly high ; this is spoken of as reaction.

The reaction of degeneration is one exhibited by muscles cut off from connexion with the nerve centres that control their nutrition.

RECTAL DOUCHE. An ordinary enema (*q.v.*) apparatus can be used for washing out the bowel, the injection being made slowly so that as large a quantity of liquid as possible may be introduced into the bowel. The patient lies on the left side with the hips somewhat raised.

Rectal douching is specially associated with the treatment at the Plombières spa, in France, but treatment such as is carried out there may be obtained at any British spa. When it is desired to wash out a considerable length of the large bowel, the patient is put into a lying position ; when the rectum only, he sits upon a specially designed stool.

See Douche ; Rectum.

RECTAL FEEDING. When feeding by the mouth is impossible or highly undesirable, an attempt may be made to get food into the system by nutrient enemata, or injections of liquid foods into the rectum. Each injection should not exceed 3 ounces, and no more than four injections should be given in the 24 hours. The ingredients may include glucose and milk that has been peptonised for 24 hours ; milk peptonised for a shorter time is quite useless.

The best apparatus for giving the injection is a glass funnel to which is attached a rubber tube with a round, blunt extremity and a lateral opening near the end. The injection should be made slowly, the temperature of the liquid being about 100° F.

Rectal feeding cannot be carried on indefinitely, however.

RECTIFIED SPIRIT. In rectified spirit, or S.V.R. (spiritus vini rectificatus) there is 90 per cent., by volume, of alcohol. This spirit is valuable as a solvent for drugs, and, either in the pure state or diluted with distilled water, is used for making tinctures and other medicinal preparations. It is very expensive, however, and other forms of spirit are generally used for making lotions and liniments.

See Alcohol ; Methylated Spirit.

RECTOCELE. The rectum in women lies just behind the back wall of the vagina, except for the lowest part, where the perineal body is interposed. Sometimes the back wall of the vagina, with the rectum behind it, prolapses through the vaginal orifice. The swelling so formed is called a rectocele. More frequently, however, the front wall of the vagina prolapses, bringing with it the urinary bladder, and forms a swelling called a cystocele. A tear through the perineum at childbirth, if not repaired, predisposes to rectocele, and an operation for repair may be necessary. Otherwise the use of a pessary might suffice. Sometimes an abdominal operation to fix up the womb is desirable.

RECTUM. The lowest part of the bowel is called the rectum, and is rather over 6 inches in length. It extends from the end of the sigmoid flexure of bowel to the anus, and lies entirely within the pelvis. Its longer part passes downwards in the hollow of the sacral bone, thus forming a convexity backwards, but the shorter terminal portion, usually called the anal canal, makes a curve with its convexity forwards. The lower end of the rectum is surrounded by two sphincter, or closing, muscles, the internal and the external anal sphincters, the former consisting of involuntary and the latter of voluntary muscle fibres. Above these muscles the rectum is dilated, this portion being called the ampulla.

In the lower part of the rectum there is an arterial plexus, or network, and a corresponding venous plexus; the blood from this drains partly into the portal vein and for the rest into the inferior vena cava. The connexion with the portal vein explains the frequency of piles when there is congestion of the liver.

The entrance of faeces into the rectum, and especially its lower part, tends to

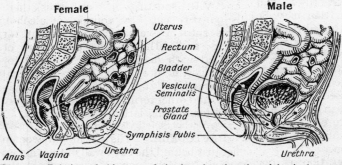

Female **Male**

Uterus
Rectum
Bladder
Vesicula Seminalis
Prostate Gland
Symphisis Pubis
Anus Vagina Urethra Urethra

Rectum. Relation of this part of the bowel to the other abdominal organs

create a desire to go to stool. If this call be neglected, however, bowel contents may accumulate in the rectum and distend it without causing much desire to empty the bowel.

The space between the rectum and bladder in the male is lined with peritoneum, and is called the recto-vesical pouch; in the female the uterus and vagina are interposed between the rectum and bladder, the space between the rectum and uterus being called the pouch of Douglas.

Diseases of the Rectum. On either side of the lower part of the rectum is a space filled with fat and called the ischio-rectal fossa. Through injury to the bowel-lining, as by a fish-bone, or through ulceration, infection may be admitted to the fossa and cause an acute ischio-rectal abscess. A chronic ischio-rectal abscess may occur in debilitated persons, and is not uncommon in those who suffer from tuberculosis of the lungs. The symptoms and treatment of an abscess are described under that heading. An abscess in this situation is often followed by a fistula (q.v.).

Inflammation of the rectum, or proctitis, may be caused by the presence of threadworms, of piles or of a polypus, or by dysentery or some other infection. It causes straining, and the faeces contain

mucus, mixed, perhaps, with pus or blood, or both. The source of irritation must be removed, the bowels kept freely open with laxatives, and sedative enemata administered.

When there is chronic straining there is a tendency to the occurrence of prolapse of the rectum, either its lining simply, or, especially in children, all the coats of the bowel, protruding through the anus. This happens particularly when the bowels move, but the prolapse may sometimes continue in the intervals unless the bowel is replaced. Here, again, the source of irritation must be removed. After a motion, the bowel is washed and gently replaced, being kept in position by a pad and a T-bandage. An operation may become necessary, however.

From chronic proctitis, associated with syphilis and numerous other causes, stricture of the rectum may arise, interfering with emptying of the bowel, and leading to the chain of symptoms caused by chronic obstruction (q.v.) of the bowel. In addition to treating the prime cause of the condition, dilatation of the stricture by the passage of instruments, or a cutting operation, will often be needed.

The commonest tumours of the rectum are polypus, which occurs most often in children, and cancer, which is found in adults. A polypus appears as a small, cherry-like growth attached to a long stalk. It is of the nature of an adenoma. It causes irritation, straining, and perhaps the presence of blood and mucus in the stools. It should be removed by operation, a simple matter as a rule.

Cancer is insidious in its onset and course, and often is far advanced before it is discovered. In the early stages it may cause a little irritation and straining, but later these symptoms become pronounced, and there are signs of partial obstruction. From an early stage a little blood may be present in the stool; this is often ascribed merely to the existence of piles. Pain hardly occurs till late in the disease. If the disease is allowed to persist sufficiently long, extension to the bladder, vagina and the neighbouring parts may occur, and dissemination to distant organs. The growth must be extirpated by an operation, the success to be expected depending largely on the stage at which the operation is done. If the disease has gone beyond an operable stage, radium may be of some use as a palliative measure.

See Anus ; Constipation ; Intestine ; Obstruction ; Piles ; Tenesmus.

REDNESS OF SKIN. *See* Blushing ; Dermatitis ; Erythema ; Rash.

REDUCTION. In surgery the replacement of broken or dislocated bones into a correct position is called reduction, as also pushing back the contents of a hernial sac into their proper position.

See Dislocation ; Fracture ; Hernia.

REFLEX ACTION. When the sole of the foot is tickled the foot is drawn away. This occurs independently of the will and is an example of a reflex action. The irritation of the skin causes a nerve stimulus to pass up to a centre in the spinal cord, which in turn liberates stimuli to cause contraction of the muscles required to drag the foot away. Very many instances of reflex action occur in the body, as part of its ordinary working or in connexion with disease.

The knee jerk, which is caused by tapping the patellar tendon, is an example of what is called a deep reflex in contrast with a superficial reflex, which is caused by irritation of the skin. A deep reflex is rather a measure of the tone of the muscles concerned in producing it than an instance of a simple reflex action, but the information derived from it is practically the same as that got from investigating a simple reflex. Both depend on the integrity of the afferent route, the centre on the cord and the efferent route, and both are exaggerated if the path from the brain to the spinal centre is blocked, thus cutting off control by the will.

See Knee Jerk ; Nervous System.

REFRACTION. The bending of rays of light when they pass from one medium into another, as, for example, from air into water or conversely, is called refraction. Its significance in connexion with vision is discussed under the heading Eye.

REGENERATION. The restoration of diseased or injured tissues to their original condition is described as regeneration. If the damage amounts to destruction of tissue to any extent actual regeneration can hardly take place ; the damage may be repaired, but ever afterwards the signs of repair are apparent. In favourable circumstances a divided nerve can become regenerated, by a fresh growth from the healthy end.

See Scar.

REGURGITATION. A back-flow of the stomach contents into the mouth without the effort associated with vomiting is called regurgitation. It is often seen in infants after a feed which they may have taken too greedily, and sometimes occurs in adults. In some circumstances bile may regurgitate through the pylorus, and in paralysis of the palate food, when being swallowed, may regurgitate through the nose. The back-flow of blood through a damaged heart-valve is also called regurgitation.

See Heart; Indigestion.

REJUVENATION. Grafting the testicle of one of the higher apes into the scrotal or abdominal cavity has apparently been successful in turning back the hands of the clock for some elderly men. The transplanted gland has acquired a connexion with the blood vessels at the site of transplantation. It pours into the blood stream an internal secretion which invigorates body and mind. The operation may fail owing to this connexion with the circulation not taking place, but even when the operation is successful the good effects do not persist for very long.

Another operation for the same purpose is to divide the vas deferens, or testicular duct, causing a consequent atrophy of the reproductive cells of the testicle, but a probable increase of the internal secretion. Good results in either sex are claimed for the administration of extracts made from the respective sexual glands, but these claims certainly require further investigation.

See Age Changes ; Endocrine.

RELAPSE. A recurrence of a disease after convalescence has apparently begun is described as a relapse. The symptoms of the relapse are the same as those of the original attack. Relapses are the rule in certain infections, such as relapsing fever and paratyphoid fever, and are occasional incidents in others.

RELAPSING FEVER. Under the general name of relapsing fever is included a group of fevers caused by species of spirochaeta, a slender, thread-like micro-organism with a wavy outline, the disorders being characterised by recurring bouts of fever lasting for several days and separated by apyrexial periods of about the same duration.

In Europe the disease is caused by spirochaeta obermeieri, or recurrentis, and this is conveyed by the louse, inoculation taking place through scratch marks on the skin. This disease was once often referred to as famine fever. In Africa it is also known as tick-fever, because the tick is responsible for conveying the parasite. This insect may also convey the parasite in the American form of the disease. Besides the louse and the tick, the bed-bug may possibly act as a carrier.

The incubation period is on the average from five to seven days and the fever begins suddenly with chills and rigors, the temperature shooting up to about 104° F., remaining high with slight remissions for five to seven days as a rule. There is severe headache but delirium is not common. There is also pain in the muscles and probably also in joints. Often there is vomiting and slight jaundice, but the bowels are constipated. There is considerable prostration. At the end of the time mentioned the fever declines by crisis, the temperature generally falling to some distance below the normal, and this is accompanied by profuse sweating and perhaps diarrhoea. There is no rash except, perhaps, sudamina, or clear blisters, accompanying the sweating.

In a few hours the patient feels well and may wish to get up. He remains well till about the fourteenth day from the beginning of the disease, when he has another attack of fever, similar to the first but usually of shorter duration. At the end of this attack he feels feeble and exhausted in contrast to his state at the end of the first attack. In the European form of the disease a third attack sometimes occurs, while in the African and other forms a series of relapses is the rule rather than the exception.

Complications are not common in relapsing fever and the mortality is low, generally speaking ; but there is a distinct risk of a fatal issue where old or debilitated persons are concerned. There is an especial danger of collapse at and shortly after the times of crisis. An obstinate form of inflammation of the eyes has followed some epidemics of the disease.

Relapsing fever is a notifiable disease.

Preventive treatment consists in vigorous measures to destroy lice, etc.

The infection may be destroyed by administering one of the organic arsenical preparations of the salvarsan type, otherwise treatment is largely that of the state of fever. Heart stimulants are often necessary.

See Fever ; Infectious Disease.

RELAXED THROAT. Chronic pharyngitis is often referred to as relaxed throat. Astringent gargles, sprays or lozenges should be used, and the general health improved by attention to the regular action of the bowels, by open-air exercise and, if necessary, by tonics.

See Pharynx.

REMITTENT. When the daily decline of a fever is considerable but does not reach normal limits, the fever is said to be of a remittent type. One form of malaria is generally referred to as remittent fever.

See Fever ; Malaria.

RENAL. Anything pertaining to the kidney may be described as renal. Thus, one speaks of the renal tissue or structure, of renal function, renal diseases and so on. A stone in the kidney is a renal calculus, and the paroxysms of pain caused by its passage down the ureter, renal colic. Renal insufficiency means a failure of the kidney to carry out its duties efficiently, as determined by the quantity of water or of solids excreted.

See Kidney.

RENNET. The gastric juice contains a ferment, or enzyme, known as rennet, or rennin, which coagulates milk. A preparation of rennet, obtained from the calf's stomach, is sold in liquid and tablet form for making curds and whey. The process is described under the heading Milk.

RESIN. From various plants there exudes a semi-solid substance which hardens on exposure and is known as a resin. In nature it may be combined with an essential oil, forming an oleo-resin, with a mucilaginous substance, forming a gum-resin, or with benzoic or cinnamic acid, forming a balsam. Various resins, including jalap, podophyllum, etc., are used in medicine.

The substance referred to in the British Pharmacopoeia simply as resin or rosin is the residue left after distilling the oil of turpentine from the crude oleo-resin, or turpentine, obtained from various species of pinus. It forms hard, brittle masses which are transparent and of a yellowish colour. It is used for making various plasters, including the ordinary resin, or adhesive, plaster, and resin ointment, which is often referred to as basilicon ointment. This is used as a stimulating application for indolent sores.

See Gum ; Turpentine.

RESORCIN. A white crystalline substance, obtained from benzene, resorcin acts as an antiseptic and antipyretic. When applied to unhealthy skin it aids materially in removing the unhealthy cells and in promoting a sound growth. It is consequently much used in skin diseases. In acne a preparation consisting of 15 grains in an ounce of Lassar's paste is useful.

In seborrhoea of the face a lotion made by dissolving 10 grains or more in an ounce of spirit is sometimes used, and also for dandruff. When resorcin is applied to the head, however, care must be taken that hair is washed clean from alkalies or soap, otherwise resorcin may stain the hair, especially in blondes. Weak solutions of resorcin are used as antiseptic lotions.

Resorcin is not often given internally, as it is poisonous, and for the same reason it should not be used over a very large surface of skin, when there would be a risk of an excessive amount being absorbed. From resorcin is prepared fluorescein.

RESPIRATION. In respiration or breathing, air is alternately drawn into the lungs and expelled from them. The drawing-in of air, or inspiration, is accomplished by the capacity of the chest being increased by the descent of the midriff, or diaphragm, and the elevation of the ribs. The flattening of the dome of the diaphragm increases the vertical diameter of the chest, the ascent of the ribs its antero-posterior diameter, and, owing to the elasticity of the ribs, there is also some increase in the transverse diameter when they are raised. The elevation of the ribs, in ordinary quiet breathing, is mainly done by the external intercostal muscles.

The chest is an airtight cavity, except for the respiratory passages, and when its capacity is increased air is bound to rush into the lungs, which expand to fill up

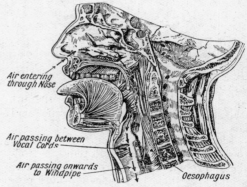

Respiration. First stage in passage of air to lungs

the increased space. At the end of inspiration the muscles which produce it relax, the diaphragm again rises, and the ribs fall. Consequently, air is forced out of the lungs, or, in other words, expiration takes place.

As compared with air that is inspired, that which is expired contains less oxygen, more carbonic acid gas, and more watery vapour ; it is also warmer. The explanation of these changes is that the alveoli, or air-cells of the lungs, have a close network of capillary blood vessels in their walls, the blood vessels being separated from the air in the cells by a thin membrane only, and an exchange of gases is constantly taking place between the blood and the alveolar air, oxygen passing into

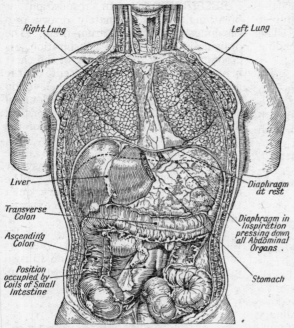

Respiration. Showing expansion of lungs by depression of the diaphragm, this increasing the chest capacity

about 100 cubic inches of residual air. The total amount of air that can be taken into the chest by a full breath and expelled by a deep expiration amounts to about 230 cubic inches. This is sometimes called the vital capacity, and a machine for measuring it is known as a spirometer; it is actually a modified gasometer.

The movements of breathing are caused by rhythmic discharges of energy by a respiratory centre in the brain, and are automatic, although they may be modified at will, as in holding the breath and in the efforts of speech, singing, and so on. Normally the movement of inspiration lasts somewhat longer than that of expiration. The combined movements of respiration occur about eighteen times per minute.

In children the diaphragm is the main factor in causing inspiration, and, as its movements cause a

the blood and carbonic acid gas passing out of it into the alveolar air. Respiration keeps up the supply of oxygen in the air-cells and gets rid of the carbonic acid gas.

Blood carries the oxygen to the tissues, to which it gives it up, and removes from them carbonic acid gas, which is a waste product of their metabolism. This process is often referred to as internal respiration. Oxygen in the blood is united with the haemoglobin, the colouring matter of the red blood corpuscles; carbonic acid gas is chiefly carried as carbonate of sodium, but a certain amount is carried by the red corpuscles.

The quantity of air which is passing in and out during ordinary breathing, and which is called the tidal air, measures about 30 cubic inches in a healthy adult man. By taking a full breath, about 100 cubic inches of additional, or complemental, air can be inspired, and, on the other hand, by a forcible expiration during ordinary breathing an additional 100 cubic inches of air can be expelled. This is called the supplemental air. The lungs cannot be quite emptied of air; there always remains after the fullest expiration

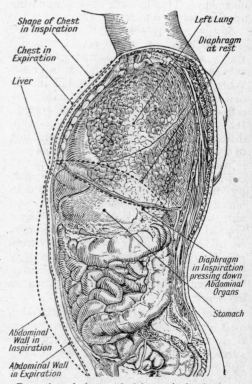

Expansion of chest and abdomen in inspiration

marked rise and fall of the abdominal wall, breathing in children is said to be abdominal. In adult males there is also a free movement of the lower part of the chest, a type of breathing referred to as the lower costal, while in women the type is commonly upper costal, that is, there are free movements of the upper part of the chest.

Cessation of breathing is called apnoea. It occurs, for example, after deep breathing for a minute or two, and lasts for a short time. It also occurs in Cheyne-Stokes breathing, in which the respiratory movements gradually increase in extent up to a point and then gradually decline. This type of breathing, which has a sinister significance, may occur in apoplexy, meningitis, uraemia and other disorders.

Difficulty in breathing is called dyspnoea. Additional muscles come into play for raising the ribs, and the internal intercostals for depressing the ribs. If the dyspnoea is such that the patient cannot breathe when lying down, the condition is described as orthopnoea.

See Artificial Respiration; Asphyxia; Breathing Exercises; Circulation of the Blood; Lung; Shortness of Breath.

RESPIRATOR. Persons who work in a dusty atmosphere should wear efficient respirators to trap the dust. The same precaution may be desirable for an elderly person or one who is subject to bronchitis when it is necessary to go out in foggy weather.

A respirator of the Burney-Yeo type is sometimes used as a means for the inhalation (*q.v.*) of drugs.

REST. All the working tissues of the body must have rest if they are to carry on their duties efficiently. Even the heart, which apparently goes on beating uninterruptedly for years, has a period of rest in each beat-cycle, a period which is ordinarily quite sufficient for its needs. The main object of rest in the case of muscle is to enable it to get rid of waste products resulting from its activities. Glandular cells require to have a rest period to accumulate the materials for the particular secretion that they produce.

Rest is an all-important part of the treatment of acute inflammatory and of febrile disorders. It is an important factor in promoting the repair of injuries. It is now realized, however, that in the old treatment of fractures and sprains, and of certain chronic disorders of joints, rest was often overdone and stiffness and impairment of function not uncommonly resulted. The time when exercise becomes necessary in such conditions, and the form that exercise should take and its amount, are matters for skilled judgement.

When a patient is ordered complete rest this implies rest of mind as well as of body, and worries and excitement should be avoided as far as possible. Complete rest in bed means that the patient should not leave his bed or sit up on any pretext, not even to relieve the bowels or bladder. A rest-cure means treatment on the lines of the Weir-Mitchell treatment (*q.v.*).

See Exercise; Fatigue.

RESTLESSNESS. While restlessness in a child usually is a perfectly natural thing, it is not so in young infants and some cause for it should be sought out. It may be induced by many causes, including too much fussing and excitement, discomfort from clothing, teething, indigestion, constipation, rickets and so on. Even in older children restlessness may be abnormal in degree, and the possibility of the existence of chorea or some other disorder should be considered. The presence of adenoids is a common cause of restlessness at night.

In adults an unusual restlessness may mark the beginning of some mental disorder.

RETINA. The sensitive membrane at the back of the eye is called the retina. Retinitis means inflammation of this membrane.

See Eye.

RHATANY. *See* Krameria.

RHEUMATISM. Acute rheumatism, or rheumatic fever, is a disease with distinctive characteristics, but the terms rheumatism, rheumatic and rheumatoid are applied to disorders which have little or no connexion with acute rheumatism, a fact which should be borne in mind when considering such disorders.

Acute rheumatism is an infective disease caused probably by a streptococcus, the route of entrance to the body being by way of the throat or the naso-pharynx. Children and young adults are mostly affected. Dampness in the home and the existence of sepsis in the tonsils are factors which strongly favour the occurrence of acute rheumatism. One attack predisposes to others.

The onset of an attack may be preceded by sore throat or general slight pain, but usually it is sudden, with fever and pain, redness and swelling of one of the large joints—the knee, elbow, wrist or ankle. Other large joints are soon affected, the pain disappearing from one as another becomes involved. The affected joint is very tender, and even to jar the bed causes severe suffering.

There is profuse sweating, and the sweat has a sour odour ; often crops of small, glistening blisters form on the skin. The fever may be high, but, as a rule, there is no delirium, unless hyperpyrexia should occur.

In about half the number of those who suffer from acute rheumatism there is inflammation of the lining of the heart, or endocarditis (*q.v.*). Sometimes there is pericarditis as well, or this may occur independently ; sometimes there is pleurisy. In some cases, especially in children, little firm, painless swellings occur beneath the skin over tendons or bones. These are called rheumatic nodules, and vary in size from that of a pin-head to that of a large pea.

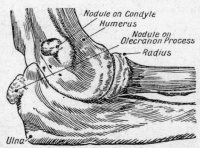

Rheumatic nodules occurring on the elbow

Nodule on Condyle Humerus
Nodule on Olecranon Process
Radius
Ulna

When the symptoms are less severe than in the above description, rheumatism is said to be subacute. There are slighter cases still which are often neglected because they are considered to be " growing pains," in ignorance of the fact that healthy growth causes no pain. In other instances acute rheumatism occurs simply in the form of sore throat, and in others the most prominent symptoms are those of chorea, or St. Vitus' dance.

It cannot be too strongly emphasised that there is the same risk of involvement of the heart in the slighter forms of acute rheumatism as in the typical disease. In fact, it is not uncommon to find rheumatic disease of the heart when other signs of the disease have been absent or are so slight as to be overlooked.

The after-effects of acute rheumatism may be very serious, from the effects on the heart, but as regards the joints complete recovery is to be expected. The joints never suppurate, and any stiffness or impairment of movement after the acute symptoms have gone is very rare.

A person who suffers from acute rheumatism should be kept absolutely in bed, however slight the disease may appear to be, not getting out of bed on any pretext whatever. He should lie between blankets and wear a flannel nightdress which opens down the front and down the sleeves, so that it can be readily taken off ; this is of great importance when the patient is sweating freely. The general treatment is that of fever (*q.v.*), but a thorough course of salicylates must be administered. Salicylates should clear away the pain and reduce the temperature in acute rheumatism within 48 hours. The joints should be covered with cotton wool, and it is desirable also to smear them with methyl salicylate. Rest for a joint can be secured by a splint (*see* Plate XXXII, 1 and 2). Complications are treated as described under individual headings. When the patient is convalescent, attention should be paid to the state of the throat, and the question of removing diseased tonsils may have to be considered. The patient, especially if a child, should be seen by a doctor from time to time for some years after an attack of acute rheumatism.

The so-called chronic rheumatism is a disease which affects adults, especially those whose occupations expose them to cold and damp. The joints may become stiff and painful, and more or less swollen. Another form is called muscular rheumatism. All these cases are instances of fibrositis (*q.v.*), and should be treated as

such. A condition described as rheumatic gout is rheumatoid arthritis when it is not true gout, and in neither case has any connexion with rheumatism.

See Endocarditis; Fibrositis; Formic Acid; Guaiacum; Heart.

RHEUMATOID ARTHRITIS. According to present usage, the name rheumatoid arthritis is applied to more than one kind of chronic inflammation of joints. In one type there are no bony changes in the joints, at any rate not until the disease is very advanced, but swelling of the synovial membrane and the soft tissues round the joint. These become contracted, and may thus cause more or less fixation of the joint, probably in a bad position.

In another type, although there is first of all synovitis, bony changes appear early. The cartilage on the ends of the bones softens and disappears, and at a later stage the exposed bone may become smooth and polished, or eburnated. Frequently there are ridges on one bony surface which fit into grooves on another with which it comes into contact. Fringes form on the synovial membrane, and in these there may be a deposition of lime salts. The bone at the margins of the joint also becomes prominent, or lipped. In some cases bony ankylosis of the joint occurs.

The changes in the type just described are similar to those found in osteoarthritis (*q.v.*), which, however, is a disease affecting elderly people, whereas the victims of rheumatoid arthritis are usually between twenty and forty when the disease begins.

Rheumatoid arthritis occurs in a series of acute attacks, lasting from four to six weeks at a time. Fever is not very high and the pulse is rapid, more so than would be expected from the height of the temperature. The first joints to be affected are those just beyond the knuckles, but later joints all over the body are involved, those of the lower jaw being common ones.

Rheumatoid Arthritis. Changes that occur in an affected knee joint

As the acute attacks follow one another, the deformity and disablement become worse. A common deformity of the hand is deflection of the fingers to the ulnar side.

The prime cause of rheumatoid arthritis is the activity of certain bacteria of low virulence. These form foci of infection, most commonly at the roots of the teeth or in the tonsils, but it may be at other situations in, or on, the body. The treatment of the disease should therefore begin with a search for some such focus and an attempt to clean it up, with, possibly, a course of vaccine treatment also.

During the acute stage the patient should be kept at rest, and, as the deformity is caused in the first place by spasm of muscles, the affected joints should be splinted in such a position as to prevent deformity. These positions are described under the heading Joint, and they must also be preserved when there is a risk of a joint becoming ankylosed.

When, however, the acute stage has passed off, the joints are freely and fully moved by the doctor or someone under his direction.

Various methods, including fomentations, baths of various kinds, diathermy and electrical treatment, are used to diminish pain and swelling. Massage, whirlpool baths and electrical stimulation are also useful in preserving the tone of the muscles.

The diet should be generous, a considerable amount of red meat being allowed, but it may be desirable to restrict carbohydrate foods. Cod-liver oil is often a useful addition to the diet. Ultra-violet rays are often used in order to increase the general resistance to infection, and guaiacol carbonate or sulphur may be given to disinfect the bowel.

See Guaiacol; Health Resort; Joint; Osteoarthritis.

RHINITIS. Inflammation of the nasal mucous membrane is called rhinitis, the commonest form being acute catarrh.

See Cold, Common; Nose.

RHINOSCOPY. An instrument for obtaining a view of the inside of the nose is called a rhinoscope, and the use of it, rhinoscopy.

RHUBARB. The root-like stem, or rhizome, of various species of rhubarb, commonly referred to as rhubarb root, contains a substance resembling cathartic acid, the active principle of senna, and also an astringent principle called rheotannic acid. Rhubarb thus acts as a purgative but is liable to be followed by some binding of the bowels. This is a useful kind of action in the event of diarrhoea, as offending matters are first swept from the bowel and the tendency to diarrhoea is then checked.

The preparations of rhubarb include the powdered root, dose 15 to 30 grains for a single dose and 3 to 10 grains for repeated doses ; compound rhubarb powder, or Gregory's mixture, 10 to 60 grains ; compound tincture of rhubarb, $\frac{1}{2}$ to 1 drachm or 2 to 4 drachms for a single dose ; infusion of rhubarb, $\frac{1}{2}$ to 1 ounce ; syrup of rhubarb, $\frac{1}{2}$ to 2 drachms ; and extract of rhubarb, 2 to 8 grains, given in a pill.

RIB. A rib, or costa, is a curved, elongated bone which is attached behind to the dorsal part of the spinal column and prolonged at its forward end into a bar of cartilage, or gristle, described as a costal cartilage. The attachment to the spine is by means of two joints. The first is formed by the thickened extremity of the rib fitting into a shallow depression, or facet, on the bodies of adjoining vertebrae, or, in the case of some of the ribs, on the body of one vertebra. The second is formed between a prominence, a short distance along the rib, and known as the tubercle of the rib, and the front of the transverse process of a vertebra. Through these two joints a rib is able to rotate on the spine, making a movement similar to that of the handle of a bucket. At some distance from

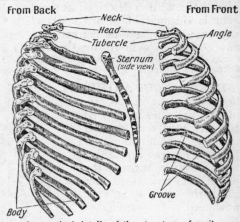
Anatomical details of the structure of a rib

its hinder end, each rib, except the last two, exhibits a bend in its shaft, which is called the angle of the rib. A fracture of the rib usually occurs near the angle. There are twelve ribs on either side, and the costal cartilages of the upper seven are directly attached to the breast bone, or sternum. These are consequently referred to as true ribs. Of the remaining five, or false ribs, the costal cartilage of each of the upper three is attached to the costal cartilage of the rib above it, that of the eighth to the cartilage of the seventh, and so on. The last two are not attached to other ribs, and are therefore called floating ribs.

Along the lower border of each rib, on its inner side, is a groove occupied by the intercostal blood vessels and nerve. The space between two ribs is called the intercostal space, and is filled in by the external and internal intercostal muscles, the fibres of the former running downwards and forwards, and those of the latter downwards and backwards. The external muscle raises the rib below, and the internal depresses the rib above.

Fracture of a rib may be due to direct violence, as by a blow, but more often is caused by indirect violence, by the chest

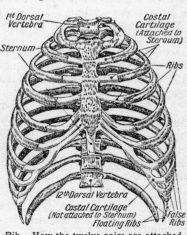
Rib. How the twelve pairs are attached

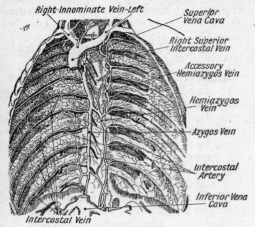

Right-Innominate Vein-Left

Superior Vena Cava

Right Superior Intercostal Vein

Accessory Hemiazygos Vein

Hemiazygos Vein

Azygos Vein

Intercostal Artery

Inferior Vena Cava

Intercostal Vein

Rib. Intercostal blood vessels and nerves

being much compressed, as when a vehicle runs over the body. There is acute pain increased by breathing. The pleura or lung may be injured by the pointed end of one of the fragments, and there may be spitting of blood. The first-aid treatment is described under the heading Fracture.

See Chest ; Respiration.

RICKETS. A nutritional disease of children, rickets, or rhachitis, usually begins in the period between the sixth and the thirtieth month. An important factor in its production is the absence, or even shortage, of the supply to the tissues of a substance described as vitamin D. This vitamin, as well as the other necessary dietetic constituents of this nature, is present in sufficient quantities in the mother's milk when this is good.

If, however, the mother's milk is thin, as is usual, for example, after nursing for over nine months, or if a child is fed on starchy foods, even with the addition of fat in the form of margarine, there will be starvation as regards this essential vitamin. This may apparently occur, also, if a child suffers from constant indigestion, especially if diarrhoea is present, a common result of giving starchy food, such as sopped bread, potatoes and cornflour, to a young infant.

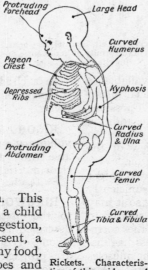

Protruding Forehead

Large Head

Curved Humerus

Pigeon Chest

Depressed Ribs

Kyphosis

Curved Radius & Ulna

Protruding Abdomen

Curved Femur

Curved Tibia & Fibula

Rickets. Characteristics of this widespread deficiency disease

A deficiency of the anti-rhachitic vitamin is made good if the body is sufficiently exposed to ultra-violet rays, either in natural sunlight or artificially produced. Fats deficient in the vitamin acquire it by being submitted to these rays, and, in exposure of the body to them, it would appear that ergosterol in the skin acquires the properties of the vitamin. The passage of the rays is arrested by clothing, however, and by ordinary window glass.

The lack of active exercise in the open air seems to have some influence in causing the disease, but is a subordinate factor as compared with those mentioned.

Rickets begins insidiously, but sooner or later the child becomes restless and peevish, with a certain amount of fever and free sweating, from the head especially, when it sleeps. There is great tenderness over the body, the slightest touch being resented. The appetite and digestion are impaired, and commonly there is constipation alternating with diarrhoea. The child tends to become pot-bellied. Teething is delayed, and the fontanelles, or spaces, between the bones of the skull are slow in filling up.

The ends of the long bones become swollen, so that the wrists and other joints are unduly large, and there are rows of enlargements down each end of the chest in front, at the junctions of the ribs and cartilages, forming the so-called rickety rosary (*see* illustration in page 143). The child is slow in beginning to walk, or, if it has done so, may lose the art ; the muscular weakness may be so great as to suggest paralysis.

As time goes on, the frontal eminences on the skull become enlarged, producing a broad, square forehead, and sometimes portions of the skull towards the back of the head become thin and papery. The bones of the legs bend, causing bow leg (*see* Plate XXXII, 3), or knock knee, and there is commonly flat foot. If the child rests much weight on the arms, these also may bend. The spine develops a hump and the walls of the chest are flattened ; the breast bone may be pushed forward, a condition described as pigeon breast. Sometimes, however, particularly if there is nasal obstruction, as from adenoids, the breast bone is depressed, forming the funnel-shaped chest. The pelvis is deformed, and in females this may be of much consequence should they subsequently become pregnant, as it may greatly increase the difficulties of childbirth.

Children suffering from rickets are prone to certain nervous troubles, such as convulsions, tetany, and a spasmodic type of choking, known as laryngismus stridulus.

It is most important to prevent rickets. This can be done by giving a child the diet, the sunshine, the fresh air and the exercise which it requires.

A list of foods containing vitamin D is given under the heading Diet. When the disease actually exists, the same hygienic requirements must be satisfied but, as the child will be kept in bed for a time, the room in which it is confined should be thoroughly ventilated day and night. Should the weather permit, the child may be allowed to lie out of doors during the day. If natural sunlight is not available, a course of treatment by artificial ultra-violet light should be procured, if possible. Cod-liver oil is a very valuable addition to the diet, but should be given in an emulsion, or with malt, in view of the difficulty of digesting the plain oil.

The child should not be allowed to get on its feet until the bones are sufficiently strong, and to prevent its doing so it may be necessary to attach long splints to either side of the body and the corresponding limb. When tenderness has disappeared, gentle massage of the muscles should be employed, however. The deformity of the limbs generally dis-

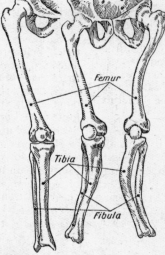

Rickets. Left, normal leg bones. Right, deformity of knock knee due to vitamin starvation

appears, but if it persists in a troublesome degree surgical treatment may be desirable.

See Bow Leg ; Convulsions ; Diet ; Light ; Vitamin.

RIGIDITY. Stiffness or rigidity of a joint may be due to a partial or complete ankylosis, but is sometimes caused by muscular spasm. This may be a reflex phenomenon, designed to protect the diseased joint from movement, and a similar thing may occur when there is inflammation in the abdomen, when the rigidity of the abdominal wall may be board-like. In some nervous diseases, such as hemiplegia and paraplegia, there is rigidity in the affected limbs from an increase in muscle-tone.

RIGOR. A severe shivering fit, such as occurs in malaria and other fevers, is called a rigor. The patient at the beginning looks blue and pinched. After a short time he commences to shiver and his movements are so violent that he shakes the bed, while his teeth chatter. This goes on from a few minutes to an hour, when the patient again begins to feel warm. Notwithstanding the sensation of cold during a rigor, the temperature is actually above normal. Treatment consists in giving hot drinks and in the use of extra blankets and of hot-water bottles.

In a child a convulsive fit often takes the place of a rigor at the beginning of a fever.

RIGOR MORTIS. The stiffness of voluntary muscles, which occurs at a variable time after death, is described as rigor mortis.

See Death.

RINGWORM. Certain affections due to the presence of parasitic fungi are described as ringworm. The fungi, which belong, of course, to the vegetable kingdom, are propagated by little round or oval bodies known as spores. The variety of the infection depends upon the size of the spores and, when it occurs in a hairy situation, upon their position, whether they are on the surface of the hair, within its substance, or both.

A fungus that produces small spores is called a microsporon ; one that produces large spores, a megalosporon, or tricophyton. Of the latter, one in which the spores are within hairs, referred to as an endothrix, and another in which they are both within and on the hairs, an endoectothrix, are, apart from the microsporon, the common parasites in human ringworm. The lesions of ringworm are commonly rounded or oval, the disease spreading out in all directions from the centre.

Ringworm may be found on the scalp, the beard, non-hairy parts of the body, and the nails.

Ringworm on the Body

Ringworm of the body, or tinea circinata, may occur in children suffering from ringworm of the head or in adults who come into close contact with domestic animals. The usual cause is a tricophyton. A reddish patch forms on the skin, and as it spreads at the edges the central part tends to heal. The margin is somewhat raised, and is covered with glistening scales. The course is rapid. Treatment consists in painting with tincture of iodine for three or four days and then applying an ointment consisting of 1 drachm of white precipitate ointment with soft paraffin to make 1 ounce, or a similar preparation. Clothing which has come into contact with the diseased skin must be carefully disinfected.

Ringworm of the beard, or tinea barbae, which is usually caused by the tricophyton ectothrix, is discussed under the heading Barber's Itch.

Ringworm of the scalp, tinea tonsurans, is almost entirely confined to children, usually such as are of school age. The commonest cause is microsporon audouini. In this type there are one or more patches, slightly reddened and covered with greyish scales. The hairs within the patch are lustreless and many of them are broken. In the type known as suppurative ringworm, or kerion, there are large, raised patches from which pus exudes at many points. This is usually caused by the endothrix parasite. In a third type, known as black dot ringworm, there are bald patches resembling those found in the variety of baldness (q.v.) called alopecia areata, but the scalp within the areas is stippled over with small black dots, representing hair stumps. This type is caused by the endothrix parasite. It is difficult to cure, but is not common.

As regards treatment, it may be said that kerion tends to cure itself, the suppuration loosening the hairs and causing them to fall out. The patch should be painted with tincture of iodine, however. Epilation can be accomplished in other forms of ringworm by exposure to X-rays, though this should be at the hands of an expert. When the hairs come away they bring the infection with them. When X-ray treatment is not available, the scalp should be shaved weekly, though if there is only one patch it may suffice to shave this and for about half an inch around it, while the remaining hair is clipped very short. The patches then have a colourless iodine ointment, such as unguentum iodi denigrescens, B.P.C., rubbed into them daily. This treatment must be continued for a long time. Other forms of treatment by drugs, if handled by experts, may produce a more rapid cure, however.

The patient should wear a cotton cap which is frequently disinfected by boiling, and should on no account use brushes or towels common to the household. Other children in the house should have their hair clipped short, and it is a useful precaution to rub the colourless iodine ointment into their heads also.

Ringworm of the nail may be due to extension from the hand or to handling other affected parts, being not uncommon, for this reason, in nurses. It is caused by a tricophyton. The nail, which becomes dull yellow in colour and ridged, is raised off its bed by a greyish-looking mass. It is very brittle, and usually looks irregular, from pieces having been broken off.

The only treatment is to remove the nail and kill the parasite in the nail-bed by painting with tincture of iodine.

See Barber's Itch ; Favus ; Sycosis.

ROCHELLE SALT. The tartrate of sodium and potassium, also known as tartarated soda and Rochelle salt, is a saline purgative and is used in doses of 120 to 240 grains.

RODENT ULCER. The usual site of a rodent ulcer, which is a variety of cancer, is the face, particularly in the neighbourhood of the root of the nose or the scalp. It is uncommon before the age of forty. It begins as a reddish papule which is paler on the top and perhaps scaly, but before long an ulcer forms, and this, in course of time, spreads outwards and also deeply into the tissues.

Its progress is slow, however, and it differs from other varieties of cancer in showing no liability to infect neighbouring lymphatic glands or distant organs, though it may become infected by septic germs and cause general poisoning in this way.

Rodent ulcer can usually be treated very successfully with radium, and also with X-rays. If quite small, it may be possible to effect a cure by means of cauterisation, carbonic acid snow, or diathermy. Many surgeons remove the growth by a cutting operation and, as is usually necessary, cover the gap in the skin by grafting.
See Cancer ; Ulcer.

ROMBERG'S SYMPTOM. Inability to stand with the eyes closed and the feet together is called Romberg's symptom. It most commonly indicates the presence of locomotor ataxia. A disorder characterised by progressive wasting of the tissues on one side of the face, facial hemiatrophy, is sometimes called Romberg's disease. Usually no cause for the disorder can be discovered and treatment is ineffectual.

ROSACEA. A red eruption on the face, with some resemblance to acne, is called rosacea, or acne rosacea (*q.v.*).

ROSEMARY. Oil of rosemary is sometimes used as a stimulant in doses of $\frac{1}{2}$ to 3 minims. More often it is used externally, as a rubefacient, in an ointment or, as the spirit of rosemary, in a lotion. It is an ingredient in stimulating preparations for the hair.

ROUND LIGAMENT. A round cord that attaches the womb to the groin on each side of the body is called the round ligament of the womb. The round ligament of the liver is actually the obliterated umbilical vein of the embryo. The name ligamentum teres, given to a ligament in the hip-joint, literally means round ligament.

ROUNDWORM. *See* Worm.

RUBEFACIENT. An agent used for reddening the skin by causing dilatation of the blood vessels is called a rubefacient. The liniment of camphor is an example.
See Counter-irritation.

RUPIA. A rash consisting of scabs having a resemblance to limpet shells is described as rupia. It occurs in syphilis.

RUPTURE. *See* Hernia.

RUSSIAN BATH. A steam-bath, usually called a Russian bath, is taken by exposing the body in a chamber in which the atmosphere is charged with hot steam. It is only suitable for the healthy, and should be followed by a cold plunge or douche.
See Baths.

SAC. A bag-like cavity enclosed by a membrane may be described as a sac, as, for example, the peritoneal sac, the sac of a hernia and the sac of a cyst or tumour. A tiny sac is called a saccule, or sacculus. The term sacculated is applied to structures having the appearance of a saccule or divided up into saccules. Thus, a sacculated aneurysm is one in which there is a bag-like expansion on one side of a blood vessel, and the expanded termination of an air tube in the lung, which has air cells opening into it all round, is said to be sacculated.

SACCHARIN. A coal-tar product, saccharin or glusidum is a white, crystalline substance, mainly used as a sweetening agent. The official preparation of glusidum is 550 times sweeter than cane-sugar, but samples of the drug on the market are considerably less sweet. Saccharin is of much service as a substitute for sugar when this is harmful, as in diabetes or obesity, and it is perfectly safe.

SACRUM. A triangular-shaped bone which closes in the pelvis behind, the sacrum really consists of the five sacral vertebrae fused together. Its expanded upper end forms a basis of support for the rest of the spine, and to its lower end, or apex, is attached the coccyx, or tail-vertebra. On either side it is jointed to the hip-bone, the joint being called the sacro-iliac synchrondrosis. Pain caused by inflammation in this joint is sometimes mistaken for sciatica.

ST. VITUS'S DANCE. Acute chorea, also called minor chorea, Sydenham's chorea and by the popular name of St. Vitus's Dance, is a nervous disorder in which there are irregular, jerky, inco-ordinated movements of voluntary muscles. It is mainly a disease of childhood, seldom beginning after the age of puberty, and is commoner in girls. In adults it is most often seen in connexion with a first pregnancy. It is more common in the lower classes, and in ill-nourished children.

There is a very important connexion between chorea and acute rheumatism ; one disease may be followed by the other, and either may cause inflammation of the heart and pericardium. Sometimes the disease has followed scarlet fever or some other of the infectious diseases. In some instances it has occurred after a severe fright, but it is not considered that this could happen unless there is already a liability to chorea. In children with this liability eye strain, adenoids, intestinal worms or some other disturbing factor may possibly excite the manifestations of the disease.

The seat of the disease is in the masses of grey matter in the base of the brain known as the corpus striatum.

As a rule the onset of chorea is insidious. A child may become awkward in handling things, liable to break dishes and peevish and irritable. For a time this alteration in behaviour may be regarded rather as a matter for disciplinary treatment. Soon, however, there are irregular jerky movements of the fingers, hands and face, which the child obviously cannot control and which, in fact, become worse when attention is drawn to them. The hands are opened and shut, the forearms jerked round, and there is shrugging of the shoulders, while various grimaces appear on the face. The trunk may be jerked round in one direction or the other, and the child may be unsteady on its feet. The spasms, however, may be more or less confined to one side of the body.

Speech may be slow and indistinct, and there may be difficulty in chewing and swallowing, sometimes so much so that it is necessary to feed through a tube. The child may become emotional and may suffer from hallucinations, while there may be weakening of the memory and other evidences of mental dullness. It may be noted here that when chorea occurs in pregnancy there may be maniacal excitement. Except in the severest cases, choreic movements cease during sleep, but when severe may interfere with it.

Usually the disease lasts for three or four months, after which there is complete recovery, but in some cases, on the other hand, there is a tendency to relapse or to drag on for a year or two. During the progress of the disease a constant watch must be kept on the heart.

A child suffering from chorea should be kept in bed, at any rate during the acute stage, and if the movements are violent the sides of the bed should be padded. Strict isolation is sometimes required. The nutrition should be improved by a liberal allowance of milk, cream, eggs, broths and other liquid nourishment, with the addition of cod-liver oil if it can be digested.

Drugs and other Remedies

Sodium salicylate, aspirin or arsenic are the drugs usually given to attack the cause of the disease, while bromides, chloral and other hypnotics may be used to exercise a sedative effect and procure sleep. A hot bath or pack is often useful for this purpose, and may be given daily.

When the acuter stage has passed, massage may be useful, and then simple exercises to improve the co-ordination of movements. Throughout the disease the child should be as much as possible in the open air, and the sick-room should be kept well ventilated.

A pregnant woman suffering from chorea requires very careful attention and constant observation.

There is a form of chorea called chronic or Huntington's chorea, which usually begins between thirty and forty years of age, and in the causation of which heredity is the main factor. In this form mental derangement is an early and marked feature and becomes progressively worse. The mischief is in the same part of the brain as in acute chorea.

As a sequel to encephalitis lethargica, there may be spasms resembling those of chorea, and this may also happen in certain cases of hemiplegia.

SAL ALEMBROTH. A combination of the chlorides of mercury and ammonium, sal alembroth, or alembroth simply, is used as an antiseptic, chiefly to impregnate gauze and other surgical dressings.

See Dressing.

SAL AMMONIAC. Chloride of ammonium (*q.v.*) is commonly called sal ammoniac.

SALICIN. A crystalline glucoside obtained from the bark of species of willow and poplar, salicin is used in the treatment of acute rheumatism. In the stomach and bowel it is converted into salicylic acid. The dose is 5 to 20 grains.

SALICYLATE. A salt of salicyclic acid is called a salicylate. Those most often used in medicine are sodium salicylate, methyl salicylate or oil of wintergreen, salol or phenyl salicylate, and bismuth salicylate.

SALICYLIC ACID. A colourless, crystalline substance, salicylic acid is found in various plant products, including oil of wintergreen and oil of sweet birch, from which it can be prepared ; but it is also prepared synthetically. It is used in treating acute rheumatism, in doses of 5 to 20 grains, but usually sodium salicylate, dose 10 to 30 grains, is preferred for this purpose.

Excessive dosage with these substances causes symptoms of poisoning, referred to as salicylism, such as fullness in the head, noises in the ears, deafness, dimness of vision, sickness, delirium and cardiac depression. Such symptoms should at once be brought to the notice of the doctor.

Salicylic acid acts as an antiseptic, and is sometimes used as such in a lotion. It assists in dissolving off the horny cells of the skin, and is used to remove corns and warts and in the treatment of skin diseases in which there is much scaling or thickening.

See Aspirin ; Gaultheria.

SALINE. Purgatives like Epsom salt and Glauber's salt are described as salines. A solution of common salt, however, is called a saline solution.

See Cathartic ; Normal Saline Solution.

SALISBURY DIET. Sometimes prescribed in gout, rheumatism, chronic psoriasis, obesity and in intestinal disorders, associated with fermentation of carbohydrates, the Salisbury diet consists exclusively of meat and hot water. The meat, of which two or three pounds are taken daily, is minced and served as underdone little cakes. Four or five pints of hot water are taken daily, a pint being sipped an hour before each meal and half an hour before bed-time. The treatment is continued over a period of two or three months. It is not suitable unless the kidneys are sound.

See Diet.

SALIVA. The saliva, or spittle, consists mainly of the secretion of the salivary glands, but receives some addition from glands in the lining of the mouth. Epithelial scales, referred to as salivary corpuscles may be found in it, and are derived from the tonsils. Saliva is a somewhat opalescent and sticky liquid, and is alkaline in reaction. It contains a ferment known as ptyalin, which converts starch into dextrine and maltose, a kind of sugar.

Besides assisting digestion, saliva aids in chewing, swallowing and speaking, and, by dissolving substances in the mouth, assists the function of taste.

A great increase in the amount of saliva is called salivation. This occurs after

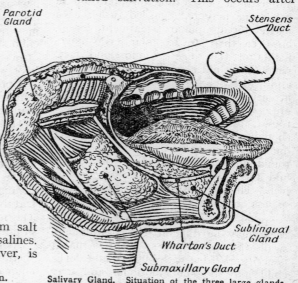

Salivary Gland. Situation of the three large glands

overdoses of mercury, for example. An agent which increases the amount of saliva is called a sialagogue, one that inhibits the secretion and causes dryness of the mouth, an antisialic. Mustard and pilocarpine are examples of the former, and belladonna an example of the latter class of remedy.

See Eating ; Digestion.

SALIVARY GLAND. There are three pairs of salivary glands, namely, the parotid, which lies in front of and below the ear ; the submaxillary, behind the lower border of the body of the lower jaw ; and the sublingual, in the floor of the mouth, beneath the forepart of the tongue. The saliva secreted by the parotid is thin and watery, and is said to be serous and albuminous ; that of the others, especially the sublingual, is thicker, and sticky from the presence of mucin. All secrete the ferment ptyalin.

See Parotid Gland.

SALOL. Phenyl salicylate, or salol, is a white, crystalline powder with a characteristic odour. It is split up into carbolic and salicylic acids in the intestine and so is given as an intestinal antiseptic. It is generally given with sugar of milk or a bismuth salt. Sometimes salol is applied as a local antiseptic.

SALPINGITIS. Inflammation of the Fallopian tube is called salpingitis. The symptoms of the disorder resemble those of perimetritis (*q.v.*).

See Genital System.

SALT. In chemistry a compound of an acid and a base is called a salt. Thus, bluestone, or copper sulphate, is a salt formed by the union of sulphuric acid and copper. In ordinary language, however, the term salt is taken to mean common salt, or sodium chloride.

See Sodium.

SALTPETRE. Potassium nitrate, or nitre, is also called saltpetre.

See Potassium.

SALTS. Saline purgatives are often referred to as salts simply. In this group are included Epsom salt, Glauber's salt, " fruit " salts, and others. Salts should be taken first thing in the morning.

See Cathartic.

SALVARSAN. An organic preparation of arsenic introduced by Ehrlich, salvarsan, which is also known as 606, arseno-benzol,

arsenobillon, diarsenol and kharsivan, is chiefly used in the treatment of syphilis, though it is also useful in yaws, relapsing fever and other diseases caused by spirochaetes, and sometimes in pernicious anaemia.

It consists of a fine, yellow powder which deteriorates rapidly on exposure to air and is given in solution, usually by injection into a vein. It causes a rapid disappearance of the symptoms of syphilis and shortens the period during which the patient is infectious, but to complete the cure of the disease the administration also of mercury or bismuth is usually necessary. A number of injections of salvarsan are needed, perhaps six or eight.

Sometimes the drug causes a severe form of dermatitis, and other occasional effects are jaundice and epileptiform convulsions, but by the use of glucose, intramine, which is an organic preparation of iron, or other drugs, the likelihood of such untoward results is much lessened.

Disease of the kidneys, heart or blood vessels and certain other disorders contraindicate treatment by salvarsan. Another organic arsenical preparation which is used for the same purposes is called neo-salvarsan, novarseno-benzol, and by other names.

See Arsenic.

SAL VOLATILE. Aromatic spirit of ammonia, or sal volatile, is a popular remedy for faintness. It is given diluted with water.

SANATOGEN. The chief constituent of sanatogen, which is an artificial food, is casein, the more abundant of the proteins contained in milk. To this is added 5 per cent. of the glycero-phosphate of sodium. Sanatogen may prove useful in convalescence from acute diseases and in other forms of debility.

SANATORIUM. The main lines of the sanatorium treatment of consumption are a combination of rest and graduated exercises, fresh air, and a suitable and generous dietary. A patient who is running a temperature, as the saying goes, requires continuous rest in bed, and is not, therefore, at the proper stage of the disease for sanatorium treatment ; at any rate, full advantage cannot be taken of this kind of treatment. On the other hand, treatment can be quite satisfactorily carried out in other types of institution, or even at home if the necessary fresh air, comfort, food and nursing are available.

The cases most suitable for sanatorium treatment are early cases after fever has disappeared and the disease has become quiescent. Treatment in a sanatorium should last at least six months, and may have to be prolonged for a year or two.

In addition to the benefits conferred during the course of treatment, a patient learns in a sanatorium how to look after himself when the disease has become arrested and he is living his ordinary life.

See Consumption.

SAND BAG. Bags of a cylindrical or pillow shape, filled with clean sand, are used to support injured limbs and for other purposes. The bag may be made of bed-ticking, and is often covered with jaconet to make it waterproof and capable of being washed with a disinfecting solution.

SAND-FLY FEVER. In tropical and subtropical countries, during the hot weather people are liable to suffer from a disease which is usually called sand-fly fever, but is also known as phlebotomus fever, three-day fever, and by other names. The infective parasite has not been discovered, but is believed to be ultra-microscopic. It is introduced into the body by the bite of a sand-fly, a minute flying insect, the species usually responsible being the phlebotomus papatasii.

The incubation period is from two to eight days, and the disease begins suddenly with a rapid rise of temperature. Headache is generally severe, and there may be backache and pain in other muscles. The eyes are injected, their appearance often being referred to as pink eye. The tongue is coated and the mouth foul. Frequently there is vomiting, but the bowels are constipated at the beginning, though later there may be diarrhoea. The temperature generally becomes normal on the third day, though it may subside earlier. The appetite then returns, but there may be a sense of feebleness for a week or two.

The preventive treatment consists in the use of netting with a very fine mesh, 45 meshes to the square inch; the sand-fly passes through ordinary mosquito netting quite easily. Failing this, the exposed parts of the body may be smeared with oil of citronella or some other pungent oil in soft paraffin. Another method is to use an electric fan. Rooms, especially their corners, should be sprayed with an antiseptic, and the ground around dwellings with tar, to a distance of 20 feet.

The treatment of the disease is simply that of fever (*q.v.*).

SANITAS. A proprietary disinfectant, sanitas has a pleasant odour, due to the aromatic substances that it contains, but its most active constituent is hydrogen peroxide. It can be used in dilution as a mouth-wash or as a lotion for sores, and is often used as a spray to freshen the air of rooms or places of entertainment.

Sanitas-Okol is quite different, being one of the coal-tar or cresol (*q.v.*) group of disinfectants.

SANITATION. Sanitary science means the same thing as Public Health (*q.v.*), and sanitation may be understood as including any measure taken in the interests of the health of the community, though the term is sometimes used with special reference to measures directed against filth and other sources of infection.

SANTONIN. The active principle of santonica, or the dried, unexpanded flower-heads of the plant artemisia maritima, santonin occurs as colourless flat crystals which become yellow on exposure to light. It is used to kill intestinal worms. It is given on an empty stomach along with castor oil or some other purgative. It colours the urine saffron or purple, and may cause yellow vision. Symptoms of poisoning have occurred in some instances.

See Worm.

SAPRAEMIA. When there is a putrefying mass anywhere about the body, poisons or toxins, manufactured by the bacteria responsible for the putrefaction, may pass into the blood and circulate throughout the body. Such an occurrence is described as sapraemia. It is found most frequently in connexion with childbirth or an abortion, when blood-clot or portions of afterbirth may be retained in the womb and putrefy. Other circumstances in which it may arise include the putrefaction of clot in any sort of wound or of a collection of pus in the pleura and gangrene of some part of the body.

Usually the patient suffers from fever, often ushered in by a rigor, and there is severe headache and delirium, especially at night. The tongue is furred and there may be vomiting and diarrhoea. There is progressive exhaustion and the typhoid state (*q.v.*) may be developed.

Treatment consists in searching, if necessary, for the offensive substance which is causing the trouble, and removing it as completely as possible. If this can be done successfully the patient will be well on the way to recovery within a few hours. The treatment otherwise is that of fever (*q.v.*).

See Ptomaine ; Pyaemia ; Septicaemia.

SARCINA. Certain organisms of the coccus type, which occur clumped together in cubical masses, are called sarcinae. They are widely distributed in Nature but are not disease-producing.

SARCOMA. There are two kinds of cancer. One is derived from epithelial tissue and is called a carcinoma, while the other is derived from the tissues developed from the mesoblastic layer of the embryo, namely, connective tissue and muscle, and is called a sarcoma. Each is what is known as a malignant tumour ; it eats into and destroys the healthy tissue by which it is surrounded, and it tends to spread to distant organs of the body. But while the chief route for the dissemination of a carcinoma is by the lymphatic vessels, and carriage through the blood vessels is relatively uncommon, the converse holds with regard to sarcoma. Another difference is that sarcoma is not uncommon in children, while carcinoma is seldom found.

An account of the different varieties of carcinoma is given under the heading Cancer.

The sarcomata are classified mainly according to the shape of the cells composing the tumour. There is the small round-celled, the large round-celled, the small spindle-celled and the large spindle-celled. Both of the small-celled varieties are very deadly, growing with great rapidity. In consequence of this rapid rate of growth it may be found that many

of the cells in the spindle variety are actually round, though an intermediate stage in this transition from the spindle to the round cell is found in cells which from their shape are described as oat-cells.

A special variety of sarcoma is called the melanotic sarcoma. Its cells contain much pigment and it arises from a mole, the retina, or perhaps from pigmented cells connected with the skin. It rapidly extends to the lymphatic glands in its neighbourhood. Another special variety, the endothelial sarcoma, or endothelioma, arises from the endothelial cells lining small blood vessels. What is called the myeloid sarcoma is so benign that it is now hardly regarded as a sarcoma at all. It is derived from the bone-marrow.

Sometimes groups of cells in a sarcoma are developed into bone, or cartilage or some other recognisable tissue, and then one speaks of an osteo-sarcoma, a chondro-sarcoma, a myxo-sarcoma, and so on.

Our knowledge of the causation of sarcomata is still very uncertain, but it may be said that the researches of Gye, an account of which is given under the heading Cancer, were mainly done in connexion with sarcomata.

Diagnosis of the Growth

A sarcoma may occur in any part of the body, but bones and the retina are common sites. When growing in the places where it can be felt, it may appear first as a slight, painless swelling, though if growing very rapidly it may cause considerable pain. Often there is difficulty in distinguishing between a sarcoma and a benign tumour or a chronic inflammatory swelling, due to syphilis or some other cause, but a microscopical examination of a small piece of the growth should reveal its true nature. If allowed to persist a sarcoma may grow out and burst through the skin. Symptoms pointing to the spread of the growth to other organs may make their appearance. Thus, spitting of blood, breathlessness or pleural effusion would be highly suggestive of involvement of the lung.

The best treatment is removal of the growth by operation, if possible, and when a limb is affected this generally means amputation. When this cannot be done, treatment by X-rays or radium may be tried, or Coley's fluid may be injected. This consists of a sterilised culture of certain micro-organisms which cause inflammation. This treatment, however, does not appear to be of use in sarcomata in bone.

See Cancer ; Cell ; Tumour.

SARSAPARILLA. The dried root known as sarsaparilla has a great popular reputation as a blood purifier. There is no foundation for this claim, however, as the drug at most is a feeble one, and any benefit which may be derived from so-called sarsaparilla preparations is due to other substances contained in them, such, for example, as potassium iodide.

SASSAFRAS. The dried, brown root of the ague-tree of North America, usually called sassafras root, has astringent, stimulating and sudorific properties. It is generally used, however, as the source of an aromatic oil, known as oil of sassafras. This substance is sometimes used as a flavouring or perfuming agent, but more frequently as a means of destroying head-lice.

See Louse.

SCAB. A crust covering an area of superficial ulceration is commonly called a scab. Blood-clot, coagulated lymph or pus may be included in its composition. Sometimes healing goes on beneath a scab, but it is often necessary to clear off scabs in order to make healing possible. They should be softened by soaking with a hot alkaline solution, or by means of a boracic or a starch poultice, or an oily application.

SCABIES. Better known by its popular name of the itch, scabies is a contagious disorder of the skin caused by the presence of a mite, known as the acarus, or sarcoptes, scabiei. The disease is usually contracted from a bedfellow, or by sleeping in a bed which has just been occupied by an affected person, but the parasites may be deposited on privy seats or may possibly be transferred by a common towel or some other kind of direct or indirect contact with an affected person.

The female parasites, after impregnation, burrow into the skin. The burrows, which may be as long as a quarter of an inch, may be straight or curved, and they exhibit black dots along their course which are formed by the excrement of the parasite. Along the burrows the eggs of the mite are also deposited. At the end of the burrow where the parasite has come to rest there is a little swelling containing a drop of fluid. The male parasites wander over the surface of the skin, generally in the neighbourhood of the burrows. When the eggs hatch out, the young parasites make their way through the roof of the burrow on to the skin.

There are several sites in which burrows are more likely to occur, including the inside of the fingers near the webs, the inside of the toes, the inside of the ankle and knee joints, the front of the armpit, beneath the breasts in females, and on the scrotum and penis in males. The disease never occurs on the face.

How Scabies May Simulate Eczema

The presence of the parasite causes intense itching all over the body, and this is worse at night when warm in bed. Sometimes it prevents sleep. The itch leads to much scratching, by which the skin is abraded, and this in turn favours infection with pus-producing bacteria, so that the skin may be the site of numerous pustules, and there may be patches of eczema. Sometimes there are crops of boils. Not uncommonly the condition is looked upon as being ordinary chronic eczema, and the existence of scabies is unsuspected.

Treatment is begun by taking a hot bath, the whole body, except the head, being freely lathered with soap, preferably soft soap. A stiff nailbrush should be used as vigorously as possible on affected parts in order to open up the burrows. The body is then dried with a soft towel, and every inch of it below the neck is anointed freely with sulphur ointment, or, if the skin is delicate, with equal parts of sulphur and zinc ointment. If there is much eczema, the following is preferable :

Beta-naphthol	15 grains
Prepared chalk..	30 grains
Green soft soap	120 grains
Soft paraffin	to 1 ounce

The patient then dresses in cotton underwear or clean night-raiment. This treatment is repeated on four successive nights, and on the fifth day a soap-and-water bath is taken, and the body is rubbed over with ordinary zinc ointment. This may have to be continued for some time to clear off any dermatitis. For children, an ointment consisting of 120 grains of sublimated sulphur and one ounce each of balsam of Peru and soft paraffin may be used. Sulphur should not be used on infants except on medical advice.

Bed clothing and any personal clothing that has come into contact with affected skin must be thoroughly disinfected. Steam disinfection, as carried out by a sanitary authority, is preferable, but, where this cannot be had, linen and cotton clothing should be boiled and flannel or wool soaked in a solution of lysol, a teaspoonful to the pint, for some hours, and then be washed thoroughly. The clothes should be dried in the open air.

See Disinfection ; Eczema.

SCALD. Inflammation or destruction of tissue from the action of hot liquids or gases is called a scald, which, apart from its causation, is exactly the same thing as a burn (*q.v.*) and is treated in the same way.

SCALE. Flakes of horny epidermis thrown off by the skin are called scales. If these are very fine they are described as branny scales.

See Desquamation ; Pityriasis.

SCALP. The soft structures covering the cranium, or brain-pan, consist of the skin, the subcutaneous fatty layer, the aponeurosis of the occipito-frontalis muscle, a layer of loose fibrous tissue and a dense membrane, known as the epicranium. It is customary to regard the scalp as being made up of the first three layers.

Owing to the looseness of the tissue beneath the occipito-frontalis aponeurosis, the scalp can be moved fairly freely by pushing it with the fingers, and some people are able to call the muscles into operation and thus move the scalp backwards and forwards. The muscle consists of the frontalis, a broad sheet of muscle over the front of the head, and another, the occipitalis, at the back, the two muscles being united to one another by a tendinous sheet or aponeurosis.

The fat beneath the skin in the scalp is not loosely packed as in most other parts of the body surface but forms a dense layer, the fat being disposed in more or less self-contained compartments.

It follows that inflammation or an abscess resulting from infectior of the scalp does not spread very far as a rule, but, as it is confined, the pain is all the more intense. If, however, a wound penetrates beneath the aponeurosis the infection can easily spread in the loose

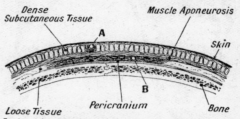

Scalp. An abscess (A) in the dense subcutaneous tissue cannot spread far ; one (B) below the muscle aponeurosis may extend freely over the skull

fibrous layer which occurs in this situation, so that almost the whole scalp might be raised off the bone by pus.

Wounds of the scalp should be cleansed very carefully, and to make it easier to maintain cleanliness the scalp should be shaved all round the wound. As the scalp is stretched over the underlying bone, a blow with a blunt instrument tends to cause a wound resembling a cut.

Scales coming from the scalp are described as dandruff (*q.v.*), and an inflammatory condition associated with dandruff is called seborrhoeic dermatitis. Cysts formed by an accumulation of secretion in sebaceous glands are fairly common on the scalp. Such a cyst is called a wen (*q.v.*).

See Baldness ; Favus ; Impetigo ; Ringworm.

SCAMMONY. From scammony root is extracted a resin which acts as a powerful cathartic, producing profuse watery motions a few hours after a dose has been taken. The dose is 3 to 8 grains, in a pill or a powder. The resin is contained in the compound colocinth pill and other pills. The purified resin is known as scammonin. The compound powder of scammony contains jalap and ginger in addition to scammony. The dose is 10 to 20 grains.

SCAPULA. Popularly known as the shoulder blade, the scapula is a plate of bone, somewhat triangular in shape, placed on the upper part of the back of the chest, to which it is firmly attached by powerful muscles, notably the serratus

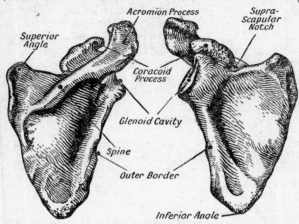

Scapula. Left, the bone seen from behind; right, front aspect

magnus. If these muscles are paralysed the edge of the scapula towards the spine tends to project backwards when the arm is pushed forwards, a condition described as winged scapula.

The bone has an inferior angle and a superior angle, but at the site of the third or external angle there is a thickened mass of bone, on which is a shallow, oval cavity, the glenoid cavity, for the head of the humerus. Projecting from the front of the mass in a forward direction is the coracoid process, a beak-like piece of bone, to which is attached one head of the biceps muscle. On the back of the scapula there is a process of bone, somewhat resembling the plate which casts the shadow on a sundial, running upwards and outwards and prolonged into a broad, thick process, the acromion process, which overhangs the shoulder joint.

To this process the clavicle, or collar-bone, is attached, to form the shoulder-girdle.

Fracture of the main part of the scapula may occur from a gun-shot wound or a severe blow, but displacement of the fragments is usually slight owing to the extensive muscular attachments. The coracoid and the acromion processes are sometimes broken off.

See Fracture; Shoulder.

SCAR. Repair of tissue destroyed by injury or disease can only take place in the form of a scar, or cicatrix. The gap caused by the loss of tissue is filled up by a mass of newly-formed cells, or granulation tissue, and this is converted into fibrous tissue. The granulation tissue is plentifully supplied with blood vessels, but as the transformation into fibrous tissue goes on the blood vessels are gradually squeezed out of existence, so that while a recent scar is pink in colour an old scar is white.

The contraction of the fibrous tissue reduces the area of scarring to smaller dimensions than what it promises to have

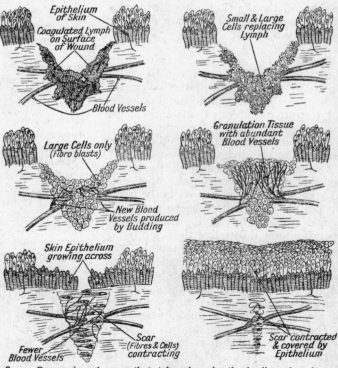

Scar. Progressive changes that take place in the healing of a clean wound, leading to the formation of a scar or cicatrix

at first, but sometimes produces deformity, especially in the neighbourhood of joints. Also, if a nerve happens to be included in a scar the pressure on it causes pain.

An overgrowth of a scar is called a keloid (*q.v.*).

SCARF SKIN. The superficial layer of the skin is sometimes called the scarf skin.

SCARIFICATION. Making superficial incisions in the skin or mucous membrane is called scarification. This is done, for example, in vaccination or as part of the operation of cupping (*q.v.*).

SCARLET FEVER. A common infectious disease, scarlet fever, or scarlatina, owes its name to the vividness of its rash. Epidemics occur from time to time and children are more commonly the subjects of the disease. The specific cause seems to be a variety of streptococcus which generally enters the body through the nose and throat ; moreover, the infection is most often communicated by the secretions from those parts. Those usually infected are therefore susceptible persons who come into close personal contact with others suffering from the disease or carrying the germs in the throat or nose.

Other discharges caused by the disease, such as a running from the ear, may be infective, and also scales thrown off from the patient's body during desquamation. In some instances infection appears to be conveyed by fomites, that is, things handled by the patient or which have otherwise been in close contact with the patient's body. Epidemics have sometimes been caused by milk.

The incubation period is usually about three or four days, but may be only one day or as many as eight. Then the patient becomes fevered and suffers from sore throat and probably vomiting, especially if it is a child. On the second day the rash appears, first on the neck and chest but in the course of a day or two usually covering the whole body, with the exception of the skin around the mouth. The contrast between the flushed face and this region of what is called circumoval pallor is often very striking.

The rash consists of tiny red spots, each being surrounded by an areola of pink, the general appearance of redness being caused by the enormous assemblage of such spots (*see* Plate XXXI,1). The rash disappears temporarily on pressure and the skin which has been pressed looks yellowish. The mouth and throat have also a vivid scarlet colour. Often there is much enlargement of the tonsils and perhaps one or more white or yellowish spots on their surface.

The tongue is furred at the beginning of the fever and may have the appearance described as the white strawberry-tongue. In this the surface is covered with white fur but is dotted over with red spots, due to swollen papillae projecting through the fur. Later on the fur is thrown off, leaving a clean red surface, but the redness of the papillae is of a different shade and they are still conspicuous ; this is called the red strawberry-tongue.

With the appearance of the rash the temperature rises further, reaching 102° to 103° F. or more, and when a hand is placed on the patient's skin it may feel what is called biting hot. The pulse-rate and breathing are increased more or less correspondingly. There is great thirst but vomiting does not usually persist.

Peeling that Follows the Rash

The rash lasts for three or four days and then fades, the temperature also gradually declining. About seven days after the appearance of the rash peeling begins, and this usually goes on for two or three weeks at least. Its appearance has procured for it the name of pin-hole desquamation, but the small bare areas so described gradually enlarge and, as the skin peels off in flakes, a lace-like pattern is produced.

The description of scarlet fever which has been given above is that of a case of moderate severity. In rare instances the toxaemia, or poisoning, may be so severe as to cause death in a day or two. In a proportion of cases, not so large as it was some years ago, what is called the septic type of scarlet fever occurs. There is severe inflammation in the throat and probably ulceration of the tonsils. The glands in the neck, which are usually enlarged to some extent in any case of the disease, are much enlarged in the septic type and probably suppurate. There is commonly a muco-purulent discharge from the nose. Fever is more pronounced and there is some degree of prostration.

This type of the disease may be the predominant one in an epidemic occurring in a community which has previously been free from the disease. In Great Britain a considerable proportion of cases are now of a slight nature. Sometimes there is but little fever and there may be so little rash that it is overlooked.

Several very important complications may occur in scarlet fever. There may be inflammation of the kidneys, or nephritis. The urine becomes scanty and contains albumin and often blood, while there is oedema of the feet, ankles and face or even more generally. In view of this risk the urine should be tested periodically during the course of the disease.

Another complication is otitis media, or inflammation of the middle ear. Infection passes up the Eustachian tubes from the nose and throat and commonly causes a suppurative discharge from the ear. Possibly the infection may pass backwards and cause mastoid disease.

A third complication is acute rheumatism, the larger joints being involved, and sometimes there is inflammation of the heart or of the pericardium. In septic cases the inflammation in the joints may be of a different character and result in suppuration.

In some cases of scarlet fever the throat becomes affected with diphtheria.

Treatment of Scarlet Fever

The general treatment of scarlet fever is that of an infectious disease (q.v.) and of the state of fever (q.v.). The mouth and throat should be kept very clean by the use of an antiseptic mouth-wash (q.v.) several times daily, and it will often be necessary to use a nasal douche as well. This should be given with great gentleness, however, otherwise there is a risk of infective material being driven into the Eustachian tubes.

Complications are dealt with as described under appropriate headings. Should otitis media occur the question of removing tonsils and adenoids when the patient is sufficiently fit must be considered, as the ear mischief might thus be cured. So long as there is any abnormal discharge the patient remains infectious.

By inoculation with a vaccine a skin reaction is obtained in persons susceptible to scarlet fever, and these can then be given a prophylactic serum or vaccine. The test is known as the Dick test. Sera are also used in treating the disease.

See Quarantine ; Rash.

SCHOTT - NAUHEIM TREATMENT. The treatment of chronic heart affections by a combination of saline baths, charged with carbonic acid gas, and Schott's exercises is called the Schott-Nauheim treatment. The aeration of the bath makes it mildly stimulating to the skin. Schott's exercises are carried out by the patient against resistance made by the physician or a nurse.

See Heart.

SCIATICA. Pain along the course of the great sciatic nerve, that is, down the back of the lower limb, is described as sciatica. Usually it is caused by inflammation of the nerve, sometimes it is caused by the presence of an overloaded bowel or of a tumour in the pelvis or by disease in the hip joint, but in other instances the pain is purely neuralgic in character. Pain resembling that of sciatica may be due to disease of the spinal cord or the vertebral column, or to disease in the sacro-iliac joint, and must be distinguished from sciatica. It is important also to recognize as early as possible the existence of pressure or other local disease as a cause of sciatica.

In the remaining cases the possibility of some kind of poisoning should be considered. Lead and alcohol, toxins from sepsis in the mouth or elsewhere in the body, the poisons of influenza and other infections, and diabetes, are possible causes of neuritis. When sciatica exists on both sides of the body the likelihood is that diabetes is the cause. As contributory causes, exposure to cold and damp and excessive muscular toil are of some importance, and the pressure of a hard seat may have something to do with the occurrence of the disease in clerks and others who may sit on uncushioned seats when at work.

Sciatica is a much commoner complaint in men than in women, and most often occurs from thirty to fifty years of age.

The pain may begin at the back of the hip, but sometimes there is first lumbago and then an extension of the pain downwards. The pain is very severe and is variously described as being of a burning, sharp or stabbing character. It abates somewhat for intervals, but acute paroxysms recur and it is made worse by jarring the body, as in coughing. Even when it has quietened down there is a sharp pain at the back of the hip if an attempt is made to straighten the leg at the knee when the thigh is bent up towards the abdomen ; this manoeuvre tends to stretch the nerve. Points of definite tenderness are found at the back of the hip and knee, over the middle of the calf and on either side of the ankle.

The severity of the attack may moderate in a week or two, but in a lesser degree the disorder may last for a month or two or in some cases for many months or for years. A victim of acute sciatica should rest in bed with a pillow below the knee, and the limb should be immobilised by sand-bags or by a well-padded splint, reaching from the armpit to below the sole of the foot, as illustrated in Plate XXXIII, 3. Pain may be relieved by the application of heat from a hot-water bag or a large poultice. A hot-air bath, baths of other kinds, and diathermy, are other methods of using heat.

Aspirin, sodium salicylate, quinine and phenacetin are some of the drugs used in this disorder ; sometimes, however, an opiate is required. The introduction of drugs into the body by ionisation may be the best form of medication.

Other methods of treatment are the application of fly-blisters along the course of the nerve, galvanism and other forms of electricity, acu-puncture, or piercing the nerve with a needle, and the application of ultra-violet rays. Massage should be started as soon as possible. When the disease is obstinate the operation of nerve stretching may have to be carried out. Chronic cases of sciatica may derive

Branches to Muscles on back of Thigh

Branches to Calf Muscles

Branches to Deep Muscles on back of Leg

Branch to Muscles on front of Leg

Branch to Muscles on Outer Side of Leg and to Skin on upper surface of foot

Branch to Skin on Back of Leg and Outer Side of Foot

Branches to Muscles and Skin of Sole of Foot

Sciatic Nerve. Its course in the lower limb

much benefit from treatment at a spa. In some cases, such as those in which gout or diabetes exists, a correct diet is an important part of the treatment.

See Neuralgia ; Neuritis.

SCIATIC ARTERY. Known also as the inferior gluteal artery, the sciatic, which is a branch of the internal iliac, artery emerges from the pelvis along with the great sciatic nerve. It is deeply placed in the buttock and so is rarely injured by ordinary accidents.

SCIATIC NERVE. The great sciatic nerve supplies the back of the thigh and the leg, both front and back, and contains motor and sensory fibres. It is about the thickness of the little finger and is the largest nerve in the body. It emerges from the pelvis about the middle of the buttock and passes downwards in the groove between the tuberosity of the ischium and the great trochanter of the femur. In the popliteal space it divides into the internal and the external popliteal nerves. The chief affection of the nerve is sciatica.

The small sciatic nerve is a sensory nerve, supplying skin over the buttock, and the back of the thigh and leg as far as the middle of the calf.

SCIRRHUS. A type of carcinomatous tumour which contains a large amount of fibrous tissue, and is therefore firm or hard, is called a scirrhus. It is especially common in the breast.

See Cancer.

SCLERA. The firm, white, outer covering of the eye (*q.v.*) is called the sclera or sclerotic coat.

SCLERODERMIA. A disease characterised by hardening of the skin, sclerodermia occurs in two forms. In one, which is very rare, it is diffuse, in the other, which is much more common, it occurs as circumscribed patches. The former is also called sclerema adultorum and "hide-bound" disease, and the latter, morphoea and Addison's keloid. Both forms usually occur in adult life, morphoea more commonly in young adults.

The cause is unknown, but disorder of the thyroid gland has been associated with some cases, and thyroid gland treatment has been beneficial, especially in the circumscribed form. In this form also the disease has sometimes followed an injury.

Diffuse sclerodermia begins as patches of oedema, often brown in colour and usually symmetrical. These often occur on the neck and arms. At the same time there may be pain in joints and muscles suggestive of rheumatism. The patches spread until considerable areas are affected, and in course of time the oedema disappears, the skin becoming shrunken and adherent to underlying tissues. If the face is involved, talking and chewing may be very difficult.

Morphoea generally appears as one or more patches on the breast or leg. The patch is ivory-white with a brownish border and outside this a violaceous zone. One whole side of the face may be affected.

The treatment of sclerodermia is to give a general tonic, iron, arsenic and cod-liver oil being useful examples. Thyroid treatment has been already mentioned. Massage and passive movements should be carried out persistently. Exposure to chill must be avoided.

SCLEROSIS. The term sclerosis means hardening, and is used for certain pathological changes in tissues which result in their becoming firmer. In the nervous system, for example, an increase of the neuroglia, or supporting tissue, may occur at some spot, and the nerve-tissue proper, that is, cells or fibres, is more or less crushed out of existence. Such is described as a patch of sclerosis. Arteriosclerosis, or hardening of arteries, is due to thickening of the inner coat of the vessels. In other organs or tissues a condition similar to sclerosis is generally called fibrosis or cirrhosis.

SCOLIOSIS. *See* Spinal Curvature.

SCORPION BITE. The scorpion belongs to the spider class of animal. It is found in warm countries. During the day it lurks in dark places, but goes abroad at night to hunt for large insects and spiders. It only attacks when cornered or molested. Though it grasps with its pincers, the real damage is done by a poisonous spine in its tail. The poison injected by this spine has some resemblance to the toxin of diphtheria and may readily prove fatal to children. The treatment is the same as that for snake-bite, described under the heading Bite.

SCROFULA. Tuberculosis of the glands or bones was at one time called scrofula.

SCROFULODERMIA. Disease of the skin caused by infection from an underlying tuberculous gland, bone or joint is called scrofulodermia, scrofuloderm or, sometimes, a tuberculous gumma.

SCROTUM. The pouch containing the testicles is called the scrotum. It consists of two compartments, lying side by side, the division being indicated by a raphe, or seam, on the surface ; and the left is the larger and hangs lower down. The skin of the scrotum is brown in colour and thin. Beneath this there is a layer called the dartos containing many plain muscle fibres, the contraction of which throws the scrotal skin into rugae, or corrugations.

A swelling of the scrotum may be caused by a hernia, a hydrocele, a haematocele, a varicocele or an enlargement of the testicle itself. Irritation by parasites or chemicals may cause eczema of the scrotum. This is an especially common occurrence in paraffin workers, tar workers, chimney-sweeps, etc., in whom also cancer may subsequently appear on the scrotum. Strict cleanliness is required in order to obviate this risk.

See Testicle.

SCURF. *See* Dandruff.

SCURVY. It has long been known that scurvy, or scorbutus, can be prevented by including fresh food, especially vegetables and fruit, in the diet, and the disease is now rare, apart from war conditions. It has been found that the difference between fresh and preserved or dried food, as regards the liability to cause scurvy, consists in the absence from the latter of a complex substance called water-soluble vitamin C. Infantile scurvy, sometimes called Barlow's disease and scurvy-rickets, although it has no connexion with rickets, has occurred in infants fed exclusively on boiled or preserved milk or patent foods.

Scurvy begins insidiously with a gradual loss of weight and strength and increasing pallor. The breath becomes offensive and the gums are soft and bleed easily, while teeth may loosen and drop out. Numerous minute haemorrhages occur into the skin, and slight injuries may be followed by large extravasations of blood beneath the skin. Bleeding may also occur from the nose, and blood may appear in the urine, stools or vomit. Owing to extensive small bleedings into skin and underlying muscle these tissues may feel solid and hard, a condition described as scurvy-sclerosis.

The patient loses his appetite and may suffer from sickness and diarrhoea. There is usually mental depression and possibly headache and other nervous symptoms.

Signs of Infantile Scurvy

In infantile scurvy there is great tenderness in the long bones, first in those of the legs, and the infant may scream when anyone approaches and appears to be going to touch it. The tenderness is caused by bleeding beneath the periosteum, or covering of the bones, and this also causes definite swelling of the limbs, which also may lie so motionless as to give an impression of paralysis. Later, the ribs and breast bone may sink back towards the spine and there may be swellings on the bones of the head.

The gums bleed readily and teeth may fall out. The child looks sallow and anaemic. The disease usually begins before the end of the first year.

The treatment of scurvy consists in giving food containing a sufficiency of vitamin C. Under the heading Diet will be found a list of foods classified according to their vitamin content. The juice of two or three lemons should also be given daily. It may be said that, failing other sources of vitamin, it can be obtained by moistening dry peas or beans, allowing them to sprout and cooking only for a very short time. Recovery is the rule unless the patient is very far gone or some accident, such as bleeding into the brain, has occurred.

An infant should be put on fresh milk and have a teaspoonful of orange juice three or four times a day.

In all cases of scurvy an antiseptic mouth wash (*q.v.*) should be used several times a day.

See Diet ; Vitamin.

SEA-SICKNESS. In the preservation of the balance of the body a very important part is played by the semi-circular canals which form part of the internal ear, and agitation of the fluid in these canals by the movements of the ship is the main cause of sea-sickness. In some people the sight of the movements of the ship and the sea is disturbing, and they feel better if they can keep the eyes shut. In others there is a psychical factor ; they make up their minds that they are bound to be sick. It may be helpful for such to keep the mind preoccupied as far as possible with literature or other interesting matters.

As a rule there is no danger to be feared from sea-sickness, but if there is much retching this may have injurious results for full-blooded people, for those suffering from heart disease, for pregnant women, or for those suffering from rupture.

When a sea journey is contemplated an attempt should be made to correct any dyspepsia or constipation that may exist. Various drugs, such as chloral, bromide, chloretone, and chlorobrom may be useful if taken before, and possibly after, going on board, but it is desirable that anything of the kind should be taken under medical guidance. A tight binder over the whole abdomen is often helpful. A person who is apprehensive of being sick should sit in a low deck-chair, either facing or with the back to the bow of the ship. The chair should preferably be on deck, but in a sheltered position, and the body should be kept warm with wraps, although it may be an advantage to have the breeze playing on the face.

A safer position still is to lie down, preferably on the right side, and bring the knees well up towards the body. It is said that packing the earholes with sterile gauze is sometimes very effective treatment, but this must be done by a doctor.

If sickness ensues ice may be sucked, or if there is much depression relief may be afforded by sipping iced champagne.

If sickness persists for several days an altered state of the blood, described as acidosis (*q.v.*), is liable to occur and further provoke sickness. To prevent this happening it would be well to take sodium bicarbonate, a teaspoonful in a little soda-water, three or four times a day.

See Ear ; Vomiting.

SEBACEOUS GLAND. To each of the hair follicles, the pits out of which the hairs grow, are attached two or more little glands which pour out an oily secretion or sebum, and are known as the sebaceous glands. The secretion greases the hairs and the superficial cells of the skin, keeping them smooth, elastic and watertight. If the duct of a gland becomes obstructed the sebum may accumulate behind the obstruction and form a sebaceous cyst or wen (*q.v.*).

See Acne ; Seborrhoea.

SEBORRHOEA. An excessive secretion by the sebaceous glands is known as seborrhoea, and is likely to occur first at puberty, when there is an increased activity of all the glands of the body. There may be an inherited tendency to seborrhoea. The skin looks greasy, and is liable to infection by different micro-organisms and hence to a variety of skin disorders, including acne vulgaris, dandruff and dermatitis of different kinds. The commonest sites of seborrhoeic complications of this sort are the scalp, the forehead, the nose, over the breastbone and between the shoulders.

Seborrhoea may be diminished by living much in the open air and by a diet in which sugar, starch and fat are restricted, and there is abundance of fresh vegetables and fruit. Preparations of sulphur are used largely in treating its complications.

See Acne ; Dandruff.

SECRETION. Certain epithelial cells, grouped together in glands or membranes, have the special function of extracting materials from the blood out of which they manufacture some substance which is known as a secretion, though if the substance is being discharged from the body—the urine, for example—it is referred to rather as an excretion.

A secretion may, like mucus, the digestive juices, etc., be discharged into some body cavity to serve some useful function ; or, like the secretions of the thyroid and supra-renal glands, it may be poured into the blood, also to perform a useful function. The latter type is called an internal secretion. Cells are excited to secrete by the action of nerves, but in some cases also by hormones (*q.v.*). Nervous action, on the other hand, may inhibit or arrest secretion.

SEDATIVE. An agent that lessens functional activity is called a depressant or, when it calms down excessive activity, a sedative. Certain agents, such as opium and the bromides, are general sedatives, but others have a more limited scope as a nervine, cardiac, gastric, respiratory, or other sedative, according to the organ affected. A remedy that relieves pain, heat or itching in skin or mucous membrane may be called a local sedative.

See Anodyne ; Antispasmodic.

SEDENTARY HABITS. The natural kind of life for man is an active outdoor occupation. A sedentary life deprives him, more or less, of the exercise which keeps his muscles hard and his bodily functions active, and often also of the stimulating effects of fresh air and sunlight. Moreover, most people who follow sedentary occupations eat more than is necessary for their actual needs.

Amongst the possible consequences of a sedentary life are feebleness of the muscles, sluggishness of functions, constipation, dyspepsia, and a tendency to run to fat. Also, a sedentary occupation often means the close association of numbers of people in an indifferent atmosphere, infections are spread and lowered bodily vigour diminishes the powers of resistance.

Against this must be put, however, the undoubted fact that the body has very considerable powers of adapting itself to new conditions and of developing resistance to infection. Also, most of the disadvantages of a sedentary occupation can be removed by adequate ventilation of workrooms and bedrooms, with such open-air exercise as might be undertaken, and limitation of food to actual needs. The inclusion in the diet of fresh fruit and vegetables, and of other foods providing sufficient roughage to stimulate the bowels and prevent constipation, is another important matter.

See Diet ; Exercise ; Light ; Ventilation.

SEIDLITZ POWDER. A saline purgative made up for taking as an effervescent drink, a seidlitz powder is the effervescent tartarated soda powder.

See Sodium.

SELENIUM. Colloidal selenium, which is an element allied to sulphur, is sometimes used in the treatment of inoperable cancer.

SELTERS WATER. Also known as Seltzers water, Selters water is a natural mineral water containing a small quantity of common salt and sodium bicarbonate, and is used as an effervescent table water.

SENEGA. The root of senega acts as a stimulating expectorant. From it are prepared tincture of senega, dose ½ to 1 drachm, and infusion of senega, dose ½ to 1 ounce. The drug is used in chronic bronchitis, especially when there is a copious, sticky sputum. The following is an example of a cough-mixture containing senega :

```
Ammonium carbonate   ..   ..  60 grains
Compound tincture of camphor  6 drachms
Syrup of ginger   ..   ..   ..  4 drachms
Infusion of senega ..   ..   to  6 ounces
A tablespoonful in a little water thrice
   daily after food.
```

SENILE DECAY. The effects of advancing years on body and mind are discussed under the heading Age Changes.

SENNA. The leaflets of Alexandrian and of East Indian, or Tinnivelly, senna contain cathartic acid and chrysarobin and have a purgative action, producing profuse, soft, but not watery, stools. There is no reaction in the shape of constipation, and senna is therefore a very useful remedy of its kind. It has the disadvantage, however, that it causes much griping, which can generally be prevented all the same by combining it with an aromatic drug. If senna is given to a nursing mother it will cause griping in the infant.

Preparations include the infusion, dose ½ to 1 ounce ; the confection, also called lenitive mixture, dose 60 to 120 grains ; the compound tincture, dose ½ to 1 drachm ; the syrup, dose ½ to 2 drachms ; and the compound mixture, or black draught, dose 1 to 2 ounces, as a draught. Senna is likewise contained in the compound liquorice powder.

Senna is sometimes taken as senna tea, which can be made by infusing three to six senna pods in a cup of boiling water and allowing to stand till cold.

SENSATION. Our knowledge of what goes on around us and within our bodies is derived through the senses. Certain of these, namely, sight, hearing, touch, taste and smell, are described as special senses, and besides these there are the senses of heat, cold and pain, the kinaesthetic, motorial or muscular sense and the visceral senses, such as hunger and thirst.

A sensation is primarily caused by the action of a stimulus on an afferent nerve-ending, in consequence of which an impulse passes along the nerve to the cortex of the brain. Here the impulse provokes activity in nerve-cells and a mental process is initiated ; there is a recognition of a certain sensation. It may be possible afterwards to recall the sensation, apart from the action of the stimulus, but as a rule the recollected sensation lacks the vividness of that primarily caused by stimulus. If it possesses such vividness as to make it appear that the stimulus is actually in operation, it is described as a hallucination.

The stimulation of the nerve-ending is associated with activities in special sense organs as regards the special senses, and there are also sense organs in connexion with the endings of the afferent nerves of muscles. Different regions of the cortex of the brain (*q.v.*) are concerned with the various special senses. One part, at the back of the parietal lobe, seems to serve the sense of what is called stereognosis, that is, the faculty of recognizing the nature of an object by handling without seeing it, say a coin or a key contained in the pocket.

A sensation may be pleasing or the reverse ; on the other hand, it may be neither. This affective quality, as it is called, of a sensation appears to be influenced by the activity of cells in the optic thalamus (*q.v.*), a mass of grey on either side at the base of the brain.

A stimulus requires to be of a certain strength before it can be appreciated at all, and the same applies to differences in the intensity of the stimulus. Thus, while the addition of one candle to a hundred others already lighting a room might be noticeable, the addition of five to a thousand others would not be so. The required amount of increased intensity varies in the different kinds of sensation. Thus for light, as in the illustration above, it is about $\frac{1}{100}$, for noise about $\frac{1}{3}$, for pressure on the skin $\frac{1}{30}$ to $\frac{1}{10}$ according to the part of the body, and so on.

A definite time, referred to as the latent period, occurs between the application of a stimulus and the recognition of a sensation. It represents the time taken by the processes initiated in the end organs by the stimulus, the passage of the impulse along the nerve and the changes in the brain cells. The latent period is longer for some sensations than for others ; it is longer for sight, for example, than it is for sound. The sensation may outlast the stimulus, a fact illustrated by the after-images which occur in vision.

The various special senses, as also hunger and thirst, are discussed under individual headings. The kinaesthetic sense is that which gives information regarding movements of parts of the body. Thus, when the eyes are closed it is possible to tell the precise position of one of the limbs. The impulses responsible for this may partly originate in the muscles concerned, but some, probably most, come from the surfaces of joints. This sense may be lost while the sense of touch remains intact, in locomotor ataxia, for example.

See Anaesthesia ; Hyperaesthesia ; Paraesthesia ; Spinal Cord.

SEPSIS. Poisoning by the products of putrefaction is called sepsis or septic poisoning. A wound invaded by pus-producing organisms is said to be septic.

SEPTICAEMIA. The form of blood-poisoning caused by bacteria gaining access to, and multiplying in, the blood is known as septicaemia. The bacteria make their way into the blood from some focus, such as an infected wound, an abscess at the root of a tooth or elsewhere, a sore throat, or a boil, etc. Occasionally septicaemia has been caused by the bite of an insect. The bacteria most commonly found in the blood in cases of septicaemia are streptococci, staphylococci and pneumococci, but gonococci, the influenza bacillus and others are sometimes found.

Generally there is high fever in septicaemia, the temperature falling considerably during the night, though not reaching normal ; the fall may be accompanied by profuse sweating. Often the existence of septicaemia is first notified by the occurrence of a rigor, and further rigors may occur in the course of the illness. Delirium is common and there may be severe headache. Sometimes there is severe diarrhoea and this may bring about a state of collapse. There may be a red rash, perhaps with minute haemorrhages, or petechiae, into the skin, and sometimes there is blood in the urine and stools. There is progressive anaemia, and the patient becomes gradually exhausted and may pass into a condition of extreme weakness, described as the typhoid state.

Treatment consists in clearing up any infective focus that can be discovered. In the search it may be necessary to use X-rays on the teeth, the chest and other parts. Sometimes the removal of offensive material will be followed by a very rapid recovery, indicating that symptoms have been caused by the presence of the toxic products of bacteria in the blood, or sapraemia, rather than by the presence of the bacteria themselves. Sometimes the injection of antistreptococcic serum causes much benefit, and if a particular organism is cultivated from the blood an appropriate anti-serum may be useful, or a vaccine made from the organism actually present may be used.

Otherwise the treatment is that of fever (*q.v.*) and of sleeplessness, headache or other troublesome symptoms.

See Sapraemia ; Pyaemia.

SEPTUM. In anatomy a partition between two cavities or between two parts of an organ is often called a septum ; for example, the septum of the nose, the septum between the auricles and between the ventricles of the heart, and that between the two sides of the tongue.

SEQUELA. A disorder that persists into convalescence or after recovery from an acute illness, or which occurs after and as a consequence of such an illness, is called a sequela of the illness in question. Thus, a running ear or nephritis may be a sequela of scarlet fever.

SEQUESTRUM. A piece of bone that has died and is lying loose in the tissues is called a sequestrum. This term is sometimes used, however, for loose, dead pieces of other tissues.
See Necrosis.

SEROUS MEMBRANE. Smooth, delicate membranes, known as serous membranes, line certain body-cavities and are reflected on to the organs contained in the cavities. The peritoneum, lining the abdomen, is an example. Each membrane is so disposed as to form a serous bag or cavity. A serous membrane is covered with flat or pavement epithelium, and in most such membranes there are little openings or stomata, through which the watery secretion, or lymph, which moistens the membrane drains into lymphatic vessels. In fact, the serous membranes form part of the lymphatic system (*q.v.*).

An accumulation of lymph in a serous cavity, caused by inflammation of the membrane, as, for example, in a wet pleurisy, is called a serous effusion or exudate.
See Pericardium ; Peritoneum ; Pleura, etc.

SERUM. The clear, straw-coloured fluid left after clotting of the blood is called serum. It contains all the constituents of blood except the corpuscles and the ingredients of the clot. The proteins in serum are called serum-albumin and serum-globulin.
See Coagulation.

SERUM SICKNESS. The injection of an animal serum into the body may produce symptoms which are referred to as serum sickness. They are caused by the protein in the serum, which is, of course, foreign to the human body, and therefore may occur even when the serum of a healthy animal is used.

There may be slight fever, a rash resembling nettle-rash, vomiting and diarrhoea. In some cases there are in addition pain and swelling of joints, and in asthmatics severe attacks of this disorder. In a few cases there is sudden collapse. Serum sickness begins about eight or nine days after the injection of the serum.

A person who has suffered from serum sickness should always mention the fact when it is again proposed to administer serum to him.

Calcium chloride and adrenalin are used, when necessary, in relieving the condition. If the breathing is very difficult artificial respiration should be employed.

SERUM THERAPY. The treatment of disease by the use of serums, or sera, which is commonly referred to as serum therapy, is based on facts observed in relation to natural processes of immunity and recovery from infectious disorders. When bacteria invade the body they discharge toxins, or poisons, but the body-cells prepare and liberate into the blood certain substances that counteract the toxins and which are therefore known as antitoxins, besides other substances that have a destructive action on the bacteria themselves.

By injecting progressively increasing doses of bacterial toxins into an animal, the antitoxin for the particular toxin injected will be developed in the animal's blood, and if some of this is drawn off and the serum separated out it will contribute antitoxin to a person suffering from the disease caused by the bacteria in question. If a serum is taken by the mouth it is altered by the action of the digestive juices and loses its virtues. The horse is usually selected as a means of procuring a serum.

Sera are used with benefit in diphtheria, tetanus, cerebro-spinal meningitis, dysentery, streptococcal infections, such as erysipelas or scarlet fever, and pneumonia. As, however, any one of four types of pneumococcus may be responsible for causing pneumonia, it is necessary that the serum administered should correspond to the type actually present in the particular case. A few sera have bactericidal properties. A serum prepared from the blood of a person recovering from an infectious disorder, and usually referred to as convalescent serum, is sometimes used. A serum of this kind has been of considerable use in measles.

Sera are used for prophylactic as well as curative purposes.
See Anaphylaxis ; Antidiphtheritic Serum ; Immunity ; Vaccine.

SESAME OIL. Also known as teel oil, sesame oil has a yellow colour and a mild, pleasant taste. It resembles olive oil and is sometimes used instead of the latter in making liniments and other preparations. Iodinol or iodipin and brominol or bromipin are preparations of sesame oil and iodine and bromine respectively; they are supposed to be very readily absorbed by the nervous system.

SETON. A piece of tape or lint, or a skein of thread passed under the skin and left, in order to keep up counter-irritation, is called a seton. It is sometimes used on the back of the neck to relieve an intractable headache. Care should be taken to keep the part clean and aseptic.

SEVEN-DAY FEVER. Several fevers are known as seven-day fever, namely, relapsing fever, Rogers' seven-day fever —which is caused by an unknown parasite, inoculated by an insect-bite. and has a peculiar saddle-back temperature curve— and Japanese seven-day fever. This last is probably a form of infective jaundice, and is caused by the leptospira hebdomadalis, inoculated by the bite of a mouse or swallowed.

SEWAGE. The water-carriage system of dealing with sewage is the rule in towns. Such sewage consists of excreta, scullery waste, waste from factories and the like, and the scourings of yards and streets. Its composition depends to some extent on the nature of the industries carried on in the place, but in any case some kind of purification is required before the sewage can be discharged into a stream or river. There are a large number of sewage purification systems in use. In some the sewage is acted upon by chemicals; in others it is thoroughly oxygenated and the resulting sludge used for manure.

In the country sewage from individual dwellings may have to be dealt with independently. A common method is to collect it in a cess-pool. This should not be nearer a dwelling than 50 feet, nor within 60, or preferably 100, feet of a water supply, and should not be in such a position that sewage could drain into the water supply.

It should be carefully cemented inside, should have an overflow pipe, and its cover should be thoroughly ventilated. There should be an efficient ventilating trap on the pipe carrying the sewage from the dwelling, otherwise gases may escape back through the pipes. The liquid sewage is generally pumped up and used as manure, and the deposit is cleaned out periodically.

Excreta can be dealt with efficiently by using an earth-closet with an arrangement of pails so that the liquid part is drained off. Dried garden soil is used for covering the excreta, and each day the contents of the pail are buried in the top soil of the garden. The liquid part is diluted with water and used for watering the garden. *See* Drains ; Flies.

SEWER GAS. From stagnant sewage there may be a large evolution of sulphuretted hydrogen, or of carbonic acid gas, and if this is contained in a confined space there is a risk of suffocation for anyone entering the space. Otherwise sewer gas is unlikely to damage health, as contamination with microbes cannot occur unless the sewage is splashed.

SHAKING PALSY. *See* Parkinson's Disease.

SHAMPOO. A good shampoo for healthy hair consists of the yolk of an egg beaten up with a gill of tepid water. This is rubbed into the hair and scalp thoroughly and the head is then douched repeatedly with warm water.

SHELL SHOCK. Various functional nervous disorders which occurred during the Great War were termed shell shock. *See* Neurosis.

SHINGLES. *See* Herpes.

SHOCK. A condition of extreme weakness which may follow an injury, especially one of a crushing nature, or an operation, is described as a surgical shock. The patient becomes pale and the skin is covered with cold perspiration, the pulse is weak and rapid, the breathing weak and irregular, and though consciousness is usually retained there is torpor or restlessness. Expert examination would reveal that the blood-pressure is very low.

When this condition follows immediately on receipt of an injury it is called primary shock, is nervous in origin and generally the patient recovers from it after a short time. When, on the other

PLATE XXXIII

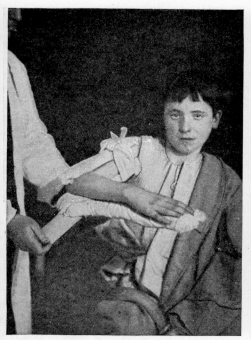

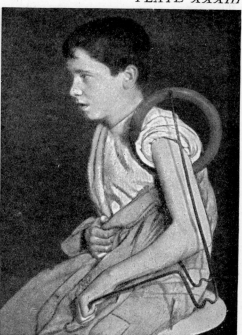

Splint. 1. In fracture near the elbow a rectangular splint is placed beneath the limb and a short one on the outer side of the arm

2. Thomas' skeleton splint for the arm. The ring fits round the shoulder and the splint is bent at right angles at the elbow

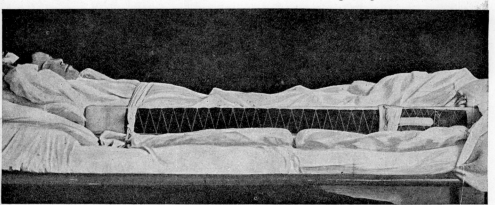

3. Long splint, reaching from the armpit to beyond the foot, to keep the limb at rest in sciatica

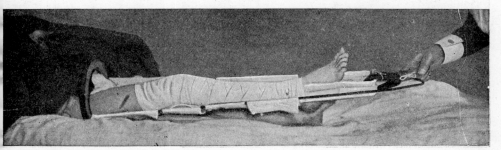

4. Thomas' splint applied for fracture of the femur, the site being indicated by a mark. The limb is supported on slings made from pieces of broad bandage, and extension is applied by a rubber elastic tube

PLATE XXXIV

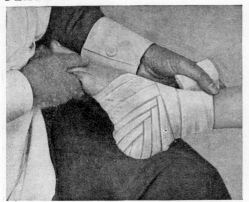

1. Sprain. Figure of 8 bandaging applied in the treatment of a sprained ankle

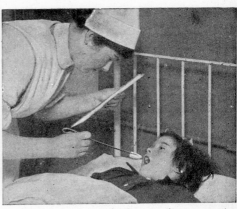

2. Swab. A sheet of glass used to prevent possible infection when swabbing the throat

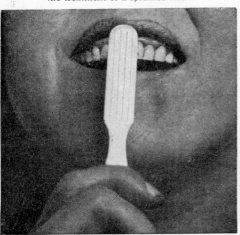

Teeth. 3. Vertical brushing is best and is essential for cleansing the backs of the teeth

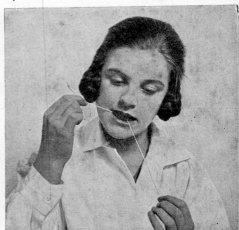

4. Closely adjoining tooth surfaces cleansed by drawing a strand of dental floss between

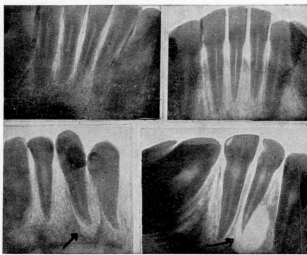

5. Infection revealed by X-rays. Top, left, normal lower teeth; right, pyorrhoea. Below, commencing and developed abscesses

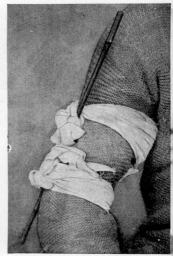

6. Tourniquet improvised with a stone, stick and bandage

To face page 601

hand, it does not occur till some hours after an injury it is called secondary shock, and is due to a somewhat complicated set of factors.

The treatment of shock is to lay the patient flat in bed with a low pillow or none at all, and to keep the head low by raising the foot of the bed. Several hot-water bottles should be placed around him, care being taken, however, to avoid any risk of burning him. Weak hot tea or coffee may be given if he can swallow, otherwise about a pint of warm coffee can be injected into the rectum, provided this is done with the minimum of disturbance. If, however, there is any possibility of bleeding going on no liquid should be given. The lighting of the room should be dimmed and absolute quiet preserved.

A doctor may attempt to improve the circulation by injecting normal saline solution, containing gum arabic, into a vein. Severe mental shock presents similar features to those above described and the treatment is the same.

SHORTNESS OF BREATH. A person is said to be short of breath when the breathing is rapid and there is a sense of difficulty or distress. This condition is also called dyspnoea. It may occur in various degrees. Thus, shortness of breath may only occur when a person undergoes moderate exertion, as in running upstairs, for example, when there may be such distress as would not be expected in a normal person and the rate of breathing also takes longer in slowing down. Matters may be worse than this, however, as the person may be short of breath on slight exertion or even when at rest. Sometimes the shortness of breath will be accompanied by cyanosis, or blueness of the lips and hands.

Acute or chronic disorders of different kinds may be accompanied by shortness of breath, but it will only be one of a number of symptoms. There are some persons, however, in whom shortness of breath is the main, or the only, complaint. In some of these the heart is not disordered at all and in most instances it is a functional and not an organic disorder ; in others the shortness of breath is caused by emphysema or some other lung affection ; in others still it is anaemia.

Shortness of breath in a young person may be due to adenoids ; or sometimes it points to the beginnings of consumption. It has been noted also that it is sometimes the first complaint of a person suffering from acute Bright's disease.

The treatment of shortness of breath depends on its cause.

SHORT SIGHT. The condition of sight in which only near objects can be clearly focussed is called short sight or myopia. *See* Eye.

SHOULDER. The roundness of the shoulder is caused by the deltoid muscle which hangs over the joint like an epaulette except that its fibres are gathered together below to be inserted into the humerus. The deltoid raises or abducts the arm as far as to make a right angle with the body, while movement above this level is brought about by the muscles that rotate the shoulder-blade, or scapula.

The squareness of the shoulder is caused by the acromion process of the scapula which projects outwards over the joint, but the outer end of this process is kept up and out by the clavicle, and if this bone is broken the shoulder sags downwards, inwards and forwards.

The chief muscle engaged in bracing the shoulder is the trapezius, and in depressing it the levator scapulae, which acts by rotating the scapula.

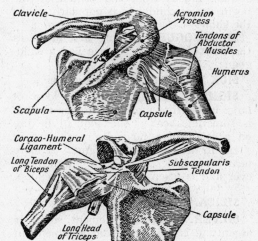

Shoulder. Back (above) and front views of the joint which is formed by the scapula, clavicle and humerus clothed with muscles and their tendons

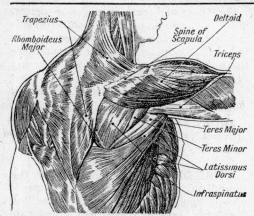

Trapezius

Rhomboideus Major

Spine of Scapula

Deltoid

Triceps

Teres Major

Teres Minor

Latissimus Dorsi

Infraspinatus

Shoulder. Powerful muscles actuating this region

The shoulder joint is made by the head of the humerus resting in the glenoid cavity of the scapula. This cavity is very shallow, and the bones are mainly held in position by the powerful muscles that surround the joint. There is no support of this kind beneath, however, and consequently a dislocation generally occurs in this direction, the usual cause being a fall on the hand, with the upper limb outstretched. The joint is of the ball-and-socket variety, and from the shallowness of the glenoid fossa movements are very free in all directions.

See Bandage ; Collar Bone ; Dislocation ; Humerus ; Joint ; Scapula.

SHOW. The slight discharge of blood-stained mucus from the vagina at the beginning of childbirth is popularly called the show.

SIALOGOGUE. A drug that increases the flow of saliva (*q.v.*) is called a sialogogue.

SICK HEADACHE. *See* Migraine.

SIGMOID FLEXURE. The loop of large bowel that empties into the rectum is sometimes called the sigmoid flexure on account of a fancied resemblance in shape to the Greek letter sigma. It more nearly resembles the Greek omega, however and is often called the omega loop.
See Intestine.

SILICA. *See* Dust Disease.

SILVER. A metallic element, silver, or argentum, is used in medicine, chiefly in the form of its compounds silver nitrate and silver oxide, its organic compounds, or as colloidal silver.

Silver nitrate occurs as flat, colourless crystals, and solutions of these of varying strength are used as lotions or injections for ophthalmia, colitis, gonorrhoea, etc. A drop or two of a solution containing 2 grains to the ounce is often put into the eyes of a new-born baby as a prophylactic measure against ophthalmia. A one per cent. solution in sweet spirits of nitre is a useful remedy for eczema of the ears or about the angles of the mouth, when painted on the patches.

A stick formed of fused crystals of silver nitrate is called lunar caustic and is used to destroy warts and for other purposes. If a little potassium nitrate is fused along with the silver, one gets the toughened caustic ; if two parts of potassium are fused with one part of silver nitrate, it is known as mitigated caustic. This is milder in its effects than the other forms.

Silver nitrate and the oxide were once used extensively in epilepsy and other nervous diseases, being given in the form of pills, and sometimes a permanent staining of the skin, known as argyria, resulted from the treatment.

Organic preparations of silver, including vitellin, or argyrol, and argentum proteinicum, or protargol, have been used as antiseptic solutions in place of silver nitrate, but it is at least very doubtful whether they are better remedies.

Colloidal silver administered in various ways has been beneficial in colitis, septicaemia and other disorders.

SINEW. *See* Tendon.

SINKING FEELING. Though the peculiar sensation in the pit of the stomach, commonly described as a sinking feeling, may be caused by a grave organic disorder of the heart or the great blood vessels, it is much more often due to a merely functional disorder of the heart or to some such disorder as gastric catarrh, flatulent dyspepsia or diminished muscular and nervous tone. Hysteria is a fairly common cause.

A hot drink or a dose of sal volatile will probably remove the feeling, but the underlying cause should be investigated and treated.

SINUS. The term sinus is used to denote a variety of spaces and passages in the body. Thus, there are the spaces in certain bones, the frontal sinus, the sphenoidal sinus and so on, and the large venous channels in the membranes of the brain, the superior longitudinal sinus, the lateral sinus and other such sinuses. The ventricle of the larynx is known also as the sinus of the larynx, and certain other cavities are also called sinuses. Lastly, a narrow suppurating tract is called a sinus.

See Abscess.

SIXTH NERVE. The sixth cranial nerve is also called the abducens because it supplies the external rectus muscle which turns the eye outwards. Paralysis of the nerve causes an internal squint (*q.v.*).

SKELETON. It is customary to describe the skeleton as consisting of an axial and an appendicular set of bones, the former comprising the skull, the vertebral column, the hyoid bone, the ribs and the breastbone, and the latter the bones of the limbs. The upper limb is attached to the axial skeleton by the clavicle and scapula, but the only joint between the two occurs at the inner end of the clavicle, the scapula being attached by muscular connexions only. The lower limb is attached by the innominate bones, which are jointed in front to one another and at the back to the sacrum, the lower part of the spine.

The two innominate bones form the pelvic girdle, which is converted into an actual rigid girdle by the sacrum. The shoulder girdle, which is formed by the scapulae and the clavicles, is incomplete in front and behind, but supported in front by the uppermost part of the breastbone.

Including the tiny bones, or ossicles, of the middle ear, there are altogether 206 bones in the adult human skeleton. The individual parts of the skeleton are described under separate headings.

See Bone.

SKIN. All over the body the skin rests on a layer, known as the subcutaneous tissue, or superficial fascia, which is composed of loose fibrous tissue in which are embedded numerous collections of fat cells. The skin itself is divided into two well-defined portions. The deeper is called the corium, dermis, cutis vera, or true skin, and consists of a dense fibrous tissue which becomes looser, however, at the level at which it merges with the subcutaneous tissue. The corium is prolonged upwards into numerous small projections, or papillae, which in the main are occupied by loops of capillary blood vessels and lymphatic capillaries. Some of the papillae are occupied by little organs concerned in the sensation of touch.

The more superficial portion of the skin is called the epidermis, cuticle, or scarf skin, and is described as consisting of a deeper and a superficial layer, the former being called the rete mucosum, or Malpighian layer, and the latter the horny layer. Each consists of layers of cells superimposed one on the other. The most superficial cells of the horny layer are constantly being shed, but as constantly are replaced by new cells formed in the rete mucosum, which become more horny in

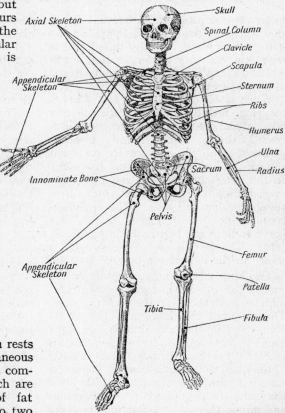

Skeleton. Two main divisions and general arrangement of the body's bony framework

character the nearer they approach the surface of the body.

The epidermis is moulded on the true skin, and shows the elevations formed by the papillae of the latter. The lines on the fingers which are so distinctive in the

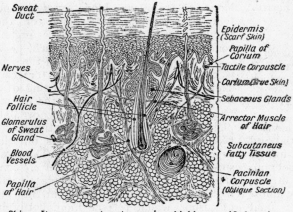

Skin. Its component parts seen in a highly magnified section

finger-print impressions used for identification consist of rows of these papillae, and if the epidermis is partially raised off the true skin the new epidermis that forms will show exactly the same arrangements of lines as formerly existed.

When a blister forms on the skin its covering includes all but the deepest layer of the epidermis. When the skin is grazed, the numerous minute bleeding points seen on the raw surface represent the tops of the papillae of the true skin. In the spaces between the papillae, however, sufficient epidermal cells remain to cover the denuded area. The epidermis contains no blood vessels, though fine nerve endings can be seen lying amidst its cells. The peripheral nerve supply is shown in the illustration in page 496.

Two kinds of openings are found on the surface of the skin, those of the hair follicles and those of the sweat glands. The roots of the hairs and the sweat glands are in the true skin and perhaps even project down into the subcutaneous fat. To the hair follicles plain muscle fibres are attached, constituting the arrectores pilorum, little muscles which erect the hairs. In the true skin of the scrotum and nipple there are similar muscle fibres without any connexion with hair follicles.

Into the hair follicles open the ducts of the sebaceous glands, the oily secretion of which keeps the hairs and the superficial horny cells glossy.

The skin forms a tough protective covering for the underlying tissues. It is very elastic, and thus is able to stretch over tumours and other swellings and resume its ordinary dimensions when the swelling has disappeared, though if the swelling is very great, as, for example, in pregnancy, there may be overstretching, and evidence of this may persist in the shape of fine linear scars. As a person grows older this elasticity diminishes, and thus are explained the loose folds and lines on the faces of the elderly.

The skin is impermeable to water, but oils and fats may be absorbed. Certain fatty preparations are advertised as being " skin foods," but there is no ground for the suggestion that the skin can be directly fed by anything used externally, as any fat that is absorbed is carried off at once by the lymphatics, and can only benefit the cells of the skin by coming back to them in the blood in the usual way.

The skin is not merely a protective covering, however, but is an important sensory organ, and is also concerned in maintaining an even body temperature by regulating the loss of heat. A small amount of carbonic acid gas is excreted through the skin, but the amount is insignificant as compared with that excreted by this route in frogs and other animals.

A dull, muddy appearance of the skin may be due to constipation or indigestion, and is common in debilitating diseases. A harsh, rough surface, liable to become red, may result from too much washing with soap, especially if this contains any excess of alkali. The various abnormalities of skin structure, induced by disease, comprise macules, papules, vesicles, pustules, bullae, tubercles and scales which are described as primary lesions, and atrophy, pigmentation, sclerosis or hardening, ulceration, crusts and other lesions, which are described as being secondary; they are consequences of some primary condition. The meaning of these terms and the various skin diseases, or dermatoses, are discussed under appropriate headings.

See Birth Mark ; Blister ; Burn ; Complexion ; Dermatitis ; Eczema ; Erysipelas ; Erythema ; Favus ; Graft ; Ichthyosis ; Impetigo ; Itching ; Lassar's Paste ; Leprosy ; Leucoderma ; Lichen ; Lupus ; Mole ; Molluscum ; Mycosis ; Nettle-rash ; Pemphigus ; Pityriasis ; Prickly Heat ; Prurigo ; Psoriasis ; Resorcin ; Ringworm ; Scabies ; Sclerodermia ; Soap ; Sweat ; Wart ; Wrinkle ; Xeroderma Pigmentosa.

SKULL. The skeleton of the head is called the skull and consists of two parts, the cranium, or brain-pan, and the face. The cranium is formed in front by the frontal bone ; behind by the occipital ; at the sides by the sphenoid, temporal and parietal bones ; and its roof, or vault, by the frontal and parietal bones. The base of the skull is formed by the occipital, temporal, sphenoid and ethmoid bones. The occipital bone is pierced by a large opening, the foramen magnum, through which the brain connects with the spinal

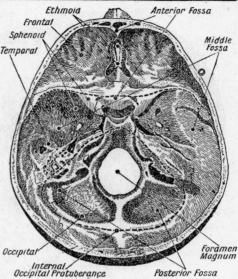

Base of the skull, exhibiting the three fossae

cord. Besides this, there are numerous other openings for the passage of nerves and blood vessels.

Folds of dura mater project into the interior of the cranium, forming partitions which separate portions of the brain from one another. The falx cerebri is interposed between the two cerebral hemispheres, the tentorium cerebelli between the cerebrum and cerebellum and the falx cerebelli between the hemispheres of the cerebellum. Within these folds are channels, or sinuses, for draining the venous blood from the skull.

The bones of the face are disposed beneath the orbits, around the nasal cavities and mouth and in the cheek.

Ethnologists classify skulls according to their cephalic index or index of breadth, that is, the proportion between the breadth and length. On this basis they are described as long or dolichocephalic, round or mesaticephalic, and broad or brachycephalic, and it is found that the type varies with the race. Examples of the first are seen in the skulls of kafirs and Australian aborigines, of the second in the skulls of Europeans and Chinese, and of the third in the skulls of Mongolians.

The bones forming the vault of the skull of a new-born child are thin and are separated at various points to form what are called fontanelles, as shown in the

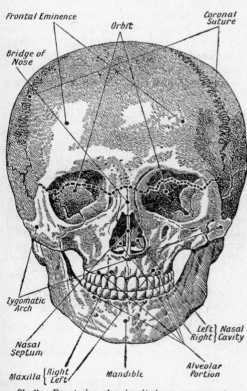

Skull. Front view showing its bony components

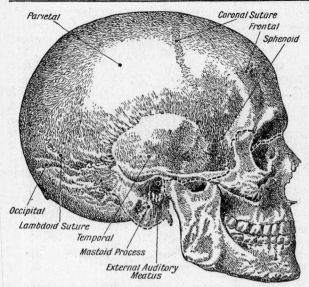

Side view of the skull, showing by a dotted line the line of separation between the bones of the cranium and those of the face

illustration in page 57. They move on one another readily so that the shape of the head is altered by moulding during birth in order to facilitate this process. The proper shape is regained very soon, however. The shape of the head may be altered later on by various diseases, such as rickets, hydrocephalus, acromegaly and osteitis deformans.

A fracture of the vault of the skull is caused by direct violence. It must be remembered that only the inner table of the bone may be broken, so that a spicule of bone may be projecting into the brain, although the outer surface of the skull appears to be sound. A fracture may be linear or star-shaped. Sometimes an oval or round piece of bone is driven down. This is called a " pond " fracture. At other times there is a " gutter " fracture.

Fracture of the base of the skull may be caused indirectly, as by a blow on the vault of the skull, or directly, as by the pressure upwards of the end of the spine when one falls on the feet or buttocks. It is generally compound, and blood appears at

various points according to the situation of the fracture. Thus, if in the forepart of the base, blood may pass into the orbit and the eyeball becomes reddened from below upwards, or in this situation the roof of the nose may be penetrated and blood may flow from the nose or down the throat. Further back the middle ear may be opened, causing a flow of blood from the ear. When blood is able to flow freely from the skull it is accompanied by the watery cerebrospinal fluid, which may escape in large quantities, soaking dressings and pillows.

The first-aid treatment of fractures of the skull is discussed under the heading Fracture.

See Brain ; Concussion ; Dura Mater ; Ethmoid Bone ; Frontal Bone ; Neck ; Occipital Bone ; Sphenoid Bone ; Temporal Bone ; Trephine.

SLEEP. A sufficiency of sleep is as essential to life as a sufficiency of food, and the need for sleep comes periodically as does hunger, though in the one case as in the other the time for satisfying the need may be partly determined by habit. An infant sleeps all the time except when feeding, a child of two or three years

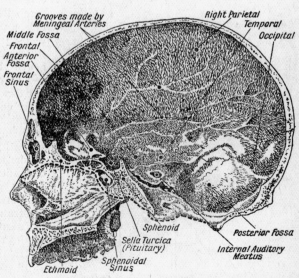

Skull. Internal view of right side, showing the division into three fossae and the situation of the frontal and sphenoidal sinuses

of age should sleep for 12 or 13 hours in the 24, and an adult, on the average, for 7 or 8 hours. During sleep the tissues build up their reserves of energy, and the longer sleep required in the early years of life is due to the large demands of the growth processes.

These demands remain considerable throughout the whole period of growth, and to ignore them by curtailing a young person's sleep in order to accomplish cramming for an examination, or to earn a little money before going to school, is to run the risk of doing serious damage to body and mind.

Sleep is a natural temporary loss of consciousness, but it is difficult to say how it is brought about. Various theories have been advanced on the subject, such as, for example, that it is due to a diminished flow of blood to the brain, that it is due to an accumulation of waste products in the blood, that it is due to fatigue, or that it is due to the diminution of stimuli reaching the brain, but no definite circumstance or group of circumstances can be proved to be the actual factors in producing sleep.

During sleep the activities of the body are lessened ; the heart beats more slowly, breathing is slower and shallower, the muscles, generally speaking, are relaxed and the body temperature is lowered. It is very doubtful if thought processes ever entirely cease even during the first two hours, when sleep is deepest. Probably dreaming goes on throughout, though, of course, we do not recall such dreams, but only such as occur when we are near the point of waking.

See Dreams ; Insomnia ; Narcolepsy ; Somnambulism.

SLEEPING DRAUGHT. A single dose of medicine for inducing sleep is called a sleeping draught. Some remedies for this purpose do not become effective for several hours, but, generally speaking, a patient should be settled down for the night before receiving his draught and the room should then be darkened and quietness preserved.

See Insomnia.

SLEEPING SICKNESS. The disease described as sleeping sickness, negro lethargy or African lethargy represents the second stage of trypanosomiasis or infection with one of the species of trypanosome, a spindle-shaped protozoal micro-organism with a wavy appearance.

Three types of human trypanosomiasis are recognized. Two of them are found in Africa, the West African and the Rhodesian types, and these resemble one another. The third type, the South American, also known as Chagas' disease, presents different features.

The cause of the West African type is trypanosoma gambiense, which is injected by a species of tsetse fly, the glossina palpalis, and of the Rhodesian type, trypanosoma rhodesiense, which is injected by another species of tsetse, the glossina morsitans.

Signs of the Infection

After an infective bite by the glossina palpalis, which may leave an inflamed swelling, there follows a latent period ranging from about two weeks to many months, after which the patient begins to suffer from irregular bouts of fever lasting from one to three weeks and separated by afebrile intervals of about one week. Lymphatic glands over the body become enlarged, and noticeably at an early stage those about the back of the neck. Europeans commonly suffer from erythematous rashes or from patches of oedema.

This state of things may go on for months or years, the patient gradually becoming weaker, thinner and anaemic, and then possibly he may recover. This event is very seldom indeed, however, and what is likely to happen is that he will become apparently lazy, lethargic and dull, and careless about his work and personal appearance. He has attacks of somnolence, and this tendency steadily increases until he has to be awakened to take food and may even fall asleep again with food in his mouth. Meanwhile he has been wasting more rapidly and become weaker. At the beginning of this stage he may complain of headache, and as the disease progresses tremors of the tongue and of the limbs and abdominal muscles commonly make their appearance.

Death may occur in a state of coma, but at any time during the course of the malady and in either stage the patient may be carried off by pneumonia, dysentery or some other intercurrent disease.

The most effective remedy so far used for the disease is known as Bayer 205. This is injected into a muscle or a vein. Other drugs which have been used are the organic compounds of arsenic, atoxyl and tryparsamide, and sodium antimony tartrate.

The Rhodesian type of the disease runs a more rapid course, death usually occurring within a year after infection. Arsenical remedies are not very satisfactory, but Bayer 205 is useful.

Chagas' disease is caused by trypanosoma cruzi, which is inoculated by the bite of a large bug, triatoma magista. The disease may occur in an acute form, but this is generally in infants under a year old, and death may occur within a month. There is slight fever, with general swelling over the body, enlargement of lymphatics and a pronounced enlargement of the thyroid gland.

The chronic form of the disease, which may follow on after the acute or occur independently, may last for several years, and different people are differently affected. Some develop myxoedema (q.v.), others suffer from irregularity and slowness of the heart's action, and still others from tremors, paralysis and other nervous symptoms.

The treatment used for the African types does not serve in Chagas' disease, but the tendency to myxoedema can be countered by giving thyroid extract.

See Trypanosome.

SLEEP WALKING. *See* Somnambulism.

SLEEPY SICKNESS. The correct designation of the malady commonly known as sleepy sickness is encephalitis lethargica.

See Encephalitis.

SLING. A bandage suspended for the support of a limb is described as a sling.

See Bandage.

SLOUGH. A dead mass of soft tissue is called a slough or sphacelus.

See Gangrene ; Necrosis.

SMALLPOX. An acute infectious disease, smallpox, or variola, is now uncommon in Great Britain, though from time to time limited epidemics break out in different parts of the country. The infective agent would appear to be either a minute bacterium or a protozoal organism, and this occurs abundantly in the pustules and crusts which form in this disease. The infection is disseminated through the air, and may be carried for long distances.

The incubation period is about twelve days, and then there is a sudden rise of temperature with severe headache and pain in the back, and often vomiting. On the second day there is often what is called a prodromal rash, and this commonly takes the form of reddening or erythema, a common site being the lower part of the abdomen. On the third day the rash proper makes its appearance in the form of red spots, usually on the forehead and wrists. These spots become elevated, forming papules, and the rash extends to other parts of the body. When the rash comes out, the fever is reduced, perhaps disappearing altogether. The rash is most profuse, as a rule, on the face and forearms, the trunk being relatively free, and this contrasts strongly with the rash of chicken-pox, in which the trunk is particularly affected, while the limbs exhibit very little. Parts subjected to irritation are more likely to display the smallpox rash.

Progressive Changes in the Rash

On the sixth day the papules become converted into vesicles, or blisters, containing a fairly clear liquid. The vesicles are depressed in the centre (Plate XXXI, 4). About the eighth day the contents of the vesicles become purulent, or, in other words, the vesicles become pustules, and, from absorption of poisonous matter from them, there is again a rise of temperature, this being described as secondary fever.

A red zone surrounds each pustule, and there is considerable swelling of the neighbouring skin, particularly on the face. There is often also intense irritation. The temperature may be very high, and there may be much depression, the patient possibly developing the typhoid state.

On the eleventh day the pustules mature, as it is called ; they rupture, and their contents dry, forming blackish scabs, which gradually fall off, leaving more or less pitting. This goes on during the third week, and the temperature also generally falls by lysis.

When the pustules are relatively few and are isolated, the rash is said to be discrete ;

when they are numerous, and so run together, it is said to be confluent, and then the general symptoms are correspondingly severe. When the disease occurs in a person who has been vaccinated, there may only be a pustule here and there. This is sometimes called the varioloid type of the disease.

In what is called the haemorrhagic type, bleeding occurs into the skin and from mucous membranes, that is, from the nose, the bladder and so on, and the outlook is extremely grave.

The rash always occurs in the mouth, and may invade the larynx, so that there may be considerable swelling of the tongue, and laryngitis. Broncho-pneumonia is a common complication. Conjunctivitis, or perhaps even deeper inflammation of the eyes, may occur, and may result in permanent blindness. Inflammation of the middle ear is not uncommon, and there are other possible complications.

One attack of the disease usually protects against further attack, though second attacks do occur.

Efficient vaccination almost always gives protection, but this diminishes in the course of years, and re-vaccination should be done at the age of ten and again in adult life.

Any person who has possibly been in contact with a person suffering from the disease should be re-vaccinated, unless there has been a successful re-vaccination during the previous five years. Vaccination may even protect when it is done during the early days of the incubation period, and in any case is likely to mitigate the disease, should it develop.

Measures to Avoid Pitting

The general treatment of smallpox is that of an infectious disease (*q.v.*). Isolation must be very strict.

In order to lessen the ravages of the disease on the skin, unremitting and careful attention is required in sponging and in the application of antiseptic and sedative ointments. Sometimes red curtains and red shades for artificial lights are used in order to protect the skin from the chemical rays of light, and thereby lessen the irritation on the skin of the face and the subsequent pitting. This may be of some use, but the flood of red light is apt to have a depressing effect on the patient.

Though the question is not definitely settled, there are grounds for believing that the disease called alastrim is identical with smallpox.

See Chicken-pox ; Quarantine ; Vaccination.

SMELL. The stimulus that provokes the sense of smell is caused by certain substances, in solution, coming into contact with special cells in the nose. Such substances usually enter the nose in the form of vapour. While this sense has not in man the importance which it has in lower animals, it has more than a mere aesthetic value, as what we call flavour in food is really a compound of taste and smell, and flavour in food is an important aid to its digestion. Moreover, the sense of smell gives warning of certain dangerous vapours and of putrefaction in food.

There would appear to be certain primary, or elementary, smells, out of which others are compounded, just as happens with colours. The sense of smell is easily fatigued ; if one smells a perfume sufficiently long the sense for it is lost, although something else may be detected readily.

Pungent substances like ammonia and strong acetic acid are not smells so much as ordinary sensation, and stimulate the ordinary sensory nerve endings in the nose rather than those of the olfactory nerves. Such substances should not be used when testing the sense of smell. What is often used for this purpose is a solution of camphor, contained in test-tubes in progressive degrees of dilution, the patient being asked to identify first the most dilute.

The loss of smell is described as anosmia and may be due to many causes. The most frequent one is nasal obstruction, and smell may be restored if the obstruction is removed. Atrophic changes in the lining of the nose also interfere with smell, and a victim of ozoena is himself unconscious of the foul stench emitted from his nose. Another cause is the action of tobacco or some other poison on the olfactory nerves. Loss of smell may also be a consequence of injuries to the brain, or of tumours or other diseases there.

A tumour towards the front of the temporal lobe may give rise to a subjective smell of some kind, but in many mental disorders there is a hallucination of some smell, with no obvious changes in the brain or elsewhere to account for it.

See Nose ; Olfactory Nerve.

SMELLING SALTS. The inhalation of pungent vapours reflexly stimulates the heart and the breathing, and a smelling-bottle is a useful thing to have at hand when anyone faints or feels faint. Mostly ammonia vapour is used, but that of strong acetic acid is also effective.

SMOKER'S HEART. Irregularity of the heart, palpitation and even syncope may result from smoking. The smoker's heart is a form of functional disease of the heart.

See Heart ; Tobacco.

SMOKER'S THROAT. An habitual over-indulgence in tobacco tends to cause chronic pharyngitis. The symptoms and treatment of this disorder are described under the heading Pharynx.

See Tobacco.

SNAKE BITE. The symptoms and treatment of the bite of an adder, which is the only poisonous snake native to Great Britain, are discussed under the heading Bite. The first-aid treatment there described should be carried out for bites of foreign poisonous snakes, but the site of the bite usually requires to be dealt with more drastically. Incisions are made through the skin over the marks of the fangs, and a strong solution of permanganate of potassium is poured into the wounds. A serum, known as anti-venine, is injected if it is at hand.

SNEEZING. The mechanism of a sneeze is similar to that of a cough. There is first of all a deep inspiration and then closure of the glottis. Following on this is a violent expiration-effort, the glottis flies open, and a blast of air is sent out through the nose. The sneeze is provoked by some irritation in the nose, and its object is to get rid of the irritant.

Paroxysmal sneezing is a feature of hay fever, but may be caused by other irritants beside pollen, and sometimes occurs when there is no evidence of any irritant at all. There is at the same time free watering of the eyes and a copious nasal discharge.

Sneezing is a symptom also of a common cold and of influenza, and its effect in these diseases may be to disseminate the germs far and wide. A sufferer from one of those diseases should have a handkerchief impregnated with some volatile antiseptic and should always sneeze into the handkerchief.

The treatment of sneezing is that of the disease underlying it, but when bouts of sneezing are frequent it is well to have the nose examined, as a septal spur or some other source of irritation may exist.

See Cold, Common ; Hay Fever.

SNORING. Caused by vibrations of the soft palate, snoring is most likely to occur when one sleeps on the back with the mouth open, especially when the air is passing in and out through both the nose and the mouth. Snoring in children is generally due to adenoids, which prevent sleeping with the mouth shut.

A drunk person or one under a general anaesthetic is prone to snore, and here there is some degree of paralysis of the soft palate, but also the base of the tongue falls backwards and obstructs breathing more or less. The same applies to the snoring in concussion or apoplexy and similar conditions. The noisy breathing in all those abnormal conditions is usually called stertor. It can generally be relieved, like snoring in health, by turning the patient on his side or by pushing forwards the lower jaw and with it the base of the tongue.

SNOW BLINDNESS. The actinic rays of sunlight reflected from the surface of snow may cause conjunctivitis (*q.v.*), which may be complicated by ulceration of the cornea. There is great intolerance of light, spasmodic contraction of the eyelids and a copious flow of tears. The condition is commonly called snow blindness. Cold compresses over the eyelids are comforting at first, and later the eye is bathed with boracic lotion. The patient must rest in a darkened room.

SNUFFLES. The nasal catarrh of infants suffering from congenital syphilis is commonly called snuffles.

SOAP. A chemical combination of a fatty acid and an alkali is described as a soap, and the process of soap-making consists in splitting up fats or oils into their constituents, which are glycerin and fatty acids, in the presence of some alkali. The character of the soap depends on the kind of fat or oil and of alkali used, and the proportions of each. Soft soap is a potash soap and hard soap a soda soap. Curd soap is made of soda and a purified animal fat. Marine soap, that is, one that can be used for washing in sea-water, is made from cocoa-nut oil and soda or potash. Some laundry soaps are made with ammonia instead of soda or potash. Silicated soap is made by adding silicate of soda, or soluble glass, to ordinary soap ; it is a useful soap when the water is hard. Yellow soap is a mixture of resin soap with hard soap.

Toilet soaps are ordinary soaps more or less purified, and perhaps with the addition of some perfume and colouring matter. A transparent soap is made by dissolving ordinary soap in alcohol and then distilling this off. Glycerin soap consists of ordinary soap with added glycerin, and in the same way powdered pumice or other substances may be incorporated in a soap.

Why Toilet Soap is Different

Most soaps contain an excess of alkali, and the greater the amount of alkali the stronger the cleansing power, as the alkali combines with greasy dirt and facilitates its removal. This is the explanation of the need of soap for a proper cleansing of the skin. On the other hand, an excess of alkali proves very irritating to the skin, and so a laundry soap should never be used for toilet purposes. Some people find even some kinds of soap often used as toilet soap too irritating, and these should use a neutral soap, that is, one with no excess of alkali. What are called super-fatted soaps may have an excess of fat, though there is a risk of such an excess causing rancidity.

As, however, any soap has a chemical as well as a physical action on the skin, frequent washing with soap may irritate a delicate skin, as Nature intends the skin to retain a certain amount of its greasy secretion.

Medicated soaps are made with olive oil, and have such drugs as carbolic acid, camphor, iodine, sulphur and salicylic acid incorporated in them.

Soaps are used in making some medicinal preparations. Both hard and curd soap are used as a basis for pills, and a piece of firm soap, properly shaped, can be used as a purgative suppository. Soap plaster contains hard soap, resin and lead plaster, and soap liniment, or opodeldoc, soft soap, camphor, oil of rosemary, alcohol and distilled water.

Soap spirit, or tincture of soap, may be made by dissolving soft soap in spirit, and is useful for removing greasy dandruff from the scalp. It is much used in cleansing the skin prior to operation. Ether soap is one in which both alcohol and methylated ether are included.

See Complexion ; Skin.

SODA. The term soda usually signifies sodium carbonate or bicarbonate, but sometimes the oxide of sodium is meant. Soda water is aerated water containing a small quantity of sodium bicarbonate.

SODIUM. A soft metallic element belonging to the alkaline group, sodium forms compounds which are wide-spread in nature, and some of which are important constituents of the body.

Sodium chloride is common salt, and is an essential item in diet. It has medicinal uses also. It is used to make normal saline solution (*q.v.*), which is injected into the tissues or blood vessels to replace fluid lost by bleeding, and for other purposes. A pinch of salt in a glass of water makes an excellent gargle or mouth wash. A tablespoonful in a glass of water serves as an emetic, and a strong solution is often used to kill thread-worms by injecting it into the bowel. A pound of common salt in three gallons of water makes a brine bath, which is used warm to relieve pain in chronic joint disorders.

Sodium bicarbonate, or baking soda, is given in doses of 5 to 30 grains or more as an antacid. If the dose is taken about half an hour before a meal, it stimulates digestion. The lozenges, each of which contains three grains, provide a convenient means of carrying the drug about when it is being taken regularly.

Large doses of sodium bicarbonate are given in acidosis (*q.v.*), a condition which may supervene in diabetes and other disorders. It helps to liquefy mucus, and a pinch in a glass of hot milk sometimes benefits a cough. A solution in water is sometimes used to cleanse the nose or other mucous surfaces. A teaspoonful of sodium bicarbonate in a pint of water is often used as a lotion to relieve itching.

Sodium carbonate, or washing soda, has the same actions and dosage as the bicarbonate, but is not often given, as it may prove irritating. It is used to make an alkaline bath.

The following salts of sodium are used as purgatives : sodium phosphate and effervescing sodium phosphate, sodium sulphate and effervescing sodium sulphate, the effervescing citro-tartrate of sodium, the dose of each of these being 120 to 240 grains for a single dose and 60 to 120 grains for repeated doses ; tartarated soda, or Rochelle salt, dose 120 to 240 grains ; and the effervescing powder of tartarated soda, which is better known as a Seidlitz powder. The last is made up in two papers, a white one containing tartaric acid and a blue one containing tartarated soda and sodium bicarbonate.

The acid phosphate of sodium, dose 30 to 60 grains, is given to make the urine acid, an important matter, for example, when hexamine is being used.

Sodium citrate, dose 5 to 10 grains, is a refrigerant. It is often used to prevent the formation of thick curds in the milk given to bottle-fed babies or invalids, one grain or more being added to each ounce of milk.

Sodium sulphite, dose 5 to 20 grains, is sometimes taken to relieve fermentation in the stomach, and for this purpose the solution of chlorinated soda, dose 10 to 20 minims, may also be taken diluted with water. Half a drachm of this solution in an ounce of water makes an excellent antiseptic gargle or mouth wash, or a lotion for bathing wounds or sores.

Sodium hypophosphite, dose 3 to 10 grains, acts as a tonic. Sodium bromide, sodium iodide, sodium arsenate, sodium benzoate and other salts owe their usefulness to the acid which they contain.

See Bromide ; Hypophosphite ; Iodide ; Potassium.

SOFTENING OF THE BRAIN. When the blood supply of a part of the brain is cut off it degenerates and becomes softened. The disturbance of the circulation is brought about by blocking of an artery by embolism or thrombosis and may occur in any part of the brain, but its situation can generally be ascertained by paying due regard to the symptoms. If the symptoms do not clear up in a few weeks they are unlikely to do so at all.

Mental deterioration, such as occurs in the aged, is often referred to popularly as softening of the brain, but in many instances of this kind there is no actual softening of brain tissue.

See Dementia ; Embolism ; Thrombosis.

SOLAR PLEXUS. Situated behind the stomach but in front of the abdominal aorta, the solar, or coeliac, plexus consists of a matted network of nerve fibres connected with a mass of nerve tissue on either side, which, from the shape, is called the semilunar ganglion, but is also known as the coeliac ganglion. The splanchnic nerves join the plexus by penetrating the diaphragm from the

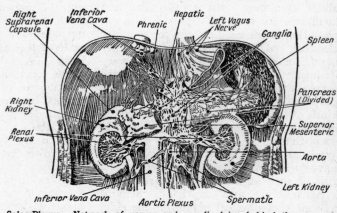

Solar Plexus. Network of nerves and ganglia lying behind the stomach

thorax, and it also receives branches from the right vagus nerve.

In connexion with this plexus are subsidiary plexuses supplying the stomach, bowel, liver and other abdominal viscera. The plexus forms part of the sympathetic nervous system (*q.v.*).

SOMNAMBULISM. Sleep-walking, or somnambulism, occurs most frequently in children. Although the senses may be acute and complicated movements be performed, nothing that happens during somnambulism can be remembered. The condition represents one form of mental dissociation, the larger portion of the mental activities that connote personality being still asleep. When there is a still greater degree of awareness the condition of double consciousness (q.v.) is reached. Somnambulism may also be described as a dream in action.

Although there is usually sufficient awareness during sleep-walking to prevent the person from injuring himself, there is a risk of his doing so if suddenly awakened. A person who is subject to sleep-walking should have someone sleeping in the same room ; if this cannot be done the door should be locked or fastened with a chain and the window should be protected. A simple expedient which is sometimes successful is to have a piece of linoleum by the bedside, as contact with its cold surface may be sufficient to awaken the sleeper when he steps on it. To remove the cause of the habit some kind of psychotherapy would be required.

SOOTHING SYRUP. Preparations are sold as soothing syrups to be given to fretful infants or children.

The indiscriminate use of nostrums of this kind is highly blameworthy, as the proper course is to discover the cause of the fretfulness and treat that.

It may be teething, indigestion, constipation or some other minor disorder, but, on the other hand, it may be some serious disorder, requiring active treatment, and time is lost by giving soothing syrups. Moreover, while, for example, a syrup containing dill or some other aromatic drug may relieve flatulence, some adjustment of diet is probably required to prevent the flatulence. The same applies to soothing syrups for coughs, sold for the use of adults.

SOPORIFIC. A drug used to induce sleep may be called a soporific.
See Hypnotic ; Sleeping Draught.

SORDES. In the state of profound weakness which may occur in acute fevers, crusts are apt to form on the lips and teeth, yellow at first, but becoming brown and then black. Such are described as sordes, and consist of epithelial débris, food particles and bacteria. An attempt should be made to prevent the occurrence of sordes by keeping the mouth clean, an ordinary duty in any case of sickness. Wiping with a piece of cotton wool soaked in a solution of glycerin of borax or of permanganate of potassium will usually serve to clear away sordes. The parts should not be allowed to become dry.
See Mouth Wash.

SORE THROAT. A sore throat may be due to pharyngitis, tonsillitis, or, sometimes, laryngitis.
See Clergyman's Throat ; Diphtheria ; Larynx ; Pharynx ; Tonsil.

SOUND. The source of sound is vibration in some body. If one of the prongs of a tuning-fork, while it is sounding, is placed in contact with a piece of paper or some other object the fact that it is vibrating will be evident at once. These vibrations are communicated to the ear by waves of air, though they may likewise be transmitted through liquids or solids, and are heard or appreciated as sounds.

When the waves come in regular succession the sounds are musical, but they are merely noises if the waves are irregular. The pitch of a musical sound depends on the rate of vibration. The loudness of a sound depends on the size of the waves ; its timbre, or quality, upon secondary waves that form on the main waves.
See Ear ; Hearing.

SOUTHEY'S TUBES. Fine silver tubes designed for withdrawing dropsical fluid through the skin are called Southey's tubes. Very large amounts may thus be got rid of, but strict antiseptic precautions must be observed while using the tubes.

SPAHLINGER TREATMENT. The treatment of consumption devised by M. Spahlinger consists of sera and vaccines which are injected into the patient, the course lasting about six months as a rule. Medical men who have observed the effects of this treatment have expressed contradictory opinions as to its value.

SPASM. An involuntary or undue contraction of a muscle is described as a spasm. It may occur in involuntary or voluntary muscles, and the usual cause is irritation of the nerve cells or nerves supplying the muscle. If the contraction is sustained the spasm is said to be a tonic one, but if contractions and relaxation rapidly succeed one another it is said to be clonic. When spasm is more or less general over the body the occurrence is called a convulsion or a fit. A localised spasm, when painful, is called a cramp. The stiff or sticky gait observed in paraplegia is described as a spastic gait and is due to chronic excess of tone in the paralysed muscles.

See Antispasmodic ; Cramp ; Gait ; Nervous System ; Tic ; Tetany ; Tremor.

SPECIFIC. A remedy that has a definite curative value for a disease is said to be a specific for that disease. Thus, quinine is a specific for malaria, mercury for syphilis, organic arsenical compounds for relapsing fever or a salicylate for acute rheumatism. A specific disease is one caused by a particular microbe, enteric fever or diphtheria being an example of such a disease. Sometimes the term specific disease is used as a euphemism for syphilis.

The specific gravity of a substance is the weight of a measured quantity of it compared with that of the same quantity of another substance, distilled water as a rule, which is taken as a standard.

SPECTACLES. Lenses, prisms or tinted glass worn in front of the eyes for some purpose are described as glasses. By spectacles is meant the particular form of glasses in which the framework includes a rigid bridge for the nose and side-pieces to go over the ears. This is the best type of glasses, generally speaking, and it is the one that should be worn by children or when the lenses are heavy. Preferably the side-pieces should have loops to go behind the ears. The framework should be as light as may be consistent with rigidity. Tortoiseshell and horn do not cut into the skin as the narrow metal frames sometimes do.

Lenses should be maintained in such a position in front of the eyes that the line of vision passes through the centre. A lens hollowed out behind is called a toric lens and permits of the glass being worn nearer the eye without touching the lashes. People who require different glasses for near and distant vision can have suitable lenses combined in one glass, an arrangement described as bifocal lenses.

To protect unduly sensitive eyes from sunlight, tinted glasses may be worn, and may be of Crookes' glass of the lighter shades. Euphos glasses, which are tinted yellowish-green, are used for the same purpose, and sometimes ordinary smoked glasses.

See Astigmatism ; Eye ; Lens.

SPECTRUM. *See* Light.

SPECULUM. An instrument for dilating one of the various body passages and thus permitting a proper view of its cavity is called a speculum. There is a variety of types for use in the nose, ear, vagina and rectum. Elaborations of the speculum are seen in such instruments as the bronchoscope and urethroscope.

SPEECH. The definition of speech as the communication of ideas by articulate sounds sets out, it will be noted, three propositions regarding it. The first is that speech is primarily a mental process. It implies the storage in the mind of a stock of names for things, qualities and actions, and an intelligent method of stringing words together. All this is accomplished in the brain, especially in certain centres in its cortex, which have been identified, and in right-handed people these centres are in the left side of the brain. An injury or disease that interferes with the cells in such centres, or with the fibres that link them together, interferes with the thought processes of speech. A speech-defect of this type is called aphasia (*q.v.*).

In the second place, speech implies the production of sound. This is effected by vibrations of the vocal cords, and these in turn by the rush of air through the larynx in consequence of breathing movements. When there is partial paresis of the vocal cords, as in laryngitis, no sound may be produced and the voice sinks to a whisper. Paralysis of the cords may also occur from a lesion of the recurrent laryngeal nerve. When the voice is lost suddenly and there is no obvious abnormality to be seen in the cords, the cause is hysteria. This usually occurs in females. Loss of voice is called aphonia.

Thirdly, the sound produced in the larynx is modified by alterations in the shape of the mouth and pharynx and by certain movements of the lips, teeth, tongue and palate. This **action** is described as articulation, and the nerve centres controlling it are situated in the bulb, or medulla, of the brain and are connected with the speech centres in the brain. Lesions affecting these centres, the nerves proceeding from them or the muscles supplied by such nerves, may cause dysarthria, that is, difficulty in articulating, or may render it impossible, a condition known as anarthria.

Paralysis of the facial muscles, the tongue or the soft palate will cause some interference with articulation, and in bulbar paralysis the speech becomes slurred and mumbling. Inflammation in or about the mouth, causing swelling of the parts, also makes speech indistinct. Scanned, syllabic or staccato speech occurs in some nervous diseases, especially disseminated sclerosis. A hesitating kind of speech may be noted in severe chorea.

A nasal quality is imported to the voice by nasal obstruction or by paralysis of the soft palate.

Inability to pronounce the letters S and Z correctly is described as lisping, and a similar difficulty may occur with the letter R. Some partial help in overcoming such difficulties may be achieved by education.

Stammering, or stuttering, is not due to actual defect in the speech mechanism but to inability to control it on account of emotional disturbance. It is an expression of anxiety hysteria, and an attempt should be made to cure it by finding out the emotional disturbance that underlies the hysteria. Voice exercises, as in declaiming, and breathing exercises may be beneficial by giving the patient confidence.

SPERMACETI. A solid, fatty substance derived from the head of the sperm whale, spermaceti occurs as pearly-white, glistening, translucent masses. It is an emollient, and is used in making ointments, cerates and bougies.

SPERMATIC CORD. The structure of the spermatic cord, which is attached to the testicle, is described under the heading Genital System. Torsion of the cord may occur from rotation of the testicle and causes strangulation of the blood vessels. There is a sudden, sickening pain in the groin, usually accompanied by vomiting and collapse. Unless the condition is

rectified at once the testicle becomes gangrenous. Inflammation of the cord is generally due to extension upwards from the testicle. The cord may be involved in a varicocele and may be the site of a localised hydrocele or haematocele. A small growth formed of fatty tissue sometimes occurs in the cord and possibly there may be a cancer, but this is almost always due to extension from the testicle.

See Haematocele; Hydrocele; Testicle; Varicocele.

SPERMATORRHOEA. The involuntary discharge of semen is called spermatorrhoea. It commonly takes the form of nocturnal emissions (*q.v.*), but may occur after micturition or when the bowels move. Sometimes the discharge is not semen at all and may be a milky discharge from other glands, when it is called urethrorrhoea. A discharge may come entirely from the prostate gland. This is called prostatorrhoea. Much harm comes from reading quack literature on this subject instead of consulting a doctor.

SPERMATOZOON. The human male germ cell, or spermatozoon, consists of a head, a neck, a middle piece, and a long, slender tail. The total length is $\frac{1}{500}$ inch. The spermatozoon progresses by an undulatory movement of the tail.

SPHAGNUM MOSS. Sheets of dried sphagnum moss are used as absorbent dressings, accouchement sheets and for other similar purposes.

SPHENOID BONE. The term sphenoid means wedge-like, and has been applied to one of the bones of the skull because it is, as it were, wedged into the centre of that structure. It forms part of the floor of the skull and also, by thin expansions called the great wings, of the sides of the skull. In its central mass are two cavities, lying side by side, called the sphenoidal sinuses. These open into the upper and back part of the cavity of the nose and are sometimes infected from the nose.

See Skull.

SPHINCTER. A circular band of muscle at the orifice of a hollow organ, a sphincter controls the passage outwards of the contents of the organ. Certain nerves cause it to contract and close the orifice, while others cause it to relax and allow the contents to pass through.

Examples are the pyloric sphincter between the stomach and bowel, the two sphincters of the anus and the sphincter at the neck of the bladder.

SPHYGMOGRAPH. An instrument for obtaining a tracing of the movements of the pulse on a strip of blackened paper is called a sphygmograph. Blood pressure is estimated by means of another instrument, the sphygmomanometer, of which there are two types, the aneroid and the mercurial, resembling the two types of barometer.

SPINA BIFIDA. In the developing embryo the spinal cord is first a groove along the back. The groove deepens and its edges grow in towards one another and finally coalesce. The cavity so formed is the central canal of the cord and is relatively large at first, but growth of the solid nervous tissue later reduces it to a minute tube. Also, the cord is continuous at first with the outer layer, or skin, but soon other cells push their way between them, and these cells ultimately become the vertebrae and the muscles of the back.

Should these various tissues fail to meet in the way just described the condition is that of spina bifida, or split-spine. When this occurs it is usually in the lower part of the back. The edges of the groove above mentioned may fail to meet and then even the spinal cord will be split. There is a raw area on the lower part of the back when the child is born, but this deformity is so serious that either the child is stillborn or dies in a day or two.

The usual appearance in spina bifida is a soft rounded tumour in the lower part of the back, which becomes more tense when the child cries, showing that it contains cerebro-spinal fluid. Generally the spinal cord, flattened out, is attached to the skin, and from defects in its functioning there is likely to be some deformity and weakness of the lower limbs, and evidence of trophic changes there.

Many cases can be successfully treated by operation, but others, especially if there is much paralysis, are best left alone, though it may be desirable to protect the swelling by a large cap.

Sometimes the bony parts fail to meet across the back, but the other tissues are sufficiently strong to prevent any protrusion of the cord or its membranes. This is called spina bifida occulta and generally requires no treatment.

See Spinal Cord.

SPINAL ACCESSORY NERVE. The 11th cranial, or spinal accessory, nerve derives its fibres both from the medulla of the brain and from the spinal cord. These unite to form a trunk which passes out of the skull along with the vagus nerve. Branches are supplied to muscles in the soft palate and to the sterno-mastoid and trapezius muscles in the neck.

SPINAL ANAESTHESIA. By injecting a solution of an anaesthetic drug, stovaine usually, into the spinal canal, parts below the navel are rendered insensitive and operations can be performed on them without causing pain, although the patient retains consciousness. This is called spinal anaesthesia.

SPINAL CORD. The medulla spinalis, or spinal cord, occupies the canal formed by the arches of the superimposed vertebrae of the spine, as shown in the illustration in page 495. It is continuous above with the medulla, or bulb, the lowest part of the brain, and extends downwards as far as the lower border of the first lumbar vertebra, where it ends in a blunt point, called the conus medullaris. Its average length in the male adult is about 18 inches and its thickness about that of the little finger. Prolonged downwards from the conus medullaris is a cord, known as the filum terminale, which is attached at its lower end to the first coccygeal vertebra.

The membranes of the brain are prolonged through the foramen magnum, the large opening in the base of the skull, and

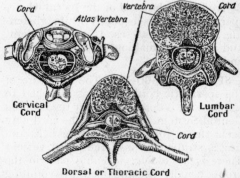

Spinal Cord. Cross sections showing the varying shape of the cord in different parts of the spine

the outermost, the dura mater, lines the spinal canal. Within this is the arachnoid, and, around the cord, the pia mater, a band of which passes across on either side attaching the cord to the inner surface of the dura; as this attachment is by means of a series of tooth-like processes, the band is called the ligamentum denticulatum.

The cord is cylindrical in shape, but somewhat flattened in front and behind, and presents two enlargements, one in the cervical region, from which the nerves to the arms go out, and another in the lower dorsal region, from which are supplied the nerves to the legs. There are thirty-one pairs of spinal nerves, namely, eight cervical, twelve dorsal or thoracic, five lumbar, five sacral and one coccygeal. The first cervical passes out above the topmost vertebrae, the axis, the others pass between adjoining vertebrae. Each nerve has an anterior motor root, its fibres actuating muscles, and a posterior sensory root bearing sensations. On the latter is a swelling formed by the posterior root ganglion.

As the cord itself reaches no lower than the first lumbar vertebrae, the lumbar, sacral and coccygeal nerves pass downwards in a bunch, somewhat resembling a horse's tail, and so called the cauda equina. The bag formed by the dura mater extends as far down as the middle of the sacrum, however. This bag contains cerebro-spinal fluid.

The cord is divided into two symmetrical halves by a fissure in front and another, or, rather, a septum, behind. On either side, also, and particularly in its upper portions, it presents two grooves, an anterior and a posterior, which divide it into anterior, lateral and posterior columns. From the anterior groove emerge the anterior roots of the nerves, while the posterior roots emerge slightly in front of the posterior groove.

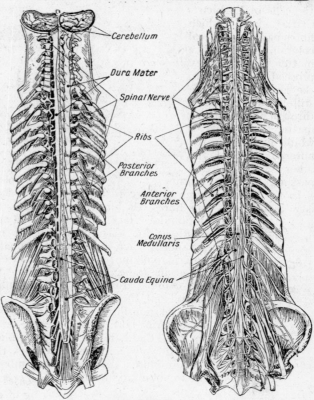

Cerebellum

Dura Mater

Spinal Nerve

Ribs

Posterior Branches

Anterior Branches

Conus Medullaris

Cauda Equina

Spinal Cord. Left, exposed from the back; right, from the front

In a cross section of the cord it will be noted that the grey matter occupies the central part, and has a shape somewhat like the letter H. The cross piece is known as the posterior commissure, and down its centre passes the central canal of the spinal cord, which is blind at its lower end, but above opens into the fourth ventricle of the brain. The projections of the H represent the anterior and the posterior cornua or horns respectively.

In the grey matter are numerous groups of nerve cells. Those in the anterior horn give origin to the fibres of the anterior roots, which are efferent fibres. The posterior root consists of afferent fibres, and these are connected with nerve cells in the root ganglia. These fibres, on entering the cord, have different destinations. Some pass into the posterior columns of white matter on the same side and upwards to the cerebrum; others pass to cells known as the cells of Lockhart-Clarke, from which fibres pass to a lateral column of white matter in which they proceed upwards to the cerebellum; while still others pass through the grey matter to columns of white matter in the anterior part of the other side; these pass up to the cerebrum.

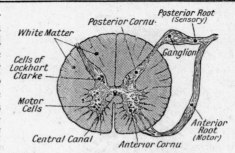

Spinal Cord. The grey matter, enclosed within the white, is roughly in the shape of the letter H

In the lateral column of the cord there is a bundle of white fibres, the crossed pyramidal tract, and another, the direct pyramidal tract, in the anterior column. The fibres in these tracts are coming from the brain, and they come into relationship with the anterior horn cells. In fact, they are the fibres down which pass the impulses giving rise to voluntary movements.

It will be seen that one important function of the cord is to serve as a conducting cable, as it were, between the brain and other parts of the body, the nerve fibres being grouped together in bundles, or tracts, according to their function and the parts they supply. The other function of the cord is to act as a reflex centre. Some of the afferent fibres pass forward in the grey matter to arborise round motor cells in the anterior horn, thus completing a reflex arc—sensory nerve endings in the skin or elsewhere, afferent fibres, nerve centres in the cord, efferent fibres, and muscles whereby the reflex action is produced.

The spinal nerves have a segmental distribution which is most clearly seen in the thoracic nerves, each of which passes round beneath a rib, thus supplying a ring of the body tissues. Below the

Horizontal emergence of upper nerve roots

seventh rib the terminations of the intercostal nerves are in the anterior abdominal wall, that of the tenth, for example, being in the region of the umbilicus. This explains why a pain in the abdomen, which may be thought to indicate appendicitis, or some other abdominal lesion, may actually be due to pleurisy. The budding-out of the limbs rather obscures the segmental distribution of some of the nerves, but it is quite easy to map out the distribution of any spinal nerve, and when symptoms of disease affect the area of this distribution inflammation of the nerve root, or radiculitis, or of its main stem, is indicated.

In three regions spinal nerves form a plexus, or network, from which branches are supplied to various parts. Thus, there is the cervical, the brachial and the lumbo-sacral plexus.

Diseases of the Spinal Cord. A severe jarring of the body may cause concussion of the spinal cord, the result of which is paralysis of the parts supplied by the affected parts of the cord. This will probably clear up, however, with complete rest. The continuity of the cord may be interrupted more or less by myelitis (*q.v.*), caused by pressure from disease

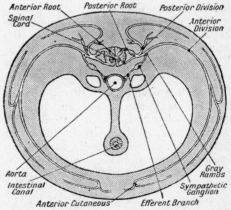

Schema of a spinal nerve. Each nerve is distributed in two divisions to skin and muscles

or dislocation of the spine, tumours or haemorrhage of the spinal canal or cord, etc. In the disease known as syringomyelia (*q.v.*), cavities form in the grey matter interrupting the fibres conducting impulses of temperature and pain, and interfering with the nutrition of parts supplied by the affected portion of the cord.

Interruption of tracts in the cord may be caused by a hardening process in the nervous tissue described as sclerosis (*q.v.*). Inflammation in the grey matter is called poliomyelitis, and is discussed under the heading Infantile Paralysis.

Spinal meningitis may be caused by extension from the meninges of the brain, as in cerebro-spinal fever, or occur independently, when the cause may be a penetrating or other injury, or infection. Tuberculous infection, for example, may extend to the spinal meninges from the vertebrae, in Pott's disease. Amongst the symptoms are pain, rigidity of the spine, paralysis and wasting of various muscles, loss of sensation, and so on.

See Ataxia ; Cerebro-spinal Fever ; Friedreich's Ataxia ; Myelitis ; Nervous System ; Progressive Muscular Atrophy ; Spina Bifida.

SPINAL CURVATURE. The structure of the spine is described under the heading Backbone, where it is noted that the spine, though straight when viewed from the back, presents four curves when viewed from the side, namely, one in the neck

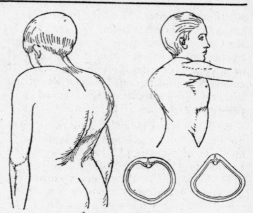

Left, kyphosis due possibly to physical toil ; right, projection associated with Pott's disease. Below, cross section of chest in each condition

and another in the lumbar region, with the convexity forwards, and one in the back, or dorsal region, and another in the sacrum with the convexity backwards.

The deformity referred to as spinal curvature may be an exaggeration of one of those curves or it may be a new curve, that is to say, in a lateral direction and visible when the spine is looked at from behind. Exaggeration of the normal backward dorsal curve is called kyphosis, or, if there is a sharp backward projection, angular curvature ; exaggeration of the forward lumbar curve, lordosis ; and lateral curvature, scoliosis.

Kyphosis, commonly known as round shoulders, may be associated with a disappearance or even reversal of the lumbar curve, producing the so-called C type of deformity, the whole spine curving backwards. This sometimes happens in rickets from softness of the bones, and in old people from thinning of the intervertebral disks. Kyphosis is sometimes due to other disorders involving the bones or joints of the spine, such as osteomalacia, osteitis deformans or osteo-arthritis, but the commonest cause is habitual stooping. This faulty posture is encouraged in school-children by short-sightedness and it is also incidental to cobbling and other trades. A factor in causing kyphosis, especially in children, is a loss of tone in the muscles of the back.

Lordosis occurs in stout people, in cases of large abdominal tumours and during pregnancy, and in these instances, by

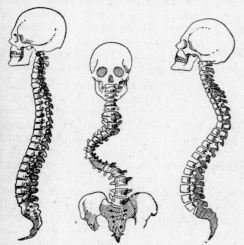

Spinal Curvature. Left, normal curves of spine ; right, kyphosis with exaggerated forward lumbar curve (lordosis) ; centre, severe kypho-scoliosis

shifting the centre of gravity further back, corrects a tendency to fall forwards. For the same reason it is seen in pseudo-hypertrophic paralysis of the calves and in atrophy of the lumbar muscles. It occurs also in congenital dislocation of the hip and hip-joint disease in order to compensate for flexion at the joints.

Scoliosis is occasionally present at birth and caused by imperfect development of one side of a vertebra. It may be caused by rickets, by shortness of one leg, by wry-neck, by hip-joint disease or by empyema, but the usual cause is a loss of tone in the muscles of the back with, sometimes, the additional factor of faulty posture (*see* Plate XXXII, 4).

In addition to the lateral curvature of the spine there is rotation of the bodies of the vertebrae so that one shoulder

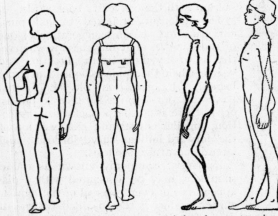

Spinal curvature resulting in young people from incorrect carriage. Correct postures are shown in the second and fourth diagrams

projects backwards or "grows out." There may also be an associated kyphosis.

The loss of tone in the muscles which counts for so much in the production of the postural spinal curvatures may result from an acute fever, or another debilitating illness, but can sometimes be attributed to chronic constipation, infection in the tonsils or ears, adenoids, or to overwork and an insufficiency of open-air exercise.

Angular curvature is oftenest due to tuberculous diseases of the spine or Pott's disease (*q.v.*), which usually begins in early life, but in older people may be caused by cancer of the spine or by an injury involving displacement of vertebrae.

The treatment of spinal curvature depends on the cause. In the postural type the first object is to restore muscular tone by cleaning up sources of toxaemia and by improving the general health by fresh air, good food and tonics, such as iron, arsenic and cod-liver oil. In addition to this the child should carry out prescribed exercises, under careful supervision. Children with short sight should be fitted with proper glasses.

It is important that this treatment should begin as early as possible; if a curvature is allowed to persist for some time the shape of the bones may alter and there can then be little hope of correcting the deformity.
When the back is very weak it may be desirable for the child to wear a spinal support during some part of the day. The best form is one with steel rods which lie along the spine and are firmly attached to a broad band which passes round the pelvis. Attached to the rods are broad curved plates which are applied to the lower part of the chest at the sides and support it as one might do with the palms of the hands. Other forms of spinal support are made of poroplastic or of leather.

In the other forms of curvature much may be done by correcting the cause, lengthening a leg by a high-heeled boot, for example, but in some cases little can be done. Pain can sometimes be relieved by exercises, but a spinal support will often be needed. It should be said, in conclusion, that before any active treatment for curvature is begun the possibility of Pott's disease must be carefully excluded.

Rigidity of the spine, with a disappearance of the normal curves, a condition often described as "poker-back," occurs when there is inflammation in the joints of the spine, or spondylitis. This may be due to gonorrhoea or to some other infection, and the first step in treatment is to get rid of any such source of poisoning. If the condition is severe, rest in bed is required, and, when the patient gets up and about, a spinal support. In mild cases heat, electrical treatment and massage may be sufficient.

See Backbone; Jacket; Pott's Disease; Rickets.

SPINE. *See* Backbone.

SPIRILLUM. A spirillum is a spiral organism which is rigid. It was confused formerly with the spirochaete, another spiral organism which, however, is not rigid but flexuous, and the organisms that cause relapsing and some other diseases, although sometimes called spirilla, are really spirochaetes (*q.v.*).

SPIRIT. The beverages classed as spirits are brandy, whisky, rum and gin, and contain about fifty per cent. of alcohol. The pharmacopoeial preparations classed as spirits are mostly alcoholic solutions of volatile oils or ethers. A common dose is 5 to 20 minims. Spirit of salt is another name for hydrochloric acid.
See Alcohol ; Methylated Spirit ; Rectified Spirit.

SPIROCHAETE. A genus of spiral bacteria, spirochaetes form many species, some of which cause diseases in man and the lower animals. Among the human diseases due to spirochaetes are included syphilis, yaws, relapsing fever, yellow fever, acute infectious jaundice or Weil's disease, rat-bite fever, Japanese seven-day fever, tropical bronchitis and Vincent's angina.

Under favourable conditions a spirochaete progresses freely by an undulatory movement. Organic preparations of arsenic of the salvarsan order are specific remedies against spirochaetosis, as infection by spirochaetes is called.

SPIROMETER. An instrument called a spirometer is used for testing the vital capacity, that is, the breathing capacity, of the lungs.
See Respiration.

SPITTING. *See* Expectoration.

SPLEEN. The largest of the ductless glands, the spleen is situated in the upper left-hand corner of the abdomen, towards the back and just below the diaphragm. It lies in front of the ninth to the eleventh ribs. Its shape somewhat resembles that of a segment of an orange, and in an adult it weighs rather less than half a pound. It is dark red in colour. Its front edge is usually notched, and when enlarged and the edge comes below the margin of the ribs, the notches can be felt.

The spleen is surrounded by a fibrous capsule from which processes, or trabe-

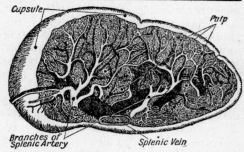

Spleen. Internal structure, showing the large blood vessels which are characteristic of this gland

culae, pass into the interior of the organ, dividing it up into numerous spaces, which are filled with a soft material— the spleen pulp. In this are to be seen numerous small round bodies, the Malpighian corpuscles, which are agglomerations of lymphoid tissue. The blood vessels of the spleen are large. The capillaries into which the artery breaks up open into blood spaces from which other capillaries take their origin and conduct the blood to the splenic vein, which is a tributary of the portal vein.

The spleen contributes new corpuscles, both white and red, to the blood, and in the spleen there is partial destruction of the effete red corpuscles. It also aids in the fight against infection, and probably has other functions. It is not essential to life, however, as there is no interference with health when the organ is removed in consequence of an injury.

The spleen may be ruptured by a crush or a blow, and more readily if it is enlarged, when, in fact, it may even rupture spontaneously. Like other abdominal organs, the spleen may sag downwards, and it has occasionally happened that the displaced organ has been twisted sufficiently to occlude its blood vessels and cause gangrene of the organ.

Enlargement of the spleen, or splenomegaly, may occur from a large number of causes. When acute, it may be associated with considerable pain and tenderness beneath the ribs on the left side, and also in the back, but when chronic the only complaint may be that of fulness or weight on the left side of the abdomen.

In the tropics an acute enlargement of the spleen is most often due to malaria, but kala-azar and other tropical diseases are other possible causes. Enteric fever, streptococcal septicaemia, pyaemia, anthrax and other infections which occur anywhere, are also causes of acute enlargement. Sometimes an abscess occurs on the organ, and this causes acute pain as a rule.

Chronic enlargement may be due to malaria, leukaemia, splenic anaemia, pernicious anaemia, Hodgkin's disease, amyloid disease, hydatid disease, and other disorders, and in some of these the organ may fill the whole of the left side of the abdomen and weigh many pounds. Cancer and other tumours may occur, but only rarely.

Treatment depends on the cause, and, except in splenic anaemia, in which removal of the spleen may cure the disease, is more concerned with other conditions than with the spleen itself.

SPLENIC ANAEMIA. A disease for which changes in the spleen appear to be primarily responsible is described as splenic anaemia. Males are frequently attacked, and usually at or before middle age. Commonly the first indication of the malady that is noticed by the patient is fullness and a sense of weight in the abdomen. There is an increasing pallor and shortness of breath on exertion, and in the course of time the legs show signs of dropsy when the patient has been up and about. There may also be bleeding from mucous membranes, so that blood may be passed in the stools or urine, or be vomited.

Later there is cirrhosis of the liver with jaundice and the accumulation of dropsical fluid in the belly, or ascites. This stage is often referred to as Banti's disease. The infantile affection known as Von Jaksch's disease is possibly of the nature of splenic anaemia.

The treatment at the beginning is usually that of anaemia (*q.v.*) simply, but removal of the spleen is necessary to a radical cure.

SPLINT. Any rigid substance applied to a part of the body in order to prevent movement may be described as a splint. The substance may be wood, metal, leather, poroplastic, plaster of Paris or anything else that answers the purpose. In an emergency, walking-sticks, umbrellas, brooms, bundles of newspapers or of twigs, and many other things may be used to improvise a splint (*see* Plates XVIII and XXXIII).

The most familiar use of splints is in the treatment of fracture, but in certain diseased states splints are equally useful. To prevent movement in a part of a limb it is necessary to fix both the joint above it and the joint below. Unless a splint is well padded it may cause serious damage by pressure, and particular care must be taken to pad over bony prominences like those at the ankle. While the bandages attaching the splints must be sufficiently tight to hold them securely, they should not be tight enough to interfere with the circulation in the limb.

Certain splints are specially named, mostly after the person who first introduced them. Perhaps the most useful of these is Thomas's splint. This is made of metal and consists of a padded ring to go round the hip or shoulder and limbs extending from the ring and united at their other ends (*see* Plate XXXIII, 2 and 4). In the arm splint the limbs are bent at an angle a short distance below the position of the patient's elbow.

A Thomas's splint allows of extension being applied to the bone or joint being treated. Liston's splint is a long splint, reaching from the armpit to below the sole of the foot, and with triangular notches cut in its lower end, thus forming a peg round which bandages can be drawn tightly. A shorter splint, with similar notches, sometimes used in treating Pott's fracture of the fibula (*q.v.*), is known as Dupuytren's splint.

See Bandage; Extension; Fracture; Ischaemia.

SPONGE. The horny skeleton of a marine animal, a sponge is very absorbent and was once much used in surgery for mopping up blood and other discharges, but as it is very difficult to clean it has been almost entirely replaced for such purposes by swabs made of sterile gauze. For toilet purposes, and especially where children are concerned, a sponge with a soft texture should be selected.

SPONGIO - PILINE. An absorbent material made of wool and sponge, spongio-piline is sometimes used for making a fomentation (*q.v.*).

SPONGY GUMS. A soft condition of the gums, with a tendency to bleed readily, is described as spongy gums. This may occur from various causes, including scurvy and over-dosage with mercury. The constitutional cause must be treated and the gums may be bathed with a mouth wash (*q.v.*).

SPORADIC. Isolated cases of infectious diseases are said to be sporadic.
See Epidemic.

SPORE. The seed or reproductive body of bacteria and other low vegetable organisms is called a spore. It is much more resistant to heat and chemicals than the mature form of an organism.

SPOTTED FEVER. Cerebro-spinal fever and typhus fever are sometimes called spotted fever.

SPRAIN. A sudden overstretching of a muscle or of the ligaments of a joint is called a strain when it stops short of actually tearing the structure, but when there is tearing it constitutes a sprain. A strain is followed by little or no swelling of the part, but swelling follows a sprain. If it occurs immediately, it is due to the effusion of blood, if after the lapse of several hours, or a longer period, to inflammatory exudation. Even a strain, however, may cause very acute pain.

When there is effusion of blood into the tissues, there is a red or livid discoloration of the skin, the colour changing to green and then yellow in the course of a few days. Inflammation in a joint may cause, in addition to local heat, pain and tenderness, a painful sense of pressure, or tension, in the joint.

It should be remembered that though an injury to a joint may cause no definite signs of fracture, or dislocation, and appear to be merely due to a sprain, nevertheless a small fragment of bone may be broken off, or there may be slight displacement of the bones. An X-ray examination is desirable when there can be any possible doubt as to the extent of the injury. Sometimes also an important nerve may be damaged.

In the process of repair following a sprain, scar tissue may form adhesions which limit the movements of the joint. The risk of this happening is increased by keeping the joint too long at rest. Another possibility is that a sprain may be followed by osteo-arthritis of the joint.

The first-aid treatment of a strain or sprain of a joint consists of rest and cold applications. If the injury can be treated as soon as it occurs, however, a firm bandage should be applied evenly and smoothly over the joint in order to limit internal bleeding, or if the accident has occurred out of doors the boot should be left on, and a bandage applied over it and wetted. As it dries the bandage shrinks and increases the pressure.

A strain of a joint is often treated by strapping with plaster, but skill is required to do this properly. Strips of plaster long enough to go round the joint and overlap at the ends are put on from below upwards, each overlapping about one-third of the width of the one below it until the whole joint is covered in, as shown in Plate II, 4.

Sprains may be treated by putting a layer of cotton-wool about one inch thick over the joint, and for an inch or two beyond it on either side, and bandaging as firmly as possible, without causing discomfort, with a flannel bandage (*see* Plate XXXIV, 1). The bandage is taken off once or twice a day. Heat may be applied to relieve pain.

The patient should be encouraged to move the joint gently from the outset, and after a few days the joint is moved by the doctor or nurse through its full range ; this is to prevent adhesions. After four or five days massage may be started. Should there be symptoms of acute inflammation, as mentioned above, no movement or massage is permissible.

Strains or sprains of muscles are treated by rest and cold or hot applications. Movements that cause dragging on the injured muscle should be avoided, and by a skilful application of plaster this may be accomplished, although other movements of the limb can be carried out.
See Joint ; Muscle ; Tendon.

SPRAY. A liquid drug or a solution of a drug may be applied to some surface of the body in the form of a spray. Here the liquid is in a state of fine subdivision.

There are different kinds of spray-producing apparatus. Some produce a spray of relatively large particles or a coarse spray, while others produce a very fine cloud-like spray. An apparatus of the latter type is called a cloudiser, nebuliser, vaporiser or atomiser (*q.v.*). In this the liquid is oily, and this type of spray is the better for applying remedies to a surface. A coarse spray is usually a watery spray, and is the best type for cleansing a surface.

A cleansing spray might consist of 5 grains each of sodium bicarbonate and common salt, half a drachm of glycerin and water to one ounce ; or of 2 grains of permanganate of potassium dissolved in an ounce of water. The latter is also antiseptic and deodorant, and is useful as a prophylactic against a common cold or influenza, and when the mouth is foul.

Ether and ethyl chloride are sometimes sprayed on the skin in order to chill it and make it insensitive for the purposes of some little operation. The drug is contained in an air-tight glass cylinder, and by its own evaporation forces a fine jet of liquid through a nozzle.

See Atomiser ; Gargle ; Inhalation.

SPRUE. People living in the tropics, especially Europeans, may suffer from sprue, a disease also known as psilosis, Ceylon sore-mouth and Indian hill diarrhoea. The symptoms at the beginning are suggestive of something that has been eaten having disagreed. There is indigestion and diarrhoea. Then superficial ulcers form in the mouth, and chewing becomes very painful. Diarrhoea occurs in the mornings, copious pale, frothy motions being passed. This may go on for months, and the patient becomes thin and anaemic.

The treatment is to take calcium lactate, 10 to 15 grains, in a cachet, or, failing this, calcium chloride or lime-water, three times a day, and $\frac{1}{10}$ grain of parathyroid extract twice a day. This treatment is kept up for several months after the disease is apparently cured. Diet at the beginning consists of milk, the daily ration of which may be gradually increased, and then light foods. Strawberries may be taken freely. Some doctors give a liberal ration of under-done meat along with milk.

SPUTUM. Substances that are coughed up are referred to as sputum, or expectoration, and usually come from the air tubes or lungs, but sometimes from the throat, when they are more likely to be hawked up. The characters of the sputum may give useful indications of the nature of a pulmonary affection, and of the stage that it has reached. In acute bronchitis the sputum is at first scanty and clear, and, if vomiting is violent, may be streaked with blood. As the disease progresses the sputum becomes more abundant and mixed with pus, or muco-purulent.

A very profuse watery and frothy sputum suggests oedema of the lungs. In bronchiectasis, consumption and even in later stages of bronchitis the sputum may contain a very large amount of pus. If it consists of pure pus, it is likely to be due to the bursting of an abscess into a bronchial tube. Sometimes parts of the sputum appear, in water used for the reception of the sputum, as rounded disks. Such is described as a nummular sputum, and occurs in consumption, but perhaps also in bronchiectasis or chronic bronchitis.

A very adhesive rust-coloured sputum is mainly suggestive of lobar pneumonia, and a prune-juice sputum of gangrene of the lung. The sputum of persons who inhale much smoke or coal-dust may be black. When a tropical abscess of the liver bursts into the lung a dark brown sputum resembling anchovy sauce is coughed up.

When the sputum contains a certain amount of pure or almost pure blood, the occurrence is described as haemoptysis (*q.v.*). The first possibility to be considered in this event is consumption, but heart disease and disease of the blood or the blood vessels are amongst other possible causes.

An offensive, foul-smelling sputum occurs in foetid bronchitis, bronchiectasis, gangrene of the lung, and sometimes in consumption.

. In bronchiectasis large quantities of sputum may be coughed up at one time, and also when there are diseased cavities in the lung, as in consumption. In these diseases it is customary to measure the daily amount of sputum in order to help in forming an opinion as to the progress of the case.

A microscopic examination of the sputum is useful in many cases. In consumption, besides pus, it may reveal fibres of elastic tissue and tubercle bacilli, and germs may also be identified in other sputa. The little pellets coughed up in asthma are revealed as convoluted structures which are known as Curschmann's spirals, and there are also crystals, pointed at each end and called Charcot-Leyden crystals.

See Cough.

SQUILL. The squill bulb contains a bitter active principle, scillitoxin, which stimulates the lining of the air-tubes and also the kidneys, so that the drug is given as an expectorant and diuretic. Its use as an expectorant should be limited to chronic bronchitis, as it is likely to aggravate acute conditions. Similarly it should not be given when there is Bright's disease, its chief use as a diuretic being in cardiac dropsy, when it is generally given in combination with digitalis and mercury. Squill is liable to upset the stomach.

The preparations of squill are the acetum or vinegar, and the tincture, the dose of each being 5 to 15 minims ; the oxymel or honey, dose $\frac{1}{2}$ to 2 drachms ; the syrup, dose $\frac{1}{2}$ to 1 drachm ; the compound pill, dose 4 to 8 grains ; and the pill of ipecacuanha and squill, which contains opium, dose 4 to 8 grains.

In India and the East, a bulb of another species of the same genus of plants is used. Its actions are the same as those of squill and it has the same preparations and doses. The preparations are described as vinegar of urginea and so on.

SQUINT. Failure to focus the vision of both eyes on the same point constitutes a squint, or strabismus. One eye is fixed on the object looked at, but the other is turned from it. If this eye turns inwards the strabismus is said to be convergent ; if outwards, divergent. The commoner type of this disorder, concomitant squint, occurs in children. It is due to some defect in the eye, usually an error of refraction, which may not induce a squint until the general health is impaired, and it is not uncommon for a squint to appear after an illness.

The child learns to ignore the image on the retina of the squinting eye, and thus avoids double vision, which is a prominent symptom in the other type of the disorder, namely, paralytic strabismus. A squint in a child may be disfiguring, however, and failure to use the squinting eye may result in the child being unable to use it for near work or even for detailed vision of large objects.

It is a duty, therefore, to take a child to a doctor as soon as any tendency to squint is observed. Possibly the squint may be cured by wearing suitable glasses, though sometimes the squinting eye must be trained to its work by preventing vision with the other for a time, or exercises with a stereoscope, or some other instrument, may be prescribed. In some cases it is necessary to operate on the muscles of the eyeball.

Paralytic squint is due to interference with the 3rd, 4th, or 6th cranial nerves, which may occur in diphtheria, syphilis and other disorders. Double vision, or diplopia, is the chief symptom, though sometimes there is considerable giddiness. One consequence of double vision is loss of judgement of the position of things. The treatment of a paralytic squint depends on the cause, and recovery can be expected in many cases.

See Binocular ; Double Vision ; Eye ; Vision.

STAMMER. *See* Speech.

STAPHYLOCOCCUS. The round form of bacterium is called a coccus, and when it grows in masses resembling a bunch of grapes, a staphylococcus. Cultures of different species are variously coloured, and white, golden and yellow forms are distinguished. Staphylococci are widely distributed in Nature and are common organisms in pus.

See Bacteria.

STAPHYLOMA. A protrusion of the cornea or of the sclerotic coat of the eye is called a staphyloma.

See Eye.

STARCH. The group of natural carbohydrates called the polysaccharides or polysaccharoses includes starch, cellulose, dextrin, glycogen and some others. Starch is widely distributed in the vegetable kingdom, especially in seeds and tubers. Wheat and other cereals contain about

60 to 70 per cent. ; rice, 75 to 80 per cent. ; tapioca, 87·5 per cent. ; and potatoes, 15 to 20 per cent. Starch occurs as granules, variously shaped according to its source, but always constructed of alternate layers of starch and cellulose around a central nucleus. This structure is plainly seen under the microscope.

Starch is insoluble in cold water but forms an opalescent solution with boiling water, which when it cools hardens into a jelly. Boiling splits the cellulose envelopes and exposes the starch, and for this reason starchy foods require cooking. The salivary ferment cannot digest uncooked starch, though amylopsin, a ferment in the pancreatic juice, can do so. In digestion starch is first converted into dextrin, the sticky substance that is put on the back of postage stamps, and then by further stages is converted into grape sugar. Starch can also be converted into dextrin by dry heat and by the action of weak acids.

Starch must be converted into sugar before it can be absorbed, but is not stored in the body as sugar, but as glycogen, a substance which is akin to starch and which is sometimes called animal starch.

In addition to its dietetic uses, starch has certain medicinal ones. It is included in the pharmacopoeias under its Latin name, amylum. Starch powder is used as a soothing powder for inflamed conditions of the skin, generally in combination with zinc oxide powder. Glycerin of starch is used for the same purpose, but occasionally causes irritation. Mucilage of starch is used as an enema to relieve irritation of the bowel and check diarrhoea, often in combination with laudanum. A solution of starch is an antidote for iodine poisoning.

See Carbohydrate ; Digestion ; Food ; Sugar.

STARVATION. When the body is deprived of food it is thrown upon its reserves of fat and the glycogen stored in the liver and muscles. There comes a time, however, when it even draws on the protein in the muscles to a considerable extent. The most vital organs, the heart and brain, suffer last and least, but on the other hand they may become exhausted from lack of food even before the store of fat is finished. Rest and warmth mitigate to some extent the effects of starvation.

The energies of all the organs are much weakened and care must be exercised in feeding a person who has been starved. The diet ordinarily prescribed for fever (*q.v.*) is the suitable one, with the addition of cod-liver oil if it can be digested.

See Emaciation ; Fasting.

STASIS. Stagnation of a body fluid may be called stasis. Thus a local stasis of the blood occurs in a stage of inflammation, and obstruction of a vein causes venous stasis. This is also called passive congestion. Stasis of lymph from obstruction of lymphatic vessels occurs in filariasis. Intestinal stasis means a very sluggish flow of the contents of the bowel. These are retained unduly long in certain segments, such as the caecum, and poisons are absorbed causing various kinds of illness.

See Constipation.

STATUS LYMPHATICUS. Infants and even older children may have an undue development of the thymus gland (*q.v.*), and probably with this enlargement of the tonsils and of other collections of lymphatic tissue throughout the body. This condition is called the status lymphaticus or lymphatism. The children are usually plump but flabby and may be anaemic, though often the general health appears to be quite satisfactory. There is a tendency to sudden death from slight shocks, and many deaths under anaesthetics are due to lymphatism. Unfortunately, its existence can rarely be recognized beforehand and is only revealed by some such tragedy.

STAVESACRE. The seeds of delphinium staphisagria, generally called stavesacre seeds, are used in the form of an ointment for killing lice and their eggs.

STEEL. Tincture of perchloride of iron is popularly known as steel drops.

STEGOMYIA. A genus of mosquitoes is called stegomyia and includes many species. One of these, stegomyia, or aëdes, fasciata, is the carrier of yellow fever, and other species are also disease carriers.

See Mosquito.

STENOSIS. Narrowing of one of the natural orifices or passages of the body is called stenosis. This may be caused by disease, such as inflammation, a tumour or scar-formation in the walls of the opening, or be due to pressure from something outside the walls. Instances are stenosis of the mitral valve of the heart, stenosis of the gullet and so on.

STENSEN'S DUCT. The main duct of the parotid gland is called Stensen's duct.

STERILISATION. By sterilisation is meant the process of freeing any substance from living micro-organisms. It is necessary to sterilise instruments, dressings, ligatures and other things likely to come into direct or indirect contact with operation or accidental wounds, or which are to be introduced into body-cavities, such as the bladder or uterus. The term wound is to be understood in its widest sense, as including, for example, the prick of a hypodermic needle.

Clothing and other things that have come into contact with a person suffering from an infectious disease must be sterilised, but the word generally used in this connexion is disinfected. To render milk absolutely safe it must be sterilised, though pasteurisation is often considered enough. It should be remembered, however, that this process only kills a proportion of the bacteria contained in milk. Other foods are sterilised to enable them to keep.

The simplest method of sterilising is by exposure to heat, moist heat being the more effective, except when an object can be actually passed through a flame, a common method of sterilising needles. If water is brought to the boil all the mature forms of organism present are killed, but prolonged boiling, probably for some hours, is required to kill the spores. Dressings, operating gowns, towels and other articles are sterilised, when possible, by super-heated steam in an auto-clave. Cutting instruments, whose edges might be blunted by heat, are kept immersed in pure carbolic acid or lysol for some time.

Milk can be sterilised by keeping it for a short time at a temperature of 230° F. This can be done at home in Cathcart's or the Soxhlet apparatus.

See Antiseptic ; Disinfection ; Milk ; Operation.

STERILITY. Barrenness, or sterility, most commonly results from some defect in the female. It may be due to some congenital malformation of the generative organs, a lack of activity in the ovaries, which may also be shown by obesity, or the cause may be some such disorder as displacement of the womb, inflammatory changes in the genital organs or a tumour. Similarly, in the male there may be congenital defects, but the most common cause of inability to procreate, a different thing from sexual impotence, is some consequence of inflammation. The most common cause of inflammation of the genital organs, male or female, it may be added, is gonorrhoea.

Sterility may occur, however, when there is no gross defect, either congenital or acquired. The use of contraceptive methods in the early years of married life and before conception has occurred may make the remaining years of the marriage sterile. The impediment to impregnation may be even more subtle, as the divorced partners of a fruitless union have each proved to be capable of obtaining children in a subsequent marriage.

From what has been said it is clear that a great deal of sterility could be prevented. When a marriage has been fruitless for two years it is desirable that the wife, and possibly the husband also, should be examined. Some of the disorders above-mentioned can be rectified by treatment, operative or otherwise, but others are hopeless.

See Genital System.

STERNUM. The breast-bone, or sternum, has been likened in shape to a Roman sword and consists of three portions. The uppermost is called the manubrium, or handle ; the middle, the gladiolus, or blade ; and the lowest, or point, the xiphoid, or ensiform, cartilage. The inner end of the collar-bone rests on the manubrium, and the upper six ribs are joined to the side of the sternum by their cartilaginous portions.

STETHOSCOPE. Auscultation, or the examination of a patient by listening over his body, is usually performed with a stethoscope, an instrument of which there are several types. One consists of a single tube with a funnel-shaped chest-piece and a broad, flat ear-piece. Another, the binaural, has two rubber tubes to conduct the sound to both ears. There are various modifications of the chest-piece with the object of multiplying the volume of the sound.

See Auscultation.

STICKING PLASTER. *See* Adhesive Plaster.

STIFF NECK. The commonest cause of stiff neck is muscular rheumatism or fibrositis, but before any active treatment is undertaken it is desirable to eliminate other possible causes.

See Fibrositis ; Wry Neck.

STILL BIRTH. A still birth must be notified to the Medical Officer of Health within 36 hours after birth. A still-born child is one with a total length of over thirteen inches, and which shows no sign of life whatever at birth. If the birth takes place after the 28th week of pregnancy it must also be registered.

STILL'S DISEASE. A rather uncommon disorder found in children, which passes under the name of Still's disease, is characterised by a subacute inflammation of the joints and enlargement of lymphatic glands and the spleen. It is believed to be due to an unidentified germ. The general health must be improved by fresh air, good feeding and sunlight. Exposure to ultra-violet rays from lamps has proved particularly beneficial. A watch must be maintained against the development of deformities.

STIMULANT. The action of a stimulant may be more or less general in its scope, or be confined to some particular organ. A general stimulant increases the sense of well-being, removing fatigue, quickening and cheering the mind and making bodily exertion easier. Such effects are commonly ascribed to alcohol, and alcoholic liquors hold a high position as stimulants in the popular estimate. The grounds for this reputation are largely illusory, however, as, although alcohol in small doses stimulates digestion and, for a short time, the heart, its main action is that of a narcotic.

Tea, coffee and other beverages containing caffeine act as true general stimulants in the sense above described, but other things than drugs may do so, such as sunshine, a sea breeze or good news.

The use of general stimulants is well-nigh universal and in moderation does no harm and probably much good, but any excess is very detrimental. Also, while the occasional use of a stimulant to tide a tired body or mind over an emergency may be allowable, stimulation when rest has become entirely necessary may have disastrous effects.

Local stimulants are classified according to the particular organ that they affect. Thus, there are cardiac stimulants, such as ammonia, camphor or even hot water ; digestive stimulants, such as condiments and bitters ; intestinal stimulants, such as aloes and salts ; and so on.

See Tonic.

STING. *See* Bee Sting.

STOMACH. The portion of the alimentary tract extending from the lower end of the oesophagus, or gullet, to the beginning of the duodenum, or first part of the small intestine, is called the stomach. Its shape differs according as it is full or empty. When full, it is somewhat pear-shaped, but the narrow, or pyloric, part is placed horizontally, running to the right, while the rest, the cardiac part, is more vertical. The uppermost part rises above and to the left of the opening of the gullet into the stomach and is known as the fundus of the stomach. It reaches as high as the left sixth costal cartilage, and is usually filled with air. When distended by flatulence, it may press on the heart and cause palpitation.

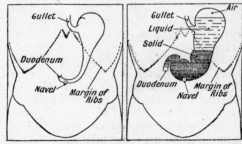

Stomach. Its outline when empty and when full

The part of the stomach between the fundus and the pyloric portion is usually called the body. The opening from the gullet into the stomach is called the cardiac opening, and from the stomach into the duodenum the pyloric opening. The part of the outline of the stomach connecting these openings on the right, or posterior side, is called the lesser curvature, and the part on the other side the greater curvature, the latter being four or five times the length of the former. When the stomach is empty it forms a tube simply, except that the bulging of the fundus persists.

The stomach is covered with peritoneum, and from the greater curvature the layers of this membrane are prolonged downwards to form the apron-like structure known as the great omentum. Similarly from the lesser curvature the membrane is prolonged upwards to the liver to form the lesser or gastro-hepatic omentum. Other folds connect the stomach with the spleen and with the diaphragm. Below, the stomach is in close relation to the pancreas.

There are three muscular coats in the stomach, an outer or longitudinal, a middle or circular, and an inner or oblique. At the pyloric opening the circular coat is greatly thickened to form what is called the pyloric sphincter, which, by contracting, is able to shut off the stomach from the bowel.

The stomach is lined by a mucous coat, between which and the muscle coats there is a layer of loose, fibrous tissue called the submucous coat. In this run blood vessels, lymphatics and nerves, branches of the right and left vagus, and fibres from the sympathetic system. When the stomach is empty the mucous coat is thrown into folds or rugae, most of them being longitudinal; these are smoothed out as the stomach fills up.

The internal surface of the stomach, when viewed through a magnifying glass, displays an immense number of small openings which represent the ducts by which the gastric glands pour their secretion into the stomach. These glands are tiny tubular structures in the mucous coat, lined with cells, which secrete the digestive ferment pepsin and the milk-curdling ferment rennin. There are no other cells in the pyloric glands, but in the glands elsewhere there are cells

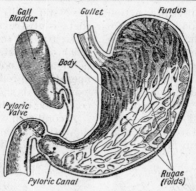

Stomach. The lining is of mucous membrane which forms folds when the organ is empty but smoothes out when it fills

which, because they are situated outside the others, are called parietal cells, and because they secrete the hydrochloric acid of the gastric juice, oxyntic cells.

In addition to these substances and water, of which it contains a very large amount, gastric juice contains some mucus and a small quantity of a fat-splitting ferment or lipase. Gastric juice is being secreted all the time, but in the intervals of digestion is neutralised, partly by regurgitation of the alkaline secretion of the duodenum and partly by an alkaline secretion from pyloric glands. An increased flow for digestion may be stimulated psychically, that is, by the thought, smell or sight of food, by the swallowing of food, and sometimes by an internal secretion known as gastrin. About every twenty seconds a wave of contraction passes along the stomach from the fundus to the pylorus, and the sensation of hunger is probably due to these contractions becoming more vigorous. During digestion the contractions cause partially digested food to pass into the duodenum in the form of chyme.

The actions of the gastric juice are discussed under the heading Digestion. Besides digesting and liquefying food,

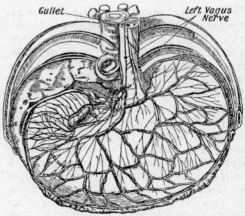

Front view, showing the larger blood vessels and the fine ramifications of the nerve supply

the gastric juice has an antiseptic action on bacteria contained in food.

Diseases of the Stomach. Indigestion, inflammation of the stomach lining or gastritis, and gastric ulcer are discussed under those headings. An increase in the amount of gastric juice causes acidity, or hyperchlorhydria. If the juice contains too little hydrochloric acid the condition is called hypochlorhydria. This may occur in gastritis and certain n e r v e disorders. An absence of hydrochloric acid, described as achlorhydria, or achylia gastrica, occurs sometimes without any evidences of indigestion. It may be found, however, in association with pernicious anaemia and other disorders, including cancer of the stomach, in which it is a very constant feature.

Dilatation of the stomach is caused by narrowing, or stenosis, of the pyloric opening, or by atony or weakness of the muscle wall, induced by constant overfilling of the organ, or otherwise. Pyloric stenosis may be due to the contraction of scars of ulceration, to cancer, or to hypertrophy of the pyloric sphincter. Congenital hypertrophic stenosis is sometimes found in infants, and causes pain, vomiting and wasting. The obstruction, however, may exist in the duodenum from scarring, gall-stones, etc., within it, or from outside pressure by growths, etc.

When the stomach is dilated it may contain large quantities of fluid in which fermentation occurs, and which is vomited from time to time, the vomited matter usually being greyish in colour, with a sour smell, and showing a frothy scum on the surface when it is allowed to stand. In thin people the peristaltic movements of the stomach may be visible. When the fact of dilatation is established, the next step will be to determine whether there is obstruction and its cause.

Treatment consists in daily lavage (*q.v.*) of the stomach, though it will be necessary to consider the question of an operation to relieve obstruction when this exists. Meals should be small and frequent, consisting chiefly of meat.

A condition which may be confused with dilatation is that of dropped stomach, or gastroptosis. This usually occurs in association with sagging of the abdominal viscera generally, or visceroptosis (*q.v.*).

Cancer of the stomach usually occurs in late middle life, and more frequently in men than in women. There is sometimes a history of a gastric ulcer, or of bouts of indigestion, but often there is nothing of the kind. It should be considered a suspicious circumstance when dyspepsia occurs in a middle-aged man, previously free from anything of the kind, particularly when the symptoms are not entirely removed by ordinary simple treatment. The suspicion may be groundless, but the possibility of cancer should be thoroughly investigated.

Cancer usually manifests itself first as dyspepsia, and there may be little or no real pain, though later on pain may be severe and more or less constant. Sometimes there is vomiting, and there may be blood in the vomit, but it is not likely to be copious, and generally will have been altered by the gastric juice and look like coffee grounds. From a fairly early stage, however, it may be possible by microscopical examination to discover blood in the stools. Later the stools may be tarry. The patient loses flesh and becomes anaemic. If the growth is at the pyloric end of the stomach, as is most often the

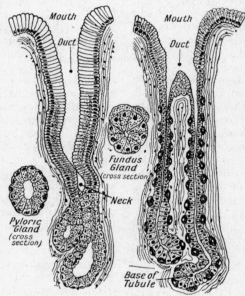

Stomach. Gastric glands, source of the juice

case, there may be evidence of dilatation of the stomach, and if at the cardiac opening, difficulty in swallowing. A microscopic examination and a chemical analysis of the stomach contents are also helpful, but early and reliable information is usually furnished by an X-ray examination.

It is important that the disease should be diagnosed at the earliest possible opportunity, as an operation then may cure it, but if time has been given for the growth to invade adjoining organs, or to be carried to distant organs, the condition is hopeless.

Rupture of the stomach may be caused by a blow when the organ is full, but this occurrence is uncommon. The usual cause of rupture is perforation of a simple or a malignant ulcer. Rupture usually causes considerable shock, but this may be recovered from in an hour or two, and the patient may complain of little more than thirst. Liquids should be withheld, however, and the patient should attempt to relieve his thirst by sucking a pebble. Immediate surgical treatment is urgently necessary.

See Digestion ; Gastric Ulcer ; Gastritis ; Indigestion.

STOMACHIC. A drug that stimulates the flow of gastric juice is called a stomachic. Most bitter, aromatic, pungent and spirituous substances, such as nux vomica, fennel, mustard and wine are stomachics. Alkalies, such as bicarbonate of sodium, when taken about 20 minutes before a meal, also act in this way.

See Appetite ; Bitters ; Indigestion.

STOMACH PUMP. A pump with a long rubber tube attached is sometimes used to draw off the contents of the stomach, but the usual instrument for this purpose is the stomach tube, which is used as a siphon. The tube is about 39 inches long and may have a funnel-shaped expansion at its upper end, or a glass funnel is fitted.

See Forcible Feeding ; Lavage.

STOMATITIS. Inflammation of the mouth (*q.v.*) is called stomatitis. There are several varieties.

STONE. *See* Calculus.

STOPPAGE OF THE BOWELS. The urgent forms of constipation, often described as stoppage of the bowels, are discussed under the heading Obstruction.

STRABISMUS. *See* Squint.

STRAIN. The causes, symptoms and treatment of strain of a muscle or joint are described under the heading Sprain. A strain of the heart, voice, etc., is in effect a muscular strain.

STRAMONIUM. The leaves of the thorn apple, datura stramonium, contain hyoscyamine and atropine. The drug is chiefly used in asthma and in the form of fumigatory powders or cigarettes, but there is also a tincture which is sometimes given. *See* Asthma.

STRANGULATION. The term strangulation is used in two senses. It may mean strangling or throttling, which is a cause of asphyxia (*q.v.*), or it may mean the cutting off of the blood supply of an organ by constriction. Unless the constriction is speedily removed the organ will die, or mortify. The commonest instance of this kind of strangulation is in a hernia (*q.v*).

STRANGURY. An urgent desire to pass urine, accompanied by severe pain, and the passage of a few drops only or none at all, is described as strangury, or vesical tenesmus. The passage of urine does not relieve the pain nor the feeling of an urgent necessity to pass more. Something of this kind may happen from the presence of gravel, but in an aggravated form is more likely to be due to stone, inflammation of the bladder or prostate, or of the urethra, as in gonorrhoea. In women it may be caused by prolapse of the womb, or some other disorder of the womb or ovaries. It also results from taking certain drugs such as turpentine and cantharides. It sometimes occurs as a nervous disorder, as in the vesical crisis of locomotor ataxy.

Hot hip baths and fomentations are helpful, and the patient should drink large quantities of bland liquids. Often, however, opiates are required. While these measures may secure much immediate relief, it is necessary at the same time to seek out the cause of the strangury and correct it when possible.

STREPTOCOCCUS. The round type of bacterium is called a streptococcus when it occurs in chains resembling tiny strings of beads. Streptococci cause many diseased conditions. They are present in spreading inflammations, like erysipelas and cellulitis, in puerperal fever, septicaemia, pyaemia and many abscesses. They are also thought to have a possible connexion with scarlet fever and acute rheumatism.

See Bacteria.

STREPTOTHRIX. A vegetable parasite which is supposed to occupy an intermediate position between bacteria and fungi, a streptothrix consists of filaments or threads. Actinomycosis and Madura foot are diseases caused by a streptothrix.

STRICTURE. A narrowing of one of the natural canals of the body is described as stricture. The commonest sites are the urethra, the gullet and the intestine. The stricture may be an organic one, that is, caused by such changes as ulceration and consequent scarring, or a new growth in the walls of the canal, or it may be simply spasmodic, the muscle fibres in or around the walls of the canal being contracted. In some situations a stricture is generally referred to as stenosis (*q.v.*).

STRIDOR. A harsh, creaking or whistling sound produced in the act of breathing is called stridor. Stridulous breathing is due to obstruction in the larynx, and this may be caused by diphtheritic membrane, oedema, paralysis or spasm of the vocal cords or something else.

See Croup ; Diphtheria ; Larynx ; Rickets.

STROKE. Generally used as a colloquial name for apoplexy, the term stroke also occurs in the name heat stroke or sunstroke and sometimes is applied to sudden attacks of illness of other kinds.

STRONTIUM. A metallic element, belonging to the group of alkaline earths, strontium is sometimes used in medicine in the form of the bromide, iodide, phosphate or some other salt. It is well tolerated by the body.

STROPHANTHUS. The seeds of strophanthus kombé contain a glucoside, strophanthin, and have medicinal actions resembling those of digitalis. The action on the heart is more powerful than that of digitalis but the diuretic action is less pronounced. There are two official preparations, the tincture and the extract.

See Digitalis.

STROPHULUS. Various skin disorders have been given the name strophulus, including the so-called gum-rash. Strophulus albidus is the condition of milium (*q.v*). Strophulus is now generally taken to mean the disease known as lichen urticatus, which is discussed under the heading Nettle-rash.

STRYCHNINE. *See* Nux Vomica.

STUPOR. The state of diminished consciousness which may be caused by poisoning, head injuries or brain diseases is described as stupor. If, however, there is profound unconsciousness, so that the patient cannot be aroused, coma is the name given to the condition.

Stupor also occurs without any organic cause in the subjects of a psycho-neurosis and in insanity. In the insane stupor may almost mimic death, the patient taking absolutely no notice of anything and requiring to be artificially fed. In others answers may be given to questions and there may be temporary awakenings. Though this may go on for many months the patient eventually recovers.

See Catalepsy ; Ecstasy.

STUTTER. *See* Speech.

STYE. A hordeolum, or stye, is a little abscess at the root of one of the eyelashes, caused by infection of the

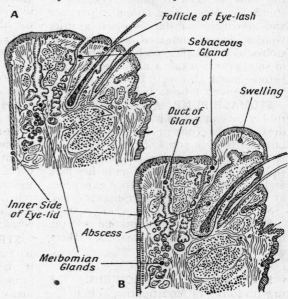

Stye. A, rim of normal eyelid, showing eyelash emerging from its follicle, and the sebaceous and meibomian glands. B, abscess in a sebaceous gland, constituting a stye

PLATE XXXV

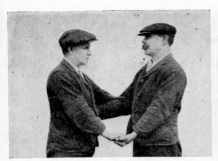

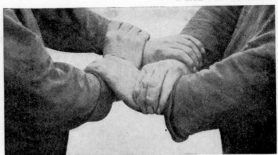

Transport of Sick and Injured.   1 (top left).   Hook-grip forming two-handed seat.   2 (above).   Four-handed seat

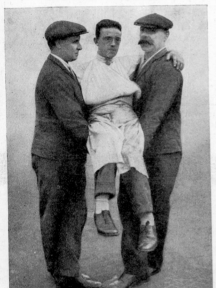

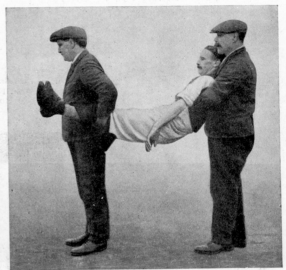

3. Patient supporting himself on a hand-seat.   4. Helpless patient carried by the fore and aft method

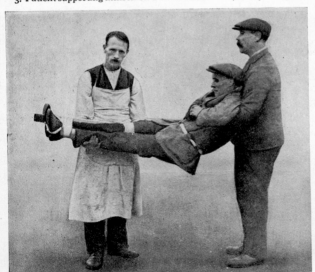

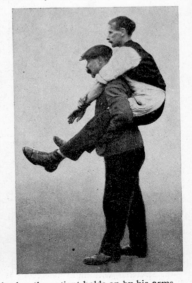

5. Variant of fore and aft method when a leg is injured.   6. Pick-a-back ; the patient holds on by his arms

PLATE XXXVI

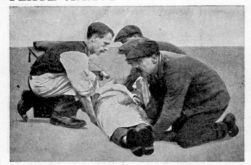

Transport of Sick and Injured. 1. Preparing to place a helpless patient on a stretcher

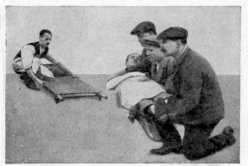

2. Patient placed on the right knees of three bearers while the fourth brings the stretcher

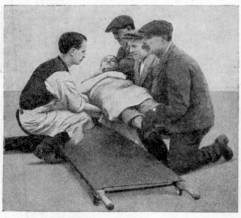

3. The stretcher is placed in position and the fourth bearer helps to lower the patient

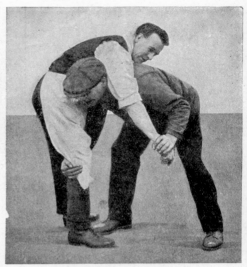

4. Fireman's Lift. A helpless patient is raised to his knees and then to his feet as shown

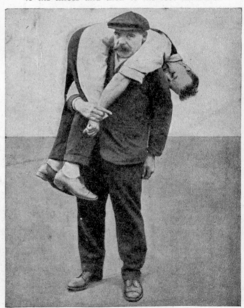

5. Final stage of fireman's lift, the bearer having one hand free to steady himself

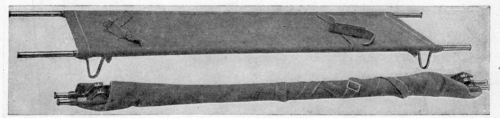

6. Stretcher with light telescopic steel frame. It folds and opens by means of self-locking steel bars

Courtesy of John Ward, Ltd.

sebaceous glands in the margin of the lid. There is first a little red and very painful swelling at the root of the lash, which in the course of a few days becomes yellowish on the top and bursts, the discharge of matter relieving all the symptoms.

Treatment consists in pulling out the affected lash and applying hot fomentations. Frequently the general health is unsatisfactory and tonics, such as syrup of iodide of iron and cod-liver oil, may be required. If the patient suffers from acne an attempt should be made to clear this up. When styes tend to recur in one who appears to enjoy good health otherwise, the eyesight should be tested, as glasses may be needed.

See Blepharitis ; Eye.

STYPTIC. A substance that arrests bleeding is called a haemostatic or styptic. The simplest and most reliable method of stopping bleeding is by pressure, but when this cannot be done readily a styptic is used.

Cold water or ice is often valuable and sometimes, as in bleeding from the womb, very hot water. Chemical styptics include vinegar, oil of turpentine, the tincture, or preferably the strong solution, of perchloride of iron, alum, copper, zinc or lead salts, tannic acid and substances containing this, such as witch-hazel, kino, krameria and red gum.

One of the most powerful styptics is adrenalin, which may be used internally or externally. Preparations of ergot are used internally. To increase the coagulability of the blood horse-serum and sometimes human serum are injected, as in haemophilia, for example.

At one time matico leaves and spiders' webs were recognized styptics, but these are now considered unclean and possibly infective. Moreover, their action was purely mechanical and can be imitated by a thin layer of cotton wool.

See Bleeding ; Ligature ; Tourniquet.

SUBCLAVIAN. The subclavian artery and vein are large, important blood vessels passing from the root of the neck out to the upper limb. On the right side the artery springs from the innominate artery ; on the left, straight from the aortic arch. It passes over the first rib, upon which it can be compressed for arresting bleeding. The vein on each side joins the corresponding innominate vein.

See Bleeding ; Collar Bone.

SUBCUTANEOUS. An adjective meaning beneath the skin, the term subcutaneous is used in various connexions, as, for example, subcutaneous fascia or subcutaneous injection. The latter is also called a hypodermic injection.

See Injection.

SUBLINGUAL GLAND. The smallest of the salivary glands, the sublingual lies in the floor of the mouth, one on either side of the middle line, beneath the fore part of the tongue. It has eight or ten ducts, which open into the floor of the mouth.

See Ranula ; Saliva ; Salivary Gland.

SUBMAXILLARY GLAND. A pair of salivary glands, lying between the tongue and lower jaw on either side, the submaxillary glands are larger than the sublinguals but smaller than the parotids. The duct of the gland is known as Wharton's duct and opens into the mouth by the side of the frenum of the tongue.

See Saliva ; Salivary Gland.

SUBSULTUS TENDINUM. An involuntary twitching, especially of the hands and feet, seen in the extreme depression that may follow typhoid and other fevers is called subsultus tendinum.

SUCCUS. The Latin word for juice, succus occurs in the technical name of the pharmacopoeial, and sometimes of the digestive, juices.

See Juice.

SUDAMINA. An eruption consisting of tiny vesicles caused by retention of sweat in the ducts of the sweat glands is sometimes called sudamina, or sudamen.

See Miliaria.

SUDORIFIC. A diaphoretic, or an agent that increases perspiration, is called a sudorific when it acts powerfully. Pilocarpine, for example, is generally sudorific in its effect.

See Diaphoretic ; Sweat.

SUFFOCATION. *See* Asphyxia.

SUFFUSION. The flow of a body-fluid into the surrounding tissues may be called suffusion. Thus, after a sprain the soft parts round the joint may be suffused with blood which has escaped from the torn blood vessels, or after crying the eyes may look puffy and swollen from an effusion of lymph into the conjunctiva and lids. The term is also applied to pouring water over a patient as a method of treatment.

SUGAR. The sweet class of carbohydrates comprises the sugars. There are different kinds of sugar, but it will suffice to mention two groups, which are of importance to health. The first is that of the hexoses, a sub-group of the monosaccharides or monosaccharoses. This includes dextrose, also called glucose and grape sugar ; laevulose, also called fruit sugar and fructose ; invert sugar, which is a mixture of dextrose and laevulose ; and galactose.

Dextrose exists in all fruits, and is prepared commercially by boiling starch with acids. Starch is converted into glucose during digestion, and sugar can only be absorbed as glucose or laevulose. It is glucose that is present in the urine in diabetes mellitus. Laevulose is present in many fruits. Invert sugar exists naturally as honey, but can be prepared by boiling cane sugar or by the action of dilute acids or of ferments on cane sugar. Thus it is formed in the stomach by the action of hydrochloric acid and in the bowel by a ferment. Galactose is formed by the digestion of lactose, or milk sugar.

The second group of sugars to be considered is that of the disaccharides or disaccharoses. To this group belongs cane sugar, sucrose or saccharose. This is obtained from the sugar cane but also from other sources, such as the beet and the maple. Barbados and Demerara sugars are unrefined forms of cane sugar, and treacle, or molasses, and golden syrup are by-products in its manufacture. In this group are also maltose, which is formed by the action of ferments on starch either in germinating grain or malt, or in the digestive tract, and lactose, or milk sugar. This is less soluble in water than the other sugars and therefore less sweet.

Sugar is a very valuable food, and in Great Britain the average annual consumption per head amounts to 90 pounds. It is a source of energy. There is a tendency, however, to take too much sugar, and the excess is responsible for indigestion and for obese flabbiness in some children.

Strong solutions of sugar are rather irritating, and the constant handling of sugar sometimes causes grocers' eczema.
See Carbohydrate ; Digestion ; Saccharin.

SUGAR OF LEAD. *See* Lead.

SUGGESTION. One of the methods of psycho-therapy is that of suggestion, making a statement of fact to a patient, which he accepts without exercising his judgement upon it.
See Auto-suggestion ; Psycho-therapy.

SULPHATE. A salt of sulphuric acid is called a sulphate. The medicinal action of a sulphate depends mainly on the substance with which the acid is combined, as, for example, iron sulphate, quinine sulphate and magnesium sulphate, or Epsom salt.

SULPHONAL. A popular hypnotic, sulphonal occurs as a powder made up of colourless crystals and is tasteless and odourless. It is only slightly soluble in cold water but dissolves fairly readily in hot water and alcohol. It is generally taken in hot milk and, as it is slow in action, preferably three or four hours before bedtime. The dose is 10 to 30 grains. It is of no avail in sleeplessness due to pain, but otherwise produces natural sleep without ill effects, except that some people feel somewhat tired and depressed on the following day. Sometimes also it brings out a rash.

Poisoning by Sulphonal. If the drug is taken regularly for some time symptoms of poisoning may appear, such as nervousness, giddiness and abdominal pain. A constant symptom of poisoning is a port-wine colour of the urine, caused by a breaking down of the red blood corpuscles. Should any such signs occur the drug should be discontinued at once. If an overdose of sulphonal has been swallowed the treatment is that of narcotic poisoning.
See Insomnia ; Poisoning.

SULPHUR. Brimstone, or sulphur, is a yellow, non-metallic element, and is used in medicine in the form of sublimed sulphur, or flowers of sulphur, a gritty greenish yellow powder, or of precipitated sulphur, or milk of sulphur, a greyish-yellow powder, which is free from grittiness. The dose of each of these is 10 to

60 grains. The sublimed form is more commonly used, and may be taken with sugar, or in molasses or marmalade.

A pleasant way of taking it is as the confection of sulphur which contains cream of tartar also, with flavouring substances, and is used in doses of 60 to 120 grains. With the exception that the sulphur is in the precipitated form, the lozenges of sulphur may have the same composition as the confection. Each contains 5 grains of sulphur, and 1 to 6 lozenges are taken as a dose. Sulphur is the principal ingredient of the compound liquorice powder.

Sulphur is used internally as a laxative, in certain skin diseases, in chronic rheumatism, etc. It is contained in an old remedy for rheumatism, known as the Chelsea pensioner, an electuary which contains guaiacum (q.v.) and other drugs also. Sulphurated lime is sometimes used in pills to prevent suppuration in acne, etc.

Applied externally, sulphur is a parasiticide, and is the best remedy for scabies, or the itch. It is generally used as sulphur ointment, but sometimes as Vleminckx's solution, which is made by boiling slaked lime and sulphur in water. Another method is to use a sulphur bath, made by mixing 5 ounces of sulphurated potassium in a large warm bath.

Sulphur is used externally for other skin diseases such as dandruff, seborrhoea or acne. For dandruff, the ointment may be used, but for other complaints about 5 grains of sulphur is incorporated with an ounce of Lassar's paste. The drug is irritating to the skin, and care must be exercised in its use. Colloidal sulphur is sometimes used internally or externally in preference to the ordinary form of the drug. A sulphur candle affords an excellent method of disinfecting by fumigation. *See* Disinfection.

SULPHURIC ACID. A heavy, colourless, oily liquid, sulphuric acid, or oil of vitriol, is a powerful caustic. Dilute sulphuric acid and aromatic sulphuric acid are sometimes given to arrest bleeding from the stomach or upper reaches of the bowel. The dose of each is 5 to 20 minims. The dilute acid is also used in the prevention and cure of lead poisoning. *See* Caustic.

SULPHUROUS ACID. A solution in water of the gas formed when sulphur is burned in air or oxygen, sulphurous acid is a colourless liquid with a strong odour of sulphur. It is given internally, in doses of $\frac{1}{2}$ to 1 drachm, as an antiseptic in gastric fermentation. Externally, it is used in a lotion for ringworm and other parasitic diseases. A good preparation for this purpose is a mixture of equal parts of the acid and glycerin. This is serviceable also for chapped hands.

Salts of the acid are called sulphites. Sodium sulphite, dose 5 to 20 grains, is used for the same purpose as the acid, and also sodium hyposulphite or thiosulphate, dose 10 to 60 grains.

SUNBURN. The tanning of the skin which follows exposure to sunlight is preceded by more or less redness, or erythema, and sometimes by swelling and blistering. Individuals differ in their susceptibility to such effects and some require the protection of suitable headgear and possibly of a simple dusting powder also. Should inflammation be pronounced calamine lotion or zinc ointment may be applied. To remove the tanning cucumber juice and almond emulsion is used.

See Complexion ; Dermatitis ; Freckles ; Light.

SUNLIGHT. The nature of sunlight is discussed under the heading Light, where there is also an account of the therapeutic uses of light, natural and artificial. Injurious effects of the sun are discussed under the headings Dermatitis and Heat Stroke. Another ill effect, but uncommon, is sun-blindness, caused by prolonged gazing at the sun. This has usually happened at the time of a solar eclipse, and sometimes permanent damage has been done to the retina.

SUNSTROKE. *See* Heat Stroke.

SUPPOSITORY. Drugs may be introduced into the rectum in a suppository. This is a cylindrical object, sharpened at one or both ends and consisting of a basis, usually of cacao butter or oil of theobroma, but sometimes of gelatin and glycerin, in which the desired drug is incorporated. There are seven official suppositories, those of carbolic acid, tannic acid, belladonna, glycerin, iodoform, and morphine, and the compound suppository of lead.

A suppository is pushed well into the bowel by a screwing movement and if there is any tendency to extrude it a folded cloth should be held firmly against the anus for a minute. In a short time the suppository melts, liberating the drug.

A suppository for the vagina is larger than the rectal type and generally is egg-shaped. It is usually called a pessary. Ichthyol and other drugs may be used in this way. A similar preparation for introducing drugs into the urethra is long and pencil-shaped. It is known as a bougie. Bougies, known as buginaria, are made for using in the nose, and there are also bougies and cones for putting into the ear ; these are called aurinaria.

SUPPRESSION. The cessation of a secretion or excretion owing to its being dried up at its source is described as suppression. There may be, for example, suppression of the urine, of the menses or of the sweat. The non-appearance of a discharge does not necessarily mean its suppression, as it may simply be retained. Thus, urine may be secreted but be retained in the bladder.

See Kidney.

SUPPURATION. The formation of pus is described as suppuration. This may occur as an abscess (*q.v.*) or on an inflamed surface.

See Ulcer ; Wound.

SUPRA-RENAL GLAND. The structure and functions of the supra-renal glands, or capsules, are described under the heading Adrenal. A secretion of the gland, adrenalin, is sometimes called supra-renal extract.

SUSPENDED ANIMATION. A death-like state, sometimes referred to as suspended animation, may occur in asphyxia, syncope, or fainting, and the condition of trance. If the patient is not soon brought round by appropriate treatment the persistence of life can be established by various tests.

See Death.

SUSPENSORY BANDAGE. A bag, attached to a strap which goes round the waist, is used for supporting the scrotum and is called a suspensory bandage. It is valuable in diseases of the testicle and in varicocele.

SUTURE. In anatomy a suture is a kind of joint, the chief examples of which occur between the bones of the skull. In surgery it means a stitch or the act of stitching.

The chief material used for deep, or buried, sutures is catgut, because it is soon absorbed, but silk is used for some purposes. For the skin, silkworm gut or catgut is generally used. Michel's suture for the skin consists of metal clips.

SWAB. A piece of cotton wool or gauze used for mopping up blood or other substances is called a swab. Formerly marine sponge was extensively used for making swabs, but it is too difficult to clean to be safe for the purpose. A swab is often fastened to a stick or to a longish instrument called a sponge-holder. The method of swabbing the throat is illustrated in Plate XXXIV, 2.

SWALLOWING. In the first of three stages of swallowing, or deglutition, the tongue passes the substance to be swallowed backwards while at the same time the soft palate is drawn upwards, shutting off the nasopharynx, and the opening of the larynx is drawn up beneath the base of the tongue, thus shutting off the lower air-passages. Then the muscles around the pharynx contract, pressing anything that is being swallowed into the opening of the gullet, down which tube it is carried by a peristaltic movement. The first stage is the only one that is properly under the control of the will. Liquids

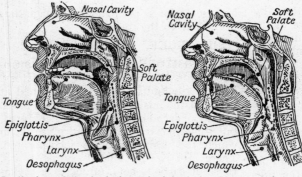

Swallowing. Left, food thrust backwards by the tongue into the pharynx, while the soft palate shuts off the entrance to the nose. Right, the entrance to the larynx is closed by being drawn up under the tongue

would appear to be shot down the gullet much more rapidly than solids.

Difficulty in swallowing, or dysphagia, may be due to some disorder of the gullet, but sometimes the fault is in the mouth, the pharynx or the larynx, and reference should be made to each of these headings for a full account of the causes and treatment of dysphagia.

See Gullet.

SWEAT. Perspiration, or sweat, is secreted by special glands, the sweat glands, or sudoriferous glands, which are situated in the deepest part of the true skin or in the subcutaneous tissue all over the body. A gland consists of a coiled tube, and outside the secreting cells are plain muscle fibres which contract and squeeze the sweat out. The duct of the gland passes up through the skin and opens on the top of one of the superficial ridges. The glands are most numerous in the palm and sole and are large in the armpit and groin.

Efferent Tube

Secreting Tube

Sweat Gland. The sweat is secreted from the blood by columnar cells lining the coiled tube, and carried off by the efferent tube or duct

Sweat is a very watery fluid, containing small amounts of salts and urea. It is acid in reaction, but usually becomes alkaline if sweating is profuse.

Sweat is being continuously discharged from the skin, but may evaporate at once. Such is described as insensible perspiration, as contrasted with the sensible perspiration that occurs when one is warm or takes exercise. The total amount of sweat excreted in 24 hours is on the average about $1\frac{1}{2}$ pints.

The evaporation of sweat cools the surface of the skin and is a factor in lowering body temperature. Poisonous substances may also be excreted in the sweat, and in uraemia (*q.v.*) the amount of urea is increased, so that in Bright's disease and in uraemia part of the treatment consists in inducing free sweating. It is desirable to keep the skin active in fevers, in order to promote coolness. Drugs that do this are called diaphoretics,

examples being sweet spirit of nitre, and the solution of Mindererus, and a drug which, like pilocarpine, causes profuse sweating, is called a sudorific.

Hyperidrosis is the name given to excessive sweating. It occurs in certain diseases such as consumption, malaria, and pyaemia. In rickets there is commonly free sweating about the head. Sometimes there is a localised hyperidrosis, perhaps limited to one side of the body, but generally this condition occurs on the hands or feet, and in the latter instance is often associated with bromidrosis, that is, a foul-smelling sweat. Unless the skin is kept as clean and dry as possible when there is excessive local sweating, it becomes sodden and inflamed.

An agent that reduces sweating is called an anhidrotic, and in this class are included belladonna, quinine, zinc oxide, etc. For local sweating, in the armpits or feet, the best thing to do is to wash the parts frequently, bathe with weak solutions of permanganate of potassium or formaldehyde and dust over with a powder containing zinc oxide and salicylic acid, or the following :

Boracic acid	60 grains
Zinc oxide	120 ,,
Powdered starch	to 1 ounce

The absence or diminution of sweating, or anhidrosis, may be associated with some skin disease like ichthyosis or sclerodermia, or a general disease like diabetes. Some people have a dryness of the skin, but otherwise show nothing peculiar. Dryness of the skin and inability to sweat increases the risk of heat stroke when circumstances favour its occurrence. Remedies for increasing sweating have already been noted, and to these may be added Dover's powder, which is sometimes called a sweating powder. Turkish baths and radiant heat baths are other useful methods.

Coloured sweat, or chromidrosis, sometimes occurs, and blue, red, green, yellow ar d black sweating have been described. In blue sweating indigo has been found in the sweat, and in red sweat, blood or haematin.

See Diaphoretic ; Skin.

SWEDISH EXERCISES. *See* Exercise.

SWEETBREAD. Two glands, the thymus and the pancreas, are sold by butchers as sweetbread. The former is called by the trade throat sweetbread, and the latter, heart or stomach sweetbread. Both glands are mainly cellular in structure and both are very digestible and nutritious, and consequently very suitable for invalids. They should not be given to gouty subjects, however, as they are rich in purin bodies.

See Invalid Cookery.

SWEET SPIRIT OF NITRE. Spirit of nitrous ether, or sweet spirit of nitre, is a transparent and almost colourless liquid with an apple-like odour and a sharp burning taste. Its uses are described under the heading Ether.

SYCOSIS. The most important disease of the beard area is technically known as sycosis. It is an inflammation due to microbic invasion of the hair follicles and sebaceous glands. It may be acquired from an infected shaving-brush, but when it begins on the upper lip is generally due to an infective discharge from the nose. It most frequently occurs on the chin and the upper lip, and consists of a number of spots, hard and shotty, which tend to run together and to form a considerable quantity of matter.

It is imperative that the disease be taken seriously, and that the patient should recognize that he is suffering from an infection that may be communicated to other people.

A further reason for paying serious attention to the trouble is that its natural course tends towards complete destruction of the roots of the hair, with a scarred and distorted skin, which produces permanent disfigurement of the face.

The treatment of sycosis can be successfully undertaken by the use of X-rays. Where this cannot be had or is not adopted, the older means of treatment are as follows : The hair must be cut short—shaving is impossible—and some antiseptic lotion must be employed several times a day. Probably the best is a

1 in 1,000 or 2,000 solution of corrosive sublimate. This contains mercury, and the same drug must also be used as an ointment, such as what is called white precipitate ointment. The fact that corrosive sublimate is a deadly poison must be kept in mind.

The ointment must be rubbed in most thoroughly, and the vigour of application must not be relaxed when some improvement has been gained, or even when only one or two patches of diseased skin remain. The patient must avoid constipation and will do well to take a course of baths, in order to stimulate the functions of the skin in general.

It is wiser not to allow the beard to grow for several months after apparent cure, so that any signs of renewed attack upon the skin may be immediately counteracted. Vaccine treatment has been helpful

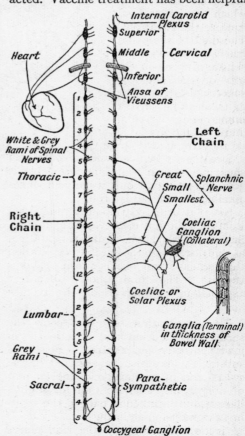

Sympathetic Nervous System. Schema showing the two main trunks and their connexions with the spinal nerves. See opposite page for text

in difficult cases. Infective conditions in the nose, if present, must of course be cleared up.

See Barber's Itch ; Ringworm.

SYMPATHETIC NERVOUS SYSTEM. On either side of the spinal column in the neck, thoracic and lumbar regions, there is a chain of nerve ganglia, or nodules containing nerve cells. These belong to the sympathetic nervous system. They are connected by fibres with the spinal cord, and with other ganglia which lie further out, some of them actually in the walls of the intestine. There are similar ganglia at various points in the head and in front of the sacrum, but these constitute another part of the nervous system, namely, the parasympathetic. The ganglia in the head receive fibres from the brain through certain of the cranial nerves. The sympathetic and parasympathetic together form the autonomic nervous system.

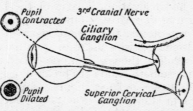

A sympathetic ganglion connects by efferent nerve fibres with the spinal cord, and by afferent fibres, through the spinal nerve, with the arteries, muscles and viscera

The sympathetic system supplies branches to the internal organs of the chest, abdomen and pelvis, to blood vessels, to the sweat glands, to the tiny muscles that raise the hairs and to other parts. The existence of this system permits of a wide distribution of impulses coming from the central nervous system, and also, although it has not been shown that reflex actions take place in its nerve cells, it is possible that they do.

Impulses through sympathetic nerve fibres cause dilatation of the pupil, sweating, quickening and augmentation of the heart beats, stoppage of the flow of gastric juice, contraction of

Example of antagonism of sympathetic and parasympathetic nerves : the pupil is dilated by the former and contracted by the latter

arteries and many other phenomena. The action of the parasympathetic system is more or less antagonistic to that of the sympathetic. Thus, it slows the heart and it stimulates the flow of gastric juice.

Raynaud's disease and other affections seem to depend on some disorder of the sympathetic system.

See Nervous System.

SYMPHYSIS. A joint in which the cartilaginous surfaces of the opposing bones are united by a broad, flat plate of fibro-cartilage is called a symphysis. Examples are the joints between the bodies of the vertebrae and the symphysis pubis. There is very little movement in such joints.

SYMPTOM. A manifestation of disease is called a symptom. If it can only be perceived by the patient himself it is called a subjective symptom, but if perceptible by an outside observer, an objective symptom, or sign. A pathognomonic symptom is one that points with certainty to a particular disease.

See Syndrome.

SYNCOPE. Swooning, or fainting, is also known as syncope. It may be noted here, however, that besides the causes of an ordinary attack of fainting noted under the heading Fainting, syncope may be due to poisons that depress the heart in overdoses, such as digitalis or aconite, or to organic disease of the heart, and may prove fatal ; the heart suddenly stops and never resumes beating. Death may occur by fainting, however, even when there is no organic cause. Signs of fainting from such serious causes resemble those of an ordinary fainting fit, and the treatment is similar.

See Collapse ; Fainting ; Heart.

SYNDROME. The aggregate of the symptoms and signs of a disease constitute its syndrome. The Stokes-Adams syndrome is the occurrence of syncopal or of epileptiform attacks with a slow pulse due to heart-block. There are other named syndromes.

SYNOVIA. The ligaments binding the bones of a joint are lined with a smooth membrane known as the synovial membrane. This secretes a glairy fluid called the synovia, or synovial fluid, which lubricates the interior of the joint. Synovial membrane also lines tendon sheaths.

See Joint ; Tendon.

SYNOVITIS. Inflammation of the synovial membrane of a joint (*q.v.*) is called synovitis, and of that lining a tendon sheath, teno-synovitis.

SYPHILIS. A highly contagious disease, syphilis is caused by the spirochaeta pallida, or treponema pallidum, a germ resembling a tiny thread twisted like a cork-screw. This is communicated by contact with an infected surface, which is generally brought about by sexual connexion, but may occur in kissing, suckling or touching syphilitic sores. Sometimes the contact is indirect, as in drinking from a glass that has been used by an infected person and not washed.

After an incubation period, lasting on the average about four weeks, though it may be as many as six, what is called the primary sore appears on the site of infection. When developed it takes the form of a round, flattened elevation, the base of which feels firm as if gristly. The surface is slightly ulcerated, and exudes a slight watery discharge which may dry into crusts or scales, though sometimes the surface is smooth and shiny, and there is no discharge. This sore is described as the hard, or Hunterian, chancre. In some situations, notably on the lip, ulceration may be more active, with a free discharge which dries into a scab. Generally there is only one sore, but there may be more. With the development of the sore the neighbouring glands become enlarged.

About six weeks after the appearance of the primary sore, the symptoms of the secondary stage make their appearance. There may be fever and this may be considerable, but often there is none. The patient may be conscious of depreciation in his general health, or may feel about as well as usual. There is a general enlargement of lymphatic glands all over the body, the superficial glands feeling like hard, shotty nodules. A rash also appears, usually having a resemblance to that of measles, but it may consist of papules or of pustules. The front of the chest and abdomen are generally first affected, but the rash usually becomes distributed over other parts of the body.

The throat feels sore, and the tonsils will be found to be enlarged with the appearance of snail-tracks upon the surface, caused by the superficial ulceration, and there will probably be mucous tubercles or patches, that is, white spots, on the tongue and the inside of the lips and cheeks. The hair falls out, producing a general thinning described as syphilitic alopecia. Within six months of the beginning of the disease there may be iritis, inflammation of the coloured curtain of the eye. One eye may be affected first, but both usually suffer. The eye looks reddened and swollen, and there is probably severe neuralgic pain.

Parasites in Second and Third Stages

In the secondary stage there is more or less copious infection of the blood with the parasites, but these gradually disappear, and this stage merges into the third, or tertiary, stage, in which, although the blood is free, parasites lurk in different parts of the body. From time to time, but perhaps as late as twenty or thirty or more years after infection, parasites in some such haunt may give rise to a swelling described as a gumma, which is liable to break down and ulcerate. As this may happen anywhere in the body, there is the possibility of a large variety of functional derangements, and when internal organs are involved symptoms may be very obscure. It can be determined, however, by the application of the Wassermann test to the patient's blood and perhaps to the cerebro-spinal fluid, whether or not syphilitic infection persists in his body. Another common tertiary lesion is degeneration of arteries.

There is a still further stage of syphilis, the quaternary, or parasyphilitic, in which the mischief affects the nervous system and may be represented by either of the two serious disorders known as locomotor ataxy and general paralysis of the insane. These developments of the disease are rare in women, however, and in the natives of tropical countries of either sex.

Congenital Form of the Disease

Parents who are syphilitic may transmit the disease to their offspring. This is described as hereditary, or congenital, syphilis. If the disease is active in the parents, the mother is likely to abort, or, at any rate, the child will probably be born dead, but as time goes on and the virulence of parental infection lessens, live children may be got, sometimes with the marks of the disease on them, but often apparently healthy. In these the disease may manifest itself after a week or two, but possibly only years after. In course of time children free from any taint of the disease may be born.

Congenital syphilis may show itself a few weeks after birth by the development of nasal catarrh, described in this connexion as snuffles. The inflammation within the nose may progress and cause destruction of tissue, so that the bridge of the nose becomes flattened out. Fissures are apt to form in the skin around the nose and the angles of the neck, and leave permanent scars. The skin generally may become shrivelled, and there may be great depression of the health. When the permanent teeth make their appearance, the upper central incisors may be peg-shaped, and have a notch cut out of the centre of the cutting edge. Such are known as Hutchinson's teeth, and are very characteristic of congenital syphilis. About this time also deafness may begin.

At puberty inflammation of the cornea of the eye may occur, and may ultimately cause blindness. It should be noted also that the nervous diseases described as parasyphilitic phenomena may occur in childhood in the subjects of congenital syphilis. A child who survives these earlier risks of the disease has a good chance of enjoying ordinary health, and

such a person may marry without fear of transmitting the disease.

In its primary stage syphilis can be eradicated by treatment with organic arsenical compounds of the salvarsan class combined with mercury or bismuth, and very probably in the secondary stage also, although the treatment must be more thorough and more prolonged. Treatment in any case should last for at least two years. In addition to the drugs above mentioned, iodide of potassium is generally given, and this drug has a marked effect in curing the gummata of the third stage. The adequacy of treatment is tested by examinations by the Wassermann method at intervals, and a patient should not neglect treatment until assured by his doctor that it is safe to do so, nor should he marry for two years after the termination of treatment, and only then if periodical tests have been negative. The same remedies are used in treating congenital syphilis as are used in the acquired disease.

See Black Wash ; Chancre ; General Paralysis of the Insane ; Locomotor Ataxia ; Salvarsan ; Wassermann Reaction.

SYRINGE. Various kinds of syringe are used in the treatment of different disorders. A very useful form is known as Higginson's syringe (Plate XXVI, 4). This consists of a rubber tube, expanded in the middle into a ball, and with a bone or glass nozzle at one end and a metal valve at the other. This syringe is mainly used for giving enemata or, with the addition of a special tube, vaginal douches ; but it has other uses.

Syringes with sharp needles are used for giving hypodermic and other injections through the skin, and also for withdrawing, or aspirating, blood or other fluids for diagnostic purposes. Such syringes must be capable of thorough sterilisation.

SYRINGOMYELIA. A nervous disease in which there is new growth in the grey matter of the spinal cord and the formation of cavities by degeneration of the growth, syringomyelia usually occurs before the age of thirty, and is more common in males. The symptoms depend to a considerable extent on the situation of the growth, but this is most often in the dorsal region, though it may extend down the cord and upwards, even into the medulla.

The sense of touch is preserved, but those of pain and temperature are lost, so the patient may burn himself seriously without feeling it. There is wasting and weakness of muscles, generally those of the upper limbs, and there may be trophic changes also in skin, bones and joints. Painless whitlows, or Morvan's disease (*q.v.*), are caused by syringomyelia.

There is no satisfactory treatment, but unless the infection is extensive, the patient may live for many years after the onset of the disease.

See Spinal Cord.

SYRUP. A syrup is a strong solution of sugar in water. Simple syrup is included amongst the official preparations and also a number of other syrups, which either contain aromatics or colouring matter, like syrup of ginger and syrup of rose, or some active drug, like syrup of chloral, syrup of squill and syrup of iron phosphate.

SYSTOLE. The contraction of the heart (*q.v.*) is described as its systole.

TABES. Formerly the general name for a wasting disease, the word tabes when used now without qualification is meant to refer to tabes dorsalis, or locomotor ataxia (*q.v.*). Tuberculous peritonitis is sometimes called tabes mesenterica.

TACHE. A bright red line which appears on the skin when the finger-nail is drawn across it, and which persists for some time, is called the tache cérébrale because it is prone to occur in meningitis. As it occurs in other conditions, however, no weight can be attached to it as a sign. A tache bleuâtre is a small bluish stain on the skin. It appears to be associated with the presence of lice. Tache is a French word meaning a stain.

TACHYCARDIA. Excessive rapidity of the pulse is called tachycardia, especially when it is not attributable to an organic cause. In the disorder known as paroxysmal tachycardia the pulse may suddenly begin to beat at a rate of 200 or more per minute.

See Heart ; Pulse.

TAENIA. A member of a family of tapeworms is known as taenia, for example, taenia solium and taenia echinococcus. In anatomy the term is applied to certain bands of nerve fibres in the brain.

See Worm.

TALC. Talcum powder, or talc, consists chiefly of magnesium silicate. It is soft and unctuous and absorbs perspiration. It is therefore used extensively as a dusting powder, though generally with other ingredients, such as salicylic acid. Talc is sometimes included in Lassar's paste (*q.v.*).

TALIPES. *See* Club Foot.

TAMARIND. The fruit of tamarindus indica contains tartaric acid and acid potassium tartrate and, preserved with sugar, is used in medicine as a laxative, the dose being $\frac{1}{2}$ to 1 ounce or more. An infusion of the fruit in water is used as a cooling drink in fevers. Tamarind is combined with senna in the official confection of senna and in tamar indien pastilles.

TAMPON. A wad of cotton wool or some other material used for plugging the nose, etc., is described as a tampon. Sometimes it is impregnated with a drug.

TANNIC ACID. The tannin, or tannic acid, of the British Pharmacopoeia is obtained from oak-galls and occurs as a pale brownish powder which is freely soluble in water and gives an acid reaction. The dose is 2 to 5 grains. There are three official preparations, namely, glycerin of tannic acid, suppository of tannic acid and the tannic acid lozenge.

The drug is an astringent and styptic, and acts also as an antidote in poisoning by alkaloids. The glycerin is used for local applications. Tannic acid is used in inflammation of the mouth and throat, in nasal catarrh, in diarrhoea and as an injection or local application in " whites." It is also given in haemorrhage from the stomach and bowel.

Tannigen, tannalbin and tannoform are other preparations of the acid which are used in the treatment of chronic diarrhoea. Tannin is also contained in catechu, kino and other drugs, and in coffee and tea. A strong infusion or decoction of tea affords a ready means of giving tannin in cases of poisoning.

TAPEWORM. *See* Worm.

TAPPING. The withdrawal of dropsical or other fluids from a body-cavity or the subcutaneous tissue is described as tapping. An aspirator, trochar and cannula or syringe may be used for this purpose. *See* Aspiration.

TAR. Coal tar is a by-product in the manufacture of coal gas. It is composed of many substances which can be distilled off from it, the ultimate residue being pitch. From coal tar are obtained, directly or indirectly, carbolic acid and cresol, picric acid, aniline and aniline dyes, phenacetin and similar drugs, and many other substances.

Prepared coal tar is used in medicine in the form of liquor picis carbonis and liquor carbonis detergens.

By the destructive distillation of the wood of pinus sylvestris and other pines is obtained Stockholm tar, which is known in pharmacy as pix liquida. From this is prepared tar ointment, tar water and syrup of tar.

Both kinds of tar may be vaporised and the fumes inhaled by patients suffering from whooping-cough or chronic bronchitis. For the latter complaint wood tar is also given, in doses of 3 grains or more, in pills or perles, or syrup of tar or tar water may be used.

Tar has a stimulating action on the skin and also relieves itching. It is used extensively in treating psoriasis and chronic eczema, either in the form of one of the liquors, as an ointment or as tar water. Sometimes a tar bath, made by adding tar solution to the bath, is used. Crude tar is sometimes applied on eczema. For skin complaints, instead of the ordinary tars, one of the following is sometimes used ; oil of cade, or juniper tar oil ; beech tar ; or birch tar, also called oleum Rusci.

TARSUS. The bones of the ankle (*q.v.*) are collectively known as the tarsus or tarsal bones. The term is also applied to the firm fibrous plate in the eyelid.

TARTAR. The deposit on the neck of a tooth, described as tartar, may consist of deposits from the saliva or from the serous exudate that occurs in this situation. It tends to press the gum off the tooth and also favours the growth of germs, so should be removed, an operation known as scaling.

The deposit of tartrate of calcium and potassium in wine casks is likewise known as tartar. Cream of tartar is acid potassium tartrate.

TARTAR EMETIC. *See* Antimony.

TARTARIC ACID. In the form of the free acid or of acid tartrate of potassium, tartaric acid is widely distributed in the vegetable kingdom, but the chief source of supply is the grape. The commercial product is prepared from acid tartrate of potassium and occurs as colourless crystals. The dose is 5 to 20 grains. It is chiefly used to make effervescing and cooling drinks.

TASTE. The sense of taste depends on stimulation of organs known as taste buds which are mostly situated in the tongue, though a few are found in the soft palate. To cause this stimulation, a substance must be in solution and the sensation it gives rise to is either sweet, sour, salt or bitter, or a combination of these. Sweetness is best appreciated at the tip of the tongue, sourness at the sides and bitterness at the back. The nerves connected with the taste buds carry impulses to a centre in the medulla, whence they are carried up to the parts of the brain towards the tip and inner side of the temporal lobe, in close relation to the area of brain concerned with the sense of smell. Indeed, flavours which are usually thought of as being purely the result of taste-sensations are really compound sensations of taste and smell.

The loss of taste, or ageusia, may occur when the tongue is too dry or its surface disordered by the presence of a copious furring or otherwise. The impairment of taste in a common cold is a reminder of the part played by smell in the discrimination of flavours. Loss of taste may also be due to disorder of the taste-nerves, that is the lingual the chorda tympani and the glosso-pharyngeal, or of their nervous connexions up to and including its centres on the brain. The chorda tympani is a branch of the facial nerve and partial loss of taste may be noted in connexion with facial paralysis.

Loss of taste may occur in hysteria, and in this disorder there may also be hallucinations of taste, though such may also occur in insanity and when there is a tumour in the neighbourhood of the taste centres in the brain.

The hallucination may be one of the simple tastes, but it may be an unpleasant one. A bad taste is common, however, in digestive disorders and when some drugs are being taken.

See Sensation ; Smell ; Tongue.

TATTOOING. In tattooing, pigments are carried by the needle right into the true skin and the only certain method of getting rid of the marks is to have them cut out, an impracticable proposition, however, if tattooing is extensive. Syphilis and other infections have occasionally been introduced into the body by tattooing. The disfigurement caused by white patches on the cornea of the eye may be lessened by tattooing them.

TEA. In the form in which we know it, tea consists of the leaves of the tea plant, dried and rolled up. The difference between green and black tea is due to the latter having been left to ferment for some time. The finer grades of tea consist of buds and the smaller leaves.

The chief constituents of tea are caffeine or theine, to which the stimulating properties are due, tannic acid and a volatile oil. Green tea contains more tannic acid than black and Indian and Ceylon tea than China.

An excessive consumption of tea or over-infused tea may cause nervous irritability and sleeplessness, dyspepsia and constipation. Tea should be infused in water just brought to the boil and not for longer than five minutes. Infusing for twenty minutes, for example, while it only slightly increases the caffeine content of the infusion, almost doubles the amount of tannic acid.

See Caffeine.

TEARS. The watery secretion of the lachrymal gland is commonly called the tears. It flows down over the surface of the eye moistening it and also the surface of the lid. The stream of tears tends to wash foreign bodies off the eye-ball, and has also an antiseptic action.

See Eye ; Lachrymal Apparatus.

TEETH. A tooth exhibits a crown, a neck and one or more roots or fangs. The roots are composed of dentine, or ivory, and this exists also beneath the crown, surrounding a hollow in the centre of the tooth, described as the pulp cavity, which is continued down into the roots. In this cavity is the pulp, consisting of blood vessels, nerves and loose connective tissue including special cells which send slender processes along with nerve fibrils into tubules which run outwards through the dentine.

The crown is formed of an intensely hard substance known as enamel ; it forms a cap for the tooth and may have two or more eminences, or cusps, on its biting surface.

The part of the jaw that carries the teeth is called the alveolus and along this are arranged the tooth-sockets. Between the root of a tooth and the wall of the socket is a substance called the cement, or crusta petrosa. This overlaps the lower edge of the enamel. The dense soft tissue, or gum, which covers the alveolus grips the neck of the tooth, a shallow groove between the crown and the root, and a portion like an inverted V occupies the interval between two teeth.

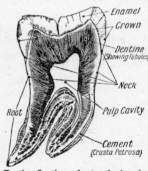

Teeth. Section of a tooth showing anatomical details

The process of cutting teeth is usually known as teething or dentition. There are two dentitions. In the first, the deciduous, temporary or milk teeth appear and consist of four incisors, two canines and four molars in each jaw. The incisors are the front cutting teeth and the two in the middle are described as the central, and those on either side as the lateral, incisors. Outside the latter are the canines, which are sharp, pointed and adapted for tearing, and outside these again the molars or grinding teeth.

The first of the milk teeth to appear are usually the lower central incisors, and this generally happens in the 6th month. In a short time the upper central, and all the lateral incisors emerge, and then follow in order the first molars in the 12th month, the canines in the 18th month, and the second molars in the 24th month. Variations of these times occur even in healthy children, and in rickets dentition may be much delayed. When the milk

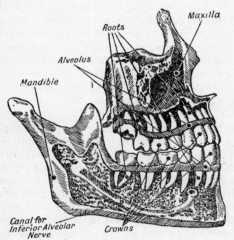

Teeth. Their relative position in the jaws

teeth emerge they have over them a thin, horny covering, called Nasmyth's membrane, but this soon wears off.

The second dentition begins about the 6th year with the appearance of the first permanent molars and each year after this the other permanent teeth are cut— the central incisors, the lateral incisors, the first premolar, the second premolar, the canines and the second molar. The premolars have two cusps on the crown, and are also known as the bicuspids ; they replace the milk molars. The third molar tooth may appear about the 17th year or not until the 25th, and is also called the wisdom tooth ; sometimes it does not erupt at all. It will be found that the cusps of the upper teeth overlap slightly those of the lower.

The first teething is sometimes a trying event for the infant and the gums may be swollen, hot and tender, and the child is feverish and restless. The digestion may be upset, and there may be constipation or diarrhoea. Sometimes there is earache, indicated by restless movements of the head and crying.

It is not uncommon also for a child to suffer from bronchitis while teething. Another possibility is that the child may have a convulsion (*q.v.*) or even several convulsions.

A child that is being suckled should not be taken off the breast while it is having difficulty in teething. Cool, boiled water may be given freely to cool the mouth and relieve thirst. If there is constipation fluid magnesia in the mornings is a useful remedy and the best remedy for diarrhoea, at any rate at the beginning, is a teaspoonful of castor oil. Earache may be treated by applying cold cloths to the ear. As the child salivates very freely it may soak the garments over the front of the chest, and care should be taken to prevent this.

There is rarely any trouble to speak of in connexion with the second dentition, except that the eruption of a wisdom tooth may occasion considerable aching. Sometimes the teeth are over-crowded and are placed irregularly. This may be due to a lack of development of the jaw or to malformation of the jaw.

The use of a baby's comforter creates a danger of infection because the comforter may be dropped on the floor and be put back in the baby's mouth without being sufficiently cleansed, but there is this further count against it that it may cause malformation of the jaws.

It is desirable that an infant should begin gnawing at crusts or rusks when it is about six months old as this practice helps to develop the jaws, and insufficient development may be due to the child not having been given firm food to gnaw ; but

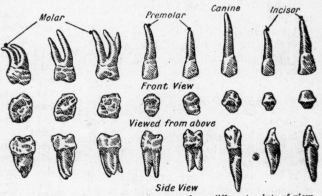

Teeth of one-half of the upper jaw seen from different points of view

this is quite a different thing from a baby keeping a comforter stuck in the side of its mouth more or less constantly.

When the teeth are overcrowded and there is no hope of their settling into a correct position one or more of them should be extracted. When a child has been debilitated by scarlet fever, measles or some other disorder, it may chance that the permanent teeth are undersized and their surface marked by pits and grooves. Such teeth may not exhibit any special tendency to decay, however.

How to Clean the Teeth

Unless teeth are efficiently cleansed there is a tendency to the deposition of tartar about the neck of the tooth, and this may separate the gum from the tooth, giving access to bacteria and possibly leading to pyorrhoea. Moreover, carbohydrate foods, such as sticky fragments of bread, may lodge in the crevices between the teeth, and ferment, giving rise to acid substances which attack and dissolve the tooth-substance. This is the beginning of caries, or decay, of a tooth.

The natural method by which teeth are cleaned is by chewing crisp foods and such as require a good deal of mastication. This acts mechanically by crushing any particles out from between the teeth, and as chewing causes a free flow of saliva it ensures that the teeth are bathed in this alkaline secretion. The teeth should also be brushed, however, twice a day at least.

The motion of the brush should be up and down and it is necessary to hold it vertically when brushing the backs of the teeth. Parts which cannot be reached with the brush can be cleansed by drawing a strand of dental floss between the teeth (*see* Plate XXXIV, 3 and 4).

A smooth dentifrice should be selected, as erosion of the teeth has followed the use of a gritty dentifrice. The tooth is worn away at the gum margin and decay is encouraged. A common cause of erosion is the little metal clip often used by dentists to keep a small denture in position. This should be avoided whenever possible, and so far as the upper jaw is concerned the use of a sufficiently large plate may make clips unnecessary.

As soon as decay begins the part should be cleaned out and stopped, and it is only prudent to have the teeth examined periodically by a dentist so that the first beginnings of caries may be discovered and dealt with.

The importance of keeping the teeth sound cannot be over-estimated. Apart from the digestive troubles that proceed from deficient or defective teeth an enormous amount of illness is caused by the absorption of poisons from defective teeth.

It should be stated in this connexion that there is a fairly general condemnation by doctors of the practice of killing the nerve of a tooth for the purpose of stopping or crowning it. If such a tooth is left in the jaws it may become seriously infected at its root without giving any warning of the fact. Persons suffering from illnesses of which the causation was obscure have been found by X-ray examination to have this condition, and have been cured by the extraction of the offending tooth (*see* Plate XXXIV, 5).

Pain in a tooth, or toothache, may be due to mischief at the root or to exposure of the pulp by caries. If there is a cavity, a little pledget of cotton wool soaked in oil of cloves may be put into the cavity and warmth applied to the jaw. A dose of opening medicine may often be given with advantage. Sometimes pain caused by a diseased tooth is referred to a sound one, a fact to be borne in mind when there is a question of extraction.

Excessive bleeding after the extraction of a tooth may be arrested by folding a part of a handkerchief into a pad and biting on it, or by plugging the socket with cotton wool.

Care of Artificial Teeth

Artificial teeth must be kept scrupulously clean. They should be taken out at night and brushed with tooth-powder, and then be left in water containing some antiseptic. For a vulcanite plate this might be hydrogen peroxide, but for a metal plate it may be necessary to use a weak solution of chlorinated soda from time to time in order to keep the metal bright.

A removable denture is much to be preferred to bridge-work as juices may lodge beneath the bridge and decompose.

See Alveolus; Dentifrice; Dentine; Pyorrhoea; Tartar.

TELANGIECTASIS. Dilatation of the minute blood vessels of the skin, producing an appearance with some resemblance to a birth-mark, is described as telangiectasis. Much exposure to the weather or to a hot sun often causes the type of this disorder known as the " spider " naevus, but this may also follow a blow or an insect bite. Telangiectasis is seen most frequently on the face and chest, but other parts may be affected and occasionally the condition occurs all over the body.

The patches, if not very large, can be removed by carbonic acid snow or radium. Caustics should not be used for this purpose.

TEMPER. Good health is generally associated with good temper. The victims of gout and of congestive disorders of the liver are notoriously prone to irascibility, but those who suffer from other diseases, and in particular chronic invalids, may be similarly affected. Sometimes the provocation is purely mental and unreasonable outbursts of anger may be early symptoms of insanity, whether or not this is associated with organic changes in the nervous system. Bad temper in a child demands a thorough investigation of the physical and mental health.

TEMPERAMENT. The ancient physicians believed that the predominance in the body of any one of four humours, namely, blood, black bile, yellow bile and phlegm, produced certain distinctive physical and mental characteristics.

Consequently they were in the habit of describing four temperaments: (1) The sanguine, comprising persons of a full-blooded appearance, ruddy, blue-eyed, with red or auburn hair, and with a hopeful and passionate disposition. (2) The melancholic, comprising those with thinner and firmer frames, black hair, dark complexion and grave and meditative disposition. (3) The choleric, comprising those with a swarthy but yet ruddy complexion, black, curling hair, a thick, rough skin, and occupying a somewhat intermediate position between the preceding two categories. (4) The phlegmatic, or lymphatic, comprising persons with a lax skin and soft muscles, fair of skin and somewhat sluggish in both their bodily and mental functions.

Later physicians added to these a nervous temperament, comprising those with a highly strung, excitable disposition and a tendency to anxiety and worry.

The humoral theory underlying the old classification has long since gone by the board, and attempts at a precise collocation of mental and physical characteristics had largely shared the same fate until recently. Some physicians now seek to distinguish types, or temperaments, caused by predominance of one of the endocrines or internal secretions, describing an adrenal, a pituitary, and a thyroid, type.

However this may be, it is permissible to distinguish as temperaments certain combinations of mental characteristics and speak, for example, of the artistic temperament, the philosophic temperament, the jealous temperament and so on, without implying any distinctive bodily characteristics.

TEMPERATURE. The intensity of the heat of anything, as measured by the thermometer, is described as its temperature. The normal temperature of the human body is 98·4° F. and climate makes no difference to this. There is a slight daily variation amounting possibly to 1° F., the higher temperature occurring in the evening. The temperature may also be raised slightly after a meal or after hard exercise, but it soon returns to normal.

The heat of the body is produced by chemical action in the muscles and in the glands, especially the liver. Heat is lost in warming the air and watery vapour expired from the lungs, in the excretions of the bladder and bowels, but chiefly by radiation and conduction from the skin and sweating. More heat is lost by sweating than by anything else.

The fact that the body temperature keeps so constant means that a strict balance must be kept between heat production and heat loss. This is accomplished by centres in the base of the brain. An instance of these centres coming into operation is seen in shivering, which is really involuntary muscular exercise intended to produce heat.

Disease of one kind and another may upset the heat-regulating mechanism, and the temperature may go up or down. If, apart from the circumstances mentioned above, it goes up beyond 99° F. a state of fever (*q.v.*) exists. If the temperature falls below 98° F. it is subnormal, and below 96° it represents collapse. This is a dangerous state of affairs, and equally so is a temperature of 105·8° F. and over. The method of taking the temperature is described under the heading Thermometer.

TEMPORAL BONE. One of the bones of the cranium, or brain-pan, the temporal is made up of several portions, and has an irregular shape. The thin, plate-like or squamous part helps to close in the lateral wall of the skull. Below and behind this part is a thicker part which is jointed to the occipital bone and which is prolonged downwards into a nipple-like projection, the mastoid process, to which is attached the upper end of the sterno-mastoid muscle.

Above and in front of the process is the orifice of the bony part of the external ear-passage, or meatus, and projecting downwards and forwards in front of this is a slender, sharp process of bone, the styloid process, which gives attachment to several muscles, the stylo-glossus, etc. Behind the root of this process is an opening, the stylo-mastoid foramen, by which the facial nerve emerges from the skull.

Projecting forwards from in front of the ear-passage is the zygomatic process which unites with a backward projection of the malar bone to form the zygomatic arch of the cheek. Beneath the back part of this process is the articular surface for the mandible or lower jaw.

A portion of the bone, known as the petrous portion, is directed inwards and forwards and forms part of the base of the skull. It is roughly pyramidal in shape and contains the internal ear and the internal ear-passage, or meatus. The internal carotid artery also runs through the petrous portion in part of its course.

See Ear ; Gasserian Ganglion ; Skull.

TENDERNESS. The sensation of pain when caused by touch, pressure or dragging, is described as tenderness. Sometimes tenderness exists without any spontaneous feeling of pain, and vice versa.

Tenderness may be hysterical in origin and may be very acute. The significance of tenderness depends on its situation, whether or not it is accompanied by other signs of inflammation, and other circumstances.

TENDON. The white fibrous tissue by which so many muscles are attached to bone is known as tendon. Its fibres are strong and, unlike those of muscle, do not stretch. In the limbs many tendons are long and slender. Where it passes over a bone a tendon often runs in a fibrous sheath which is lined with synovial membrane. In some tendons little bones, known as sesamoid bones, develop. The knee-cap is the largest of these, but others exist in the tendons of the thumb and elsewhere.

A tendon may be snapped by a sudden strain, as, for example, the Achilles tendon in dancing ; or a tendon may be cut across, an accident which is most common on the front of the wrist or of the fingers. The muscle usually contracts and pulls the severed ends apart. The ends may be brought and kept together sometimes by adjusting the position of the limb, but it is generally advisable to suture the ends together.

On the other hand, it may be necessary for the correction of a deformity to divide a tendon, an operation called tenotomy; sometimes the tendon is separated by a Z-shaped incision, dividing it half-way across above and below but on opposite sides, and the two ends are dragged partially apart and stitched together so that the tendon is lengthened.

A tendon-jerk, or tendon-reflex, is the name given to contraction of a muscle if the tendon is smartly tapped

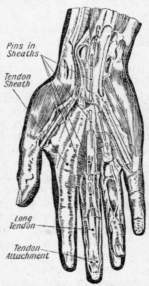

Pins in Sheaths

Tendon Sheath

Long Tendon

Tendon Attachment

Tendon. Fibrous sheaths in which some tendons run

when it is on the stretch. The knee jerk (*q.v.*) is an example of such a reflex.

See Aponeurosis ; Muscle.

TENESMUS. A frequent, painful straining but ineffectual effort to empty the bowel is described as tenesmus. Little or no faeces is passed, but there may be a little blood and mucus. This occurs in acute dysentery and in other forms of acute diarrhoea. It may also occur in intussusception and in other disorders inside or outside the bowel, such as impacted faeces, fissure of the anus, polypus, cancer of the rectum, inflammation of the rectum, enlarged prostate, stone in the bladder and, in women, retroversion of the womb. The treatment depends on the cause.

A similar condition in the bladder is sometimes called vesical tenesmus, but the usual name for it is strangury (*q.v.*).

TENNIS ELBOW. *See* Elbow.

TENT. An instrument used for dilating an orifice of the body by absorbing moisture and expanding is called a tent. It is usually made of tupelo-wood or of sea-tangle.

TERATOMA. Certain tumours are found to contain tissues derived from all of the three primitive layers of the embryo, such as teeth, hairs, glandular structure and muscle. A tumour of this kind is called a teratoma and may occur in the sacral region, in the genital organs, and elsewhere.

TEREBENE. A colourless liquid with a pleasant aromatic taste and smell, terebene is obtained by the action of sulphuric acid on turpentine. It is used as a stimulating expectorant and antiseptic in chronic bronchitis, pulmonary tuberculosis and whooping-cough, and may be used as a spray or inhalation or, in doses of 5 to 15 minims, may be given in an emulsion, in capsules or on sugar.

In the same doses it is given as an intestinal antiseptic in dysentery and other infectious disorders of the bowel. As a spray it is used as a deodorant to freshen the air of a room. While terebene is being taken inwardly the urine should be tested regularly for albumin, as the drug may cause irritation of the kidneys.

TERTIAN FEVER. *See* Malaria.

TESTICLE. The sexual gland in the male is called the testicle, or testis. There is a pair of these glands, a right and a left, and each occupies a separate compartment in the scrotum or bag in which it is suspended by the spermatic cord. The gland consists of two portions, the body or testis proper, and the epididymis.

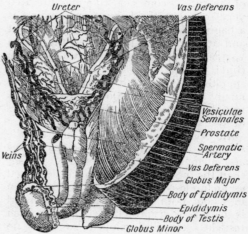

Testicle. Parts of the male generative gland

The shape of the body is somewhat like that of a kidney bean, the convex border being directed forwards. It has a tough, fibrous covering, known as the tunica albuginea, from the inner surface of which partitions or septa project and divide the cavity into a number of spaces, or loculi. In these spaces are contained the seminiferous tubules in which the spermatozoa are produced. The spermatozoa make their way along a number of ducts into the upper part or epididymis, which consists really of a long, convoluted tube, and are discharged into the main duct of the testis, the vas deferens.

In addition to spermatozoa, however, the testicle produces a secretion which does not pass out through its duct but goes into the blood stream. This internal secretion, which is produced by special cells, is responsible for the existence of the sexual characteristics, both bodily and mental. The falsetto voice, the hairless face, and the change in the general conformation of the body to a more feminine type which follow castration are due to the loss of this internal secretion and are associated with a diminution of the robust, energetic and courageous qualities of mind.

The testicles are developed within the abdominal cavity and do not pass out until just before birth. The testicle passes through the inguinal canal carrying with it a tube-like process of the peritoneal lining of the abdomen. The upper part of this tube becomes closed and obliterated very soon but the lower part remains as a bag which covers in the testicle in front and at the sides. It is called the tunica vaginalis and ordinarily its walls are in contact with one another, but being smooth they diminish any friction which might arise from movements of the testicle. Sometimes fluid accumulates in the bag and forms a hydrocele.

In some male children one of the testicles, or both, may not leave the abdomen, or may not get any farther than the inguinal canal. This is described as an undescended testicle, and a person in whom both testicles are undescended is called a cryptorchid. Usually such testicles are ill-developed so that no useful purpose is served in bringing them down into the scrotum, even should this be possible.

Association with a Hernia

Frequently an undescended testicle is accompanied by a hernia, and in order to ensure a cure of the hernia by operation it will probably be necessary to remove the testicle. In any case it is desirable to remove it, especially if there is a sound testicle on the other side, because an undescended testicle is probably liable to develop a malignant growth.

Inflammation of the testis proper is called orchitis and of the epididymus, epididymitis. Acute orchitis is not uncommon in mumps and sometimes occurs in other infectious fevers. It may also occur by extension of gonorrhoeal infection from the epididymis. The testis beomes swollen, painful and very tender. Chronic orchitis may follow acute attacks or be caused by syphilis or by extension of tuberculosis from the epididymis. The testis is swollen but there may be little pain. The gland is softened and may become adherent to the scrotum, when the abscess may burst through the skin.

The treatment of acute orchitis is to rest in bed and support the testicle by raising it on a pillow or by a suspensory bandage. Cold or hot applications are put on according to which gives more relief. It is advisable to take a sharp purge. The treatment of chronic orchitis is mainly that of the cause. In tuberculosis it may be possible to remove the diseased tissue, but sometimes it is necessary to take away the whole gland.

A tumour of the testis is usually either a sarcoma or a carcinoma. If a simple tumour occurs it is generally of a cystic nature.

Bruising of the testis by kicks, etc., causes a sickening pain and very considerable shock.

See Epididymis ; Genital System ; Haematocele ; Hydrocele ; Scrotum ; Spermatic Cord ; Varicocele.

TEST MEAL. A meal given for the purpose of examining digestive capacity is called a test meal. Before a test breakfast is given a stomach tube is passed and the contents of the stomach are drawn off and set aside for examination. The patient is then given two slices of dry toast and two cups of weak tea. After the lapse of an hour the contents of the stomach are again drawn off and subjected to a chemical and microscopical examination. Another method is to draw off portions of the contents every 15 minutes ; this is called the fractional test method. Meals consisting of bread, milk, cornflour or mucilage mixed with bismuth carbonate or oxychloride or barium sulphate, are given before X-ray examinations of the digestive organs ; such are called opaque meals.

TETANUS. *See* Lockjaw.

TETANY. A spasmodic nervous disorder, tetany may occur in either sex and at any age. In children it is associated with rickets and in adults with disturbance of the digestion. Frequently there is gastroptosis or sagging of the stomach, and dilatation of this organ. Removal of the parathyroid glands, which are tiny structures at the back of the thyroid gland, is followed by tetany. These glands are supposed to be concerned with the calcium metabolism of the body and it is significant that in tetany there is a diminution of the calcium content of the blood. Possibly the functioning of the glands is disturbed by the presence in the blood of toxins resulting from gastro-intestinal stasis.

The notable thing in tetany is excessive excitability of the nerves. This manifests itself in tonic spasms, mostly of the limbs, but sometimes of the head and trunk. The elbows and wrists are bent and also the fingers at the knuckle joints, but at the other joints the fingers are extended. The thumb is flexed and drawn into the palm of the hand. The toes are flexed and the ankle and knee extended. These spasms may occur spontaneously or may be brought on by slight irritation of the nerves as by pressing on the nerves, or even the artery, in the arm.

Tetany is treated by giving large doses of calcium chloride and by attention to the general health. Child patients are given cod-liver oil, and exposure to natural or artificial sunlight is useful. In adults the digestive apparatus should be brought into as good working order as possible. *See* Rickets.

TETRONAL. A hypnotic belonging to the same group as sulphonal, tetronal is more powerful than the latter. It has a bitter taste. *See* Sulphonal.

TETTER. Many and diverse skin diseases of man and lower animals are popularly called tetter.

THEOBROMA. Cacao butter, or oil of theobroma, is a fixed oil expressed from the warmed crushed seeds of theobroma cacao. It is a yellowish, solid oil with an odour resembling that of cocoa, and is used in making suppositories. Theobromine is the alkaloid contained in cacao seeds and resembles caffeine in its actions, but is a more powerful diuretic. Compounds of theobromine are therefore used to promote the flow of urine and diminish dropsy. *See* Diuretic.

THERMO-CAUTERY. In the instrument known as Pacquelin's thermo-cautery there is a platinum point which is first heated over a spirit-lamp and then kept hot by pumping benzine vapour through it. This cautery can be used for the removal of polypi or other growths, for arresting bleeding and for other purposes. *See* Cautery.

THERMOMETER. An instrument for measuring temperature is known as a thermometer. In its construction the principle of the expansion of matter by heat is utilised. The substance most commonly employed is mercury, but when very low temperatures have to be measured it is necessary to use alcohol. When extreme accuracy is needed an air-thermometer may be used.

A thermometer in which mercury or alcohol is used generally consists of a glass bulb connected with a long, fine tube. When heat is applied to the bulb the liquid contained in it rises in the tube to a height varying with the amount of heat applied. On the tube there is marked a graduated scale and the mark reached by the fluid indicates the degree of temperature.

In graduating a thermometer two points are first obtained, namely, freezing point and boiling point. The graduation between those points and beyond them may be done according to one of three recognized scales. The one which is adopted for ordinary purposes in Great Britain is called the Fahrenheit scale. In this freezing point is marked as 32° and boiling point as 212°, the intervening scale thus representing 180°. In the Centigrade scale, which is that used on the Continent and for scientific purposes all over the world, freezing point is marked 0°, or zero, and boiling point 100°, and in the Réaumur scale, which is used in some parts of the Continent, freezing is also zero, but boiling point is at 80°.

To convert the Fahrenheit scale into the Centigrade subtract 32, divide by 9 and multiply by 5 ; to convert Centigrade into Fahrenheit divide by 5, multiply by 9 and add 32. In the following examples 104° F. and 36·9° C. are converted into their equivalents in the other scale : (1) 104° F.—32=72 ; 72÷9=8 ; 8×5=40° C. (2) 36·9° C.÷5=7·38 ; 7·38×9=66·4 ; 66·4+32=98·4° F.

Meteorologists use what is called the maximum and minimum thermometer, which records the highest temperature reached during the day and the lowest that is reached at night.

The instrument used for taking the temperature of the body is known as the clinical thermometer. On the Fahrenheit scale it is usually graduated between 95° and 110°, each degree also being subdivided into fifths, corresponding to the decimal 0·2. The normal temperature of the body, 98·4°, is generally indicated by an arrow. In some of these instruments the glass in front is prism-shaped so that a magnified view of the mercury column can be obtained and reading is thus made easier.

Before proceeding to take a temperature the mercury must be shaken down well below the normal mark, and this can be done in several ways. One is to grasp the stem firmly between the thumb and forefinger and flick the instrument forcibly in the air, and another is, while holding the stem in the same way, to strike the inner side of the wrist on the knee. A third method is to whirl the instrument in a patent case provided for the purpose.

The temperature is usually taken in the mouth or in the armpit, but that of a young child is commonly taken in the groin, the thigh being brought up against the abdominal wall. It can be taken in the bowel also, and this method is often resorted to when a patient is unconscious.

Before a thermometer is put into the mouth it should be thoroughly washed. When the temperature is being taken regularly it is customary to leave the thermometer in a jar containing an antiseptic solution, a piece of cotton wool being placed in the bottom of the jar to prevent breakage of the instrument. If the patient has just had a hot or a cold drink a few minutes should be allowed to elapse before proceeding, in order to give the mouth time to resume its ordinary temperature. The patient is directed to raise the tip of the tongue, the bulb of the thermometer is placed beneath it and he is then told to keep the lips tightly closed.

Before placing a thermometer in the armpit or the groin the part should be thoroughly dried and care should be taken when placing the instrument that it lies between two skin surfaces ; sometimes clothing is allowed to interpose between the bulb and the skin. For introduction into the bowel the bulb of a thermometer is smeared with a little vaseline and manipulations must be very gentle.

A thermometer should be left in the mouth or the bowel for two or three minutes, and in the armpit or groin for seven to ten minutes or perhaps even longer.

See Temperature.

THIGH. The part of the lower limb between the hip and the knee is described as the thigh. In the skeleton it is represented by the femur, commonly known as the thigh-bone, and in the clothed skeleton the femur is surrounded by massive muscles. On the front there is the quadriceps extensor group, the function of which is to straighten the knee, on the back the group of hamstrings, which flexes, or bends, the knee, and on the inner side the adductor group, which draws the knee towards the middle line of the body.

Crossing the front of the thigh, obliquely downwards and inwards, is a long, straplike muscle, which is known as the sartorius, or tailor's muscle, because its action is to draw the leg into the position assumed by tailors when sitting at work. All the muscles of the thigh are enclosed by a strong tube of fascia, which ensheaths them like a sleeve and from the inner surface of which partitions of fascia pass between the various muscles.

This sheath presents a specially strong band on the outer surface of the thigh, and here also there is a muscle, the tensor fasciae femoris, which drags on the fascia and keeps it taut. The fascial sheath has an opening on its

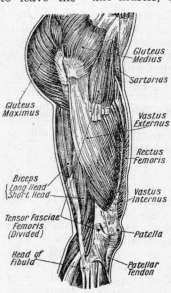

Gluteus Medius

Sartorius

Gluteus Maximus

Vastus Externus

Rectus Femoris

Biceps { Long Head Short Head

Vastus Internus

Tensor Fasciae Femoris (Divided)

Patella

Head of Fibula

Patellar Tendon

Thigh : its powerful musculature

upper and inner aspect, the saphenous opening, through which the long, or inner, saphenous vein passes in to join the femoral vein. Through this opening a femoral hernia may emerge.

The main artery of the thigh, the femoral, enters about the middle of the groin and runs downwards to the inner side of the back of the knee where it passes into the popliteal space. Running down the back of the thigh is the large nerve known as the great sciatic, which is sometimes affected by the painful disorder called sciatica (*q.v.*). The course of the principal blood vessels and nerves is shown in the illustration in page 428.

See Biceps ; Femur ; Hip ; Knee.

THINNESS. In many people thinness is constitutional and is consistent with perfect health. In fact, those who retain their thinness after middle life have a better chance of reaching a ripe old age than those who, as the saying goes, run to fat. At the same time it will be prudent to scrutinise the digestion and diet of anyone who is unduly lean, and supplement the carbohydrates and fats if necessary.

When a person is losing weight a scrutiny of the various organs and functions of the body is an urgent matter, and the possibility of the existence of consumption, diabetes, a malignant growth, or some other disorder must be considered.

THIRST. The sensation of thirst is associated with dryness of the pharynx, and, though in general thirst is an expression of the need for replenishment of the body with liquid, it may be provoked by dryness of the pharynx when no such need exists. Mouth-breathers, for example, and those who suffer from chronic pharyngitis may have a desire to drink when liquid is not actually required for the general needs of the body, and their thirst might be relieved by simply gargling with water or even sucking a pebble. The last expedient may be successful also in relieving the intense thirst associated with rupture of the stomach.

When there is a serious drain of liquid from the body there is great thirst. This happens after a large bleeding, after profuse watery diarrhoea, as in cholera, after profuse sweating and when there is a copious discharge of urine, as in diabetes. In fevers also, thirst is usually a prominent symptom.

Those engaged in hot occupations generally find oatmeal water or barley water a more efficient thirst-quencher than plain water, and the reason is that these mucilaginous drinks hinder the pharynx from becoming dry so quickly as when plain water is used. More than a very moderate use of iced drinks is harmful as the digestion gets upset.

See Beverages.

THOMSEN'S DISEASE. In Thomsen's disease, which is technically known as myotonia congenita, there is a delay in carrying out movements because the first attempt causes the muscles to become rigid. In from five to thirty seconds the stiffness passes off, however, and the movement is carried out, nor is there any difficulty about the subsequent movements, so that the patient can take a long walk for example, or dance. The arms and legs are most affected. Sometimes there is mental dullness. The disease is hereditary and appears in childhood. There is no cure, but warmth and freedom from excitement may lessen the severity of the condition.

THORACIC DUCT. The main lymphatic channel of the body, the thoracic duct begins in the upper part of the abdominal cavity, passes through the diaphragm along with the aorta, ascends through the thorax and passes out into the root of the neck on the left side, where it joins the angle of junction of the left internal jugular and subclavian veins. Its average length in the adult is about 18 inches.

At its commencement it presents a dilatation, about 2 inches long and $\frac{1}{4}$ inch broad, this portion being called the receptaculum chyli (*see* diagram, p. 212). The thoracic duct drains the lower part of the body, including the intestine, the left side of the chest, the left upper extremity and the left side of the head and neck.

A short tube that gathers up the lymph from the right side of the upper part of the body is called the right lymphatic duct. This joins the angle of junction of the right internal jugular and subclavian veins.

See Lymphatic System.

THORAX. In anatomy the chest is referred to as the thorax. Puncturing the chest-wall in order to withdraw pleural fluid is called thoracentesis. In consumption and other lung diseases an operation known as thoracoplasty is sometimes performed for the purpose of causing collapse of the lung and allowing healing to take place. A portion of each of the upper ten ribs is removed and the chest-wall falls in. The collapse of the lung is permanent, but life may be prolonged.

See Chest; Empyema; Lung.

THREADWORM. *See* Worm.

THROAT. The fauces, pharynx and larynx, which are collectively described as the throat, are discussed under those headings. The term is also applied to the front of the neck.

THROBBING. *See* Pulsation.

THROMBOSIS. Clotting of the blood in the heart or a blood vessel during life is called thrombosis, and the clot that is formed, a thrombus. It should be noted, however, that while the thrombus sometimes consists of the whole blood, and thus resembles an ordinary clot, at other times it is composed mainly of fibrin and occasionally mainly of white cells.

The primary event in thrombosis would appear to be an accumulation of the very minute particles in blood, known as the blood platelets, at some point on the wall of the heart or of a blood vessel, and it is upon the mass so formed that the clot is laid down. The circumstance that determines the adhesion of the platelets to the wall of the vessel is some injury to the lining endothelium of the latter, and their adhesion is favoured by slowing down of the blood stream.

Thus, thrombosis tends to occur in diseased arteries, but more particularly when there is an aneurysmal dilatation on an artery or when from debility or some other cause the circulation is feeble. Its occurrence in a vein is favoured by inflammation of the vein, or phlebitis, and more particularly when the vein is dilated and varicose.

The symptoms and consequences of thrombosis depend upon its site. In an artery it may shut off all the blood supply to some part of the body, though in other cases the part may be supplied by other arteries taking on the duty. If the blood supply is quite shut off the part dies.

If thrombosis occurs in a vein the venous circulation below the thrombus will be obstructed, and if the blood cannot easily make its way along other veins, as when the main vein of a limb is affected, signs of dropsy will shortly appear. Thrombosis of the main vein of the leg is a not uncommon event after childbirth or enteric fever. The formation of the thrombus causes inflammation, with pain and tenderness, and if the vessel can be felt it is found to be hard and cord-like.

A thrombus may become softened, and there is then a risk that a part of the clot may be detached and cause embolism (*q.v.*) somewhere. On the other hand, a thrombus may become organized, that is to say, it is converted into fibrous or scar-like tissue and in this event the lumen of the vessel is obliterated. A natural cure of a varicose vein sometimes comes about in this way.

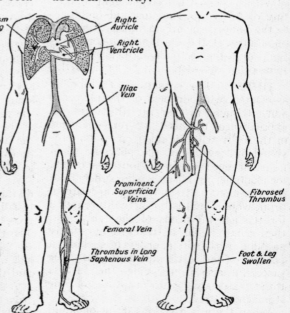

Thrombosis. Left, thrombus in a vein of the left leg; a portion of it has been carried to the right lung, causing embolism. Right, a thrombus in the right femoral vein has become fibrosed and so blocks the circulation.

To obviate the risk of embolism as far as possible, complete rest for six or eight weeks may be required when thrombosis has occurred. Pain may be relieved by cold or hot applications. Any general or local disorder which predisposes to thrombosis must also be treated.

See Embolism ; Pyaemia.

THRUSH. The growth of a fungus, oidium albicans, on a mucous membrane constitutes thrush. The patches usually occur in the mouth, but may spread to the throat and even to the bowel. In rare instances they have appeared in the vagina. The disorder is most common in children, but debilitated persons of any age may be affected with it.

See Borax ; Furred Tongue ; Mouth.

THUMB. Although there are only two phalanges, or segments, in the thumb as contrasted with three in the fingers, the thumb is much the more mobile because its metacarpal bone moves freely on the carpal bones and those of the fingers do not. Besides the muscles in the forearm that move the thumb there are others in the hand, which together form the fleshy mass known as the thenar eminence, or ball of the thumb. Most of these small muscles are supplied by the median nerve, but others are supplied by the ulnar nerve.

The thumb can be extended and flexed, that is to say, straightened and bent at its middle joint ; it can be abducted, or drawn back from the hand, and adducted, or drawn across the palm ; and it can be opposed or brought across to touch the other fingers with its tip. In paralysis of the median nerve this movement of opposition is lost.

In dislocation the thumb is generally displaced backwards. Sometimes there is considerable difficulty in reducing the dislocation.

See Finger ; Hand.

THYMOL. A crystalline substance obtained from the essential oil of thyme and other plants, thymol has the odour of thyme and a burning taste. It is a powerful antiseptic and in doses of $\frac{1}{2}$ to 2 grains is used to combat infective organisms in the bowel. In doses of 15 to 30 grains it is used to kill hook-worm. When such large doses are administered no oil or alcohol should be taken, otherwise too much thymol may be absorbed into the blood and cause poisoning, the symptoms of which rather resemble those caused by poisonous doses of turpentine.

Thymol is used to make antiseptic lotions, gargles and mouth-washes. It is contained in the compound solution of thymol of the B.P.C., which is used diluted with 3 or 4 parts of water.

THYMUS GLAND. Behind the upper part of the breastbone and projecting above it into the root of the neck, is a structure called the thymus gland. The base rests upon the pericardium, and behind the gland is the trachea. There are two lobes, a right and a left, but there are no ducts, so that if there is any secretion formed, it is an internal one. Under the microscope the thymus is seen to consist of lymphoid tissue, but scattered throughout this are little bodies, composed of epithelial cells concentrically arranged, and known as Hassall's corpuscles.

The gland grows up to the time of puberty, after which it withers, becoming replaced by fatty and fibrous tissue, but portions of the original structure sometimes persist into old age.

Like other masses of lymphoid tissue, the thymus takes part in producing white blood corpuscles. As regards other functions, our knowledge is rather uncertain, and it cannot be said that Hassall's corpuscles do anything. It would appear, however, that there is some connexion between the thymus and the sex glands, as removal of the testes delays the disappearance of the thymus, and removal of the thymus, on the other hand, causes precocious development of the testes. Moreover, there may be some connexion with general development, as in some instances of poor bodily development and muscular weakness, the thymus has been found to be prematurely atrophied.

An overgrowth of the thymus occurs in what is called the status lymphaticus, and also in some other disorders. Such overgrowth may easily be dangerous owing to pressure on the windpipe, and such pressure is the cause of thymic asthma, this being the name given to urgent attacks of difficulty in breathing which occur in infants and sometimes cause sudden death. The only treatment for this condition is removal of the thymus, but this is a difficult operation. In rare instances the thymus is the seat of cancer.

See Status Lymphaticus.

THYROID CARTILAGE. The largest of the cartilaginous structures forming the larynx is called the thyroid cartilage. It is the projection of this cartilage that forms the Adam's apple.

See Larynx.

THYROID EXTRACT. From the thyroid gland of the sheep a powder is prepared which is known as dry thyroid or thyroid "extract." It is commonly given in the form of a tablet, the dose being ½ to 4 grains. There is also a solution of thyroid the dose of which is 5 to 15 minims. Thyroid preparations provide a specific remedy for myxoedema and cretinism, but are useful in obesity and certain other disorders. It is a powerful drug, and over-dosage must be avoided.

See Endocrine ; Thyroid Gland.

THYROID GLAND. One of the important group of structures known as the endocrine glands, the thyroid consists of two lobes connected together by a narrow portion called the isthmus. Each lobe is about 2 inches long and lies by the side of the larynx (*q.v.*) and the upper part of the trachea; the isthmus usually covers the second, third and fourth rings of the trachea. The gland is attached to the cricoid cartilage of the larynx and moves upwards with the larynx in the act of swallowing. The blood supply of the organ is unusually liberal for its size.

The minute structure of the thyroid is seen to consist of a multitude of small spaces, or alveoli, lined with cubical cells and filled with colloid substances. In infancy and at other times when the gland is exceptionally active, the contents of the alveoli are watery. From this thyroid secretion a crystalline substance known as thyroxin, and containing about 60 per cent. of iodine, has been extracted.

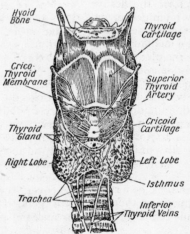

Thyroid Gland. Important two-lobed ductless gland lying in front of the trachea

The thyroid secretion is absorbed by the lymphatics and blood vessels. Its great importance in controlling the metabolism and growth of the body is demonstrated by the fact that a congenital deficiency in the thyroid causes cretinism, while a deficiency occurring in adult life leads to myxoedema. A cretin is a dwarf and an idiot, and the subject of myxoedema becomes heavy and coarse in appearance and dull and stupid in mind. Fortunately any such deficiency in the thyroid gland can be made good by feeding the patient on the extract of the thyroid gland of animals. The extract is even effectual in reducing the weight in ordinary obesity, but as it is a very powerful agent, has to be handled very carefully. Overdosage causes restlessness, headache, insomnia, a very rapid pulse and other symptoms, the ensemble of symptoms being referred to as thyroidism. An excessive activity of the gland occurs in the disorder known as exophthalmic goitre, which is characterised by nervousness, tremor, rapidity of the pulse, wasting of the body, and in typical instances by protrusion of the eyeballs.

A diminishing functioning of the thyroid gland is called hypothyroidism, an excessive functioning, hyperthyroidism, and it is necessary to remember that instances of either of insufficient degree to constitute such patent manifestations as myxoedema or exophthalmic goitre may occur, and sometimes in the slighter degrees the significance of the symptoms may be overlooked. Any enlargement of the thyroid gland is commonly referred to as goitre.

See Cretinism ; Endocrine ; Exophthalmic Goitre; Goitre ; Myxoedema.

TIBIA. The shin-bone, or tibia, is the larger of the two bones of the leg. The shaft is prismatic in shape, one of the edges being directed forwards and forming the shin. This and the inner edge can be easily felt as the surface of the bone between them is covered by skin simply. The bone is expanded at its ends, especially the upper one which with the lower end of the femur forms the knee joint. The fibula takes no part in forming this joint but it forms the outer boundary of the ankle joint, where it swells into a prominence known as the external malleolus. A similar prominence on the inside of the ankle is formed by the tibia and is called the internal malleolus. The bone is shown in the illustration in page 427.

On account of its position and the thinness of its coverings the tibia is very liable to injury from kicks and knocks and periostitis not infrequently follows the bruising of the bone. From the thinness of its covering also a fracture of the tibia is likely to be a compound one.

A forward bending of the tibia in rickets causes what is called sabre-shin. Deformity of the tibia may also be found in congenital syphilis and in other diseases which affect bones.

See Fibula ; Leg.

TIC. A recurring twitch of a muscle or a group of muscles may be an instance of a habit spasm, or tic. Such occurs in a child, usually one with a nervous constitution, and is more common in girls. It begins most frequently between the ages of seven and fourteen. It may follow some acute disease or a fright and is sometimes induced apparently by nasal obstruction, eye trouble, decayed teeth, or some other kind of local irritation. At the beginning, in fact, it may represent some action that might naturally be expected in connexion with such irritation, such as sniffing to clear the nose, or blinking in consequence of irritation in the eye caused by a foreign body or by conjunctivitis.

These are two common forms of tic, but in other cases it may be jerking up the angle of the mouth, shrugging the shoulders, jerking the thigh forward or something else.

The tic can generally be suppressed by force of will but this causes considerable distress and often the tic is aggravated after such an experiment. It is increased also by excitement. In the early stages a tic can usually be cured without great difficulty but if it persists for some time

it is doubtful if anything can be done to prevent its going on throughout life.

The general health should be improved where necessary, and any source of irritation should be dealt with appropriately. It is necessary also to investigate the mental condition, as help can probably be afforded here. Sometimes hypnotism is beneficial. In any event, the child should be trained in controlling the movement.

In adults spasmodic contortions of the face sometimes occur, the trouble usually beginning about the outer angle of the eye. This disorder, which is described as mimic tic, is incurable.

Grimacing may also occur in muscles that have recovered from facial paralysis and in chorea.

See Spasm.

TIC DOULOUREUX. A painful type of neuralgia occurring in branches of the 5th cranial nerve is known as tic douloureux, or trigeminal neuralgia. Most often the first, or ophthalmic, division of the nerve is affected and there is pain above or below the eye or in the eyeball itself, but the second or maxillary division, or the third or mandibular division may be affected, with pain in the upper or the lower jaw. Wherever the pain begins, however, it commonly spreads into other branches of the nerve. Generally the disorder is on one side only.

The paroxysms are very severe and cause twisting of the face on the affected side. There may be a free flow of tears or of saliva and there may be flushing and a sensation of fullness. Paroxysms may succeed one another every few seconds or at much longer intervals. They may be excited by attempts at talking or swallowing or even by a breath of wind on the face.

The disease almost always begins after thirty-five years of age and its causation is obscure. Some local source of irritation is sometimes blamed, such, for example, as carious teeth, but often enough even good teeth have been extracted without the slightest benefit. The usual remedies for neuralgia (*q.v.*) are tried ; aspirin, phenacetin, arsenic or quinine or combinations of these are sometimes of use. Gelsemium and butyl-chloral hydrate are even more powerful. Alcohol and opiates are dangerous remedies as a craving for either may be created. The injection of alcohol into branches of the nerve or even into the Gasserian ganglion may be adopted when the disease is intractable, or the ganglion may even be removed by operation. *See* Neuralgia ; Trigeminal Nerve.

TICK. In the spider class of animal are included the ticks, creatures which lurk in undergrowth and herbage but make their way from time to time on to the bodies of men or the lower animals for the purpose of feeding on blood. Not only mammals but birds and reptiles are thus laid under tribute. The female tick becomes engorged and swells, becoming like a reddish or purplish berry.

Relapsing fever in Equatorial Africa and Madagascar is called tick fever, as it is carried from one person to another by a tick. Mountain fever, or the spotted fever of the Rocky Mountains, which seems to be identical with typhus, is also carried by a tick, and so is the Texas fever in cattle. This, however, does not by any means exhaust the list of the infections so carried.

A tick should not be dragged off the skin by main force, otherwise a nasty sore will probably result. The spontaneous detachment of the creature will be provoked by bathing the part with petrol or with a weak solution of carbolic acid, or some other antiseptic. The bite should be dabbed over with iodine.

TIGHT LACING. A downward displacement of the abdominal organs is caused by tight lacing and leads to dyspepsia and constipation. Another possible consequence is that the venous circulation in the abdomen may be obstructed and result in varicose veins, piles, and congestion in the pelvic organs. A notable improvement in health amongst women generally has followed the adoption of a more rational style of dress, though a larger amount of open-air exercise, made possible by the freer clothing, shares in the credit for the improvement.

TIN. A mixture of pure tin and tin oxide, or the latter substance alone, has been found to have a curative effect in boils, acne and similar complaints.

Acute poisoning by tin has been caused by the acids of preserved fruits dissolving off a considerable quantity of the metal from containers. The symptoms are those of acute irritant poisoning.

TINCTURE. Alcoholic solutions of drugs, tinctures may contain only one drug or several. The former, described as simple tinctures, are represented by such tinctures as those of aconite, belladonna, digitalis, nux vomica, opium, etc., and the latter, or compound tinctures, by such as those of benzoin camphor and gentian, the ammoniated tinctures of quinine and opium and the tincture of chloroform and morphine. In the ethereal tincture of lobelia ether is used as the menstruum instead of alcohol.

As regards dosage, tinctures can be grouped in two classes, those with a dose of $\frac{1}{2}$ to 1 drachm and those with a dose of 5 to 15 minims or less. Tincture of pyrethrum and the strong tincture of iodine are not used internally at all.

TINEA. A generic name for a group of skin diseases caused by fungi, the term tinea is qualified in the names of the various diseases by an adjective indicative of the particular parasite present. the site of the disease or the appearance of the eruption. Examples are tinea trico-phytina or ringworm caused by the tricophyton fungus, tinea barbae or ringworm of the beard, and tinea favosa or honeycomb ringworm, properly called favus.

TINNITUS. *See* Noises in the Ears.

TISSUE. A considerable number of different tissues go to the make-up of the body, but they can all be included in four groups, namely, nervous tissue, muscular tissue, epithelial tissue and connective tissue. Essentially, any tissue consists of cells and an intercellular substance, though the characters and the relative proportions of each of these may vary. Thus, epithelium consists almost entirely of cells with very little intercellular substance, while in some kinds of connective tissue the opposite is found.

A cell consists of a mass of protoplasm containing a nucleus. The protoplasm is composed of a more solid element in the form of a network, known as the spongioplasm, in the interstices of which is a more liquid part, the hyaloplasm. The nucleus is surrounded by a membrane and its substance also consists of a spongy part, the nuclear reticulum, and a more liquid part, the nuclear lymph. ❧ Within the nucleus there is contained a tiny rounded body known as the nucleolus ; sometimes there is more than one. The membrane, the reticulum, and the nucleolus contain a substance which takes on certain stains and is therefore described as chromatin.

Cells multiply by dividing and occasionally the division is a simple process, but almost always it is a complicated process called karyokinesis. Here there is first a definite rearrangement of the chromatin filaments and then a division through these.

Nervous tissue is discussed under the heading Nervous System, muscular tissue under that of Muscle, and epithelial tissue under that of Epithelium.

There are several varieties of connective tissue, including jelly-like tissue, fibrous tissue, cartilage, bone and blood. In these the cells and the intercellular tissue differ in character. In blood the latter is constituted by the plasma. In the jelly-like tissue, which occurs in the umbilical cord and forms the vitreous humour of the eye, a clear, soft substance forms the great bulk of the tissue, while in fibrous tissue most of the bulk consists of white fibres which have been laid down in a homogeneous matrix, or ground substance.

How Bone and Cartilage are Formed

Cartilage, or gristle, consists of a ground substance in which numerous cells and sometimes fibres, white or yellow elastic, are disposed. Cartilage containing fibres is called fibro-cartilage, white fibro-cartilage or yellow elastic fibro-cartilage as the case may be. Cartilage with a clear matrix is called hyaline cartilage. Bone is developed from hyaline cartilage. Fibres first form in the matrix and round these lime salts are deposited. In the dentine, of which teeth are formed, and which resembles bone, mineral salts have also been laid down.

A type of connective tissue, known as areolar tissue, which occurs in the subcutaneous tissue, in the sheaths of organs, nerves and blood vessels and elsewhere, consists of cells, ground substance and fibres, both white and yellow. Adipose or fatty tissue consists of areolar tissue in which cells have become swollen with fat.

A tissue composed of a network made up of white fibres and an odd yellow one, and a rather fluid matrix, is called retiform tissue. When the spaces are filled with lymph corpuscles it is called lymphoid tissue. This occurs in the tonsil and elsewhere.

In the developing embryo there are three primitive layers, an outer one, known as the epiblast, or ectoderm ; an inner, known as the hypoblast, or entoderm ; and a middle one, called the mesoblast, or mesoderm. From the first are developed the surface epithelium and the nervous tissues ; from the second most of the epithelial lining of the alimentary and respiratory tracts ; and from the third, the muscular and connective tissues.
See Blood ; Bone ; Cell.

TOBACCO. The tobacco leaf contains an oily alkaloid known as nicotine which is freely soluble in water and alcohol and is volatilised by heat so that it occurs in tobacco smoke. Most occurs when tobacco is damp, so that a bigger dose of alkaloid is obtained from the smoke of a dirty pipe, in addition to what is swallowed in the moisture sucked from the pipe. There is more of the alkaloid in cigar smoke than in cigarette smoke ; but if a long holder is used and the cigarette is smoked to the end the effect is more or less that of smoking a pipe.

When tobacco is burned certain volatile substances are produced, the most important being carbon monoxide, pyridine and ammonia. Pyridine is not very toxic, but it and the ammonia irritate the air passages. The carbon monoxide unites with the haemoglobin of the red blood corpuscles.

The poisonous effects of tobacco are due to the nicotine and the carbon monoxide and may manifest themselves on a first trial of the drug in giddiness, nausea, vomiting, and profuse sweating and perhaps diarrhoea. There is also general relaxation of the muscles, a fact of which advantage has sometimes been taken to facilitate the reduction of a dislocation.

With continued use of tobacco, however, tolerance is acquired and there are no such unpleasant effects; on the other hand, there may be a stimulating effect on the brain and at the same time a sedative one, so that work may be done more easily and worry and excitability may be lessened. Some people find that a smoke after breakfast is a useful aid to securing an action of the bowels. It is possible that some of the comfort derived from smoking is due to the sight of the smoke, as the habit is usually given up if for any reason a smoker loses his sight. Sometimes the ritual of smoking may also contribute; some people, for example, find little pleasure in smoking unless they roll their own cigarettes or fill the pipe for themselves.

Although for the mature smoking may have undoubted advantages, there is an almost unanimous medical opinion against juvenile smoking. The use of tobacco by growing persons is believed to hinder growth and development and there are good grounds for thinking that the habit may induce a desire for alcohol.

Even adults may sustain damage if they use tobacco immoderately. Tobacco diminishes the sense of hunger and an excessive use may impair appetite and digestion. It may also cause spasm of the pyloric end of the stomach and hyperchlorhydria, which in turn may lead to the development of a duodenal ulcer. Sometimes also spasm in the lower bowel may cause an obstinate constipation which disappears when tobacco is given up. Hiccough is occasionally due to excessive smoking.

Excess in tobacco may cause instability of the heart and a quickening of its action, a condition sometimes described as the tobacco heart. It may give rise to painful attacks resembling angina pectoris, and may even cause syncope, and this has been fatal in some instances.

It is the cause also of the spasmodic contraction of the arteries of the limbs in some of the victims of the disorder known as intermittent claudication. Excessive smoking may cause the

onset of headache and perhaps induce a habit of insomnia.

The smoke from cigarettes may get into the eyes and cause a catarrhal conjunctivitis; but much more serious than this is the effect of an excess of tobacco on the optic nerves, causing an impairment of vision which is referred to as tobacco amblyopia. There is first a diminution in the power to distinguish the colours of small objects, and a blunting of the sharpness of outlines. If tobacco is given up before the condition has lasted very long there may be complete recovery, but sometimes ability to read and do similar near work is permanently lost.

Excessive smoking may cause inflammation of the mouth, nose, and throat, and there may be a serious diminution of the sense of smell. Pharyngitis may occur, and this results in an irritating cough, frequently troublesome on first getting up in the morning. Catarrh in the lower air tubes may result from inhaling tobacco smoke and may be accompanied by wheezing. The appearance of any of the consequences of excessive smoking should be taken as a hint to reduce the allowance. Sometimes, however, the only possible course is to give up tobacco altogether.

TOE. Each of the toes consists of three segments, or phalanges, except the first, or great, toe, which has only two. The joints between the phalanges are called the inter-phalangeal joints, and those between the toe and the remainder of the foot, the metatarso-phalangeal joints (*see* illustration in page 314).

Disorders and deformities of the toes are mainly due to improperly designed boots and especially to the pointed boot. By this the great toe is pressed outwards

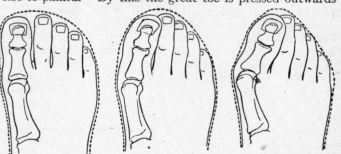

Toe. Deformity of the great toe, leading to the formation of a bunion, due to wearing a pointed shoe instead of one made in a natural shape (left)

and in time remains in this position, described as hallux valgus (*q.v.*). To relieve pressure on the head of the metatarsal bone to which the toe is jointed a bursa forms, but this may become inflamed and swollen, forming a bunion.

Hallux rigidus is the name applied to the great toe when there is immobility or stiffness at the metatarso-phalangeal joint. This usually occurs in young adults with flat foot, but here again the boot is probably responsible. There is more or less disability in walking. Correction of the flat foot and the provision of a proper boot is necessary, while the joint may be dressed with the compound mercury or with the colourless iodine ointment. Sometimes, however, an operation will be required.

A common accompaniment of hallux valgus is overcrowding of the other toes, which may actually overlap one another. A hammer toe (*q.v.*) is one that is over-extended at the metatarso-phalangeal joint and flexed at the first inter-phalangeal joint, so that the first two segments make a V with the point directed upwards.

An X-ray photograph showing dislocation of the great toe is given in Plate XIV, 5.

See Corn ; Foot ; Hallux Valgus ; Hammer Toe.

TOLERANCE. Persons who take certain drugs regularly may be able to take with impunity doses which would cause poisonous effects in one not so habituated. They are said to have acquired a tolerance for the drug. This happens, for example, with opium, arsenic and tobacco. There may even be a natural tolerance for some drug with, however, the ordinary, or perhaps an excessive, susceptibility to the action of other drugs.

Tolerance towards the activities of bacteria and their poisons is described as immunity (*q.v.*).

See Dose.

TOLU. Balsam of tolu is a fragrant substance which is used as an expectorant. There is a syrup and a tincture, the dose of each being $\frac{1}{2}$ to 1 drachm. Tolu is contained in Friar's balsam.

TONE. Normally a muscle is always prepared for action and there is no need to gather in any slack before it begins to contract. This preparedness is described as tone, and it depends on the integrity of the reflex arc that connects the muscle with the spinal cord. It is the existence of tone that accounts for the tendon reflexes of which the knee jerk (*q.v.*) is an example. Tone exists in the involuntary muscles as well as in the voluntary, and dyspepsia and constipation are sometimes due to lack of tone in the musculature of the stomach and bowel

TONGUE. The substance of the tongue consists almost entirely of interlaced bundles of muscle-fibres, some of them passing from side to side, others from before backwards, and others still from above downwards. These are called the intrinsic muscles of the tongue. The other muscles of the tongue, the extrinsic set, connect the organ to the lower jaw, the hyoid bone and the soft palate. The tongue is covered with mucous membrane.

The upper surface of the tongue is called the dorsum, and presents towards the back a V-shaped formation of red spots, slightly elevated. The apex of the V is directed backwards, and is formed by a depression, called the foramen caecum, which represents the upper end of a tube,

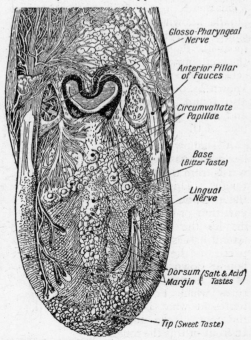

Glosso-Pharyngeal
Nerve

Anterior Pillar
of Fauces

Circumvallate
Papillae

Base
(Bitter Taste)

Lingual
Nerve

Dorsum (Salt & Acid)
Margin (Tastes)

Tip (Sweet Taste)

Tongue. The upper surface is studded with **papillae**

the thyro-glossal duct, by which in the embryo the thyroid gland opens into the throat, but which is subsequently obliterated.

About two-thirds of the dorsum of the tongue lie in front of the V, and its mucous covering has a different appearance from that of the remaining third. This is studded with lymphoid nodules, the total collection of which is often referred to as the lingual tonsil, but the mucous membrane of the anterior two-thirds is thick and rough from the presence of an immense number of elevations, or papillae. Most of these are little conical elevations, but dotted over the surface are larger and redder papillae, known on account of their mushroom shape as fungiform papillae. In other papillae the end of the cone is prolonged into a bunch of thread-like projections ; these are called filiform papillae.

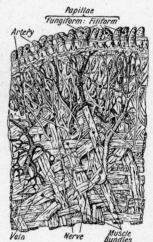

Tongue. Section showing interlaced intrinsic muscles

The red spots of the V-formation represent still another kind of papilla known as the circumvallate, because each is surrounded by a tiny, moat-like depression. In the covering of these circumvallate papillae are specialised cells, grouped in bundles, which are known as taste-buds, but taste-buds are also found dotted here and there on the front part of the tongue.

A shallow furrow will be seen passing backwards from the tip of the tongue. This represents the position of a fibrous partition, or raphe, which divides the tongue into lateral halves. The back part of the tongue is bound down to the floor of the mouth by structures which together represent what is called the root of the tongue. In front of this the tongue is free and presents an

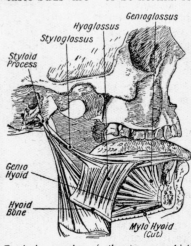

Extrinsic muscles of the tongue which connect it to the jaw and actuate it

under surface which has a smooth covering, however, as contrasted with what obtains on the dorsum. Part of the smooth covering is prolonged forwards in the middle line to make a fold, and this is known as the frenum of the tongue. Sometimes it comes too far forward and is shorter than usual, so that the movements of the tip of the tongue are hampered. This condition is popularly called tongue-tied, and can easily be remedied.

The tongue is freely supplied with blood, a large artery, the lingual, passing up into the organ from the neck. All the muscles are supplied by the 12th cranial, or hypo-glossal nerve. Ordinary sensation in the anterior two-thirds of the tongue depends on the lingual branch of the trigeminal nerve and taste on the chorda tympani, which is a branch of the facial nerve. The posterior third is supplied, both for touch and taste, mainly by the glosso-pharyngeal nerve.

The tongue takes an active part in chewing, swallowing and talking, and is the organ of the sense of taste.

The tongue is normally pink in colour, moist and clean and, although it seems to be normal for some individuals to have a little fur on the tongue, the presence of fur points, as a rule, to indigestion, bad teeth or some other local or general disorder. Fur consists of moulds and other organisms with epithelial débris and particles of food. The colour may be white, yellow, brown or even black.

The appearance of the tongue may be a useful guide in diagnosis, and sometimes in prognosis. What is called the strawberry tongue usually points to scarlet fever, for example, and a dry, brown, tremulous tongue in a late state of fevers is a bad sign.

Injuries and Diseases of the Tongue. A wound of the tongue may give rise to free bleeding. It may be possible to arrest this by grasping the tongue with the fingers and stitching the wound, but it is sometimes necessary to tie the lingual artery in the neck.

Inflammation of the tongue is called glossitis, and may be superficial or deep. If the latter, the swelling may be considerable, more particularly if an abscess should form, and breathing may be obstructed. An immediate free incision is required to liberate any pus.

Acute superficial glossitis may be caused by excessive smoking, drinking hot or pungent liquids or some infection. There is swelling and pain, interfering more or less with the functions of the organ. Diet should be restricted to bland, cool liquids, and a bland mouth wash used, say a weak solution of borax or of permanganate of potassium. Smoking should be discontinued until the tongue has recovered.

Chronic superficial glossitis may follow acute attacks, or may come on insidiously. Syphilis is the commonest cause. White patches occur on the tongue, constituting what is called leukoplakia, but later these peel off, leaving the tongue red and glazed. Later still, cracks and fissures tend to appear, and in one of these an epitheliomatous cancer may occur. Aphthous patches may form on the tongue, or patches of thrush. Ulceration of the tongue is often caused by a jagged tooth, but may be due to syphilis or tuberculosis, or to cancer. Naevi and other simple tumours may form in the tongue, but are not common. Cancer occurs fairly frequently, especially in men. Its appearance may be preceded by chronic superficial glossitis, or an ulcer caused by a tooth or otherwise, but it may appear apart from any such circumstances. At the beginning it may resemble a wart or only a slight thickening of the surface of the tongue, and may be quite painless. Later it ulcerates, and probably becomes infected by bacteria. The glands under the jaw become enlarged. The growth

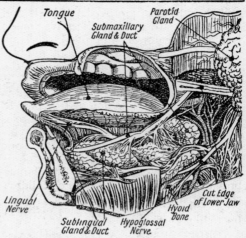

Tongue. All the tongue muscles are served by the hypoglossal nerve, and sensation supplied to the anterior two-thirds by the lingual nerve

should be removed by operation, and also any glands which might possibly be affected, and this must be done at the earliest stage to afford much hope of a cure. Radium may have great usefulness here.

Sometimes a black patch forms on the tongue, usually at the back. It is referred to as black tongue, hairy tongue, or nigrites, and is caused by overgrowth of the filiform papillae with degeneration of the surface epithelium or growth of a fungus called aspergillus niger. The patch should be rubbed over with glycerin containing 5 grains of salicylic acid to the ounce.

See Hyoid Bone ; Radium ; Ranula ; Salivary Gland ; Speech ; Taste.

TONIC. In a literal sense a tonic is an agent that improves muscular tone or tension, but the term has come to have a more extended meaning and is applied, for example, to agents that improve the quality of the blood or of the nerves. Nevertheless, the purpose in view in giving a tonic is actually that of increasing the tone of the muscles and thus developing vigour. Iron is given as a blood tonic, for instance, and when it improves the quality of the red blood corpuscles there is necessarily an improvement in the nutrition and therefore in the tone of muscles whenever this is at all possible.

Similarly, strychnine is given as a nerve tonic, but if the activity of the motor centres in the spinal cord is stimulated by this drug the muscles share in the benefit and their tone is improved. Bitters and other drugs are given as digestive tonics, and here again an improved digestion makes for a better nutrition of muscles in common with the other tissues of the body and an increase of tone.

Digitalis is given as a heart tonic and is entitled to the designation as it definitely improves the tone of the heart muscle. During convalescence or in debility induced by excessive application to work Easton's Syrup, which contains the phosphates of quinine, iron and strychnine, provides an excellent tonic. For children chemical food is a suitable tonic.

See Bitters; Digitalis; Easton's Syrup; Iron; Nux Vomica.

TONIC SPASM. A continuous spasmodic contraction of a muscle is called a tonic spasm. A general tonic spasm is illustrated in the first stage of an epileptic fit in which the whole body becomes rigid as contrasted with the rapid, tumultuous movements, or clonic spasms, of the second stage. A localised tonic spasm is seen in lockjaw.

TONSIL. A mass of lymphoid tissue situated between the pillars of the fauces (*q.v.*) on either side, the tonsil varies in shape and size in different individuals. It

Tonsil. Left, relative position of the tonsils. Right, tonsils cut across, showing the crypts which may harbour infective microbes

is relatively large in childhood, but in elderly people usually shrinks to very small dimensions. On its surface there are from twelve to fifteen depressions representing the openings into the passages, or crypts, that run more or less deeply into its substance. The tonsil does not fill the space between the pillars of the fauces right to the top, and the unoccupied space is known as the supratonsillar recess; it contains fibrous tissue.

For its size the tonsil is very freely supplied with blood vessels, and its main function appears to be that of trapping toxic material as it passes backward from the mouth. The organ drains into the upper group of lymphatic glands in the neck. It often happens, however, that the tonsil is overwhelmed by the toxins and becomes itself chronically infected, when it is a source of danger rather than a protection.

Diseases of the Tonsil. The tonsil is the usual first site of diphtheritic infection and is probably the usual door of entrance of the germs of scarlet fever and of acute rheumatism. It is one of the routes by which tuberculosis invades the system. The tonsil may be the site of a sarcomatous growth, and is sometimes invaded by a carcinoma from the mouth or throat, or such a tumour may originate in the organ. Unless it is very small a malignant growth in the tonsil is very difficult to eradicate.

Inflammation of the tonsil, or tonsillitis, may assume a variety of forms. The tonsils may be involved in the simple catarrhal inflammation of the throat that occurs in a common cold, but types of acute inflammation also occur in the tonsil itself. The first type is called acute follicular, or lacunar, tonsillitis. The inflammation is superficial and the tonsil is swollen and reddened, but dotted over it are yellowish spots, caused by the accumulation of inflammatory products in the crypts. Generally both tonsils are affected. It is sometimes impossible, without a bacteriological test, to say that the deposit on the tonsil is not due to diphtheria.

The second type is called parenchymatous tonsillitis, that is, inflammation in the substance of the tonsil, and a third is called peritonsillitis, as the inflammation occurs mainly in the connective tissue around the tonsil. These two types are sometimes called quinsy. Peritonsillitis usually ends in suppuration, and the matter presses the already swollen tonsil inwards. Suppuration occasionally occurs also in the parenchymatous and lacunar varieties.

PLATE XXXVII

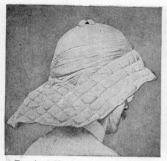
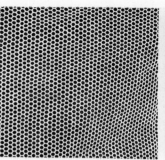
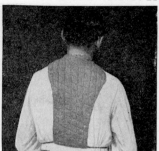

Tropical Hygiene. 1. Sun helmet. 2. Mosquito netting, actual size. 3. Quilted pad for spinal protection

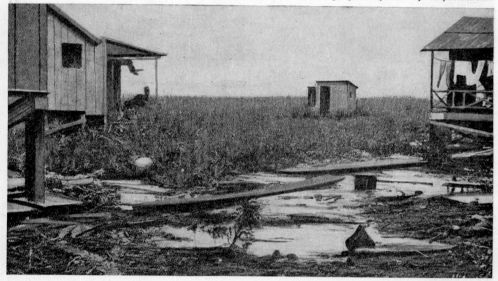

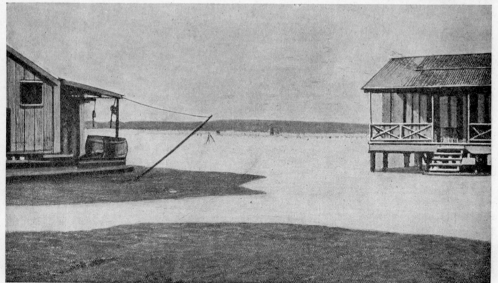

4. Huts in a labourers' camp in Costa Rica, the undrained land affording ideal breeding-places for mosquitoes, with much resulting sickness. 5. Site after the land had been drained and the surface concreted

PLATE XXXVIII

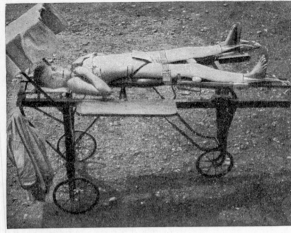
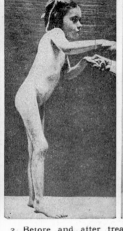
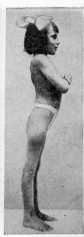

Tuberculosis.   1. Open-air treatment for hip disease   2. Before and after treatment at Alton

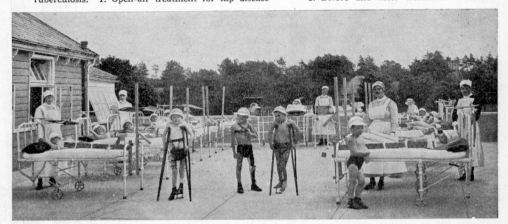

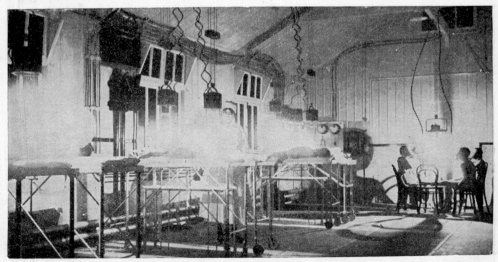

3. (Above) Treatment by natural sunlight. 4. Light department where patients are exposed to ultra-violet rays

1, *Courtesy of Princess Mary's Hospital for Children, Margate;* 2—4, *Courtesy of Treloar Cripples' Hospital and College, Alton*

To face page 665

The fourth type is that of acute ulcerative tonsillitis, but in this there are various sub-types, as the ulceration is sometimes superficial and sometimes deep, and, moreover, the cause varies in different instances. Vincent's angina is a form of ulcerative tonsillitis in which a membrane appears on the tonsil and the ulceration may extend to adjoining parts and even involve its bone. It is caused by a spirillum working in conjunction with a bacillus. Ulceration also occurs in secondary syphilis and in diphtheria.

Acute tonsillitis begins with stiffness in the throat and pain in swallowing. The temperature shoots up and is usually high ; sometimes there is chill or even a definite rigor. There may be headache and pains in the back and limbs. The tongue is furred, and there is constipation. Pain increases, especially in quinsy, and may shoot into the ear. Also, on account of the pain and the swelling of the tonsils and neighbouring parts, swallowing becomes difficult and, in quinsy. may be well nigh impossible. The glands below the angle of the jaw become swollen and painful.

Measures to Relieve Pain

As regards treatment, certain things may be done to relieve pain and difficulty in swallowing, whatever the nature of the disorder, but tonsillitis cannot be properly treated unless a correct diagnosis has been made, and the possibility of diphtheria ruled out.

The abscess in quinsy will burst in time, but it should not be allowed to do so, as the patient's sufferings can be curtailed by opening it. Moreover, there is a definite risk of pus being drawn into the windpipe, should the abscess burst when the patient is asleep.

To relieve pain, hot fomentations or poultices may be put to the throat, and steam may be inhaled from a jug of hot water. The addition of a teaspoonful of Friar's balsam to the water in the jug is a distinct advantage. Sprays containing menthol are soothing. Ice may be sucked, especially before the patient drinks as swallowing will be rendered easier. The bowels should be kept freely open by salines in the morning. Doses of sodium salicylate, or of aspirin, help to relieve pain and are necessary if there is any question of acute rheumatism.

In follicular tonsillitis the following gargle should be used :

Potassium chlorate..	90 grains
Tincture of perchloride of iron	2 drachms
Glycerin	4 drachms
Chloroform water	to 6 ounces

A tablespoonful in a little water to be gargled and swallowed thrice daily. This is the dose for an adult.

When the tonsillitis is severe, a swab examination should be made to determine the nature of the infecting organism, as the injection of an appropriate serum may be very beneficial.

If there has been a recurrence of attacks of acute tonsillitis, the tonsils should be removed when the patient has properly recovered from the attack.

A chronic enlargement of the tonsils is common in children, and is generally associated with adenoids. If the diseased structures are allowed to persist, not only do they interfere with breathing, but they act as foci of infection. A frequent result is enlargement of the glands in the neck owing to tuberculous infection. Chronic disease may exist in adults also, although the tonsils are not greatly swollen, and may also poison the system, giving rise to rheumatism and other disorders. The correct treatment for diseased tonsils is to have them removed, an operation described as tonsillectomy. This generally means that the structures must be dissected out, as it is undesirable that even a small portion of diseased tonsil should be left.

See Adenoids ; Angina ; Atomiser ; Diphtheria ; Fauces ; Inhalation.

TOPHUS. A chalk-like deposit that occurs in gout is known as a tophus. Despite its appearance and its popular name of chalkstone a tophus does not consist of chalk but of biurate of sodium. The commonest site of a tophus is the external ear and then the joints of the fingers and toes, but a tophus may form in other situations.

See Gout.

TORPOR. A sluggish condition of body and mind is described as torpor. This occurs, for example, after a heavy meal and is a not uncommon event in old people. Torpidity of the liver is generally just constipation and can be relieved by attention to the bowels and restriction of the diet.

TORSION. The term torsion, which simply means twisting, is applied to the method of arresting bleeding from small arteries by grasping them with forceps and twisting them. This causes the inner coat of the artery to curl up. Torsion is also said to take place when the stalk of a pedunculated tumour becomes twisted or when the bowel becomes twisted and produces volvulus.

TORTICOLLIS. *See* Wry Neck.

TOUCH. Knowledge of something being in contact with a surface of the body, irrespective of the temperature of the touching object or of its causing any pain, is derived through the special tactile, or touch, sense. Special nerve endings receive the tactile impressions, and the nerve-impulses run along special fibres and in special tracts in the spinal cord. One is able to say, without looking, what part of the body is being touched, and if two objects are touching a part of the body at the same time, to recognize that there are two, but only if they are sufficiently far apart.

The distance required for this discrimination varies for different parts. Thus, at the tip of the tongue it is only $\frac{1}{25}$ inch, at the tip of a finger it is about $\frac{1}{12}$ inch, but on the back of the hand it is 1 inch, and on the back of the trunk about $2\frac{1}{2}$ inches. This test is made by means of an instrument called an aesthesiometer. This resembles a pair of calipers, but the points are blunted sufficiently to prevent them from pricking. Hairy parts are specially sensitive to touch, as the hair convey the impressions of contact to the skin very accurately.

Certain minute areas on the skin are concerned with tactile reception, while others are concerned with receiving sensations of temperature or pain.

Loss of the sense of touch, or anaesthesia, may be noted in many disorders. In syringomyelia, however, the sense of touch may be preserved, although the sense of temperature and of pain have been lost. Excessive sensibility to touch, that is, a sensation of considerable pressure

from a very light object, may be present in hysteria, but generally what occurs in this and other disorders is a heightened sensibility to pain, or hyperalgesia. Unusual sensations, such as numbness, tingling, are described as paraesthesia.
See Hyperaesthesia ; Sensation.

TOURNIQUET. An instrument used for arresting or preventing bleeding, a tourniquet consists essentially of a pad for placing over the artery and an appliance for pressing the pad down on the artery. This appliance may be a rubber tube, which is drawn tightly round the limb, as in the elastic tourniquet ; a rigid band, as in the field tourniquet ; or a screw, as in Petit's tourniquet.

An improvised tourniquet is made by tying a folded handkerchief or triangular bandage loosely on the limb, placing a pad beneath the bandage and over the artery and passing a stick under the bandage and screwing it round until the pad is pressing sufficiently tight on the artery. The stick is prevented from slipping by tying another bandage round it and the limb (*see* Plate XXXIV, 6). A sufficient amount of pressure has been applied when the bleeding stops or there is a cessation of pulsation in the arteries below the tourniquet.

A tourniquet must be applied where it is possible to compress an artery, that is, on the thigh for the lower limb and on the arm for the upper. To prevent bleeding during an operation it is customary to make several turns with a pure rubber or a woven elastic bandage round the limb. A tourniquet should not be left tightly applied for longer than half-an-hour at a time, otherwise the tissues that are deprived of blood may die.
See Bleeding ; Ligature ; Styptic.

TOXAEMIA. Poisoning of the blood by substances formed by bacteria or by perverted activities of the body cells themselves is called toxaemia. Apart from more definite diseases this often happens from sepsis in the mouth or from constipation or a malignant growth.

TOXICOLOGY. The branch of medical science dealing with poisons, their nature, their detection, their effects on the body, and the treatment of poisoning, is called toxicology.

TOXIN. The poisonous substances produced by bacteria are known as toxins. Some of these substances are set free in the blood or any other medium in which the organisms can thrive, while others are contained in the protoplasm of the organisms themselves, but are liberated when the protoplasm is disintegrated. The former are called exotoxins and the latter endotoxins. The tissues of the body form substances that neutralise the circulating toxins and are therefore known as antitoxins. The effects of the toxin of one species of bacterium may differ from those caused by that of another just as the active principles in the higher plants differ in their actions.

See Antibody ; Antitoxin.

TRACHEA. The main airway into the lungs, the trachea, extends from the lower border of the cricoid cartilage of the larynx to the level of the second piece of the breast-bone and is about $4\frac{1}{2}$ inches in length. It consists of a membranous tube which is strengthened by the inclusion of about twenty cartilaginous rings. These are not complete, however, but have a considerable gap behind where the tube is represented by membrane simply.

Behind the trachea is the gullet. In front of the 2nd, 3rd and 4th rings is the isthmus of the thyroid gland, the lateral lobes of which are applied to the sides of the tube, and between the trachea and the first part of the breast bone is the thymus gland. Any considerable enlargement of either of those glands is liable to compress the trachea and cause difficulty in breathing.

The tube may be obstructed by compression from without in strangling or garrotting ; or by a foreign body which manages to pass through the larynx ; or by a foreign body in the gullet, which, on account of the gap in the rings, is able to compress the tube by projecting forwards into it. The trachea forks at its lower end into the right and left bronchial tubes, as shown in the illustration in p. 119. By means of an instrument known as the bronchoscope, it is possible to examine the interior of the trachea and of the upper parts at least of the bronchial tubes. In the operation called tracheotomy a vertical opening is made into the trachea, either above or below the isthmus of the thyroid gland, and through this opening a tracheotomy tube is passed.

TRAGACANTH. A gummy exudation from certain leguminous trees, tragacanth occurs as thin, curved transparent flakes resembling the peelings of corns. It swells up and forms a mucilage on the addition of water. It may be used as a demulcent in sore throat, but is chiefly used for suspending a heavy powder in a mixture and for making pills. There are three official preparations, namely the glycerin, the mucilage and the compound powder. The dose of the last is 10 to 60 grains.

TRAINING. The aims in training for athletics are to develop as far as possible the necessary muscles for the feat that is aimed at, and to get rid of superfluous fat. The exercise must be graduated for a person whose condition is only fair to begin with and, throughout the training, must be kept within bounds.

The chief changes in the diet are an increase in proteins and a diminution of carbohydrates. Proteins are chiefly taken in the form of meat, and especially beef steaks. Pastries, jams and sweets were formerly cut out, but there is a tendency nowadays to relax this régime in so far as sugar is concerned, as a ration of sugar, preferably as glucose, minimises fatigue in men doing arduous muscular toil. The usual aim is a diet furnishing about 4,000 calories. Liquids are restricted and the use of tobacco is barred.

See Exercise.

Trachea or windpipe. Principal air tube of the body

TRANCE. A condition that simulates death very closely is described as a trance. The patient makes no movement whatever and cannot be roused by any kind of external stimulus. It may be impossible to feel the pulse or even to hear the heart, and there may be no signs of breathing. The body remains warm, however, the muscles respond to electrical stimulation, and there is no evidence of decomposition. These facts should enable a correct diagnosis to be made.

A trance generally comes on suddenly, often after a convulsion, and may persist for many weeks. Recovery is also sudden, as a rule. Sometimes the condition is not quite so pronounced as in the description just given, for the heart may be heard and there may be slight dimming of a mirror held in front of the mouth. The patient may even make some resistance to interference. A state of this kind can be induced by hypnotism.

Trance is hysterical in origin and occurs most often in young women. While it lasts the patient should be kept warm and must be fed through a tube, if necessary. After the awakening psychotherapeutic treatment is required for the hysteria.

See Catalepsy ; Death ; Ecstasy.

TRANSFUSION. After a severe haemorrhage, or in serious forms of anaemia, it may be considered necessary to transfuse blood into the patient. This is done by withdrawing blood from a volunteer, described as the donor, into a vessel in which clotting is prevented by oiling the inside or by the addition of a solution of sodium citrate, and then allowing the blood to run into one of the patient's veins.

It has been found that the blood of one person may not be compatible with that of another in that it causes a destruction of the red corpuscles, and it has likewise been shown that what matters is the fate of the red blood corpuscles of the donor's blood. If these are not affected by being injected into the blood of the patient, then there is compatibility, although some red blood cells of the patient may be broken down.

From tests it would appear that in this respect human beings can be divided into four classes. There is a class which can take blood from any other person, and these are known as universal recipients. There is another class whose blood is compatible with that of any other person, and these are known as universal donors Then there are two classes whose blood is only compatible with that of their own class or with that of a universal recipient.

It cannot be presumed that the blood from members of the same family will be compatible. Frequently it is not, and the only way to determine the matter is by making tests by means of the blood serum of the patient with a drop of blood from a volunteer.

Often it is considered sufficient to transfuse with normal saline solution instead of blood.

See Normal Saline Solution.

TRANSPORT OF THE SICK AND INJURED. Not only does a proper method of carriage make a patient more comfortable, but a haphazard and unskilful method may aggravate his condition, perhaps to the extent of endangering life. The choice of a method will depend on the nature of the injury or illness, the number of bearers available, the appliances at hand, the nature of the route and the distance to be traversed.

Should the injury or sickness be of a serious nature, it is desirable that a patient should be seen by a doctor before he is moved at all beyond what is necessary to keep him clear of risks from machinery or otherwise. When a bone has been broken the fracture should be secured by splints or bandages, when such will suffice, before any attempt is made to move the patient.

When there is a fracture of a lower limb or an injury to the spine, it is necessary to use a rigid stretcher ; that is, one that will not sag from the weight of the patient. Though, if the patient must be carried along a narrow passage, and the fracture is only in the lower limb and securely splinted, three bearers, all facing in the same direction, might carry the patient pillowed in their arms. If there is a spinal injury, however, the patient must lie on a board, as the spine could not be kept sufficiently rigid by side splints.

When a patient is unconscious, and must be moved at once, owing to fire or some other danger, and there is only one bearer, or it is necessary to go down a ladder, the best method is that known as the fireman's lift. The patient should be lying on the face. The bearer stoops opposite the patient's head and raises him into a kneeling position. He now places his right shoulder against the patient's body about the middle and carries the patient's right arm behind his own neck. Then he places his right arm between the patient's thighs—or, if it is a woman, round both thighs—grasps the patient's right wrist and rises. The bearer's left hand is thus left free to grip a ladder, or otherwise afford support (*see* Plate XXXVI, 4 and 5).

When the Patient can Help Himself

When a patient is able to walk, a single bearer can afford him assistance by taking the patient's right or left arm over his own shoulders and grasping him round the middle with his other hand. By inclining his body away from the patient, the bearer can take much of the weight off the patient's legs. Another method of removal by a single bearer is to carry the patient pickaback (Plate XXXV, 6). The patient is put in a sitting position with his legs apart, and the bearer stands between his legs and stoops with his back to the patient, who then puts his arms round the bearer's neck. The bearer grasps the patient's thighs and rises up. A stout bandage looped round the bearer's shoulders and below the patient's buttocks makes this method considerably easier.

When two bearers are available, the fore-and-aft method may be adopted. One bearer supports the head and trunk by placing his hands beneath the patient's armpits and clasping them in front of his chest, while the other places himself between, and carries, the thighs (Plate XXXV, 4). Should a leg have been injured a splint is put on, the legs tied together and carried in the arms of the first bearer (Plate XXXV, 5).

If, however, the patient can sit up, he may be carried by making one of the so-called seats. The bearers face each other. To make a two-handed seat, the right bearer bends the fingers of his right hand to make a hook, and the left bearer does the same with his left hand. They then hook the hands together and each places his free hand on the haunch of the other, thus making a back to the seat (Plate XXXV, 1). To make a three-handed seat, the right bearer grasps his left forearm with his right hand and with his left hand the left forearm of the other bearer, who, with his left hand, grasps the right forearm of the right bearer. The left bearer then puts his free hand on the shoulder of the right bearer. To make a four-handed seat, each bearer grasps his own left wrist and the right wrist of his neighbour (Plate XXXV, 2). In carrying the patient, the bearer crosses his legs one in front of the other, the right bearer moving off with the left foot, and the left bearer with the right foot (Plate XXXV, 3).

All the methods above described are suitable for fairly short distances only, and for longer distances resort must be had to a stretcher. There are various models, but each consists of two poles, made of light wood as a rule, between which canvas, usually tarred, is stretched, and with hinged iron bars, or traverses, beneath the poles, to keep these apart when the stretcher is loaded with a patient. The poles are from 6 feet 9 inches to 7 feet long, and the canvas is 6 feet long and about 2 feet wide. The stretcher is mounted on wheels or on V-shaped steel runners, which raise it about 6 inches off the ground (Plate XXXVI, 6).

How to Improvise a Stretcher

A stretcher may be improvised by rolling up poles of suitable length in the sides of a blanket until a width of the blanket of about 2 feet remains (Plate XXVII, 1 and 2), and fixing the corners of the blanket to the poles by tying with bandages or handkerchiefs. Another method is to turn the sleeves of two coats outside in, pass the poles through the sleeves and button up the coats. In either case cross-pieces of wood must be tied on at the ends in order to keep the poles apart. A hurdle, or a door taken off its hinges, will serve very well as a stretcher when occasion requires.

When the patient suffers from a spinal injury, it is necessary to pass boards between the traverses of the stretcher and the canvas in order to secure rigidity, or if a stretcher is improvised, it should be a door or a strong hurdle. The same precaution may also be necessary in fractures of the lower limb.

For loading a stretcher, three bearers place themselves on the left side of the patient, kneel on the left knee, and raise the patient on to their right knees. Another bearer then places the stretcher beneath the patient, and he is gently lowered on to it (Plate XXXVI, 1-3). Some stretchers have a movable piece of canvas for a pillow, or a pillow may be provided. Otherwise, a folded coat may be placed beneath the patient's head if a pillow is desirable. A patient with a broken leg is placed so as to incline somewhat towards the injured side, but a patient with an injured arm should incline towards the sound side. A patient with a wound across the abdomen should have his legs well bent up at the knees, one with a vertical wound should have them stretched out. These positions prevent gaping of the wound in the respective injuries.

Crossing a Ditch with a Stretcher

The front bearer steps off with the left foot and the rear bearer with the right, and the broken step must be maintained, as it minimises swinging of the stretcher. The stretcher must not be carried on the shoulders, nor must any attempt be made to pass it over a wall, as the patient might fall off the stretcher and gravely aggravate his injuries. If a broad ditch must be crossed, the stretcher is lowered at its edge, and the front bearer gets down and pulls the stretcher across until the head-end is resting on the bank, when the rear bearer gets down in turn. A similar procedure is adopted for getting out of the ditch.

Generally speaking, the patient is carried feet foremost, but when ascending a hill, or going upstairs, the head-end of the stretcher should go first unless where the patient has a broken leg, as the weight of the body in this instance might cause displacement of the fragments of the bone. A stretcher should always be kept as level as possible, and to secure this the bearers should be as nearly as possible of the same height. Properly adjusted strings attached to the handles of the stretcher, and placed over the shoulders of the bearers will also help in this direction, besides taking much of the strain off the arms of the bearers.

A carrying-chair forms a convenient means of taking a patient about the house or out-of-doors. One can be improvised by procuring two stout poles, sufficiently long to project about 18 inches in front of and behind a light easy chair, and attaching the poles to the legs of the chair just below the seat by loops made of straps or bandages. When a patient must be removed a long distance, and an ambulance or a car sufficiently roomy to take a stretcher is not available, the bottom of a cart may be thickly covered with branches and the stretcher laid on these. *See* First Aid ; Fracture.

TRAUMA. A wound or other injury is sometimes called a trauma. The results of a trauma may be called traumatism, the corresponding adjective being traumatic. Thus, epilepsy due to an injury to the head is called traumatic epilepsy. Fever occurring within thirty-six hours after an injury is called simple traumatic fever and is due presumably to the absorption of damaged tissue and inflammatory products. When it is due to sepsis it is called symptomatic traumatic fever. A traumatic neurosis is one following an injury, but the physical damage is not the cause of the nervous disorder ; this is purely due to emotional disturbance.

TREMOR. A more or less persistent quivering or trembling of voluntary muscles is called tremor. It is said to be fine or coarse according to the extent of the movements. Tremor may occur for a short time after a severe muscular effort and is common in nervous people during excitement. It may be caused by the excessive use of tea, coffee, tobacco or alcohol, and by poisoning with mercury, lead and other substances.

It occurs in nervous diseases, both functional and organic. In disseminated sclerosis and sometimes also in other disorders there is what is called intention tremor, that is, a tremor that only begins, or becomes worse, when a voluntary movement is made, say carrying a glass of water to the mouth. Tremor of the eyeball is called nystagmus.

TRENCH DISEASES. During the Great War men serving in the field, especially in the trenches, were particularly liable to certain diseases Trench fever was the name given to an acute infectious disease probably caused by a virus and disseminated by lice. After an incubation period lasting for a week or longer the patient suddenly becomes ill, with shivering, pain in the limbs, headache and, occasionally, vomiting and diarrhoea. The temperature rises quickly, possibly to 103° F. or more. A characteristic feature of the disease is severe pain in the shinbones, which may interfere with sleep.

There may be continued fever for one or two weeks and then recovery by lysis, or the fever may be intermittent and there may be relapses. The disease is never fatal but may be followed by prolonged debility, associated perhaps with irritability of the heart. The treatment is that of fever (*q.v.*).

Trench foot resembled frost bite except that the feet were sodden and frequently became infected with septic organisms. It was caused by continuous immersion of the feet in cold mud. A daily change of socks and the use of gum-boots reduced the risk to the feet very considerably.

Trench, or war, nephritis was the name given to nephritis occurring in soldiers in the field, amongst whom it was considerably more common than it was amongst the general population. It is now supposed by most people not to have been a special disease but simply the ordinary type made more common by the fatigue, exposure and infections which were the lot of soldiers in the field. In a large number of cases there was complete recovery.

TREPHINE. A cylindrical saw used for cutting out a disk of bone, usually from the skull, is known as a trephine. The operation of trephining is a very ancient one and was practised by man when he had nothing better than flint instruments for the purpose.

Trephining is required when there is a depressed fracture of the skull, an abscess of the brain, bleeding from the middle meningeal artery or any other intra-cranial artery that can be reached, and is also used to obtain access to brain tumours and for other reasons. When the disk of bone has been lifted out the opening can be enlarged by means of other instruments.

TREPONEMA PALLIDUM. The organism that causes syphilis is called treponema pallidum. It is also known as spirochaeta pallida.
See Syphilis.

TRICHIASIS. The eyelashes grow normally outwards, away from the eye, but from inflammation of the lids they may come to be directed inwards so that they rub against the cornea. This condition is called trichiasis and causes inflammation of the eye. The offending lashes should be pulled out but it may be necessary to destroy their roots by electrolysis.

TRICHINOSIS. The disease caused by the presence in the body of a tiny round worm, trichina spiralis, is called trichinosis, or trichinelliasis. It is contracted by eating infected pork that has not been sufficiently cooked.
See Worm.

TRICHOPHYTON. *See* Ringworm.

TRICUSPID VALVE. The valve between the right auricle and ventricle of the heart is called the tricuspid valve as it has three cusps.
See Heart.

TRIGEMINAL NERVE. The 5th cranial, or trigeminal, nerve contains both sensory and motor fibres, which arise from separate nuclei in the part of the brain known as the pons. The motor fibres activate the muscles of mastication. On the sensory part of the nerve is a large ganglion, the Gasserian, situated within the skull behind the orbit, and from this ganglion three main divisions of the nerve pass out, each furnishing numerous branches The first, or ophthalmic, division passes into the orbit, supplying ordinary sensation to the eye and to the forehead and scalp as far back as the top of the skull. The second, or maxillary, division supplies the lower eyelid, the upper part of the face, the upper teeth and the tonsil. The third, or mandibular, division supplies the lower part of the face, the salivary glands, the lower teeth and the anterior two-thirds of the tongue.

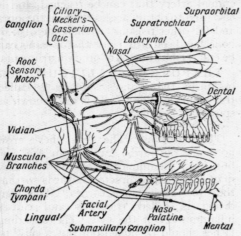

Ganglion { Ciliary / Meckel's / Gasserian / Otic

Supraorbital

Supratrochlear

Lachrymal

Nasal

Root { Sensory / Motor

Dental

Vidian

Muscular Branches

Chorda Tympani

Lingual

Facial Artery

Submaxillary Ganglion

Naso-Palatine

Mental

Trigeminal Nerve : its wide facial distribution

Irritation of one branch of the nerve may cause pain to be referred to the distribution of some other branch. Thus, a carious tooth may cause pain in the ear or at the temple. In the severe form of neuralgia known as tic douloureux (*q.v.*) pain may be felt in the sockets of the teeth which are perfectly sound, the irritation apparently being in the Gasserian ganglion, and it may be necessary to remove or paralyse the ganglion to obtain relief.

Paralysis of the trigeminal nerve causes loss of sensation on the same side of the face and in the tongue, as well as loss of taste in the part of the tongue supplied by the nerve. There is also a loss of ordinary sensation in the nasal cavity on the same side, although smell, which is subserved by another nerve, is retained.

In herpes zoster a vesicular eruption may appear on the forehead, the cornea, and the side of the nose, areas supplied by branches of the ophthalmic division of the nerve.

See Brain ; Gasserian Ganglion ; Herpes.

TRIONAL. A hypnotic drug resembling sulphonal in its effects, but more powerful, trional occurs as a colourless, crystalline powder with a bitter taste. The symptoms caused by poisonous doses are like those of sulphonal poisoning, and the treatment is the same.

See Sulphonal.

TRISMUS. A spasmodic closure of the lower jaw is known as trismus. It occurs in lockjaw, but may be present in other diseases, such as meningitis and tetany. Even irritation about the teeth may sometimes cause it.

TROCAR. An instrument for perforating body-cavities and giving exit to fluids, a trocar consists of a stilette, or perforator, which fits into a tube, or cannula. Only the sharp point of the stilette projects beyond the end of the cannula. When the trocar has been plunged into a cavity the stilette is withdrawn and the fluid runs out. Usually a straight trocar is used, but there is also a curved pattern.

TROCHANTER. *See* Femur.

TROCHLEAR NERVE. The 4th cranial, or trochlear, nerve supplies the superior oblique muscle, the action of which is to turn the eyeball downwards and outwards. *See* Eye.

TROPHIC. Certain nerves are known as trophic nerves because they control the nutrition of tissues. If such nerve fibres are damaged by injury or disease there is a wasting of the muscles and changes in the skin supplied by the fibres. The skin becomes glossy and there are alterations in the hairs and nails. Whether trophic nerve fibres influence nutrition without affecting other functions has not yet been decided. *See* Nervous System.

TROPICAL ABSCESS. *See* Dysentery ; Liver.

TROPICAL HYGIENE. For the maintenance of health in the tropics not only must the ordinary hygienic laws regarding diet, clothing, housing, etc., be observed, but extra precautions must be taken against possible dangers from the excessive sunlight and heat, from uncooked food and water, and from insect bites.

Clothing must be light for the sake of coolness, but it must be absorbent in order to minimise the risk of chilling from dampness of the clothing. This risk is increased by the quick and extensive changes of temperature that may occur and by a sensitiveness to even slight changes which Europeans develop by residence in hot countries. Thin woollen, mixed wool and cotton or cellular cotton garments should always be worn next the skin, and an abdominal belt should be worn at night.

A solar topee should be worn when in the sun, and sometimes a spinal pad will also be necessary (*see* Plate XXXVII, 1 and 3). The nape of the neck should be shaded. The eyes should be protected from the glare of the sun by tinted glasses.

A hot, dry climate is more easily borne than a hot, moist one even though the temperature of the latter be not as high. Alcohol is dangerous when the sun is up, and although what is called a " sun-downer," a glass of spirits and water, may be innocuous, greater temperance is required in the tropics than in a temperate climate. There is no foundation for the notion that soaking in alcohol is a protection against mosquitoes, and grave harm is done to the health by the practice.

All the water used for drinking or for washing food utensils should be boiled, and when water is drawn from pools it should be boiled even for personal washing as there is a risk of acquiring bilharzia from bathing in such water. It may be added here that cold baths are not safe for tropical residents owing to the increased susceptibility to chill. On the other hand, frequent bathing is desirable in order to keep the skin clean and active.

Salads are inadmissible as a rule, and care must be taken that fresh fruit is sufficiently, but not over, ripe, as diarrhoea may be caused by unsuitable fruit and expose to a risk of dysentery and, in some parts of the tropics, to cholera.

The increased perspiration, by raising the concentration of solids in the urine, creates a tendency to the formation of urinary calculi, and this must be prevented by drinking water freely. This is required also to prevent constipation, to which tropical residents are the more prone from the fact that many take too little exercise.

In some parts of the tropics it is unsafe to walk about rooms or verandahs with bare feet as jigger fleas may be picked up. *See* Acclimatisation ; Climate ; Malaria ; Mosquito ; Tick.

TRUSS. One of the instruments used for retaining a hernia, or rupture, is called a truss. The common type consists of a piece of flat steel spring, covered with leather and with a firm pad at one end to fit over the opening through which the hernia would emerge. On the outer side of the truss the leather is prepared leather but on the inner side it is wash leather. The pad is shaped according to the variety of hernia being treated, and the angle at which the pad is fixed on the truss also varies for the same reason.

Variations in the pad of a truss may also be required to meet some special condition. Thus, a truss used for inguinal hernia is triangular in shape, and in order to give sufficient support it may be necessary to prolong the apex. This variety, on account of its shape, is described as a " rat-tail " truss. For an irreducible hernia a truss with a hollow pad may be worn.

Care should be taken in the fitting of a truss. If it is too small the pad may fail to retain the hernia and if too large the pad presses on the pubic bone and causes pain. The truss should lie well down at the back and should come forward just below the prominent point at the front end of the curve of the haunch bone. The perineal strap should be fixed just behind the centre of the curve of the truss on the affected side.

For children an all-rubber truss with an inflatable bag instead of a pad is the most comfortable, though a truss improvised from a skein of wool often suffices The truss must always be kept clean and should remain on the infant during its bath. It may be removed while the infant is being dried and a dry one is applied, but while the truss is off the nurse must keep her hand over the rupture so as to prevent its coming down should the infant cry. A truss for an umbilical hernia has a round pad which is attached to a broad band.

See Abdominal Belt ; Hernia.

TRYPANOSOMA. A genus of animal micro-organism, belonging to the protozoa, is known as trypanosoma, and species are found living as parasites in man and the lower animals, both vertebrate and invertebrate. A trypanosoma has a worm-like body from the fore end of which projects a whip-like process, or flagellum, which is attached to an undulating membrane, this membrane reaching along the body almost to the hinder end. By movements of the flagellum the creature can propel itself either backwards or forwards. Multiplication can occur by simple division of the organism, but in the body of the tsetse fly, which is an intermediate host, there is a sexual multiplication.

Some trypanosomes appear to be harmless but others cause sleeping sickness in man and surra and other diseases in lower animals. Infection with the parasites is called trypanosomiasis.

See Sleeping Sickness. (

TRYPSIN. The ferment in the pancreatic juice that digests proteins is called trypsin. It can carry the digestive process further than the pepsin of the gastric juice and convert the simpler proteins resulting from gastric digestion into amino-acids. As secreted into the bowel it occurs as trypsinogen and cannot affect the proteins, but enterokinase, a ferment in the intestinal juice, liberates the captive trypsin from trypsinogen.

Preparations of the fresh pancreas of the pig are used as peptonising agents and are included in some pre-digested foods.

See Digestion ; Pancreas.

TSETSE FLY. The glossina or tsetse group of flies inhabits Africa, especially the more central parts, and south-western Arabia. The species vary in size, some being about $\frac{1}{4}$ inch long while others are as much as $\frac{1}{2}$ inch. They are blood-sucking insects and usually feed during the middle part of the day. They act as intermediate hosts of trypanosomes, which undergo a stage of sexual development in the bodies of the flies.

See Trypanosoma.

TUBAL PREGNANCY. Gestation occurring in the Fallopian tube is called tubal pregnancy. It constitutes a dangerous state of affairs as the sac ruptures sooner or later, causing shock and severe internal bleeding.

TUBERCLE. The term tubercle is used in various connexions in medicine. It is applied to the small, rounded collections of new cells that occur in tuberculosis and to which this disease owes its name. It is also applied to one of the types of lesion in diseases of the skin, an elevation of the skin resembling an over-grown papule or pimple. Finally, it is applied in anatomy to certain rounded prominences on bones.

TUBERCULOSIS. An infectious disease, characterised by the occurrence of minute rounded bodies known as tubercles, to which circumstance it owes its name, tuberculosis is caused by an organism known as the tubercle bacillus. In human tuberculosis two types of bacillus are found, the human and the bovine, but other types are found in birds, reptiles, and fish. The bovine type is the one found in cattle.

A tubercle consists of a mass of cells of different kinds, and generally bacilli are found in it. The cells accumulate, in fact, around bacilli, and in consequence of the irritation caused by the latter. Tubercles tend to aggregate and form considerable masses which replace the healthy tissues. Soon, however, the cells in tuberculous tissue begin to degenerate, and it comes to form a yellowish-white cheesy mass. This is described as caseation (*see* Plate XI, 2). Then this caseous matter may soften and give rise to a tuberculous abscess. Should, however, the resistance of the body to the disease process be sufficient, the caseous matter may not form, or may disappear, and be replaced by fibrous tissue (Plate XI, 3), or lime salts may be deposited in the mass. This is called calcification. When a tuberculous abscess bursts or is opened, an ulcerated surface, covered with unhealthy granulations, is left.

The chief sources of tuberculous infection are the sputum of persons suffering from consumption, and cow's milk. Infection from sputum may occur through kissing, inhaling the spray ejected by a consumptive when coughing, inhaling the dust formed by dried sputum, or consuming food contaminated by such dust or by tubercle bacilli which have been carried by flies.

Much of the cow's milk that is purveyed to the public contains the bovine type of bacillus, and is a source of a large proportion of the tuberculosis occurring in young children.

Meat may also contain bacilli, but is much less dangerous, as it is cooked before being consumed.

Tubercle bacilli that are inhaled may pass directly into the lungs, but usually are absorbed through the lining of the mouth or throat, and especially through the tonsils, or are swallowed and absorbed through the lining of the bowel. The last happens also when infected food is swallowed. The passage of the bacilli causes little or no change in the lining itself, although when a consumptive swallows his sputa the disease may occur in the lining of the bowel and cause ulceration. Occasionally tubercle bacilli are absorbed through the skin, the so-called butcher's wart being an instance of this.

Bacilli Carried by Lymphatic Glands

When bacilli are absorbed, they are carried to the nearest lymphatic glands, and if they are in sufficient numbers, they cause inflammation and swelling of the glands. If their entrance is from the mouth, the glands in the neck become enlarged, if through the bowel, the mesenteric glands, and so on. From one set of glands the bacilli proceed to the next in the chain, and so onward to the main lymphatic drainage channels, through which they are poured into the blood stream. By the blood they are carried to various organs, where they may settle and form tubercles. Very frequently this happens to be the lung. In children the peritoneum is frequently affected, but also bones and joints.

Sometimes there are such swarms of bacilli in the blood as to constitute a septicaemia, and tubercles are formed all over the body. This is called acute miliary tuberculosis, and it may cause different types of illness according to the organs principally affected. Thus, it may suggest typhoid fever in some instances, in others it may cause acute lung disease, which is sometimes referred to as galloping consumption, while in others it may take the form of meningitis. When there is a focus of tuberculous infection anywhere in the body, there is always a risk of a generalised infection taking place, or of extension to some other organ, say, from the bones to the lungs.

Tubercle bacilli set free a poison which causes local irritation, but more or less of it is carried throughout the body, and produces fever, anaemia, loss of flesh, and other symptoms. Should the tubercles be converted into fibrous tissue, the bacilli are walled off from the general circulation, and their toxin ceases to enter the blood. The disease is then said to be in a quiescent stage. When a tuberculous abscess opens on to any body surface or into the lung, there is a risk of infection with pus-forming microbes also, and should this occur, the toxaemia is aggravated, as the toxins of such microbes are added to those of the tubercle bacilli, and the local irritation from toxins is similarly increased. The symptoms of tuberculous infection consist of those due to the toxaemia, and of those proceeding from the damage to particular organs, and the latter will vary with the acuteness of the attack and the amount of the damage. Thus, when the lungs are affected, there may be symptoms of acute bronchial catarrh or pneumonia, of acute pleurisy, or of the more chronic changes described under the heading Consumption (q.v.).

Age Incidence in Tuberculous Infection

Tuberculosis of the lungs most commonly manifests itself first in adolescence or the early years of adult life. Abdominal tuberculosis is most common between the ages of two and three, gradually declining from then onwards, an age incidence which fixes the chief responsibility for causation on infected milk. Meningitis is most common between the ages of two and five, and generally runs its course in from two to six weeks. Disease of bone and joints (see Plate VII, 8) is commonest between the ages of three and fifteen, and the spine is frequently affected. Some skin diseases, like lupus and scrophulodermia, are caused by the actual invasion of the skin by bacilli, but others, like lichen scrophulosorum, are due simply to the irritation of the toxins.

The problem of the prevention of tuberculosis must be attacked along various lines. Persons suffering from the disease in an infectious stage must dispose of their sputa in such a way as to prevent danger to others. When the accommodation at home is insufficient to permit of precautions being taken against the spread of infection, the patient should be treated in a suitable institution. Attempts must be made to secure a pure milk supply, though any risk from this source can be removed by boiling milk before use. It has been found that tuberculosis is more prevalent in districts with a wet subsoil, and great improvement follows a thorough drainage of such places.

An adequate supply of good food at a price that can be afforded by the humblest is an end which should be strenuously striven for, as this has a lot to do with the matter.

Notification, disinfection of premises, meat inspection, the destruction of flies, and other activities also contribute towards the prevention of the disease. In the general treatment of tuberculosis, sunshine, fresh air and feeding are the important elements, but in the acute stage of the disease, wherever it occurs, rest is equally important. Details of the treatment of pulmonary tuberculosis are given under the heading Consumption, and many of them are applicable to the treatment of tuberculosis in other parts of the body.

A vaccine prepared from the tubercle bacillus is known as a tuberculin. There is a large number of tuberculins, some of them containing the toxin set free by the germs, that is to say, the exotoxin, others the poison contained in the germs themselves, the endotoxin, while a third class contains both toxins. Sometimes the use of a tuberculin has valuable results, but, if used unskilfully, a remedy of this kind is capable of doing very great harm.

Tuberculosis of the glands, bones and joints is sometimes referred to as surgical tuberculosis because surgical treatment was at one time the rule for such, but nowadays the surgeon is more inclined to stay his hand and trust to rest and light, either natural or artificial (*see* Plate XXXVIII) for a time, contenting himself with aspirating abscesses or other operations which may become necessary, and only operating for the removal of glands or other diseased structures when a sufficient trial of the other methods has proved ineffectual. On the other hand, operative treatment on a tuberculous lung is now being undertaken in certain circumstances. *See* Consumption; Light; Lupus; Pott's Disease.

TUFFNELL'S DIET. A diet sometimes used in aneurysm is known as Tuffnell's diet. It consists of 2 ounces of bread and butter and 2 ounces of milk or cocoa for breakfast; 3 ounces of cooked meat, 3 ounces of bread or potato and 4 ounces of water or light claret for dinner; and 2 ounces of bread and butter and 2 ounces of milk, tea or cocoa for supper. It is seldom, however, that a patient can endure this restriction of liquids for long.

TUMOUR. The literal meaning of the word tumour is a swelling, but in pathology its application is restricted to those swellings formed of cells resembling ordinary tissue cells but developed independently of the factors regulating normal development and serving no useful purpose. Such a swelling is also described as a new growth or a neoplasm.

The scope of this definition will be better understood if a few examples of fresh development of tissue are considered. Thus, in syphilis, tuberculosis, actinomycosis and some other diseases a swelling formed of new cells is a common event, but the cells do not resemble any of the normal cells of the body and although such a swelling is called a granuloma or an infective new-growth it is not classed as a tumour. Again, if one kidney be removed the other will probably become much enlarged, beyond the normal plan for the size of a kidney, but the new tissue serves the normal purpose of kidney tissue and is therefore not a tumour.

A tumour is usually named by adding the suffix oma (plural omata) to the Greek or Latin root of the name of the tissue in question; thus, an angioma is a tumour made up of newly-formed blood vessels, a fatty tumour is a lipoma, a cartilaginous tumour is a chondroma, and so on. A sarcoma is so named because its substance resembles to the naked eye a fleshy mass, and in the term carcinoma the name-root means a crab, and the reference is to the processes which grow out from such a tumour into the surrounding tissues.

A tumour may develop in tissue which it resembles, as, for example, an osteoma or bony tumour in bone, or an adenoma or glandular tumour in the breast; but tumours composed of alien tissues may occur in certain structures, as for example, a cartilaginous or a fatty tumour in the substance of the parotid gland.

The causation of tumours is not understood. It has been shown that irritation is a common antecedent to cancer and, recently, evidence has been adduced to suggest that cancer may be caused by a virus acting in conjunction with a complementary substance, but the evidence still requires verification, and should the hypothesis be established it still remains to discover the source of the complementary substance. It would also remain to explain the causation of tumours other than cancers.

There is a large class of tumours which exercise no harmful effects on the body except by the pressure caused by their growth. A tumour of this kind is called a simple, benign or innocent tumour and can generally be left alone, removal only being required when it is disfiguring or presses on a vital organ, or when it is in such a position that it is being irritated by friction.

The other class of tumour comprises the malignant tumours. A tumour of this type not only presses on neighbouring tissues but actually invades and destroys them. Moreover, small portions of the tumour-tissue make their way along lymphatics or veins into other tissues or organs, a phenomenon described as metastasis. Also the growth of such tumours causes a depreciation of health, and in time proves fatal.

In this class, commonly described as cancer, are included the carcinomata and the sarcomata. Such tumours should be removed at the earliest possible moment, as should metastasis occur it may not be possible to save life even by removing the whole of the original growth.

See Cancer ; Polypus ; Sarcoma ; Teratoma.

TURKISH BATH. *See* Baths.

TURMERIC. Papers soaked in tincture of turmeric, which contains a yellow vegetable dye known as curcumin, are used for testing for alkalies, which turn the colour into reddish-brown. Turmeric is sometimes used for colouring ointments and other pharmaceutical preparations.

See Litmus.

TURPENTINE. Oil of turpentine is distilled from an oleo-resin obtained from pinus sylvestris and other pines. It is a colourless liquid with a characteristic smell and a pungent taste. There are two official preparations, turpentine liniment and acetic turpentine liniment, and if either is thoroughly rubbed into the skin it is quickly reddened and a sense of warmth is produced. Pain may thus be relieved in muscles or joints or the discomfort in the chest caused by bronchitis. Another way to use turpentine is to sprinkle it on a fomentation.

Turpentine is sometimes used in half-ounce doses, with an equal quantity of castor oil, as a means of killing and dislodging tapeworms, but there is a risk in giving turpentine inwardly as it may cause severe inflammation of the kidneys with the appearance of large quantities of albumin and blood in the urine. Large doses cause lethargy, vertigo, and possibly coma and sensory paralysis.

If an overdose has been taken an emetic should be given and, when it has acted, a dessertspoonful of Epsom salts in half a glass of water. Demulcent drinks are given to relieve irritation in the stomach, and hot poultices are applied over the kidneys to relieve congestion and pain.

Old oil of turpentine is used as an antidote in phosphorus poisoning, half-drachm doses being given every hour.

See Resin.

TYMPANITES. Distension of the abdomen with gas or air is called tympanites ; it also goes by the name of meteorism. The gas or air may be in the intestine or in the peritoneal cavity. It gains admission to this cavity through a rupture of the stomach or gut. It is more likely to accumulate in the gut if the muscle fibres in the wall of the latter are weakened or paralysed. Hence tympanites occurs in general peritonitis and in the intestinal paralysis that sometimes follows an abdominal operation. Tympanites is common also in typhoid fever. Occasionally it is a manifestation of hysteria.

There is always a certain amount of gas in the bowel and the amount may be increased if there is constipation, or after taking beans or some other articles of diet, but the accumulation from such causes is rarely sufficient to constitute tympanites. Here the abdominal wall is arched and tense and a drum-like note is obtained all over it on percussion. If the distension is extreme there may be serious embarrassment of the heart and lungs.

If there is definite tympanites it means, as a rule, that there is something seriously wrong, and medical advice should therefore be obtained without delay. Meanwhile an attempt may be made to relieve the patient by putting turpentine stupes on the abdomen and, if necessary, giving an enema of soap and water containing a tablespoonful of oil of turpentine. Aromatics by the mouth may also be useful, and peppermint, sal volatile or oil of cinnamon may be tried. Sometimes a long tube has to be passed up into the bowel.

TYMPANUM. ‗ The middle ear, or tympanum, is an air-filled cavity in the temporal bone. The lower part of the cavity, or the tympanum proper, lies behind the drum-head or tympanic membrane and above this level is the attic. The tympanum contains the ossicles and communicates in front, through the Eustachian tube, with the throat, and behind with the tympanic antrum and the mastoid cells.

See Ear.

TYPHOID FEVER. An acute infectious disease in which the small intestine is specially affected, typhoid or enteric fever is caused by an organism known as the typhoid bacillus, or bacillus typhosus, or Eberth. This is a rod-shaped organism with a number of whip-like processes, or flagella, projecting from all round its body. By the lashing of these flagella it makes its way through any liquid in which it occurs.

The bacillus is found in the blood and in numerous organs of persons suffering from the disease. It is also found in the faeces and urine, and may persist in those discharges for many years after recovery from the disease. A person who harbours the bacilli in this way is called a typhoid carrier, and a common place for the bacilli to persist and multiply is in the gall bladder.

The chief source of infection is water that has been polluted with the discharges of a typhoid patient or carrier. If polluted water is used to wash milk containers or utensils, the bacilli multiply readily in the milk ; this becomes highly infectious and also the cream or cheese made from such milk. Freezing does not kill the typhoid bacillus, and ice-cream made with infected milk or cream can readily communicate the disease. Salads polluted by sewage or washed with infected water are also dangerous. Another common source of typhoid infection is the oyster, as these molluscs are sometimes bred in water which is polluted with sewage. For the same reason mussels are sometimes implicated. Flies and other insects may likewise be agents of infection by feeding on sewage or excreta and afterwards visiting food or food utensils.

Persons who handle typhoid patients or their clothing may have their hands contaminated or may inhale the germs in the dust of excrement which has dried on bedding or utensils.

Symptoms of the Infection

After infection has occurred there is an incubation period of from seven to twenty-eight days ; usually it is about twelve days. Fever then begins ; occasionally it is high from the onset, but usually it is not very high for the first few days though it is progressively increasing, the temperature each evening being higher than on the preceding one. During this time the patient probably keeps getting about, but suffers from loss of appetite, headache, vague abdominal pain and slight diarrhoea or, perhaps, constipation. Frequently there is epistaxis or bleeding from the nose, and bronchitis is not uncommon.

The temperature reaches its acme on the fifth to the seventh day, when it may be 103° to 105° F., and, if he has not done so before, the patient now feels compelled to take to his bed. For the next ten to fourteen days the temperature, beyond dropping a little in the mornings, does not vary very much, but after this, in favourable cases, it begins to come down gradually day by day, or, in other words, it ends by lysis. Sometimes, however, the high level of temperature is maintained for several weeks.

When the patient takes to his bed, diarrhoea is generally established, with thin motions, which, from their appearance, are described as pea-soup stools. Sometimes the character changes to what is called the chopped parsley stool. In any case these are usually very foul. There is some distension of the abdomen and pain. The tongue is covered with a yellowish fur in the centre, but is red at the tip and edges. The eye is clear, and the mind is usually alert, though sometimes headache is severe, or there is dulness and apathy. Frequently sleep is disturbed and the patient tends to be wakeful at night. The rate of the pulse and respirations corresponds as a rule with the elevation of temperature. The spleen is enlarged.

Characteristic Appearance of the Rash

On the seventh or eighth day a characteristic rash usually appears, first on the abdomen, chest and back, but later it may be found on the limbs and face. It consists of small rose spots, slightly elevated above the level of the skin, and these appear in crops, the older spots beginning to disappear as the new ones come out (*see* Plate XXXI, 11).

By the end of the second week the patient is beginning to feel exhausted. The tongue is probably dry. The pulse is rapid and weak. The abdomen is more distended, sometimes very much, a condition described as meteorism or tympanites. This may cause embarrassment to the heart and lungs. There has been considerable loss of flesh, and the face is thin.

If the temperature begins to decline, there is a gradual improvement in other respects also, but if the fever continues, the patient tends to develop what is called the typhoid state (*q.v.*).

In typhoid fever there is inflammation of Peyer's patches, the collections of lymphoid tissue in the lining of the small intestine, particularly towards its lower end. These become swollen, and project above the surface of the bowel. Then the superficial part of a patch dies, forming a slough which is thrown off and leaves an ulcerated surface. The ulcer becomes deeper and may reach the peritoneal lining. Blood vessels in the bowel wall are also liable to be opened by the ulcerative process. There is a general catarrhal condition along the lining of the bowel.

From the end of the second week there is a possibility of two serious complications occurring. One of these is severe hæmorrhage from the bowel. Should this happen, the temperature drops to subnormal, and there are signs of collapse.

The other is perforation of the bowel. This also causes signs of collapse, and probably pain, though sometimes pain is absent, and after a short time signs of peritonitis appear.

Amongst other possible complications are pneumonia, pleurisy, meningitis, parotitis, and inflammation of joints or bones. A stiff or painful condition in the backbone, sometimes referred to as typhoid spine, is caused by inflammation of the inter-vertebral disks. Thrombosis (*q.v.*) in a vein, usually in one of those of the lower limb, sometimes occurs, but generally during convalescence. Typhoid fever may be followed by prolonged physical weakness, and sometimes by mental derangement.

Illnesses resembling typhoid fever, but generally of less severity, are caused by bacilli which are akin to the typhoid bacillus. These illnesses are described as paratyphoid fever A, and paratyphoid fever B. Relapses occasionally occur in typhoid fever, being more frequent in some epidemics than in others ; they are fairly common in paratyphoid A.

There may be some difficulty in diagnosing typhoid fever in its early stages, and it is sometimes mistaken for pneumonia, acute tuberculosis, appendicitis and other disorders. After a few days, however, it may be possible to cultivate the typhoid bacillus from a sample of the blood, and after ten days the Widal test, which is based on the agglutination (*q.v.*) of the bacilli, is generally found to be positive. Other tests may be applied.

How to Prevent the Disease

The main method of preventing typhoid fever is to provide a supply of pure water for households, and now that this has been pretty well accomplished, at any rate for the towns, typhoid fever is a relatively uncommon disease. There is always a danger, however, when water is drawn from shallow wells or in a casual way from streams. Considerable attention is also being given to the oyster and mussel industries, and dangers from these sources are being lessened. Another method of lessening the prevalence of typhoid fever is the control of flies (*q.v.*). An important preventive measure is to discover human carriers of the disease and sterilise them, if possible. This can sometimes be done by removing the gall bladder. In any case, such persons should not be allowed to have anything to do with preparing or handling food. Also, during an epidemic, a watch must be maintained for instances in which the disease is so mild that the patient can get about all the time. This type is called ambulant typhoid.

When typhoid fever is prevalent, all water used for drinking or for washing kitchen utensils, and all milk, should be boiled. Protection is afforded by inoculation with anti-typhoid vaccine, and preferably one which deals not only with typhoid but paratyphoid also; this is usually referred to as the T.A.B. vaccine. This gives protection for about two years and if, in spite of inoculation, the disease is contracted, it is likely to follow a milder course.

Extreme Importance of Good Nursing

The issue of typhoid fever depends to a large extent on the quality of the nursing and in most cases it is desirable that a patient suffering from this disease should be treated in an institution, as the accommodation and wealth of appliances provided in such a place make nursing easier and more efficient. The treatment is in general that described under the headings Fever and Infectious Disease. As typhoid is such a protracted disease, however, special care is necessary in keeping the mouth clean, and in preventing bed sores.

The patient should be encouraged to drink a large quantity of water, and some of this may usefully be in the form of home-made lemonade. At the same time sufficient food should be taken, mainly milk but also eggs, beaten up or as albumen water, sugar, butter, bread and cornflour, or arrowroot. A watch should be kept on the motions and if large, or many, milk-curds appear, the milk should be citrated or even peptonised.

Typhoid is one of the diseases in which the control of the temperature by cold or cool baths is much practised in some parts of the world.

Drugs, with the exception of intestinal antiseptics, such as beta-naphthol and oil of cinnamon, are little used in uncomplicated typhoid. For haemorrhage styptics are employed, but for perforation the only useful treatment is immediate operation. Tympanites, or distension of the bowels with gas, is treated by giving oil of cinnamon, 2 to 5 minims in capsules, and by applying turpentine stupes to the abdomen. Constipation occurring during the course of the disease, or in early convalescence, should be corrected by enemata and not purgatives.

Stimulants should not be given as a matter of routine, but only when they appear to be necessary. Sometimes in the later stages whisky or brandy is invaluable, and large quantities may be required.

TYPHOID STATE. In severe febrile diseases, especially if protracted, and in some instances of profound poisoning, the patient may pass into a condition of extreme prostration, which is referred to as the typhoid, or typhic, state.

He lies on his back with the eyes open but apparently is unconscious of anything. The tongue is tremulous, dry, brown or black and cracked, the lips and teeth tend to become covered with sordes unless sedulously cleaned, the pulse is very rapid and feeble and the breathing shallow. There is low, muttering delirium going on constantly, and the patient may keep on picking at the bed-clothes or make passes in the air as if catching flies. There are jerky movements of muscles, especially of the hands and feet, this being called subsultus tendinum. The bowels and bladder are likely to be emptied involuntarily and the patient slips further and further down the bed.

This state of affairs, although highly dangerous, is not necessarily fatal, but very efficient nursing is required. Stimulants should be given skilfully, especially in the small hours of the morning when vitality is at its lowest ebb.

TYPHUS FEVER. An acute infectious disease, typhus now occurs but rarely wherever there is enlightened sanitary supervision. Formerly epidemics were frequent and so constantly in association with overcrowding that the disease was known by such names as gaol fever, hospital fever, camp fever and ship fever, overcrowding in such institutions and places being notoriously the rule in former times. Even more recently in times of stress during and following on the Great

War, overcrowding has resulted in epidemics of typhus.

It has long been recognized that a lack of personal cleanliness was associated with overcrowding in causing the disease, and it is now clear that the explanation is that such conditions favour the presence and communication of lice. The infection of typhus exists in the blood, and lice extract it when feeding and carry it to other people. It is not known which organism is responsible, but several, including the so-called Rickettsia bodies and the Weil-Felix bacillus, have been isolated from the blood of persons suffering from the disease.

It is considered that the disease known in America as mountain fever is really typhus, and this disease is propagated by ticks and other blood-sucking creatures.

Early Appearance of Mental Symptoms

The incubation period in typhus is about twelve days and symptoms begin suddenly, often with a rigor. In a day or two the temperature reaches its maximum of about 105° F., and there it remains with only a slight fall in the mornings for about twelve days, when, in favourable cases, it may decline somewhat, and on the fourteenth day reach the normal by crisis. The face is flushed and swollen, and the eyes are commonly bloodshot. Mental dulness usually occurs early and, with this, delirium which may be violent in the beginning. The patient may be roused to answer questions, but does so stupidly, especially as the days run on. Sleeplessness is a notable feature of the disease. At the beginning there is much complaint of headache and of pain in the back and limbs.

The tongue is large, pale and covered with white fur, which soon becomes brown, however, and the tongue becomes dry and tremulous, while the lips and teeth become covered with sordes. The pulse and respirations are rapid, and as the disease progresses, the pulse becomes very weak.

On the fourth or sixth day, as a rule, the rash appears, usually first on the abdomen, or on the folds of the armpits, but later on any part of the body except the face. It consists of small, mulberry-coloured spots, which in a few days become brown. Commonly also, and certainly in severe cases, there are darker spots which do not, like the others, fade on pressure. These are called petechiae, and represent bleeding into the skin. There is a third element in the typical rash, and this consists of a pinkish flush with clear areas throughout it.

As the disease runs on, the patient becomes rapidly weaker, and may pass into the typhoid state. A favourable termination to the disease is usually indicated by the patient falling into a natural sleep from which he awakes with his mind considerably cleared. The fall in the temperature may be accompanied by profuse sweating or a copious flow of urine. Convalescence is generally rapid.

The complications which may occur in typhus include bronchitis, pneumonia, parotitis, bed sores, thrombosis in one of the veins of the leg, and gangrene of the fingers, toes, ears or nose.

The preventive treatment of typhus consists in the prevention and destruction of lice, and the prompt isolation of persons suffering from the disease, or who have been in contact with such. The usual period for contacts is sixteen days after lice have been destroyed. All the clothing of patient and contacts should be disinfected in order to kill lice and their eggs.

Desirability of Hospital Treatment

Whenever it is possible, a person suffering from the disease should be taken to an isolation hospital. The general treatment of the disease is laid down under the headings Fever and Infectious Disease. The sick room should be kept cool and very freely ventilated. Usually hypnotics, such as paraldehyde, are needed, and their use should be begun early. A constant watch must be kept on the patient night and day, as he may get out of bed and injure himself. There should be no undue haste in giving stimulants. To relieve headache, it may be desirable to shave the head, so that cold applications may be more effective. Sometimes warm applications are more grateful. Care must be taken that the urine is passed, and the use of the catheter will sometimes be necessary. The prospect of recovery is greater, generally speaking, the younger the age of the patient.

ULCER. A sore that involves the true skin is described as an ulcer. It is kept open and extends by the death of minute particles of tissue which are liquefied and removed in a discharge. A similar process may affect a mucous membrane and cause an ulcer there. Many different types of ulcer are described, but each consists of an area more or less depressed below the general surface of the skin or mucous membrane, which is known as its floor, and around this a margin, or edge. From the surface of the ulcer there exudes a discharge which may be purulent or watery and profuse or scanty; sometimes it is mixed with blood.

The body is instant in its attempts to repair breaches in the continuity of its tissues and repair of an ulcer takes place by the floor becoming filled up and covered with a layer of granulation tissue (q.v.), which gives the surface of the ulcer a pink, granular appearance. At the same time new epithelium grows in from the edges over the surface of the granulations and can be readily seen as a thin blue margin. The discharge is scanty and is of a watery, or serous, character. When healing has been completed a scar remains.

Subdivisions based on Causation

As regards causation, ulcers fall into three main groups, namely, those due to mechanical, chemical or septic irritation, those due to specific micro-organisms, such as the tubercle bacillus and the spironema of syphilis, and those due to malignant new growths.

In the causation of an ulcer belonging to the first group the nutrition of the affected skin or mucous membrane may be compromised, and this may be a predominant factor in keeping an ulcer going. The explanation of this nutritional defect may be found in some local disturbance such as varicose veins or Raynaud's disease, or it may have to be sought for in some constitutional disorder such as anaemia, diabetes, chronic Bright's disease or locomotor ataxia.

An inflamed ulcer discharges freely and there is redness and swelling of the skin around the ulcer. If considerable portions of dead tissue appear on the ulcer it is called a sloughing or phagedaenic ulcer. An irritable ulcer is one in which a nerve is included in the floor of the ulcer, a circumstance that gives rise to great pain.

A callous, or indolent, ulcer is a chronic ulcer with a thickened rounded edge, the floor being pale. The discharge is scanty as a rule, but may be offensive. This kind of ulcer is most common on the leg and in elderly people who suffer from varicose veins. A trophic, or perforating, ulcer is one that occurs in locomotor ataxia, diabetes, or some other condition in which there is disease of nerves. An ulcer of this kind is quite painless. The most frequent site is on the ball of the great toe.

Ulcers due to Micro-organisms

A tuberculous ulcer has a ragged, irregular margin, which is undermined and its floor is covered with pale granulations amongst which tiny yellow tubercles may be visible. Ulceration occurs in the first and second stages of syphilis, but when one speaks of a syphilitic ulcer what is generally meant is the sore that is left when a gumma, a swelling that forms in the tertiary stage, softens and ruptures, discharging its contents. The margin of the ulcer is sharply-cut and steep, and the floor has the appearance of wash-leather.

Ulcers that are caused by the growth of a malignant tumour are represented by the rodent ulcer (q.v.), by epitheliomata, and by the sores produced by malignant tumours, in structures like the breast, breaking through the skin.

Ulcers belonging to all the three groups which have been mentioned occur on the lining of the various cavities and hollow organs of the body and are discussed in connexion with these.

The treatment of an ulcer depends on its cause. If this should be malignant disease, an attempt should at once be made by operation to remove all the diseased tissues and any glands which may possibly be infected. A tuberculous ulcer may be removed by operation or treated by artificial sunlight, while the general treatment of tuberculosis is carried out. A syphilitic ulcer requires in the first place general anti-syphilitic treatment, and so for any specific infection, while local treatment is used to keep the ulcer clean.

In the treatment of ulcers belonging to the first group the main considerations are rest and cleanliness and, where necessary, the removal of any constitutional factor in so far as this is at all possible. Satisfactory healing of an ulcer can hardly be expected, for example, if anaemia is allowed to persist, or diabetes is untreated. Rest can only be secured for a lower limb by the patient lying up, though it may be sufficient to support an upper limb on a sling.

If the floor of an ulcer is sloughy or very dirty it may be necessary for a doctor to treat it with a strong antiseptic, such as pure carbolic acid, or to scrape it. Commonly, however, an ulcer can be cleaned up by applying boracic fomentations. The fomentation is made by wringing a double thickness of boracic lint lightly out of hot water, applying it and covering with gutta-percha tissue so as to overlap the lint at least half an inch all round. At the beginning it may be necessary to renew the fomentations three or four times daily, and each time the fomentation is taken off the ulcer should be washed with an antiseptic lotion.

Special Dressings to Prevent Adhesion

When the ulcer is clean treatment may be continued with the moistened lint without the gutta-percha tissue, but if the lint adheres it may injure the delicate epithelium that is growing in to cover the ulcer, and to obviate this a piece of oiled silk perforated with a number of openings to let out the discharge may be applied beneath the lint. The silk is first of all left for a short time in an antiseptic lotion.

An alternative treatment is to apply lint smeared with a thickish layer of boracic ointment.

When the area of ulceration is considerable skin-grafting will hasten healing very considerably, but this can only be carried out when the surface of the ulcer is thoroughly clean. An irritable ulcer is treated by cutting across its floor so as to divide the nerve and then proceeding as above described. Incisions may also be required in order to start the healing of a callous ulcer.

When the granulations are exuberant, forming what is called proud flesh, they may usefully be rubbed over lightly with blue stone. If on the other hand they are forming but slowly it will be well to bathe them with a stimulating lotion, such as red lotion.

To obtain healing of varicose ulcers it is necessary to support the limb by applying a pure rubber bandage, a woven elastic bandage or a crêpe bandage. The pure rubber bandage is liable to cause irritation by imprisoning the sweat. A useful application for varicose ulcers is found in Unna's paste (q.v.). When the ulcer has healed it may be desirable to operate for the cure of the varicose veins.

See Antiseptic ; Basilicon Ointment ; Duodenum ; Gastric Ulcer ; Phagedaena ; Rodent Ulcer ; Varicose Vein.

ULNA. The inner of the two bones of the forearm is called the ulna. Its shaft is somewhat prismatic in shape but the bone is enlarged at the upper end where it forms a notch to grasp the lower end of the humerus. The notch is called the greater sigmoid cavity and extends between the olecranon process above and the coronoid process below. Illustrations showing the bone are given in pages 44 and 565, and a radiogram showing infection with tuberculosis in Plate VII, 8.

On the outer side of the coronoid process is a shallow depression, the lesser sigmoid cavity, for articulation with the head of the radius. The lower end of the shaft is cylindrical and is prolonged on the inner side into a peg-shaped projection, the styloid process. The lower end of the bone articulates with the radius and with the wrist bones. The ulna can be readily felt from one end to the other and a fracture of the bone is easily recognized.

See Forearm ; Radius.

ULNAR NERVE. A branch of the brachial plexus, the ulnar nerve lies near the brachial artery in the upper part of the arm but leaves it to reach the back of the elbow where it lies in the groove between the inner prominence, or condyle, of the lower end of the humerus and the olecranon process of the ulna, as shown in the illustration in page 456. It passes, however, on to the front of the forearm, down the inner side of which it runs, for the greater part of its course in company with the ulnar artery. It ends in branches to the back and front of the hand.

It supplies one of the muscles of the forearm and the interossei muscles and other small muscles in the hand. It supplies sensation to the palm and back of the hand on the inner side and to the little finger and half of the ring finger. Paralysis of the nerve results in anaesthesia of those areas and in wasting of the hand except for the ball of the thumb. The fingers also assume a characteristic position, being bent backwards at the joint by which they are attached to the hand and bent forwards, or flexed, at the other joints. This condition is described as claw-hand, or main-en-griffe.

The nerve is quite superficial at the back of the elbow and a blow on it or on the bone causes a peculiar sensation to shoot down the forearm, a fact which has given the name funny-bone to this part. Long continued violent exercise with the arms may irritate the nerve at this point and it may become inflamed and thickened, with more or less paralysis of its functions. *See* Arm; Median Nerve; Musculo-spiral Nerve; Neuritis.

ULTRA-VIOLET RAYS. The nature and actions of ultra-violet rays are discussed under the heading Light.

UMBILICUS. The navel, or umbilicus, is a depressed scar left after the separation of the umbilical cord. A hernia sometimes occurs in this situation and should be prevented from emerging by applying a circular pad, kept in position by a broad band, though sometimes an operation will be necessary. A congenital fistula is another abnormality occasionally found.

UNCONSCIOUSNESS. If a person is found unconscious, or becomes so, he should be placed on his back, with the head to one side and slightly raised or not according as the face is flushed or pale. The clothing about the neck and chest should be loosened. The nature of the first-aid to be rendered further will depend on the circumstances in each case but a doctor should be summoned at once or as soon as a messenger is available.

The state of consciousness may be tested by opening the eyelids and touching the white of the eye. If the patient is at all conscious he will wince and make some attempt to close the eye.

The causes of unconsciousness may be summarised briefly as follows : (1) Death ; there is no evidence of the beating of the heart or of breath. (2) Fainting or syncope ; the condition resembles death, but there is quick recovery from simple fainting. (3) Asphyxia ; the face shows some lividity and the circumstances suggest the nature of the condition, as when a body has been taken from the water or from a gas-filled room, etc. (4) Apoplexy ; the breathing is stertorous and relative weakness may be discernible on one side of the body. (5) Epilepsy ; there may be signs of the patient having had a fit, such as marks on the ground or foam and blood on the lips. (6) Heat stroke ; the atmospheric temperature will be suggestive and the skin will feel burning hot ; this will also be found when the unconsciousness is due to excess of fever. (7) Poisoning by narcotics, such as alcohol, opium, etc. (8) Injuries to the head ; there may be concussion, in which consciousness is not often completely lost, or compression of the brain by fragments of bone or by blood-clot. (9) Shock or collapse ; there may be evidence of injury or of internal bleeding, which causes extreme pallor and a very rapid, thready pulse. (10) Poisoning in diabetes or uraemic poisoning from kidney disease ; such conditions could only be recognized by an expert, as also unconsciousness due to meningitis or other diseases of the brain. (11) Cold ; in cold countries this is always a possible cause. (12) Shock from lightning or electricity ; the circumstances would be suggestive. (13) Hysteria, including the death-like condition known as trance.

Possible Errors in Diagnosis

It is necessary to guard against certain possible errors when proposing to identify any of those causes in a particular instance. In the first place, it should not be too readily assumed that a person is dead, as other conditions simulate death very closely. In the second place, a smell of alcohol from the patient should be ignored unless the possibility of some other cause of unconsciousness is definitely excluded. In the third place, a scalp wound does not necessarily mean that unconsciousness is due to a brain injury, as a person who becomes suddenly unconscious may strike his head in falling.

As regards a number of the causes enumerated above, a clue will probably be furnished by the circumstances in which the patient is found. A bottle or the wrapping of a package in the vicinity of the person might put one on the track of poison. If an apoplectic seizure or an epileptic or hysterical convulsion is actually witnessed, the diagnosis of the subsequent unconsciousness will present little difficulty. A hysterical convulsion will often be preceded by emotional manifestations, and the patient will usually be a female.

No attempt should be made to give an unconscious person alcohol, and this should be withheld even if the patient recovers sufficiently to be able to swallow, unless possibly after a simple faint.

Not even water should be given until the patient can swallow, and his ability to do so should be first tested by giving a few drops at a time. If breathing ceases artificial respiration should be carried out, but the mouth should first be opened to ensure that the throat is clear. If the patient begins to vomit the head should be turned well to one side and the opposite shoulder should be raised. Warmth should be maintained when necessary by extra coverings and by hot-water bottles at the feet.

An examination should be made to ensure that no bone is broken, and if there is any such thing the patient should not be moved until the fracture is properly controlled by splints. An unconscious patient should be carried in a recumbent position and should be handled with great gentleness. If there has been bleeding from a wound the possibility of a recurrence should be borne in mind, and someone should therefore be watchful and ready to control it should it happen.

See Apoplexy ; Collapse ; Death ; Epilepsy ; Fainting ; Fit ; Hysteria ; Poisoning ; Shock.

UNDER-FEEDING. Among the poor, and especially the children, under-feeding is a common cause of ill-health. It could be prevented, however, to a considerable extent by a wiser choice of food-stuffs. Advice regarding this is given under the headings Diet and Food.

UNNA'S PASTE. A preparation consisting of zinc oxide, 5 parts ; gelatin, 5 parts ; boracic acid, 1 part ; glycerin, 8 parts ; and water, 6 parts, is called Unna's paste. Ichthyol, 1 or 2 parts, is often incorporated in it. The paste is

mixed with the aid of heat and sets on cooling, so that it has to be warmed each time it is proposed to apply it. It is used in the treatment of varicose eczema and ulcers and other skin disorders. The part is cleansed as well as possible and the paste is smeared over it and covered with a layer of gauze. Then another layer of the paste and of gauze are applied, for as many layers as are desired. A layer of cotton wool is then put on, and over this a bandage (see Plate XXXIX, 1 and 2).

URAEMIA. When the kidneys are disabled waste substances, which should be excreted, accumulate in the blood and either these or substances resulting from a perverted body-chemistry, caused by their presence, give rise to symptoms of poisoning. This state of affairs is known as uraemia, and may occur in an acute or a chronic form.

Headache is a common symptom, and there may be giddiness and vomiting. Sometimes the most notable thing is shortness of breath. There may be a transient impairment of vision or deafness. Acute symptoms may occur after premonitory symptoms, such as have just been described, or without warning the patient has a convulsion. This resembles an epileptic fit and is followed by coma or profound unconsciousness. In some cases coma comes on without the convulsion. There are instances where acute mania is caused by uraemia.

There is always a diminution of urea in the urine of persons suffering from this disorder, but it has been decided that it is not urea that causes the poisoning. Uraemia is liable to supervene in nephritis, either acute or chronic, and in other diseases of the kidneys.

The treatment of chronic uraemia is that of the chronic forms of Bright's disease (*q.v.*). When the acute condition occurs an attempt should be made to get rid of waste matter from the blood by inducing free sweating and free purgation. Sweating may be caused by putting the patient in a hot pack or a hot air bath. Under expert supervision a hot bath and an injection of pilocarpine nitrate are sometimes used. As regards the bowels, the object is to obtain copious watery motions, and this may be obtained by giving ½ ounce of Epsom salts dissolved in as little water as can take up the salt. When the patient is unconscious a drop of croton oil in a little pat of butter may be placed on the back of the tongue.

Another method of diminishing the poison in the blood is to bleed the patient and then perform a transfusion of blood or saline, or inject the saline solution under the skin or into the bowel.

A convulsion or fit is treated like an epileptic one. It may be desirable to administer chloroform in order to control the fits, however. In expert hands certain drugs, especially morphine, are of great value.

See Bright's Disease ; Kidney ; Normal Saline Solution.

URATE. A salt of uric acid is called a urate. In the blood and urine uric acid occurs as sodium urate.

See Uric Acid.

UREA. The most abundant solid in the urine is a nitrogenous substance called urea. This is formed in the liver from the nitrogenous waste substances and is found in the blood and lymph. About an ounce is excreted in the urine in the 24 hours and there is also a trace in the sweat. When the kidneys are not functioning properly urea accumulates in the blood, but is not the cause of the poisonous symptoms that occur in kidney disease.

Urea is prepared synthetically in the laboratory and is obtained as a colourless, crystalline solid, which is freely soluble in water at body temperature. It is administered as a diuretic, and in conjunction with quinine has been used as a local anaesthetic.

Urea is the source of the group of hypnotic and sedative drugs which includes barbitonum, or veronal, proponal, dial, luminal, etc. Urea is also known as carbamide.

URETER. The tube that conducts urine from the pelvis of the kidney into the bladder is called the ureter. It is about 10 to 12 inches long, and has a thick wall containing muscle fibres, by the contraction of which urine is forced down the tube. The ureters pass obliquely downwards and inwards, and enter the bladder at the upper angles of the space known as the trigone. The passage through the wall of the bladder is in an oblique direction, and the obliquity creates a valve-like mechanism at the orifices of the tubes, preventing regurgitation of urine from the bladder under ordinary circumstances. The position of the ureters is shown in the Frontispiece.

A calculus in the ureter is forced down the latter by the contraction of its muscle-fibres, and this is the cause of renal colic. Sometimes a stone may become impacted in the ureter, however, and require to be cut out. Kinking of the ureter by displacement of a movable kidney causes the attacks of pain and other symptoms referred to as Dietl's crisis. Rupture of the ureter by violence has occurred on some occasions.

See Bladder ; Hydronephrosis ; Kidney.

URETHRA. The passage by which urine is discharged from the bladder is called the urethra. It is lined with mucous membrane throughout, and its narrowest part is its external orifice, or meatus. In the male the urethra is about 8 inches long and consists of three portions, which are continuous, however. The first, or prostatic portion, begins at the neck of the bladder and traverses the prostate gland. Opening on its floor are the prostatic ducts, by which prostatic secretion is discharged, and the ejaculatory ducts, by which semen is discharged.

The second, or membranous, portion lies between the layers of the triangular ligament. It is very short, and except for the meatus is the narrowest part of the tube. The third portion is called the cavernous or spongy portion and traverses the corpus spongiosum of the penis. Opening into it are ducts of various glands and there are also recesses, or lacunae, opening off it. If infection invades the urethra it is apt to lodge in these ducts and lacunae, and hence the difficulty often met with in overcoming the infection.

From developmental defects the meatus may be found to open on the upper or on the lower surface of the penis. In the former event the condition is described as epispadias, and in the latter hypospadias.

By kicks or by falling astride on a hard object the urethra may be ruptured and the urine may flow through the opening into the surrounding tissues and perhaps further afield. This is called extravasation of urine. The accident may also be followed by a stricture, or narrowing, of the tubes, from the contraction of scar tissue.

Inflammation of the urethra, or urethritis, is usually caused by gonorrhoea (*q.v.*) and frequently is followed by stricture. When it has this origin a stricture occurs in the cavernous portion of the urethra. It causes difficulty in passing water and the stream becomes smaller ; sometimes it is forked or has a spiral form. If congestion of the lining of the urethra occurs, as after an alcoholic bout or from chill, there may be complete stoppage of the urine.

When a stricture has existed for some time dilatation and hypertrophy of the bladder occur and the effects of the obstruction may even extend to the ureters and kidneys. Occasionally the urethra becomes blocked by a stone, or calculus, or by a foreign body, either of which may have to be cut out.

A stricture should be dilated periodically with a gum-elastic or metal bougie. Sometimes it is necessary to divide the stricture either by cutting from the inside, internal urethrotomy, or from the outside, external urethrotomy. An examination of the lining of the tube can be made by means of an instrument called the urethroscope.

In the female the urethra is about $1\frac{1}{2}$ inches long, and is wider and more dilatable than it is in the male. A small red swelling, about the size of a pea, is sometimes found at the meatus, and is known as a urethral caruncle. It tends to cause slight bleeding but may be painless, though in some instances it causes a burning pain when the urine is passed and is very tender. If painless it is best left alone, otherwise it can be cut out or destroyed by the use of a cautery.

See Bladder ; Gonorrhoea ; Prostate.

URIC ACID. A nitrogenous substance occurring in the tissues, blood and urine, uric acid has a neutral reaction but is nevertheless able to form salts with bases. It occurs in the body as sodium urate and is excreted in the urine as such, from 7 to 10 grains being thus got rid of in the 24 hours. Uric acid is formed in the tissues by the destruction of nucleo-proteins.

These are converted by various ferments into substances known as purin bases, which by other ferments are converted into uric acid. Some foods, such as meat, are rich in purin bases and the consumption of such foods increases the uric acid in the body and urine.

In gout sodium urate is thrown out of solution in the joints and tophi, and in certain circumstances the acid may be thrown out of solution in the urine and form gravel or stones in the urinary tract. Such calculi usually form in the kidney (*see* Plate XXI, 1) rather than in the bladder. A tendency to the accumulation of uric acid in the body is described as the uric acid diathesis. The importance of uric acid as a cause of disease, however, is now considered to be very considerably less than was formerly thought to be the case.

Uric acid crystals may occur as a deposit in urine. The crystals have various shapes and are almost always stained by the urinary pigment.

See Gout ; Lithaemia ; Purin.

URINARY SYSTEM. In the urinary system are included the two kidneys, the ureters, the bladder and the urethra. These various parts are described under their respective headings.

URINE. A watery solution of waste substances excreted by the kidneys, the urine flows down the ureters into the bladder, from which it is voided by the act of urination, or micturition. An adult excretes on the average about 50 to 60 ounces of urine in the 24 hours, most of it during the day, though in chronic nephritis a large amount may be excreted at night.

Urine is a clear liquid with a straw or a light amber colour. The colour is due to a pigment known as urochrome. There may also be a small quantity of another pigment, urobilin, but this is not usual in health. Urine has a somewhat aromatic odour. The reaction, as tested by litmus paper, is faintly acid, but after a meal, and in vegetarians, may be definitely alkaline. The specific gravity is from 1015 to 1025, but may be greater or less, according to the concentration of the urine. The specific gravity is taken when the urine has been allowed to cool to room temperature.

When urine stands, a filmy deposit of mucus forms at the bottom of the receptacle. In a concentrated acid urine there may be a brick-red deposit of amorphous urates, or, in an alkaline urine, a white deposit of phosphates. Neither of these deposits has any special significance. It may be noted that while heating the urine favours the phosphatic deposition, it causes the urates to dissolve and disappear. When urine stands for some time ammonia is produced and is easily recognized by its odour.

Chemical Constituents of Urine

In 1000 parts of urine there are about 960 parts of water and 40 parts of solids. Of the latter urea constitutes more than a half, and common salt, or sodium chloride, rather more than a quarter. Urea is a nitrogenous waste product, though not the only one, as there are small quantities of uric acid, which occurs in the form of urates, creatin and creatinine, and also the pigment. Besides sodium, there are present potassium, calcium, magnesium, and ammonium, and, in addition to hydrochloric acid, sulphuric, phosphoric and oxalic acids, but these acids and bases are combined to form salts.

The daily quantity of urine may vary in health. Thus, it may be increased in cold weather, or by taking large quantities of liquids, and, conversely, may be diminished in hot weather, when sweating is profuse. The quantity is also greatly affected in some diseases. In diabetes it may amount to many pints daily, and in hysteria and other disorders there may be a notable increase. In fevers and in acute nephritis there may be a great diminution.

If urine has an ammoniacal odour when passed, it has undergone decomposition, and this generally occurs with chronic inflammation of the bladder. In diabetes the odour may be that of new-mown hay, and after taking turpentine it resembles that of violets.

The colour becomes deeper as the urine becomes more concentrated. If bile is present in considerable quantity, the colour is mahogany brown, if there is less it is greenish yellow ; the froth has a green tint. A small quantity of blood gives the urine a smoky appearance, and larger quantities make it pink or bright red. In haemoglobinuria the urine may resemble porter, or be almost black, and in haematoporphyrinuria, which occurs from overdoses of sulphonal and other causes, the colour is that of port wine. Rhubarb, senna and logwood impart a red or orange colour, and santonin a bright yellow colour. Methylene blue causes a vivid green, or a blue colour, and carbolic acid and similar drugs, if taken in excess, make the urine a dark greenish-brown.

The acidity of the urine is increased by taking much meat in the diet, and, on the other hand, a large amount of vegetable food makes it alkaline. There may also be alkalinity in dyspepsia.

The specific gravity depends upon the concentration, but is considerably raised in diabetes mellitus, when it may be 1035 to 1045 or more, the normal being from 1015 to 1025. In diabetes insipidus, on the other hand, it is very low, and it is low also in cirrhosis of the kidney.

In the examination of a sample of urine, it is necessary to exclude the presence of at least two abnormal constituents, namely, albumin and sugar. A simple test for albumin is to boil a little of the urine in a test tube. If a white cloud forms, it may be due to albumin, but, on the other hand, it might be phosphates, and to determine the question, a drop or two of dilute acetic acid is put into the urine. If the cloud is phosphatic, it clears up on the addition of the acid. Albumin in the urine may be indicative of nephritis, or some other disorder, but sometimes it is physiological, as explained under the heading Albuminuria.

Testing for Sugar and Blood

To test for sugar, take 30 minims of Benedict's solution in a test tube, add 4 drops of urine, boil for 2 minutes, and allow the liquid to cool. If there is sugar present, a yellowish-red precipitate will form. The test for blood is to put urine in the test-tube to the height of about $\frac{1}{2}$ inch, add a drop of tincture of guaiacum, fill up to a height of about 2 inches with ozonic ether, and shake vigorously. The presence of blood is indicated by the development of a blue colour. The existence of blood corpuscles can quickly be discerned by the use of the microscope.

and this is a good method for finding out whether there is pus in the urine, a condition known as pyuria.

In addition to the deposits already mentioned as possibly occurring when urine is allowed to stand, there are others, some of which can be identified with the naked eye, but others only by microscopical examination. Sometimes there is what is called a cayenne-pepper deposit, tiny brown granules appearing in the urine, or on its surface. This deposit consists of crystals of uric acid. Another deposit is called the powdered-wig deposit, because it consists of white granules which are sprinkled, as it were, on the surface of the mucous deposit at the bottom of the urine-glass. This deposit consists of crystals of oxalate of calcium. While the appearance of one of these deposits may mean that there is an excessive amount of the substance in question in the urine, it must not be assumed that this is so. A quantitative analysis would be required to ascertain the precise amount.

Amongst other deposits sometimes found are crystals of urates, leucin and tyrosin, bilharzia eggs and tube-casts. The last, as their name implies, consist of various substances which have accumulated in, and been shaped by, the renal tubules. These occur in nephritis and amyloid disease of the kidney.

In certain circumstances it is necessary to determine the quantity of some normal or abnormal constituent of the urine. This is often done with regard to urea. There is a diminution of urea in nephritis and some other disorders.

See Bacilluria ; Diuretic ; Kidney ; Oxalic Acid ; Urea ; Uric Acid.

URINOMETER. An instrument for ascertaining the specific gravity of urine, a urinometer consists of an air-filled glass cylinder, drawn out at its lower end into a little bulb and at the upper end into a narrow stem. The bulb contains mercury in order to weight the instrument, and in the stem is a graduated scale. The graduations are between zero, which, however, is read as 1000, and 55, or 1055. The smallest marks represent units, thus, 1001, 1005, 1015 and so on. The specific gravity of distilled water at room temperature is taken to be 1000.

When testing the specific gravity of urine a sufficient quantity must be taken to float the urinometer properly and this must be kept away from the sides of the container, as it may adhere to the latter and give an incorrect reading. The point on the scale which is on a line with the upper level of the urine represents the specific gravity.

See Urine.

URTICARIA. *See* Nettle-rash.

UTERUS. *See* Genital System ; Womb.

UVULA. The small fleshy projection from the middle of the lower border of the soft palate is called the uvula. If it is too long it tickles the back of the throat and gives rise to a troublesome cough.

See Palate.

VACCINATION. Human beings can be protected against smallpox by being inoculated with cowpox, or vaccinia, a disease of the cow in which vesicles appear on the teats and udder, and the practice is based on the fact that milk-maids and other persons who contracted cowpox accidentally were generally immune from smallpox. There are strong grounds for believing that cowpox is actually the same disease as smallpox but attenuated, or weakened in severity, from having passed through cattle.

When vaccination is successful and vesicles appear, lymph taken from these will reproduce vaccinia in another susceptible individual, and this arm-to-arm vaccination, as it was called, was once extensively practised. It has been blamed for transmitting other diseases besides cowpox from one person to another, and although the risk of such an occurrence has been very much exaggerated, arm-to-arm vaccination has been almost entirely replaced by vaccination with lymph obtained from the calf. This, since it is subsequently treated with glycerin, is referred to as glycerinated lymph.

It is stored in little glass tubes and, when about to be used, a tube is broken at each end so that the lymph can run out. The skin is thoroughly cleaned, and a number of scratches are made with a lancet or needle at four places about an inch apart and the lymph is rubbed into these. In scratching it is not necessary to go deep enough to draw blood.

In about three days a papule with a red areola appears, and on the fifth or sixth day this becomes a vesicle, or blister, which increases in size until about the eighth day. On the tenth day the contents

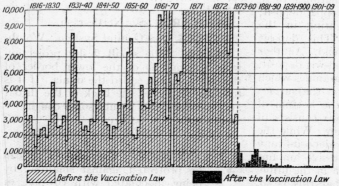

| 1816-1830 | 1831-40 | 1841-50 | 1851-60 | 1861-70 | 1871 | 1872 | 1873-80 | 1881-90 | 1891-1900 | 1901-09 |

▨ *Before the Vaccination Law*   ▮ *After the Vaccination Law*

Vaccination. Chart showing remarkable results of compulsory vaccination in the German Empire, the smallpox mortality falling from 10,000 in 1872 to about 1,500 in 1875 (the year of introduction) and later almost to zero

of the vesicle become turbid from the presence of pus, or matter, and the blister is now called a pustule. The liquid contents quickly begin to dry up and form a scab while the surrounding redness lessens, and from the fourteenth to the twenty-first day the scab drops off, leaving a depressed scar.

Vaccination is usually done on the arm but in girls the leg may be preferred in order to avoid disfigurement. After vaccination the part should be kept scrupulously clean until the scabs have dropped off. The amount of inflammation around the vesicles differs in various individuals, and also the amount of constitutional disturbance. It may be noted that the wire arm-guard sometimes used for protecting the pocks is extremely liable to rub against them and actually is more a danger than a protection.

If a first vaccination is unsuccessful another attempt should be made, but not until about four weeks after the first one. A successful vaccination almost always confers immunity from smallpox for a number of years, and in some instances for life, but re-vaccination should be done about the tenth year and again at the

twenty-first, and always when smallpox makes its appearance in the neighbourhood unless successful vaccination has been performed fairly recently.
See Smallpox.

VACCINE. The term vaccine is applied to preparations containing disease germs which are injected beneath the skin in the treatment or prevention of diseases caused by those germs. Occasionally vaccines with living germs are used, but as a rule a vaccine contains dead germs. The preparations are made in such a way that a given quantity of the liquid contains a certain number of germs, five, twenty or 1000 millions as the case may be, so that accurate dosage can be carried out.

When the germs are grown from secretions or blood taken from the patient so that the vaccine contains the strain of germs actually responsible for his disease, the vaccine is called an autogenous one. It often suffices, however, to use a stock vaccine, that is, one containing the kind of germ that is known to cause the disease from which a patient suffers. Very often a mixed vaccine is used, that is, one containing a variety of germs. Such are used, for example, in prophylactic vaccines against a common cold or influenza. A vaccine usually causes more or less reaction, both local and general, the former in the shape of inflammation and the latter as feverishness.
See Immunity.

VAGINA. The female genital passage is called the vagina. Inflammation of the passage, or vaginitis, may be due to gonorrhoea or to septic infection in connexion with an abortion or otherwise. It may also be caused by a retained pessary or some other foreign body in the passage, or by irritating injections. It sometimes occurs as a complication or sequela of measles, scarlet fever or some other infectious disease.

It may cause a sense of weight and pain in the lower part of the body, and the passage may be very painful and tender. On the other hand, if the condition is not very acute the symptoms may be slight. There is more or less discharge, the characters of which vary according to the severity of the inflammation. A certain amount of pus is nearly always present, however. The vaginal discharge is commonly referred to as leucorrhoea (*q.v.*), or whites.

Vaginismus is the name given to a painful spasmodic contraction of the muscles at the entrance to the vagina which causes difficulty in sexual connexion. It may be due to such causes as excessive tightness of the orifice, inflammation of the parts, urethral caruncle, anal fissure or disorders of the womb or ovaries. Treatment depends on the cause, but when, as not infrequently happens, no definite cause can be assigned, gradual dilatation of the orifice, sedative remedies and the relinquishment for a time of any attempts at sexual intercourse will probably be beneficial.

The anterior or posterior wall of the vagina may prolapse and form a cystocele or rectocele as the case may be. Sometimes after a difficult labour a fistulous opening between the bladder and vagina may be left, so that urine runs out through the latter. An attempt should be made to close up the breach as soon as possible. A fistula may also occur between the rectum and the vagina, but this is less common.

See Douche; Genital System; Leucorrhoea.

VAGUS. *See* Pneumogastric Nerve.

VALERIAN. From valerian root can be distilled a volatile oil which after exposure to the air develops a highly disagreeable odour. It has also an unpleasant taste. It exerts a slightly depressant effect on the central nervous system and has a reputation in the treatment of hysteria. There is one official preparation, the ammoniated tincture, the dose of which is $\frac{1}{2}$ to I drachm, and several non-official ones.

VALVE. In the heart, veins and lymphatics there are flaps that have the effect of permitting the blood or lymph, as the case may be, to flow in one direction only. If the liquid tends to flow backwards the flap opens out and blocks its passage. Such a flap, or arrangement of flaps, is called a valve. The smaller flaps consist of a double thickness of the lining of the vessel, but in the valves of the heart there is a considerable reinforcement by fibrous tissue.

A similar flap occurs at the junction of the ileum, the lowest part of the small bowel, and the caecum, and is called the ileo-caecal valve. There are also other instances of this kind of valve to be met with in the body.

In the expression valvular disease the reference is to disease of the valves of the heart (*q.v.*).

VARICELLA. *See* Chicken-pox.

VARICOCELE. A swelling in the scrotum caused by dilatation and tortuosity of veins in the spermatic cord is described as a varicocele. The veins affected are those of the pampiniform plexus, which drain the testicle and its coverings. The condition occurs most frequently on the left side and in young men. Its occurrence is favoured by constipation.

The swelling, which feels like a bag of worms, disappears almost completely when the patient lies down, as the veins are more or less emptied. There may be no symptoms, but often there is a sense of weight, and perhaps dull pain.

Occasionally there is acute neuralgia of the testicle. Discomfort is likely to be greater after vigorous exercise and during hot weather.

A slight degree of varicocele should be disregarded, but if larger a suspensory bandage should be worn. A cold bath in the mornings is helpful on account of its bracing effect. Regularity of the bowels should be secured. When the condition is irksome, a radical cure by operation should be undergone, and this will be required of any candidate for the public services. Ligatures are tied around the plexus about an inch apart, and the intervening portion is cut out, the two ends then being stitched together.

See Testicle.

VARICOSE VEIN. When a vein is dilated, knotty and tortuous, it is said to be varicose. The tortuosity is due to the fact that the vein has become lengthened. Such a fate may come to veins in many situations, but the most frequent is the lower limb, and, in fact, when one mentions varicose veins, it is almost always the veins of the lower limb that are meant. The vessel which is usually affected is the long saphenous vein which passes up on the inner side of the leg and thigh.

Many people are predisposed to the development of varicose veins by an inherent weakness in the venous walls, so that relatively slight degrees of the causes about to be mentioned are sufficient to damage the veins. Speaking generally, anything that impedes the circulation in the veins is apt to cause varicosity. The weight of the blood itself in a long vein is considerable, and in persons who have to stand a great deal, such as shop assistants and policemen, this often causes varicose veins. The risk is very considerably increased if tight garters are worn instead of suspenders.

Pregnancy is a common cause in women, as the enlarged womb presses on the great veins through which blood from the lower limbs is drained. A tumour in the pelvis or lower abdomen might have a similar effect, and even constipation, in so far as the left limb is concerned, as the overloaded bowel is capable of causing enough pressure. The circulation in the veins is much assisted by the existence of the valves, which resist back pressure, but when a vein dilates the valves become useless, and the vein becomes more and more stretched.

Even before there is much sign of varicosity to be seen, there may be a sense of weight and fulness in the limb, but these symptoms are marked when the condition is developed, and especially after standing about or a long walk. When varicosity has developed, the veins bulge out beneath the skin and are seen to be tortuous. At some points, for example, behind the knee, there may be considerable venous knots. The skin over these and over the more dilated parts of the veins tends to become thin.

The obstruction to the venous flow tends to cause dropsy, and this is especially marked about the ankle. The nutrition

Garter

Internal Saphenous Vein

Varicose vein resulting from a tight garter

of the skin consequently suffers, and it is easily irritated, so that eczematous patches may develop. Slight irritation also may cause a breach in the skin, and this may be the beginning of a varicose ulcer. Another complication that may occur is thrombosis (*q.v.*), or clotting of the blood in the veins ; this may be caused by slight knocks on the limb, or it may happen during some infectious disease. Yet another risk is rupture of a vein and of the thin skin covering, and the occurrence of very free, and possibly fatal, bleeding.

The compulsory provision of seats for shop assistants and others similarly employed, on which they can rest at intervals, should do something to lessen the risk that they run. Another beneficial reform is the fairly general substitution of suspenders for garters. During pregnancy the weight on the veins may be relieved by lying down with the legs elevated on a cushion at intervals during the day, and by the improvement of the circulation by massage and bandaging.

When the veins have become varicose, an elastic bandage (*q.v.*) or stocking should be worn. It should be put on before getting out of bed in the morning, and should not be taken off till the patient is again in bed. The object of this is to prevent a large column of blood from collecting in the vessels and pressing on their walls and valves. It may be useful also to massage the limb at night. This should consist of gentle rubbing in an upward direction, so as to propel the blood towards the heart. Gentleness is necessary because of the risk of injury to the vein and consequent thrombosis. If the skin becomes reddened, it should be powdered freely with a dusting powder containing zinc oxide and boracic acid.

Eczema and an ulcer are treated by the methods described under those headings. A method that is sometimes used is the application of Unna's paste (*q.v.*), as shown in Plate XXXIX, 1 and 2. When varicosity is severe, or there is a risk of rupture, or ulcers have occurred, it is desirable that a radical cure for the condition should be sought.

This may be procured by an operation, ligaturing or actually removing the veins. Most people prefer, however, to have their veins treated by the injection method. This consists of injections of sodium salicylate, quinine or some other substance into the veins with the object of producing a firm clot in the vein and thus closing it. The vein eventually is converted into a fibrous cord. A number of injections are required but it is not necessary for the patient to lie up. In some cases, however, this form of treatment cannot be adopted.
See Vein.

VARIOLA. *See* Smallpox.

VARIX. A dilated and tortuous vein is called a varix, or varicose vein. The expression aneurysmal varix is applied to a varix caused by a vein communicating directly with an artery, while a varicose aneurysm means a vein that communicates with an aneurysmal sac. Each is caused by a wound that penetrates an adjoining artery and vein.
See Aneurysm ; Varicose Vein.

VASA VASORUM. The tiny blood-vessels that supply the walls of the arteries and veins themselves are called vasa vasorum.

VAS DEFERENS. The main excretory duct of the testicle (*q.v.*) is called the vas deferens.

VASELINE. A proprietary brand of soft paraffin (*q.v.*), vaseline is an excellent emollient and forms the basis of many ointments.

VASOMOTOR NERVE. Branches of sympathetic nerves pass to blood vessels. They cause contraction of the muscle fibres in the vessel-wall and so constrict the arteries or, on the other hand, cause relaxation of the arteries, and are therefore called vasomotor nerves. They play an important part in controlling blood-pressure. There is a principal vasomotor centre in the medulla of the brain that controls such nerves throughout the body.
See Sympathetic Nervous System.

VEGETABLE FOODS. The characteristics of vegetable foods are that they are poor in protein and fat and rich in carbohydrate, while they contain a large amount of indigestible material. The protein is in the form of globulin but is of inferior quality to the protein found in animal foods, such as meat, fish, milk, cheese and eggs. The largest amount of protein is contained in dried pulses, and the largest amount of fat in nuts. Vegetable fat is more oily than the animal type.

Some vegetable foods, such as beet and ripe fruits, contain sugar, but in most the carbohydrate is in the form of starch. The starch granules are contained, however, in envelopes of cellulose, another carbohydrate but an indigestible one, and the starch is only available when the envelopes have been ruptured by cooking. The cellulose gives bulk to the intestinal contents and stimulates them, so that the inclusion of vegetable foods with a large amount of cellulose is of advantage to persons who are liable to constipation. Green vegetables and turnips contain very little actual nutriment.

Vegetable foods are an important source of mineral salts required by the body, and which in these foods are mainly salts of potassium. Vegetable foods, especially green vegetables and fruits, are also an important source of vitamin.
See Diet ; Food ; Vitamin.

VEGETARIANISM. A strict vegetarian diet is not to be recommended, as it lacks sufficient protein and in particular does not contain the protein which is built up of the amino-acids required by the body. Competent observers have traced some cases of mental disorder to this shortage. The addition of eggs and milk to a vegetarian diet may make all the difference, however, and the only criticism that can be made against such a diet is that it is so bulky that it may cause gastric and intestinal distension in some persons. Some people who suffer from chronic headache, obesity, constipation, gout and some chronic skin disorders may do much better on a vegetarian diet, with milk and eggs ; but the ideal diet for the ordinary person is one in which animal and vegetable foods are balanced.
See Diet ; Food.

VEGETATION. A small inflammatory outgrowth on a valve of the heart is called a vegetation. It may prevent the proper closure of the valve or it may be broken off and form an embolus.
See Embolism ; Heart.

VEIN. A vessel that returns blood to the heart is called a vein. It has the same three coats as an artery, but the middle one is less developed and the wall of a vein is therefore thinner. Many veins are provided with valves which are semi-lunar folds which open out when the blood attempts to flow backwards. Often there are two such folds opposite one another. The veins of the lower limbs are especially well provided with valves, but the branches of the portal vein, the veins of the brain and spinal cord and other veins, have no valves at all.

The blood in veins is of a dark purplish colour, except that contained in the pulmonary veins, which is pure blood in transit from the lungs to the heart. All the venous blood from the body, except that from the heart itself, is poured into the heart through two large veins called the superior and the inferior vena cava, the former receiving the blood from the head and upper limbs through the innominate veins, which are formed by the internal jugular and subclavian veins on each side, and the latter beginning at the junction of the two common iliac veins and receiving branches in its upward course through the abdomen and thorax.

A vein begins as a tiny vessel, or venule, which gathers up blood from the capillaries. Several venules pour their blood into a larger vein, and this into one still larger, until the main venous trunks are reached.

The portal vein, which drains the blood from the stomach, bowel, spleen, p a n c r e a s and gall-bladder, is peculiar in that it breaks up into capillaries. This happens when the vein has entered the liver.

Veins as a general rule follow the course of the arteries, and many are named after the arteries they accompany. A wound of a vein is, generally speaking, less dangerous than a wound of an artery, as bleeding is more easily controlled. Bleeding from a varicose vein may be very profuse, however, and possibly fatal. A wound of one of the large veins of the neck or in the armpit is dangerous, as, apart from the loss of blood, air may be sucked

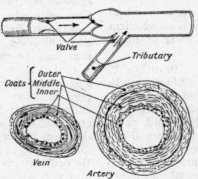

Vein. The three coats of a vein are thin and inelastic compared with those of an artery. Above, diagram of vein valves

into the vessel and form an air-embolus. This causes great distress and breathlessness, and death may occur in a few seconds.

Veins that are dilated and tortuous are called varicose veins (*q.v.*).

Inflammation of a vein, or phlebitis, may be of a septic or a simple character. Septic phlebitis may be caused by organisms circulating in the blood or by such organisms being introduced through a wound or making their way into the vein from septic tissues which surround it. It is a very dangerous condition as clotting, or thrombosis, occurs in the vein, and the clot becomes infected. Small portions of the clot are likely to break off into the circulation and cause pyaemia (*q.v.*).

Simple phlebitis is more prone to occur in the gouty and in those who are anaemic. It is more likely also to occur in veins that have been in a varicose condition for a long time, or in veins in which the circulation has been sluggish for a long time, as in those of the legs after a protracted illness such as typhoid fever. In these instances acute phlebitis may occur without any other assignable cause. Phlebitis may also be caused by injury to the vein or by thrombosis (*q.v.*) occurring within it. On the other hand, simple phlebitis may be followed by thrombosis.

The occurrence of phlebitis is marked by pain and tenderness in the line of the affected vein, which is felt to be firm and cord-like. If the vein is superficial, the skin over it is reddened and somewhat swollen. Usually there is some degree of fever, and this may precede the appearance of local signs by a day or two. If a large deep vein of a limb is involved, the limb below the site of the mischief becomes progressively swollen, and brawny to the touch.

A person suffering from phlebitis should rest in bed, and if the affection is in one of the veins of a lower limb, as it most commonly is, the limb should be swathed in cotton wool and elevated on a pillow.

Pain may be relieved by smearing glycerin of belladonna along the line of tenderness. The weight of the bedclothes should be taken off the limb by using a bed-cradle. The patient must avoid sudden or jerky movements of the limb, which should always be handled very gently.

The diet at the beginning should be light, and regularity in the action of the bowels should be maintained throughout. Large doses of sodium or potassium citrate are sometimes given in order to lessen the risk of thrombosis.

This treatment should be carried out until all signs have been gone for at least a fortnight, and if no thrombosis has occurred, the patient may be able to get up at the end of a month, but if there has been thrombosis, not till six or eight weeks have elapsed. Before he gets up, the limb should be massaged and moved gently, but the suitable time when massage and movements can be undertaken, and their regulation, are matters for expert judgement.

See Bleeding ; Circulation of the Blood ; Thrombosis ; White Leg.

VENA CAVA. Two great veins gather up the blood from all over the body and pour it into the heart, and are known as the inferior and the superior vena cava.

See Vein.

VENEREAL DISEASE. A disease acquired through sexual intercourse is called a venereal disease, and the diseases in this category are syphilis, gonorrhoea, and soft chancre. The infection of such diseases can be acquired in other ways, however ; that of gonorrhoea may be conveyed to the eyes, for example, and syphilis may be contracted from drinking vessels, etc., which have been just used by an infected person.

VENESECTION. Opening a vein to allow blood to escape for some therapeutic purpose is called venesection. This operation is discussed under the heading Bleeding or Blood-letting.

VENOM. The poisonous substance produced by a snake is usually referred to as venom. This varies in appearance, chemical composition, and effects on the human body in different kinds of snake, but is always of a complex nature, and is always acid. The term venom is sometimes applied to the poison produced by a scorpion, an insect and other creatures.

See Bite ; Snake Bite.

VENTILATION. The movement of fresh air through rooms and other spaces, in or out of doors, is described as ventilation. If free access of air to dwellings

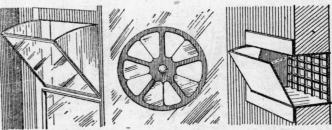

Ventilation. Left, Hopper window ventilation; centre, Cooper's disk for a window that does not open; right, Sheringham ventilator for an outside wall

is prevented by their being crowded together, or anything prevents its passage through the dwellings, ill health is bound to follow.

When air is left to make its way into and out of a room through ordinary or special openings, ventilation is said to be natural, but if air is forced in or extracted by a fan or any such apparatus, it is said to be artificial.

The principal agent in natural ventilation is a fireplace with the chimney. The wind blowing across the top of the chimney sucks air out and a fire or lamp below heats the air and sends it upwards. There is thus a strong upward draught carrying air out of the room, and this loss must be replenished through windows and doors.

A window should be constantly open, as air coming in by this route must obviously be fresher than that coming in through an inner doorway.

The complaint is often made that an opened window causes a draught, but this happens because the window is not opened sufficiently far.

If air must make its way through a narrow chink it will enter with greater force than when there is a larger opening, just as water comes with increased

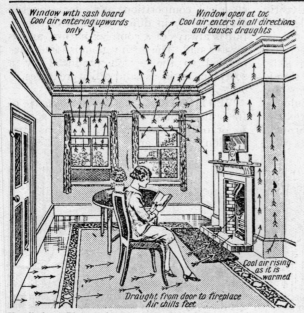

Window with sash board
Cool air entering upwards only

Window open at top
Cool air enters in all directions and causes draughts

Cool air rising as it is warmed

Draught from door to fireplace
Air chills feet

Ventilation. Right and wrong ways of admitting cool air to a room

force through the nozzle of a hosepipe, and it will travel farther as a definite stream before it becomes diffused.

One method of preventing draught, therefore, is to open the window widely. Another method is to give the current of air an upward direction as it comes through the window. One way of doing this, devised by Hinckes Bird, is to place a closely fitting board, 3 or more inches high, beneath the lower sash, this raising the sash correspondingly. The current of air flows up in the space between the two sashes. Another method is to have the upper sash hinged below so that it can be allowed to slant backwards. This arrangement is more efficient if there are side pieces to the opening when the window is down, making a sort of hopper. A third method is to have a louvred pane on the window. When a window cannot be opened a Cooper's disk may be fitted. This has openings through it which can be brought over similar openings cut in the window, or horizontal slits may be cut in the window.

Special openings are sometimes used, especially in halls, shops, and places of the kind. For the admission of air Tobin's tube or Sherringham's valve may be used. The former is a rectangular tube, usually about 6 feet high, which stands against the inside of the wall, and to which air is admitted by a perforated plate in the outside of the wall and at floor level. Sherringham's valve is a metal box which is placed in the thickness of the wall at a suitable height. Air is admitted through a grating or a perforated brick, and there is a movable side with side checks which slant upwards and which can be opened or closed as desired. Gratings may be placed in the roof or at the top of the walls for carrying off the heated air.

Several methods of artificial ventilation are in vogue. In the Plenum system air is forced by a large fan, mechanically driven, through large tubes into the various rooms of a building. The air is filtered and can be moistened and warmed. In the balance system air is driven in by fans placed at opposite ends of the room and extracted by a fan placed on the roof. The windows must be kept sealed in order to preserve the balance of incoming and outgoing air.

To secure efficient ventilation it is essential that there should be sufficient cubic space in a room according to the number of persons occupying it. When it can be obtained there should be at least 1000 cubic feet per head but many people have to be content with less. In special hospitals, regulations insist on 2000 to 3000 cubic feet per head.

See Air ; Death Rate ; Housing.

VENTRICLE. The term ventricle, which literally means a little stomach, is applied to the two lower chambers of the heart and to certain spaces in the brain and in the larynx.

VERATRINE. A mixture of alkaloids extracted from the seeds of a plant belonging to the natural order liliaceae, veratrine is a very poisonous drug and is rarely given internally. Applied to the skin as the ointment of veratrine, however, it is often of great use in neuralgia.

VERMIFUGE. A drug, such as jalap, that may expel worms from the bowel, although unable to kill them, is called a

PLATE XXXIX

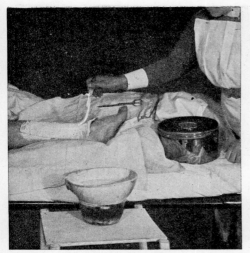 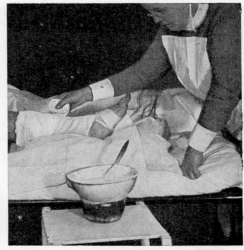

Unna's Paste.   1. A varicose ulcer may be treated by applying successive layers of Unna's paste and thin gauze.   2. The final gauze layer is covered with lint and the limb bandaged from below upwards

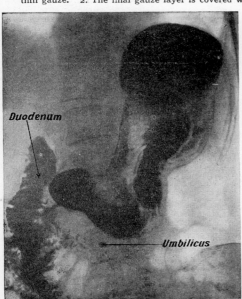 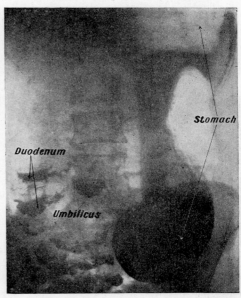

Visceroptosis.   3. Radiogram taken after an opaque meal, the patient lying down, showing outline of stomach
4. Remarkable dropping of stomach when the patient stands up, the lower end being far below the umbilicus

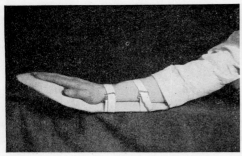 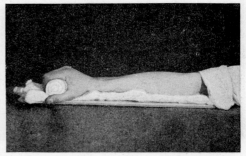

5 and 6. Wrist Drop.   Two preventive methods both of which consist in keeping the hand bent backwards

PLATE XL

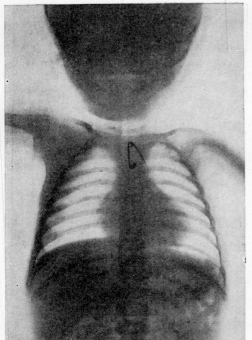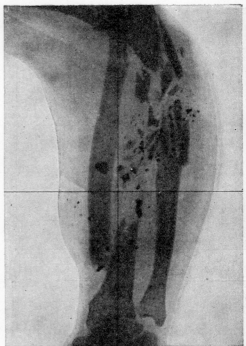

X-rays. 1. Detection of a foreign body in the gullet   2. Extent of bone injuries from a bullet wound

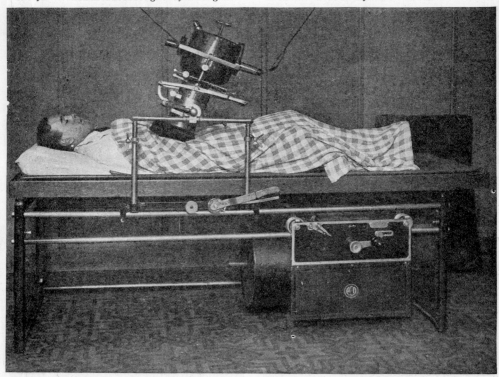

3. X-ray apparatus in use ; here the stomach is being photographed. The tube is contained in the lead-glass case above the patient, and a sensitive plate or film is placed beneath his body

vermifuge. On the other hand a drug that can kill worms is called a vermicide, though some additional drug may be required to carry the parasite out of the bowel. Oil of male fern and santonin are examples of a vermicide.

See Worm.

VERONAL. A derivative of urea, veronal, or barbitonum, is a powerful hypnotic drug which occurs as a white crystalline powder. It is usually given in hot milk and produces a natural type of sleep. It sometimes causes a measly rash and a dark discoloration of the urine. Poisonous doses produce coma with great depression of the heart.

If an over-dose has been taken and the patient is still conscious an emetic of mustard and water should be given at once, and then strong hot coffee freely. The patient should be kept warm by blankets and hot-water bottles. If the patient is unconscious a pint of warm coffee should be injected into the bowel.

See Hypnotic; Poisoning.

VERSION. Turning an unborn child so as to convert one presentation (*q.v.*) into a more suitable one is called version.

VERTEBRA. The backbone is built up of a number of separate bones, one superimposed on another, and each of these bones is called a vertebra (Plate VII, 2). Typically it consists of two parts, a body and an arch. The body consists of a more or less massive disk of spongy bone and is placed in front, the series of bodies with the fibrous disks between each pair making a solid but yet flexible column (*see* illustrations in pp. 62-63).

The series of arches, with the ligaments that fill in the gaps between them, build up the spinal canal which contains the spinal cord. From the middle of the arch of a vertebra a piece of bone projects backwards and in some of the vertebrae downwards also. It is called the spinous process and its termination may be pointed, as in the dorsal vertebrae, or bifurcated, as in

most of the neck vertebrae. Projecting from either side of the arch near the body is a transverse process. In the neck this is perforated for the passage of the vertebral artery. There are also articular processes by which the arch of one vertebra is jointed to that of another.

Several of the vertebrae are atypical. The uppermost of all, which supports the head, does not possess a body and merely forms a ring. It is called the atlas vertebra. The next, known as the axis, has a peg-shaped process of bone projecting from the upper surface of its body. This process fits into the front part of the ring of the atlas. The sacral vertebrae are fused together to form a solid triangular mass and the coccygeal vertebrae are mere nodules of bone.

See Backbone; Pott's Disease; Spinal Cord.

VERTIGO. *See* Dizziness.

VESICAL. The word vesical denotes something pertaining to the bladder. Thus, a vesical calculus is a stone in the bladder.

VESICANT. *See* Blister.

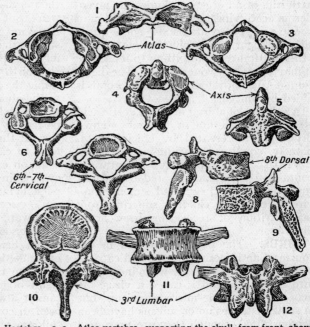

Vertebra. 1–3. Atlas vertebra, supporting the skull, from front, above and below. 4–5. Axis vertebra, supporting the atlas, from above and front. 6–7. Neck vertebrae from above. 8–9. Back vertebra, side view and in section, showing its structure. 10–12. Lumbar vertebra, from front above, front and behind

VESICLE. *See* Blister.

VIBURNUM. The bark of the black haw, viburnum prunifolium, is used in medicine in the form of the official liquid extract, dose 1 to 2 drachms, and other preparations. It has a sedative action on the nervous system and relieves and prevents spasms. It is used chiefly in menstrual disorders.

VILLUS. The lining membrane of the small intestine is studded all over with tiny finger or club-shaped processes, which give it the appearance of velvet-pile. These processes are called villi and each villus represents the beginning of a lacteal, the tube which carries off the fat absorbed from the intestine (*q.v.*).

The name villus is also given to the little processes on the outer surface of the chorion, one of the membranes that surround the embryo in the womb. In one region the villi take part in forming the placenta, or after-birth, through which the embryo is nourished.

VINCENT'S ANGINA. *See* Angina.

VINEGAR. An acid liquid, prepared by the oxidation of alcohol through the activities of an organism known as myco-derma aceti, vinegar is a dilute solution of acetic acid, but contains also small quantities of sugar, gum, colouring matter and other substances. According to its source it may be malt or wine vinegar. The digestion of salads, oysters, mussels and crab is aided by vinegar.

A solution of a drug in dilute acetic acid is called an acetum or vinegar. Three drugs are represented by official aceta, namely, squill, cantharidin and urginea.

VIROL. A proprietary preparation, containing bone marrow, red bone marrow, malt extract, eggs and lemon syrup, virol is useful to children suffering from mal-nutrition or recovering from acute illnesses.

VIRUS. The poison produced in the course of an infective disease and capable of reproducing the disease when inoculated into another person is called a virus. It may contain visible micro-organisms, but in some instances no organisms have been demonstrated, though they are presumed to exist. When the infective virus can pass through a porcelain filter it is called a filterable virus. A virus which has had its potency diminished by chemical or other means is called an attenuated virus. *See* Bacteria.

VISCERA. The internal organs are called viscera, a single organ being described as a viscus.

VISCEROPTOSIS. Sagging of the abdominal organs is known as visceroptosis, abdominal ptosis or Glenard's disease. Sagging of an individual organ is described by a name indicative of the organ. Thus, sagging of the stomach is called gastroptosis ; of the intestine, enteroptosis ; of the kidney, nephroptosis, and so on. The condition is most common in women, and the years between twenty-five and fifty is the usual age-period.

In the causation of visceroptosis, lessening of the forward curve of the lumbar region of the spine and weakness of the muscles of the anterior abdominal wall take a prominent part. The straightening of the back may be determined by heredity in some instances, but in others it is part of a poor skeletal development due to lack of exercise in girlhood, often combined with underfeeding. From the same causes the muscles of the abdominal wall are also weak, but they may also be weakened by frequent pregnancies and other circumstances that stretch them unduly. Stretching or rupture of the pelvic floor during childbirth may also contribute by diminishing the support which it normally gives to the abdominal and pelvic contents.

The abdominal viscera are partly supported by pads of fat, and a rapid loss of this fat through some wasting disease will tend to cause visceroptosis. This is the common cause in elderly men. Constant overloading of the bowel is another possible factor. Tight-lacing also tends to cause visceroptosis by pressing the viscera downwards.

In association with visceroptosis peritoneal bands may be found, fixing the intestine down to the abdominal wall. It has been taught that such bands are the result of inflammatory changes, but this cannot always be the case as they have been discovered to have existed in some children prior to birth. It would appear that visceroptosis is only likely to produce symptoms when such bands are also present, and many persons have visceroptosis without experiencing discomfort, at any rate until their attention is drawn to the existence of the condition.

Such as do suffer complain of a feeling of weight and probably of a dull pain in the lower abdomen. These sensations are caused by dragging on the nerves contained in the peritoneal attachments of the organs. Also the sagging of the digestive tube at some parts is apt to cause kinking at the parts firmly fixed in position, and hence more or less obstruction to the flow of the contents of the tube. So from gastroptosis there may arise dilatation of the stomach with dyspepsia and vomiting, and from kinking of parts of the gut, constipation. Headache and dyspepsia are common symptoms in visceroptosis apart from dilatation of the stomach, and with the sense of weight and pain in the abdomen are relieved by lying down.

Sagging of the liver may cause kinking of the bile-ducts and jaundice, while colicky attacks may result from twisting of a prolapsed kidney or spleen. In some instances visceroptosis has imitated appendicitis, both acute and chronic, gallstones, and other abdominal disorders.

When the condition has persisted for some time a neurasthenic habit supervenes and adds to the difficulties in treatment.

When visceroptosis is suspected the patient is examined both in the recumbent and upright positions, and the altered sites of the organs may be made out. It

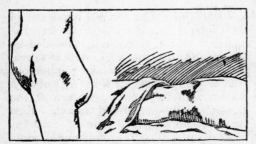

Visceroptosis. Contour of the abdomen when the patient stands compared with that when lying down

may be found that although the abdominal wall is quite flat when the patient is lying down, there is a definite bulging of the lower part when the patient is upright. If there is any difficulty in diagnosis

X-ray examination after an opaque meal will quickly settle the question (*see* Plate XXXIX, 3 and 4).

In the early stages of the disorder much good may be done by rest, combined with graduated general and abdominal exercises. The diet should be easily digestible and the bowels should be kept moving regularly. A belt that supports the lower part of the abdominal wall is also useful. When such methods fail after a thorough trial the advisability of an operation should be considered, but it may be said that an operation which simply consists in stitching an organ to the posterior abdominal wall, nephropexy or fixation of the kidney, for example, is not likely to be satisfactory. It may give relief for a time, but this is mainly due to rest and to suggestion.

See Abdomen ; Belt ; Intestine.

VISION. The sense of sight, or vision, furnishes us with knowledge regarding the form, colour, solidity, position, distance and movement or stillness of external objects. The mechanism of vision is discussed under the heading Eye.

The acuity of vision, that is the ability to see objects and recognize their shape, is usually noted by means of test types. These are black letters printed on a white board, the size of the letters being such as should be easily visible to the normal eye at distances from 6 metres upwards.

The size of those to be read at a distance of 6 metres represents a visual angle of one minute. The visual angle is the angle formed by lines drawn from the extremities of an object to the nodal point of the eye. This point lies about one-fifth of an inch behind the cornea, and all lines of light pass through it without being refracted. The smallest object that can be seen is one represented by a visual angle of rather less than one minute.

There are different theories accounting for the perception of colour, that most favoured being Koenig's, which is that there are separate cones for distinguishing red, green and violet. Red and green are not seen towards the periphery of the field of vision (*q.v.*), unless when occupying a large surface which is brilliantly illuminated. There are various kinds of colour blindness (*q.v.*).

Impressions of the solidity of objects are acquired through stereoscopic vision, that is, the super-imposition of the vision of each eye on the other. The visual judgement of distance is a complex act including an interpretation of muscular efforts in moving the eyes and in accommodation, and the results of experience as to the size and clearness of objects. Thus in the tropics a European is liable to misjudge distance owing to the clearness of the light until he has revised his experience.

See Asthenopia ; Binocular ; Eye ; Field of Vision ; Nyctalopia ; Optic Nerve.

VITAL STATISTICS. Statistics dealing with such matters as the birth, death and marriage rates, and the causes of death, are described as vital statistics.

See Birth Rate ; Death Rate.

VITAMIN. Certain complex substances which exercise a profound influence on the metabolism of the body are known as vitamins. Six are definitely known to exist, and are described as vitamin A, B1, B2, C, D and E respectively. Vitamin A and vitamin D, which appears to occur in close association with it, are not soluble in water but dissolve in fats. They are not easily destroyed by heat. The former promotes growth and the latter prevents rickets, and to a lesser extent promotes growth. Vitamins B1, B2 and C are soluble in water and are more easily destroyed by heat, especially vitamin C. The absence of vitamin B1 from a diet leads to the development of beri-beri, a disease in which inflammation of the nerves occurs, the absence of B2 to the development of pellagra, while the absence of vitamin C results in scurvy. The absence of vitamin E has been found to interfere with the fertility of rats fed on an otherwise correct diet.

The vitamins originate in plant life and are present in the fresh tissues of animals that live on plants, so that they occur in varying proportions in both animal and vegetable foods. Under the heading Diet there appears a list of foods with the vitamins they contain, and the amounts. It will be understood that vitamin D is included with fat-soluble vitamin A.

It has been found possible to create vitamin D by exposing cholesterol, which is chemically an alcohol, to ultra-violet rays. Cholesterol is found throughout the body. The other vitamins have not yet been isolated, however, though it has been possible to obtain them in a highly concentrated form.

See Diet.

VITRIOL. *See* Sulphuric Acid.

VIVISECTION. The experiments on living animals which are described as vivisection, although in very many of them there is no cutting, are strictly controlled by a system of licensing. The benefits that have accrued to mankind from such experiments are incalculable. A very great deal of our knowledge of the normal working of the body and of our capacity for preventing and curing diseases, including some of the most deadly, would have been impossible without such experiments.

VOCAL CORDS. Two pairs of bands stretch across the larynx. The upper pair are called the " true," and the lower the " false," vocal cords.

See Larynx.

VOICE. The manner in which the voice is produced and the various disorders of voice are discussed under the heading Speech.

VOLVULUS. Twisting of a loop of bowel so as to cause obstruction is called volvulus. This happens most often to the sigmoid loop of the large bowel.

See Intestine ; Obstruction.

VOMER. The small bone, shaped like a plough-share, which helps to form the middle partition of the nose is called the vomer.

See Nose.

VOMITING. The forcible expulsion of the contents of the stomach through the mouth, vomiting is generally preceded by nausea and with this a free flow of saliva. It is a complex act involving numerous muscles and nerves. There is first of all a deep breath followed by closure of the glottis. The abdominal muscles then contract briskly, and the stomach is pressed up against the diaphragm, while at the same time the upper opening of the stomach relaxes, and the stomach contents are shot up through the gullet. The muscular wall of the stomach takes comparatively little part in the act of vomiting.

The first thought on the occurrence of vomiting will generally be that it is due to some disturbance of the stomach itself caused by the ingestion of unsuitable food or of some irritant poison, but there is a very large list of possible causes, many of which have no connexion whatever with the digestive apparatus. Those that have such a connexion, apart from gastric affections themselves, include irritation in the pharynx, irritation or obstruction of the intestine, appendicitis, gall-stone, and other affections of the liver and gall-bladder, and pancreatic affections. Occasionally, for example, it is due to a strangulated hernia, which is not suspected for some time.

On the other hand, vomiting may occur in the eye disorder known as glaucoma, and even in ocular headache caused by errors of refraction ; it occurs in some ear disorders in which there is disturbance of the apparatus concerned with preserving balance ; it is a common incident in pregnancy ; it usually occurs when there is renal colic ; it may be an early symptom of meningitis, and is caused by tumours in the brain.

It is obvious, therefore, that irritation in many scattered situations can cause vomiting, and it does so reflexly through a vomiting centre which is situated in the medulla, or bulb, of the brain, although in meningitis and other brain disorders there may be some direct irritation of the centre. When vomiting is caused by brain disorders, it is often unaccompanied by nausea.

Conditions that may Provoke Vomiting

The vomiting centre can also be provoked to activity by substances circulating in the blood. Thus, a hypodermic injection of apomorphine brings on vomiting very quickly. In certain diseased states vomiting is also common for the same reasons, as, for example, in fever, chronic kidney disease and the condition of acidosis. In the last there is a diminution in the alkalinity of the body fluids, and amongst the various instances of vomiting from this cause is what is called the cyclical vomiting of children. Very disagreeable smells, or even the mere remembrance of such smells, or of disgusting sights, may be sufficient to excite vomiting.

Information regarding the cause of vomiting may be derived from an examination of the vomitus, or vomited matter.

Frequently this will consist of undigested food simply, but when vomiting is caused by corrosive poisons, the vomitus may contain shreds of stomach-lining and blood. In gastric ulcer and cancer there is also blood, but there are other causes for blood vomiting, or haematemesis, as it is called. After severe vomiting from any cause there may be a streak of blood in the vomit, merely from the effects of straining. Blood may colour the vomit red, but sometimes it gives it a dirty brown, or coffee, colour.

Reason for the Appearance of Bile

Bile is often found in the vomit, and sometimes wrongly supposed to be the cause of the vomiting, but what happens is that bile is either forced out of the duodenum into the stomach by the muscular contractions that cause vomiting, or it is sucked into the stomach. It gives a yellow or green colour to the vomit.

A considerable amount of mucus occurs in the vomit of chronic gastritis, particularly when the cause is alcoholism. In dilatation of the stomach large quantities of vomit are brought up from time to time, and it has a frothy appearance and a yeasty smell. In obstruction of the bowel, the vomit after a time begins to be of a definitely faecal character. Roundworms, fragments of tapeworms, and other parasites may also be found in the vomit.

The treatment of vomiting depends on the cause, and in many of the conditions above mentioned treatment will have to be directed to other things than the vomiting, which is merely incidental and relatively unimportant. When the cause is irritating food or something of the kind, it is desirable to give large draughts of tepid water. This washes the stomach out, and makes the act of vomiting less distressing. Sips of hot water may check vomiting, though sometimes sips of iced soda water are more successful. In persistent vomiting during fevers, sips of iced champagne often prove beneficial when other remedies have failed. Counter-irritation over the pit of the stomach by applying a mustard plaster is another useful measure in some instances.

Many drugs, including bismuth, morphine, dilute hydrocyanic acid, and others are used in treatment. A convenient remedy may be found in a single drop of tincture of iodine in a tablespoonful of water, the dose to be repeated every 15 minutes for five or six doses.

See Emetic ; Indigestion ; Poisoning ; Seasickness.

VULVA. The external genital organs in the female are collectively described as the vulva. Inflammation of the vulva, or vulvitis, is characterised by redness, swelling, burning and irritation, and more or less discharge, the symptoms varying according to the intensity of the inflammation. Gonorrhoea is a common cause, but a lack of cleanliness or the irritation of threadworms may be responsible, especially in children.

The treatment will depend on the cause, but rest in bed is necessary if the condition is at all acute. The parts should be bathed frequently with an antiseptic lotion and at night the labia should be separated by a piece of lint smeared with an antiseptic and soothing ointment.

See Genital System ; Urethra.

WARBURG'S TINCTURE. A remedy sometimes used in malaria, Warburg's tincture contains quinine sulphate, aloes, rhubarb, white agaric, opium and aromatics. It is also called tinctura antiperiodica. The dose is 1 to 4 drachms and is taken after the bowels have been cleared.

WART. There are various kinds of wart, or verruca, but each consists of an overgrowth of skin-papillae and the overlying epidermis and so belongs to the type of tumour described as a papilloma.

The common wart occurs most frequently in children, favourite sites being the back of the hand, the fold between the fingers and the knuckles, but they may also occur on the face, the sole of the foot and elsewhere. Naturally it is yellowish in colour but frequently is brown or black from ingrained dirt ; this happens when the surface of the wart is roughened. But the surface may be smooth, and then the wart is generally flattened ; otherwise it rises abruptly from the sound skin.

The common wart is contagious, but the virus that produces it has not been identified. The period of incubation may last as long as six months. Warts on the hand may infect the sole of the foot, the face and other parts.

In children a wart frequently disappears without treatment. A recent wart may be treated with an ordinary corn plaster or by painting on collodium callosum daily for some time. Older warts are best treated by applying glacial acetic acid daily for a short time. This can be done with the end of a match. If the skin around becomes inflamed the application should be interrupted for a day or two. Fuming nitric acid and lunar caustic are also used for this purpose, but are unsatisfactory in inexpert hands.

If a wart resists simple treatment it can be removed by a doctor by freezing with carbonic acid snow, electrolysis, ionisation, the cautery, or X-rays.

A seborrhoeic wart occurs in elderly people or in those with a greasy skin. Its nature is different from that of the common wart. It is flattened and brownish or black in colour and most often appears on the trunk, although it can occur elsewhere. If irritated it may become cancerous in character. These warts can be removed by carbonic acid snow, radium or X-rays. Any attempt to remove them by caustics is dangerous.

Venereal warts are such as occur about the external genital organs. They are soft and vascular, and bleed easily. They may give rise to an offensive discharge. The parts should be kept very clean and strong alum solutions or some other astringent remedy may be used, but treatment by X-rays is much more comfortable.

The cadaveric, anatomical or butcher's wart is caused by an invasion of the skin by the tubercle bacillus. It should be cut out. This is the best treatment also for the warts that occur in paraffin and tar workers.

WASH. Certain lotions are described as washes. Thus the black lotion of mercury is called black wash and the yellow lotion of mercury, yellow wash.

WASP STING. *See* Bee Sting.

WASSERMANN REACTION. A complicated test used to determine the presence or absence of syphilitic infection is known as the Wassermann reaction.

The test is applied to the blood-serum and sometimes to the cerebro-spinal fluid also. It is used for diagnostic purposes and also to check the results of treatment. A few other infections, such as yaws and trypanosomiasis, give a positive reaction, but generally speaking a positive reaction is indicative of syphilis.

See Syphilis.

WASTING. *See* Atrophy ; Emaciation.

WASTING PALSY. *See* Progressive Muscular Atrophy.

WATER. A chemical combination of hydrogen and oxygen gases, water is essential to animal and vegetable life. It forms at least two-thirds of the weight of the human body and at least three-fourths of the substance of protoplasm, which constitutes the body-cells. Water is removed from the body by the kidneys, the sweat glands, the lungs and the bowels, the total amount in the 24 hours averaging about 4½ pints for an adult.

This waste is replenished to a certain extent by water contained in food, but the greater proportion must be made up by drinking water and other liquids. It is of the greatest importance, therefore, that a sufficient supply of wholesome water should be available. It has been estimated that the minimum daily ration of water in towns should be 30 gallons per head. This includes the amount needed for drinking, personal ablutions and other purposes in the home, and general municipal purposes such as flushing of sewers, street washing, provision for extinguishing fires, and so on.

The source of the domestic water supply may be rain-water, a pond, a lake, a spring, a stream, a river, or a deep or shallow well. It should be noted that the distinction between a deep and a shallow well is not simply a matter of depth. The earth is disposed in layers, or strata, some of which, such as sand or gravel, are permeable by water ; while others, like clay and rock, are impermeable. The upper layer is commonly permeable, but by digging down to a certain depth an impermeable layer is reached, and if, on going through this, another permeable layer is found, water will probably collect at the bottom of the hole, or, in other words, a deep well has been made.

A shallow well, on the other hand, is one that descends no further than the superficial layer of soil which it drains and into which, therefore, surface water also drains. In order to prevent this water from getting into a deep well a cement or other impermeable lining is given to the well as far down as the impermeable layer. There is then no possibility of surface water running into the well if the opening is also surrounded by a wall.

Rain-water is collected off roofs and led into a cistern or storage-tank which should not be constructed of wood. In the country it receives comparatively little contamination from the air, but in towns it may receive so much as to become distinctly acid. In any case, pollution is likely to be washed off the roof ; and although by the use of an arrangement such as the Roberts' rain-water separator, the first washings may not be permitted to enter the storage tank, rain-water ought to be purified before it is used for drinking. Moreover, rain-water is distinctly unpalatable.

How a Spring is Formed

As a rule, the water in ponds is simply rain-water that has drained off from the surrounding ground surface, and if there is sewage contamination of the surface the water will be polluted. A spring is formed by rain-water sinking through permeable soil until it reaches an impermeable layer where it collects, and, when it has reached a certain level, breaks through the surface of the soil on a hillside or declivity. When it comes from the deeper permeable layers it is pure water, and can generally be depended upon to give a continuous supply. To preserve its purity, however, the spring must be surrounded by a wall in order to keep out surface water.

As it sinks through the soil water dissolves carbonic acid gas, and this enables it to dissolve calcium carbonate which is present as lime or chalk. It may also dissolve calcium sulphate and magnesium salts. Some natural mineral waters contain considerable quantities of these, and many contain iron, sulphuretted hydrogen or other constituents. Water which contains no more than a small amount of dissolved salts lathers easily with soap and is called soft water, and in this category is included any water containing no more than 10 parts of chalk, or its equivalent in other salts, in 100,000. If it contains 15 parts, or more, it is definitely a hard water, and uses up a lot of soap before a lather begins to form. If the amount exceeds 25 parts, the water is unfit for general purposes.

Temporary and Permanent Hardness

It has been pointed out above that calcium carbonate is held in solution by carbonic acid in water, and the same may apply to magnesium carbonate and iron carbonate. When the water containing such substances is heated, however, the carbonic acid is driven off and the carbonates are thrown down. They constitute the " fur " that forms in kettles and boilers. The water has been correspondingly softened, and any hardness that can be got rid of in this way is called temporary hardness. When it is caused by sulphates or other salts that are not affected by boiling it is called permanent hardness.

The water in streams, in so far as it is derived from springs, is likely to have some degree of hardness, but in so far as it is derived from surface water and marshes, it will be soft. This also applies to rivers and to lakes when there is a free outflow from the latter. If the outflow is not free, the salts become concentrated in the water in consequence of evaporation. The water in wells is also likely to have some degree of hardness, more especially that in deep wells. A deep well in which the pressure of water is such that the water rises to the surface and overflows is called an artesian well, but this name is sometimes also used, though improperly, for any well obtained by a deep boring.

The surface of the earth is likely to be polluted with sewage, particularly in the neighbourhood of habitations, and the sewage is washed off the soil by rain into ponds and streams. Some is also carried into the soil, but after a sufficient time the soil purifies itself. If there is much sewage, however, or if heavy rain falls, sewage is readily washed into shallow wells. Unless proper precautions are taken, a shallow well may be readily contaminated by sewage from a cess-pool. The water in streams, rivers, or lakes may also be contaminated by sewage, deliberately run in from villages or towns.

Sewage contamination of water may possibly cause its infection with the germs of typhoid fever, diarrhoea and other diseases. At certain times, and especially in hot countries, the germs of cholera or dysentery may be present. Sewage-polluted water may also contain the eggs of various parasitic worms.

A further risk of pollution of water is created by the lead pipes which conduct it into dwellings and the receptacles in which it is stored. If water pipes are too near sewage pipes, and both are defective, a leakage from a sewer may find its way into water pipes. Lead poisoning may occur from solution of the lead by the water. This is not likely when water contains carbonates, and especially carbonate of lime, but may happen even then in hot water pipes. There is a special risk of solution of lead by peaty waters and those that are soft.

The household supply may be drawn direct from the main or may be received into a cistern. This should be constructed of galvanised iron, or porcelain. Sometimes slate is used, but it is very heavy. The cistern should be in a light airy position, and be protected from dust. It should be cleaned out every three months. It should not connect directly with the stool of the W.C., but through a special cistern, and its over-flow pipe should be at some distance from soil pipes.

How to Soften Hard Water

Hard water has been blamed for giving rise to dyspepsia, diarrhoea, constipation, and other internal disorders, and for causing irritation of a sensitive skin when used for washing. It may be softened by boiling and passing through filter-paper, or by the addition of lime, or of washing soda. A very effective method is to instal a Permutit apparatus. The softening medium in this case can be reconstituted when it becomes stale by adding a strong solution of common salt.

Drinking water should be clear, sparkling and odourless, and have a pleasant taste. It should not be forgotten, however, that water may possess all these qualities and yet contain dangerous disease-germs. Nowadays a public water supply can generally be depended upon to be free from such risks, but when water is drawn from ponds or shallow wells, or privately, from streams, lakes or rivers, steps must be taken to free it from possible infection.

This can be done in various ways. A large measure of safety is secured by the use of an efficient domestic type of filter (*q. v.*). Boiling the water from 10 to 15 minutes will kill most microbes, but a second boiling is sometimes required. Boiling makes water insipid to the taste, however, and the same applies to distilled water, which is the purest of all water, being also free from dissolved salts, but the insipidity can be corrected by aerating the water by carbonic acid gas.

Purifying Water by Chemicals

Chemical methods of purification are also used. Fresh bleaching powder, which evolves chlorine, is a useful agent. A stock solution of this may be made by adding half a teaspoonful of the powder to a pint of cold water, and a teaspoonful of this solution added to 10 gallons of water will generally make it safe after acting for half an hour. The unpleasant taste of chlorinated water can be removed by adding sodium hyposulphite, and tablets of this substance and of bleaching powder can be obtained for treating water of doubtful purity.

Acid sodium sulphate, in a strength of 15 grains to the quart, and allowed to act for 15 minutes, is also effective. Tablets of this drug are sold, and are valuable for casual use, when camping out, etc. Another method is to add sufficient permanganate of potassium to make the water pink, and allow to stand for half an hour. The sterilisation of water on a large scale is also carried out by using ozone or ultra-violet rays.

An unpleasant taste is sometimes given to water by algae growing in tanks and pipes. This can be removed by adding permanganate of potassium, as above.

In some places there is a definite connexion between the water supply and the prevalence of goitre (*q.v.*).

See Drains; Filter; Infectious Disease; Sewage.

WATER-BED. A large rubber bag or mattress for containing water, and known as a water-bed, is used to lessen the risk of bed-sores and otherwise promote the comfort of helpless and chronic invalids (*see* Plate XXVII, 3).
See Nursing.

WATER-BRASH. The regurgitation of a hot, acid liquid into the mouth is described as water-brash. It is generally accompanied by heartburn and is a symptom of indigestion (*q.v.*).

WATER-HAMMER PULSE. In disease of the aortic valve, accompanied by regurgitation of blood, the pulse may have a thumping character while the artery collapses in the intervals of the beats. This is called the water-hammer, or Corrigan's, pulse.
See Heart.

WATER ON THE BRAIN. *See* Hydrocephalus.

WAX. *See* Ear.

WAXY DISEASE. *See* Amyloid Disease.

WEANING. *See* Breast-feeding.

WEBBED TOES. When adjacent toes are united by a fold of skin they are said to be webbed. This may also occur in the fingers, and while webbing of toes is of little consequence, in the fingers it causes a definite disability. This can be put right, however, by dividing the web. A similar condition sometimes occurs in fingers as a result of burns and is treated in the same way.

WEIGHT. There is a correspondence between the weight and the height of a person, as is shown in the table under the heading Growth; but weight also varies with age, habits of diet and exercise, and other factors. A progressive loss of weight which is not due to training or changes in diet suggests that some disease process is sapping the resources of the body.

WEIGHTS AND MEASURES. *See* Apothecaries' Weights and Measures; Domestic Measures.

WEIL'S DISEASE. A febrile disorder accompanied by jaundice and commonly by haemorrhages also, Weil's disease is caused by infection with a spirochaete, known as leptospira ictero-haemorrhagica.

The disease occurs in rats, and the micro-organisms are discharged in their urine and can infect earth and water. The infection may be acquired from food or drinking water polluted by rats or otherwise, but can also be acquired by bathing in infected water.

The symptoms come on abruptly with high fever. Jaundice appears on the fourth day and increases until the tenth day. There may be haemorrhages into the skin, and blood may be vomited or coughed up. The spirochaetes are found in the blood during the first week, and during the second in the urine, in which they may persist for a long time. Recovery is the rule in Weil's disease.

The treatment includes that of fever (q.v.), but the bowels should be kept freely open by means of calomel and salines, or the latter alone. A specific anti-serum has been used successfully.

See Jaundice.

WEIR MITCHELL TREATMENT. The régime introduced by Dr. Weir Mitchell for the treatment of hysteria and similar disorders consists of isolation, rest, a generous diet and massage. The treatment lasts for several weeks, and at the beginning rest and isolation are absolute; the patient is not allowed out of bed on any pretext whatever, and is not permitted to indulge in reading, knitting or any other occupation, nor may letters be sent or received. At first the diet consists of milk only, three ounces every three hours; but gradually the amount of milk is increased and solid food is added. Massage begins after two or three days, and is given for a period of twenty minutes morning and evening. The patient's weight is ascertained each week, and generally shows a notable and progressive increase.

WEN. A sebaceous cyst is popularly known as a wen. It is formed by the accumulation of the secretion of one of the sebaceous glands which pour out an oily secretion on the skin, and the cause of the accumulation is obstruction of the duct through which the secretion is discharged. The commonest sites for a wen are the scalp, the face and the back, and women are more often affected with this type of cyst than men.

A small, soft swelling forms and gradually enlarges, reaching the size of a hazel nut as a rule, but sometimes much larger dimensions. The skin over the wen becomes thinned, and very often is reddened. Frequently, from rubbing or other kinds of irritation, inflammation occurs, and this may be followed by suppuration. If a wen is ruptured also, it becomes infected and pours out a very offensive discharge.

Treatment consists of opening the cyst, evacuating the contents and removing the entire cyst-wall.

WHEAT. A grain of wheat consists of the germ, out of which a new plant would grow; the endosperm, which makes up most of the bulk of the grain; and the bran or husk, which encloses the other parts. The germ contains fat and is rich in protein; the endosperm, protein and a large proportion of starch; and the bran, mineral salts. In making white flour the germ and the bran are discarded, and this involves the loss of vitamins, in addition to the loss of food constituents.

See Bread.

WHEY. The watery liquid that remains when the clot formed in milk by the action of rennet is removed is called whey. It contains about $4\frac{1}{2}$ per cent. of sugar and small quantities of protein, fat and salts. It also contains vitamins.

The treatment of disease by giving large quantities of this liquid, and no other food but vegetables and fruit, is described as the whey cure. This is chiefly used in dyspepsia from overfeeding and some cases of chronic bronchial catarrh; but whey is a useful beverage also in fevers, kidney diseases and some other complaints. In the cure a tumblerful is taken morning and evening at first, but the amount is gradually increased up to about five pints daily.

Wine whey is made by adding half a glass of sherry to a teacupful of milk in a clean saucepan, heating until clotting has occurred, and straining. If desired the milk may be sweetened by adding a little sugar.

WHIPWORM. *See* Worm.

WHITE LEG. Swelling of the leg, which at the same time becomes of a dead white colour, sometimes occurs in the mother after childbirth and is popularly known as white leg. It most commonly affects the left leg. The swelling, which is usually first noticed in the second week after the baby is born, begins in the thigh but extends to the rest of the limb. The limb feels hard and brawny and does not pit on pressure like an ordinary dropsy. The swelling is due to inflammation in the lymphatics and obstruction to the drainage through these vessels. The inflammation is caused by septic infection, which often gains entrance to the tissues through a tear in the neck of the womb.

White leg is treated by rest in bed with the limb elevated on pillows, and the application of belladonna and glycerin for the relief of pain. The swelling may disappear after a few weeks, but sometimes it does not do so entirely or it swells up after the patient has been up and about for a short time. In such events massage is likely to prove useful.

A lower limb may also swell from clotting, or thrombosis, in the deep veins. This may occur after childbirth but it may also happen after pneumonia, typhoid fever and other diseases.

See Lymphatic System ; Thrombosis.

WHITES. *See* Leucorrhoea.

WHITLOW. Septic inflammation going on to suppuration in a finger or thumb, and caused by the prick of a thorn, pin or something of the kind, is described as a whitlow, or paronychia. The whitlow is said to be subcuticular when it occurs beneath the scarf skin only, subcutaneous or parenchymatous when it is in the cellular tissue beneath the true skin, thecal when it involves the sheath of the tendons, which always means the flexor tendons, and subperiosteal when it exists beneath the periosteum, or the covering of the bone.

A whitlow at those deeper levels may be caused by the prick going sufficiently far into the tissues or by a more superficial infection passing down into the deeper tissues.

A subcuticular whitlow occurs first as a painful, tender red spot but this soon becomes the site of a blister filled with matter. If the mischief is situated more deeply the finger swells, the extent of the swelling depending on that of the

sepsis, and becomes reddened. In the deeper forms the glands in the armpit become inflamed and swollen and may

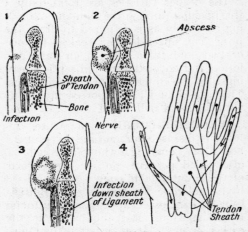

Whitlow : various degrees of infection.   1. Pus superficial.   2. Abscess pressing on nerve.   3. Abscess infecting tendon sheath.   4. Connexion of tendon sheaths with large sheath at wrist

suppurate. Moreover, if there is infection in the tendon sheath it may extend into the hand, or, if the whitlow is in the thumb or little finger, to the wrist and forearm, and abscesses may form in those situations.

There are fever and other constitutional symptoms, the severity of which depend largely on the extent of the local mischief. When the infection is beneath the skin, pain is very severe and interferes with sleep.

Suppuration in the tendon sheath is likely to be followed by sloughing of portions of the tendon, with resulting stiffness and deformity of the finger, and further mischief may be wrought by suppuration in the joints or death of portions of bone. If the infection extends to the wrist it may even be necessary to sacrifice the hand. Nor is the risk confined to local damage, for there is always a possibility of septicaemia occurring, and this may easily prove fatal.

It follows, therefore, that prompt and skilful treatment is required for a whitlow. *It is dangerous to continue poulticing a whitlow for some days without consulting a doctor.*

For the subcuticular variety all that is needed is to open the blister, clear out the contents and snip off the loose skin.

This is a painless operation. The part is then dressed with boracic lint until the raw surface has healed.

The deeper varieties are treated by a free opening through the skin and extending as deeply as is required to drain the pus. The finger is then soaked for one or two hours at a time in an antiseptic lotion and covered with antiseptic dressings in the intervals of the soakings. The arm should be supported in a sling with the hand well raised.

WHOOPING-COUGH. An acute, infectious disease characterised by peculiar bouts of coughing, whooping-cough is also called pertussis and, in some parts of the country, chin-cough. It is caused by a microbe known as the Bordet-Gengou bacillus. This is generally found in the sputum, most abundantly in the earlier weeks. It is usually communicated by close personal association with an infected person but may also be carried by the toys of the patient or by other fomites.

The disease is most common in young children, but adults are sometimes affected with it. A child suffering from measles may contract whooping-cough also, and vice versa. Whooping-cough also creates a susceptibility to the activities of the tubercle bacillus. One attack of the disease usually confers a life-long immunity against further attacks.

The incubation period is from seven to fourteen days, after which symptoms appear and are generally such as suggest that the patient is suffering from a cold, with more or less feverishness as a rule, and a hard cough. The characteristic cough may occur after a few days or not for two or three weeks. It consists of a series of short, quick coughs succeeded by a long drawn out crowing sound. This constitutes the whoop and is caused by a deep inspiration while the vocal cords are contracted. This is repeated several times and the attack usually ends with the expulsion of some sticky mucus, although often it ends in vomiting.

During the attack the child's face becomes dusky red and the eyes bulge and may become bloodshot. The child commonly stoops forward with the hands on the thighs or sides in order to assist the expulsive effort. The nose may bleed and occasionally bleeding takes place into the membranes of the brain, the symptoms resulting from this varying with the site of the bleeding. In young children the paroxysms may induce convulsions.

The paroxysms occur on the average every two or three hours during the day, but there may be fewer or many more, and generally they are more frequent at night. Interference with sleep causes depression, and insufficient nourishment from lack of appetite, and often from frequent vomiting, leads to wasting.

The severe paroxysms may keep on recurring for three or four weeks, after which they decline in frequency and severity, but for some months there may possibly be an occasional return of the cough.

The chief complication of whooping-cough is broncho-pneumonia, and this is more likely to occur in very young or weakly children. Haemorrhages and convulsions have already been mentioned. The disease is rarely fatal after ten years of age.

Isolation Periods of Patient and Contacts

To prevent spread of the contagion a person suffering from whooping-cough should be isolated for six weeks from the onset of the whoop, and infants who have been in contact with the disease for three weeks from the last date of contact. Children who have not suffered from the disease and who show signs of a cold during an epidemic of the disease should be isolated until the real nature of their complaint is apparent.

The room occupied by a patient suffering from whooping-cough should be well ventilated, but the temperature should not be allowed to fall below 65 deg. F. If there is feverishness the child should be kept in bed, but when the temperature is normal it may be allowed up and even out of doors for short spells under supervision if the weather is fine. The clothing should be warm. Food must be light and often must consist mainly of milk and eggs, beaten up with milk or as a light custard. If vomiting is frequent a little food should be given as soon as a bout is over, and in any case meals should be small and frequent.

Someone should be at hand to help the child during a paroxysm and to reassure it, and a basin should be put down to receive the sputum which should be at once disinfected or burnt.

Cresolin vaporised by heat and other inhalations are sometimes used. In order to loosen the sputum, a simple cough mixture containing paregoric is often given, and to lessen the severity of the paroxysms resort may be had to belladonna, the bromides or other drugs. The use of an appropriate vaccine is very often successful in protecting children against the disease and may mitigate it if used in the early stages.

See Bromide ; Broncho-pneumonia ; Disinfection ; Fever ; Infectious Disease.

WIDAL TEST. A test for typhoid fever depending on the agglutination of typhoid bacilli is known as the Widal test. A similar test is used in the discrimination of some other infective diseases.

See Agglutination.

WILL MAKING. The fact that a person suffers from delusions does not render him incapable of making a valid will so long as he has a reasonable remembrance of what property he possesses and of those related to him and the relative strength of the natural claim that each might have on his bounty. Delusions on any such subjects, however, would invalidate a will.

WIND. *See* Flatulence.

WINDPIPE. *See* Trachea.

WINTER COUGH. *See* Bronchitis.

WINTERGREEN. *See* Gaultheria.

WITCH HAZEL. The bark of witch hazel, hamamelis virginiana, contains tannic acid, and the leaves tannic acid and a volatile oil. From the former is prepared tincture of hamamelis, dose ½ to a drachm, and from the latter, liquid extract of hamamelis, dose 5 to 15 minims ; liquor, or solution, of hamamelis ; and the ointment of hamamelis. Those are the official preparations, but there are also others. Liquid extracts are also sold as hazeline and Pond's extract.

Preparations of witch hazel are used as astringents and for the arrest of bleeding. The tincture or the liquid extract, diluted, may be used for bleeding from the nose, mouth or stomach or in a lotion for injection into the vagina or bowel. The ointment is an excellent remedy for piles.

WOMB. The uterus or womb is a hollow organ with a thick wall composed of an admixture of plain muscle fibres and ordinary fibrous tissue. It is pear-shaped but flattened from before backwards, measuring, in the adult virgin, about 3 inches long, 2 inches at its widest part, and 1 inch at its thickest part. It consists of an upper part, or body, and a lower part, the cervix, or neck, the junction of the two parts being marked by a slight constriction called the isthmus.

Through the cervix runs a spindle-shaped canal, the outer and inner narrowed parts of which are called the os externum and os internum, respectively. This canal is lined with mucous membrane, which unites with that lining the vagina at the os externum. The mucous membrane lining the body of the womb is of a special type. It undergoes alterations before each menstrual period to fit it for the reception of a fertilised ovum, and when this event does not take place, is stripped off and discharged in the menstrual flow.

The womb is situated in the middle of the pelvis between the rectum and bladder, and its position is affected by the fulness or emptiness of those organs, and especially the bladder. The body of the organ is covered with peritoneum which is reflected behind on to the rectum and in front on to the bladder, forming so-called ligaments. A double fold also passes out on either side to the pelvic wall, forming the broad

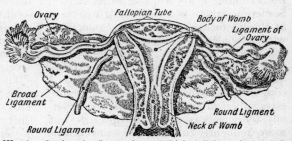

Womb. Section showing cavity and thick wall formed of muscle and fibrous tissue, also situation of ligaments

ligament. At the top of the fold runs the Fallopian tube, and between the layers of the fold are two other ligaments, one attaching the ovary to the womb and the other, the round ligament, attaching the womb to the front wall of the pelvis.

The body of the womb may bend at the isthmus, forming an angle with the cervix. This is called flexion of the womb, and may be antero-flexion, retroflexion, or latero-flexion, according as the body of the womb bends forwards, backwards or towards one or other side. The axis through the cervix may be considered to run upwards and downwards. If it runs downwards and backwards, the womb is said to be anteverted, if downwards and forwards, retroverted. The normal position in the origin, when the womb is empty, is one of considerable anteversion and slight anteflexion.

The womb may be displaced in various directions by the pressure of tumours or other swellings, adhesions to other organs, which drag upon it, or by its own weight. This will take place more readily when there is weakness in the ligaments attaching it to other parts, or weakness in the floor of the pelvis. The usual cause of the last condition is tearing during childbirth, though the floor may be weakened merely by stretching from frequent pregnancies. The weight of the womb may be increased by a failure to revert to its ordinary dimensions when childbirth is over. The pregnant womb grows during pregnancy to a length of 12 inches, but within a few weeks after childbirth it should have reverted to a size approaching that of the virgin womb.

Some Causes of Displacement

The weight of the womb may be increased also by congestion in its walls, or by a tumour in its walls or in its cavity. Sometimes there is a congenital weakness of the ligaments of the womb, associated with a tendency to sagging of the abdominal viscera, a condition described as visceroptosis. Frequent straining, in consequence of chronic constipation or a chronic cough, tends to displacement of the womb, especially if other factors exist. Occasionally the womb is displaced upwards, but more frequently the displacement is downwards, constituting what is called prolapse

of the womb, or if the organ descends sufficiently far to protrude more or less through the vaginal orifice, procidentia. In other instances there is retroversion, retroflexion, or both, or anteflexion.

Slight degrees of displacement may cause no symptoms, but when the condition is more pronounced, there is a sensation of weight and dragging in the lower part of the abdomen, the menstrual flow may be excessive and painful, and there is leucorrhoea, or whites. A considerable degree of anteflexion tends to cause irritability of the bladder, and backward displacements may cause constipation. If conception occurs in the womb when it is displaced backwards, abortion is likely to occur about the 3rd or 4th month. Retention of urine sometimes occurs in the same circumstances. In procidentia the neck of the womb is irritated, and sooner or later becomes ulcerated.

How to Treat the Condition

The treatment of a displacement will depend upon its cause. Sometimes it will suffice to replace the organ and maintain it in its correct position by means of a pessary (*q.v.*). In other instances treatment will be required to produce a healthier condition of the womb, or some kind of operation, to repair a torn perineum, for example, to remove a tumour, or to tack up the organ more securely. Sometimes the top of the womb becomes indented and projects into the cavity of the organ, and this may go on until the whole organ is turned outside in. This is described as inversion of the womb, and may occur in an acute form after the expulsion of the child in labour. When this takes place the patient becomes collapsed and there is very free bleeding. Inversion may also occur as a chronic condition, and tends to be accompanied by frequent and free bleedings. The treatment is to push back the inverted portion, if possible, but sometimes it is necessary to remove the womb.

The commonest tumour of the womb is what is called a fibroid, or a fibro-myoma. This rarely occurs before the age of thirty, and is commoner in unmarried and in childless women. The tumour may grow within the wall of the organ, when it is called an intramural fibroid, or it may grow just beneath the inner lining, a submucous fibroid, or may bulge out beneath the peritoneum, a subserous fibroid. In the latter two instances it may develop a stalk.

There is usually more than one fibroid. If quite small, a subserous growth may cause no symptoms, but if sufficiently large, it will cause pressure on various organs. From the other two tumours there is likely to be an excessive menstrual flow, and possibly bleeding in the intervals of the periods, and there may be pain with the periods and a more or less constant leucorrhoea. There may also be pressure symptoms.

A fibroid may disappear spontaneously after pregnancy, and tends to atrophy at the menopause, but, on the other hand, it may take on active growth at this time. Fibroids are always liable to undergo certain degenerative changes.

Treatment of a Fibroid Tumour

If a fibroid is causing no symptoms, it may be left alone, but its progress should be kept under observation by a doctor. If it is causing bleeding or other symptoms, and the patient is in the child-bearing period of life, the growth should be removed. Otherwise, X-ray or radium treatment may be suitable, especially if there is bleeding, but this kind of treatment will induce an artificial change of life prematurely in women who have not reached the age for the natural change.

A submucous fibroid may form a polypus of the womb, but a polypus need not be of this nature. The growth should be removed.

Cancer of the womb much more commonly affects the cervix, and in this situation is almost always found in women who have borne children. It causes irregular bleeding, and may cause no pain until a late stage. Bleeding after the menopause, or after sexual intercourse, should always be reported to a doctor.

A sarcoma occasionally occurs in the womb, and may occur in young girls. Another malignant growth of the womb is called deciduoma malignum. It is due to overgrowth of the villi of the chorion,

one of the membranes that surround the embryo.

See Endometritis ; Genital System ; Haematocele ; Menstruation ; Parametritis ; Perimetritis ; Pessary ; Visceroptosis.

WORD BLINDNESS. *See* Aphasia.

WORM. A large number of species of worm have been found leading a parasitic existence in the human body, some of them in the digestive tract, and others in the blood or elsewhere. They belong to two main groups, namely, the round worms or nematodes, and the flat worms, these again being of two classes, the cestodes, or tapeworms, and the trematodes, or flukes.

The round worms most commonly found in the digestive tract are oxyuris vermicularis, commonly called the thread, pin, or seat, worm ; ascaris lumbricoides, commonly called the roundworm ; and tricocephalus dispar, commonly called the whipworm.

The threadworm is very common in children, but is also found in adults. The female is about $\frac{1}{2}$ inch long, and the male only $\frac{1}{6}$ inch. The worm gets into the body by the eggs being swallowed. The eggs hatch out in the intestine, and the worms mature. In some instances a large number of young threadworms has been found in the vermiform appendix, and this suggests that eggs may hatch out there. The impregnated female worm makes her way into the rectum, where she discharges her eggs, and is voided in the stools.

Threadworms also wriggle their way out through the anus, around which they cause considerable irritation. This happens especially at night. They may also make their way into the vulva and vagina and cause irritation and a discharge there. Children, when scratching in order to relieve this irritation, receive the eggs of the worm on their fingers and beneath the nails and the eggs may thus be conveyed to the mouth and swallowed, so bringing about a fresh infection. Infection may also be acquired from fresh vegetables, such as salads and water-cress.

Children suffering from threadworms may be restless and peevish, the appetite may be poor, and they may complain of colicky pains. They may suffer from night terrors, and sometimes from convulsions. The worms can readily be seen on inspection of the motions. They resemble, as one of their names implies, tiny wriggling pieces of white thread.

To get rid of the worms an enema may be given twice a week for a few weeks, and also a few doses of santonin by the mouth, but as santonin may cause poisoning, it should only be given to young children under medical observation. The enema may consist of a solution of common salt, a tablespoonful to the half pint, or of infusion of quassia. A young child should receive about 6 ounces, and older ones up to ¾ pint. The anus should be washed on rising and after the bowels move, and should be kept smeared with an ointment consisting of equal parts of soft paraffin and white precipitate ointment. To prevent a child from scratching the parts during the night a close pair of knickers may be put on. The bowels should be kept moving regularly, and doses of Gregory's powder or liquid paraffin may be given if necessary.

Ascaris lumbricoides, or the roundworm, resembles the ordinary earth worm, but is more pointed at each end, and has a whitish colour. Its length varies from 4 to 12 or more inches. It inhabits the small intestine, but may make its way into the stomach and even up the gullet and so may get into the trachea and air tubes. It may also make its way into the bile ducts, and has been known to perforate the wall of the intestine and cause peritonitis. As a rule, only two or three worms are present, but occasionally there are great numbers. The female worm discharges thousands of eggs each day. When only two or three worms are present, there may be no symptoms, and the first indication of their existence may be the appearance of one or more of them in the stools. Sometimes, how-

ever, there is restlessness, and, in young children, convulsions. There may also be a capricious appetite, itching at the nose and anus, nausea, vomiting and diarrhoea, sometimes with bloody stools.

The most effective drug in killing roundworms is santonin, and an adult might take a powder consisting of 3 grains of santonin and 2 grains of calomel at bedtime, and follow this with a dessertspoonful of salts in half a glass of water in the morning. The dose might have to be repeated on one or two nights. It should be noted that after taking santonin the urine is tinted orange or red, and that there may be green or yellow vision for a short time. The eggs are swallowed in polluted water or on fresh vegetables.

The whipworm owes its name to the fact that it has a small head and a long slender neck with a considerably thicker hind part, or body, so that it actually resembles a tiny whip. It is usually found in the caecum, but occasionally wanders to other parts of the intestine. It attaches itself to the mucous membrane by its head, the rest of the worm swinging free. It may cause appendicitis, or, by piercing the bowel, may give rise to peritonitis. There is no reliable anthelmintic against this parasite, but the possibility of infection by it is one reason for boiling all questionable drinking water. The eggs of the whipworm must remain for a long time in water before the young parasite is

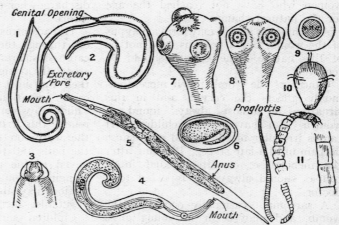

Worm : diagrams of three intestinal species. Roundworm : 1, male ; 2, female ; 3, head seen from above. Threadworm : 4, male ; 5, female ; 6, egg. Tapeworm : 7 and 8, head of taenia solium ; 9, egg ; 10, embryo ; 11, portion of taenia solium, showing segments

sufficiently developed to be capable of existence in a fresh host.

A tapeworm consists of a head, or scolex, a narrow portion, or neck, and a succession of flat segments, or proglottides. There may be only three proglottides, as in taenia echinococcus, the parasite of hydatid disease, or several thousands, when the total length of the worm may extend to 30 feet, or exceptionally, to many more feet than this. A tapeworm has no digestive apparatus, but depends for its nourishment on digested foods which are absorbed into its tissues from its host, but each proglottis has both male and female sexual organs, and, when mature, produces fertilised eggs. From time to time a proglottis, or even a string of the segments is passed out of the bowel, and the eggs are set free. These are consumed by some animal, sometimes man himself, and in the alimentary canal the covering of the egg is dissolved or otherwise removed and the embryo emerges. By means of hooklets it bores its way through the wall of the intestine and reaches the muscles, lungs, brain, or some other tissue.

Tapeworms in Animal Food-stuffs

Here it discards its hooklets and develops a head like that of the adult worm, which is enclosed, however, in a sac, containing fluid. At this stage the worm is known as a cysticercus. The cysticercus found in the meat of the pig is that of taenia solium, in the meat of an ox, that of taenia saginata, and in the meat of the pike, salmon and perch, that of dibothriocephalus latus. These are the three tapeworms most commonly found in human beings, and they occur where it is the habit to eat the food-stuffs mentioned either uncooked, or imperfectly cooked. That most likely to be encountered in Great Britain is taenia solium, which is got through eating measly pork, the mottling of the pork being due to the cysticerci which are dotted throughout it. When the meat is consumed the cyst is dissolved, and the head, or scolex, fastens itself to the mucous lining of the small intestine, being furnished with four suckers and a circle of horny hooklets for this purpose. Proglottides are then produced, and at first are broader than

they are long, but in the maturer segments the reverse holds, and on an average they come to measure about $\frac{1}{2}$ inch in length and about $\frac{1}{4}$ inch across.

The immature form of this worm, known as cysticercus cellulosae, is sometimes found as a cystic growth in the human being, in the brain, eye, or elsewhere.

The nervous symptoms which have already been noted as occurring from the presence of other worms may sometimes be caused by a tapeworm also, but as a rule the symptoms are indefinite and the first indication of the existence of the parasite is the passage of proglottides in the stools, or, in the case of taenia saginata, in the bed or on the clothing, as the proglottis of this worm has a habit of making its way out of the intestine by its own efforts.

Some Useful Anthelmintics

A number of drugs are used for killing tapeworms, but the one most often used is oil of male fern, 30 to 40 minims of the liquid extract of male fern being taken in milk and peppermint water. Other drugs are oil of turpentine, half an ounce of which is taken with the same quantity of castor oil, and pelleticrine. A dose of one of these drugs is taken in the morning on an empty stomach, and two hours after a dose of saline, and if the bowels have not moved in four or five hours after the anthelmintic is given, a dose of castor oil should be taken. A milk diet only should be taken on the day preceding the treatment. More elaborate methods of treatment are also in vogue.

A close watch must be kept on the stools in order to see whether the head comes away, and to facilitate inspection it is well to wash the stools through a strainer made of crape. The parasite narrows to a fine strand at the end of which is the head, about the size of the head of a pin.

The three tapeworms which have just been discussed inhabit the human body in their adult stage as a rule, existing during their immature stage in some other animal. In contrast to this is taenia echinococcus which, when present in the human body is in the immature form, giving rise to what is called hydatid disease, but passes through its adult stage in the body of the dog.

The only trematode, or fluke, that is common in man is that called bilharzia haematobia, or distomum haematobium, which causes the disease known as bilharziasis, though the liver-fluke, or distomum hepaticum, which in sheep causes the disorder called sheep rot, is sometimes found in man.

Important roundworms, in addition to those which infest the intestine, are the filaria sanguinis hominis, described under the heading Filariasis, the guinea worm and the trichina, or trichinella, spiralis, the immature form of which is found encysted in the voluntary muscles and certain other tissues of man and other animals. Human beings usually derive this parasite from infected, or, as it is called, trichinised pork, and the disease resulting from such infection is described as trichinosis, or trichinelliasis.

When infected pork, which has not been thoroughly cooked, is eaten, the coverings of the cysts are dissolved and the young parasites set free. They quickly reach sexual maturity and the female becomes impregnated and increases in size, attaining about an eighth of an inch in length. She bores her way out of the intestine into a lymphatic in which she begins to discharge the young worms in enormous swarms. These reach the blood stream, by which they are carried to the muscles, where they come to rest, coil up and become encysted. They really give rise to a form of inflammation of the muscle, or myositis.

Symptoms after Eating Infected Pork

Shortly after partaking of trichinised pork there may be sickness and diarrhoea, but in any case, at about the end of a week, there is pain in the muscles and high fever. The intercostal muscles and the diaphragm are commonly affected and there may be difficulty in breathing, and, from involvement of the muscles concerned, there may also be difficulty in chewing and swallowing, and perhaps loss of voice. Usually there are signs of dropsy, beginning first in the face. The patient may become very ill, and may die, but if the disease takes a favourable course, convalescence usually begins about the fifth or sixth week. The worms in the muscles remain alive, however, and perhaps for many years.

There is no satisfactory treatment for trichinelliasis. If suspicion is attached to pork shortly after it has been eaten it is desirable to give an emetic, and afterwards a dose of calomel in order to clear the alimentary tract. Otherwise the treatment is largely that of fever (*q.v.*). Prevention consists in refraining from eating pork unless it is thoroughly cooked, and, as the rat is suspected of having something to do with harbouring and spreading the worms, this is one of the many reasons that make the destruction of these pests a duty.

See Bilharziasis; Filariasis; Guinea Worm; Hydatid Disease; Santonin.

WOUND. Any breach of the continuity of a tissue, caused by violence, constitutes a wound, and such an injury as a fracture or a bruise is in fact a wound, though it is customary to restrict the application of this term to a breach involving one of the surfaces of the body. It may be internal, as when the lining of the stomach is wounded by a foreign body, but it is proposed to deal here with external wounds, whether of the skin or a mucous membrane, though much that will be said applies equally to wounds of internal surfaces.

It is usual to distinguish between incised, lacerated, contused, punctured and gun-shot wounds.

An incised wound is one made by the slash of a cutting instrument. The tissues are simply divided without being bruised. A deep cut on a limb may possibly divide tendons or nerves as well as blood vessels and bleeding may be free. It should be remembered that a sharp blow on skin stretched over a bone causes a wound resembling an incised one, but the surrounding tissues are bruised by the blow, so that it is really a contused wound. This may happen on the scalp, for example, or on the skin over the knee-cap.

A lacerated wound is one caused by tearing, by machinery or something of the kind. Sometimes the bite of an animal causes a lacerated wound. The edges of the wound are irregular and bruised more or less; as the instrument that causes it is commonly foul the wound is likely to be septic, and infection is favoured by the vitality of the tissues being lowered by the bruising. Bleeding may not be as free as in an incised wound, as the vessels are torn rather than cut.

Dangers of a Punctured Wound

A punctured wound is a stab and may be caused by such small instruments as thorns, splinters of wood or the sting of an insect, or by large objects such as the spike of a railing or a dagger. From the point of view of infection a minute punctured wound may be as dangerous as a large one. A whitlow on the finger is caused by a tiny prick from some object admitting infection, and blood poisoning has resulted from this and from the sting of an insect. When the wound is made by a larger insect there is the added risk of important organs and structures being damaged. Pieces of clothing may be carried deeply into the tissues on the point of a stabbing instrument.

By a gun-shot wound is meant a wound caused by a missile impelled by the discharge of an explosive. It may be a bullet, a fragment of a bomb, a piece of masonry broken off by the violence of the concussion, or some other object.

The missile is travelling with great speed and even although its entrance may only be marked by a small puncture it may cause much laceration of the tissues beneath. Sometimes it does not, however, but bores a clean hole through the part. As with a punctured wound, though probably more frequently, pieces of clothing may be carried deeply into the wound. In a gun-shot wound also there may be some scorching of the tissues. In the radiogram of a bullet wound given in Plate XL, 2, the soft tissues are badly torn and bruised and the bone shattered.

The immediate treatment of a wound consists in the arrest of bleeding and the relief of shock if such are present, and in cleansing and protecting the wound from further risk of infection. If a wound occurs in the street or elsewhere in the open the best thing to do is to cover it with an antiseptic dressing if such is available or, if not, with a clean handkerchief or something of the kind. If tincture of iodine can be secured it should be dabbed over the edges of the wound and surrounding skin. As soon as possible the patient should be taken somewhere for a proper cleansing of the wound. A suitable antiseptic lotion can be made by mixing a teaspoonful of tincture of iodine in a pint of water. For swabbing the wound cotton wool or gauze should be used or, failing either, soft clean cotton or linen rags. A piece of one of these moistened with the lotion is placed on the wound and the surrounding skin is thoroughly cleansed first with soap and water and then with the lotion (*see* Plate II, 5). A sufficient amount of the lotion is then squeezed into the wound to wash it out, or, if the wound is on the hand or the foot, the part may be put into a basin containing the lotion and allowed to soak for some minutes.

If there is a possibility of clothing or any other foreign matter being at the bottom of a wound, or if there is grit in the wound that cannot be washed off, it will be necessary to have it cleansed under an anaesthetic. If there is any possibility of earth-soiling of the wound the patient should receive anti-tetanic serum to prevent any risk of lockjaw developing.

When the wound has been cleansed the skin around is dried and a dressing of boracic lint or cyanide gauze is put on, then a layer of cotton wool and lastly a bandage (*see* Plate II, 6).

See Antiseptic; Bandage; Bite; Bleeding; Bruise; Burn; Collodion; Cut; Dressing; Graft; Granulation Tissue; Iodine: Iodoform; Lockjaw; Shock; Septicaemia; Tourniquet.

WRINKLE. The three factors in the causation of wrinkles are the loss of elasticity in the skin as one gets older, a diminution of the subcutaneous fat and the habitual movements of the facial muscles. Wrinkles about the eyes, for example, are likely to be numerous and to occur early in people who suffer from some visual defect and screw up their eyes when making an effort to see clearly. The elasticity of the skin is better preserved in those who maintain good general health.

The use of a so-called " skin-food " is much vaunted as a local treatment, but the most that any such preparation can do is to produce an emollient effect. This can be obtained with cold cream, almond oil, almond pastes or something of the kind.

See Skin.

WRIST. The structures of the wrist, or carpus, include an upper and a lower row of four small bones, the joint between the upper row and the radius and ulna, which is the wrist joint proper, and the joints between the lower row and the meta-carpal bones. The adjacent bones of the carpus, which are referred to as the carpal bones, glide on one another and add to the movement that takes place at the wrist joint.

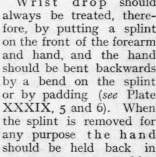

Wrist. Structure of the joint. A synovial cavity separates the end of the radius from the carpal bones

The movements which can be made at the wrist are flexion, or forward bending ; extension, or backward bending ; adduction, or bending to the little finger side ; and abduction, or bending to the thumb side. But as a forward or backward movement may be combined with a lateral one the wrist possesses great flexibility. Therefore dislocation does not often occur at this part though a sprain is a common event. The tendons proceeding to the hand on the back and front of the wrist strengthen this part considerably.

Fracture of one of the carpal bones may be caused by injury, the trapezium, to which the thumb is attached, being especially liable to be broken, from the thumb being forced backwards. As there is little or no displacement of the fragments as a rule, the existence of the fracture might only be revealed by an X-ray examination. The main risk in this and other injuries, and in inflammatory diseases of the wrist, is that the products of inflammation may become organized into new fibrous tissue which anchors one tendon to another or to bone, thus producing more or less interference with movement. It is necessary therefore that movements should be carried out as soon as the more acute symptoms of the disease or injury have abated.

The muscles that extend the hand are supplied by the musculo-spiral nerve (*q.v.*) and when the nerve is sufficiently damaged by disease or injury there is wrist drop, that is, the hand is flexed and cannot be raised out of this position. Wrist drop also may occur in hemiplegia, or paralysis of one side of the body, or, again, may have a hysterical origin. The muscles on the front of the forearm are more powerful than those on the back, and when there is any weakness in the latter they tend to draw the hand down.

Wrist drop should always be treated, therefore, by putting a splint on the front of the forearm and hand, and the hand should be bent backwards by a bend on the splint or by padding (*see* Plate XXXIX, 5 and 6). When the splint is removed for any purpose the hand should be held back in order to avoid even a momentary stretching of the weakened muscles. The hand should be put up in the same way during inflammatory disease or after injuries of the wrist.

See Forearm ; Ganglion ; Hand ; Joint ; Radius ; Sprain.

WRITER'S CRAMP. The affection known as writer's cramp, or scrivener's palsy, is an instance of what is called an occupational neurosis. This occurs in people whose occupation involves continuous, rapid manipulations, and besides writers, typists, telegraphists, violinists, pianists and others may suffer. The muscles of the hands and arms become subject to cramps and later on are enfeebled, painful and tremulous. The particular occupation becomes impossible, and also any other in which manipulations are required.

A rest from all work of this kind for six months or longer, combined with tonic treatment and massage, may bring about sufficient improvement to permit of work being resumed, but as a rule there is a quick relapse. It is thought that the disorder is more than a mere disturbance of the muscle and nerve apparatus concerned in making the manipulations and has also a psychical origin. There is a sense of incapacity for the work in question which expresses itself as a neurosis. Consequently it is advantageous to combine psychotherapy with the other kinds of treatment. Even so, however, the outlook is rarely very hopeful.

See Neurosis.

WRY NECK. Bending of the neck to one or other side, when due to spasm or shortening of the muscles, is called wry neck, or torticollis. Besides being bent, the neck is more or less rotated so that the face is directed towards the sound side and a little upwards. The muscle that is chiefly concerned in causing wry neck is the sterno-mastoid.

Wry neck may appear soon after birth and seems then to be due to a birth injury though sometimes there may be some other explanation. If manipulation of the neck is undertaken as soon as the deformity is noticed, a cure may be effected. Sometimes an apparatus is worn at the same time to keep the head in a correct position.

If wry neck has existed for some time, however, it will be necessary to divide the shortened structures ; but though this may correct the wry neck it is unlikely to remove the atrophy of the face, which usually accompanies this early form of the deformity.

Wry neck may be caused by rheumatism in the muscles of the neck, by inflammation of glands in the neck, by irritation in the teeth or elsewhere or by spasm, sometimes of a hysterical character. The spasmodic variety occurs mostly in women and at first is intermittent and the spasms are clonic in type but later on there is a constant fixation. This variety is very resistant to treatment. The rheumatic variety is treated by giving sodium salicylate or aspirin and by gentle massage, preferably with a liniment containing methyl salicylate. When irritation is the cause the obvious course is to clear up the source of irritation as far as possible.

XANTHELASMA. The occurrence of yellowish deposits on the eyelids due to fatty degeneration of the muscle fibres is described as xanthelasma.

XANTHINE. One of the substances to which the term purin (*q.v.*) is applied, xanthine is found in many animal tissues and in many plants. It is obtained as a colourless powder, but its nitrate is yellow and hence the name xanthine. It acts as a heart stimulant. It may occur in minute quantities in the urine and on rare occasions has been found in considerable amount in renal stones.

XANTHOMA. In diabetes mellitus yellowish swellings sometimes form in the skin. Such a swelling is called a xanthoma. It is surrounded by a zone of reddened skin. There is another form of xanthoma which is usually associated with liver disease.

XANTHOPSIA. Yellow vision is technically called xanthopsia. It occurs in people who have taken santonin, a drug used for killing roundworms.

XERODERMA PIGMENTOSA. A rare disease of the skin, which begins in early childhood, xeroderma pigmentosa first manifests itself in little brown spots, like freckles, that cover the exposed parts but later on the covered parts also. These may deepen in colour and become quite black. After a time little red marks resembling birth-marks make their appearance, interspersed amongst the other spots, and also white spots, which represent areas of atrophied skin.

Numbers of these white spots may coalesce, forming scar-like patches. At the site of the brown spots a shallow ulceration develops, the ulcers being covered with yellow or greenish crusts, and these ulcers soon assume a frankly cancerous character. Several members of a family may be affected and it is thought that the disease may be due to an undue sensitiveness of the skin to the chemical rays of sunlight. It may delay the fatal issue if the cancerous patches are cut out or treated with radium, but the disease is quite incurable.

X-RAYS. The X-rays, which are also known as the Roentgen rays, consist of undulations in the ether, like those of light, but of a much shorter wave-length. They are produced by passing an electric current through a glass tube in which there is a more or less complete vacuum. From the cathode, or negative electrode in the tube, a stream of electrons, constituting what are called cathodal rays, is made to impinge on a plate of platinum, or tungsten, let into the tube on a part of the apparatus, called the anti-cathode.

The impact of the electrons generates X-rays and heat, and as the plate is set at an angle of $45°$, the rays are directed through the side of the tube. To make the passage of the electrons possible, it is necessary to have a small residuum of air in the tube or, as in the Coolidge type of tube, the cathode must resemble the filament in the thermionic valve used in wireless, and be capable of being heated, as the heated metal gives off electrons.

X-rays are able to penetrate solid substances, but their capacity to do so varies. Such as are capable of passing through dense substances like metal, are described as " hard " rays, and those with less power of penetration, " soft " rays. Hard rays are produced in a tube with an almost complete vacuum ; otherwise the rays are soft. To produce X-rays, a current of high potential is required, for the softest rays as much as 40,000 volts, and for the hardest, 250,000 volts.

How an X-ray Film is Made

The power of X-rays to penetrate the tissues of the body varies with the density of the latter, and where penetration does not take place, or only partially, shadows are cast, the depth of which depends on the extent to which the passage of the rays has been blocked. An imprint of these shadows can be obtained on a screen, rendered fluorescent by coating it with such substances as platino-cyanide of barium or tungstate of calcium, or on a photographic plate or film. The screen or plate is placed on the other side of the patient from the one on which the X-rays are falling (see Plate XL, 3). Screening is used for the immediate examination of the patient, and the action of the heart, lungs and other viscera may be observed. The record on a photographic film or plate is required for a more prolonged and detailed study. It should be noted that what is recorded is a picture of shadows, and therefore the forms and position of an organ or a foreign body will vary according to the direction of the X-rays.

There is a very wide field for the use of X-rays in diagnosis, embracing, amongst other things, fractures and other lesions of bone, diseases of joints, disease in the lungs, heart, alimentary tract and in other viscera, the position of foreign bodies in the viscera and tissues, and the state of the roots of the teeth. For the investigation of disorders of the alimentary tract what is called an opaque meal,

that is, one containing barium or bismuth salts, is given, and the progress of the meal along the tract is studied. Opaque substances are injected into other hollow viscera in order to obtain a better view of them. Examples of radiograms made for diagnostic purposes have been included in the Plates in this volume and the reader is referred to the following : VII, 8 ; XIV, 5 and 6 ; XXI, 1 and 2 ; XXXII, 3 and 4 ; XXXIV, 5 ; XXXIX, 3 and 4 ; and XL, 1 and 2.

X-rays are also used as a therapeutic agent. When the skin is subjected to a sufficient dose, it is stimulated to activity, as is shown by its subsequently becoming reddened. If an over-dose is given, there may be blistering, or even sloughing, signs of an X-ray burn. The stimulation of the skin may be of benefit in chronic eczema and other chronic skin diseases, and although bacteria may not be affected directly, the stimulation of the tissues assists them in their fight against bacteria. By a sufficient exposure to X-rays, epilation of hair may be accomplished in ringworm and other diseases, and the hair will grow again, though an unskilful application of the rays may cause permanent baldness. This method is not recommended for the removal of superfluous hairs, however. Another use of the rays is the treatment of pruritus, or itching.

Curative Value in Treating Growths

Some disorders of the blood and blood-producing tissues are successfully treated by X-rays, and benefit is also derived by some who suffer from exophthalmic goitre. X-rays have the power of destroying many new growths, and, whether or not they can remove malignant tumours, they can at least reduce their activities very considerably and stay their progress for a time. For the treatment of deeply-seated growths, chiefly those in the pelvic organs in women, rays of great penetrating power have recently been used, with a metallic filter to cut off the softer rays and lessen the effects on the skin.

Frequent exposure of the skin to X-rays tends to cause a chronic dermatitis, which later on may lead to cancer, and some X-ray workers have had unfortunate experiences of this kind. Another consequence of frequent exposures is sterility, from the action of the rays on the sexual glands. To obviate such risks, X-ray tubes are enclosed in metal boxes, and special gloves and aprons are worn by those who handle them.

See Barium ; Bismuth ; Cancer ; Electricity in Medicine.

YAWS. In many parts of the tropics there occurs a disease which is known as yaws or framboesia and by a number of local names given to it in places where it is prevalent. The name framboesia was given to the disease because many of the lesions on the skin may have a resemblance to a raspberry. The cause of the disease is a micro-organism called treponema pertenue, which is related to treponema pallidum, the parasite in syphilis. For many years, in fact, yaws was considered to be but a form of syphilis, but the two diseases are now known to be quite distinct. The most numerous victims of yaws occur amongst coloured children, apparently because the liability to contagion is greatest.

To permit of infection there must be some abrasion of the skin, and on this the treponema may be implanted by direct contact with a yaws sore or through the agency of flies or other insects. The site of inoculation is most commonly on the lower part of the leg. There is a period of incubation lasting from 12 to 20 days or longer, during which there may be irregular fever, with pains in muscles and joints and disturbances of digestion, but these symptoms cease, as a rule, when the initial lesion forms at the site of inoculation. This consists of a papule, tiny at first, but growing to the size of a pea. The skin of the papule cracks, exposing a raw, red surface, from which oozes a yellowish-white discharge. This sore may heal, leaving a pigmented scar, or it may become enlarged and covered with masses of granulation tissue.

From six weeks to three months after the appearance of this primary sore similar sores break out on the face and limbs, occasionally on the back, and rarely on the scalp. The occurrence of this rash is preceded by symptoms of illness similar to those that precede the primary sore. This secondary stage may last from a few months to a few years, and there may be no further trouble, but in some instances there is a tertiary stage, characterised by painful swellings on bones and by deep ulceration in various parts, perhaps in the nose and throat.

Yaws can be cured by intravenous or intramuscular injections of salvarsan and other organic arsenical compounds. Bismuth and mercury may also be used, by injection, or mercury and potassium iodide by the mouth.

YELLOW FEVER. An acute fever occurring in tropical and subtropical countries, and particularly in South America, yellow fever, also known as black vomit and yellow jack, is caused by infection with a micro-organism called leptospira icteroides. This consists of a fine filament thrown into a very fine spiral formation. It is carried by a mosquito known as stegomyia fasciata, or aëdes argenteus. If this insect bites a person suffering from yellow fever during the first three days of the illness, it will very probably pick up the infection, and after an interval of twelve days will inject the organisms into any person it may chance to bite.

The incubation period lasts from three to five days, and the disease usually begins abruptly, though sometimes the patient may have been out of sorts for a day or two. The temperature shoots up, and there is headache and perhaps pain in muscles and in the joints of the legs. The face is flushed and the eyes injected. There is uneasiness or pain in the pit of the stomach and perhaps vomiting. The pulse is raised more or less in correspondence with the temperature.

Albumin may appear in the urine as early as the second day.

On the second or third day there is a decline in the severity of the symptoms and, in favourable cases, this may go on to recovery, but in other cases there is again a rise of temperature, and a return of the vomiting which increases in severity, the vomited matter containing altered blood and constituting the so-called black vomit. Large quantities of albumin may be present in the urine, which may become very scanty. It is a remarkable fact, however, that though the temperature may be stationary or even rising, the pulse rate drops, perhaps as much as 20 per minute in a space of 24 hours. Jaundice becomes apparent when the face loses its flush at the remission and increases in intensity from day to day. Death is commonest about the sixth or seventh day, and may be due to sudden heart failure, toxaemia or uraemia. When the patient recovers convalescence is slow.

The incidence of yellow fever has been considerably diminished by preventing the access of mosquitoes to water in the neighbourhood of dwellings. The stegomyia lives in or near dwellings and in coastal or riverside regions. Houses that are known to harbour the insect should be thoroughly fumigated. People suffering from the disease should be screened so that mosquitoes may be unable to get at them. A person who has suffered from yellow fever is rendered immune, but during an outbreak others should receive preventive inoculations.

As regards those who are suffering from the disease, it is likely that the disease will be cured if they receive injections of Noguchi serum during the first day or two of the disease ; after the third day the serum does not seem to have any effect. The treatment otherwise is largely that of fever (*q.v.*) and of the troublesome symptoms.

See Mosquito ; Tropical Hygiene.

ZINC. A number of zinc compounds are used in medicine, some of them very extensively as outward remedies. Zinc is not used much as an internal remedy nowadays, but zinc oxide is still sometimes given to diminish night sweats, usually in combination with belladonna, or as a nervine tonic. Zinc sulphate is used as an emetic in doses of 10 to 30 grains in a little water, and is safe except for young children.

The salt occurs as small, colourless, prismatic crystals, very like those of Epsom salt. It has a sharp, astringent taste, and is used in a solution in water as an astringent and antiseptic lotion, the strength varying according to the purpose in view. Thus, in a lotion for conjunctivitis there is generally 1 grain to the ounce, and in an injection for leucorrhoea or gonorrhoea, 3 grains to the ounce. A solution of this salt is also used, generally in the form of red lotion, to stimulate sluggish ulcers.

Zinc chloride is a powerfully corrosive salt. The official solution of zinc chloride, or Burnett's fluid which resembles it, is sometimes used to disinfect the stools in typhoid fever and other disorders, or otherwise as a disinfectant.

Zinc oxide and zinc carbonate, particularly the prepared native carbonate, or calamine (*q.v.*), are used to make lotions, creams, ointments, pastes and powders. All are insoluble in water, and a lotion containing one or more of them must be thoroughly shaken just before it is applied. The official zinc ointment consists of zinc oxide and benzoated lard. It is slightly astringent and very soothing in its action, and is much used in inflammation of the skin. It may be made creamy by adding almond oil. The ointment of oleate of zinc is also a good ointment. Zinc oxide is contained in Lassar's paste (*q.v.*). Zinc oxide is generally combined with starch or talc in a powder, commonly with some boracic acid also. Sixty grains each of zinc oxide and boracic acid might be made up to an ounce with the starch or powdered talc.

Poisoning by Zinc. In acute poisoning by a preparation of zinc an emetic should not be used, but a weak solution of washing soda or some strong tea. Afterwards, egg, milk or olive oil can be given.

ZOSTER. *See* Herpes.

ZYGOMA. The bony arch that lies beneath the cheek is called the zygoma, or zygomatic arch. It is formed by a backward projection of the malar bone and a forward projection of the temporal bone, and gives attachment to some of the muscles of mastication.

See Jaw.

ZYMOTIC DISEASE. An infectious disease is sometimes called a zymotic disease. The term zymotic is derived from a Greek word meaning ferment. The agent is always a living organism.

See Infectious Disease.

THE END

€ 63.94